An Invitation to Health

DIANNE HALES

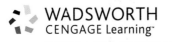

WADSWORTH
CENGAGE Learning

Australia • Brazil • Japan • Korea • Mexico • Singapore • Spain • United Kingdom • United States

WADSWORTH
CENGAGE Learning

An Invitation to Health, 2009–2010 Edition
Dianne Hales

Publisher: Yolanda Cossio

Development Editors: Nedah Rose, Pat Brewer

Assistant Editor: Elesha Feldman

Editorial Assistant: Elizabeth Momb

Marketing Manager: Jennifer Somerville

Marketing Assistant: Katy Malatesta

Marketing Communications Manager:
Belinda Krohmer

Project Manager, Editorial Production:
Trudy Brown

Creative Director: Rob Hugel

Art Director: John Walker/Caryl Gorska

Print Buyer: Judy Inouye

Permissions Editor: Bob Kauser

Production Service: Lachina Publishing Services

Text Designer: Brian Salisbury

Photo Researcher: Terri Miller

Copy Editor: Lachina Publishing Services

Cover Designer: Robin Terra

Cover Image: ©Ben Welsh/zefa/Corbis

Compositor: Lachina Publishing Services

For product information and technology assistance, contact us at
Cengage Learning Customer & Sales Support, 1-800-354-9706

For permission to use material from this text or product,
submit all requests online at **cengage.com/permissions**
Further permissions questions can be emailed to
permissionrequest@cengage.com

Library of Congress Control Number: 2007943555

ISBN-13: 978-0-495-38855-5

ISBN-10: 0-495-38855-6

Wadsworth Cengage Learning
10 Davis Drive
Belmont, CA 94002-3098
USA

Cengage Learning is a leading provider of customized learning solutions with office locations around the globe, including Singapore, the United Kingdom, Australia, Mexico, Brazil, and Japan. Locate your local office at **international .cengage.com/region**.

Cengage Learning products are represented in Canada by Nelson Education, Ltd.

For your course and learning solutions, visit **academic.cengage.com**

Purchase any of our products at your local college store or at our preferred online store **www.ichapters.com**

Printed in the United States of America
1 2 3 4 5 6 7 12 11 10 09 08

To my husband Bob and my daughter Julia,
who make every day an invitation to joy

Brief Contents

Contents

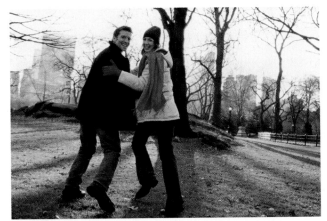

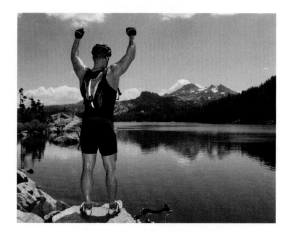

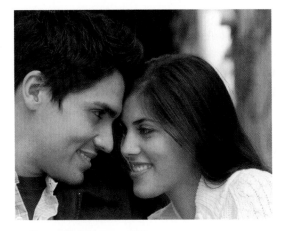

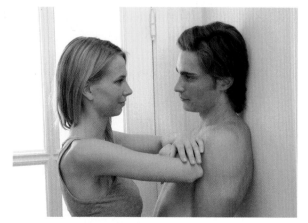

SECTION
4
Avoiding
Health Risks   301

CHAPTER 12   Alcohol Use, Misuse, and Abuse   339

CHAPTER 13   Tobacco Use, Misuse, and Abuse   371

SECTION 5   Protecting Your Health   393

CHAPTER 14   Preventing Major Diseases   395

CHAPTER 15   Avoiding Infectious Diseases   435

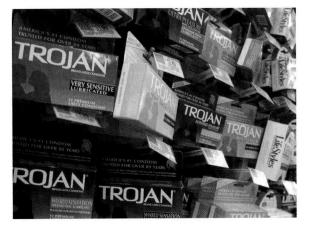

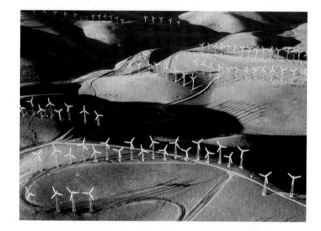

Key Features

POINT COUNTERPOINT

Savvy Consumer

Preface

To the Student

This textbook is an invitation to you—an invitation to a healthier, happier, fuller life. Every day you make choices that can affect both how long and how well you live. The knowledge you acquire in this course will help you make better choices, ones that will have a direct impact on how you look, feel, and function—now and for decades to come.

Perhaps you are in good health and think you know all you need to know about how to take care of yourself. If so, take a minute and ask yourself some questions:

- How well do you understand yourself? Are you able to cope with emotional upsets and crises? Do you often feel stressed out?

- How nutritiously do you eat? Are you always going on—and off—diets?

- Do you exercise regularly?

- How solid and supportive are your relationships with others? Are you conscientious about birth control and safe-sex practices?

- Do you occasionally get drunk or high? Do you smoke?

- What do you know about your risk for infectious diseases, heart problems, cancer, or other serious illnesses?

- Are you a savvy health-care consumer? Do you know how to evaluate medical products and health professionals?

- How much do you know about complementary and alternative medicine?

- If you needed health care, do you know where you'd turn or how you'd pay?

- Have you taken steps to ensure your personal safety at home, on campus, and on the streets?

- Can you improve your odds for living a long and healthy life?

- What are you doing today to prevent physical, psychological, social, and environmental problems in the future?

As you consider these questions, chances are there are some aspects of health you haven't considered before— and others you feel you don't have to worry about for years. Yet the choices you make and the actions you take now will have a dramatic impact on your future.

Your health is your personal responsibility. Over time, your priorities and needs will inevitably change, but the connections between various dimensions of your well-being will remain the same: The state of your mind will affect the state of your body, and vice versa. The values that guide you through today can keep you mentally, physically, and spiritually healthy throughout your lifetime. Your ability to cope with stress will influence your decisions about alcohol and drug use. Your commitment to honest, respectful relationships will affect the nature of your sexual involvements. Your eating and exercise habits will determine whether you develop a host of medical problems.

The 2009–2010 Edition of *An Invitation to Health* is packed with information, advice, recommendations, and research, and provides the first step in taking full charge of your own well-being. An important theme of this book is prevention. Ultimately, the power of prevention belongs to you—and it's a lot easier than you might think. You could simply add a walk or workout to your daily routine. You could snack on fruit instead of high-fat foods. You could cut back on alcohol. You could buckle your seat belt whenever you get in a car. These things may not seem like a big deal now, yet they could make a crucial difference in determining how active and fulfilling the rest of your life will be.

Knowledge alone can't assure you a lifetime of well-being. The rest depends on you. The skills you acquire, the habits you form, the choices you make, the ways you live day by day will all shape your health and your future. You cannot simply read this book and study health the way you study French or chemistry. You must decide to make it part of your daily life.

This is our invitation to you.

—*Dianne Hales*

To the Instructor

I am writing to invite you to something new. Yes, *An Invitation to Health* has been the leading college health textbook for years, and the 2009–2010 Edition once again presents up-to-date, comprehensive, research-based coverage of personal health. However, this edition goes beyond the standard themes and topics to introduce a new dimension: an integrated approach to learning and living personal health.

Integration appears in many ways throughout this new edition:

- Mind-body integration, a theme throughout the book that is best encapsulated by a new chapter on Emotional and Spiritual Well-Being.
- Integration of concepts within each chapter, such as the focus on the new medical frontier of cardiometabolic health in the chapter on major diseases.
- Integration of behavioral change, which extends beyond our popular "Your Strategies for Change" and "Your Life Change Coach" to a breakthrough supplement, *An Invitation to Personal Change,* which lays out step-by-step blueprints for directing change, eliminating unhealthy habits, and developing healthier behaviors.
- Integration of the newest research, such as the American College of Sports Medicine's most recent exercise guidelines and the most current recommendations for HPV vaccination.

As always, this edition defines health in the broadest sense of the word—not as an entity in itself but as an integrated process for discovering, using, and protecting all possible resources within the individual, family, community, and environment.

New in the 2009–2010 Edition

This edition of *An Invitation to Health* includes four new chapters:

- Chapter 1, "Your Invitation to Healthy Change," outlines the dimensions of health, reports on the state of college students' health, and provides a primer in behavioral change, including topics such as the transtheoretical model of change, the stages of change, and the keys to successful change.
- Chapter 2, "Emotional and Spiritual Well-Being," broadens and deepens our coverage of the latest research findings from positive psychology, extends our coverage of spiritual health, and includes practical information on sleep and sleep problems on campus.
- Chapter 14, "Preventing Major Disease," introduces the state-of-the-science concept of "cardiometabolic health" and provides guidance on identifying and reducing cardiometabolic risk factors. It includes in-depth coverage of metabolic syndrome, diabetes mellitus, cardiovascular diseases, stroke, and cancer.
- Chapter 16, "Lowering Your Risk of Sexually Transmitted Infections," extends and deepens our

coverage of STIs in society and on campus, including an in-depth discussion of human papilloma virus infection and vaccination, and an even greater emphasis on safer-sex practices.

Every chapter includes a provocative new feature called "Reality Check," which invites students to test the accuracy of their social norms by asking questions such as how many students they think feel overwhelmed by all they have to do, are on diets, have never had vaginal intercourse, use drugs, practice safer sex, and so on. The answers, mainly from the authoritative American College Health Association National College Health Assessment, appear on the pages following the "Reality Check."

Another new feature, "Point/Counterpoint," presents opposing viewpoints and invites discussion of timely and often controversial topics, such as "Generation Me or We," "Sports Doping on Campus," "Same-Sex Marriages," "Advocating for Abstinence," "Is Spreading an STI a Crime?" and "Who Should Pay for the Uninsured?"

The 2009–2010 Edition also features a Running Glossary that provides a concise definition on the same page that a term is first used in context.

Many chapters have been extensively revised, updated, and reorganized. Here are some examples:

- "Your Mental Health" (Chapter 4): updated sections on mental health on campus, depression, anxiety, attention disorders, and suicide.
- "The Joy of Fitness" (Chapter 5): the latest exercise guidelines from the American College of Sports Medicine and the American Heart Association, a totally revised section on working out on campus, and updates on the benefits of exercise, stretching, warming up, and body composition.
- "Taking Control of Your Weight" (Chapter 7): the latest findings on social networks and genetic influences on weight, as well as a new review of popular weight loss diets.
- "Reproductive Choices" (Chapter 10): completely reorganized in a more reader-friendly format, with coverage of new contraceptive options, such as the "no-period" pill and emergency contraception.
- "Avoiding Addictive Behaviors and Drug Abuse" (Chapter 11): totally revised, with extensive coverage of prescription drug abuse, including a new table of commonly abused prescription medications and new sections on why students do and don't use drugs.
- "Alcohol Use, Misuse, and Abuse" (Chapter 12): completely reorganized with new emphasis on student behavior, including sections on choosing not to drink, safe and unsafe drinking, high-risk

student drinking, why students stop drinking, college alcohol problems, and changing the culture of college drinking.

- "Protecting Yourself from Injury, Violence, and Victimization" (Chapter 18): adds or expands coverage of hot topics such as recognizing potentially violent people, guns on campus, hazing, consequences of campus violence, and halting sexual violence.

Within chapters we've retained, updated, and enhanced popular features, including "Your Strategies for Change/ Your Strategies for Prevention," "Your Life Change Coach," "Savvy Consumer" and "Learn It/Live It" sections.

At the end of each chapter is a Self Survey, followed by a Health Action Plan. Other end-of-chapter resources include Review Questions, Critical Thinking Questions, and Key Terms. At the end of the book are a full Glossary and the Hales Health Almanac, which includes a directory of resources, emergency procedures, and a guide to common medical tests.

 This edition includes gender-specific information in every chapter, flagged with icons representing men and women. As in previous editions, icons also indicate material related to students and campus life and to cultural or racial diversity. Because the health sciences advance so rapidly, all of the chapters have been updated with the most current research, including many citations published in 2007 and incorporating the latest available statistics. The majority come from primary sources, including professional books, medical, health, and mental health journals, health education periodicals, scientific meetings, federal agencies and consensus panels, publications from research laboratories and universities, and personal interviews with specialists in a number of fields. In addition, "Internet Connections" presents reliable Internet addresses where students can turn for additional information.

As I tell students, *An Invitation to Health* can serve as an owner's manual to their bodies and minds. By using this book and taking your course, they can acquire a special type of power—the power to make good decisions, to assume responsibility, and to create and follow a healthy lifestyle. This textbook is our invitation to them to live what they learn and make the most of their health and of their lives.

This textbook also is an invitation to you as an instructor. I invite you to share your passion for education and to enter into a partnership with the editorial team at Wadsworth Cengage Learning. We welcome your feedback and suggestions. Please let us hear from you at academic.cengage.com/health. I personally look forward to working with you toward our shared goal of preparing a new generation for a healthful future.

An Overview of the 2009–2010 Edition

Following is a chapter-by-chapter listing of some of the key topics that have been added, expanded, or revised for this 2009–2010 edition:

Chapter 1: Your Invitation to Healthy Change

New section: A National Report Card on Student Health, with the latest data from ACHA-NCHA

New section: Student Health Norms

New: Reality Check (cigarettes, alcohol, marijuana)

New section: Staying Healthy on Campus

New section: Understanding Risky Behaviors

New section: A Report Card on the Nation's Health

New section: Healthy People 2010: How Are We Doing?

New section: Living Longer, Healthier Lives

New section: Overcoming Health Disparities

Revised section: Making Healthy Changes

New section: Models of Behavioral Change

New section: The Health Belief Model

Chapter 2: Emotional and Spiritual Well-Being

Expanded sections on positive psychology, spiritual health, and sleep

New section: The New Science of Happiness

Revised and expanded Spiritual Health section

New Your Life Change Coach: Enriching Your Spiritual Life

New section: Sleepless on Campus

New section: Sleep's Impact on Health

New Savvy Consumer: Straight Talk on Sleeping Pills

New Learn It/Live It: Keys to a Fulfilling Life

Chapter 3: Personal Stress Management

Updated section on Stress and Physical Health

New section: Racism and Discrimination

New section: Some College Responses (to Minorities Under Stress)

Updated section on Job Stress, with expanded new subsection: Burnout

New Your Strategies for Change: How to Cope with Distress After a Trauma

Expanded and updated section on Posttraumatic Stress Disorder (PTSD) (includes info on Iraq veterans)

Chapter 4: **Your Mental Health**

New anatomical art for the brain

Updated section: Who Develops Mental Disorders?

Updated section: Mental Health on Campus

All Depression sections updated

New Savvy Consumer: Weighing the Risks and Benefits of Antidepressants

New Your Strategies for Prevention: Helping Someone Who Is Depressed

Updated section: Anxiety Disorders

Updated section: Attention Disorders

Updated section: Suicide

New Your Life Change Coach: Preventing Suicide

New section in Types of Therapy: Other Approaches (on solution-focused therapy and behavioral activation)

New Self Survey: Are You Depressed?

New Health Action Plan for Getting Help for a Psychological Problem

Chapter 5: **The Joy of Fitness**

New exercise recommendations from the American College of Sports Medicine and the American Heart Association

Functional fitness—definition added

Updated section: Toll of Sedentary Living

Totally revised section: Working Out on Campus: Student Bodies in Motion

Revised and updated section on benefits of exercise: Why Exercise?

New Your Life Change Coach: Motivating Yourself to Move

Revised and updated section: How Much Exercise Is Enough?

New figure on good walking technique

New section: Stretching and Warming Up

Complete Discussion of body composition: BMI, Waist Circumference, Waist-to-Hip Ratio, Measuring Body Fat

New section on Sports Drinks

Chapter 6: **Personal Nutrition**

All nutrition sections updated with latest research findings

New section: Dietary Supplements

New figures illustrating USDA Guidelines

New section: His Plate, Her Plate: Gender and Nutrition

New section: Campus Cuisine: How College Students Eat

New table on Fast Food Choices

New section: You Are What You Drink

New section: What Is Organic?

New section: Avoiding *E. coli* Infections

Chapter 7: **Taking Control of Your Weight**

Updated section: How Did We Get So Fat? Includes latest research on social networks and on the obesity gene

Revised and updated section: Weight and the College Student

Updated section: Health Dangers of Excess Weight

Completely revised section: Weight Loss Diets: What Works, What Doesn't with new comparison table on Atkins, Ornish, and Weight Watchers

New section: Low-Glycemic-Load Diets

Updated section: Over-the-Counter Diet Pills

Revised section: Obesity Surgery covering gastric bypass and banding

Chapter 8: **Communicating and Relating**

Updated section: Dating on Campus

Updated section: Hooking Up

Updated section: Emotional Abuse

Updated section: Living Arrangements

Completely revised section: Same-Sex Marriage

Chapter 9: **Personal Sexuality**

Updated section: Circumcision with information on risk reduction for HIV

Updated section: Teen Sexual Behaviors

Updated section: Sex on Campus

New section: Why People Have Sex

Updated section: Transgenderism and Transsexuality

Updated section: Abstinence

Updated section: Erectile Dysfunction (ED)

Chapter 10: **Reproductive Choices**

Contraceptive methods reorganized: barrier, hormonal, IUD, fertility awareness, emergency contraception, sterilization

Table of options updated

New table by type and accessibility

All methods updated

Revised section: Contraceptive Sponge

Revised section: Vaginal Spermicides

New section: Seasonale

New section: Lybrel, the "No-Period" Pill

Revised and updated section: Emergency Contraception

Updated section: Abortion

Completely revised section: A Cross-Cultural Perspective

Updated section: Assisted Reproductive Technology

Chapter 11: Avoiding Addictive Behaviors and Drug Abuse

Totally revised section: Drug Use on Campus

New section: Why Students Do Use Drugs

New section: Why Students Don't Use Drugs

Revised and updated section: Caffeine, with the latest positive health effects of caffeine

New section: Prescription Drug Abuse, with the new table on commonly abused prescription medications

New section: Prescription Drug Abuse on Campus

All sections on Common Drugs of Abuse updated

Updated section: Treating Substance Abuse

Chapter 12: Alcohol Use, Misuse, and Abuse

Chapter reorganized to put behavior first: Drinking in America, then Drinking on Campus, with many new sections

New section: Choosing Not to Drink

New section: Safe and Unsafe Drinking

Completely revised and updated section: Drinking on Campus

New section: Why Students Don't Drink

Completely revised section: Why Students Do Drink

New section: High-Risk Student Drinking

New section: Why Students Stop Drinking

New section: College Alcohol-Related Problems

New section: Changing the Culture of Campus Drinking

Revised section: Alcohol Poisoning

Updated subsections in the Impact of Alcohol on the Body, with latest research

Alcohol, Gender, and Race: new table on how alcohol discriminates

New subsection in Alcoholism Treatments section: Harm Reduction Therapy

Chapter 13: Tobacco Use, Misuse, and Abuse

Totally revised section: Tobacco Use on Campus, new art

Updated section: Health Effects of Cigarette Smoking

New section: Health Effects on Students

Quitting sections updated

Updated section: The Risks of Secondhand Smoke

Chapter 14: Preventing Major Diseases

First sections all based on concept of cardiometabolic health

New section: The Power of Prevention

New section: Your Cardiometabolic health

New section: Cardiometabolic Risk Factors

New section: Risk Factors You Can Control

New section: Risk Factors You Can't Control

New Your Life Change Coach: Lowering Your Cardiometabolic Risk Factors

All sections updated with the latest research: diabetes, hypertension, lipoprotein profile, lowering high blood pressure

New section: Heart Risks on Campus

New section: Hearts and Minds: Psychological Risk Factors, with new subsections Depression, Anger and Hostility, Personality Types

New section: The Heart of a Woman

New section: Cardiac Arrest

Cancer sections updated

Chapter 15: Avoiding Infectious Diseases

New section: Immunity and Gender

Updated section: Allergies

Revised section: Autoimmune Disorders

Updated section: Common Cold, with new research on vitamin C, *Echinacea*

New Your Life Change Coach: Cold Comfort

Revised and expanded section: Meningitis

Hepatitis sections updated

Updated section: Chronic Fatigue Syndrome

New section: The "Superbug" Threat: MRSA

Updated section: Lyme Disease

Updated section: Avian Influenza

New section: The Threat of a Pandemic

Chapter 16: Lowering Your Risk of Sexually Transmitted Infections

This chapter is a new addition to ITH

New section: Sexually Transmitted Infections and Diseases

New section: STIs in Society

Updated section: STIs on Campus

New Your Life Change Coach: The ABCs of Safer Sex

New section: STIs and Gender

Revised section: Risk Continuums

Completely revised section: Human Papilloma Virus

New Savvy Consumer: Who Should Get the HPV Vaccine?

Revised section: Herpes Simplex

Revised section: Chlamydia

Updated section: HIV/AIDS

Chapter 17: Getting Quality Traditional and Nontraditional Health Care

New section: Quality Health Care

Updated section: Oral Health

Updated section: Getting Quality Health Care, new art

New section: Preventing Medical Errors

All CAM sections revised and updated

Updated section: Paying for Health Care

Updated section: The Uninsured

Chapter 18: Protecting Yourself from Injury, Violence, and Victimization

New Your Strategies for Prevention: What to Do in an Emergency

New section: Cell Phones and Safety

Updated section: Living in a Dangerous World

New Your Strategies for Prevention: How to Recognize Potentially Violent People

Updated section: Crime and Violence on Campus

New section: Consequences of Campus Violence

New section: Hazing

New section: Murders and Assaults

New Your Life Change Coach: Preventing Rape

Updated section: Halting Sexual Violence

Chapter 19: Working Toward a Healthy Environment

New section: Climate Change

New section: The Air You Breathe

Expanded and updated section: Ozone

New section: Particle Pollution

Updated Your Life Change Coach: Going Green

New section: Cigarette Smoke

Sections on asbestos and mercury updated

Updated Savvy Consumer: Are Cell Phones Safe to Use?

Chapter 20: A Lifetime of Health

New section: The Aging of America

Updated section: Successful Aging

Updated section: Women at Midlife

Updated section: Men at Midlife

Updated section: Sexuality and Aging

Updated section: Alzheimer's Disease

Updated section: Osteoporosis

Reorganized and updated section: Advance Directives

Updated section: Grief

Supplemental Resources

An Invitation to Personal Change

A key part of our integrated *An Invitation to Health* approach to lifelong healthy choices is a new supplement, *An Invitation to Personal Change (IPC)*, coauthored by Dianne Hales and Kenneth W. Christian, Ph.D., a psychologist with more than 30 years of experience in personal change and maximum potential. Based on decades of psychological research and clinical practice, *IPC* serves as a curriculum for change, inviting students to take appropriate action in simple, compellingly straightforward ways.

The *IPC* icons throughout this book signal links to *Labs for An Invitation to Personal Change*, which present step-by-step blueprints for creating healthier habits, eliminating harmful behaviors, maximizing performance, and achieving greater physical, psychological, and spiritual well-being. The labs focus on key dimensions of personal health, including:

- Psychological and spiritual well-being ("The Grateful Thread," "Soul Food," "Your Psychological Self-Care Pyramid," "Defusing Test Stress," "Rx: Relax," "Taming a Toxic Temper," "Finity").

- Healthy habits ("Excise Exercise Excuses," "Thinking Thinner," "Mind over Platter," "Sleep Power").
- Behavioral Choices ("Do It Now," "Don't Go There," "Your Alcohol Audit," "Butt Out," "The Seduction of Safer Sex," "To Have or Have Not").
- Communication skills ("Listen Up," "Help Yourself," "What's Your Intimacy Quotient?").
- Social Dimensions of health ("Health Assurance," "Your Guardian Angel," "YourSpace").

We invite you to sample *An Invitation to Personal Change* by going to servicedirect.cengage.com

CengageNow™   Class-tested and student-praised, CengageNow™ offers a variety of features that support course objectives and interactive learning. This online tutorial for students, available with new texts, offers a Personalized Change Plan, pre- and post-tests, a wellness journal, and a variety of activities, all designed to get students involved in their learning progress and to be better prepared for class participation and class quizzes and tests. Students log on to CengageNow by using the access code available with the text.

Instructor's Manual and Test Bank   These two essential ancillaries are bound together for your convenience. The Instructor's Manual provides chapter outlines, learning objectives, classroom handouts, discussion questions, a video list, a resource integration guide, and more. The Test Bank was thoroughly revised to include test questions that are linked to the book's Chapter Objectives. Questions within the Test Bank are categorized according to Bloom's taxonomy, and are broken down by types: remembering/fact recall, understanding, applying, and analyzing.

JoinIn® on Turning Point™   Enhance how your students interact with you, your lecture, and each other using JoinIn® content for Response Systems tailored to this text. Thomson's exclusive agreement to offer TurningPoint™ software lets you pose book-specific questions and display students' answers seamlessly within the Microsoft® PowerPoint® slides of your own lecture, in conjunction with the "clicker" hardware of your choice.

ExamView Computerized Testing   Create, deliver, and customize the thorough Test Bank in minutes with this easy-to-use assessment and tutorial system. *ExamView* offers both a *Quick Test Wizard* and an *Online Test Wizard* that guide you step-by-step through the process of creating tests, while it allows you to see the test you are creating on the screen exactly as it will print or display online. You can build tests of up to 250 questions using up to 12 question types. Using *ExamView*'s complete word-processing capabilities, you can enter an unlimited number of new questions or edit existing questions.

PowerLecture for Health, Fitness, and Wellness: A Microsoft® PowerPoint® Link Tool   This teaching tool contains lecture presentations that feature more than 100 PowerPoint® slides, including a text outline, art, and resources such as the Instructor's Manual with Test Bank, all on one convenient CD-ROM. PowerLecture also includes JoinIn® on TurningPoint™ content, which allows you to enhance your students' interaction with you, your lecture, and each other using JoinIn® content for Response Systems tailored to this text.

InfoTrac® College Edition Student Guide for Health   This 24-page booklet offers detailed guidance for students on how to use the *InfoTrac College Edition* database. Includes log-in help, a complete search tips "cheat sheet," and a topic list of key word search terms for health, fitness, and wellness. Available *free* when packaged with the text.

Health, Fitness, and Wellness Internet Explorer   A handy trifold brochure contains dozens of useful health, fitness, and wellness Internet links.

Personal Daily Log   The Personal Daily Log contains an exercise pyramid, study and exercise tips, a goal-setting worksheet, cardiorespiratory exercise record form, strength training record form, a daily nutrition diary, helpful Internet links, and more.

Careers in Health, Physical Education, and Sport   This is the essential manual for majors who are interested in pursuing a position in their chosen field. It guides them through the complicated process of picking the type of career they want to pursue, suggests how to prepare for the transition into the working world, and offers information about different career paths, education requirements, and reasonable salary expectations. The supplement also describes the differences in credentials found in the field and testing requirements for certain professions.

Diet Analysis Plus 8.0   is the market-leading diet assessment program used by colleges and universities that allows students to create their own personal profiles based on height, weight, age, sex, and activity level. Its new dynamic interface makes it easy for students to track the types and serving sizes of the foods they consume, from one day to 365 days! Now including even more exciting features, the updated 8.0 version includes a 10,000 food database, nine reports for analysis, a new food recipe feature, the latest Dietary References, and goals and actual percentages of essential nutrients, vitamins, and minerals.

Students can use this information to adjust their diet and gain a better understanding of how nutrition relates to their personal health goals. Thoroughly revised and updated, the software is available online or on a new Windows/Mac® compatible CD-ROM.

academic.cengage.com/health When you adopt the 2009–2010 edition of *An Invitation to Health,* you and your students will have access to a rich array of teaching and learning resources that you won't find anywhere else. This outstanding site features both student resources for the text—including quizzes, web links, suggested online readings, and discussion forums—and instructor resources—including downloadable supplementary resources and multimedia presentation slides. You will also find an online catalog of Wadsworth/Cengage Learning's health, fitness, wellness, and physical education books and supplements.

Relaxation: A Guide to Personal Stress Management This 30-minute video shows students how to manage their stress and what a healthy stress level is in their lives. Experts explain relaxation techniques and guide the student through progressive relaxation, guided imagery, breathing, and physical activity.

Testwell This online assessment tool allows you to complete a 100-question wellness inventory related to the dimensions of wellness. Complete the personal assessments in order to evaluate your personal health status related to nutrition, emotional health, spirituality, sexuality, physical health, self-care, safety, environmental health, occupational health, and intellectual health.

Behavior Change Workbook *The Behavior Change Workbook* includes a brief discussion of the current theories behind making positive lifestyle changes, along with exercises to help students effect those changes in their everyday lives.

Health and Wellness Resource Center at gale.cengage .com Gale's Health and Wellness Resource Center is a new comprehensive website that provides easy-to-find answers to health questions.

Walk4Life® Elite Model Pedometer This pedometer tracks steps, elapsed time, distance, and includes a calorie counter. Whether to be used as an activity in class or as a tool to encourage students to simply track their steps and walk toward better fitness awareness, this is a valuable item for everyone.

Readings in Healthy Living As a frequent author of health-related articles produced by Parade® Magazine, Dianne Hales has published numerous articles that students will find useful and interesting. This 12-article reader is a collection of key articles, including *Take Your Meds—The Right Way* and *You Can Think Yourself Thin.*

ABC Videos for Health and Wellness These videos allow you to integrate the newsgathering and programming power of the ABC News networks into the classroom to show students the relevance of course topics to their everyday lives. The videos include news clips correlated directly with the text and can help you launch a lecture, spark a discussion, or demonstrate an application. Students can see firsthand how the principles they learn in the course apply to the stories they hear in the news.

Acknowledgments

One of the joys of writing *An Invitation to Health* is the opportunity to work with a team I consider the very best of the best in textbook publishing.

I thank Peter Adams, our fearless leader, for his unwavering support. Nedah Rose, our Senior Development Editor, has been endlessly supportive and enthusiastic and has made every step of the process of creating this edition go smoothly.

My deepest thanks go to Pat Brewer, the developmental editor on this edition, whose contributions always extend far beyond the demands of duty. I consider her a partner, co-conspirator, and friend.

I thank Elizabeth Momb, our editorial assistant, who provided endless help—with endless patience and good humor. Thanks to Trudy Brown, Project Manager, for expertly shepherding this edition from conception to production, to Brian Salisbury for his vibrant new design, and to Lachina Publishing Services for art. Terri Miller, our photo researcher, has provided us with dazzling, dynamic images that capture the diversity and energy of today's college students. I appreciate the skill and dedication of copy editor Amy Mayfield.

My thanks to Jennifer Somerville, Managing Marketing Manager, for her enthusiastic support, to Talia Wise for her work on the promotional materials, to Jake Warde, who guided the ancillaries, and to Stephanie Thiel, my student intern.

Finally, I would like to thank the reviewers whose input has been so valuable through these many editions. For the 2009–2010 Edition, I thank the following for their comments and helpful assistance:

Daniel Adame, *Emory University*

Carol Allen, *Lane Community College*

Elain Bryan, *Georgia Perimeter College*

Carla Gilbreath, *University of Central Arkansas*

John Kowalczyk, *University of Minnesota, Duluth*

Sophia Munro, *Palm Beach Community College*

Stephen Sansone, *Chemetka Community College*

Ronda Sturgill, *Marshall University*

Rosmarie Tarara, *High Point University*

For their help with earlier editions I offer my gratitude to:

Ghulam Aasef, *Kaskaskia College*

Andrea Abercrombie, *Clemson University*

Judy Baker, *East Carolina University*

Marcia Ball, *James Madison University*

Jeremy Barnes, *Southeast Missouri State University*

Rick Barnes, *East Carolina University*

Lois Beach, *SUNY-Plattsburg*

Liz Belyea, *Cosumnes River College*

Betsy Bergen, *Kansas State University*

Nancy Bessette, *Saddleback College*

Carol Biddington, *California University of Pennsylvania*

David Black, *Purdue University*

Jill M. Black, *Cleveland State University*

Cynthia Pike Blocksom, *Cincinnati Health Department*

James Brik, *Willamette University*

Mitchell Brodsky, *York College*

Jodi Broodkins-Fisher, *University of Utah*

Elaine Bryan, *Georgia Perimeter College*

James G. Bryant, Jr., *Western Carolina University*

Marsha Campos, *Modesto Junior College*

Richard Capriccioso, *University of Phoenix*

James Lester Carter, *Montana State University*

Peggy L. Chin, *University of Connecticut*

Patti Cost, *Weber State University*

Maxine Davis, *Eastern Washington University*

Lori Dewald, *Shippensburg University of Pennsylvania*

Julie Dietz, *Eastern Illinois University*

Robert Dollinger, *Florida International University*

Gary English, *Ithaca College*

Melinda K. Everman, *The Ohio State University*

Michael Felts, *East Carolina University*

Lynne Fitzgerald, *Morehead State University*

Kathie C. Garbe, *Kennesaw State College*

Gail Gates, *Oklahoma State University*

Dawn Graff-Haight, *Portland State University*

Carolyn Gray, *New Mexico State University*

Mary Gress, *Lorain County Community College*

Janet Grochowski, *University of St. Thomas*

Jack Gutierrez, *Central Community College*

Stephen Haynie, *College of William and Mary*

Ron Heinrichs, *Central Missouri State University*

Michael Hoadley, *University of South Dakota*

Harold Horne, *University of Illinois at Springfield*

Linda L. Howard, *Idaho State University*

Mary Hunt, *Madonna University*

Kim Hyatt, *Weber State University*

Dee Jacobsen, *Southeastern Louisiana University*

John Janowiak, *Appalachian State University*

Peggy Jarnigan, *Rollins College*

Jim Johnson, *Northwest Missouri State University*

Chester S. Jones, *University of Arkansas*

Herb Jones, *Ball State University*

Jane Jones, *University of Wisconsin, Stevens Point*

Lorraine J. Jones, *Muncie, Indiana*

Becky Kennedy-Koch, *The Ohio State University*

Mark J. Kittleson, *Southern Illinois University*

Darlene Kluka, *University of Central Oklahoma*

John Kowalczyk, *University of Minnesota, Duluth*

Debra A. Krummel, *West Virginia University*

Roland Lamarine, *California State University, Chico*

David Langford, *University of Maryland, Baltimore County*

Terri Langford, *University of Central Florida*

Beth Lanning, *Baylor University*

Norbert Lindskog, *Harold Washington College*

Loretta Liptak, *Youngstown State University*

David G. Lorenzi, *West Liberty State College*

S. Jack Loughton, *Weber State University*

Rick Madson, *Palm Beach Community College*

Ashok Malik, *College of San Mateo*

Michele P. Mannion, *Temple University*

Jerry Mayo, *Hendrix College*

Jessica Middlebrooks, *University of Georgia*

Esther Moe, *Oregon Health Sciences University*

Kris Moline, *Lourdes College*

Rosemary Moulahan, *High Point University*

Richard Morris, *Rollins College*

John W. Munson, *University of Wisconsin–Stevens Point*

Anne O'Donnell, *Santa Rosa Junior College*

Randy M. Page, *University of Idaho*

Carolyn P. Parks, *University of North Carolina*

Anthony V. Parrillo, *East Carolina University*

Miguel Perez, *University of North Texas*

Pamela Pinahs-Schultz, *Carroll College*

Rosanne Poole, *Tallahassee Community College*

Janet Reis, *University of Illinois at Urbana-Champaign*

Pamela Rost, *Buffalo State College*

Sadie Sanders, *University of Florida*

Steven Sansone, *Chemeketa Community College*

Debra Secord, *Coastline College*

Behjat Sharif, *California State University–Los Angeles*

Andrew Shim, *Southwestern College*

Steve Singleton, *Wayne State University*

Larry Smith, *Scottsdale Community College*

Teresa Snow, *Georgia Institute of Technology*

Carl A. Stockton, *Radford University*

Linda Stonecipher, *Western Oregon State College*

Laurie Tucker, *American University*

Emogene Johnson Vaughn, *Norfolk State University*

David M. White, *East Carolina University*

Sabina White, *University of California— Santa Barbara*

Robert Wilson, *University of Minnesota*

Roy Wohl, *Washburn University*

Martin L. Wood, *Ball State University*

Sharon Zackus, *City College of San Francisco*

About the Author

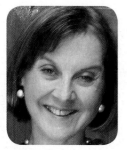

Dianne Hales, a contributing editor for *Parade*, has written more than 2,000 articles for national publications. Her trade books include *Think Thin, Be Thin; Just Like a Woman: How Gender Science Is Redefining What Makes Us Female* and the award-winning compendium of mental health information, *Caring for the Mind: The Comprehensive Guide to Mental Health.*

Dianne Hales is one of the few journalists to be honored with national awards for excellence in magazine writing by both the American Psychiatric Association and the American Psychological Association. She also has won the EMMA (Exceptional Media Merit Award) for health reporting from the National Women's Political Caucus and Radcliffe College, and numerous writing awards from various organizations, including the Arthritis Foundation, California Psychiatric Society, CHAAD (Children and Adults with Attention-Deficit Disorders), Council for the Advancement of Scientific Education, National Easter Seal Society, and the New York City Public Library.

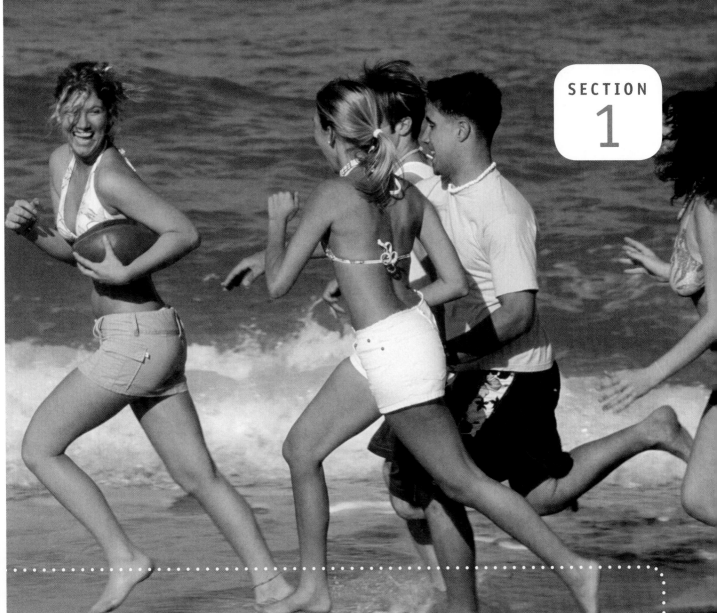

Taking Charge of Your Health

HEALTH may be a science; living is an art. The principles that can help you understand the science and practice the art are simple and timeless and form the basic premise of this book: You have more control over your life and well-being than anything or anyone else does. Through the decisions you make and the habits you develop, you can influence how well-and perhaps how long-you will live. This section defines health and wellness and provides the information you need to take charge of your well-being now and in the years to come.

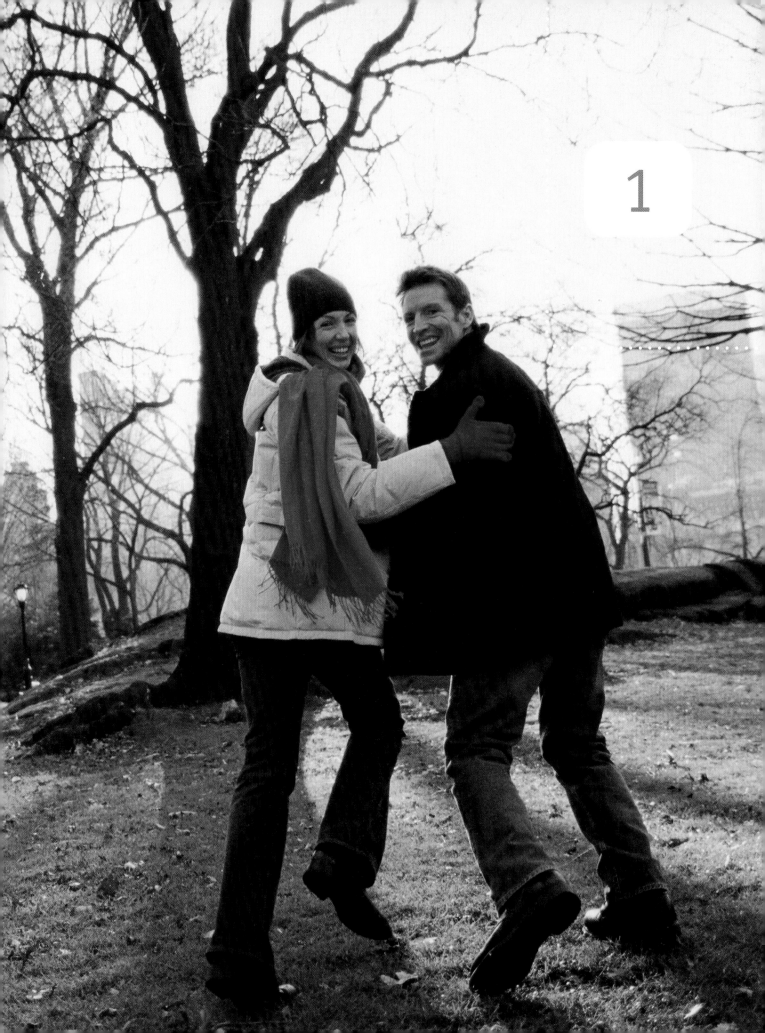

Your Invitation to Healthy Change

ANGELA always thought of health as something you worry about when you get older. Then her twin brother developed a health problem she'd never heard of: prediabetes (discussed in Chapters 7 and 16), which increases his risk of diabetes and heart disease. At a health fair on campus, she learned that her blood pressure was higher than normal. "Maybe I'm not too young to start thinking about my health," she concluded. Neither are you-whether you're a traditional-age college student or older, like an ever-increasing number of undergraduates.

An Invitation to Health asks you to go beyond thinking about your health to taking charge and making healthy choices for yourself and your future. This book is both *about* and *for* you: It includes material on your mind and your body, your spirit and your social ties, your needs and your wants, your past and your potential. It will help you explore options, discover possibilities, and find new ways to make your life worthwhile. If you don't make the most of what you are, you risk never discovering what you might become.

Being healthy, as you'll learn in this chapter, means more than not being sick or in pain. Health is a personal choice that you make every day when you decide on everything from what to eat to whether to exercise to how to handle stress. Sometimes making the best choices demands making healthy changes in your life. This chapter will show you how.

This chapter also extends an invitation to live more fully, more happily, and more healthfully. It is an offer that you literally cannot afford to refuse. The quality of your life depends on it.

After studying the material in this chapter, you should be able to:

- **Define** health and wellness.
- **Name** the dimensions of health and **describe** how they relate to total wellness.
- **Define** the three factors that shape health behaviors.
- **Name** the three key components of the transtheoretical model of change.
- **Describe** the stages of change and give an example of each.
- **Make** a decision about a lifestyle behavior you want to change.

CENGAGENOW™ Log on to HealthNow at **academic.cengage.com/login** to find your Behavior Change Planner and to explore self-assessments, interactive tutorials, and practice quizzes.

Health and Wellness

By simplest definition, **health** means being sound in body, mind, and spirit. The World Health Organization defines health as "not merely the absence of disease or infirmity," but "a state of complete physical, mental, and social well-being."[1] Health is the process of discovering, using, and protecting all the resources within our bodies, minds, spirits, families, communities, and environment.

Health has many dimensions: physical, psychological, spiritual, social, intellectual, and environmental. This book integrates all these dimensions within a *holistic* approach that looks at health and the individual as a whole, rather than part by part. Your own definition of health may include different elements, but chances are you and your classmates agree that it includes at least some of the following:

- A positive, optimistic outlook.
- A sense of control over stress and worries; time to relax.
- Energy and vitality; freedom from pain or serious illness.
- Supportive friends and family and a nurturing intimate relationship with someone you love.
- A personally satisfying job.
- A clean environment.

Wellness can be defined as purposeful, enjoyable living or, more specifically, a deliberate lifestyle choice characterized by personal responsibility and optimal enhancement of physical, mental, and spiritual health. Health professionals use other definitions to encompass this broad, active meaning of wellness:

- As a decision you make to move toward optimal health.
- As a way of life you design to achieve your highest potential.
- As a process of developing awareness that health and happiness are possible in the present
- As the integration of body, mind, and spirit.
- As the belief that everything you do, think, and feel has an impact on your state of health and the health of the world.[2]

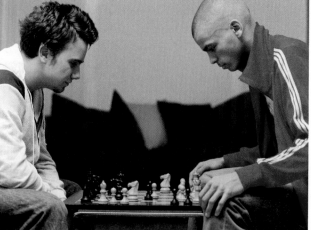

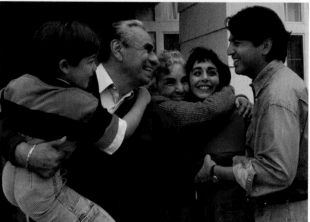

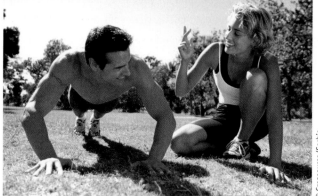

Health is the process of discovering, using, and protecting all the resources within our bodies, minds, spirits, families, communities, and environment.

"The 'well' person is not necessarily the strong, the brave, the successful, the young, the whole, or even the illness-free being," notes John Travis, M.D., author of The Wellness Workbook. "No matter what your current state of health, you can begin to appreciate yourself as a growing, changing person and allow yourself to move toward a happier life and positive health."

Dr. Travis, who created the Wellness Inventory (see Self Survey on page 25) uses the analogy of an iceberg (Figure

health A state of complete well-being, including physical, psychological, spiritual, social, intellectual, and environmental dimensions.

wellness A deliberate lifestyle choice characterized by personal responsibility and optimal enhancement of physical, mental, and spiritual health.

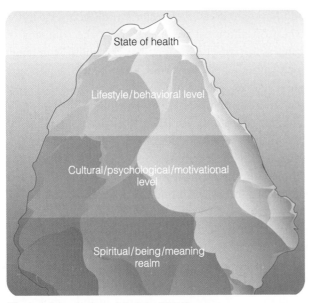

Figure 1.1 Iceberg Model of Wellness

Like an iceberg, only a small part of your total wellness is visible: your current state of health. Just as important are hidden dimensions, including lifestyle habits, cultural and psychological factors, and the realm of spiritual meaning and being.

Source: Reprinted with permission, *The Wellness Workbook*, 3rd edition, John W. Travis, MD, and Regina Sara Ryan, Celestial Arts, Berkeley, CA. ©1981, 1988, 2004 by John W. Travis. www.wellnessbook.com

1.1) to describe optimal health and wellness. Only about one-tenth of the mass of an iceberg is visible; the rest is submerged. Your current state of health is like the tip of the iceberg—the part that shows.

"To understand all that creates and supports your current state of health," says Dr. Travis, "you have to look 'underwater.'" The first hidden level—the "lifestyle/behavioral" level—consists of what you eat, how active you are, how you manage stress, and how you protect yourself from hazards. Below this dimension is the "cultural/psychological/ motivational" level, the often invisible influences that lead us to choose a certain lifestyle. The foundation of the iceberg is the "spiritual/being/meaning" realm, which encompasses issues such as your reason for being, the meaning of your life, and your place in the universe. "Ultimately," says Dr. Travis, "this realm determines whether the tip of the iceberg, representing your state of health, is one of disease or wellness."[3]

In wellness, health, and sickness, there is considerable overlap of the functions of the mind, body, and spirit. As scientists have shown again and again in recent decades, psychological factors play a major role in enhancing physical well-being and preventing illness, but they also can trigger, worsen, or prolong physical symptoms. Similarly, almost every medical illness affects people psychologically as well as physically.

The Dimensions of Health

By learning more about the six dimensions of health, you can explore the hidden levels of the iceberg.

Physical Health

The various states of health can be viewed as points on a continuum (Figure 1.2). At one end is early and needless death; at the other is optimal wellness, in which you feel and perform at your very best. In the middle, individuals are neither sick enough to need medical attention nor well enough to live each day with zest and vigor.

What matters even more than your place on the continuum is the direction in which you are moving: toward high-level wellness or toward premature death. Individuals in physical good health who are always worrying or not working to develop more fully may be on the right of the neutral point but facing left. Others who may be disabled or have a chronic health problem may have a positive outlook and a network of mutually supportive relationships that keeps them focused toward wellness.[4]

For the sake of optimal physical health, we must take positive steps away from illness and toward well-being. We must feed our bodies nutritiously, exercise them regularly, avoid harmful behaviors and substances, watch out for early signs of sickness, and protect ourselves from accidents.

Psychological Health

Like physical well-being, psychological health is more than the absence of problems or illness. Psychological health refers to both our emotional and mental states—

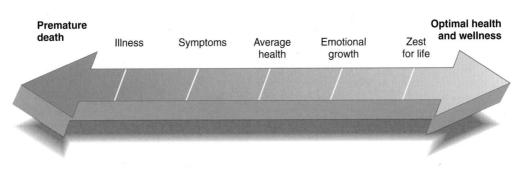

Figure 1.2 Wellness–Illness Continuum

that is, to our feelings and our thoughts. It involves awareness and acceptance of a wide range of feelings in oneself and others, the ability to express emotions, to function independently, and to cope with the challenges of daily stressors.

Spiritual Health

Spiritually healthy individuals identify their own basic purpose in life; learn how to experience love, joy, peace, and fulfillment; and help themselves and others achieve their full potential. As they devote themselves to others' needs more than their own, their spiritual development produces a sense of greater meaning in their lives. (See Chapter 2 for an in-depth discussion of spiritual and emotional well-being.)

Many studies have confirmed health benefits for individuals who pray, attend religious services, and engage in spiritual practices. However, the largest-ever study of "intercessory" prayer (praying for other individuals) found no benefits for coronary bypass patients. In fact, the patients who knew strangers were praying for them fared significantly worse than those who received no prayers.[5] These findings are "not an indictment of prayer or prayer's potential power," notes Dr. Mitchell Krucoff, a pioneer in spirituality research, but a call for more vigorous study and thinking about the complexity of the interactions between mind, body, and spirit.[6]

Social Health

Social health refers to the ability to interact effectively with other people and the social environment, to develop satisfying interpersonal relationships, and to fulfill social roles. It involves participating in and contributing to your community, living in harmony with fellow human beings, developing positive interdependent relationships (discussed in Chapter 8), and practicing healthy sexual behaviors.

"Far more than we are consciously aware," says psychologist Daniel Goleman, Ph.D., author of *Social Intelligence*, "our daily encounters with others—family, friends, coworkers, even strangers—shape our brains and affect cells throughout our body for good or ill."[7]

In times of crisis, social connections provide comfort and support. Even in tranquil times, social isolation increases the risk of sickness and mortality. People with spouses, friends, and a rich social network may outlive isolated loners by as much as 30 years.

Social connections make us feel good psychologically as well as physically. "If there's one thing that separates happy people from ridiculously happy people, it's the quality of their social relationships," says psychologist

Todd Kashdan, Ph.D., who teaches a college course in the science of emotional well-being. Even the company of strangers can affect your mood. As he notes, "you laugh much harder when you're with other people in a theatre than when you watch a movie by yourself."[8] (See Chapter 2 for an in-depth discussion of happiness.]

Health educators are placing greater emphasis on social health in its broadest sense as they expand the traditional individualistic concept of health to include the complex interrelationships between one person's health and the health of the community and environment. This change in perspective has given rise to a new emphasis on **health promotion,** which educators define as "any planned combination of educational, political, regulatory, and organizational supports for actions and conditions of living conducive to the health of individuals, groups, or communities." Examples on campus include smoke-free policies for all college buildings, residences, and dining areas, prohibiting tobacco advertising and sponsorship of campus social events, and promoting safety at parties and enforcing alcohol laws and policies.

How socially aware and responsible are today's college students? As you'll find in Point/Counterpoint: "Generation 'Me' or 'We'?" on page 7, some research suggests that today's undergraduates are more narcissistic than previous generations, while others view them as community-minded and generous. Where do you stand?

Intellectual Health

Your brain is the only one of your organs capable of self-awareness. Every day you use your mind to gather, process, and act on information; to think through your values; to make decisions, set goals, and figure out how to handle a problem or challenge. Intellectual health refers to your ability to think and learn from life experience, your openness to new ideas, and your capacity to question and evaluate information. Throughout your life, you'll use your critical thinking skills, including your ability to evaluate health information, to safeguard your well-being.

Environmental Health

You live in a physical and social setting that can affect every aspect of your health. Environmental health refers to the impact your world has on your well-being. It means protecting yourself from dangers in the air, water, and soil, and in products you use—and also working to preserve the environment itself. (Chapter 19 offers a thorough discussion of environmental health.)

A National Report Card on Student Health

Most undergraduates assume they are healthy. According to the American College Health Association National College Health Assessment (ACHA-NCHA)—the most comprehensive survey of student health and behaviors—more than nine in ten students describe their health as good, very good, or excellent.[9]

Your personal health depends on many factors, including your age, gender, race, and ethnic background. If you're in your late teens or early twenties, you are in a potentially risky transition. According to a longitudinal study that followed 10,000 young Americans from adolescence into adulthood, health risks increased significantly as they came of age. Young men and women of every race and ethnic group are more likely to eat fast food, not exercise, be obese, and smoke cigarettes. Many do not have health insurance, do not get regular physical or dental examinations, and do not receive health care when they need it. Drug abuse and sexually transmitted infections (STIs) are widespread in this age group.[10]

No single race or ethnic group leads or falters in health across all of the health indicators studied. White Americans, who have the best health in adolescence, experience the greatest decline in early adulthood. Native Americans face higher health risks both as teens and adults. Individuals in minority groups are most likely to need care but to be unable to pay for it.

An estimated 7.1 million college students—43 percent of the undergraduates in U.S. institutes of higher education-are age 24 or older.[11] If you're among them, think back to how your habits have changed since you were a teenager. Have they improved or deteriorated over time? Remember that many health problems are not inevitable, and it's never too soon or too late to improve and safeguard your health.

Student Health Norms

Psychologists use the term *norm*, or **social norm,** to refer to a behavior or attitude that a particular group expects, values, and enforces. Norms influence a wide variety of human activities, including health habits. However, perceptions of social norms are often inaccurate. Only anonymous responses to a scientifically designed questionnaire can reveal what individuals really do—the *actual* social norms—as compared to what they may say they do to gain social approval.

Undergraduates are particularly likely to misjudge what their peers are—and aren't—doing. In recent years colleges have found that publicizing research data on behaviors such as drinking, smoking, and drug use helps students get a more accurate sense of the real health norms on campus.[12]

The gap between students' misperceptions and accurate health norms can be enormous. For example, undergraduates in the ACHA-NHCA survey estimated that 54 percent of students had smoked cigarettes one or two days in the previous month. In fact, only 5 percent had. Similarly, students guessed that about a third (34 percent) of their peers drank alcohol every day. In reality, only .5 percent did.[13] Providing accurate information on drinking norms on campus has proven effective in changing students' perceptions and in reducing alcohol consumption by both men and women.[14]

A new feature in every chapter of this book, Reality Check, tests the accuracy of your perceptions of health norms by asking what you think is normal for college students and then providing the latest data from the National College Health Assessment. You can get started on page 9.

health promotion An educational and informational process in which people are helped to change attitudes and behaviors in an effort to improve their health.

social norms The unwritten rules regarding behavior and conduct expected or accepted by a group.

Staying Healthy on Campus

College students generally don't get good grades for their health habits. Often on their own for the first time, college students leave behind their family's ways of eating, sleeping, and relaxing and develop new habits and routines—usually not healthier ones. Many simply don't get enough sleep or keep irregular schedules that throw their sleep patterns off. Often it seems that there aren't enough hours in the day for all the things undergraduates need or want to do—study, socialize, pursue extracurricular activities, surf the Internet, work at part-time jobs, participate in community service. Sleeping less and juggling more, students can quickly end up exhausted—and at greater risk for colds, flus, digestive problems, and other maladies.

Students also become more sedentary in college, as they log more hours in classes and in front of computers. The combination of a high-fat diet and a sedentary lifestyle in college can set the stage for the development of health problems that include obesity, diabetes, metabolic syndrome, heart disease, and certain cancers.

In the National College Health Assessment survey, undergraduates rank stress as the number-one impediment to academic performance. Sleep difficulties, an epidemic on most campuses, further undermine well-being. More undergraduates are seeking psychological counseling to deal with the strain they feel as well as for mental disorders such as anxiety and depression.

Yet health problems are not inevitable. You can do more than anyone else to prevent or overcome them because when it comes to your health, you call the shots. You decide which foods to eat, whether to take vitamins, when to sleep or exercise. You determine when to see a doctor, what kind of doctor, and with what sense of urgency. You decide what to tell the physician and whether to follow his or her advice, take a prescribed medication as directed, or seek further help or a second opinion. The entire process of maintaining or restoring health depends on your decisions. It cannot start or continue without them.

Simply by acquiring more years of schooling, you are increasing your chance of a long and healthful life. Many risk factors for disease—including high blood pressure, elevated cholesterol, and cigarette smoking—decline steadily as education increases, regardless of how much money people make. Education may be good for the body as well as the mind by influencing lifestyle behaviors, problem-solving abilities, and values. People who earn college degrees acquire positive attitudes about the benefits of healthy living, learn how to gain access to preventive health services, join peer groups that promote healthy behavior, and develop higher self-esteem and greater control over their lives.

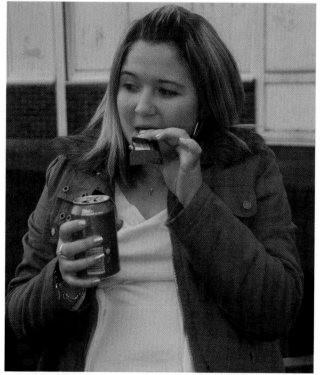

Your choices and behaviors during your college years can influence how healthy you will be in the future.

This course in itself may be good for your health. In studies on the impact of health and wellness courses, students reported that they not only learned about the many dimensions of health but made changes to improve their health. Many changed their diet and eating habits, began exercising at a campus gym, developed schedules for better time management, engaged in stress-releasing activities, or altered a dangerous habit, such as smoking or drinking.

Figure 1.3 shows the top ten physical and mental problems that students experienced in the last year. Some are occasional or one-time events (such as sinus and ear infections), but the two most common—back pain and allergies—could be long-term health issues.

Preventing Health Problems

College students often think they are too young to worry about serious health conditions. Yet many chronic problems begin early in life. Two percent of college-age women already have osteoporosis, a bone-weakening disease; another 15 percent have osteopenia, low bone densities that put them at risk of osteoporosis. Many college students have several risk factors for heart disease, including high blood pressure and high cholesterol. Others increase their risk by eating a high-fat diet and not exercising regularly. The time to change is now.

No medical treatment, however successful or sophisticated, can compare with the power of **prevention.** Two out of every three deaths and one in three hospitalizations in the United States could be prevented by changes in six main risk factors: tobacco use, alcohol abuse, accidents, high blood pressure, obesity, and gaps in screening and primary health care. Prevention remains the best weapon against cancer and heart disease.

Prevention can take many forms. Primary, or before-the-fact, prevention efforts might seek to reduce stressors and increase support to prevent problems in healthy people. Consumer education, for instance, provides guidance about how to change our lifestyles to prevent problems and enhance well-being. Other preventive programs identify people at risk and empower them with information and support so they can avoid potential problems. Prevention efforts may target an entire community and try to educate all of its members about the dangers of alcohol abuse or environmental hazards, or they may zero in on a particular group (for instance, seminars on safer sex practices offered to teens) or an individual (such as one-on-one counseling about substance abuse).

Protecting Yourself

There is a great deal of overlap between prevention and **protection.** Some people might think of immunizations (discussed in Chapter 15) as a way of preventing illness; others see them as a form of protection against dangerous diseases. In many ways, protection picks up where prevention leaves off. You can prevent STIs or unwanted pregnancy by abstaining from sex. But if you decide to engage in potentially

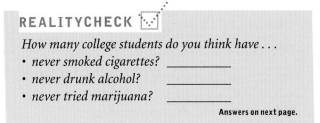

risky sexual activities, you can protect yourself with condoms and spermicides (discussed in Chapter 10). Similarly, you can prevent many automobile accidents by not driving when road conditions are hazardous. But if you do have to drive, you can protect yourself by wearing a seat belt and using defensive driving techniques (discussed in Chapter 18). What can *you* do? See "Your Strategies for Prevention" on page 10.

The very concept of protection implies some degree of risk—immediate and direct (for instance, the risk of intentional injury from an assailant or unintentional harm from a fire) or long-term and indirect (such as the risk of heart disease and cancer as a result of smoking). To know how best to protect yourself, you have to be able to realistically assess risks.

Colleges and universities take varied steps to protect students' well-being. These range from requiring vaccination against meningitis to banning alcohol at athletic and social events. Find out what your school is doing to protect your health. Would you like to see more programs and policies to safeguard student well-being?

Informing Yourself

Reliable health information can help you take better care of yourself. In the ACHA-NCHA survey discussed in the previous section, 73 percent of students turned to parents for health-related information.

The second most common source of health information is the Internet, although only about one in four consider it believable.[15] In a recent survey at two schools, three in four students reported getting health information online, and more than 40 percent frequently searched the Internet for health-related materials. As discussed in Chapter 17, you can find reliable, reputable health advice online—if you know where to look and if you remain skeptical about news or breakthroughs that seem too good to be true (see Savvy Consumer: "Too Good to Be True?").

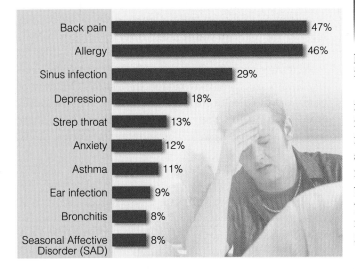

Back pain	47%
Allergy	46%
Sinus infection	29%
Depression	18%
Strep throat	13%
Anxiety	12%
Asthma	11%
Ear infection	9%
Bronchitis	8%
Seasonal Affective Disorder (SAD)	8%

Figure 1.3 Top Ten Physical and Mental Problems on Campus (last 12 months)

Source: American College Health Association. "American College Health Association National College Health Assessment Spring 2006 Reference Group Data Report (Abridged)." *Journal of American College Health*, Vol. 55, No. 4, January–February 2007 pp. 195–206.

prevention Information and support offered to help healthy people identify their health risks, reduce stressors, prevent potential medical problems, and enhance their well-being.

protection Measures that an individual can take when participating in risky behavior to prevent injury or unwanted risks.

About half of students turn to health educators for information, and most rank them and health center medical staff as believable. Although students regularly get information from flyers, pamphlets, magazines, and television, they are less likely to consider these as authoritative, believable sources.

Colleges and universities also provide health-related information to students. The most commonly covered topics are alcohol and drug use prevention, sexual assault/relationship violence prevention, sexually transmitted infections, physical activity and fitness, HIV/AIDS prevention, and nutrition and dietary behaviors.

Understanding Risky Behaviors

 Risky behaviors are not new or unusual on campus, but today's students face different- and potentially deadlier-risks than undergraduates did a generation or two ago. The problem is not that students who engage in risky behavior do not know the danger or feel invulnerable. Young people, according to recent research, actually overestimate the risk of some outcomes. However, they also overestimate the benefit of immediate pleasure when for instance, engaging in unsafe sex, and underestimate the negative consequences, such as a sexually transmitted infection.[16]

 College-age men are more likely than women to engage in risky behaviors—to use drugs and alcohol, to have unprotected sex, and to drive dangerously. Men also are more likely to be hospitalized for injuries and to commit suicide. Three-fourths of the deaths in the 15- to 24-year age range are men.

Drinking has long been part of college life and, despite the efforts across U.S. college campuses to curb alcohol abuse, two out of five students engage in binge drinking-consumption of five or more drinks at a single session for men, four for women. Heavy drinking increases the likelihood of other risky behaviors, such as smoking cigarettes, using drugs, or having multiple sexual partners.

Some behaviors are riskier than students realize. "Body art"—piercings and tattoos—may seem harmless, but health officials warn of hidden risks, including hepatitis B and C infection and transmission of HIV (see Chapter 15).

Personalizing Your Health Care

Thanks to advances in genomics (the study of the entire set of human genes), physicians are tailoring tests and treatments to individual patients. "Personalized" medicine can alert your doctor to potential threats that might be prevented, delayed, or detected at an earlier, more treatable stage and, if you do develop a disease, pinpoint the medications that will do the most good and cause the least harm.

But "personalizing" health care is also a personal responsibility. You can take charge of your own health by compiling a family health history and informing yourself about risks related to your gender, race, and ethnicity.

Your Family Health History

Someday a DNA scan from a single drop of blood may tell you the diseases you're most likely to develop. A family history can do the same—now.

Mapping your family medical history can help identify health risks you may face in the future. One way of charting your health history is to draw a medical family "tree" that includes your parents and siblings (who share half your genes), as well as grandparents, uncles, aunts,

---

YOUR STRATEGIES FOR PREVENTION *Smart Steps to Take Now*

- To lower your risk of heart disease, get your blood pressure and cholesterol checked. Don't smoke. Stay at a healthy weight. Exercise regularly.

- To lower your risks of major diseases, get regular checkups. Make sure you are immunized against infectious illnesses.

- To lower your risks of substance abuse and related illnesses and injuries, don't drink, or limit how much you drink. Avoid illegal drugs.

- To lower your risk of sexually transmitted infections (STIs) or unwanted pregnancy, abstain from sex. If you engage in risky sexual activities, protect yourself with contraceptives, condoms, and spermicides.

- To prevent car accidents, stay off the road in hazardous circumstances, such as bad weather. Wear a seat belt when you drive, and use defensive driving techniques.

Ask yourself these questions:

- What healthy change can I make in my life today?
- This week?
- This month?
- This term?

Write your answers in your HealthNow Journal.

▼ *Savvy* Consumer Too Good to Be True?

Almost every week you're likely to come across a commercial or an ad for a new health product that promises better sleep, more energy, clearer skin, firmer muscles, lower weight, brighter moods, longer life—or all of these combined. As the Savvy Consumer throughout this book points out, you can't believe every promise you read or hear. Keep these general guidelines in mind the next time you come across a health claim:

- If it sounds too good to be true, it probably is. If a magic pill could really trim off excess pounds or banish wrinkles, the world would be filled with thin people with unlined skin. Look around and you'll realize that's not the case.

- Look for objective evaluations. If you're watching an infomercial for a treatment or technique, you can be sure that the enthusiastic endorsements have been skillfully

scripted and rehearsed. Even ads that claim to be presenting the science behind a new breakthrough are really sales pitches in disguise.

- Consider the sources. Research findings from carefully controlled scientific studies are reviewed by leading experts in the field and published in scholarly journals. Just because someone has conducted a study doesn't mean it was a valid scientific investigation.

- Check credentials. Anyone can claim to be a scientist or a health expert. Find out if advocates of any type of therapy have legitimate degrees from recognized institutions and are fully licensed in their fields.

- Do your own research. Check with your doctor or with the student health center. Go to the library or do some online research to gather as much information as you can.

---

and cousins. Depending on how much information you're able to obtain for each relative, your medical family tree can include health issues each family member has faced, including illnesses with a hereditary component, such as high blood pressure, diabetes, some cancers, and certain psychiatric disorders. Although having a relative with a certain disease may increase your risk, your likelihood of ending up with the same condition also depends on your health habits, such as diet and exercise. Knowing now that you're at risk can motivate you to change any unhealthy behaviors. Realizing that you have a relative with, say, colon cancer could mean that you should start screening tests ten years before others because you're at risk of developing a tumor at an earlier age.

For guidance on creating a family history, check these websites: **www.mayoclinic.com** or **www.ashg.org/genetics/ashg/educ/007.shtml.**

Why Gender Matters

"Sex does matter. It matters in ways that we did not expect. Undoubtedly, it also matters in ways that we have not begun to imagine." This was the conclusion of the Institute of Medicine Committee on Understanding the Biology of Sex and Gender Differences in the first significant review of the status of sex and gender differences in biomedical research.

Sex, the committee stated, is "a classification, generally as male or female, according to the reproductive organs and functions that derive from the chromosomal complement." *Gender* refers to "a person's self-representation as male or female or how that person is responded to by social institutions on the basis of the individual's gender presentation." Rooted in biology, gender is shaped by environment and experience.

The experience of being male or female in a particular culture and society can and does have an effect on physical and psychological well-being. In fact, sex and gender may have a greater impact than any other variable on how our bodies function, how long we live, and the symptoms, course, and treatment of the diseases that strike us.

This realization is both new and revolutionary. For centuries, scientists based biological theories solely on a male model and viewed women as shorter, smaller, and rounder versions of men. Even modern medicine is based on the assumption that, except for their reproductive organs, both sexes are biologically interchangeable. We now know that this simply isn't so (Figure 1.4). Sex begins in the womb, but sex and gender differences affect behavior, perception, and health throughout life.

Recognition of these gender differences is transforming medical research and practice. Gender-specific medicine is replacing one-size-fits-all health care with new definitions of what is normal in both men and women, more complex concepts of disease, more precise diagnostic tests, and more effective treatments.

A Report Card on the Nation's Health

Americans are healthier and are living longer than ever before in history. Nearly 7 in 10 persons report good or excellent health; fewer than 1 in 10 are in fair or poor health. Higher percentages of white (37 percent) and Asian (36 percent) Americans report excellent health than African Americans (30 percent).[17]

Both education and income increase the likelihood of good health. College graduates are more than twice as likely as those who did not graduate from high school to be in excellent health. People with family incomes of $75,000 or more are almost twice as likely as those with family incomes of less than $20,000 to be in excellent health.

Individuals with private health insurance are also more likely to be in excellent health than those with other types of insurance or the uninsured. About 42 million Americans under age 65 do not have health insurance coverage.[18]

Healthy People 2010: How Are We Doing?

Healthy People 2010 is the prevention agenda for the nation. Every decade the federal government identifies the most significant preventable threats to health and creates leading indicators that assess the health of Americans.

Based on data from the first years of this decade, Americans are moving forward on 70 percent of the 507 objectives and subobjectives set by *Healthy People 2010.*[19] However, progress on its two main goals—improving life expectancy and eliminating health disparities—has been mixed.

Living Longer, Healthier Lives

Americans are living longer and healthier lives than ever before in history. Life expectancy has reached a new high of 77.8 years, increasing for both men and women. Life expectancy for African Americans, though increasing, is five years lower than for whites.[20]

The gender gap between male and female life expectancies has narrowed to five years, but women are living longer than men across almost all the world. The age-adjusted death rate has hit an all-time low of 801 deaths per 100,000 people, with declines in mortality from stroke, heart disease, cancer, and accidents.

The top leading causes of preventable death are tobacco use and poor diet and inactivity. Others include alcohol and drug abuse, motor vehicle accidents, sexually transmitted infections (STIs), and firearms.

Overcoming Health Disparities

Despite great improvements in the overall health of the nation, Americans who are members of racial and ethnic groups—including black or African Americans, American Indians, Alaska Natives, Asian Americans, Hispanics, Latinos, and Pacific Islanders—are more likely than whites to suffer poor health and die prematurely. Many factors, including genetic variations, environmental influences, and specific health behaviors, contribute to these disparities.[21]

Why Race Matters

We live in the most diverse nation on Earth, one that is becoming increasingly diverse. For society, this variety can be both enriching and divisive. Tolerance and acceptance of others have always been part of the American creed. By working together, Americans have created a country that remains, to those outside our borders, a symbol of opportunity. Yet members of different ethnic groups still have to struggle against discrimination.

Black Americans lose substantially more years of potential life to homicide (nine times as many), stroke (three times as many), and diabetes (three times as many) as whites. Hispanics suffer more fatal injuries, chronic liver disease, and cirrhosis of the liver.

He:

- averages 12 breaths a minute
- has lower core body temperature
- has a slower heart rate
- has more oxygen-rich hemoglobin in his blood
- is more sensitive to sound
- produces twice as much saliva
- has a 10 percent larger brain
- is 10 times more likely to have attention deficit disorder
- as a teen, has an attention span of 5 minutes
- is more likely to be physically active
- is more prone to lethal diseases, including heart attacks, cancer, and liver failure
- is five times more likely to become an alcoholic
- has a life expectancy of 75.2 years

She:

- averages 9 breaths a minute
- has higher core body temperature
- has a faster heart rate
- has higher levels of protective immunoglobulin in her blood
- is more sensitive to light
- takes twice as long to process food
- has more neurons in certain brain regions
- is twice as likely to have an eating disorder
- as a teen, has an attention span of 20 minutes
- is more likely to be overweight
- is more vulnerable to chronic diseases, like arthritis and autoimmune disorders, and age-related conditions like osteoporosis
- is twice as likely to develop depression
- has a life expectancy of 80.4 years

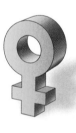

Figure 1.4 Men and women *are* different in many ways.

Caucasians are prone to osteoporosis (progressive weakening of bone tissue); cystic fibrosis; skin cancer; and phenylketonuria (PKU), a metabolic disorder that can lead to mental retardation.

Native Americans, including those indigenous to Alaska, are more likely to die young than the population as a whole, primarily as a result of accidental injuries, cirrhosis of the liver, homicide, pneumonia, and the complications of diabetes. The suicide rate among American Indians and Alaska Natives is 50 percent higher than the national rate. The rates of co-occurring mental illness and substance abuse (especially alcohol) are also higher among Native American youth and adults.

The Department of Health and Human Services has identified several areas in which racial and ethnic minorities experience significant disparities in health access and outcomes. These include the following.

Cancer Screening and Management Overall, black Americans are more likely to develop cancer than persons of any other racial or ethnic group. Black women have higher rates of colon, pancreatic, and stomach cancer. Black men have higher rates of prostate, colon, and stomach cancer.

African Americans have the highest death rates for lung cancer of any racial or ethnic group in the United States. Medical scientists have debated whether the reason might be that treatments are less effective in blacks or whether many are not diagnosed early enough or treated rigorously enough. A recent study of men with lung cancer has shown that equal treatment leads to equal outcomes. African American patients who received the same treatments as whites were just as likely to survive.[22] African American women are more than twice as likely to die of cervical cancer than are white women and are more likely to die of breast cancer than are women of any other racial or ethnic group. Native Hawaiian women have the highest rates of breast cancer. Women from many racial minorities, including those of Filipino, Pakistani, Mexican, and Puerto Rican descent, are more likely to be diagnosed with late-stage breast cancer than white women.

Cardiovascular Disease Heart disease and stroke are the leading causes of death for all racial and ethnic groups in the United States, but rates of death from heart disease and from stroke are higher among African American adults than among white adults. African Americans also have higher rates of high blood pressure (hypertension), develop this problem earlier in life, suffer more severe hypertension, and have higher rates of stroke.

Diabetes American Indians and Alaska Natives, African Americans, and Hispanics are twice as likely to be diagnosed with diabetes compared with non-Hispanic whites. Native Americans have the highest rate of diabetes in the world.

Infant Mortality African American, American Indian, and Puerto Rican infants have higher death rates than white infants.

Mental Health American Indians and Alaska Natives appear to suffer disproportionately from depression and substance abuse. Minorities have less access to mental health services and are less likely to receive needed high-quality mental health services.

Infectious Diseases Asian Americans and Pacific Islanders have much higher rates of hepatitis B. Black teenagers and young adults become infected with hepatitis B three to four times more often than those who are white. Black people also have a higher incidence of hepatitis C infection than white people. Almost 80 percent of reported cases affect racial and ethnic minorities.

HIV and Sexually Transmitted Infections Although African Americans and Hispanics represent only about a quarter of the U.S. population, they account for about two-thirds of adult AIDS cases and more than 80 percent of pediatric AIDS cases. The rate of syphilis infection for African Americans is nearly 30 times the rate for whites.

Are these increased susceptibilities the result of genetics, an unhealthy lifestyle, lack of access to health services, poverty, or the stress of living with discrimination? It is hard to say precisely. In some cases, both genetic and environmental factors may play a role. Take, for example, the high rates of diabetes among the Pima Indians. Until 50 years ago, these Native Americans were not notably obese or prone to diabetes. After World War II, the tribe started trading handmade baskets for lard and flour. Their lifestyle became more sedentary and their diet higher in fats. In addition, researchers have discovered that many Pima Indians have an inherited resistance to insulin that increases their susceptibility to diabetes. The combination of a hereditary predisposition and environmental factors may explain why the Pimas now have epidemic levels of diabetes.

But race itself isn't the primary reason for the health problems faced by minorities in the United States. Poverty is. Without adequate insurance or the ability to pay, many cannot afford the tests and treatments that could prevent illness or overcome it at the earliest possible stages. One in three Hispanics under age 65 has no health insurance. According to public health experts, low income may account for one-third of the racial differences in death rates for middle-aged African American adults. High blood pressure, high cholesterol, obesity, diabetes, and smoking are responsible for another third. The final third has been blamed on "unexplained factors," which may well include

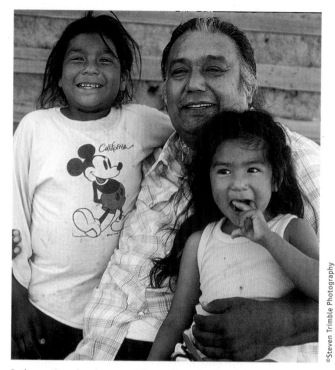

Both genetic and environmental factors have contributed to the increase in diabetes among the Pima tribe. Half of all Pima adults have diabetes.

poor access to health care and the stress of living in a society in which skin color remains a major barrier to equality.

If Your Racial Background Puts You at Risk

As a risk factor for certain health conditions, race is beyond anyone's control. However, classifications such as "black" or "Hispanic" may be overly broad. Among Hispanics, for instance, Puerto Ricans suffer disproportionately from asthma, HIV/AIDS, and high infant mortality, while Mexican Americans have higher rates for diabetes. If, like many Americans, you come from a racially mixed background, your health profile may be complex.[23]

Awareness of potential risks is the first step to protecting your health. If you do face greater health threats because of your race or ethnicity, it is up to you to educate yourself, take responsibility for the risks within your control, and become a savvy, assertive consumer of health-care services. The federal Office of Minority Health (**www.cdc.gov/omh**), which provides general information and the latest research and recommendations, is a good place to start.

Certain health risks may be genetic, but behavior influences their impact. If you are African American, for instance, you are significantly more likely to develop high blood pressure, diabetes, and kidney disease. Being overweight or obese adds to the danger. The information in Chapters 5, 6, and 7 can help you lower your risk by keeping in shape, making healthy food choices, and managing your weight.

Because diabetes and high blood pressure run in families, knowing your family history is crucial (see page 10). The National Kidney Disease Education Program has launched an initiative to encourage African Americans, who have a four-times greater risk of kidney disease, to share information about these conditions at holiday gatherings or family reunions.

Hispanics and Latinos have disproportionately high rates of respiratory problems, such as asthma, chronic obstructive lung disease, and tuberculosis. To protect your lungs, stop smoking and avoid secondary smoke. Learn as much as you can about the factors that can trigger or worsen lung diseases.

As discussed earlier in this chapter, research in personalized medicine has led to development of medications tailored to an individual's genetic make-up, including his or her race and ethnicity. One such drug, BiDil, has been approved to treat heart failure, a potentially life-threatening condition, in black patients. If you or a family member require treatment for a chronic illness, ask your doctor whether any medications have proved particularly effective for your racial or ethnic background.

Besides genetics or biology, poverty, lack of health insurance, limited or no access to preventive care, and language and cultural barriers also play a role in health disparities in the United States. Use the information in Chapter 17 to learn about your rights as a health-care consumer and to ensure that you get the best possible care. Here are more suggestions that may help when you see a doctor:

- Ask if you are at risk for any medical conditions or disorders based on your family history, racial, or ethnic background.

- Find out if there are tests that could determine your risks. Discuss the advantages and disadvantages of such testing.

- Bring someone else with you for support and to help you remember what you learn.

Healthy Campus 2010

The American College Health Association has adapted the federal *Healthy People 2010* for college and universities. Its *Healthy Campus 2010* initiative has identified 28 focus areas (and 310 objectives) particularly relevant for students. Schools that participate in the program can compare data on their students to national norms and identify the key targets that would most improve health on their campuses.

Find out if your school is participating in *Healthy Campus 2010.* If it is, what are the target objectives for your campus?

©Steven Trimble Photography

Making Healthy Changes

The stakes for modifying student behavior are high. Four in ten are binge-drinkers; one in four smokes. Among those who are sexually active, almost three in four say they've engaged in unprotected sex. Only about a third of undergraduates exercise regularly. Their nutrition is notoriously poor. Weights-and weight problems-are rising on campus. By graduation, one in four students has at least one major risk factor for diabetes, metabolic syndrome, or heart disease. Yet even students who recognize the risks and want to change their behavior often have no idea how to begin.

Fortunately, our understanding of change has itself changed. Thanks to decades of research, we now know what sets the stage for change, the way change progresses, and the keys to lasting change. We also know that personal change is neither mysterious nor magical but a methodical science that anyone can master. (See "Part I: The New Science of Personal Change" in *An Invitation to Personal Change (IPC)* for a comprehensive review.)[24] **IPC**

Understanding Health Behavior

Your choices and behaviors affect how long and how well you live. Nearly half of all deaths in the United States are linked to behaviors such as tobacco use, improper diet, abuse of alcohol and other drugs, use of firearms, motor vehicle accidents, risky sexual practices, and lack of exercise.

If you would like to improve your health behavior, you have to realize that change isn't easy. Between 40 and 80 percent of those who try to kick bad health habits lapse back into their unhealthy ways within six weeks. To make lasting beneficial changes, you have to understand the three types of influences that shape behavior: predisposing, enabling, and reinforcing factors (Figure 1.5).

Predisposing Factors

Predisposing factors include knowledge, attitudes, beliefs, values, and perceptions. Unfortunately, knowledge isn't enough to cause most people to change their behavior; for example, people fully aware of the grim consequences of smoking often continue to puff away. Nor is attitude—one's likes and dislikes—sufficient; an individual may dislike the smell and taste of cigarettes but continue to smoke regardless.

Beliefs are more powerful than knowledge and attitudes, and researchers report that people are most likely to change health behavior if they hold three beliefs:

- **Susceptibility.** They acknowledge that they are at risk for the negative consequences of their behavior.
- **Severity.** They believe that they may pay a very high price if they don't make a change.
- **Benefits.** They believe that the proposed change will be advantageous to their health.

There can be a gap between stated and actual beliefs, however. Young adults may say they recognize the very real dangers of casual, careless sex in this day and age. Yet, rather than act in accordance with these statements, they may impulsively engage in unprotected sex with individuals whose health status and histories they do not know. The reason: Like young people everywhere and in every time, they feel invulnerable, that nothing bad can or will happen to them, that if there were a real danger, they would somehow know it. Often it's not until something happens—a former lover may admit to having a sexually transmitted infection—that their behaviors become consistent with their stated beliefs.

Enabling Factors

Enabling factors include skills, resources, accessible facilities, and physical and mental capacities. Before you initiate a change, assess the means available to reach your goal. No matter how motivated you are, you'll become frustrated if you keep encountering obstacles. That's why breaking a task or goal down into step-by-step strategies is so important in behavioral change.

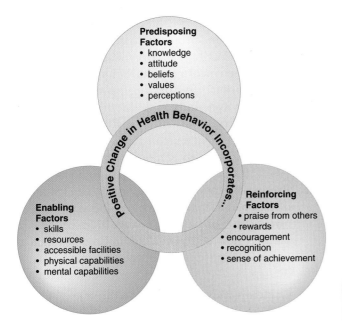

Figure 1.5 Factors That Shape Positive Behavior

predisposing factors The beliefs, values, attitudes, knowledge, and perceptions that influence our behavior.

enabling factors The skills, resources, and physical and mental capabilities that shape our behavior.

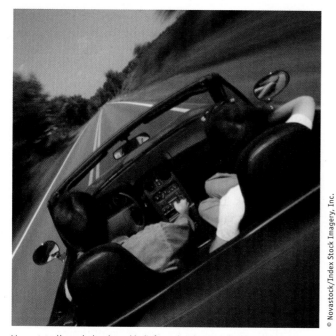

© Novastock/Index Stock Imagery, Inc.

Your *stated* knowledge-based belief may be that unsafe driving can cause accidents. Your *actual* belief is that it won't happen to you.

Reinforcing Factors

Reinforcing factors may be praise from family and friends, rewards from teachers or parents, or encouragement and recognition for meeting a goal. Although these help a great deal in the short run, lasting change depends not on external rewards but on an internal commitment and sense of achievement. To make a difference, reinforcement must come from within.

A decision to change a health behavior should stem from a permanent, personal goal, not from a desire to please or impress someone else. If you lose weight for the homecoming dance, you're almost sure to regain pounds afterward. But if you shed extra pounds because you want to feel better about yourself or get into shape, you're far more likely to keep off the weight.

Models of Behavioral Change

Change can simply happen. You get older. You put on or lose weight. You have an accident. Intentional change is different: A person consciously, deliberately sets out either to change a negative behavior, such as chronic procrastination, or to initiate a healthy behavior, such as daily exercise. For decades psychologists have studied how people intentionally change and have developed various models that reveal the anatomy of change.

In the moral model, you take responsibility for a problem (such as smoking) and its solution; success depends on adequate motivation, while failure is seen as a sign of character weakness. In the enlightenment model, you submit to strict discipline to correct a problem; this is the approach used in Alcoholics Anonymous. The behavioral model involves rewarding yourself when you make positive changes. The medical model sees the behavior as caused by forces beyond your control (a genetic predisposition to being overweight, for example) and employs an expert to provide advice or treatment. For many people, the most effective approach is the compensatory model, which doesn't assign blame but puts responsibility on individuals to acquire whatever skills or power they need to overcome their problems.

The Transtheoretical Model

This theoretical model of behavioral change, developed by psychologist James Prochaska and his colleagues, focuses on the individual's decision making rather than on social or biological influences on behavior.[25] It is the foundation of programs for smoking cessation, exercise, healthy food choices, alcohol abuse, weight control, condom use, drug abuse, mammography screening, and stress management. However, conclusive scientific evidence for its usefulness in lifestyle change remains limited.

These key components of the **transtheoretical model of change** are described in the following sections:

- **Stages of Change.**
- **Processes of Change**-cognitive and behavioral activities that facilitate change.
- **Self-Efficacy**-the confidence people have in their ability to cope with challenge.

The Stages of Change

According to the transtheoretical model of change, individuals progress through a sequence of stages as they make a change (Figure 1.6). No one stage is more important than another, and people often move back and forth between them. Most "spiral" from stage to stage, slipping from maintenance to contemplation or from action to precontemplation before moving forward again.

People usually cycle and recycle through the stages several times. Smokers, for instance, report making three or four serious efforts to quit before they succeed.

The six stages of change are:

1. **Precontemplation.** Whether or not they're aware of a problem behavior, people in this stage have no intention of making a change in the next six months. Busy college students in good health, for instance, might never think about getting more exercise.

2. **Contemplation.** Individuals in this stage are aware they have a problem behavior and are considering changing it within the next six months.

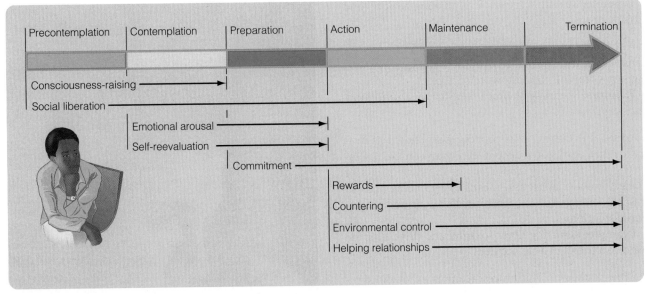

Figure 1.6   The Stages of Change and Some Change Processes
These change processes can help you progress through the stages of change. Each may be most useful at particular stages.

However, they may be torn between the positives of the new behavior and the amount of energy, time, and other resources required to change. Students in a health course, for instance, may start thinking about exercising but struggle to balance potential benefits with the effort of getting up early to jog or go to the gym.

3. **Preparation.** People in this stage intend to change a problem behavior within the next month. Some focus on a master plan. For instance, they might look into fitness classes, gyms, or other options for working out. Others might start by making small changes, such as walking to classes rather than taking a campus shuttle bus.

4. **Action.** People in this stage are modifying their behavior according to their plan. For instance, they might be jogging or working out at the gym three times a week.

5. **Maintenance.** In this stage, individuals have continued to work at changing their behavior and have avoided relapse for at least six months. New exercisers are likely to stop during the first three to six months. One reason that researchers have identified: the temptation not to exercise. However, follow-up, whether by mail, e-mail, or phone calls from supportive friends, family, or a counselor, can help maintain physical activity levels.

6. **Termination.** While it may take two to five years, a behavior becomes so deeply ingrained that a person can't imagine abandoning it. More than eight in ten college seniors who exercised regu-larly remain as active, or even more active, after graduation.

As research on college students has shown, attitudes and feelings are related to stages of change. Smokers who believe that continuing to smoke would have only a minor or no impact on their health remain in the precontemplation stage; those with respiratory symptoms move on to contemplation and preparation. In a study at Ohio State University, researchers classified student heavy drinkers according to the stages of change: Nearly two-thirds of the "precon-templators" continued to drink heavily and had no intention of changing their behavior. In the maintenance stage, students drank an average of one alcoholic drink a month even though they felt that heavy drinking was the norm on their campus.

The Processes of Change

Anything you do to modify your thinking, feeling, or behavior can be called a change process. The nine included in the transtheoretical model are shown in Figure 1.6 in their corresponding stages:

Consciousness-Raising   The most widely used change process involves increasing knowledge about yourself or the nature of your problem. As you learn more, you gain understanding and feedback about your behavior.

reinforcing factors   Rewards, encour-agement, and recognition that influ-ence our behavior in the short run.
transtheoretical model of change   A model of behavioral change that focuses on the individual's decision making; it states that an individual progresses through a sequence of six stages as he or she makes a change in behavior.

Example: Reading Chapter 5 on making healthy food choices.

Social Liberation This process takes advantage of alternatives in the external environment that can help you begin or continue your efforts to change.

Example: Spending as much time as possible in nonsmoking areas.

Emotional Arousal This process, also known as dramatic relief, works on a deeper level than consciousness-raising and is equally important in the early stages of change. Emotional arousal means experiencing and expressing feelings about a problem behavior and its potential solutions.

Example: Resolving never to drink and drive after the death of a friend in a car accident.

Self-Reevaluation This process requires a thoughtful reappraisal of your problem, including an assessment of the person you might be once you have changed the behavior.

Example: Recognizing that you have a gambling problem and imagining yourself as a nongambler.

Commitment This process acknowledges—first privately and then publicly—that you are responsible for your behavior and the only one who can change it.

Example: Joining a self-help or support group.

Countering Countering, or counterconditioning, substitutes healthy behaviors for unhealthy ones.

Example: Chewing gum rather than smoking.

Environmental Control This action-oriented process restructures your environment so you are less likely to engage in a problem behavior.

Example: Getting rid of your stash of sweets.

Rewards This process reinforces positive behavioral changes with self-praise or small gifts.

Example: Getting a massage after a month of consistent exercise.

Helping Relationships This process recruits individuals—family, friends, therapist, coach—to provide support, caring, understanding, and acceptance.

Example: Finding an exercise buddy.

Self-Efficacy and Locus of Control

Do you see yourself as master of your fate, asserting control over your destiny? Or do so many things happen in your life that you just hang on and hope for the best? The answers to these questions reveal two important characteristics that affect your health: your sense of **self-efficacy** (the belief in your ability to change and to reach a goal) and your **locus of control** (the sense of being in control of your life). See Chapter 2 in *IPC* for a detailed discussion and assessment of your locus of control. **IPC**

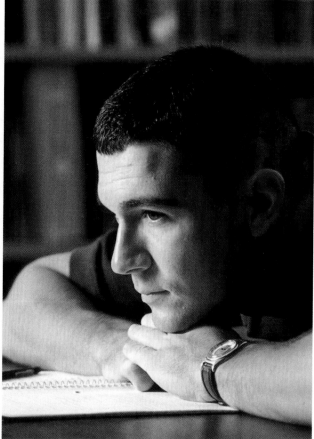

© Karim Shamsi-Basha/The Image Works

Do you picture yourself as master of your own destiny? You are more likely to achieve your health goals if you do.

Your confidence in your ability to cope with challenge can determine whether you can and will succeed in making a change. In his research on self-efficacy, psychologist Albert Bandura of Stanford University found that the individuals most likely to reach a goal are those who believe that they can. The stronger their faith in themselves, the more energy and persistence they put into making a change. The opposite is also true, especially for health behaviors. Among people who begin an exercise program, those with lower self-efficacy are more likely to drop out.

If you believe that your actions will make a difference in your health, your locus of control is internal. If you believe that external forces or factors play a greater role, your locus of control is external. Hundreds of studies have compared people who have these different perceptions of control. "Internals," who believe that their actions largely determine what happens to them, act more independently, enjoy better health, and are more optimistic about their future. "Externals," who perceive that chance or outside forces determine their fate, find it harder to cope with stress and feel increasingly helpless over time. When it comes to weight, for instance, they see themselves as destined to be fat.

The Health Belief Model

Psychologists developed the **health belief model (HBM)** about 50 years ago to explain and predict health behaviors by focusing on the attitudes and beliefs of individuals. (Remember that your attitudes and beliefs are predisposing influences on your capacity for change.) According to this model, people will take a health-related action (e.g., use condoms) if they:

· **Feel that they can avoid a negative consequence,** such as a sexually transmitted infection (STI).

· **Expect a positive outcome** if they take the recommended advice, for instance, that condoms will protect them from STIs.

· **Believe that they can successfully take action,** for example, use condoms comfortably and confidently.

Readiness to act on health beliefs, in this model, depends on how vulnerable individuals feel, how severe they perceive the danger to be, the benefits they expect to gain, and the barriers they think they will encounter. Another key factor is self-efficacy, their confidence in their ability to take action.

Over the years the health belief model has been used to help people change unhealthy behaviors, such as smoking, overeating, and inactivity, or to encourage them to take positive health actions, such as using condoms and getting needed vaccinations and medical checkups.

Changing a Bad Health Habit

When you decide to change a behavior, you have to give up something familiar and easy for something new and challenging. Change always involves risk—and the prospect of rewards.

Before they reach the stage where they can and do take action to change, most people go through a process comparable to religious conversion. First, they reach a level of accumulated unhappiness that makes them ready for change. Then they have a moment of truth that makes them want to change. One pregnant woman, for instance, felt her unborn baby quiver when she drank a beer and swore never to drink again. As people change their behavior, they change their lifestyles and identities as well. Ex-smokers, for instance, may start an aggressive exercise program, make new friends at the track or gym, and participate in new types of activities, like racquetball games or fun runs.

(See "Choosing a Change" in *IPC* to get started.) **IPC** Identify the behavior you want to change. Now think about which of the six stages of change you are in with

TABLE 1.1   Stages of Lifestyle Change

Stage of Change	Appropriate Change Goal
1. **Percontemplation:** You are not truly convinced about the importance of the lifestyle goal.	Get more information about the value of the lifestyle change goal.
2. **Contemplation:** You have no definite plan for when to begin but would like to change.	Set a date for making the change.
3. **Preparation:** You have set a date to begin the new behavior and are planning the best strategy to carry out the change.	Develop a plan and tell others about the change.
4. **Action:** You are engaged in making changes.	Adjust to new lifestyle and manage unexpected emotional and physical reactions.
5. **Maintenance:** You are working to integrate the lifestyle change into normal day-to-day life.	Continue to pay attention tothe behavior and work through any relapse. Help others achieve similar lifestyle goals.
6. **Termination/Moving On:** You have maintained the change for six months to a year and are ready to move on to other lifestyle interests.	Set new health-enhancing goals. Move on from support systems that are focused exclusively on the prior lifestyle goal.

Source: Human Resources Institute, www.healthyculture.com/Articles/mentorarticle.html. Reprinted with permission.

regard to that behavior. Table 1.1 lists some appropriate change goals for each stage. Set your goal and go for it! The next section provides more keys on how to make this change successful, and then Your Life Change Coach talks about goal-setting.

The Keys to Successful Change

Awareness of a negative behavior is always the first step toward changing it. Once you identify what you'd like to change, keep a diary for one or two weeks, noting what you do, when, where, and what you're feeling at the time. If you'd like, enlist the help of friends or family to call attention to your behavior. Sometimes self-observation in itself proves therapeutic: Just the act of keeping a diary

self-efficacy Belief in one's ability to accomplish a goal or change a behavior.

locus of control An individual's belief about the sources of power and influence over his or her life.

health belief model (HBM) A model of behavioral change that focuses on the individual's attitudes and beliefs.

can be enough to help you lose weight or kick the smoking habit.

In making a change, you have to weigh its potential pluses and minuses. **Decisional balance** involves consideration of the consequences of change to yourself and others and the reactions of both yourself and others as a result of change. These can be both positive and negative.

For instance, if your target health behavior goal is to stop smoking, you will definitely benefit in many ways, such as breathing more easily and lowering your risk of heart disease and cancer. But you may gain a few pounds or miss the camaraderie of hanging out with fellow smokers. You are more likely to make—and maintain—a health change if you see the pros of the change outweighing the cons.

Once you've identified the situations, moods, thoughts, or people that act as cues for a behavior, identify the most powerful ones and develop a plan to avoid them. For instance, if you snack continuously when studying in your room, try working in the library, where food is forbidden.

Some people find it helpful to sign a "contract," a written agreement in which they make a commitment to change, with their partner, parent, or health educator. Spelling out what they intend to do, and why, underscores the seriousness of what they're trying to accomplish.

Reinforcements—either positive (a reward) or negative (a punishment)—also can play a role. Plan a pleasant reward as an incentive for every week you stick to your new behavior—sleeping in on a Saturday morning, going out with some friends, or spending a sunny afternoon outdoors. Small, regular rewards are more effective in keeping up motivation than one big reward that won't come for many months.

Your Life Change Coach

Going for Your Goals

Think of goals as road maps that give you both a destination and a planned itinerary for getting there. "To set goals means to set a course for your life," says psychologist James Fadiman, author of *Unlimit Your Life: Setting and Getting Goals*. "Without goals, you remain what you were. With goals, you become what you wish." As studies of performance in students, athletes, and employees have shown, the one single characteristic that separates high- and low-achievers is having a clear, specific goal. The following sections describe the most effective strategies for using goals to map your way to the life you want. (See "Going for Your Goals" in *IPC*.) **IPC**

Set Your Sights on a Destination or Target

The more vividly that you can see, feel, touch, and taste what you want, the more likely you are to achieve it. The reason, explains psychologist Kenneth W. Christian, author of *Your Own Worst Enemy*, is that a destination goal transforms your brain into a satellite dish picking up the signals that are most relevant to your quest. "You begin to see possibilities that pull you closer to your goal. You meet people who can help you. It can seem magical, but it's not. Your unconscious mind is working on your goal while you go on with your life."[26]

Take a Step and a Stretch

With your target goal in sight, set "step-and-stretch" goals. Think of them like stair steps that lift you out of your comfort zone and keep you moving forward. It doesn't matter how many there are. In some instances, it may be six; in others, sixty. Every goal should be a reach from where you are that will bring you to the next level.

Break down each step goal into projects and every project into tasks. Ask yourself the following questions, and write down the answers.

- What skills do I need to achieve this?
- What information and knowledge must I acquire?
- What help, assistance, or resources do I need?
- What can block my progress? (For each potential barrier, list solutions.)
- Whom can I turn to for support?
- Who or what is likely to get in my way?
- How am I most likely to sabotage myself?

YOUR STRATEGIES FOR CHANGE *Is Your Goal S.M.A.R.T.?*

Many professional coaches use the following questions to help clients set effective goals:

- **Specific?** Identifying exactly what you want to accomplish helps you plan the steps that lead to your goal.

- **Measurable?** Your goal should be concrete enough so that both you and others can see the progress you're making.

- **Attainable?** Set goals that are slightly out of your immediate grasp but not so far that there is no hope of achieving them.

- **Realistic?** Maybe you dream of being an Olympian, but a realistic goal might be to try out for the rowing team.

- **Targeted?** A clear objective, such as quitting smoking, encourages laserlike focus.

Answer these questions in your HealthNow Journal. If you need more help in formulating your goals, consult "Your Life Change Coach" on page 20 or "The Power Tools of Personal Change" in *IPC*. **IPC**

Use an Affirmation

Once you've pictured your goal in detail, express it in an **affirmation,** a single positive sentence. As decades of psychological research have shown, affirmations serve as powerful tools for behavioral change. Make sure to use the present tense. For example, tell yourself "I am not a smoker" daily—even though you may still light up occasionally.

Once you've polished your affirmation, put it on paper. By putting it in writing, you become more committed to making your words come true. Some people post their affirmations on their computers and night stands or carry them in their wallets. Wherever you jot yours, look at your affirmation often—ideally at least once a day.

Go All the Way

Despite good intentions and considerable progress, many people give up their goals just before the rainbow's end—and congratulate themselves for getting that far. "Would you ever board a plane for Chicago and say, 'Well, we got three-quarters of the way there!' as if that were good?" asks psychologist Christian, who urges goal-seekers to persist, persevere, and "not settle for almost-there." If you stall on the final stretch, do a quick reality check. Maybe you need to add some smaller-step goals, seek more support, or simply allow yourself more time.

Whenever you achieve a goal, acknowledge it, tell a friend, or just raise your hands above your head like a runner crossing the finish line. This is what builds your sense of, "I can do it. I AM doing it. Look how far I've come!"

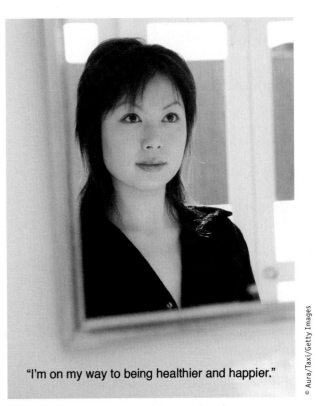

"I'm on my way to being healthier and happier."

© Aura/Taxi/Getty Images

An affirmation is a powerful tool to help you make a change.

decisional balance Weighing the positive and negative consequences of change to yourself and to others.

reinforcement Reward or punishment for a behavior that will increase or decrease one's likelihood of repeating the behavior.

affirmation A single positive sentence used as a tool for behavior change.

Recovering from a Relapse

Once you are ready to change, getting started is not the greatest challenge you'll face. That usually comes weeks or months later, when your progress hits a wall or you return to your old, unhealthy habits. Rather than looking for someone or something to help you get back on track, try the following:

- **Gather data.** Keep a detailed log of your behavior for a week, including a weekend. If your goal is to get into better shape, keep track of how much time you spend on sedentary pursuits, what derails your plans to exercise, the types of activities you most enjoy, and so forth.

- **Reassess your goals.** Are your expectations too high? Is your timetable unrealistic? Have you been derailed by finals, stress, the flu, a family crisis?

- **Check with your doctor.** Various medical conditions, such as infections, depression, diabetes, and medications (including corticosteroids and hormones) can undermine your energy and ability to pursue your wellness goals.

- **Autopsy setbacks.** If you blow your diet or slide back into couch-potato habits, analyze what went wrong and why. Start with the following questions:
  - What blindsided, distracted, demoralized, or otherwise derailed you?
  - What excuses did you use?
  - Who were the saboteurs who undermined your efforts?
  - How did they sidetrack you?

Now focus on the future.
  - What potential pitfalls do you anticipate?
  - How will you overcome them?
  - What are your back-up plans in case something or someone unexpectedly tries to sabotage your current efforts to change a health behavior?

Learn It Live It

Making Healthy Changes

Ultimately you have more control over your health than anyone else. Use this course as an opportunity to zero in on at least one less-than-healthful behavior and improve it. Here are some suggestions for small steps that can have a big payoff:

- **Use seat belts.** In the last decade, seat belts have saved more than 40,000 lives and prevented millions of injuries.

- **Eat an extra fruit or vegetable every day.** Adding more fruit and vegetables to your diet can improve your digestion and lower your risk of several cancers.

- **Get enough sleep.** A good night's rest provides the energy you need to make it through the following day.

- **Take regular stress breaks.** A few quiet minutes spent stretching, looking out the window, or simply letting yourself unwind are good for body and soul.

- **Lose a pound.** If you're overweight, you may not think a pound will make a difference, but it's a step in the right direction.

- **If you're a woman, examine your breasts regularly.** Get in the habit of performing a breast self-examination every month after your period (when breasts are least swollen or tender).

- **If you're a man, examine your testicles regularly.** These simple self-exams can spot the early signs of cancer when they're most likely to be cured.

- **Get physical.** Just a little exercise will do some good. A regular workout schedule will be good for your heart, lungs, muscles, bones—even your mood.

- **Drink more water.** Eight glasses a day are what you need to replenish lost fluids, prevent constipation, and keep your digestive system working efficiently.

- **Do a good deed.** Caring for others is a wonderful way to care for your own soul and connect with others.

SELFSURVEY : *Wellness Inventory*

What Is Wellness?*
by John W. Travis, M.D.

CENGAGENOW™ Go to HealthNow for more activities.

Most of us think in terms of illness and assume that the absence of illness indicates wellness. There are actually many degrees of wellness, just as there are many degrees of illness. The Wellness Inventory is designed to stir up your thinking about many areas of wellness.

While people often lack physical symptoms, they may still be bored, depressed, tense, anxious, or generally unhappy with their lives. Such emotional states often set the stage for physical and mental disease. Even cancer may be brought on through the lowering of the body's resistance from excessive stress. These same emotional states can also lead to abuse of the body through smoking, overdrinking, and overeating. Such behaviors are usually substitutes for other, more basic human needs such as recognition from others, a more stimulating environment, caring and affection from friends, and greater self-acceptance.

Wellness is not a static state. High-level wellness involves giving good care to your physical self, using your mind constructively, expressing your emotions effectively, being creatively involved with those around you, and being concerned about your physical, psychological, and spiritual environments.

Instructions
Set aside a half hour for yourself in a quiet place where you will not be disturbed while taking the Inventory. Record your responses to each statement in the columns to the right where:

2 = Yes, usually
1 = Sometimes, maybe
0 = No, rarely

Select the answer that best indicates how true the statement is for you presently.

After you have responded to all the appropriate statements in each section, compute your average score for that section and transfer it to the corresponding box provided around the Wellness Inventory Wheel on page 24. Your completed Wheel will give you a clear presentation of the balance you have given to the many dimensions of your life.

You will find some of the statements are really two in one. We do this to show an important relationship between the two parts-usually an awareness of an issue, combined with an action based on that awareness. Mentally average your score for the two parts of the question.

Each statement describes what we believe to be a wellness attribute. Because much wellness information is subjective and "unprovable" by current scientific methods, you (and possibly other authorities as well) may not agree with our conclusions. Many of the statements have further explanation in a footnote. We ask only that you keep an open mind until you have studied available information, then decide.

This questionnaire was designed to educate more than to test. All statements are worded so that you can easily tell what we think are wellness attributes (which also makes it easy to "cheat" on your score). This means there can be no trick questions to test your honesty or consistency—the higher your score, the greater you believe your wellness to be. Full responsibility is placed on you to answer each statement as honestly as possible. It's not your score but what you learn about yourself that is most important.

If you decide that a statement does not apply to you, or you don't want to answer it, you can skip it and not be penalized in your score.

Transfer your average score from each section to the corresponding box around the Wheel. Then graph your score by drawing a curved line between the "spokes" that define each segment. (Use the scale provided—beginning at the center with 0.0 and reaching 2.0 at the circumference.) Last, fill in the corresponding amount of each wedge-shaped segment, using different colors if possible.

*Abridged from the Wellness Index in *The Wellness Workbook*, Travis & Ryan, Ten Speed Press, 1988. Used with the permission of John W. Travis, M.D., www. wellnessworkbook.com.

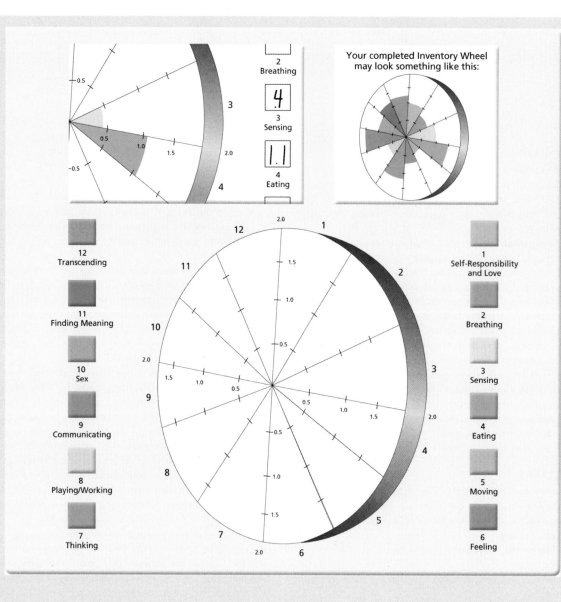

Your completed Inventory Wheel may look something like this:

Sample Questions

	Yes, usually	Sometimes, maybe	No, rarely
	2	**1**	**0**
1. I am an adventurous thinker.	✔		
2. I have no expectations, yet look to the future optimistically.		✔	
3. I am a nonsmoker.	✔		✔
4. I love long, hot baths.			
Total points for this section = 5	4	1	0

Divided by __4__ (number of statements answered) __1.3__ Average score for this section.

Section 1 WELLNESS, SELF-RESPONSIBILITY, AND LOVE

	Yes, usually 2	Sometimes, maybe 1	No, rarely 0
1. I believe how I live my life is an important factor in determining my state of health, and I live it in a manner consistent with that belief.	_____	_____	_____
2. I vote regularly.[1]	_____	_____	_____
3. I feel financially secure.	_____	_____	_____
4. I conserve materials/energy at home and at work.[2]	_____	_____	_____
5. I protect my living area from fire and safety hazards.	_____	_____	_____
6. I use dental floss and a soft toothbrush daily.	_____	_____	_____
7. I am a nonsmoker.	_____	_____	_____
8. I am always sober when driving or operating dangerous machinery.	_____	_____	_____
9. I wear a safety belt when I ride in a vehicle.	_____	_____	_____
10. I understand the difference between blaming myself for a problem and simply taking responsibility (ability to respond) for that problem.	_____	_____	_____

Total points for this section = ☐ _____ + _____ + _____

Divided by _____ (number of statements answered) = _____ Average score for this section.
(Transfer to the Wellness Inventory Wheel on p. 24.)

Section 2 WELLNESS AND BREATHING

	Yes, usually 2	Sometimes, maybe 1	No, rarely 0
1. I stop during the day to become aware of the way I am breathing.	_____	_____	_____
2. I meditate or relax myself for at least 15 to 20 minutes each day.	_____	_____	_____
3. I can easily touch my hands to my toes when standing with knees straight.[3]	_____	_____	_____
4. In temperatures over 70°F (21°C), my fingers feel warm when I touch my lips.[4]	_____	_____	_____
5. My nails are healthy and I do not bite or pick at them.	_____	_____	_____
6. I enjoy my work and do not find it overly stressful.	_____	_____	_____
7. My personal relationships are satisfying.	_____	_____	_____
8. I take time out for deep breathing several times a day.	_____	_____	_____
9. I have plenty of energy.	_____	_____	_____
10. I am at peace with myself.	_____	_____	_____

Total points for this section = ☐ _____ + _____ + _____

Divided by _____ (number of statements answered) = _____ Average score for this section.
(Transfer to the Wellness Inventory Wheel on p. 24.)

[1] Voting is a simple measure of your willingness to participate in the social system, which ultimately impacts your state of health.
[2] Besides recycling glass, paper, aluminum, and other recyclables, if you purchase products that are reusable rather than disposable, and are packaged with a minimum of material, you will reduce the drain of resources and the toxic load on the environment caused by the disposal of wastes.
[3] A lack of spinal flexibility is usually a symptom of chronic muscle tension as well as indicative of a poor balance of physical activities.
[4] If your hand temperature is below 85°F (30°C) in a warm room, you're cutting off circulation to your hands via an overactive sympathetic nervous system. You can learn to warm your hands with biofeedback and to thereby better relax.

Section 3 WELLNESS AND SENSING

	Yes, usually 2	Sometimes, maybe 1	No, rarely 0
1. My place of work has mostly natural lighting or full-spectrum fluorescent lighting.[5]	_____	_____	_____
2. I avoid extremely noisy areas or wear protective ear covers.[6]	_____	_____	_____
3. I take long walks, hikes, or other outings to actively explore my surroundings.	_____	_____	_____
4. I give myself presents, treats, or nurture myself in other ways.	_____	_____	_____
5. I enjoy getting, and can acknowledge, compliments and recognition from others.	_____	_____	_____
6. It is easy for me to give sincere compliments and recognition to other people.	_____	_____	_____
7. At times I like to be alone.	_____	_____	_____
8. I enjoy touching or hugging other people.[7]	_____	_____	_____
9. I enjoy being touched or hugged by others.[8]	_____	_____	_____
10. I get and enjoy backrubs or massages.	_____	_____	_____

Total points for this section = ☐ _____ + _____ + _____

Divided by _____ (number of statements answered) = _____ Average score for this section.
(Transfer to the Wellness Inventory Wheel on p. 24.)

Section 4 WELLNESS AND EATING

	Yes, usually 2	Sometimes, maybe 1	No, rarely 0
1. I am aware of the difference between refined carbohydrates and complex carbohydrates and eat a majority of the latter.[9]	_____	_____	_____
2. I think my diet is well balanced and wholesome.	_____	_____	_____
3. I drink fewer than five alcoholic drinks per week.	_____	_____	_____
4. I drink fewer than two cups of coffee or black (nonherbal) tea per day.[10]	_____	_____	_____
5. I drink fewer than five soft drinks per week.[11]	_____	_____	_____
6. I add little or no salt to my food.[12]	_____	_____	_____
7. I read the labels for the ingredients of all processed foods I buy and I inquire as to the level of toxic chemicals used in production of fresh foods-choosing the purest available to me.	_____	_____	_____
8. I eat at least two raw fruits or vegetables each day.	_____	_____	_____
9. I have a good appetite and am within 15 percent of my ideal weight.	_____	_____	_____
10. I can tell the difference between "stomach hunger" and "mouth hunger," and I don't stuff myself when I am experiencing only "mouth hunger."[13]	_____	_____	_____

Total points for this section = ☐ _____ + _____ + _____

Divided by _____ (number of statements answered) = _____ Average score for this section.
(Transfer to the Wellness Inventory Wheel on p. 24.)

---

[5] Full-spectrum light, like sunlight, contains many different wavelengths. Most eyeglasses, and the glass windows in your home or car, block the "near" ultraviolet light neede-by your body. Special bulbs and lenses are available.

[6] Loud noises that leave your ears ringing cause irreversible and cumulative nerve damage over time. Ear plugs/muffs, obtained in sporting goods stores, should be worn around power saws, heavy equipment, and rock concerts!

[7,8] Long recognized by hospitals as therapeutic, touch can be a powerful preventative as well.

[9] Refined carbohydrates (white flour, sugar, white rice, alcohol, and others) are burned up by the body very quickly and contain no minerals or vitamins. Complex carbohydrates (fruits and vegetables) burn evenly and provide the bulk of dietary nutrients.

[10] Coffee and nonherbal teas contain stimulants that, when overused, abuse your body's adrenal glands.

[11] Besides caffeine, the empty calories in these chemical brews may cause a sugar "crash" shortly after drinking. Artificially sweetened ones may be worse. Consider the other nutrients you won't be getting, and the prices!

[12] In addition to having a presumed connection with high blood pressure, the salting of foods during cooking draws out minerals, which are lost when the water is poured off.

[13] Stomach hunger is a signal that your body needs food. Mouth hunger is a signal that it needs something else (attention/acknowledgment), which you are not getting, so it asks for food, a readily available "substitute."

Section 5 WELLNESS AND MOVING

	Yes, usually 2	Sometimes, maybe 1	No, rarely 0
1. I climb stairs rather than ride elevators.[14]	____	____	____
2. My daily activities include moderate physical effort.[15]	____	____	____
3. My daily activities include vigorous physical effort.[16]	____	____	____
4. I run at least 1 mile three times a week (or do equivalent aerobic exercise).[17]	____	____	____
5. I run at least 3 miles three times a week (or do equivalent aerobic exercise).	____	____	____
6. I do some form of stretching/limbering exercise for 10 to 20 minutes at least three times per week.[18]	____	____	____
7. I do some form of stretching/limbering exercise for 10 to 20 minutes at least six times per week.	____	____	____
8. I enjoy exploring new and effective ways of caring for myself through the movement of my body.	____	____	____
9. I enjoy stretching, moving, and exerting my body.	____	____	____
10. I am aware of and respond to messages from my body about its needs for movement.	____	____	____

Total points for this section = [ ] ____ + ____ + ____

Divided by _____ (number of statements answered) = _____ Average score for this section.
(Transfer to the Wellness Inventory Wheel on p. 24.)

Section 6 WELLNESS AND FEELING

	Yes, usually 2	Sometimes, maybe 1	No, rarely 0
1. I am able to feel and express my anger in ways that solve problems, rather than swallow anger or store it up.[19]	____	____	____
2. I allow myself to experience a full range of emotions and find constructive ways to express them.	____	____	____
3. I am able to say "no" to people without feeling guilty.	____	____	____
4. I laugh often and easily.	____	____	____
5. I feel OK about crying and allow myself to do so when appropriate.[20]	____	____	____
6. I listen to and consider others' criticisms of me rather than react defensively.	____	____	____
7. I have at least five close friends.	____	____	____
8. I like myself and look forward to the rest of my life.	____	____	____
9. I easily express concern, love, and warmth to those I care about.	____	____	____
10. I can ask for help when needed.	____	____	____

Total points for this section = [ ] ____ + ____ + ____

Divided by _____ (number of statements answered) = _____ Average score for this section.
(Transfer to the Wellness Inventory Wheel on p. 24.)

[14] If a long elevator ride is necessary, try getting off five flights below your destination. Urge building managers to keep stair doors unlocked.

[15] Moderate = rearing young children, gardening, scrubbing floors, brisk walking, and so on.

[16] Vigorous = heavy construction work, farming, moving heavy objects by hand, and so on.

[17] Aerobic exercise (like running) should keep your heart rate at about 60 percent of its maximum (120-150 bpm) for 12-20 minutes. Brisk walking for 20 minutes every day can produce effects similar to aerobic exercise.

[18] The stretching of muscles is important for maintaining maximum flexibility of joints and ligaments. It feels good, too.

[19] Learning to take charge of your emotions and using them to solve problems can prevent disease, improve communications, and increase your self-awareness. Suppressing emotions or using them to manipulate others is destructive to all.

[20] Crying over a loss relieves the body of pent-up feelings. In our culture males often have a difficult time allowing themselves to cry, while females may have learned to cry when angry, using tears as a means of manipulation.

Section 7 WELLNESS AND THINKING

	Yes, usually 2	Sometimes, maybe 1	No, rarely 0
1. I am in charge of the subject matter and the emotional content of my thoughts and am satisfied with what I choose to think about.[21]	_____	_____	_____
2. I am aware that I make judgments wherein I think I am "right" and others are "wrong."[22]	_____	_____	_____
3. It is easy for me to concentrate.	_____	_____	_____
4. I am conscious of changes (such as breathing pattern, muscle tension, skin moisture, and so on) in my body in response to certain thoughts.[23]	_____	_____	_____
5. I notice my perceptions of the world are colored by my thoughts at the time.[24]	_____	_____	_____
6. I am aware that my thoughts are influenced by my environment.	_____	_____	_____
7. I use my thoughts and attitudes to make my reality more life-affirming.[25]	_____	_____	_____
8. Rather than worry about a problem when I can do nothing about it, I temporarily shelve it and get on with the matters at hand.	_____	_____	_____
9. I approach life with the attitude that no problem is too big to confront, and some mysteries aren't meant to be solved.	_____	_____	_____
10. I use my creative powers in many aspects of my life.	_____	_____	_____

Total points for this section = ☐ _____ + _____ + _____

Divided by _____ (number of statements answered) = _____ Average score for this section.
(Transfer to the Wellness Inventory Wheel on p. 24.)

Section 8 WELLNESS AND PLAYING/WORKING

	Yes, usually 2	Sometimes, maybe 1	No, rarely 0
1. I enjoy expressing myself through art, dance, music, drama, sports, or other activities and make time to do so.	_____	_____	_____
2. I regularly exercise my creativity "muscles."	_____	_____	_____
3. I enjoy spending time without planned or structured activities and make the effort to do so.	_____	_____	_____
4. I can make much of my work into play.	_____	_____	_____
5. At times I allow myself to do nothing.[26]	_____	_____	_____
6. At times I can sleep late without feeling guilty.	_____	_____	_____
7. The work I do is rewarding to me.	_____	_____	_____
8. I am proud of my accomplishments.	_____	_____	_____
9. I am playful and the people around me support my playfulness.	_____	_____	_____
10. I have at least one activity, hobby, or sport that I enjoy regularly but do not feel compelled to do.	_____	_____	_____

Total points for this section = ☐ _____ + _____ + _____

Divided by _____ (number of statements answered) = _____ Average score for this section.
(Transfer to the Wellness Inventory Wheel on p. 24.)

[21] When you are unconscious of the content of your thoughts, they are more likely to control you. Observing them objectively develops self-awareness and strengthens your ability to take charge.

[22] Rather than trying to completely stop yourself from judging, you can observe your judgments as efforts by your ego to avoid getting on with life and hiding behind "right/wrong" game playing.

[23] Both biofeedback and the field of psycho-neuro-immunology have shown the connections between the mind, nervous system, and body. The more you become consciously aware of that connection, the greater responsibility you can take for your health.

[24] Being aware of your internal distortion of perceptions can allow you to step back and reassess a situation more objectively.

[25] Honesty, tempered with care and concern, clears out many negative thoughts that can clutter up your mind, thus making your reality more fun. "Positive thinking" without honesty and truthfulness can backfire by suppressing valid concerns that must be addressed.

[26] Doing "nothing" can give us access to the more creative and nonverbal aspects of our being, so from another perspective, doing nothing becomes doing much more.

Section 9 WELLNESS AND COMMUNICATING

	Yes, usually 2	Sometimes, maybe 1	No, rarely 0
1. In conversation I can introduce a difficult topic and stay with it until I've gotten a satisfactory response from the other person.	_____	_____	_____
2. I enjoy silence.	_____	_____	_____
3. I am truthful and caring in my communications with others.	_____	_____	_____
4. I assert myself (in a nonattacking manner) in an effort to be heard, rather than be passively resentful of others with whom I don't agree.[27]	_____	_____	_____
5. I readily acknowledge my mistakes, apologizing for them if appropriate.	_____	_____	_____
6. I am aware of my negative judgments of others and accept them as simply judgments-not necessarily truth.[28]	_____	_____	_____
7. I am a good listener.	_____	_____	_____
8. I am able to listen to people without interrupting them or finishing their sentences for them.	_____	_____	_____
9. I can let go of my mental "labels" (for example, this is good, that is wrong) and judgmental attitudes about events in my life and see them in light of what they offer me.	_____	_____	_____
10. I am aware when I play psychological "games" with those around me and work to be truthful and direct in my communications.[29]	_____	_____	_____

Total points for this section = ☐ _____ + _____ + _____

Divided by _____ (number of statements answered) = _____ **Average score for this section.**
(Transfer to the Wellness Inventory Wheel on p. 24.)

Section 10 WELLNESS AND SEX

	Yes, usually 2	Sometimes, maybe 1	No, rarely 0
1. I feel comfortable touching and exploring my body.	_____	_____	_____
2. I think it's OK to masturbate if one chooses to do so.	_____	_____	_____
3. My sexual education is adequate.	_____	_____	_____
4. I feel good about the degree of closeness I have with men.	_____	_____	_____
5. I feel good about the degree of closeness I have with women.	_____	_____	_____
6. I am content with my level of sexual activity.[30]	_____	_____	_____
7. I fully experience the many stages of lovemaking rather than focus only on orgasm.[31]	_____	_____	_____
8. I desire to grow closer to some other people.	_____	_____	_____
9. I am aware of the difference between needing someone and loving someone.	_____	_____	_____
10. I am able to love others without dominating or being dominated by them.	_____	_____	_____

Total points for this section = ☐ _____ + _____ + _____

Divided by _____ (number of statements answered) = _____ **Average score for this section.**
(Transfer to the Wellness Inventory Wheel on p. 24.)

[27] Attacking others rarely accomplishes your goals in the long run. Persisting in your convictions without using force is more effective and usually solves the problem without creating new ones.
[28] It is important to recognize that our internal judgments of others are based on personal biases that often have little objective basis.
[29] Psychological games, as defined by Eric Berne in *Games People Play*, are complex unconscious manipulations that result in the players getting negative attention and feeling bad about themselves.
[30] Including the choice to have no sexual activity.
[31] A common problems for many people is an overemphasis on performance and orgasm, rather than on enjoying a close sensual feeling with their partner whether or not they experience orgasm.
[32] Seeing your death as a stage of growth and preparing yourself consciously is an important part of finding meaning in your life.

Section 11 WELLNESS AND FINDING MEANING

	Yes, usually 2	Sometimes, maybe 1	No, rarely 0
1. I believe my life has direction and meaning.	___	___	___
2. My life is exciting and challenging.	___	___	___
3. I have goals in my life.	___	___	___
4. I am achieving my goals.	___	___	___
5. I look forward to the future as an opportunity for further growth.	___	___	___
6. I am able to talk about the death of someone close to me.	___	___	___
7. I am able to talk about my own death with family and friends.	___	___	___
8. I am prepared for my death.	___	___	___
9. I see my death as a step in my evolution.[32]	___	___	___
10. My daily life is a source of pleasure to me.	___	___	___

Total points for this section = [ ] ___ + ___ + ___

Divided by _____ **(number of statements answered) =** _____ **Average score for this section.**
(Transfer to the Wellness Inventory Wheel on p. 24.)

This portion of the Inventory goes beyond the scope of most generally accepted "scientific" principles and expresses the values and beliefs of the authors. It is intended to stimulate interest in these areas. If you have strong beliefs to the contrary, you can skip the questions or make up your own.

Section 12 WELLNESS AND TRANSCENDING

	Yes, usually 2	Sometimes, maybe 1	No, rarely 0
1. I perceive problems as opportunities for growth.	___	___	___
2. I experience synchronistic events in my life (frequent "coincidences" seeming to have no cause–effect relationship).[33]	___	___	___
3. I believe there are dimensions of reality beyond verbal description or human comprehension.	___	___	___
4. At times I experience confusion and paradox in my search for understanding of the dimensions referred to above.	___	___	___
5. The concept of God has personal definition and meaning to me.	___	___	___
6. I experience a sense of wonder when I contemplate the universe.	___	___	___
7. I have abundant expectancy rather than specific expectations.	___	___	___
8. I allow others their beliefs without pressuring them to accept mine.	___	___	___
9. I use the messages interpreted from my dreams.	___	___	___
10. I enjoy practicing a spiritual discipline or allowing time to sense the presence of a greater force in guiding my passage through life.	___	___	___

Total points for this section = [ ] ___ + ___ + ___

Divided by _____ **(number of statements answered) =** _____ **Average score for this section.**
(Transfer to the Wellness Inventory Wheel on p. 24.)

[33] Modern physics reveals that the idea of cause and effect may be as limited as Newton's theory of a mechanical universe. It suggests that we must expand our view to see that everything in the universe is connected to everything else. (Synchronicity describes that experience.)

Your Health Action Plan for Maximum Wellness

When you have completed the Wellness Inventory, study your wheel's shape and balance. How smoothly would it roll? What does it tell you? Are there any surprises in it? How does it feel to you? What don't you like about it? What do you like about it?

We recommend that you use colored pens to go back over the questions, noting the ones on which your scores were low and choosing some areas on which you are interested in working. It is easy to overwhelm yourself by taking on too many areas at once. Ignore, for now, those of lower priority to you. Remember, if you don't enjoy at least some aspects of the changes you are making, they probably won't last.

Here are some guidelines to help you:

- Get support from friends, but don't expect them to supply all the reinforcement you need. You may join a group of overweight individuals and rely on their encouragement to stick to your diet. That's a great way to get going, but in the long run your own commitment to losing weight has got to be strong enough to help you keep eating right and light.

- Focus on the immediate rewards of your new behavior. You may stop smoking so that you'll live longer, but take note of every other benefit it brings you—more stamina, less coughing, more spending money, no more stale tobacco taste in your mouth.

- Remind yourself of past successes you've had in making changes. Give yourself pep talks, commending yourself on how well you've done so far and how well you'll continue to do. This will boost your self-confidence.

- Reward yourself regularly. Plan a pleasant reward as an incentive for every week you stick to your new behavior—sleeping in on a Saturday morning, going out with some friends, or spending a sunny afternoon outdoors. Small, regular rewards are more effective in keeping up motivation than one big reward that won't come for many months.

- Expect and accept some relapses. The greatest rate of relapse occurs in the first few weeks after making a behavior change. During this critical time, get as much support as you can. In addition, work hard on self-motivation, reminding yourself daily of what you have to gain by sticking with your new health habit.

Making This Chapter Work

Review Questions

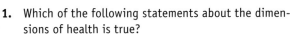
for YOU

1. Which of the following statements about the dimensions of health is true?
   a. Spirituality provides solace and comfort for those who are severely ill, but it has no health benefits.
   b. The people who reflect the highest levels of social health are usually among the most popular individuals in a group and are often thought of as the life of the party.
   c. Intellectual health refers to one's academic abilities.
   d. Optimal physical health requires a nutritious diet, regular exercise, avoidance of harmful behaviors and substances, and self-protection from accidents.

2. The term for a behavior or attitude that a particular group expects is
   a. social health.
   b. self-efficacy.
   c. social norm.
   d. reinforcement.

3. In the National College Assessment Survey, undergraduates rank this as the number-one health-related impediment to academic performance:
   a. sleep difficulties.
   b. stress.
   c. relation difficulties.
   d. cold/flu/sore throat.

4. A group of students is discussing the differences between the sexes. Whose statement is *incorrect*?
   a. Matt: "Men breathe faster but have a slower heart rate—and have a larger brain."
   b. Elena: "But women have more neurons in certain brain regions."
   c. Kristin: "And women are less likely to get arthritis."
   d. Rick: "Got me there—Men *are* more likely to have heart attacks and to get cancer."

5. Health risks faced by different ethnic and racial groups include all of the following *except*
   a. whites have higher rates of hypertension, lupus, liver disease, and kidney failure than African Americans.
   b. Native Americans have a higher rate of diabetes than other racial and ethnic groups.
   c. infant mortality is higher for African American babies than for white babies.
   d. Asian Americans have a higher rate of hepatitis B.

6. The development of health behaviors is influenced by all of the following *except*
   a. reinforcing factors, which involve external recognition for achieving a goal.
   b. preexisting health factors, which take into account the individual's current position on the wellness continuum.
   c. predisposing factors, which include knowledge, attitudes, and beliefs.
   d. enabling factors, which are related to an individual's skills and capabilities to make behavioral changes.

7. Change processes, cognitive and behavioral activities that facilitate change, include all of these *except*
   a. consciousness-raising.
   c. health awareness.
   b. countering.
   d. helping relationships.

8. According to the stages of change in the transtheoretical model of change, which statement is *incorrect?*
   a. In the maintenance stage, individuals have avoided relapse for six months.
   b. In the contemplation stage, individuals are considering changing a problem behavior in the next six months.
   c. In the action stage, individuals are actually modifying their behavior according to their plan.
   d. In the preparation stage, individuals intend to change a problem behavior in the next six months.

9. If you want to change unhealthy behavior, which of the following strategies is *least* likely to promote success?
   a. Believe that you can make the change.
   b. Reward yourself regularly.
   c. Remind yourself about all your faults.
   d. Accept that you are in control of your health.

10. Relapses are common (you're human, aren't you?), but don't let them keep you from your goal. Which of these strategies might help you recover from a relapse?
    a. Have a hot fudge sundae.
    b. Decide to think about it after finals.
    c. Analyze what went wrong and why.
    d. Put yourself back into contemplation stage.

    Answers to these questions can be found on page 583.

Critical Thinking

1. Where are you on the wellness—illness continuum? What variables might affect your place on the scale? What do you consider your optimum state of health to be?

2. Talk to classmates from different racial or ethnic backgrounds than yours about their culture's health attitudes. Ask them what is considered healthy behavior in their cultures. For example, is having a good appetite a sign of health? What kinds of self-care practices did their parents and grandparents use to treat colds, fevers, rashes, and other health problems? What are their attitudes about the health-care system?

3. Think about a behavioral change you have made in your life in the past three years in any of the dimensions of health (physical, psychological, spiritual, social, intellectual, environmental). Can you remember going through each of the six stages of the transtheoretical model of change?

4. In what ways would you like to change your present lifestyle? What steps could you take to make those changes?

Media Menu

CENGAGENOW™ Go to the HealthNow website at **academic.cengage .com/login** that will:
- Help you evaluate your knowledge of the material.
- Allow you to take an exam-prep quiz.
- Provide a Personalized Learning Plan targeting resources that address areas you should study.
- Coach you through identifying target goals for behavioral change and creating and monitoring your personal change plan throughout the semester.

INTERNET CONNECTIONS

Go Ask Alice

www.goaskalice.columbia.edu/index.html

Sponsored by Columbia University, this site offers questions and answers as well as an interactive service on a wide variety of health-related topics.

Lifescan Health Risk Appraisal

http://wellness.uwsp.edu/Other/lifescan

This site, created by Bill Hettler, M.D., of the National Wellness Institute, helps you identify specific lifestyle factors that can impair your health and longevity. Take the health questionnaire to determine your personal lifestyle risks. Your results provide a score for general results, nutrition results, and height/weight results. Your ranking among the top ten causes of death is provided, as well as suggestions on how to improve.

Transtheoretical Model—Cancer Prevention Research Center

www.uri.edu/research/cprc/TTM/detailedoverview.htm

This site describes the transtheoretical model of change, including descriptions of effective interventions to pro-mote health behavior change, focusing on the individual's decision-making strategies.

Key Terms

The terms listed are used and defined on the page indicated. Definitions are also found in the Glossary at the end of this book.

affirmation	21
decisional balance	21
enabling factors	15
health	4
health belief model (HBM)	19
health promotion	7
locus of control	19
predisposing factors	15
prevention	9
protection	9
reinforcement	21
reinforcing factors	17
self-efficacy	19
social norms	7
transtheoretical model of change	17
wellness	4

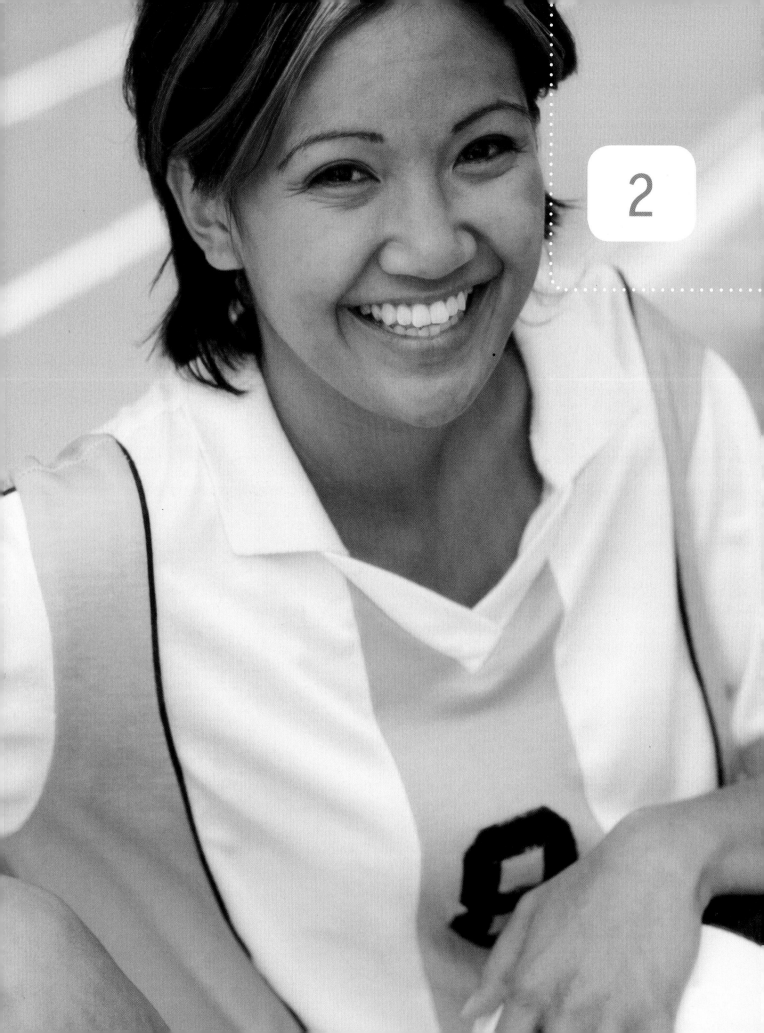

Emotional and Spiritual Well-Being

ADAM never considered himself a spiritual person until he enrolled in a class on the science of personal well-being. For a homework assignment he had to pursue different paths to happiness. As part of his experiment, he went to a Mardi Gras celebration and partied all night to see if having fun made him happier. To test whether doing good makes a person happy, Adam volunteered to help build a house for a homeless family. "I can't remember the name of a single person I met at the party," he says. "But I'll never forget the look on the family's faces when we handed them the keys to their new home."

For his final project, Adam, who did not have a religious upbringing, focused on developing a richer spiritual life. "The spirituality didn't end with the term," he says, "I continue to meditate, do yoga, and read religious texts because I believe a more spiritual life will help me in the long run with happiness and health."

The quest for a more fulfilling and meaningful life is attracting more people of all ages. The reason? As the burgeoning field of positive psychology has resoundingly proved, people who achieve emotional and spiritual health are more creative and productive, earn more money, attract more friends, enjoy better marriages, develop fewer illnesses, and live longer.

This chapter reports the latest findings on making the most of psychological strengths, enhancing happiness, and developing the spiritual dimension of your health and your life. It also explores an often overlooked dimension of physical and emotional well-being: sleep.

After studying the material in this chapter, you should be able to:

- **Identify** the characteristics of emotional and mental health.

- **Name** the two pillars of authentic happiness.

- **Explain** the health value of connecting with others.

- **Discuss** some of the health benefits of prayer.

- **Describe** four ways that sleep affects well-being.

- **Assess** your spiritual health and make a decision to enrich it in at least two ways.

CENGAGENOW Log on to HealthNow at **academic.cengage.com/login** to find your Behavior Change Planner and to explore self-assessments, interactive tutorials, and practice quizzes.

Psychological Well-Being

Unlike physical health, psychological well-being cannot be measured, tested, X-rayed, or dissected. Yet psychologically healthy men and women generally share certain characteristics: They value themselves and strive toward happiness and fulfillment. They establish and maintain close relationships with others. They accept the limitations as well as the possibilities that life has to offer. And they feel a sense of meaning and purpose that makes the gestures of living worth the effort required.

Psychological health encompasses both our emotional and mental states—that is, our feelings and our thoughts. **Emotional health** generally refers to feelings and moods, both of which are discussed later in this chapter. Characteristics of emotionally healthy persons, identified in an analysis of major studies of emotional wellness, include the following:

- Determination and effort to be healthy.
- Flexibility and adaptability to a variety of circumstances.
- Development of a sense of meaning and affirmation of life.
- An understanding that the self is not the center of the universe.
- Compassion for others.
- The ability to be unselfish in serving or relating to others.
- Increased depth and satisfaction in intimate relationships.

- A sense of control over the mind and body that enables the person to make health-enhancing choices and decisions.

Mental health describes our ability to perceive reality as it is, to respond to its challenges, and to develop rational strategies for living. The mentally healthy person doesn't try to avoid conflicts and distress but can cope with life's transitions, traumas, and losses in a way that allows for emotional stability and growth. The characteristics of mental health include:

- The ability to function and carry out responsibilities.
- The ability to form relationships.
- Realistic perceptions of the motivations of others.
- Rational, logical thought processes.
- The ability to adapt to change and to cope with adversity.

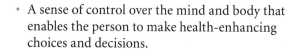 **Culture** also helps to define psychological health. In one culture, men and women may express feelings with great intensity, shouting in joy or wailing in grief, while in another culture such behavior might be considered abnormal or unhealthy. In our diverse society, many cultural influences affect Americans' sense of who they are, where they came from, and what they believe. Cultural rituals help bring people together, strengthen their bonds, reinforce the values and beliefs they share, and provide a sense of belonging, meaning, and purpose.

Where are you on the psychological well-being scale? Take the Self Survey on p. 52.

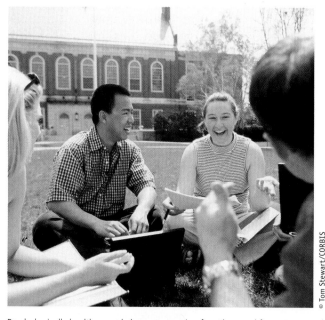

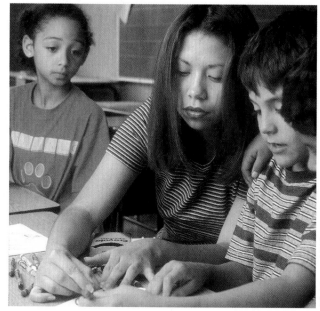

Psychologically healthy people have compassion for others and form strong and deep relationships. They adapt to a variety of circumstances, overcome challenges, and strive to achieve their full potential.

Positive Psychology 101

Psychology, a field that traditionally concentrated on what goes wrong in our lives and in our minds, has shifted its focus to the study of human strengths, virtues, and positive emotions. The three major areas of positive psychology are the study of positive emotions, such as hope and trust; positive traits, such as wisdom and courage; and positive institutions, such as strong families and democracy.

According to psychologist Martin Seligman, Ph.D., who started the positive psychology movement almost a decade ago, everyone, regardless of genes or fate, can achieve a happy, gratifying, meaningful life. The goal is not simply to feel good momentarily or to avoid bad experiences, but to build positive strengths and virtues that enable us to find meaning and purpose in life.[1]

"Psychology is not just the study of weakness and damage," Seligman argues, "it is also the study of strength and virtue. Treatment is not just fixing what is broken, it is nurturing what is best within ourselves." The traits that may well protect us from physical and mental illness include courage, optimism, hope, interpersonal skills, a work ethic, responsibility, future-mindedness, honesty, and perseverance.

Emotional Intelligence

A person's "IQ"—or intelligence quotient—was once considered the leading predictor of achievement. However, psychologists have determined that another "way of knowing," dubbed **emotional intelligence,** makes an even greater difference in a person's personal and professional success.

"EQ" (for emotional quotient) is the ability to monitor and use emotions to guide thinking and actions. Strong social or interpersonal skills are one measure of EQ. As more than a decade of research has shown, people with high EQ are more productive at work and happier at home. They're also less prone to stress, depression, and anxiety and bounce back quicker from serious illnesses.

 Men and women, who vary more in the intensity of their emotional experiences than in the nature of their emotions, are equally capable of cultivating greater emotional intelligence. Emotional intelligence isn't fixed at birth, nor is it the same as intuition. Among the emotional competencies that most benefit students are focusing on clear manageable goals and identifying and understanding emotions rather than relying on "gut" feelings.

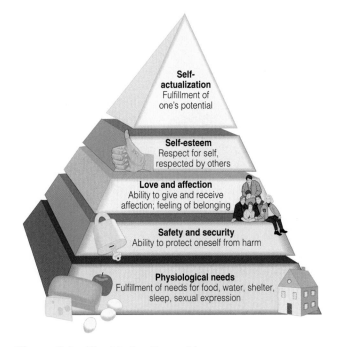

Figure 2.1 The Maslow Pyramid

To attain the highest level of psychological health, you must first satisfy your needs for safety and security, love and affection, and self-esteem.

Source: Maslow, A. *Motivation and Personality*, 3rd ed.,© 1997. Reprinted by permission of Pearson Education, Inc.

Knowing Your Needs

Newborns are unable to survive on their own. They depend on others for the satisfaction of their physical needs for food, shelter, warmth, and protection, as well as their less tangible emotional needs. In growing to maturity, children take on more responsibility and become more independent. No one, however, becomes totally self-sufficient. As adults, we easily recognize our basic physical needs, but we often fail to acknowledge our emotional needs. Yet they, too, must be met if we are to be as fulfilled as possible.

The humanist theorist Abraham Maslow believed that human needs are the motivating factors in personality development. First, we must satisfy basic physiological needs, such as those for food, shelter, and sleep. Only then

emotional health The ability to express and acknowledge one's feelings and moods and exhibit adaptability and compassion for others.

mental health The ability to perceive reality as it is, respond to its challenges, and develop rational strategies for living.

culture The set of shared attitudes, values, goals, and practices of a group that are internalized by an individual within the group.

emotional intelligence A term used by some psychologists to evaluate the capacity of people to understand themselves and relate well with others.

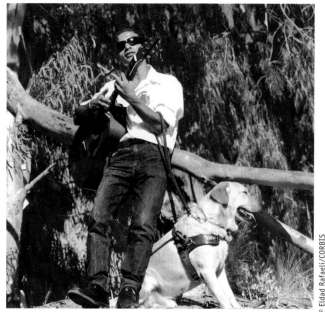

© Eldad Rafaeli/CORBIS

Health and wealth don't equal happiness. People with disabilities report almost the same level of life satisfaction as people without disabilities.

can we pursue fulfillment of our higher needs—for safety and security, love and affection, and self-esteem. Few individuals reach the state of **self-actualization,** in which one functions at the highest possible level and derives the greatest possible satisfaction from life (Figure 2.1).

The Power of Self-Esteem

Each of us wants and needs to feel significant as a human being with unique talents, abilities, and roles in life. A sense of **self-esteem,** of belief or pride in ourselves, gives us confidence to dare to attempt to achieve at school or work and to reach out to others to form friendships and close relationships. Self-esteem is the little voice that whispers, "You're worth it. You can do it. You're okay."

Self-esteem is based not on external factors like wealth or beauty, but on what you believe about yourself. It's not something you're born with; self-esteem develops over time. It's also not something anyone else can give to you, although those around you can either help boost or diminish your self-esteem.

The seeds of self-esteem are planted in childhood when parents provide the assurance and appreciation youngsters need to push themselves toward new accomplishments: crawling, walking, forming words and sentences, learning control over their bladder and bowels.

Adults, too, must consider themselves worthy of love, friendship, and success if they are to be loved, to make friends, and to achieve their goals. Low self-esteem is more common in people who have been abused as children and in those with psychiatric disorders, including depression, anxiety, alcoholism, and drug dependence.

Feeling a lack of love and encouragement as a child can also lead to poor self-esteem. Adults with poor self-esteem may unconsciously enter relationships that reinforce their self-perceptions and may prefer and even seek out people who think poorly of them.

One of the most useful techniques for bolstering self-esteem and achieving your goals is developing the habit of positive thinking and talking. While negative observations—such as constant criticisms or reminders of the most minor faults—can undermine self-image, positive affirmations—compliments, kudos, encouragements—have proved effective in enhancing self-esteem and psychological well-being. Individuals who fight off negative thoughts fare better psychologically than those who collapse when a setback occurs or who rely on others to make them feel better.

 Self-esteem has proved to be one of the best predictors of college adjustment. Students with high self-esteem report better personal, emotional, social, and academic adjustment.

The New Science of Happiness

"Imagine a drug that causes you to live eight or nine years longer, to make $15,000 more a year, to be less likely to get divorced," says Martin Seligman, the "father" of positive psychology. "Happiness seems to be that drug."[2] But even if just about everyone might benefit by smiling more and scowling less, can almost anyone learn to live on the brighter side of life?

Skeptics who dismiss "happichondria" as the latest feel-good fad are dubious. (See Point/Counterpoint: "Learning' Happiness?" on page 40.) "The notion that behavior modification can bring about true happiness is as bogus as can be," says psychiatrist Charles Goodstein, M.D., of New York University, "Happiness enhancement correlates with a sort of smug self-satisfaction because people think they're doing something real, but they're not."[3]

Happiness researchers, now backed by thousands of scientific studies, cite mounting evidence to the contrary. "Happiness is measurable, and it's buildable," says Seligman. "We're not talking about just feeling good but about something more substantial and durable. The newest finding of positive psychology is that simple, proven strategies can make you lastingly happier. However, it's not easy, and it's not obvious how to go about it."

Genetics, as research on thousands of sets of twins has demonstrated, accounts for about 50 percent of your happiness quotient. But even if you inherited the family frown rather than its joy genes, you're not fated to a life of gloom. Just don't pin your hopes on advantages like fitness, fortune, education, or good looks. The healthy, the wealthy, the bookish, and the beautiful report only somewhat greater happiness than those who are less blessed. Unless you're extremely poor or gravely ill, life circumstances account for only about 10 percent of happiness. The other 40 percent depends on what you do to make yourself happy.[4]

Unfortunately, most of us look for happiness in all the wrong places. We assume that external things—a bigger house, a better job, a winning lottery ticket—will gladden our lives. While they do bring temporary delight, the thrill invariably fades. "After 18 years studying happiness, I fell into the same trap as everyone else," says psychologist Sonja Lyubomirsky, Ph.D., author of *The How of Happiness: A Scientific Approach to Getting the Life You Want.* "I was so excited to get a new car, a hybrid I'd wanted for a long time, but within two months driving it became routine. Happiness is like weight loss. We all know how to take off a few pounds but the trick is maintaining it."[5]

In cutting-edge research, Lyubomirsky and her colleagues have fine-tuned proven strategies into practical prescriptions to enhance happiness. "Different methods are a better 'fit' for different people," she explains. "Keeping a daily gratitude journal seems hokey to some people, but writing a letter of gratitude may be very meaningful." Timing and "doses" also matter. Performing five acts of kindness on a single day, she's found, yields a greater halo effect than a single daily altruistic gesture. "But to sustain happiness you have to make the effort and commitment every day for the rest of your life," she emphasizes. For enduring joy, the key is looking beyond fleeting pleasures to the two pillars of "authentic" happiness: engagement with family, work, or a passionate pursuit and finding meaning from some higher purpose.

 Education, intelligence, gender, and race do not matter much for happiness. African Americans and Hispanics have lower rates of depression than white Americans, but they do not report greater happiness. Neither gender is clearly happier, but in different studies women are both happier and sadder than men.

 Relationships are key to happiness among undergraduates. In a survey of 222 college students, psychologists found that the "happiest" 10 percent, as determined by six different rating scales, shared one distinctive characteristic: a rich and fulfilling social life. Almost all were involved in a romantic relationship as well as in rewarding friendships. The happiest students spent the least time alone, and their friends rated them as highest on good relationships.[6]

After even the most joyous childhood, happiness typically plummets through the teens and twenties before hitting rock bottom in the forties, our most doleful decade. By age 50, happiness rises steadily and keeps soaring well into old age. The reason may be that we become mellower. Older adults don't react as intensely to life events, and they report fewer negative emotions and more positive ones. Young people, as research has consistently shown, tend to focus on the negative. They pay more attention to the bad than the good and overestimate the downside of any situation. As we get older, we learn to regulate and overcome this reaction. Age also brings other happiness advantages: Older people generally know what they want and are more likely to go after it.

Becoming Optimistic

The dictionary defines **optimism** as "an inclination to anticipate the best possible outcome." For various reasons—because they believe in themselves, because they trust in a higher power, because they feel lucky—optimists expect positive experiences from life. When bad things happen, they tend to see setbacks or losses as specific, temporary incidents. In their eyes, a disappointment is "one of those things" that happens every once in a while, rather than the latest in a long string of disasters. And rather than blaming themselves ("I always mess things up," pessimists might say), optimists look at all the different factors that may have caused the problem.

Individuals aren't born optimistic or pessimistic; in fact, researchers have documented changes over time in the ways that individuals view the world and what they expect to experience in the future. The key is disputing the automatic negative thoughts that flood our brains and choosing to believe in our own possibilities.

self-actualization A state of wellness and fulfillment that can be achieved once certain human needs are satisfied; living to one's full potential.

self-esteem Confidence and satisfaction in oneself.

optimism The tendency to seek out, remember, and expect pleasurable experiences.

Positive psychologist Martin Seligman provides "optimism training" to freshmen at the University of Pennsylvania. According to his follow-up data, those trained to look on the bright side suffered fewer illnesses throughout college than those who were not. Optimism may even help people live longer, healthier lives.

Managing Your Moods

Feelings come and go within minutes. A **mood** is a more sustained emotional state that colors our view of the world for hours or days. According to surveys by psychologist Randy Larsen of the University of Michigan, bad moods descend upon us an average of three out of every ten days. "A few people—about 2 percent—are happy just about every day," he says. "About 5 percent report bad moods four out of every five days."[7]

 There are gender differences in mood management: Men typically try to distract themselves (a partially successful strategy) or use alcohol or drugs (an ineffective tactic). Women are more likely to talk to someone (which can help) or to ruminate on why they feel bad (which doesn't help). Learning effective mood-boosting, mood-regulating strategies can help both men and women pull themselves up and out of an emotional slump.

The most effective way to banish a sad or bad mood is by changing what caused it in the first place—if you can figure out what made you upset and why. "Most bad moods are caused by loss or failure in work or intimate relationships," says Larsen. "The questions to ask are What can I do to fix the failure? What can I do to remedy the loss? Is there anything under my control that I can change? If there is, take action and solve it." Rewrite the report. Ask to take a makeup exam. Apologize to the friend whose feelings you hurt. Tell your parents you feel bad about the argument you had.

If there's nothing you can do, accept what happened and focus on doing things differently next time. "In our studies, resolving to try harder actually was as effective in improving mood as taking action in the present," says Larsen. You also can try to think about what happened in a different way and put a positive spin on it. This technique, known as *cognitive reappraisal,* or *reframing,* helps you look at a setback in a new light: What lessons did it teach you? What would you have done differently? Could there be a silver lining or hidden benefit?

If you can't identify or resolve the problem responsible for your emotional funk, the next-best solution is to concentrate on altering your negative feelings. For example, try setting a quick, achievable goal that can boost your spirits with a small success. Clean out a drawer; sort through the piles of paper on your desk; send an e-mail or text message to an old friend.

Another good option is to get moving. In studies of mood regulation, exercise consistently ranks as the single most effective strategy for banishing bad feelings. Numerous studies have confirmed that aerobic workouts, such as walking or jogging, significantly improve mood. Even nonaerobic exercise, such as weight lifting, can boost spirits; improve sleep and appetite; reduce anxiety, irritability, and anger; and produce feelings of mastery and accomplishment.

Looking on the Light Side

Humor, which enables us to express fears and negative feelings without causing distress to ourselves or others, is one of the healthiest ways of coping with life's ups and downs. Laughter stimulates the heart, alters brain wave patterns and breathing rhythms, reduces perceptions of pain, decreases stress-related hormones, and strengthens the immune system. In psychotherapy, humor helps channel negative emotions toward a positive effect. Even in cases of critical or fatal illnesses, humor can relieve pain and help people live with greater joy until they die.

Joking and laughing are ways of expressing honest emotions, of overcoming dread and doubt, and of connecting with others. They also can defuse rage. After all, it's almost impossible to stay angry when you're laughing. To tickle your funny bone, try keeping a file of favorite cartoons or jokes. Go to a comedy club instead of a movie. If you get an e-mail joke that makes you laugh out loud, don't keep it to yourself—multiply the mirth by sharing it with a friend.

Feeling in Control

Although no one has absolute control over destiny, we can do a great deal to control how we think, feel, and behave. By assessing our life situations realistically, we can make plans and preparations that allow us to make the most of our circumstances. By doing so, we gain a sense of mastery. In nationwide surveys, Americans who feel in control of their lives report greater psychological well-being than those who do not, as well as extraordinarily positive feelings of happiness.

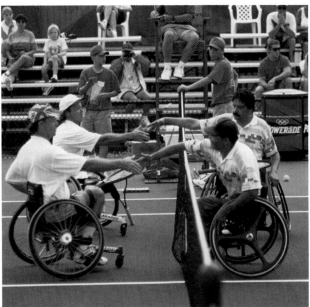

You may not have complete control over your destiny, but you can control how you respond to challenges.

© Robert W. Ginn/PhotoEdit

Developing Autonomy

One goal that many people strive for is **autonomy,** or independence. Both family and society influence our ability to grow toward independence. Autonomous individuals are true to themselves. As they weigh the pros and cons of any decision, whether it's using or refusing drugs or choosing a major or career, they base their judgment on their own values, not those of others. Their ability to draw on internal resources and cope with challenges has a positive impact on both their psychological well-being and their physical health, including recovery from illness.

Those who've achieved autonomy may seek the opinions of others, but they do not allow their decisions to be dictated by external influences. For autonomous individuals, their **locus of control**—that is, where they view control as originating—is *internal* (from within themselves) rather than *external* (from others). (See Chapter 1.)

Asserting Yourself

Being **assertive** means recognizing your feelings and making your needs and desires clear to others. Unlike

aggression, a far less healthy means of expression, assertiveness usually works. You can change a situation you don't like by communicating your feelings and thoughts in nonprovocative words, by focusing on specifics, and by making sure you're talking with the person who is directly responsible.

Becoming assertive isn't always easy. Many people have learned to cope by being passive and not communicating their feelings or opinions. Sooner or later they become so irritated, frustrated, or overwhelmed that they explode in an outburst—which they think of as being assertive. However, such behavior is so distasteful to them that they'd rather be passive. But assertiveness doesn't mean screaming or telling someone off. You can communicate your wishes calmly and clearly. Assertiveness is a behavior

mood A sustained emotional state that colors one's view of the world for hours or days.

autonomy The ability to draw on internal resources; independence from familial and societal influences.

locus of control An individual's belief about the sources of power and influence over his or her life.

assertive Behaving in a confident manner to make your needs and desires clear to others in a nonhostile way.

that respects your rights and the rights of other people even when you disagree.

Even at its mildest, assertiveness can make you feel better about yourself and your life. The reason: When you speak up or take action, you're in the pilot seat. And that's always much less stressful than taking a back seat and trying to hang on for dear life.

Connecting with Others

At every age, people who feel connected to others tend to be healthier physically and psychologically. This is certainly true in college when young adults, often living independently for the first time, need to form new relationships.

 In a study at a large Midwestern university, the students—particularly the women—who felt the greatest sense of belonging reported fewer physical symptoms than those who had not forged close friendships.

 The research also revealed a gender difference: Female students seek out, forge, and maintain more supportive ties than men, rely on friends more in times of stress, and provide more support than men.[8]

The opposite of *connectedness* is **social isolation**, a major risk factor for illness and early death. Individuals with few social contacts face two to four times the mortality rate of others. The reason may be that their social isolation weakens the body's ability to ward off disease. Medical students with higher-than-average scores on a loneliness scale had lower levels of protective immune cells. The end of a long-term relationship—through separation, divorce, or death—also dampens immunity.

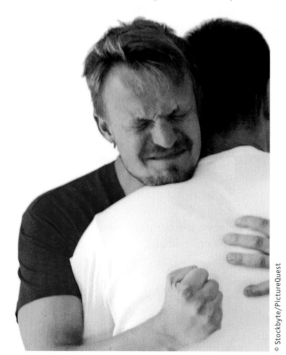

Giving and getting support from others is fundamental to good psychological health and emotional wellbeing.

It is part of our nature as mammals and as human beings to crave relationships. But invariably we end up alone at times. Solitude is not without its own quiet joys—time for introspection, self-assessment, learning from the past, and looking toward the future. Each of us can cultivate the joy of our own company, of being alone without crossing the line and becoming lonely.

Overcoming Loneliness

More so than many other countries, we are a nation of loners. Recent trends—longer work hours, busy family schedules, frequent moves, high divorce rates—have created even more lonely people. Only 23 percent of Americans say they're never lonely. Loneliest of all are those who are divorced, separated, or widowed and those who live alone or solely with children. Among single adults who have never been married, 42 percent feel lonely at least sometimes. However, loneliness is most likely to cause emotional distress when it is chronic rather than episodic.

To combat loneliness, people may join groups, fling themselves into projects and activities, or surround themselves with superficial acquaintances. Others avoid the effort of trying to connect, sometimes limiting most of their personal interactions to chat groups on the Internet.

The true keys to overcoming loneliness are developing resources to fulfill our own potential and learning to reach out to others. In this way, loneliness can become a means to personal growth and discovery.

Facing Shyness and Social Anxiety

Many people are uncomfortable meeting strangers or speaking or performing in public. In some surveys, as many as 40 percent of people describe themselves as shy or socially anxious. Some shy people—an estimated 10 to 15 percent of children—are born with a predisposition to shyness. Others become shy because they don't learn proper social responses or because they experience rejection or shame.

Some people are "fearfully" shy; that is, they withdraw and avoid contact with others and experience a high degree of anxiety and fear in social situations. Others are "self-consciously" shy. They enjoy the company of others but become highly self-aware and anxious in social situations.

 In one study of college students, men reported somewhat more shyness than women. African Americans were less shy than either Asian Americans or Caucasians.[9] Students may develop symptoms of shyness or social anxiety when they go to a party or are called on in class. Some experience symptoms when they try to perform any sort of action in the presence of others, even such everyday activities as eating in public, using a public restroom, or writing a check.

About 7 percent of the population could be diagnosed with a severe form of social anxiety, called **social phobia,** in which individuals typically fear and avoid various social situations. Childhood shyness, as reported by parents, and chronic illness increase the likelihood of this problem.[10] Adolescents and young adults with severe social anxiety are at increased risk of major depression. Phobias are discussed in Chapter 4. The key difference between these problems and normal shyness and self-consciousness is the degree of distress and impairment that individuals experience.

If you're shy, you can overcome much of your social apprehensiveness on your own, in much the same way as you might set out to stop smoking or lose weight. For example, you can improve your social skills by pushing yourself to introduce yourself to a stranger at a party or to chat about the weather or the food selections with the person next to you in a cafeteria line. Gradually, you'll acquire a sense of social timing and a verbal ease that will take the worry out of close encounters with others. Those with more disabling social anxiety may do best with psychotherapy and medication, which have proved highly effective.

Loving and Being Loved

"One can live magnificently in this world if one knows how to work and how to love, to work for the person one loves and to love one's work," Leo Tolstoy wrote. You may not think of love as a basic need like food and rest, but it is essential for both physical and psychological well-being.

Mounting evidence suggests that people who lack love and commitment are at high risk for a host of illnesses, including infections, heart disease, and cancer. "Love and intimacy are at the root of what makes us sick and what makes us well," says cardiologist Dean Ornish, author of *Love & Survival: The Scientific Basis for the Healing Power of Intimacy.* "No other factor in medicine—not diet, not smoking, not exercise—has a greater impact." (See Chapter 8 for more on relationships.)[11]

Spiritual Health

Whatever your faith, whether or not you belong to any formal religion, you are more than a body of a certain height and weight occupying space on the planet. You have a mind that equips you to learn and question. And you have a spirit that animates everything you say and do. **Spiritual health** refers to this breath of life and to our ability to identify our basic purpose in life and to experience the fulfillment of achieving our full potential. Spiritual readings or practices can increase calmness, inner strength, and meaning; improve self-awareness; and enhance your sense of well-being. Religious support has also been shown to help lower depression and increase life satisfaction beyond the benefits of social support from friends and family.

Spirituality is a belief in what some call a higher power, in someone or something that transcends the boundaries of self. It gives rise to a strong sense of purpose, values, morals, and ethics. Throughout life you make choices and decide to behave in one way rather than another because your spirituality serves as both a compass and a guide.

The term *religiosity* refers to various spiritual practices. That definition may seem vague, but one thing is clear. According to thousands of studies on the relationship between religious beliefs and practices and health, religious individuals are less depressed, less anxious, and better able to cope with crises such as illness or divorce than nonreligious ones. The more that a believer incorporates spiritual practices, such as prayer, meditation, or attending services, into daily life, the greater their sense of satisfaction with life.

Even when age, health, habits, demographics, and other factors are considered, individuals who pray regularly and attend religious services stay healthier and live longer than those who rarely or never do. In studies at several medical centers, prayer and faith speeded recovery from alcoholism, hip surgery, drug addiction, stroke, rheumatoid arthritis, heart attacks, and bypass surgery.[12]

According to a recent survey, most physicians believe that religion and spirituality have "much" or "very much" influence on health, but few feel that they often change "hard" medical outcomes. Physicians who are themselves highly religious are more likely to report that patients often mention spiritual issues, to believe that spirituality strongly influences health, and to interpret spiritual and religious influences in a positive way.[13]

In one study, researchers assessed religiosity and symptoms of depression in 104 intercollegiate athletes at a public university in the Southeast. The greater the athletes' intrinsic religiosity, the less likely they were to suffer depressive symptoms. "Perhaps intrinsic religious beliefs provide a sense of hope and security that protect against distressing events," the researchers speculated. "It may also be that unconditional love by one's God provides a stable sense of self worth" that buffers against stress.[14]

---

social isolation A feeling of unconnectedness with others caused by and reinforced by infrequency of social contacts.

social phobia A severe form of social anxiety marked by extreme fears and avoidance of social situations.

spiritual health The ability to identify one's basic purpose in life and to achieve one's full potential.

spirituality A belief in someone or something that transcends the boundaries of self.

YOUR STRATEGIES FOR CHANGE *Being True to Yourself*

- Take the tombstone test: What would you like to have written on your tombstone? In other words, how would you like to be remembered? Your honest answer should tell you, very succinctly, what you value most.

- Describe yourself, as you are today, in a brief sentence. Ask friends or family members for their descriptions of you. How would you have to change to become the person you want to be remembered as?

- Try the adjective test: Choose three adjectives that you'd like to see associated with your reputation. Then list what you've done or can do to earn such descriptions.

Spiritual Intelligence

Mental health professionals have recognized the power of **spiritual intelligence,** which some define as "the capacity to sense, understand, and tap into the highest parts of ourselves, others, and the world around us." Spiritual intelligence, unlike spirituality, does not center on the worship of a God above, but on the discovery of a wisdom within.

All of us are born with the potential to develop spiritual intelligence, but most of us aren't even aware of it—and do little or nothing to nurture it. Part of the reason is that we confuse spiritual intelligence with religion, dogma, or old-fashioned morality. "You don't have to go to church to be spiritually intelligent; you don't even have to believe in God," say Reverend Paul Edwards, a retired Episcopalian minister and therapist in Fullerton, California. "It is a scientific fact that when you are feeling secure, at peace, loved, and happy, you see, hear, and act differently than when you're feeling insecure, unhappy, and unloved. Spiritual intelligence allows you to use the wisdom you have when you're in a state of inner peace. And you get there by changing

---

Your Life Change Coach

Enriching Your Spiritual Life

Do you attend religious services? Pray or meditate on a weekly basis? In a national survey, a majority of the members of the Class of 2009 answered yes: Eight in ten went to religious services frequently or occasionally, while a third prayed or meditated every week. These percentages are somewhat lower than in the past, but a growing number of students report frequent discussions of religion.[16]

Whatever role religion plays in your life, you have the capacity for deep, meaningful spiritual experiences that can add great meaning to everyday existence. You don't need to enroll in theology classes or commit to a certain religious preference. The following simple steps can start you on an inner journey to a new level of understanding:

- **Sit quietly.** The process of cultivating spiritual intelligence begins in solitude and silence. "There is an inner wisdom," says Dr. Dean Ornish, the pioneering cardiologist who incorporates spiritual health into his mind–body therapies, "but it speaks very, very softly." To tune into its whisper, you have to turn down the volume in your busy, noisy, complicated life and force yourself to do nothing at all. This may sound easy; it's anything but.

    Start small. Create islands of silence in your day. Don't reach for the radio dial as soon as you get in the car. Leave your earpods on as you walk across campus but turn off the music. Shut the door to your room, take a few huge deep breaths, and let them out very, very slowly. Don't worry if you're too busy to carve out half an hour for quiet contemplation. Even ten minutes every day can make a difference.

- **Step outside.** For many people, nature sets their spirit free. Being outdoors, walking by the ocean, or looking at the hills gives us a sense of timelessness and puts the little hassles of daily living into perspective. As you wait for the bus or for a traffic light to change, let your gaze linger on silvery ice glazing a branch or an azalea bush in wild bloom. Follow the flight of a bird; watch clouds float overhead. Gaze into the night sky and think of the stars as holes in the darkness letting heaven shine through.

- **Use activity to tune into your spirit.** Spirituality exists in every cell of the body, not just in the brain. As a student, mental labor takes up much of your day. To tap into your spirit,

the way you think, basically by listening less to what's in your head and more to what's in your heart."[15]

Clarifying Your Values

Your **values** are the criteria by which you evaluate things, people, events, and yourself; they represent what's most important to you. In a world of almost dizzying complexity, values can provide guidelines for making decisions that are right for you. If understood and applied, they help give life meaning and structure.

There can be a large discrepancy between what people say they value and what their actions indicate about their values. That's why it's important to clarify your own values, making sure you understand what you believe so that you can live in accordance with your beliefs.

When you confront a situation in which you must choose different paths or behaviors, follow these steps:

1. Carefully consider the consequences of each choice.
2. Choose freely from among all the options.
3. Publicly affirm your values by sharing them with others.
4. Act out your values.

Values clarification is not a once-in-a-lifetime task, but an ongoing process of sorting out what matters most to you. If you believe in protecting the environment, do you shut off lights, or walk rather than drive, in order to conserve energy? Do you vote for political candidates who support environmental protection? Do you recycle newspapers, bottles, and cans? Values are more than ideals we'd like to attain; they should be reflected in the way we live day by day.

Praying

Prayer, a spiritual practice of millions, is the most commonly used form of complementary and alternative medicine. However, only in recent years has science launched rigorous investigations of the healing power of prayer.

try a less cerebral activity, such as singing, chanting, dancing, or drumming. Alternative ways of quieting your mind and tuning into your spirit include gardening, walking, arranging flowers, listening to music that touches your soul, or immersing yourself in a simple process like preparing a meal.

- **Ask questions of yourself.** Some people use their contemplative time to focus on a line of scripture or poetry. Others ask open-ended questions, such as What am I feeling? What are my choices? Where am I heading? Dr. Ornish ends his own daily meditations by asking, "What am I not paying attention to that's important?"

  In her meditations, one minister often paints a lush scene with a golden meadow, a shade tree, and a gentle brook and invites the divine spirit to enter. "Rarely do I get an immediate answer or solution, but later that day something may happen—often just a random conversation—and I suddenly find myself thinking about a problem from a perspective I never considered before."

- **Trust your spirit.** While most of us rely on gut feelings to alert us to danger, our inner spirit usually nudges us, not away from, but toward some action that will somehow lead to a greater good—even if we can't see it at the time. You may suddenly feel the urge to call or e-mail a friend you've lost touch with—only to discover that he just lost a loved one and needed the comfort of your caring. If you ignore such silent signals, you may look back and regret the consequences. Pay a little more attention the next time you feel an unexpected need to say or do something for someone.

- **Develop a spiritual practice.**
  - **If you are religious:** Deepen your spiritual commitment through prayer, more frequent church attendance, or joining a prayer group.
  - **If you are not religious:** Keep an open mind about the value of religion or spirituality. Consider visiting a church or synagogue. Read the writings of inspired people of deep faith, such as Rabbi Harold Kushner and Rev. Martin Luther King, Jr.
  - **If you are not ready to consider religion:** Try nonreligious meditation or relaxation training. Research has shown that focusing the mind on a single sound or image can slow heart rate, respiration, and brain waves; relax muscles; and lower stress-related hormones—responses similar to those induced by prayer. (See "Soul Food" in *IPC*.) **IPC**

spiritual intelligence The capacity to sense, understand, and tap into ourselves, others, and the world around us.

values The criteria by which one makes choices about one's thoughts, actions, goals and ideals.

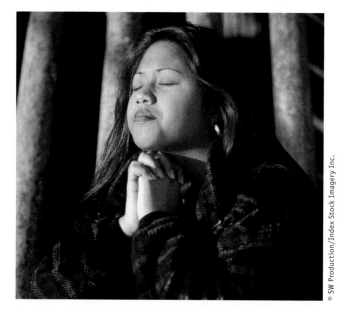

Prayer enhances physical health as well as spiritual and psychological well-being

Petitionary prayer—praying directly to a higher power—affects both the quality and quantity of life, says Dr. Harold Koenig, director of Duke University's Center for the Study of Religion/Spirituality and Health. "It boosts morale, lowers agitation, loneliness, and life dissatisfaction and enhances ability to cope in men, women, the elderly, the young, the healthy, and the sick."[17]

People who pray regularly have significantly lower blood pressure and stronger immune systems than the less religious, says Dr. Koenig. They're also less prone to alcoholism, less likely to smoke heavily, and are hospitalized less often. Science cannot explain the physiological mechanisms for what happens in human beings when they pray, but in cultures around the world throughout recorded history when people or their loved ones are sick, they pray.

In a national survey, 35 percent of Americans prayed for health concerns, with 75 percent of these praying for wellness and 22 percent praying for alleviation of specific medical conditions, such as chronic headaches, depression, back or neck pain, and digestive problems. Among those who prayed because of a medical condition, 69 percent found prayer very helpful. Only 11 percent of patients using prayer discussed it with their physicians.[18]

Some scientists speculate that prayer may foster a state of peace and calm that could lead to beneficial changes in the cardiovascular and immune systems. Sophisticated brain imaging techniques have shown that prayer and meditation cause changes in blood flow in particular regions of the brain that may lead to lower blood pressure, slower heart rate, decreased anxiety, and an enhanced sense of well-being. Membership in a faith community provides an identity as well as support, although individuals vary in their religious practices and observances.

In recent research, praying for others has not improved their symptoms or recovery. In a study of patients undergoing heart procedures, prayers (whether by Christian, Muslim, Jewish, or Buddhist groups) and other complementary bedside therapies, such as imaging and therapeutic touching, did not measurably improve their outcome.[19]

Will science ever be able to prove the power of prayer? No one is certain. "While I personally believe that God heals people in supernatural ways, I don't think science can shape a study to prove it," says Duke's Dr. Koenig. "But we now know enough, based on solid scientific research, to recommend prayer, much like exercise and diet, as one of the best and most cost-effective ways of protecting and enhancing health."

Expressing Gratitude

A grateful spirit brightens mood, boosts energy, and infuses daily living with a sense of glad abundance. Although giving thanks is an ancient virtue, only recently have researchers focused on the "trait" of gratitude—appreciation, not just for a special gift, but for everything that makes life a bit better.[20]

"Gratitude is an emotional and intellectual phenomenon that rises out of recognition that someone has treated you benevolently," says psychologist Michael McCullough of Southern Methodist University, a pioneer in gratitude research. "It's not feeling happy because something good happens, but realizing that someone who didn't have to deliberately did something of value to you."[21]

Since gratitude is not just a feeling but a mental outlook, we can consciously become more grateful—with practice. "Volunteers on college campuses who are asked to list things they're grateful for every day report more positive feelings," says McCullough. "They have more energy. They sleep better. They feel richer, regardless of how much money they have. Even their families notice visible, positive changes."

How can you help your gratitude grow? Here are some suggestions:

- Write a "gratitude letter," a belated thank you to someone in your life whom you've never properly thanked for a kindness.
- Build a time for thankfulness into your day. Some people write nightly in a gratitude journal or log.
- Develop a "good" memory, one that stores the kindnesses and comforts that have come your way.
- Pass on simple kindnesses. Open the door for a student juggling a backpack and an umbrella. Flash a smile at a server in the cafeteria. Pitch in on a beach or park cleanup. Give others a reason to savor a moment of gratitude.

See the "Grateful Thread" in *IPC*. **IPC**

YOUR STRATEGIES FOR CHANGE *How to Forgive*

- Compose an apology letter. Address it to yourself, and write it from someone who's hurt you. This simple task enables you to get a new perspective on a painful experience.
- Leap forward in time. In a visualization exercise imagine that you are very old, meet a person who hurt you long ago, and sit down together on a park bench on a

beautiful spring day. You both talk until everything that needs to be said finally is. This allows you to benefit from the perspective time brings without having to wait for years to achieve it.

- Talk with "safe" people. Vent your anger or disappointment with a trusted friend or a counselor without the danger of saying or doing anything you'll regret

later. And if you can laugh about what happened with a friend, the laughter helps dissolve the rage.

- Forgive the person, not the deed. In themselves, abuse, rape, murder, or betrayal are beyond forgiveness. But you can forgive people who couldn't manage to handle their own suffering, misery, confusion, and desperation.

Forgiving

While "I forgive you" may be three of the most difficult words to say, they are also three of the most powerful—and the most beneficial for the body as well as the soul. Being angry, harboring resentments, or reliving hurts over and over again is bad for your health in general and your heart in particular. The word *forgive* comes from the Greek for letting go, and that's what happens when you forgive: You let go of all the anger and pain that have been demanding your time and wasting your energy.

To some people, forgiveness seems a sign of weakness or submission. People may feel more in control, more powerful, when they're filled with anger, but forgiving instills a much greater sense of power. When you forgive, you reclaim your power to choose. It doesn't matter whether someone deserves to be forgiven; you deserve to be free.

However, forgiveness isn't easy. It's not a one-time thing but a process that takes a lot of time and work. Most people pass through several stages in their journey to forgiveness. The initial response may involve anger, sadness, shame, or other negative feelings. Later, there's a reevaluation of what happened, then reframing to try to make sense of it or to take mitigating circumstances into account. This may lead to a reduction in negative feelings, especially if the initial hurt turns out to be accidental rather than intentional.

Doing Good

Altruism—helping or giving to others—enhances self-esteem, relieves physical and mental stress, and protects psychological well-being. Hans Selye, the father of stress research, described cooperation with others for the self's sake as altruistic egotism, whereby we satisfy our own needs while helping others satisfy theirs. This concept is essentially an updated version of the golden rule: Do unto others as you would have them do unto you. The important difference is that you earn your neighbor's love and help by offering them love and help.

 Volunteerism helps those who give as well as those who receive. People involved in community organizations, for instance, consistently report a surge of well-being called *helper's high*, which they describe as a unique sense of calmness, warmth, and enhanced self-worth. College students who provided community service as part of a semester-long course reported changes in attitude (including a decreased tendency to blame people for their misfortunes), self-esteem (primarily a belief that they can make a difference), and behavior (a greater commitment to do more volunteer work).

The options for giving of yourself are limitless: Volunteer to serve a meal at a homeless shelter. Collect donations for a charity auction. Teach in an illiteracy program. Perform the simplest act of charity: Pray for others.

Sleepless on Campus

You stay up late cramming for a final. You drive through the night to visit a friend at another campus. You get up for an early class during the week but stay in bed until noon on weekends. And you wonder: "Why am I so tired?" The answer: You're not getting enough sleep.

You're hardly alone. According to a recent report by the Institute of Medicine, 50 to 70 million Americans have chronic sleep problems that jeopardize their ability to function at their best as well as their health and longevity. The cumulative long-term effects of sleep loss and sleep disorders include an increased risk of hypertension, diabetes, obesity, depression, heart attack, and stroke. Drowsy drivers are responsible for almost 20 percent of all serious car crash injuries.[22]

altruism Acts of helping or giving to others without thought of self-benefit.

YOUR STRATEGIES FOR CHANGE *How to Sleep Better*

- Keep regular hours for going to bed and getting up in the morning. Stay as close as possible to this schedule on weekends as well as weekdays.

- Develop a sleep ritual—such as stretching, meditation, yoga, prayer, or reading a not-too-thrilling novel— to ease the transition from wakefulness to sleep.

- Don't drink coffee late in the day. The effects of caffeine can linger for up to eight hours. And don't smoke. Nicotine is an even more powerful stimulant—and sleep saboteur—than caffeine.

- Don't rely on alcohol to get to sleep. Alcohol disrupts normal sleep stages, so you won't sleep as deeply or as restfully as you normally would.

- Although experts generally advise against daytime napping for people who have problems sleeping at night, a recent study of college students found that a 30-minute "power nap" lowers stress and refreshes energy with no disruption in nighttime sleep.

See the Sleep Power Lab in *IPC*. **IPC**

Sleep problems start young. Nearly one-half of adolescents sleep less than eight hours on school nights; more than half report feeling sleepy during the day.[23] College students are notorious for staying up late to study and socialize during the week and sleeping in on weekends. Only 11 percent of college students report good quality sleep, while 30 percent suffer chronic sleep difficulties.

On average college students go to bed 1 to 2 hours later and sleep 1 to 1.6 hours less than students of a generation ago.[24] When compared to exhaustion levels reported by workers in various occupations, college students score extremely high.[25]

Among the most common causes of sleep problems among college students are stress, bad sleep habits, poor time management, and a disruptive environment. More female than male students report problems staying asleep and morning tiredness; college men are more likely to ignore sleep problems.[26] Students taking stimulant medications for attention disorders (discussed in Chapter 4) may experience more sleep difficulties.[27]

Fortunately, college students can learn to sleep better. In an experiment with introductory psychology students—mostly freshmen—those who learned basic sleep skills (including the Strategies for Change on this page) significantly improved their overall sleep quality compared with students who did not receive such training. They took fewer naps, went to bed hungry less frequently, and consumed less caffeine. Over time they fell asleep more quickly and woke less often in the night.[28]

Sleep's Impact on Health

Sleep is essential for functioning at your best—physically and psychologically. The following are some of the key ways in which your nighttime sleep affects your daytime well-being.

- **Learning and memory.** When you sleep, your brain helps "consolidate" new information so you are more likely to retain it in your memory. In one study, healthy young adults between ages 18 and 30 learned 20 pairs of words and had to recall them 12 hours later. Those who learned the words in the evening and "slept on them" remembered significantly more words in the morning than those who stayed awake after learning the same material.

 In another study, undergraduates studied pairs of elaborately decorated ovals and were told that in each pair one oval won out over the other. They were not told that the ovals were also part of broader pattern. The undergraduates who had the opportunity to sleep afterward scored better than those who did not sleep. The sleeping brain, the researchers concluded, may help people make inferences from bits of knowledge that may at first appear random.[29]

- **Metabolism and weight.** The less you sleep, the more weight you may gain. Chronic sleep deprivation may cause weight gain by altering metabolism (for example, changing the way individuals process and store carbohydrates) and by stimulating excess stress hormones. Loss of sleep also reduces levels of the hormones that regulate appetite (discussed in Chapter 7), which may encourage eating.

- **Safety.** People who don't get adequate nighttime sleep are more likely to fall asleep during the daytime. Daytime sleepiness can cause falls, medical errors, air traffic mishaps, and road accidents.

- **Mood/quality of life.** Too little sleep—whether just for a night or two or for longer periods—can cause psychological symptoms, such as irritability, impatience, inability to concentrate, and moodiness. Poor sleep also affects your motivation and ability to work effectively. Growing evidence suggests that disturbed sleep is associated with increased rick of psychiatric disorders. [30]

Sleep-deprived university students score lower on life-satisfaction scales. Students who get eight hours of sleep but shift their sleep schedules by as little as two hours suffer more depressive symp-

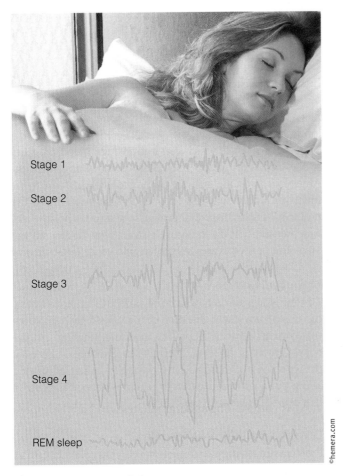

©hemera.com

Figure 2.2 Stages of Sleep

Differences in brain wave patterns characterize the various stages of sleep.

toms, lower sociability, and more frequent attention and concentration problems. They even get lower grades.

- **Cardiovascular health.** Serious sleep disorders such as insomnia and sleep apnea have been linked to hypertension, increased stress hormone levels, irregular heartbeats, and increased inflammation (which, as discussed in Chapter 16, may play a role in heart attacks).

- **Immunity/cancer prevention.** Sleep deprivation alters immune function, including the activity of the body's killer cells. For example, inadequate sleep at the time of a flu vaccination can reduce the production of flu-fighting antibodies. Keeping up with sleep may also help fight cancer. Harvard researchers have shown that women who work at night are at increased risk for breast and colon cancer, possibility because light at night alters production of melatonin, a hormone that helps put us to sleep.[31]

What Happens When We Sleep?

A normal night of sleep consists of several distinct stages of sleep, divided into two major types: an active state,

characterized by **rapid eye movement (REM)** and called **REM sleep** (or dream sleep), and a quiet state, referred to as non-REM or NREM sleep, that consists of four stages:

- **In Stage 1,** a twilight zone between full wakefulness and sleep, the brain produces small, irregular, rapid electrical waves. The muscles of the body relax, and breathing is smooth and even.

- **In Stage 2,** brain waves are larger and punctuated with occasional sudden bursts of electrical activity. The eyes are no longer responsive to light. Bodily functions slow still more.

- **Stages 3 and 4** constitute the most profound state of unconsciousness. The brain produces slower, larger waves, and this is sometimes referred to as "delta" or slow-wave sleep (Figure 2.2).

After about an hour in the four stages of non-REM sleep, sleepers enter the time of vivid dreaming called REM sleep, when brain waves resemble those of waking more than those of quiet sleep. The large muscles of the torso, arms, and legs are paralyzed and cannot move—possibly to prevent sleepers from acting out their dreams. The fingers and toes may twitch; breathing is quick and shallow; blood flow through the brain speeds up; men may have partial or full erections.

Sleep Disorders

Three of four Americans struggle to get a good night's sleep at least a few nights a week. According to the National Commission on Sleep Disorders Research, 40 million adults suffer from a specific sleep disorder, such as chronic insomnia or sleep apnea; an additional 20 to 30 million have occasional sleep difficulties.

Insomnia

Individuals with insomnia—a lack of sleep so severe that it interferes with functioning during the day—may toss

rapid-eye-movement (REM) sleep Regularly occurring periods of sleep during which the most active dreaming takes place.

and turn for an hour or more when they get into bed, wake frequently in the night, wake up too early, or not be able to sleep long enough to feel alert and energetic the next day. Most often insomnia is transient, typically occurring before or after a major life event (such as a job interview) and lasting for three or four nights. During periods of prolonged stress (such as a marriage breakup), short-term insomnia may continue for several weeks. Chronic or long-term insomnia, which can begin at any age, may persist for months or years.

For about a third of those with chronic insomnia, the underlying problem is a mental disorder, most often depression or an anxiety disorder. Many substances, including alcohol, medications, and drugs of abuse, often disrupt sleep. About 15 percent of those seeking help for chronic insomnia suffer from "learned" or "behavioral" insomnia. While a life crisis may trigger their initial sleep problems, each night they try harder and harder to get to sleep, but they cannot—although they often doze off while reading or watching a movie.

Sleeping pills may be used for a specific, time-limited problem—always with a physician's supervision. (See Savvy Consumer: "Straight Talk on Sleeping Pills.") In the long term, behavioral approaches, including the following, have proved more effective:

- Relaxation therapy, which may involve progressive muscle relaxation, diaphragmatic breathing, hypnosis, or meditation.

- Cognitive therapy, which challenges misconceptions about sleep and helps shift a poor sleeper's mind away from anxiety-inducing thoughts.

- Stimulus control therapy, in which individuals who do not fall asleep quickly must get up and leave their beds until they are very sleepy.

- Sleep restriction therapy, in which sleep times are sharply curtailed in order to improve the quality of sleep.

Breathing Disorders (Snoring and Sleep Apnea)

Although most people snore in certain positions or when they have stuffed-up noses, snoring can be a sign of a serious problem. Caused by the vibration in tissues in the mouth and throat as a sleeper tries to suck air into the lungs, snoring can be so loud that it disrupts a bed partner or others in the same house. In young people, the cause is most likely to be enlarged

tonsils or adenoids. In adults, extreme snoring may be a symptom of sleep apnea.

Translated from the Greek words meaning "no" and "breath," apnea is exactly that: the absence of breathing for a brief period. People with sleep apnea may briefly stop breathing dozens or even hundreds of times during the night. As they struggle for breath, they may gasp for air, snore extremely loudly, or thrash about.

Although apnea, which can lead to high blood pressure, stroke, and heart attack, may affect as many as 10 million Americans, most are unaware of the problem. Effective treatments include weight loss (if obesity is contributing to the problem), a nasal mask that provides continuous positive airway pressure (CPAP) to ensure a steady flow of air into the lungs and, in severe cases, surgery to enlarge the upper airway.

Movement Disorders

Restless legs syndrome, which may affect 12 million Americans, is a movement disorder characterized by symptoms that patients describe as pulling, burning, tingling, creepy-crawly, grabbing, buzzing, jitteriness, or gnawing. Many people with these symptoms have difficulty falling or staying asleep but do not realize that the cause is a medical disorder that can be treated with medications.

Circadian Rhythm Sleep Disorders

Problems involving the timing of sleep are called circadian rhythm disorders because they affect the basic circadian ("about a day") rhythm that influences many biological processes. The most common causes are jet lag and shift work. Jet lag generally improves on its own within two to seven days, depending on the length of the trip and the individual's response. Avoiding caffeine and alcohol and immediately switching to the new time zone's schedule can help in overcoming jet lag.

A "shift work" circadian rhythm disorder consists of any inability to sleep when one wants or to stay alert when needed because of frequently changing work shifts. Behavioral strategies and good sleep habits can help. In addition, phototherapy—exposure to bright light for periods ranging from 30 minutes to two hours—has shown promise as an experimental treatment to help shift workers adjust to their changing schedules.

How Much Sleep Do You Need?

Over the last century, we have cut our average nightly sleep time by 20 percent. More than half of us try to get by with less than seven hours of shut-eye a night. College students are no exception, with an average sleep time was slightly less than seven hours, with little difference between men and women.

No formula can say how long a good night's sleep should be. Normal sleep times range from five to ten hours; the average is seven and a half. About one or two people in a hundred

▼ *Savvy* Consumer Straight Talk on Sleeping Pills

Chances are you've used some form of sleep aid. After aspirin, sleeping pills are the most widely used drugs in the United States. The use of prescription sleeping pills has more than doubled since 2000, and increasing numbers of teenagers and young adults use these medications either occasionally or regularly. An even greater number buy nonprescription or over-the-counter (OTC) sleep inducers. Others rely on herbal remedies, antihistamines, and other medications to get to sleep.

In the long run, good sleep habits, regular exercise, and a tranquil sleep environment are the cornerstones of high-quality sleep. But if circumstances, travel, injury, or illness have disrupted your sleep, you may consider sleep medications. Here is what you need to know about them:

Over-the-counter medications. Various over-the-counter sleeping pills, sold in any pharmacy or supermarket, contain antihistamines, which induce drowsiness by working against the central nervous system chemical histamine. They may help for an occasional sleepless night, but the more often you take them, the less effective they become.

Dietary supplements. The most widely publicized dietary supplement is the hormone melatonin, which may help control your body's internal clock. The melatonin supplements most often found in health food stores and pharmacies are synthetic versions of the natural hormone. Although these supplements may help some people fall asleep or stay asleep and may sometimes help prevent jet lag, there are many unanswered questions about melatonin. Reported side effects include drowsiness, headaches, stomach discomfort, confusion, decreased body temperature, seizures, and drug interactions. The optimal dose isn't certain, and the long-term effects are unknown. Other supplements—such as valerian, chamomile, and kava—have yet to be fully studied for safety or effectiveness in relieving insomnia.

Prescription medications. The newest sleep drugs—nonbenzodiazepine hypnotic medications such as Lunesta (eszopiclone), Ambien/Ambien CR (zolpidem), and Sonata (zaleplon)—quiet the nervous system, which helps induce sleep. They're metabolized quickly, which helps reduce the risk of side effects the next day. These medications are mainly intended for short-term or intermittent use.

Benzodiazepines, such as Halcion (triazolam) and Restoril (temazepam), belong to an older class of sleeping pills that are more likely to cause drowsiness or headaches the next morning. They also may become habit forming.

The FDA has required stronger language about the potential risks of both nonbenzodiazepine and benzodiazepine sleeping pills. These include severe allergic reactions and complex sleep-related behaviors, including sleep-driving (driving while not fully awake after taking a sleeping pill with no memory of the driving).

If sleeping pills seem the best option at a certain time in your life, here are some guidelines for using them safely:

- **Check with your doctor.** He or she can make sure the sleeping pills won't interact with other medications or medical conditions. Your doctor can also help you determine the best dosage. If your problems are chronic, your doctor may refer you to a sleep specialist.

- **Read carefully.** Take time to read through the informational materials and warnings on pill containers. Make sure you understand the potential risks and the behaviors to avoid.

- **Take it one day at a time.** Sleeping pills are a temporary solution for insomnia. Most over-the-counter varieties should be used for only two to three nights at a time. Taken too often, some sleeping pills may cause rebound insomnia—sleeplessness that returns in full force when you stop taking the medication.

- **Avoid alcohol.** Never mix alcohol and sleeping pills. Alcohol increases the sedative effects of the pills. Even a small amount of alcohol combined with sleeping pills can make you feel dizzy, confused, or faint.

- **Quit carefully.** When you're ready to stop taking sleeping pills, follow your doctor's instructions or the directions on the label. Some medications must be stopped gradually.

- **Watch for side effects.** If you feel sleepy or dizzy during the day, talk to your doctor about changing the dosage or discontinuing the pills.

---

can get by with just five hours; another small minority needs twice that amount.[32] Each of us seems to have an innate sleep *appetite* that is as much a part of our genetic programming as hair color and skin tone.

To figure out your sleep needs, keep your wake-up time the same every morning and vary your bedtime. Are you groggy after six hours of shut-eye? Does an extra hour give you more stamina? What about an extra two hours? Since too much sleep can make you feel sluggish, don't assume that more is always better. Listen to your body's signals, and adjust your sleep schedule to suit them.

Are you better off pulling an all-nighter before a big test or closing the books and getting a good night's sleep? According to researchers, that depends on the nature of the exam. If it's a test of facts—Civil War battles, for instance—cramming all night works. However, if you will have to write analytical essays in which you compare, contrast, and make connections, you need to sleep in over to make the most of your reasoning abilities.

Learn It : Live It

Keys to a Fulfilling Life

Just like physical health, psychological well-being involves more than an absence of problems. By developing your inner strengths and resources, you become the author of your life, capable of confronting challenges and learning from them. As positive psychologists have discovered, you have greater control over how happy, optimistic, upbeat, and lovable you are than anyone or anything else. But only by consciously taking charge of your life can you find happiness and fulfillment. (See "Your Perfect Balance Point" in *IPC*.) **IPC**

- **Up your appreciation quotient.** Regularly take stock of all the things for which you are grateful. To deepen the impact, write a letter of gratitude to someone who's helped you along the way.

- **String beads.** Think of every positive experience during the day as a bead on a necklace. This simple exercise focuses you on positive experiences, such as a cheery greeting from a cashier or a funny e-mail from a friend, and encourages you to act more kindly toward others.

- **Cultivate memories.** If you have to choose between buying a new car and studying abroad, pack your bags. Cars inevitably break down. International study pays the dividend of memories you can cherish for decades.

- **Look on the lighter side.** "Humor is like salt on meat," observes psychologist Martin Seligman. "It amplifies everything." Watch reruns of the classic shows that never fail to make you laugh. Smile at the absurdities of daily nuisances.

- **Create a virtual DVD.** Visualize several of your happiest memories with as much detail as possible. Smell the air. Feel the sun. Hear the sea. Play this video in your mind when your spirits slump.

- **Fortify optimism.** Whenever possible, see the glass as half-full. Keep track of what's going right in your life. Imagine and write down your vision for your best possible future and track your progress toward it.

- **Immerse yourself.** Find activities that delight and engage you so much that you lose track of time. Experiment with creative outlets. Look for ways to build these passions into your life.

- **Do good.** Acts of kindness, however small, bring as much pleasure to the giver as the recipient. Give time, money or both to worthy causes. At the least, offer a smile or a prayer.

- **Don't isolate yourself.** Even spending time with strangers bolsters your sense of well-being. You laugh much harder when you're with other people in a theatre than when you watch a movie at home.

- **Seize the moment.** Rather than waiting to celebrate big birthday-cake moments, savor a bite of cupcake every day. Delight in a child's cuddle, a glorious sunset, a lively conversation. Cry at movies. Cheer at football games. This life is your gift to yourself. Open it!

SELFSURVEY : *Well-Being Scale*

PART I

The following questions contain statements and their opposites. Notice that the statements extend from one extreme to the other. Where would you place yourself on this scale? Place a circle on the number that is most true for you at this time. Do not put your circles between numbers.

Life Purpose and Satisfaction

1. During most of the day, my energy level is	very low	1 2 3 4 5 6 7	very high
2. As a whole, my life seems	dull	1 2 3 4 5 6 7	vibrant
3. My daily activities are	not a source of satisfaction	1 2 3 4 5 6 7	a source of satisfaction
4. I have come to expect that everyday will be	exactly the same	1 2 3 4 5 6 7	new and different
5. When I think deeply about life	I do not feel there is any purpose to it	1 2 3 4 5 6 7	I feel there is a purpose to it
6. I feel that my life so far has	not been productive	1 2 3 4 5 6 7	been productive
7. I feel that the work* I am doing	is of no value	1 2 3 4 5 6 7	is of great value
8. I wish I were different than who I am.	agree strongly	1 2 3 4 5 6 7	disagree strongly

*The definition of work is not limited to income-producing jobs. It includes childcare, housework, studies, and volunteer services.

9. At this time, I have   no clearly defined goals for my life   1 2 3 4 5 6 7   clearly defined goals for my life

10. When sad things happen to me
or other people   I cannot feel positive about life   1 2 3 4 5 6 7   I continue to feel positive about life

11. When I think about what I have done
with my life, I feel   worthless   1 2 3 4 5 6 7   worthwhile

12. My present life   does not satisfy me   1 2 3 4 5 6 7   satisfies me

13. I feel joy in my heart   never   1 2 3 4 5 6 7   all the time

14. I feel trapped by the circumstances of my life.   agree strongly   1 2 3 4 5 6 7   disagree strongly

15. When I think about my past   I feel many regrets   1 2 3 4 5 6 7   I feel no regrets

16. Deep inside myself   I do not feel loved   1 2 3 4 5 6 7   I feel loved

17. When I think about the problems
that I have   I do not feel hopeful about solving them   1 2 3 4 5 6 7   I feel very hopeful about solving them

PART II

Self-Confidence During Stress (Answer according to how you feel during stressful times.)

1. When there is a great deal of pressure being placed on me   I get tense   1 2 3 4 5 6 7   I remain calm

2. I react to problems and difficulties   with a great deal of frustration   1 2 3 4 5 6 7   with no frustration

3. In a difficult situation, I am confident
that I will receive the help that I need.   disagree strongly   1 2 3 4 5 6 7   agree strongly

4. I experience anxiety   all the time   1 2 3 4 5 6 7   never

5. When I have made a mistake   I feel extreme dislike for myself   1 2 3 4 5 6 7   I continue to like myself

6. I find myself worrying that something bad
is going to happen to me or those I love   all the time   1 2 3 4 5 6 7   never

7. In a stressful situation   I cannot concentrate easily   1 2 3 4 5 6 7   I can concentrate easily

8. I am fearful   all the time   1 2 3 4 5 6 7   never

9. When I need to stand up for myself   I cannot do it   1 2 3 4 5 6 7   I can do it easily

10. I feel less than adequate in most situations.   agree strongly   1 2 3 4 5 6 7   disagree strongly

11. During times of stress, I feel isolated and alone.   agree strongly   1 2 3 4 5 6 7   disagree strongly

12. In really difficult situations   I feel unable to respond in positive ways   1 2 3 4 5 6 7   I feel able to respond in positive ways

13. When I need to relax   I experience no peace—only thoughts and worries   1 2 3 4 5 6 7   I experience a peacefulness— free of thoughts and worries

14. When I am frightened   I panic   1 2 3 4 5 6 7   remain calm

15. I worry about the future   all the time   1 2 3 4 5 6 7   never

Scoring

The number you circled is your score for that question. Add your scores in each of the two sections and divide each sum by the number of questions in the section.

- Life Purpose and Satisfaction: _____ ÷ 17 = _____.____
- Self-Confidence During Stress: _____ ÷ 15 = _____.____
- Combined Well-Being:
(add scores for both) _____ ÷ 32 = _____.____

Each score should range between 1.00 and 7.00 and may include decimals (for example 5.15).

Interpretation

VERY LOW: 1.00 TO 2.49
MEDIUM LOW: 2.50 TO 3.99
MEDIUM HIGH: 4.00 TO 5.49
VERY HIGH: 5.50 TO 7.00

These scores reflect the strength with which you feel these positive emotions. Do they make sense to you? Review each scale and each question in each scale. Your score on each item gives you information about the emotions and areas in your life where your psychological resources are strong, as well as the areas where strength needs to be developed.

If you notice a large difference between the LPS and SCDS scores, use this information to recognize which central attitudes and aspects of your life most need strengthening. If your scores on both scales are very low, talk with a counselor or a friend about how you are feeling about yourself and your life.

Source: © 1989. Kass, Jared. *Inventory of Positive Psychological Attitudes*. The Well-Being Scale is the self-test version of the Inventory of Positive Psychological Attitudes (IPPA-32) developed by Dr. Jared D. Kass. Reprinted with author's permission. For information, contact: Dr. Jared Kass, Division of Counseling and Psychology, Graduate School of Arts and Social Sciences, Lesley College, Cambridge, MA 02138.

Your Health Action Plan for Psychological Well-Being

Just as you can improve your physical well-being, you can enhance the state of your mind. Here are some suggestions:

- **Recognize and express your feelings.** Pent-up emotions tend to fester inside, building into anger or depression.

- **Don't brood.** Rather than merely mulling over a problem, try to find solutions that are positive and useful.

- **Take one step at a time.** As long as you're taking some action to solve a problem, you can take pride in your ability to cope.

- **Spend more time doing those activities you know you do best.** For example, if you are a good cook, prepare a meal for someone.

- **Separate what you do, especially any mistakes you make, from who you are.** Instead of saying, "I'm so stupid," tell yourself, "That wasn't the smartest move I ever made, but I'll learn from it."

- **Use affirmations**, positive statements that help reinforce the most positive aspects of your personality and experience. Every day, you might say, "I am a loving, caring person," or "I am honest and open in expressing my feelings." Write some affirmations of your own on index cards and flip through them occasionally.

- **List the things you would like to have or experience.** Construct the statements as if you were already enjoying the situations you list, beginning each sentence with "I am." For example, "I am feeling great about doing well in my classes."

- **When your internal critic**—the negative inner voice we all have—starts putting you down, force yourself to think of a situation that you handled well.

- **Set a limit on self-pity.** Tell yourself, "I'm going to feel sorry for myself this morning, but this afternoon, I've got to get on with my life."

- **Volunteer.** A third of Americans—some 89 million people—give of themselves through volunteer work. By doing the same, you may feel better too.

- **Exercise.** In various studies around the world, physical exertion ranks as one of the best ways to change a bad mood, raise energy, and reduce tension.

CENGAGENOW™ If you want to write your own goals to enhance your state of mind, go to the Wellness Journal at HealthNow: **academic.cengage.com/login.**

Making This Chapter Work for YOU

Review Questions

1. Psychological health is influenced by all of the following except
   a. emotional health.
   b. physical agility.
   c. culture.
   d. a firm grasp on reality.

2. Which of these statements about self-esteem is *false*?
   a. Self-esteem is determined by genetics.
   b. Parents influence a child's self-esteem.
   c. A person's sense of self-esteem can change over time.
   d. Self-esteem is boosted by achievement.

3. Enduring happiness is most likely to come from
   a. winning a sweepstakes.
   b. work you love.
   c. a trip to the place of your dreams.
   d. having more money than your friends and neighbors.

4. Individuals who have developed a sense of mastery over their lives are
   a. skilled at controlling the actions of others.
   b. usually passive and silent when faced with a situation they don't like.
   c. aware that their locus of control is internal, not external.
   d. aware that their locus of control is external, not internal.

5. Normal shyness can usually be overcome by
   a. medication.
   b. psychotherapy.
   c. retail therapy.
   d. working at improving social skills.

6. Which of the following activities can contribute to a lasting sense of personal fulfillment?
   a. becoming a Big Sister or Big Brother to a child from a single-parent home
   b. volunteering at a local soup kitchen on Thanksgiving
   c. being a regular participant in an Internet chat room
   d. negotiating the price on a new car

7. People who pray regularly
   a. are less likely to get cancer.
   b. never get sick.
   c. recover from heart attacks more quickly.
   d. get better grades.

8. Which activity is probably *not* enriching the student's spiritual life?
   a. Claire goes dancing with her friends.
   b. James takes a solo 15-minute walk along the river trail everyday.
   c. Kate keeps a gratitude journal.
   d. Charlie goes to a taize music group with friends.

9. Lack of sleep
   a. improves memory and concentration.
   b. may cause irritability.
   c. may cause weight loss.
   d. enhances the immune system.

10. Which statement about sleep is correct?
   a. People cannot learn to sleep better.
   b. People dream during REM sleep.
   c. Drinking alcohol helps most people sleep better.
   d. Snoring may be a symptom of insomnia.

Answers to these questions can be found on page 583.

Critical Thinking

1. Would you say that you view life positively or negatively? Would your friends and family agree with your assessment? Ask two of your closest friends for feedback about what they perceive are your typical responses to a problematic situation. Are these indicative of positive attitudes? If not, what could you do to become more psychologically positive?

2. Were you raised in a religious family? If yes, have you continued the same religious practices from your childhood? Why or why not? If no, have you been to places of worship to explore religious practices? Why or why not?

3. What is your personal experience with lack of sleep? Have you suffered effects described in the text? Has cramming all night ever worked for you? Why or why not?

Media Menu

CENGAGENOW Go to the HealthNow website at **academic.cengage.com/login** that will:

- Help you evaluate your knowledge of the material.
- Allow you to take an exam-prep quiz.
- Provide a Personalized Learning Plan targeting resources that address areas you should study.
- Coach you through identifying target goals for behavioral change and creating and monitoring your personal change plan throughout the semester.

Internet Connections

Positive Psychology Center

www.ppc.sas.upenn.edu
This positive psychology website at the University of Pennsylvania has questionnaires on authentic happiness and gratitude.

American Psychological Association

www.apa.org
The APA is the scientific and professional organization for psychology in the United States. Its website provides up-to-date information on psychological issues.

Spirituality and Health

www.spiritualityhealth.org
Developed by the Publishing Group of Trinity Church, Wall Street in New York City, this website offers self-tests, guidance on spiritual practices, resources for people on spiritual journeys, and subscriptions to a bimonthly print magazine.

www.spirituality.org
Spirituality for Today is an interactive monthly magazine dedicated to current themes and questions concerning faith in this postmodern age.

www.newvision-psychic.com/bookshelf
A comprehensive list of books dealing with women and spirituality.

www.beliefnet.com
An eclectic, informative guide to different forms of religion and spirituality.

Key Terms

The terms listed are used and defined on the page indicated. Definitions are also found in the Glossary at the end of this book.

altruism	47
assertive	41
autonomy	9
culture	37
emotional health	37
emotional intelligence	37
locus of control	41
mental health	37
mood	39
optimism	39
rapid-eye-movement (REM) sleep	49
self-actualization	39
self-esteem	39
social isolation	43
social phobia	43
spiritual health	43
spiritual intelligence	45
spirituality	43
values	45

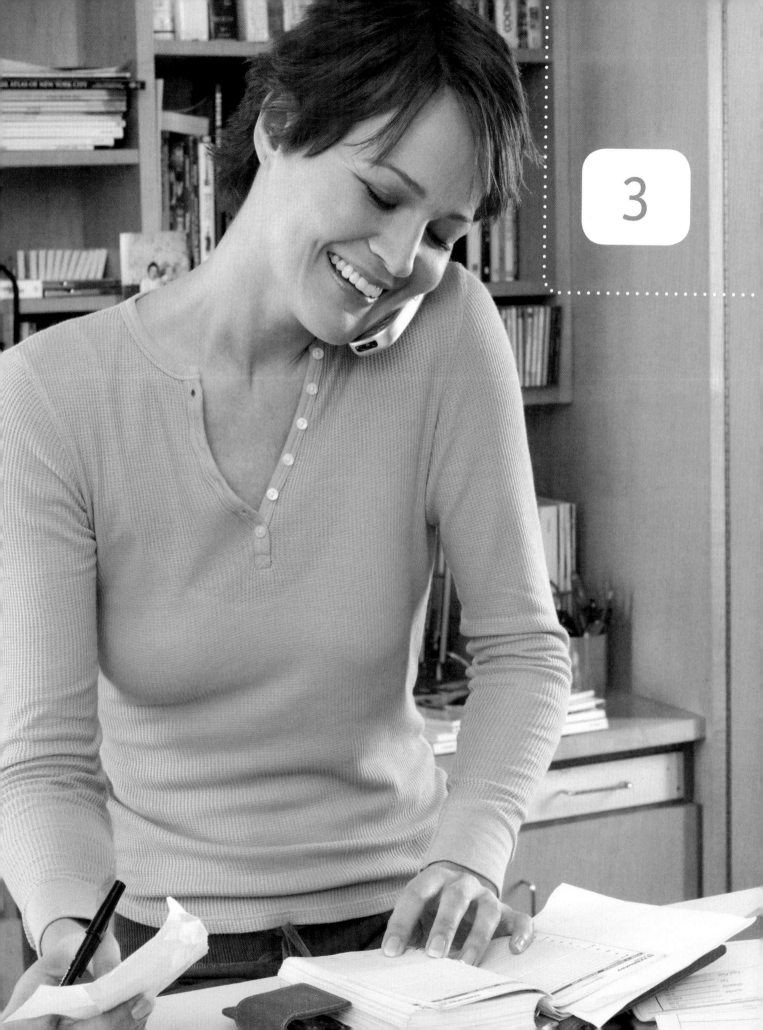

3

Personal Stress Management

TWO months into her freshman year, Ana feels as if a tornado has torn through her life. She is living thousands of miles from her family and the friends who share her culture and ethnic background. Her dormmates range from different to downright difficult. Her professors expect her to read and learn more in a week than in an entire month of high school. After blowing her budget decorating her room, she took on a part-time job—only to end up so exhausted that she dozes off in lectures. Stress? Ana considers it a way of life.

Like Ana, you live with stress every day, whether you're studying for exams, meeting people, facing new experiences, or figuring out how to live on a budget. You're not alone. College students rank stress as the top impediment to their academic performance.[1] Everyone, regardless of age, gender, race, or income, has to deal with stress—as an individual and as a member of society.

As researchers have demonstrated time and again, stress has profound effects, both immediate and long-term, on our bodies and minds. While stress alone doesn't cause disease, it triggers molecular changes throughout the body that make us more susceptible to many illnesses. Its impact on the mind is no less significant. The burden of chronic stress can undermine one's ability to cope with day-to-day hassles and can exacerbate psychological problems like depression and anxiety disorders.

Yet stress in itself isn't necessarily bad. What matters most is not the stressful situation itself, but an individual's response to it. By learning to anticipate stressful events, to manage day-to-day hassles, and to prevent stress overload, you can find alternatives to running endlessly on a treadmill of alarm, panic, and exhaustion. As you organize your schedule, find ways to release tension, and build up coping skills, you will begin to experience the sense of control and confidence that makes stress a challenge rather than an ordeal.

After studying the material in this chapter, you should be able to:

- **Define** stress and stressors and **describe** how the body responds to stress according to the general adaptation syndrome theory.
- **List** the physical changes associated with frequent or severe stress and **discuss** how stress can affect the cardiovascular, immune, and digestive systems.
- **Describe** some personal stressors, especially those experienced by students, and **discuss** how their effects can be prevented or minimized.
- **Describe** some techniques to help cope with stress.
- **Explain** how stressful events can affect psychological health and **describe** the factors contributing to posttraumatic stress disorder.
- **Identify** ways of managing time more efficiently.
- **List** the main causes of stress in your life, and **name** a strategy for managing each of them.

CENGAGENOW™ Log on to HealthNow at **academic.cengage.com/login** to find your Behavior Change Planner and to explore self-assessments, interactive tutorials, and practice quizzes.

What Is Stress?

People use the word stress in different ways: as an external force that causes a person to become tense or upset, as the internal state of arousal, and as the physical response of the body to various demands. Dr. Hans Selye, a pioneer in studying physiological responses to challenge, defined **stress** as "the nonspecific response of the body to any demand made upon it." In other words, the body reacts to **stressors**—the things that upset or excite us—in the same way, regardless of whether they are positive or negative.

Based on nearly 300 studies over four decades, researchers have distinguished five categories of stressors:

- **Acute time-limited stressors** include anxiety-provoking situations such as having to give a talk in public or work out a math problem, such as calculating a tip or dividing a bill, under pressure.

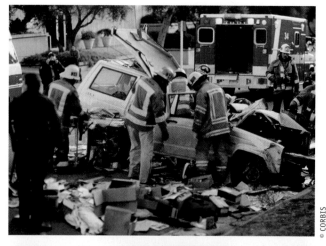

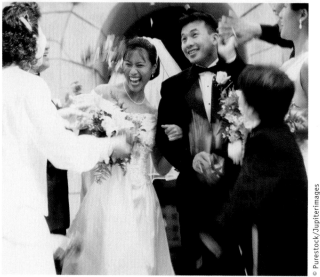

An automobile accident is an acute negative stressor. Getting married is an example of a positive stressor that triggers both joy and apprehension.

- **Brief naturalistic stressors** are more serious challenges such as taking SATs or meeting a deadline for a big project.

- **Stressful event sequences** are the difficult consequences of a natural disaster or another traumatic occurrence, such as the death of a spouse. The individuals involved recognize that these difficulties will end at some point in the future.

- **Chronic stressors** are ongoing demands caused by life-changing circumstances, such as permanent disability following an accident or caregiving for a parent with dementia, that do not have any clear end point.

- **Distant stressors** are traumatic experiences that occurred long ago, such as child abuse or combat, yet continue to have an emotional and psychological impact.

Not all stressors are negative. Some of life's happiest moments—births, reunions, weddings—are enormously stressful. We weep with the stress of frustration or loss; we weep, too, with the stress of love and joy. Selye coined the term **eustress** for positive stress in our lives (*eu* is a Greek prefix meaning "good"). Eustress challenges us to grow, adapt, and find creative solutions in our lives. **Distress** refers to the negative effects of stress that can deplete or even destroy life energy. Ideally, the level of stress in our lives should be just high enough to motivate us to satisfy our needs and not so high that it interferes with our ability to reach our fullest potential.

What Causes Stress?

Of the many biological theories of stress, the best known may be the **general adaptation syndrome (GAS),** developed by Hans Selye. He postulated that our bodies constantly strive to maintain a stable and consistent physiological state, called **homeostasis.** Stressors, whether in the form of physical illness or a demanding job, disturb this state and trigger a nonspecific physiological response. The body attempts to restore homeostasis by means of an **adaptive response.**

Selye's general adaptation syndrome, which describes the body's response to a stressor—whether threatening or exhilarating—consists of three distinct stages:

1. **Alarm.** When a stressor first occurs, the body responds with changes that temporarily lower resistance. Levels of certain hormones may rise; blood pressure may increase (Figure 3.1). The body quickly makes internal adjustments to cope with the stressor and return to normal activity.

2. **Resistance.** If the stressor continues, the body mobilizes its internal resources to try to sustain homeostasis. For example, if a loved one is seriously hurt in an accident, we initially respond intensely and feel great anxiety. During the subsequent stressful period of recuperation, we struggle to carry on as normally as possible, but this requires considerable effort.

3. **Exhaustion.** If the stress continues long enough, we cannot keep up our normal functioning. Even a small amount of additional stress at this point can cause a breakdown.

Among the nonbiological theories is the cognitive-transactional model of stress, developed by Richard Lazarus, which looks at the relation between stress and health. As he sees it, stress can have a powerful impact on health. Conversely, health can affect a person's resistance or coping ability. Stress, according to Lazarus, is "neither an environmental stimulus, a characteristic of the person, nor a response, but a relationship between demands and the power to deal with them without unreasonable or destructive costs."[2] Thus, an event may be stressful for one person but not for another, or it may seem stressful on one occasion but not on another. For instance, one student may think of speaking in front of

the class as extremely stressful, while another relishes the chance to do so—except on days when he's not well-prepared.

At any age, some of us are more vulnerable to life changes and crises than are others. The stress of growing up in families troubled by alcoholism, drug dependence, or physical, sexual, or psychological abuse may have a life-long impact—particularly if these problems are not recognized and dealt with. Other early experiences, positive and negative, also can affect our attitude toward stress–and our resilience to it. Our general outlook on life, whether we're optimistic or pessimistic, can determine whether we expect the worst and feel stressed or anticipate a challenge and feel confident. The when, where, what, how, and why of stressors also affect our reactions. The number and frequency of changes in our lives, along with the time and setting in which they occur, have a great impact on how we'll respond.

"Perceived" stress—an individual's view of how challenging life is—undermines a sense of well-being in people of all ages and circumstances. However, good self-esteem, social support, and internal resources buffer the impact of perceived stress.

Our level of ongoing stress affects our ability to respond to a new day's stressors. Each of us has a breaking point for dealing with stress. A series of too-intense pressures or too-rapid changes can push us closer and closer to that point. That's why it's important to anticipate potential stressors and plan how to deal with them.

Stress experts Thomas Holmes, M.D., and Richard Rahe, M.D., devised a scale to evaluate individual levels of stress and potential for coping, based on *life-change units* that estimate each change's impact. The death of a partner or parent ranks high on the list, but even changing apartments is considered a stressor. People who accumulate more than 300 life-change units in a year are more likely to suffer serious health problems. Scores on the scale, however, represent "potential stress"; the actual impact of the life change depends on the individual's response. (See Self Survey: "Student Stress Scale," p. 77.)

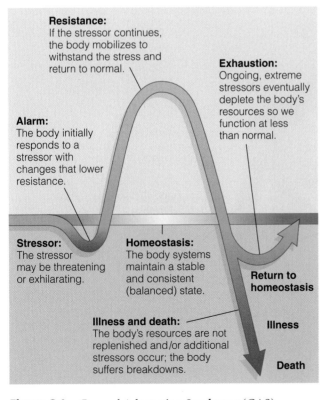

Resistance:
If the stressor continues, the body mobilizes to withstand the stress and return to normal.

Exhaustion:
Ongoing, extreme stressors eventually deplete the body's resources so we function at less than normal.

Alarm:
The body initially responds to a stressor with changes that lower resistance.

Stressor:
The stressor may be threatening or exhilarating.

Homeostasis:
The body systems maintain a stable and consistent (balanced) state.

Return to homeostasis

Illness and death:
The body's resources are not replenished and/or additional stressors occur; the body suffers breakdowns.

Illness

Death

Figure 3.1 General Adaptation Syndrome (GAS)
The three stages of Selye's GAS are alarm, resistance, and exhaustion.

stress The nonspecific response of the body to any demands made upon it; may be characterized by muscle tension and acute anxiety, or may be a positive force for action.

stressor Specific or nonspecific agents or situations that cause the stress response in a body.

eustress Positive stress, which stimulates a person to function properly.

distress A negative stress that may result in illness.

general adaptation syndrome (GAS) An anxiety disorder characterized as chronic distress.

homeostasis The body's natural state of balance or stability.

adaptive response The body's attempt to reestablish homeostasis or stability.

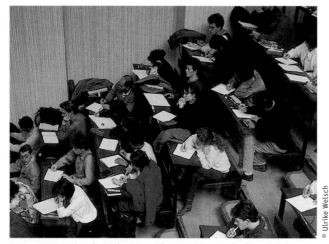

Tests are acute time-limited stressors that provoke your body's adaptive stress response.

Holmes has evaluated variations in life events among many groups, including college students, medical students, football players, pregnant women, alcoholics, and heroin addicts. Heroin addicts and alcoholics have the highest totals of life-change units, followed by college students. In general, younger people experience more life changes than do older people; factors such as gender, education, and social class also have a strong impact. Marriage seems to promote greater stability and fewer changes.

If you score high on the Student Stress Scale, think about the reasons your life has been in such turmoil. Of course, some events, such as your parents' divorce or a friend's accident, are beyond your control. Even then, you can respond in ways that may protect you from disease. Review the Health Action Plan at the end of the Self Survey (p. 78).

Stress and Physical Health

These days we've grown accustomed to warning labels advising us of the health risks of substances like alcohol and cigarettes. Medical researchers speculate that another component of twenty-first-century living also warrants a warning: stress. In recent years, an ever-growing number of studies has implicated stress as a culprit in a range of medical problems. While stress itself may not kill, it clearly undermines our ability to stay well.

While stress alone doesn't cause disease, it triggers molecular changes throughout the body that make us more susceptible to many illnesses. Severe emotional distress—whether caused by a divorce, the loss of a job, or caring for an ill child or parent—can have such a powerful effect on the DNA in body cells that it speeds up aging, adding the equivalent of a decade to biological age.

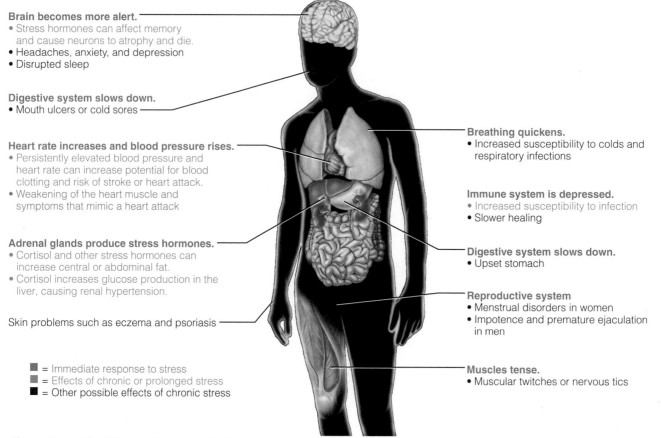

Brain becomes more alert.
• Stress hormones can affect memory and cause neurons to atrophy and die.
• Headaches, anxiety, and depression
• Disrupted sleep

Digestive system slows down.
• Mouth ulcers or cold sores

Heart rate increases and blood pressure rises.
• Persistently elevated blood pressure and heart rate can increase potential for blood clotting and risk of stroke or heart attack.
• Weakening of the heart muscle and symptoms that mimic a heart attack

Adrenal glands produce stress hormones.
• Cortisol and other stress hormones can increase central or abdominal fat.
• Cortisol increases glucose production in the liver, causing renal hypertension.

Skin problems such as eczema and psoriasis

Breathing quickens.
• Increased susceptibility to colds and respiratory infections

Immune system is depressed.
• Increased susceptibility to infection
• Slower healing

Digestive system slows down.
• Upset stomach

Reproductive system
• Menstrual disorders in women
• Impotence and premature ejaculation in men

Muscles tense.
• Muscular twitches or nervous tics

■ = Immediate response to stress
■ = Effects of chronic or prolonged stress
■ = Other possible effects of chronic stress

Figure 3.2   The Effects of Stress on the Body

This occurs because of a shortening of structures called telomeres in the chromosomes of cells. An enzyme called telomerase maintains these structures but declines with age. Every time a cell divides, which is a continuous process, the telomeres shorten. The shorter your telomeres, the more likely you are to die.

Stress also triggers complex changes in the body's endocrine, or hormone-secreting, system. When you confront a stressor, the adrenal glands, two triangle-shaped glands that sit atop the kidneys, respond by producing stress hormones, including catecholamines, cortisol (hydrocortisone), and epinephrine (adrenaline), that speed up heart rate and raise blood pressure and prepare the body to deal with the threat. This "fight-or-flight" response prepares you for quick action: Your heart works harder to pump more blood to your legs and arms. Your muscles tense, your breathing quickens, and your brain becomes extra alert. Because it's nonessential in a crisis, your digestive system practically shuts down (Figure 3.2).

Cortisol speeds the conversion of proteins and fats into carbohydrates, the body's basic fuel, so we have the energy to fight or flee from a threat. However, stress increases the amount of time required to clear triglycerides, a type of fat linked to heart disease, from the bloodstream.

Cortisol can cause excessive central or abdominal fat, which heightens the risk of diseases such as diabetes, high blood pressure, and stroke. Even slender, premenopausal women faced with increased stress and lacking good coping skills are more likely to accumulate excess weight around their waists, thereby increasing their risk of heart disease and other health problems.

 In one study, African American college students who scored low in coping skills had higher levels of cortisol than those better equipped to cope with stress.[3] Challenges that seem uncontrollable or unpredictable have a greater impact on cortisol than others.

Figure 3.2 illustrates how persistent or repeated increases in the stress hormones can be hazardous throughout the body. Prolonged or severe stress can damage the brain's ability to remember and can actually cause brain cells, or neurons, to atrophy and die. Recent research has implicated stress in both contributing to the development of cancer and reducing the effectiveness of cancer treatment. The stress hormone epinephrine, scientists have found, makes prostate and breast cancer cells more resistant to cell death. [4]

Hundreds of studies over the last 20 years have shown that stress contributes to approximately 80 percent of all major illnesses: cardiovascular disease, cancer, endocrine and metabolic disease, skin rashes, ulcers, ulcerative colitis, emotional disorders, musculoskeletal disease, infectious ailments, premenstrual syndrome (PMS), uterine fibroid cysts, and breast cysts. As many as 75 to 90 percent of visits to physicians are related to stress.

Stress and the Heart

Stress may be the most significant inherited risk factor in people who develop heart disease at a young age. According to behavioral researchers, family transmission of emotional and psychosocial stress, specifically anger in males, greatly increases the likelihood of early heart disease. Young adults whose blood pressure spikes in response to stress may be at risk of hypertension as they get older.

In the 1970s, cardiologists Meyer Friedman, M.D., and Ray Rosenman, M.D., compared their patients to individuals of the same age with healthy hearts and developed two general categories of personality: Type A and Type B. Hardworking, aggressive, and competitive, Type As never have time for all they want to accomplish, even though they usually try to do several tasks at once. Type Bs are more relaxed, though not necessarily less ambitious or successful.

The degree of danger associated with Type-A behavior remains controversial. Of all the personality traits linked with Type-A behavior, the most sinister are anger and chronic hostility. People who are always mistrustful, cynical, and suspicious are twice as likely to suffer blockages of their coronary arteries. Social isolation, depression, and stress may be even stronger risk factors for men.

Stress and Immunity

The immune system is the network of organs, tissues, and white blood cells that defend against disease. Impaired immunity makes the body more susceptible to many diseases, including infections (from the common cold to tuberculosis) and disorders of the immune system itself.

A recent "meta-analysis"—a study of studies in peer-reviewed scientific journals—confirmed earlier findings that stress alters immunity, but the effects differ between short-term and long-term stress. In the short term, stress "revs up" the immune system, a way of preparing for injury or infection. Acute time-limited stressors, the type that produce a "fight-or-flight" response, prompt the immune system to ready itself for the possibility of infections resulting from bites, punctures, or other wounds.

However, long-term, or chronic, stress creates excessive wear and tear, and the system breaks down. Chronic stressors, so profound and persistent that they seem endless and beyond a person's control, suppress immune responses the most. The longer the stress, the more the immune system shifts from potentially adaptive changes to potentially harmful ones, first in cellular immunity and then in broader immune function. Traumatic stress, such as losing a loved one through death or divorce, can impair immunity for as long as a year.

 Minor hassles that aren't related to trauma do take a toll. Under exam stress, students experience a dip in immune function and a higher rate of infections. Ohio State University researchers found that during exam periods, there is a significant drop in the immune cells that normally ward off infection and cancer in medical students.

Age and overall health also affect immune response. The immune systems of individuals who are elderly or ill are more vulnerable to acute and chronic stressors, possibly because their bodies find it more difficult to regulate their reactions.

Stress and Digestion

Do you ever get butterflies in your stomach before giving a speech in class or before a big game? The digestive system is, as one psychologist quips, "an important stop on the tension trail." No studies have ever demonstrated that stress alone causes ulcers, but it may make people more vulnerable to infection with *Helicobacter pylori* bacteria, a known culprit in many cases.[5] To avoid problems, pay attention to how you eat. Eating on the run, gulping food, or overeating results in poorly chewed foods, an overworked stomach, and increased abdominal pressure.

Some simple strategies can help you avoid stress-related stomachaches. Many people experience dry mouth or sweat more under stress. By drinking plenty of water, you replenish lost fluids and prevent dehydration. Fiber-rich foods counteract common stress-related problems, such as cramps and constipation. Do not skip meals. If you do, you're more likely to feel fatigued and irritable.

Be wary of overeating under stress. Some people eat more because they scarf down meals too quickly. Others reach for snacks to calm their nerves or comfort themselves.

 In a study of college women, higher stress increased the risk of binge eating.[6] Watch out for caffeine. Coffee, tea, and cola drinks can make your strained nerves jangle even more. Also avoid sugary snacks. They'll send your blood sugar levels on a roller coaster ride—up one minute, down the next.

Other Stress Symptoms

The first signs of stress include muscle tightness, tension headaches, backaches, upset stomach, and sleep disruptions (caused by stress-altered brain-wave activity). Some people feel fatigued, their hearts may race or beat faster than usual at rest, and they may feel tense all the time, easily frustrated and often irritable. Others feel sad; lose their energy, appetite, or sex drive; and develop psychological problems, including depression anxiety and panic attacks (Chapter 4).

Stress also is closely linked to skin conditions. If you break out the week before an exam, you know firsthand that skin can be extremely sensitive to stress. Skin conditions worsened by stress include acne, psoriasis, herpes, hives, and eczema.[7] With acne, increased touching of the face, perhaps while cramming for a test, may be partly responsible. Other factors, such as temperature, humidity, and cosmetics and toiletries, may also play a role.

Stress on Campus

Being a student—full-time or part-time, in your late teens, early twenties, or later in life—can be extremely stressful. You may feel pressure to perform well to qualify for a good job or graduate school. To meet steep tuition payments, you may have to juggle part-time work and coursework. You may feel stressed about choosing a major, getting along with a difficult roommate, passing a particularly hard course, or living up to your parents' and teachers' expectations. If you're an older student, you may have children, housework, and homework to balance. Your days may seem so busy and your life so full that you worry about coming apart at the seams. One thing is for certain: You're not alone. (See Reality Check, p. 63.)

According to surveys of students at colleges and universities around the country and the world, stressors are remarkably similar. Among the most common are:

- **Test pressures.**
- **Financial problems.**
- **Frustrations,** such as delays in reaching goals.
- **Problems in friendships** and dating relationships.
- **Daily hassles.**
- **Academic failure.**
- **Pressures** as a result of competition, deadlines, and the like.
- **Changes,** which may be unpleasant, disruptive, or too frequent.
- **Losses,** whether caused by the breakup of a relationship or the death of a loved one.

Many students bring complex psychological problems with them to campus, including learning disabilities and mood disorders like depression and anxiety. "Students arrive with the underpinnings of problems that are brought out by the stress of campus life," says one counselor. Some have grown up in broken homes and bear the scars of family troubles. Others fall into the same patterns of alcohol abuse that they observed for years in their families or suffer lingering emotional scars from childhood physical or sexual abuse.

Students aren't the only ones complaining about stress on campus. Professors working toward tenure also report high stress levels—particularly women. The reason for this gender difference may be that women take on more responsibility for mentoring female students and for teaching independent study courses with individual students.[8]

Students Under Stress

 More than a quarter of freshmen feel overwhelmed by all they have to do at the beginning of the academic year; by the year's end, 44 percent feel overwhelmed. In research at three universities, underclassmen were most vulnerable to negative life events, perhaps because they lacked experience in coping with stressful situations. Freshmen had the highest levels of depression; sophomores had the most anger and hostility. Seniors may handle life's challenges better because they have developed better coping mechanisms. In the study, more seniors reported that they faced problems squarely and took action to resolve them, while younger students were more likely to respond passively, for instance, by trying not to let things bother them.

First-generation college students—those whose parents never experienced at least one full year of college—encounter more difficulties with social adjustment than freshmen whose parents attended college. Second-generation students may have several advantages: more knowledge of college life, greater social support, more preparation for college in high school, a greater focus on college activities, and more financial resources.

The percentage of students seeking psychological help because of stress or anxiety has risen dramatically in the last 15 years (see Chapter 4). Students say they react to stress in various ways: physiologically (by sweating, stuttering, trembling, or developing physical symptoms); emotionally (by becoming anxious, fearful, angry, guilty, or depressed); behaviorally (by crying, eating, smoking, being irritable or abusive); or cognitively (by thinking about and analyzing stressful situations and strategies that might be useful in dealing with them).

A supportive network of friends and family makes a difference. Undergraduates with higher levels of social support and self-efficacy reported feeling less stressed and more satisfied with life than others.

Does stress increase drinking among college students? Many assume so, since life stress is a recognized risk for alcohol use, particularly for people with a family history of alcoholism.[9] The relationship between drinking and stress is more complex. For some, drinking occasions were times to discuss problems with friends, regardless of the day's stress. On average, students tended to drink more on days when they were feeling good—possibly because of what the researchers called the "celebratory and social"

nature of college drinking. Drinking—and positive emotions—also peaked on weekends. (See Chapter 12 for more on student drinking.)

Campuses are providing more frontline services than they have in the past, including career-guidance workshops, telephone hot lines, and special social programs for lonely, homesick freshmen. Undergratudates who learn relaxation and stress-reduction techniques report less stress, anxiety, and psychological distress than other students.

Coping with Test Stress

 For many students, midterms and final exams are the most stressful times of the year. Studies at various colleges and universities found that the incidence of colds and flu soared during finals. Some students feel the impact of test stress in other ways—headaches, upset stomachs, skin flare-ups, or insomnia.

Because of stress's impact on memory, students with advanced skills may perform worse under exam pressure than their less skilled peers.[10] Sometimes students become so preoccupied with the possibility of failing that they can't concentrate on studying. Others, including many of the best and brightest students, freeze up during tests

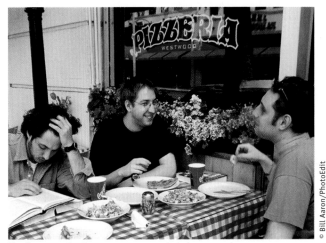

The first year of college can seem overwhelming as you learn your way around the campus, meet new people, and strive to succeed.

© Bill Aaron/PhotoEdit

and can't comprehend multiple-choice questions or write essay answers, even if they know the material.

The students most susceptible to exam stress are those who believe they'll do poorly and who see tests as extremely threatening. Unfortunately, such negative thoughts often become a self-fulfilling prophecy. As they study, these students keep wondering: What good will studying do? I never do well on tests. As their fear increases, they try harder, pulling all-nighters. Fueled by caffeine, munching on sugary snacks, they become edgy and find it harder and harder to concentrate. By the time of the test, they're nervous wrecks, scarcely able to sit still and focus on the exam.

Can you do anything to reduce test stress and feel more in control? Absolutely. (See "Defusing Test Stress" in *IPC.*) Another way is through relaxation. Students taught relaxation techniques—such as controlled breathing, meditation, progressive relaxation, and guided imagery (visualization)—a month before finals tend to have higher levels of immune cells during the exam period and feel in better control during their tests.

Minorities Under Stress

Regardless of your race or ethnic background, college may bring culture shock. You may never have encountered such a degree of diversity in one setting. You probably will meet students with different values, unfamiliar customs, entirely new ways of looking at the world-experiences you may find both stimulating and stressful.

Mental health professionals have long assumed that minority students may feel a double burden of stress. Many undergraduates experience emotional difficulties (see Chapter 4), and researchers have theorized that students from a racial or ethnic minority would be especially likely to develop psychological symptoms, such as anger, anxiety, and depression, as a result of increased stress.

Racism and Discrimination

Racism has indeed been shown to be a source of stress that can affect health and well-being. In the past, some African American students have described predominately white campuses as hostile, alienating, and socially isolating and have reported greater estrangement from the campus community and heightened estrangement in interactions with faculty and peers. However, the generalization that all minority students are more stressed may not be valid. Some coping mechanisms, especially spirituality, can buffer the negative effects of racism.

All minority students do share some common stressors. In one study of minority freshmen entering a large, competitive university, Asian, Filipino, African American, and Native American students all felt more sensitive and vulnerable to the college social climate, to interpersonal tensions between themselves and nonminority students and faculty, to experiences of actual or perceived racism, and to racist attitudes and discrimination. Despite scoring above the national average on the SAT, the minority students in this study did not feel accepted as legitimate students and sensed that others viewed them as unworthy beneficiaries of affirmative action initiatives. While most said that overt racism was rare and relatively easy to deal with, they reported subtle pressures that undermined their academic confidence and their ability to bond with the university. Balancing these stressors, however, was a strong sense of ethnic identity, which helped buffer some stressful effects.

YOUR STRATEGIES FOR PREVENTION *How to Handle Test Stress*

- **Plan ahead.** A month before finals, map out a study schedule for each course. Set aside a small amount of time every day or every other day to review the course materials.

- **Be positive.** Picture yourself taking your final exam. Imagine yourself walking into the exam room feeling confident, opening up the test booklet, and seeing questions for which you know the answers.

- **Take regular breaks.** Get up from your desk, breathe deeply, stretch, and visualize a pleasant scene. You'll feel more refreshed than you would if you chugged another cup of coffee.

- **Practice.** Some teachers are willing to give practice finals to prepare students for test situations, or you and your friends can test each other.

- **Talk to other students.** Chances are that many of them share your fears about test taking and may have discovered some helpful techniques of their own. Sometimes talking to your adviser or a counselor can also help.

- **Be satisfied with doing your best.** You can't expect to ace every test; all you can and should expect is your best effort. Once you've completed the exam, allow yourself the sweet pleasure of relief that it's over.

POINT COUNTERPOINT *Should Schools Help with Stress?*

POINT

Students identify stress as the number-one barrier to better academic performance. Colleges have been trying to help students cope by providing more mental health services, training students to be peer counselors, and providing on-campus relaxation and stress management programs.

COUNTERPOINT

Some view today's students as overly pampered and argue that stress is a personal challenge, not a university problem. While students should have access to support and counseling, they should assume primary responsibility for meeting the demands of their classes and finding balance in their lives.

YOUR VIEW

Do you think colleges should do more to address the stress of undergraduates? Do you feel stressed out? What could your school do to help you cope with stress in your life? What are you doing on your own to manage stress?

Hispanic students have identified three major types of stressors in their college experiences: academic (related to exam preparation and faculty interaction, social (related to ethnicity and interpersonal competence), and financial (related to their economic situation). Some students who recently immigrated to the United States report feeling ostracized by students of similar ancestry who are second- or third-generation Americans.

Some College Responses

Because racism and discrimination can be hard to deal with individually, they are particularly sinister form of stress. By banding together, however, those who experience discrimination can take action to protect themselves, challenge the ignorance and hateful assumptions that fuel bigotry, and promote a healthier environment for all.

In the last decade, there have been reports of increased intolerance among young people and greater tolerance of expressions and acts of hate on college campuses. To counteract this trend, many schools have set up programs and classes to educate students about each other's backgrounds and to acknowledge and celebrate the richness diversity brings to campus life. Educators have called on universities to make campuses less alienating and more culturally and emotionally accessible, with programs and policies targeted not only at minority students but also at the university as a whole.

Men, Women, and Stress

 Women, who make up 56 percent of today's college students, also shoulder the majority of the stress load. In a nationwide survey of students in the class of 2010, more women than men reported feeling depressed, insecure about their physical and mental health, and worried about paying for college. More men than women considered themselves above average or in the top 10 percent of people their age in terms of emotional health.[11]

The immune and hormonal systems of men and women may respond differently to stressors. In psychological experiments men under stress display higher aggression, for example, delivering more shocks to another volunteer, than women.[12]

Gender differences in lifestyle also may explain why women feel so stressed. College men spend significantly more time doing things that are fun and relaxing: exercising, partying, watching TV, and playing video games. Women, on the other hand, tend to study more, do more volunteer work, and handle more household and child-care chores.

Where can stressed-out college women turn for support? The best source, according to University of California research, is other women. In general, the social support women offer their friends and relatives seems more effective in reducing the blood-pressure response to stress than that provided by men.

At all ages, women and men tend to respond to stress differently. While males (human and those of other species) react with the classic fight-or-flight response, females under attack try to protect their children and seek help from other females—a strategy dubbed *tend and befriend.*

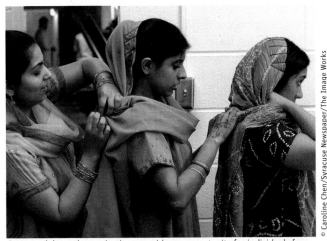

Campus clubs and organizations provide an opportunity for individuals from different ethnic backgrounds to celebrate their culture and educate others about it. These undergraduates are preparing to perform an Indian dance at a special evening sponsored by Asian Students in America.

© Caroline Chen/Syracuse Newspaper/The Image Works

YOUR STRATEGIES FOR CHANGE *How to Deal with an Angry Person*

- **Become an impartial observer.** Act as if you were watching someone else's two-year-old have a temper tantrum at the supermarket.
- **Stay calm.** Letting your emotions loose only adds fuel to fury. Talk quietly and slowly; let the person know you understand that he or she is angry.
- **Refuse to engage.** Step back to avoid invading his or her space. Retreat farther if need be until the person is back in control.
- **Find something to agree upon.** Look for common ground, if only to acknowledge that you're both in a difficult situation.

When exposed to experimental stress (such as a loud, harsh noise), women show more affection for friends and relatives; men show less. When working mothers studied by psychologists had a bad day, they coped by concentrating on their children when they got home. Stressed-out fathers were more likely to withdraw.

Other Personal Stressors

At every stage of life, you will encounter challenges and stressors. Among the most common are those related to anger, work, and illness.

The Anger Epidemic

In recent years, violent aggressive driving—which some dub *road rage*—has exploded. Sideline rage at amateur and professional sporting events has become so widespread that a Pennsylvania midget football game ended in a brawl involving more than 100 coaches, players, parents, and fans.

No one seems immune. Women fly off the handle just as often as men, although they're less likely to get physical. The young and the infamous, including several rappers and musicians sentenced to anger management classes for violent outbursts, may seem more volatile. However,

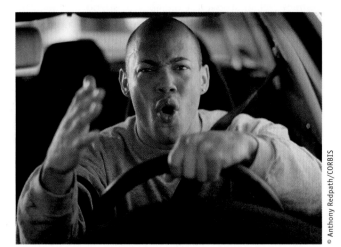

How you manage your anger has consequences for your health and for your interactions with others.

© Anthony Redpath/CORBIS

ordinary senior citizens have erupted into "line rage" and pushed ahead of others simply because they feel they've "waited long enough" in their lives.

"Everyone everywhere seems to be hotter under the collar these days," observes Sybil Evans, a conflict resolution expert who singles out three primary culprits: time, technology, and tension. "Americans are working longer hours than anyone else in the world. The cell phones and pagers that were supposed to make our lives easier have put us on call 24–7–365. Since we're always running, we're tense and low on patience, and the less patience we have, the less we monitor what we say to people and how we treat them."[13]

Getting a Grip

For years therapists encouraged people to "vent" their anger. However, research now shows that letting anger out only makes it worse. "Catharsis is worse than useless," says psychology professor Brad Bushman of Iowa State University, whose research has shown that letting anger out makes people more aggressive, not less. "Many people think of anger as the psychological equivalent of the steam in a pressure cooker that has to be released or it will explode. That's not true. People who react by hitting, kicking, screaming, and swearing aren't dealing with the underlying cause of their anger. They just feel more angry."[14]

Over time, temper tantrums sabotage physical health as well as psychological equanimity. By churning out stress hormones, chronic anger revs the body into a state of combat readiness, multiplying the risk for stroke and heart attack—even in healthy individuals.

To deal with anger, you have to figure out what's really making you mad. Usually the jammed soda machine is the final straw that unleashes bottled-up fury over a more difficult issue, such as a recent breakup or a domineering parent. Also monitor yourself for early signs of exhaustion and overload. While stress alone doesn't cause a blowup, it makes you more vulnerable to overreacting.

Conflict Resolution

Disagreements are inevitable; disagreeable ways of dealing with them are not. One of the most important skills in any setting—from family room to staff meeting to corporate boardroom—is resolving conflicts. Although many assume that you can't reason with someone who's furious, psychologists have shown that angry people are capable of processing and analyzing information, depending on how it is presented to them.[15]

The key is to focus on the problem, not the individual. Try to put aside unconscious biases, such as assuming a person is difficult to deal with, or preconceived notions about what others really want. Rather than planning what you might say, focus your attention on what others are saying.

Professionals recommend the following steps:

- **Listen.** To work through a conflict, you need to understand the other person's point of view. This demands careful listening in a quiet, private setting, away from activity and background noise. If conflict erupts in a public place, move the discussion elsewhere.

- **Assimilate.** Rather than taking a position and focusing only on defending it, try not to shut yourself off to other possibilities. Keep open the possibility that no one party is completely right or completely wrong. To get a fresh perspective, consider the situation from the "third person." If you were seeing the conflict from the outside, what would you think about the information? Once you've taken in all available information, ask yourself: What do I know now about the overall situation? Has my opinion changed?

- **Respond.** Especially if another person is responding in anger, give a calm, well-reasoned response. It will help defuse a highly emotional situation. Try to find a common goal that will benefit you both. Restate the other person's position when both of you are finished speaking so you both know you've been heard and understood.

Job Stress

More so than ever, many people find that they are working more and enjoying it less. Many people, including working parents, spend 55 to 60 hours a week on the job. More people are caught up in an exhausting cycle of overwork, which causes stress, which makes work harder, which leads to more stress. Even the workplace itself can contribute to stress. A noisy, open-office environment can increase levels of stress without workers realizing it.

High job strain—defined as high psychological demands combined with low control or decision-making ability over one's job—may increase blood pressure, particularly among men. In a recent study, blood pressure was highest at work but remained elevated at home and even during sleep.[16]

People who become obsessed by their work and careers can turn into workaholics, so caught up in racing toward the top that they forget what they're racing toward and

why. In some cases they throw themselves into their work to mask or avoid painful feelings or difficulties in their own lives.

Burnout

Burnout is a state of physical, emotional, and mental exhaustion brought on by constant or repeated emotional pressure. No one—regardless of age, gender, or job—is immune. Mothers and managers, fire fighters and flight attendants, teachers and telemarketers feel the flames of too much stress and not enough satisfaction. Many people, especially those caring for others at work or at home, get to a point where there's an imbalance between their own feelings and dealing with difficult, distressful issues on a day-to-day basis. If they don't recognize what's going on and make some changes, their health and the quality of their work suffer.

"Burnout doesn't stem from the job or the person but from both," says psychologist Christina Maslach, Ph.D., author of *Banishing Burnout,* "What matters is the relationship you have with work rather than with the work that you do."[17] As with other long-term commitments, it takes time, attention, and effort to keep this relationship healthy—and to repair it if it breaks down.

Early signs of burnout include exhaustion, sleep problems or nightmares, increased anxiety or nervousness, muscular tension (headaches, backaches, and the like), increased use of alcohol or medication, digestive problems, such as nausea, vomiting, or diarrhea, loss of interest in sex, frequent body aches or pain, quarrels with family or friends, negative feelings about everything, problems concentrating, job mistakes and accidents, and feelings of depression, hopelessness, or helplessness.

The hallmark of burnout is a shift to the negative," says Maslach. "You begin to detach and dislike your job. You become cynical, critical, hostile. You blame other people. Rather than doing your very best, you try to get by with the bare minimum." Ultimately the one-two punch of exhaustion and cynicism culminates in what she calls "inefficacy," a sense of inadequacy that saps a person's strength and spirit.

Research in the new field of social neuroscience is providing fresh insight into this process. "Our brains are designed to reflect and catch the state of the person we're with, which works to our advantage in most situations by helping us understand each other better," says psychologist Daniel Goleman, Ph.D., author of *Social Intelligence.* However, constant interaction with people who are anxious, angry, stressed, or traumatized floods the brain with

burnout A state of physical, emotional, and mental exhaustion resulting from constant or repeated emotional pressure.

negative emotions and activates its stress centers.[18] As a protective mechanism, your brain shuts down. Simply acknowledging burnout can mark a turning point. Once you see what's happening, you can't continue to approach your work in the same way.

Age is the one variable most consistently associated with burnout: Younger employees between ages 30 and 40 report the highest rates. Both men and women are susceptible to burnout. Unmarried individuals, particularly men, seem more prone to burnout than married workers. Single employees who've never been married have higher burnout rates than those who are divorced.

Illness and Disability

Just as the mind can have profound effects on the body, the body can have an enormous impact on our emotions. Whenever we come down with the flu or pull a muscle, we feel under par. When the problem is more serious or persistent—a chronic disease like diabetes, for instance, or a lifelong hearing impairment—the emotional stress of constantly coping with it is even greater.

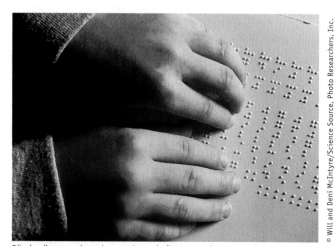

Blind college students have unique challenges and stressors that sighted students do not.

© Will and Deni McIntyre/Science Source, Photo Researchers, Inc.

A common source of stress for college students is a learning disability, which may affect one of every ten Americans. Most learning-disabled people have average or above-average intelligence, but they rarely live up to their ability in school. Some have only one area of difficulty, such as reading or math. Others have problems with attention, writing, communicating, reasoning, coordination, and social skills.

Not all students with learning disabilities experience greater stress. In one in-depth study comparing 34 undergraduates with and without learning disabilities, the learning-disabled (LD) students reported significantly fewer college stressors and demonstrated a higher need for achievement. The LD students also scored significantly higher in resiliency and initiative in solving problems and working toward goals.

Societal Stressors

Centuries ago the poet John Donne observed that no man is an island. Today, on an increasingly crowded and troubled planet, these words seem truer than ever. Problems such as discrimination and terrorism can no longer be viewed only as economic or political issues. Directly or indirectly, they affect the well-being of all who inhabit Earth—now and in the future.

The deliberate use of physical force to abuse or injure is a leading killer of young people in the United States—and a potential source of stress in all our lives. If you or someone you know has been a victim of a violent crime, a sense of vulnerability may add to the stress of daily living. See Your Strategies for Change below.

Responses to Stress

Sometimes we respond to stress or challenge with self-destructive behaviors, such as drinking or using drugs. These responses can lead to psychological problems,

---

YOUR STRATEGIES FOR CHANGE *How to Cope with Distress After a Trauma*

Senseless acts of violence or terrorism can trigger a variety of emotions, including shock, sorrow, fear, anger, and grief. You may have problems sleeping, concentrating, or going about simple chores. Because the world seems more dangerous, it may take a while for you to regain your sense of equilibrium. The following recommendations from the American Psychological Association can help:

- **Talk about it.** Ask for support from people who will listen to your concerns. It often helps to speak with others who have shared your experience so you do not feel so different or alone.

- **Strive for balance.** Remind yourself of people and events that are meaningful and comforting, even encouraging.

- **Take a break.** While you may want to keep informed, limit your exposure to news on television, the Internet, newspa-

pers, or magazines. Schedules breaks to focus on something you enjoy.

- **Take care of yourself.** Engage in healthy behaviors, such as exercise, that will enhance your ability to cope. Avoid alcohol and drugs because they can suppress your feelings rather than help you to manage your distress.

- **Help others or do something productive.** Try volunteering at your school or within your community. Helping someone else often helps you feel better too.

such as anxiety or depression, and physical problems, including psychosomatic illnesses.

Defense Mechanisms

Defense mechanisms, such as those described in Table 3.1, are another response to stress. These psychological devices are mental processes that help us cope with personal problems. Such responses also are not the answer to stress—and learning to recognize them in yourself will enable you to deal with your stress in a healthier way.

TABLE 3.1 Common Defense Mechanisms Used to Alleviate Anxiety and Eliminate Conflict

Defense Mechanism	Example
Denial: the refusal to accept a painful reality.	You don't accept as true the news that a loved one is seriously ill.
Displacement: the redirection of feelings from their true object to a more acceptable or safer substitute.	Instead of lashing out at a coach or a teacher, you snap at your best friend.
Projection: the attribution of unacceptable feelings or impulses to someone else.	When you want to end a relationship, you project your unhappiness onto your partner.
Realization: the substitution of "good," acceptable reasons for the real motivations for our behavior.	You report a classmate who has been mean to you for cheating on an exam and explain that cheating is unfair to other students.
Reaction formation: adopting attitudes and behaviors that are the opposite of what we feel.	You lavishly compliment an acquaintance whom you really despise.
Repression: the way we keep threatening impulses, fantasies, memories, feelings, or wishes from becoming conscious.	You don't "hear" the alarm after the late night, or you "forget" to take out the trash.

Relaxation

A more positive response to stress is relaxation—the physical and mental state opposite that of stress. Rather than gearing up for fight or flight, our bodies and minds grow calmer and work more smoothly. We're less likely to become frazzled and more capable of staying in control. The most effective relaxation techniques include progressive relaxation, visualization, meditation, mindfulness, and biofeedback. (Also see the Rx: Relax Lab in *IPC.*) **IPC**

Progressive relaxation works by intentionally increasing and then decreasing tension in the muscles. While sitting or lying down in a quiet, comfortable setting, you tense and release various muscles, beginning with those of the hand, for instance, and then proceeding to the arms, shoulders, neck, face, scalp, chest, stomach, buttocks, genitals, and so on, down each leg to the toes. Relaxing the muscles can quiet the mind and restore internal balance.

Visualization, or **guided imagery,** involves creating mental pictures that calm you down and focus your mind. Some people use this technique to promote healing when they are ill. Visualization skills require practice and, in some cases, instruction by qualified health professionals.[19]

Meditation has been practiced in many forms over the ages, from the yogic techniques of the Far East to the Quaker silence of more modern times. Brain scans have shown that meditation activates the sections of the brain in charge of the autonomic nervous system, which governs bodily functions, such as digestion and blood pressure, that we cannot consciously control.[20] Although many studies have documented the benefits of meditation for overall health, it may be particularly helpful for people dealing with stress-related medical conditions such as high blood pressure and heart problems.[21]

Meditation helps a person reach a state of relaxation, but with the goal of achieving inner peace and harmony. There is no one right way to meditate, and many people have discovered how to meditate on their own, without even knowing what it is they are doing.

Increasing numbers of college students are turning to meditation as a way of coping with stress. Most forms of meditation have common elements: sitting quietly for 15 to 20 minutes once or twice a day, concentrating on a word or image, and breathing slowly and rhythmically. If you wish to try meditation, it often helps to have someone guide you through your first sessions. Or try tape recording your own voice (with or without favorite music in the background) and playing it back to yourself, freeing yourself to concentrate on the goal of turning the attention within.

Mindfulness is a modern form of an ancient Asian technique that involves maintaining awareness in the present moment. You tune in to each part of your body,

defense mechanism A psychological process that alleviates anxiety and eliminates mental conflict; includes denial, displacement, projection, rationalization, reaction formation, and repression.

progressive relaxation A method of reducing muscle tension by contracting, then relaxing, certain areas of the body.

visualization, or **guided imagery** An approach to stress control, self-healing, or motivating life changes by means of seeing oneself in the state of calmness, wellness, or change.

meditation A group of approaches that use quiet sitting, breathing techniques, and/or chanting to relax, improve concentration, and become attuned to one's inner self.

mindfulness A method of stress reduction that involves experiencing the physical and mental sensations of the present moment.

scanning from head to toe, noting the slightest sensation. You allow whatever you experience—an itch, an ache, a feeling of warmth—to enter your awareness. Then you open yourself to focus on all the thoughts, sensations, sounds, and feelings that enter your awareness. Mindfulness keeps you in the here and now, thinking about what is rather than about *what if* or *if only*.

Biofeedback is a method of obtaining feedback, or information, about some physiological activity occurring in the body. An electronic monitoring device attached to the body detects a change in an internal function and communicates it back to the person through a tone, light, or meter. By paying attention to this feedback, most people can gain some control over functions previously thought to be beyond conscious control, such as body temperature, heart rate, muscle tension, and brain waves. Biofeedback training consists of three stages:

1. Developing increased awareness of a body state or function.
2. Gaining control over it.
3. Transferring this control to everyday living without use of the electronic instrument.

The goal of biofeedback for stress reduction is a state of tranquility, usually associated with the brain's production of alpha waves (which are slower and more regular than normal waking waves). After several training sessions, most people can produce alpha waves more or less at will.

Stress and Psychological Health

Traumatic events (such as a robbery, assault, or sudden death of a loved one) always take a toll on an individual, and it's normal to feel sad, tense, overwhelmed, angry, or incapable of coping with the ordinary demands of daily living. Usually such feelings and behaviors subside with time. The stressful event fades into the past, and those whose lives it has touched adapt to its lasting impact. But sometimes individuals remain extremely distressed and unable to function as they once did. While the majority of individuals who survive a trauma recover, at least a quarter of such individuals later develop serious psychological symptoms.

Your Life Change Coach

Coping with Stress

The key to coping with stress is realizing that your *perception* of and *response* to a stressor are crucial. Changing the way you interpret events or situations—a skill called *reframing*—makes all the difference. An event, such as a move to a new city, is not stressful in itself. A move becomes stressful if you see it as a traumatic upheaval rather than an exciting beginning of a new chapter in your life.

In times of stress, the following simple exercises can stop the stress buildup inside your body and help you regain a sense of calm and control.

- **Breathing.** Deep breathing relaxes the body and quiets the mind. Draw air deeply into your lungs, allowing your chest to fill with air and your belly to rise and fall. You will feel the muscle tension and stress begin to melt away. When you're feeling extremely stressed, try this calming breath: Sit or lie with your back straight and place the tip of your tongue on the roof of your mouth behind your teeth. Exhale completely through the mouth, then inhale through the nose for 4 seconds. Hold the breath for 7 seconds, then exhale audibly through the mouth for 8 seconds. Repeat four times.

- **Refocusing.** Thinking about a situation you can't change or control only increases the stress you feel. Force your mind to focus on other subjects. If you're stuck in a long line, distract yourself. Check out what other people are buying or imagine what they do for a living. Imagine that you're in a hot shower and a wave of relaxation is washing your stress down the drain.

- **Serenity breaks.** Build moments of tranquility into your day. For instance, while waiting for your computer to start up or a file to download, look at a photograph of someone you love or a poster of a tropical island. If none is available, close your eyes and visualize a soothing scene, such as walking in a meadow or along a beach.

- **Stress signals.** Learn to recognize the first signs that your stress load is getting out of hand: Is your back bothering you? Do you have a headache? Do you find yourself speeding or

biofeedback A technique of becoming aware, with the aid of external monitoring devices, of internal physiological activities in order to develop the capability of altering them.

misplacing things? Whenever you spot these early warnings, force yourself to stop and say, I'm under stress. I need to do something about it.

- **Reality checks.** To put things into proper perspective, ask yourself: Will I remember what's made me so upset a month from now? If I had to rank this problem on a scale of 1 to 10, with worldwide catastrophe as 10, where would it rate?

- **Stress inoculation.** Rehearse everyday situations that you find stressful, such as speaking in class. Think of how you might make the situation less tense, for instance, by breathing deeply before you talk or jotting down notes beforehand. Think of these small "doses" of stress as the psychological equivalent of allergy shots: They immunize you so you feel less stressed when bigger challenges come along.

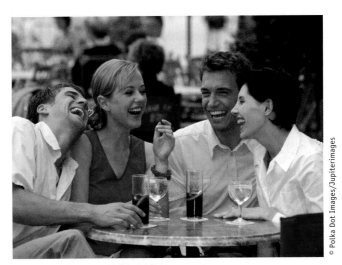

Shared laughter is a powerful antidote to stress.

- **Rx: Laughter.** Humor counters stress by focusing on comic aspects of difficult situations and may, as various studies have shown, lessen harmful effects on the immune system and overall health. However, humor may have different effects on stress in men and women.

 In a study of undergraduates, humor buffered stress-related physical symptoms in men and women. However, it reduced stress-linked anxiety only in men. The researchers theorized that men may prefer humor as a more appropriate way of expressing emotions such as anxiety, whereas women are more likely to use self-disclosure, that is, to confide in friends.

- **Spiritual coping.** Saying a prayer under stress is one of the oldest and most effective ways of calming yourself. Other forms of spiritual coping, such as putting trust in God and doing for others (for instance, by volunteering at a shelter for battered women) also can provide a different perspective on daily hassles and stresses.

- **Sublimation.** This term refers to the redirection of any drives considered unacceptable into socially acceptable channels. Outdoor activity is one of the best ways to reduce stress through sublimation. For instance, if you're furious with a friend who betrayed your trust or frustrated because your boss rejects all of your proposals, you might go for a long run or hike to sublimate your anger.

- **Exercise.** Regular physical activity can relieve stress, boost energy, lift mood, and keep stress under control. Young adults who adopt and continue regular aerobic exercise show less intense cardiovascular responses to stress, which may protect them against coronary heart disease as they age. Strength training may have similar benefits.

 In one study, college students who engaged in an eight-week weight training reported lower stress levels than those who participated in an aerobic dance program.

- **Journaling.** One of the simplest, yet most effective, ways to work through stress is by putting your feelings into words that only you will read. The more honest and open you are as you write, the better. College students who wrote in their journals about traumatic events felt much better afterward than those who wrote about superficial topics. Focus on intense emotional experiences and "autopsy" them to try to understand why they affected you the way they did. Rereading and thinking about your notes may reveal the underlying reasons for your response. See the chapter on "Power Journaling" in *IPC*. **IPC**

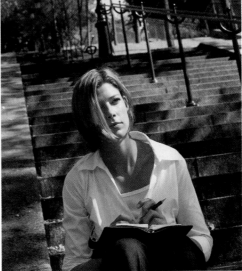

Writing in your journal about feelings and difficulties is a simple and effective way to help control your stress. You don't need to be a journalist. Just write about *you*.

Posttraumatic Stress Disorder (PTSD)

In the past, **posttraumatic stress disorder (PTSD)** was viewed as a psychological response to out-of-the-ordinary stressors, such as captivity or combat. However, other experiences can also forever change the way people view themselves and their world. Thousands of individuals experience or witness traumatic events, such as fires or floods.

 Women are, on average, twice as vulnerable as men to PTSD, but not because they experience more traumatic events. Childhood traumas occur equally in both sexes. Adult men encounter more traumas—accidents, violence, combat, terrorism, disas-

ters, injuries—than adult women. Women experience more sexual assaults and abuse.[22] PTSD is especially high in women who have served in the military. Sexual trauma ranks as the most distressing for female veterans, followed by physical assault and war zone experience.[23]

Veterans of combat in Iraq and Afganistan have high rates of PTSD, along with other problems such as substance abuse. The majority have experienced high-intensity guerilla warfare as well as the chronic threat of roadside bombs and improved explosive devices.[24] In the long term, veterans with PTSD face an increased risk of developing coronary heart disease.[25]

Savvy Consumer Can Stress-Relief Products Help?

You're stressed out, and you see an ad for a product—an oil, candle, cream, herbal tea, pill, or potion—that promises to make all your cares disappear. Should you soak in an aromatic bath, have a massage, try kava, squeeze foam balls? In most cases, you're probably not doing yourself much harm, but you aren't necessarily doing yourself much good either. Keep these considerations in mind:

- Be wary of instant cures. Regardless of the promises on the label, it's unrealistic to expect any magic ingredient or product to make all your problems disappear.

- Focus on stress-reducing behavior, rather than a product. An aromatic candle may not bring instant serenity, but if you light a candle and meditate, you may indeed feel more at peace. A scented pillow may not be a cure for stress, but if it helps you get a good night's sleep, you'll cope better the next day.

- Experiment with physical ways to work out stress. Exercise is one of the best ways to lower your stress levels. Try walking, running, swimming, cycling, kickboxing—anything physical that helps you release tension.

- Don't make matters worse by smoking (the chemicals in cigarettes increase heart rate, blood pressure, and stress hormones), consuming too much caffeine (it speeds up your system for hours), eating snacks high in sugar (it produces a quick high followed by a sudden slump), or turning to drugs or alcohol (they can only add to your stress when their effects wear off).

- Be cautious when trying "alternative" products. "Natural" products, such as herbs and enzymes, claim to have psychological effects. However, because they are not classified as drugs, these products have not undergone the rigorous scientific testing required of

psychiatric medications, and little is known about their safety or efficacy. "Natural" doesn't mean risk-free. Opium and cocaine are "natural" substances that have dramatic and potentially deadly effects on the mind.

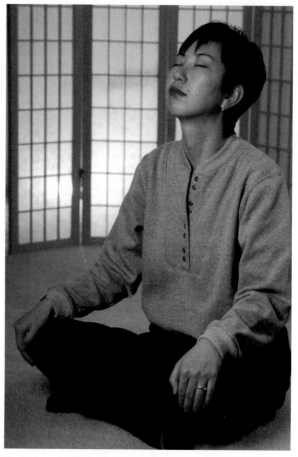

© Garry Conner/PhotoEdit

Meditation calms both mind and spirit. Sit quietly for 15 minutes and concentrate on your breath. Imagine a candle flame. Any distracting thought is a breeze that causes it to flicker.

According to research, almost half of car accident victims may develop PTSD. Individuals who were seriously injured are especially vulnerable. The main symptoms are re-experiencing the traumatic event, avoiding the site of the accident, refraining from driving in weather and road conditions similar to those on the day of the accident, and feeling a general increase in distress.

In PTSD, individuals re-experience their terror and helplessness again and again in their dreams or intrusive thoughts. To avoid this psychic pain, they may try to avoid anything associated with the trauma. Some enter a state of emotional numbness and no longer can respond to people and experiences the way they once did, especially when it comes to showing tenderness or affection. Those who've been mugged or raped may be afraid to venture out by themselves.

The sooner trauma survivors receive psychological help, the better they are likely to fare. Often talking about what happened with an empathic person or someone who's shared the experience as soon as possible—preferably before going to sleep on the day of the event—an help an individual begin to deal with what has occurred. Group sessions, ideally beginning soon after the trauma, allow individuals to share views and experiences. Behavioral, cognitive, and psychodynamic therapy sometimes along with psychiatric medication, (described in Chapter 4) can help individuals suffering with PTSD.

The words people use to express their feelings after a traumatic event may reveal whether they will develop lasting symptoms of PTSD. In a study of college students asked to describe in as much detail as possible how they had heard about the attacks of September 11, 2001, those who used fewer words, expressed less negative emotion, and included more references to death and religion were more likely to report PTSD symptoms five months after the attacks.[26]

Resilience

Adversity—whether in the form of a traumatic event or chronic stress—has different effects on individuals. Some people never recover and continue on a downward slide that may ultimately prove fatal. Others return, though at different rates, to their prior level of functioning. In recent years researchers have focused their attention on a particularly intriguing group: those people who not only survive stressful experiences but also thrive, that is, who actually surpass their previous level of functioning. See the chapter on "Shock Absorption" in *IPC*.
IPC

Resilience can take many forms. A father whose child is kidnapped and killed may become a nationwide advocate for victims' rights. A student whose roommate dies in a car crash after a party may campaign for tougher laws against drunk driving. A couple whose premature baby spends weeks in a neonatal intensive care unit may find that their marriage has grown closer and stronger. Even though their experiences were painful, the individuals often look back at them as bringing positive changes into their lives.

Researchers have studied various factors that enable individuals to thrive in the face of adversity. These include:

- **An optimistic attitude.** Rather than reacting to a stressor simply as a threat, these men and women view stress as a challenge—one they believe they can and will overcome. Researchers have documented that individuals facing various stressors, including serious illness and bereavement, are more likely to report experiencing growth if they have high levels of hope and optimism.

- **Self-efficacy.** A sense of being in control of one's life can boost health, even in times of great stress.

- **Stress inoculation.** People who deal well with adversity often have had previous experiences with stress that toughened them in various ways, such as

posttraumatic stress disorder (PTSD) The repeated reliving of a trauma through nightmares or recollection.

teaching them skills that enhanced their ability to cope and boosting their confidence in their ability to weather a rough patch.

- **Secure personal relationships.** Individuals who know they can count on the support of their loved ones are more likely to be resilient.
- **Spirituality or religiosity.** Religious coping may be particularly related to growth and resilience. In particular, two types seem most beneficial: spiritually based religious coping (receiving emotional reassurance and guidance from God) and good-deeds coping (living a better, more spiritual life that includes altruistic acts).

Resilience sometimes means developing new skills simply because, in order to get through the stressful experience, people had to learn something they hadn't known how to do before—for instance, wrangling with insurance companies or other bureaucracies. By mastering such skills, they become more fit to deal with an unpredictable world and develop new flexibility in facing the unknown.

Along with new abilities comes the psychological sense of mastery. "I survived this," an individual may say. "I'll be able to deal with other hard things in the future." Such confidence keeps people actively engaged in the effort to cope and is itself a predictor of eventual success. Stress also can make individuals more aware of the fulfilling aspects of life, and they may become more interested in spiritual pursuits. Certain kinds of stressful experiences also have social consequences. If a person experiencing a traumatic event finds that the significant others in his or her life can be counted on, the result can be a strengthening of their relationship.

Organizing Your Time

We live in what some sociologists call hyperculture, a society that moves at warp speed. Information bombards us constantly. The rate of change seems to accelerate every year. Our "time-saving" devices—pagers, cell phones, modems, faxes, palm-sized organizers, laptop computers—have simply extended the boundaries of where and how we work.

As a result, more and more people are suffering from "timesickness," a nerve-racking feeling that life has be-come little more than an endless to-do list. The best antidote is time management, and hundreds of books, seminars, and experts offer training in making the most of the hours in the day. Yet these well-intentioned methods often fail, and sooner or later most of us find ourselves caught in a time trap. (See the chapter on "Time Control" in *IPC*.) **IPC**

Are You Running Out of Time?

Every day you make dozens of decisions, and the choices you make about how to use your time directly affect your stress level. If you have a big test on Monday and a term paper due Tuesday, you may plan to study all weekend. Then, when you're invited to a party Saturday night, you go. Although you set the alarm for 7:00 a.m. on Sunday, you don't pull yourself out of bed until noon. By the time you start studying, it's 4:00 p.m., and anxiety is building inside you.

How can you tell if you've lost control of your time? The following are telltale symptoms of poor time management:

- **Rushing.**
- **Chronic inability to make choices or decisions.**
- **Fatigue or listlessness.**
- **Constantly missed deadlines.**
- **Not enough time for rest** or personal relationships.
- **A sense of being overwhelmed** by demands and details and having to do what you don't want to do most of the time.

One of the hard lessons of being on your own is that your choices and your actions have consequences. Stress is just one of them. But by thinking ahead, being realistic about your workload, and sticking to your plans, you can gain better control over your time and your stress levels.

Managing Your Time

Time management involves skills that anyone can learn, but they require commitment and practice to make a difference in your life. It may help to know the techniques that other students have found most useful:

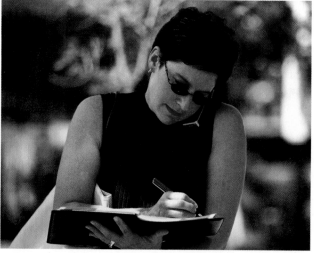

A calendar or planner is an important tool in time management. You can use it to keep track of assignment due dates, class meetings, and other "to do's."

- **Schedule your time.** Use a calendar or planner. Beginning the first week of class, mark down deadlines for each assignment, paper, project, and test scheduled that semester. Develop a daily schedule, listing very specifically what you will do the next day, along with the times. Block out times for working out, eating dinner, calling home, and talking with friends as well as for studying.

- **Develop a game plan.** Allow at least two nights to study for any major exam. Set aside more time for researching and writing papers. Make sure to allow time to revise and print out a paper—and to deal with emergencies like a computer breakdown. Set daily and weekly goals for every class. When working on a big project, don't neglect your other courses. Whenever possible, try to work ahead in all your classes.

- **Identify time robbers.** For several days keep a log of what you do and how much time you spend doing it. You may discover that disorganization is eating away at your time or that you have a problem getting started. (See the following section on "Overcoming Procrastination.")

- **Make the most of classes.** Read the assignments before class rather than waiting until just before you have a test. By reading ahead of time, you'll make it easier to understand the lectures. Go to class yourself. Your own notes will be more helpful than a friend's or those from a note-taking service. Read your lecture notes at the end of each day or at least at the end of each week.

- **Develop an efficient study style.** Some experts recommend studying for 50 minutes, then breaking for 10 minutes. Small incentives, such as allowing yourself to call or visit a friend during these 10 minutes, can provide the motivation to keep you at the books longer. When you're reading, don't just highlight passages. Instead, write notes or questions to yourself in the margins, which will help you retain more information. Even if you're racing to start a paper, take a few extra minutes to prepare a workable outline. It will be easier to structure your paper when you start writing.

- **Focus on the task at hand.** Rather than worrying about how you did on yesterday's test or how you'll ever finish next week's project, focus intently on whatever you're doing at any given moment. If your mind starts to wander, use any distraction—the sound of the phone ringing or a noise from the hall—as a reminder to stay in the moment.

- **Turn elephants into hors d'oeuvres.** Cut a huge task into smaller chunks so it seems less enormous. For in-stance, break down your term paper into a series of steps, such as selecting a topic, identifying sources of research information, taking notes, developing an outline, and so on.

- **Keep your workspace in order.** Even if the rest of your room is a shambles, try to keep your desk clear. Piles of papers are distracting, and you can end up wasting lots of time looking for notes you misplaced or an article you have to read by morning. Try to spend the last ten minutes of the day getting your desk in order so you get a fresh start on the new day. (See the "Do It Now" lab in *IPC*.) **IPC**

Overcoming Procrastination

Putting off until tomorrow what should be done today is a habit that creates a great deal of stress for many students. It also takes a surprising toll. In studies with students taking a health psychology course, researchers found that although procrastinating provided short-term benefits, including periods of low stress, the tendency to dawdle had long-term costs, including poorer health and lower grades. Early in the semester, the procrastinators reported less stress and fewer health problems than students who scored low on procrastination. However, by the end of the semester, procrastinators reported more health-related symptoms, more stress, and more visits to health-care professionals than nonprocrastinators. Students who procrastinate also get poorer grades in courses with many deadlines.

The three most common types of procrastination are putting off unpleasant things, putting off difficult tasks, and putting off tough decisions. Procrastinators are most likely to delay by wishing they didn't have to do what they must or by telling themselves they "just can't get started," which means they never do.

To get out of the procrastination trap, keep track of the tasks you're most likely to put off, and try to figure out why you don't want to tackle them. Think of alternative ways to get tasks done. If you put off library readings, for instance, is the problem getting to the library or the reading itself? If it's the trip to the library, arrange to walk over with a friend whose company you enjoy.

Do what you like least first. Once you have it out of the way, you can concentrate on the tasks you enjoy. Build time into your schedule for interruptions, unforeseen problems, and unexpected events, so you aren't constantly racing around. Establish ground rules for meeting your own needs (including getting enough sleep and making time for friends) before saying yes to any activity. Learn to live according to a three-word motto: Just do it!

Learn It | Live It

De-Stress Your Life

College is a perfect time to learn and practice the art of stress reduction. You can start applying the techniques and concepts outlined in this chapter immediately. You may want to begin by doing some relaxation or awareness exercises. They can give you the peace of mind you need to focus more effectively on larger issues, goals, and decisions.

You needn't see stress as a problem to solve on your own. Reach out to others. As you build friendships and intimate relationships, you may find that some irritating problems are easier to put into perspective. Don't be afraid to laugh at yourself and to look for the comic or absurd aspects of a situation. In addition, you might try some simple approaches that can help boost your stress resistance and resilience, including the following:

- **Focusing.** Take a strain inventory of your body every day to determine where things aren't feeling quite right. Ask yourself, What's keeping me from feeling terrific today? Focusing on problem spots, such as stomach knots or neck tightness, increases your sense of control over stress.

- **Reconstructing stressful situations.** Think about a recent episode of distress; then write down three ways it could have gone better and three ways it could have gone worse. This should help you see that the situation wasn't as disastrous as it might have been and help you find ways to cope better in the future.

- **Self-improvement.** When your life feels out of control, turn to a new challenge. You might try volunteering at a nursing home, going for a long-distance bike trip, or learning a foreign language. As you work toward your new goal, you'll realize that you still can cope and achieve.

If stress continues to be a problem in your life, you may be able to find help through support groups or counseling. Your school may provide counseling services or referrals to mental health professionals; ask your health instructor or the campus health department for this information. Remember that each day of distress robs you of energy, distracts you from life's pleasures, and interferes with achieving your full potential.

SELFSURVEY | *Student Stress Scale*

The Student Stress Scale, an adaptation of Holmes and Rahe's Life Events Scale for college-age adults, provides a rough indication of stress levels and possible health consequences.

In the Student Stress Scale, each event, such as beginning or ending school, is given a score that represents the amount of readjustment a person has to make as a result of the change. In some studies, using similar scales, people with serious illnesses have been found to have high scores.

To determine your stress score, add up the number of points corresponding to the events you have experienced in the past 12 months.

1.	Death of a close family member	100
2.	Death of a close friend	73
3.	Divorce of parents	65
4.	Jail term	63
5.	Major personal injury or illness	63
6.	Marriage	58
7.	Getting fired from a job	50
8.	Failing an important course	47
9.	Change in the health of a family member	45
10.	Pregnancy	45
11.	Sex problems	44
12.	Serious argument with a close friend	40
13.	Change in financial status	39
14.	Change of academic major	39
15.	Trouble with parents	39
16.	New girlfriend or boyfriend	37
17.	Increase in workload at school	37
18.	Outstanding personal achievement	36
19.	First quarter/semester in college	36

20. Change in living conditions	31
21. Serious argument with an instructor	30
22. Getting lower grades than expected	29
23. Change in sleeping habits	29
24. Change in social activities	29
25. Change in eating habits	28
26. Chronic car trouble	26
27. Change in number of family get-togethers	26
28. Too many missed classes	25
29. Changing colleges	24
30. Dropping more than one class	23
31. Minor traffic violations	20

Total Stress Score _____

Here's how to interpret your score: If your score is 300 or higher, you're at high risk for developing a health problem. If your score is between 150 and 300, you have a 50-50 chance of experiencing a serious health change within two years. If your score is below 150, you have a 1 in 3 chance of a serious health change.

Source: Mullen, Kathleen, and Gerald Costello. *Health Awareness Through Discovery*. Minneapolis: Burgess Publishing Company, 1981.

Your Health Action Plan for Stress Management

- **Strive for balance.** Review your commitments and plans and, if necessary, scale down.
- **Get the facts.** When faced with a change or challenge, seek accurate information, which can bring vague fears down to earth.
- **Talk with someone you trust.** A friend or a health professional can offer valuable perspective as well as psychological support.
- **Exercise.** Even when your schedule gets jammed, carve out 20 or 30 minutes several times a week to walk, swim, bicycle, jog, or work out at the gym.
- **Help others.** One of the most effective ways of dealing with stress is to find people in a worse situation and do something positive for them.
- **Cultivate hobbies.** Pursuing a personal pleasure can distract you from the stressors in your life and help you relax.
- **Master a form of relaxation.** Whether you choose meditation, yoga, mindfulness, or another technique, practice it regularly.

CENGAGENOW™ If you want to write your own goals for stress management, go to the Wellness Journal at HealthNow:**academic.cengage.com/login**.

Making This Chapter Work for YOU

Review Questions

1. In this text we define stress as
   a. a negative emotional state related to fatigue and similar to depression.
   b. the physiological and psychological response to any event or situation that either upsets or excites us.
   c. the end result of the general adaptation syndrome.
   d. a motivational strategy for making life changes.

2. According to the general adaptation syndrome theory, how does the body typically respond to an acute stressor?
   a. The heart rate slows, blood pressure declines, and eye movement increases.
   b. The body enters a physical state called eustress and then moves into the physical state referred to as distress.
   c. If the stressor is viewed as a positive event, there are no physical changes.
   d. The body demonstrates three stages of change: alarm, resistance, and exhaustion.

3. Over time, increased levels of stress hormones have been shown to increase a person's risk for which of the following conditions?
   a. high blood pressure, memory loss, and skin disorders
   b. stress fractures, male pattern baldness, and hypothyroidism
   c. hemophilia, AIDS, and hay fever
   d. none of the above

4. Stress levels in college students
   a. may be high due to stressors such as academic pressures, financial concerns, learning disabilities, and relationship problems.
   b. are usually low because students feel empowered living independently of their parents.

c. are typically highest in seniors because their self-esteem diminishes during the college years.

d. are lower in minority students because they are used to stressors such as a hostile social climate and actual or perceived discrimination.

5. Which of the following illustrates the defense mechanism of displacement?
   a. You have a beer in the evening after a tough day.
   b. You act as if nothing has happened after you have been laid off from your job.
   c. You start an argument with your sister after being laid off from your job.
   d. You argue with your boss after he lays you off from your job.

6. Which of the following situations is representative of a societal stressor?
   a. Peter has been told that his transfer application has been denied because his transcripts were not sent in by the deadline.
   b. Nia's daughter is mugged on the way home from her after-school job.
   c. Kelli's boyfriend drives her car after he had been drinking and has an accident.
   d. Joshua, who is the leading basketball player on his college varsity team, has just been diagnosed with diabetes.

7. If you are stuck in a traffic jam, which of the following actions will help reduce your stress level?
   a. deep, slow breathing
   b. honking your horn
   c. berating yourself for not taking a different route
   d. getting on your cell phone and complaining to a friend

8. A relaxed peaceful state of being can be achieved with which of the following activities?
   a. an aerobic exercise class
   b. playing a computer game
   c. meditating for 15 minutes
   d. attending a rap concert

9. A person suffering from posttraumatic stress disorder may experience which of the following symptoms?
   a. procrastination
   b. constant thirst
   c. drowsiness
   d. terror-filled dreams

10. To develop an efficient studying style:
    a. Schedule your study time on a calendar or planner, have a friend go to class and take notes for you, and join the chess club.
    b. Schedule your study time on a calendar or planner, write notes or questions about the material in the margins of the book, and give yourself a small break after every study hour.
    c. Read assignments before class, call a friend before studying, and plan on working for four continuous hours.
    d. Read assignments before class, skip class when studying for an exam, and have snacks on hand.

Answers to these questions can be found on page 583.

Critical Thinking

1. What reasons can you think of to account for high stress levels among college students? Consider possible social, cultural, and economic factors that may play a role.

2. Identify three stressful situations in your life and determine whether they are examples of eustress or distress. Describe both the positive and negative aspects of each situation.

3. Can you think of any ways in which your behavior or attitudes might create stress for others? What changes could you make to avoid doing so?

4. What advice might you give an incoming freshman at your school about managing stress in college? What techniques have been most helpful for you in dealing with stress? Suppose that this student is from a different ethnic group than you. What additional suggestions would you have for this student?

Media Menu

CENGAGENOW™ Go to the HealthNow website at **academic.cengage .com/login** that will:
- Help you evaluate your knowledge of the material.
- Allow you to take an exam-prep quiz.
- Provide a Personalized Learning Plan targeting resources that address areas you should study.
- Coach you through identifying target goals for behavioral change and creating and monitoring your personal change plan throughout the semester.

INTERNET CONNECTIONS

Stress Management: A Review of Principles
http://cehs.unl.edu/stress/resources.html
This online series of lectures on stress management is presented by Wesley E. Sime, Ph.D., M.P.H., Professor of Health and Human Performance at the University of Nebraska–Lincoln. It features information on the psychobiology of stress and relaxation, as well as the pathophysiology of stress.

How to Survive Unbearable Stress

www.teachhealth.com

This comprehensive website is written specifically for college students by Steven Burns, M.D. It features the following topics: signs of how to recognize stress, two stress surveys for adults and college students, information on the pathophysiology of stress, the genetics of stress and stress tolerance, and information on how to best manage and treat stress.

Mind Tools

www.mindtools.com/smpage.html

This site covers a variety of topics on stress management, including recognizing stress, exercise, time management, coping mechanisms, and more. The site also features a free comprehensive personal self-assessment with questions pertaining to work and home stressors, physical and behavioral signs and symptoms, as well as personal coping skills and resources.

Key Terms

The terms listed are used and defined on the page indicated. Definitions are also found in the Glossary at the end of this book.

adaptive response	59
biofeedback	70
burnout	67
defense mechanisms	71
distress	59
eustress	59
general adaptation syndrome (GAS)	59
homeostasis	59
meditation	71
mindfulness	69
posttraumatic stress disorder (PTSD)	73
progressive relaxation	71
stress	59
stressor	59
visualization, or **guided imagery**	71

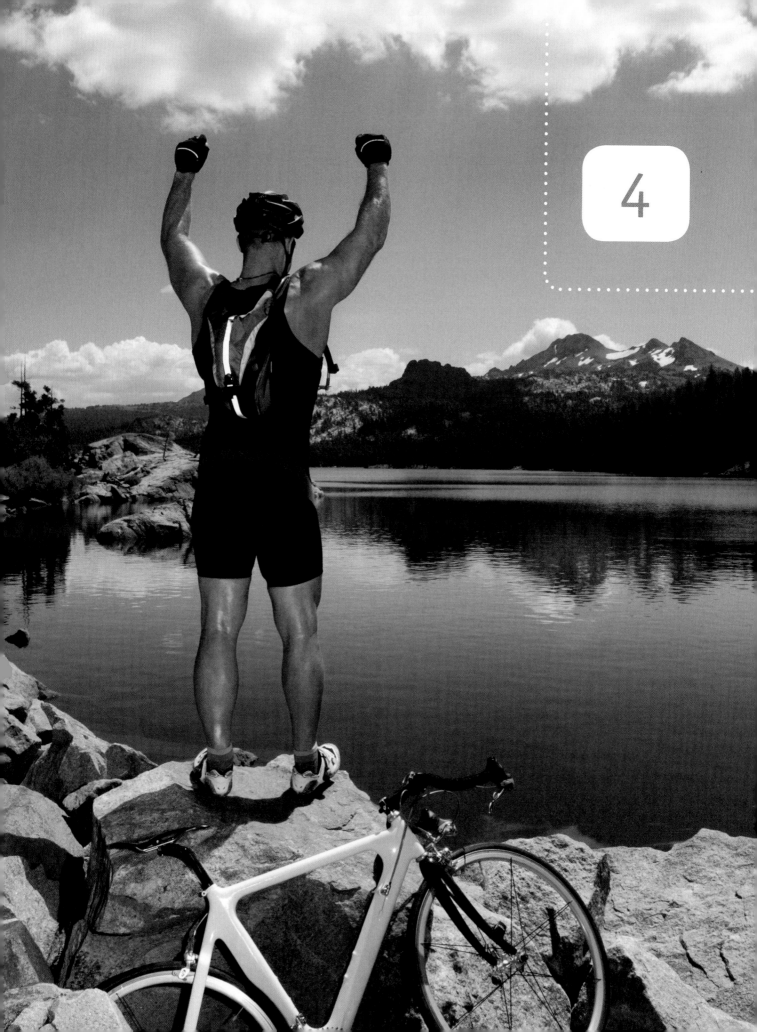

4

Your Mental Health

FOR years, Travis put on his "happy face" around his friends and family. Popular and athletic in high school, he never let anyone know how desperately unhappy he actually felt. "Whatever I was doing during the day, nothing was on my mind more than wanting to die," he recalls. On a perfectly ordinary day in his senior year, Travis tried to kill himself with an overdose of pills. Rushed to a hospital, Travis recovered, resumed his studies, and entered college. By the middle of his freshman year, he was struggling once more with feelings of hopelessness. This time he realized what was happening and sought help from a therapist. "I thought college was supposed to be the happiest time of your life," he said. "What went wrong?"

This is a question many young people might ask. Although youth can seem a golden time, when body and mind glow with potential, the process of becoming an adult is a challenging one in every culture and country. Psychological health can make the difference between facing this challenge with optimism and confidence or feeling overwhelmed by expectations and responsibilities.

This isn't always easy. At some point in life almost half of Americans develop an emotional disorder. Young adulthood—the years from the late teens to the mid-twenties—is a time when many serious disorders, including bipolar illness (manic depression) and schizophrenia, often develop. The saddest fact is not that so many feel so bad, but that so few realize they can feel better. Only a third of those with a mental disorder receive any treatment at all.[1] Yet 80 to 90 percent of those treated for psychological problems recover, most within a few months.

By learning about psychological disorders, you may be able to recognize early warning signals in yourself or your loved ones so you can deal with potential difficulties or seek professional help for more serious problems.

After studying the material in this chapter, you should be able to:

- **List** the key structures of the brain and **describe** the role of neurons in communication within the brain.

- **Explain** the differences between mental health and mental illness and **list** some effects of mental illness on physical health.

- **Name** the major mental illnesses and their characteristic symptoms.

- **Discuss** some of the factors that may lead to suicide, as well as strategies for prevention.

- **Describe** the treatment options available for those with psychological problems.

- **Name** the option you will consider if you have a mental health problem, and **describe** the reasons for your choice.

CENGAGENOW™ Log on to HealthNow at **academic.cengage.com/login** to find your Behavior Change Planner and to explore self-assessments, interactive tutorials, and practice quizzes.

The Brain: The Last Frontier

The brain has intrigued scientists for centuries, but only recently have its explorers made dramatic progress in unraveling its mysteries. Leaders in **neuropsychiatry**—the field that brings together the study of the brain and the mind—remind us that 95 percent of what is known about brain anatomy, chemistry, and physiology has been learned in the last 25 years. These discoveries have reshaped our understanding of the organ that is central to our identity and well-being and have fostered great hope for more effective therapies for the more than 1,000 disorders—psychiatric and neurologic—that affect the brain and nervous system.

Inside the Brain

The human brain, the most complex organ in the body, controls the central nervous system (CNS) and regulates virtually all our activities, including involuntary, or "lower," actions like heart rate, respiration, and digestion, and conscious, or "higher," mental activity like thought, reason, and abstraction. More than one hundred billion **neurons,** or nerve cells, within the brain are capable of electrical and chemical communication with tens of thousands of other nerve cells.

The neurons are the basic working units of the brain. Like snowflakes, no two are exactly the same. Each consists of a cell body containing the **nucleus;** a long fiber called the **axon,** which can range from less than an inch to several feet in length; an **axon terminal,** or ending; and multiple branching fibers called **dendrites** (Figure 4.2). The **glia** serve as the scaffolding for the brain, separate the brain from the bloodstream, assist in the growth of neurons, speed up the transmission of nerve impulses, and engulf and digest damaged neurons.

Until quite recently scientists believed no new neurons or synapses formed in the brain after birth. This theory

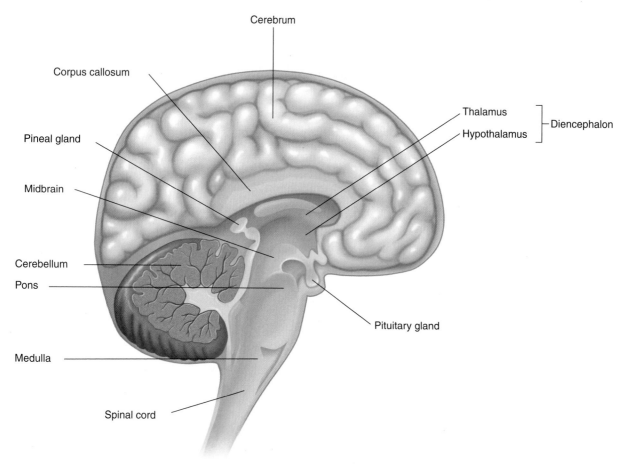

Figure 4.1 The Brain

The three major parts of the brain are the cerebrum, cerebellum, and brainstem (medulla). The cerebrum is divided into two hemispheres—the left, which regulates the right side of the body, and the right, which regulates the left side of the body. The cerebellum plays the major role in coordinating movement, balance, and posture. The brainstem contains centers that control breathing, blood pressure, heart rate, and other physiological functions.

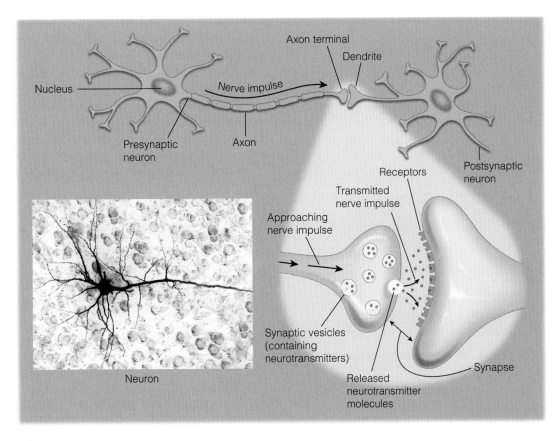

Figure 4.2 Brain Messaging: Anatomy of a Neuron

This figure shows how nerve impulses are transmitted from one neuron to another within the brain.

has been soundly disproved. The brain and spinal cord contain stem cells, which turn into thousands of new neurons a day. The process of creating new brain cells and synapses occurs most rapidly in childhood but continues throughout life, even into old age. Whenever you learn and change, you establish new neural networks.

Anatomically, the brain consists of three parts: the forebrain, midbrain, and hindbrain. The forebrain includes the several lobes of the cerebral cortex that control higher functions, while the mid- and hindbrain are more involved with unconscious, autonomic functions. The normal adult human brain typically weighs about three pounds.

Communication Within the Brain

Neurons "talk" with each other by means of electrical and chemical processes (see Figure 4.2). An electric charge, or impulse, travels along an axon to the terminal, where packets of chemicals called **neurotransmitters** are stored. When released, these messengers flow out of the axon terminal and cross a **synapse,** a specialized site at which the axon terminal of one neuron comes extremely close to a dendrite from another neuron. On

the surface of the dendrite are **receptors,** protein molecules designed to bind with neurotransmitters. It takes only about a ten-thousandth of a second for a neurotransmitter and a receptor to come together. Neurotransmitters that do not connect with receptors may remain in the synapse until they are reabsorbed by the

neuropsychiatry The study of the brain and mind.

neuron A nerve cell; the basic working unit of the brain, which transmits information from the senses to the brain and from the brain to specific body parts; each neuron consists of a cell body, an axon terminal, and dendrites.

neucleus The central part of a cell, contained in the cell body of a neuron.

axon The long fiber that conducts impulses from the neuron's nucleus to its dendrites.

axon terminal The ending of an axon, from which impulses are transmitted to a dendrite of another neuron.

dendrites Branching fibers of a neuron that receive impulses from axon

terminals of other neurons and conduct these impulses toward the nucleus.

glia Support cells for neurons in the brain and spinal cord that separate the brain from the bloodstream, assist in the growth of neurons, speed transmission of nerve impulses, and eliminate damaged neurons.

neurotransmitters Chemicals released by neurons that stimulate or inhibit the action of other neurons.

synapse A specialized site at which electrical impulses are transmitted from the axon terminal of one neuron to a dendrite of another.

receptors Molecules on the surface of neurons on which neurotransmitters bind after their release from other neurons.

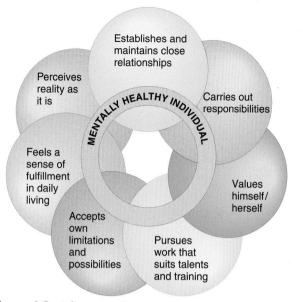

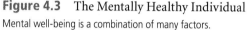

Figure 4.3 The Mentally Healthy Individual

Mental well-being is a combination of many factors.

cell that produced them—a process called **reuptake**—or broken down by enzymes.

A malfunction in the release of a neurotransmitter, in its reuptake or elimination, or in the receptors or secondary messengers may result in abnormalities in thinking, feeling, or behavior. Some of the most promising and exciting research in neuropsychiatry is focusing on correcting such malfunctions. The neurotransmitter serotonin and its receptors have been shown to affect mood, sleep, behavior, appetite, memory, learning, sexuality, and aggression and to play a role in several mental disorders. The discovery of a possible link between low levels of serotonin and some cases of major depression has led to the development of more precisely targeted **antidepressant** medications that boost serotonin to normal levels. (See "Psychiatric Drugs" later in the chapter.)

Sex Differences in the Brain

 From birth, male and female brains differ in a variety of ways. Overall, a woman's brain, like her body, is 10 to 15 percent smaller than a man's, yet the regions dedicated to higher cognitive functions such as language are more densely packed with neurons—and women use more of them. When a male puts his mind to work, neurons turn on in highly specific areas. When females set their minds on similar tasks, cells light up all over the brain.

Male and female brains perceive light and sound differently. A man's eyes are more sensitive to bright light and retain their ability to see well at long distances longer in life. A woman hears a much broader range of sounds, and her hearing remains sharper longer.

The female brain responds more intensely to emotion. According to neuroimaging studies, the genders respond differently to emotions, especially sadness, which activates, or turns on, neurons in an area eight times larger in women than men.

Neither gender's brain is "better." Intelligence per se appears equal in both. The greatest gender differences appear both at the top and bottom of the intelligence scales. Nevertheless, more than half the time, regardless of the type of test, most women and men perform more or less equally—even though they may well take different routes to arrive at the same answers. Cognitive skills show greater variability both among women and among men than between the genders. The best evaluation may have come from essayist Samuel Johnson. When asked whether women or men are more intelligent, he responded, "Which man? Which woman?"

Understanding Mental Health

Mentally healthy individuals value themselves, perceive reality as it is, accept their limitations and possibilities, carry out their responsibilities, establish and maintain close relationships, pursue work that suits their talent and training, and feel a sense of fulfillment that makes the efforts of daily living worthwhile (Figure 4.3).

According to a national report by the Centers for Disease Control (CDC), American adults spend an average of three days a month feeling "sad, blue, or depressed." Individuals who spend more time down in the dumps are more likely to report unhealthy behaviors such as cigarette smoking and physical inactivity.

 College-age young adults (18 to 24 years old) report the most days with depressive symptoms. Women had more gloomy days than men (3.5 compared to 2.4). College graduates and those earning more than $50,000 reported half as many sad, bad days as those without a high school diploma or earning less than $15,000. Regular exercisers had 1.3 fewer days with symptoms of depression than those who did not work out regularly. Those who smoked a pack or more of cigarettes a day had more down days than those who never smoked.[2] (See "Your Psychological Self-Care Pyramid" lab in *IPC*.) **IPC**

What Is a Mental Disorder?

While lay people may speak of "nervous breakdowns" or "insanity," these are not scientific terms. The U.S. government's official definition states that a serious mental illness is "a diagnosable mental, behavioral, or emotional disorder that interferes with one or more major activities in life, like dressing, eating, or working."

The mental health profession's standard for diagnosing a mental disorder is the pattern of symptoms, or diagnostic criteria, spelled out for the almost 300 disorders in the

American Psychiatric Association's Diagnostic and Statistical Manual, 4th edition (DSM-IV). Psychiatrists define a **mental disorder** as a clinically significant behavioral or psychological syndrome or pattern that is associated with present distress (a painful symptom) or disability (impairment in one or more important areas of functioning) or with a significantly increased risk of suffering death, pain, disability, or an important loss of freedom.[3]

Who Develops Mental Disorders?

In the course of their lifetime, almost half of all Americans experience a diagnosable psychological problem. The most common mental disorders are substance abuse (discussed in Chapters 11 and 12), mood disorders such as depression and bipolar disorder, and anxiety disorders such as phobias and panic disorder.[4] (See Table 4.1.)

In a recent community survey, almost 30 percent of individuals needed mental health services, but less than a third received adequate treatment.[5] In the past, many people did not seek help for mental disorders because of widespread stigma about these disorders. Attitudes toward mental health treatment have changed over the last decade, particularly among younger adults. However, the majority of Americans surveyed in a recent poll did not feel very comfortable talking with a professional about personal problems and said they would feel embarrassed if others found out about it.[6] Stigma is even greater for seeking help for a child with a mental disorder such as depression.[7]

Unlike most disabling physical diseases, mental illness starts early in life. Half of all lifetime cases begin by age 14; three-quarters by age 24. Adverse childhood experiences, such as abuse, increase the risk.[8]

Anxiety disorders often begin in late childhood, mood disorders in late adolescence, and substance abuse in the early twenties. Researchers describe such problems as "the chronic diseases of the young," striking when men and women are in their prime. The prevalence of mental disorders increases from early adulthood (ages 18 to 29) to the next-oldest age group (ages 30 to 44) and then declines. Women have higher rates of depressive and anxiety disorders; men have higher rates of substance abuse and impulse disorders.[9]

About 80 percent of those with mental disorders eventually seek treatment, but many suffer for years, even decades. The median delay for all disorders is nearly 10 years. Those with social phobia and separation anxiety disorders may not get help for more than 20 years. The earlier in life that a disorder begins, the longer that individuals tend to delay treatment.

Without treatment, mental disorders take a toll on every aspect of life, including academics, relationships, careers, and risk-taking. Symptoms or episodes of a disorder typically become more frequent or severe. Individuals with one mental disorder are at high risk of having a second one (this is called comorbidity).

About 6 percent of Americans have a "severe" mental disorder, one that significantly limits their ability to work or carry out daily activities or that has led to a suicide attempt or psychosis (a gross impairment of a person's perception of reality). On average, they are unable to function for nearly three months of the year.

Mental Health on Campus

The emotional difficulties of college students have become more complex and more severe than in the past. In one national survey, more than 80 percent of directors of counseling centers reported an increase in the number of students with serious psychological disorders. However, studies that tested students seeking help at counseling centers show that they are not more disturbed and do not have more or more serious psychiatric problems than in the past.[10] (Eating disorders, which are common among college students, are discussed in Chapter 7.)

About one in eight undergraduates seeks counseling during college. In the past students were most likely to have trouble with dating and other relationships. More recently stress and anxiety have become more common reasons for seeking help.

Many college students experience a broad range of psychological symptoms and disorders. The most common are adjustment disorders (the abnormal persistence of otherwise normal emotional or behavioral symptoms) and various forms of **depression,** which are discussed later in this chapter. According to the most recent findings from the American College Health Association National College Health Assessment, more than a third of students

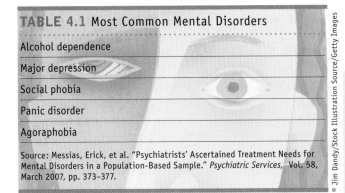

TABLE 4.1 Most Common Mental Disorders

Alcohol dependence
Major depression
Social phobia
Panic disorder
Agoraphobia

Source: Messias, Erick, et al. "Psychiatrists' Ascertained Treatment Needs for Mental Disorders in a Population-Based Sample." *Psychiatric Services,* Vol. 58, March 2007, pp. 373–377.

© Jim Dandy/Stock Illustration Source/Getty Images

reuptake Reabsorption by the originating cell of neurotransmitters that have not connected with receptors and have been left in synapses.

antidepressant A drug used primarily to treat symptoms of depression.

mental disorder Behavioral or psychological syndrome associated with distress or disability or with a significantly increased risk of suffering death, pain, disability, or loss of freedom.

depression In general, feelings of unhappiness and despair; as a mental illness, also characterized by an inability to function normally.

POINT COUNTERPOINT *Behavior Police?*

POINT

Concerned about identifying and treating students who might pose a danger to themselves or others, some campuses have set up websites or phone lines students can use to report their concerns about a classmate who seems troubled. Teachers and counselors are being urged to look for signs of mental disorders such as depression as well as signs of aggression and violence.

COUNTERPOINT

Programs that encourage observation and reporting of odd behaviors could violate a student's privacy. They also might lead to discrimination, overt or subtle, against individuals who do not conform to certain standards of acceptable behavior. Until and unless a

student threatens harm to himself or others, campuses should encourage a live-and-let-live tolerance of others.

YOUR VIEW

Should colleges do more to identify potentially troubled students? Or should individual privacy and confidentiality be the top priority? How would you respond if a classmate or friend shows signs of a serious mental disorder? How do you think campus authorities should respond?

felt hopeless at least once or twice during the academic year; a higher percentage reported episodes of sadness.[11]

Researchers at the University of Michigan have identified three key contributors to depression in college students: stress, substance abuse, and sleep loss. As they adjust to campus life, undergraduates face the ongoing stress of forging a new identity and finding a place for themselves in various social hierarchies. This triggers the release of the so-called stress hormones (discussed in Chapter 3), which can change brain activity. Drugs and alcohol, widely used on campus, also affect the brain in ways that make stress even harder to manage. Too little sleep adds another ingredient to this dangerous brew. Computers, the Internet, around-the-clock television, and the college tradition of pulling all-nighters can conspire to sabotage rest and increase vulnerability to depression. Among the most vulnerable students are those being treated for mental disorders.

 The few studies that have looked into ethnic differences in psychological health have yielded conflicting or inconclusive results: Some found no differences; others suggested higher rates of depression among Korean and South Asian students.

Some colleges offer seminars, movies, and 24-hour hot lines that students can call to talk about everything from stress to substance abuse. At the University of California, Berkeley, for example, green stickers showing a figure with hunched shoulders being comforted by a confidant mark the doors of faculty, staff, and students trained to deal with psychological problems. (See Point-Counterpoint: "Behavior Police?") A few schools have redesigned dormitories to decrease isolation and foster more interaction.

The Mind-Body Connection

According to a growing number of studies, mental attitude may be just as important a risk factor for certain diseases as age, race, gender, education, habits, and

health history.[12] Positive states like happiness and optimism have been linked with longer lifespans as well as lower risk of cardiovascular and lung disease, stroke, diabetes, colds, and upper respiratory infections. Mental disorders, on the other hand, can undermine physical well-being. Anxiety can lead to intensified asthmatic reactions, skin conditions, and digestive disorders. Stress can play a role in hypertension, heart attacks, sudden cardiac death, and immune disorders in the young as well as in older individuals.

Depression has increasingly been recognized as a serious risk factor for physical illness. According to large-scale studies on depression, depressed individuals are up to four times more likely to develop heart problems. In still unknown ways, depression may increase risk factors for heart disease, such as high blood pressure, and for premature death. Together, depression and heart disease worsen a patient's prognosis more than either condition alone.

 Major depression is associated with lower bone density in young men, but not in women. A history of depression increases the risk of physical problems such as headache and shoulder and neck pain in women as they reach middle age.

The Mind-Exercise Connection

Imagine a drug so powerful it can alter brain chemistry, so versatile it can help prevent or treat many common mental disorders, so safe that moderate doses cause few, if any, side effects, and so inexpensive that anyone can afford it. This wonder drug, proved in years of research, is exercise.

In addition to its head-to-toe physical benefits, discussed in Chapter 5, exercise may be, as one therapist puts it, the single most effective way to lift a person's spirits and to restore feelings of potency about all aspects of life. People who exercise regularly report a more cheerful mood, higher self-esteem, and less stress. Their sleep and appetite also tend to improve. In clinical studies, exercise has proved effective as a treatment for depression and anxiety disorders.[13] But remember: Although exercise can help prevent and ease problems for many people, it's no substitute for professional treatment of serious psychiatric disorders.

Depressive Disorders

 Depression, the world's most common mental ailment, affects the brain, the mind, and the body in complex ways. An estimated 8–17 percent of adults experience depression at some point in their lives.[14] The relationship between depression and race is complex. Rates of depression are higher among whites than African American and Caribbean blacks. However, depression is more likely to be unrecognized, untreated, severe, and disabling among blacks. On average 57 percent of all adults with depression get treatment, compared to 45 percent of those who are African American and 24 percent of those who are Caribbean blacks.[15] After a single episode, the risk of a recurrence, or second episode, is about 50 percent. After a third, the risk of a fourth is about 90 percent. Stress-related events may trigger half of all depressive episodes; great trauma in childhood can increase vulnerability to depression later in life.

In a study of young adults ages 18 to 23, those who'd experienced the most adversity were at greatest risk of depression or an anxiety disorder.[16] An estimated 15 to 40 percent of college-age men and women (18- to 24-year-olds) may develop depression. (See Self-Survey "Recognizing Depression" in this chapter.)

Depression in the Young

Once young people were considered immune to sadness. Now mental health professionals know better. An estimated 5 to 10 percent of American teenagers suffer from a serious depressive disorder; girls are twice as susceptible as boys. Prior to puberty, girls and boys are equally likely to develop depression.

 According to a survey of more than 2,000 young women ages 16 to 23, white girls become less depressed as they age while black girls continue feeling the same. The reason may be that white girls tend to be unhappy with their bodies in their teens and may develop symptoms of depression as a result. Over time they become more satisfied with their shapes and sizes and less depressed. African American girls tend to accept their bodies from early adolescence into adulthood.[17]

The risks of depression in the young are high. Four in ten depressed adolescents think about killing themselves; two in ten actually try to do so. Every year an estimated 11 to 13 in every 100,000 teens take their own lives, twice as many as the number who die from all natural causes combined.

"Depression is the most common emotional problem in adolescence and the single greatest risk factor for teen suicide," says child psychiatrist Peter Jensen, M.D., director for the Center for the Advancement of Children's Mental Health at Columbia University, who notes that depression rates have been rising over the last half century.[18]

No one knows the reason for this steady surge in sadness, but experts point to the breakdown of families, the pressures of the information age, and increased isolation. A family history of depression greatly increases a young person's vulnerability. A mother's anxiety and depression during early childhood can increase the risk that adolescents will develop symptoms of anxiety and depression.

However, the strongest predictor of depression is cigarette smoking. Depressed teens may smoke because they think smoking will make them feel better, but nicotine alters brain chemistry and actually worsens symptoms of depression.

The link between tobacco and depression continues during college. Students diagnosed with or treated for depression are 7.5 times as likely as other students to use tobacco, possibly because of nicotine's stimulating effects.[19] Young women with symptoms of depression and those who do not feel connected with a peer group are more likely to smoke. Individuals with other mental illnesses also are more likely to smoke.

Depression can be hard to recognize in the young, who may not look or act sad. Rather than crying, they may snap grouchily at parents or burst into angry tirades. Some turn to alcohol or drugs in hopes of feeling better; others become depressed after they start abusing these substances. As they drop out of activities and pull away from friends, depressed teens spend more time alone. Their schoolwork suffers, and many are labeled as underachievers. Those whose anger explodes in public are branded as troublemakers.

Only in the last decade have researchers in mental health specifically studied treatments for teen depression. They now know that 60 to 75 percent of teenagers—the same percentage as adults—respond to treatment with the medications called SSRIs (a group of antidepressants that includes Prozac and Paxil). The use of these antidepressants in children and teenagers has increased three- to fivefold in recent years, but there is controversy over a potential increase in the risk of suicide. (See Savvy Consumer: "Weighing the Risks and Benefits of Antidepressants.")

According to a landmark study of therapies for depression in adolescents, the most effective treatment is a combination of antidepressant medication and cognitive-behavioral therapy (CBT), which teaches problem-solving skills and ways to change negative thinking (discussed later in this chapter).

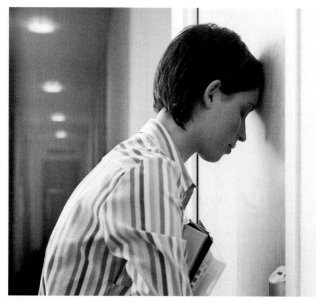

Factors that can contribute to the development of depression in college include stressful events, poor academic performance, loneliness, and relationship problems.

Gender and Depression

Female Depression

Depression is twice as common in women as men, a gender gap found through most of the world. Some have argued that women are simply more willing than men to admit to being depressed or more likely to seek help. But even when these factors are accounted for, the sex difference persists. Others contend that men in distress drown their problems in alcohol rather than becoming sad, tearful, and hopeless. In studies of the Amish, who prohibit alcohol use, and of Jewish Americans, who also drink less than other groups, women and men are equally likely to develop depression. Yet these data do not mean that fewer women among teetotalers become depressed but that more men do.

Genes may make both men and women more vulnerable to depression. Brain chemistry and sex hormones also may play a role. Women produce less of certain metabolites of serotonin, a messenger chemical that helps regulate mood. Their brains also register sadness much more intensely than men's, and they are more sensitive to changes in light and temperature. Women are at least four times more likely than men to develop seasonal affective disorder (SAD) and to become depressed in the dark winter months.

Some women also seem more sensitive to their own hormones or to the changes in them that occur at puberty, during the menstrual cycle, after childbirth, or during perimenopause and menopause. Pregnancy, contrary to what many people assume, does not "protect" a woman from depression, and women who discontinue treatment when they become pregnant are at risk of a relapse. Women and their psychiatrists must carefully weigh the risks and benefits of psychiatric medications during pregnancy.[20]

Childhood abuse also contributes to female vulnerability. In epidemiological studies, 60 percent of women diagnosed with depression—compared with 39 percent of men—were abused as children. In adulthood, relationships may protect women from depression, while a lack of social support increases vulnerability to depression.[21] Women with at least one "confiding relationship," as researchers put it, are physically and psychologically more resilient.

Male Depression

More than six million men in the United States—1 in every 14—suffer from this insidious disorder, many without recognizing what's wrong. Experts describe male depression as an "under" disease: underdiscussed, underrecognized, underdiagnosed, and undertreated.

Depression "looks" different in men than women. Rather than becoming sad, men may be irritable or tremendously fatigued. They feel a sense of being dead inside, of worthlessness, hopelessness, helplessness, of losing their life force. Physical symptoms, such as headaches, pain, and insomnia, are common, as are attempts to "self-medicate" with alcohol or drugs.

Genes may make some men more vulnerable, but chronic stress of any sort plays a major role in male depression, possibly by raising levels of the stress hormone cortisol, and lowering testosterone. Men also are more likely than women to become depressed following divorce, job loss, or a career setback. Whatever its roots, depression alters brain chemistry in potentially deadly ways. Four times as many men as women kill themselves; depressed men are two to four times more likely to take their own lives than depressed women.

Minor Depression

Minor depression is a common disorder that is often unrecognized and untreated, affecting about 7.5 percent of Americans during their lifetime. Its symptoms are the same as those of major depression, but less severe and fewer in number. They include either a depressed mood most of the day, nearly every day, or diminished interest or pleasure in daily activities.

Psychotherapy is remarkably effective for mild depression. In more serious cases, antidepressant medication can lead to dramatic improvement in 40 to 80 percent of depressed patients. Exercise also works—several studies have shown that exercise effectively lifts mild to moderate depression.

Dysthymic Disorder

Dysthymia is a depressive disorder characterized by a chronically depressed mood. Symptoms include feelings of inadequacy, hopelessness, and guilt; low self-esteem;

low energy; fatigue; indecisiveness; and an inability to enjoy pleasurable activities.

Major Depression

The simplest definition of **major depression** is sadness that does not end. The incidence of major depression has soared over the last two decades, especially among young adults. Major depression can destroy a person's joy for living. Food, friends, sex, or any form of pleasure no longer appeals. It is impossible to concentrate on work and responsibilities. Unable to escape a sense of utter hopelessness, depressed individuals may fight back tears throughout the day and toss and turn through long, empty nights. Thoughts of death or suicide may push into their minds.

The characteristic symptoms of major depression include:

- **Feeling depressed,** sad, empty, discouraged, tearful.
- **Loss of interest** or pleasure in once-enjoyable activities.
- **Eating more or less** than usual and either gaining or losing weight.
- **Having trouble sleeping** or sleeping much more than usual.
- **Feeling slowed down** or restless and unable to sit still.
- **Lack of energy.**
- **Feeling helpless,** hopeless, worthless, inadequate.
- **Difficulty concentrating,** forgetfulness.
- **Difficulty thinking clearly** or making decisions.
- **Persistent thoughts of death** or suicide.
- **Withdrawal from others,** lack of interest in sex.
- **Physical symptoms** (headaches, digestive problems, aches and pains).

As many as half of major depressive episodes are not recognized because the symptoms are "masked." Rather than feeling sad or depressed, individuals may experience low energy, insomnia, difficulty concentrating, and physical symptoms. An episode of major depression can trigger a relapse in individuals with substance abuse problems.

Treating Depression

Treatment with psychotherapy, medication, or both relieves depression for 80 percent of sufferers—yet only half of those with depression seek help and only 10 to 15 percent get optimal care.

Psychotherapy helps individuals pinpoint the life problems that contribute to their depression, identify negative or distorted thinking patterns, explore behaviors that contribute to depression, and regain a sense of control and pleasure in life. Two specific psychotherapies—cognitive-behavioral therapy and interpersonal therapy (described later in this chapter)—have proved as helpful as antidepressant drugs, although they take longer than medication to achieve results.

Antidepressants help about 70 percent of individuals feel better within six to ten weeks. According to long-term studies, treatment should continue for at least nine months after a single acute episode of depression, longer for chronic or recurrent depression.

The FDA has ordered warning labels on antidepressants stating that they increase the risk of suicidal thinking and behavior in young adults ages 18 to 24 during initial treatment. Young people treated with antidepressants are less likely to take their own lives than depressed individuals who are not taking medications, but they are at increased risk of nonfatal suicide attempts.[22] The risk of a suicide attempt is highest in those under age 20.[23] However, recent large-scale studies have shown that treatment of depression, either with medication or psychotherapy, reduces the risk of suicide in all age groups.[24] Some fear that the new labels will discourage individuals from taking antidepressants, even though the risk of suicide is much greater in individuals with untreated depression.[25] (See Savvy Consumer: "Weighing the Risks and Benefits of Antidepressants.")

When either medication or psychotherapy fails to lift depression, switching from one to the other or adding a second antidepressant can be highly effective.[26] Medications have proved effective for patients who did not recover with psychotherapy alone, and psychotherapy can help those who do not benefit from medication alone.

Exercise also has proved beneficial in both the short- and long-term for both men and women. Although walking and jogging have been studied most extensively, all forms of exercise decrease depression to some degree. The greater the length of the exercise program and the larger the total number of sessions, the greater the decrease in depression.

For individuals who cannot take antidepressant medications because of medical problems, or who do not improve with psychotherapy or drugs, *electroconvulsive therapy* (ECT)—the administration of a controlled electrical current through electrodes attached to the scalp—remains the safest and most effective treatment. About 70 to 90 percent of depressed individuals improve after ECT.[27] Experimental new techniques are using electrical and magnetic stimulation to treat depression.

Even without treatment, depression generally lifts after six to nine months. However, in more than 80 percent of people, it recurs, with each episode lasting longer

dysthymia Frequent, prolonged mild depression.

major depression Sadness that does not end; ongoing feelings of utter helplessness.

YOUR STRATEGIES FOR PREVENTION *Helping Someone Who Is Depressed*

- **Express your concern,** but don't nag. You might say: "I'm concerned about you. You are struggling right now. We need to find some help."
- **Don't be distracted** by behaviors like drinking or gambling, which can disguise depression in men.

- **Encourage the individual to remain in treatment** until symptoms begin to lift (which takes several weeks).
- **Provide emotional support.** Listen carefully. Offer hope and reassurance that with time and treatment, things will get better.

- **Do not ignore remarks about suicide.** Report them to his or her doctor or, in an emergency, call 911.

---

and becoming more severe and difficult to treat. "All the while the depression goes untreated, it is causing ongoing damage that shrivels important regions of the brain" says John Greden, M.D., director of the University of Michigan Depression Center. "The exciting news is that, as brain scans show, treatment turns the destructive process around and stops depression in its tracks."[28]

Bipolar Disorder (Manic Depression)

Bipolar disorder, or manic depression, consists of mood swings that may take individuals from manic states of feeling euphoric and energetic to depressive states of utter despair. In episodes of full mania, they may become so impulsive and out of touch with reality that they endanger their careers, relationships, health, or even survival.[29] One percent of the population—about 2 million American adults—suffer from this serious but treatable disorder. Men tend to develop bipolar disorder earlier in life (between ages 16 to 25), but women have higher rates overall. About 50 percent of patients with bipolar illness have a family history of the disorder.

The characteristic symptoms of bipolar disorder include:

- **Mood swings** (from happy to miserable, optimistic to despairing, and so on).
- **Changes in thinking** (thoughts speeding through one's mind, unrealistic self-confidence, difficulty concentrating, delusions, hallucinations).
- **Changes in behavior** (sudden immersion in plans and projects, talking very rapidly and much more than usual, excessive spending, impaired judgment, impulsive sexual involvement).
- **Changes in physical condition** (less need for sleep, increased energy, fewer health complaints than usual).

During "manic" periods, individuals may make grandiose plans or take dangerous risks. But they often plunge from this highest of highs to a horrible, low depressive episode, in which they may feel sad, hopeless, and helpless and develop other symptoms of major depression. The risk of suicide is very real.

▼Savvy Consumer Weighing the Risks and Benefits of Antidepressants

Millions of individuals have benefited from the category of antidepressant drugs called selective serotonin reuptake inhibitors (SSRIs). However, like all drugs, they can cause side effects that range from temporary physical symptoms, such as stomach upset and headaches, to more persistent problems, such as sexual dysfunction. The most serious—and controversial—risk is suicide. In every case, physicians have to weigh the potential benefits against the possible risks.

- The FDA has issued a "black box" warning about the risk of suicidal thoughts, hostility, and aggression in both children and young adults. The danger is greatest just after pill use begins.

- This risk of suicide while taking an antidepressant is about 1 in 3,000; the risk of a serious attempt is 1 in 1,000.

- Untreated depression can be fatal: The lifetime suicide rate for people with major depression is 15 percent. Depression also increases the risk of heart disease and other serious illnesses.

- While the use of SSRIs in adolescents soared in the 1990s, the suicide rate declined. With the recent warnings, antidepressant use has decreased and the youth suicide rate may be on the rise.

- Recent reviews of antidepressant use have found that the risk of suicide for both children and adults was *higher* in the month *before* starting treatment, dropped sharply in the month after it began, and tapered off in the following months.

Professional therapy is essential in treating bipolar disorders. Mood-stabilizing medications are the keystone of treatment, although psychotherapy plays a critical role in helping individuals understand their illness and rebuild their lives. Most individuals continue taking medication indefinitely after remission of their symptoms because the risk of recurrence is high.

Anxiety Disorders

Anxiety disorders are as common as depression but are often undetected and untreated.[30] They may involve inordinate fears of certain objects or situations (**phobias**), episodes of sudden, inexplicable terror (**panic attacks**), chronic distress (**generalized anxiety disorder, or GAD**), or persistent, disturbing thoughts and behaviors (**obsessive-compulsive disorder, or OCD**). These disorders can increase the risk of developing depression. Over a lifetime, as many as one in four Americans may experience an anxiety disorder. More than 40 percent are never correctly diagnosed and treated.[31] Yet most individuals who do get treatment, even for severe and disabling problems, improve dramatically.

Phobias

Phobias—the most prevalent type of anxiety disorder—are out-of-the-ordinary, irrational, intense, persistent fears of certain objects or situations. About two million Americans develop such acute terror that they go to extremes to avoid whatever it is that they fear, even though they realize that these feelings are excessive or unreasonable. The most common phobias involve animals, particularly dogs, snakes, insects, and mice; the sight of blood; closed spaces (*claustrophobia*); heights (*acrophobia*); air travel and being in open or public places or situations from which one perceives it would be difficult or embarrassing to escape (*agoraphobia*).

Although various medications have been tried, none is effective by itself in relieving phobias. The best approach is behavioral therapy, which consists of gradual, systematic exposure to the feared object (a process called *systematic desensitization*). Numerous studies have proved that exposure—especially in vivo exposure, in which individuals are exposed to the actual source of their fear rather than simply imagining it—is highly effective. Medical hypnosis—the use of induction of an altered state of consciousness—also can help.

Panic Attacks and Panic Disorder

Individuals who have had panic attacks describe them as the most frightening experiences of their lives. Without reason or warning, their hearts race wildly. They may become light-headed or dizzy. Because they can't catch their breath, they may start breathing rapidly and hyperventilate. Parts of their bodies, such as their fingers or toes, may tingle or feel numb. Worst of all is the terrible sense that something horrible is about to happen: that they will die, lose their minds, or have a heart attack. Most attacks reach peak intensity within ten minutes. Afterward, individuals live in dread of another one. In the course of a lifetime, your risk of having a single panic attack is 7.2 percent.

Panic disorder develops when attacks recur or apprehension about them becomes so intense that individuals cannot function normally. Full-blown panic disorder occurs in about 1.6 percent of all adults in the course of a lifetime and usually develops before age 30. Women are more than twice as likely as men to experience panic attacks, although no one knows why. Parents, siblings, and

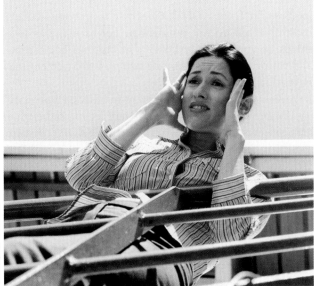

© Stockbyte/Photolibrary

Systematic desensitization is one behavioral approach to treating a fear of heights and other phobias.

bipolar disorder Severe depression alternating with periods of manic activity and elation.

anxiety disorders A group of psychological disorders involving episodes of apprehension, tension, or uneasiness, stemming from the anticipation of danger and sometimes accompanied by physical symptoms, which cause significant distress and impairment to an individual.

phobia An anxiety disorder marked by an inordinate fear of an object, a class of objects, or a situation, resulting in extreme avoidance behaviors.

panic attack A short episode characterized by physical sensations of light-headedness, dizziness, hyperventilation, and numbness of extremities, accompanied by an inexplicable terror, usually of a physical disaster such as death.

generalized anxiety disorder (GAD) An anxiety disorder characterized as chronic distress.

obsessive-compulsive disorder (OCD) An anxiety disorder characterized by obsessions and/or compulsions that impair one's ability to function and form relationships.

panic disorder An anxiety disorder in which the apprehension or experience of recurring panic attacks is so intense that normal functioning is impaired.

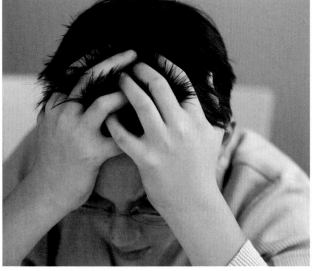

Worry is a normal part of daily life, but individuals with generalized anxiety disorder worry constantly about everything and anything that might go wrong.

children of individuals with panic disorders also are more likely to develop them than are others.

The two primary treatments for panic disorder are (1) cognitive-behavioral therapy (CBT), which teaches specific strategies for coping with symptoms like rapid breathing, and (2) medication. Treatment helps as many as 90 percent of those with panic disorder either improve significantly or recover completely, usually within six to eight weeks.[32] Individuals with a greater internal locus of control (discussed in Chapter 1) may respond better to CBT.[33]

Generalized Anxiety Disorder

About 10 million adults in the United States suffer from a generalized anxiety disorder (GAD), excessive or unrealistic apprehension that causes physical symptoms and lasts for six months or longer. It usually starts when people are in their twenties. Unlike fear, which helps us recognize and avoid real danger, GAD is an irrational or unwarranted response to harmless objects or situations of exaggerated danger. The most common symptoms are faster heart rate, sweating, increased blood pressure, muscle aches, intestinal pains, irritability, sleep problems, and difficulty concentrating.

Chronically anxious individuals worry—not just some of the time, and not just about the stresses and strains of ordinary life—but constantly, about almost everything: their health, families, finances, marriages, potential dangers. Treatment for GAD may consist of a combination of psychotherapy, behavioral therapy, and antianxiety drugs.

Obsessive-Compulsive Disorder

As many as 1 in 40 Americans has a type of anxiety called obsessive-compulsive disorder (OCD). Some of these individuals suffer only from an *obsession,* a recurring idea, thought, or image that they realize, at least initially, is senseless. The most common obsessions are repetitive thoughts of violence (for example, killing a child), contamination (becoming infected by shaking hands), and doubt (wondering whether one has performed some act, such as having hurt someone in a traffic accident). Most people with OCD also suffer from a *compulsion,* a repetitive behavior performed according to certain rules or in a stereotyped fashion. The most common compulsions involve handwashing, cleaning, hoarding useless items, counting, or checking (for example, making sure dozens of times that a door is locked). Individuals with OCD realize that their thoughts or behaviors are bizarre, but they cannot resist or control them. Eventually, the obsessions or compulsions consume a great deal of time and significantly interfere with normal routines, job functioning, or usual social activities or relationships with others. A young woman who must follow a very rigid dressing routine may always be late for class, for example; a student who must count each letter of the alphabet as he types may not be able to complete a term paper.

Treatment may consist of cognitive therapy to correct irrational assumptions, behavioral techniques such as progressively limiting the amount of time someone obsessed with cleanliness can spend washing and scrubbing, and medication. About 70 to 80 percent of those with OCD improve with treatment.

Attention Disorders

Attention-deficit/hyperactivity disorder (ADHD) is the most common mental disorder in childhood. About 10 percent of boys and 5 percent of girls between ages 5 to 18 suffer from ADHD. Contrary to previous beliefs, most children do not outgrow it. For as many as two-thirds of youngsters, ADHD persists into adolescence and young adulthood. Among adults, 4 to 5 percent may have ADHD.

ADHD looks and feels different in adults. Hyperactivity is more subtle, an internal fidgety feeling rather than a physical restlessness. As youngsters with ADHD mature, academic difficulties become much more of a problem. Students with ADHD may find it hard to concentrate, read, make decisions, complete complex projects, and meet deadlines. The academic performance and standardized test scores of college students with ADHD are significantly lower than those of their peers.[34]

Relationships with peers also can become more challenging. Young people with ADHD may become frustrated easily, have a short fuse, and erupt into angry outbursts. Some become more argumentative, negative, and defiant than most other teens. Sleep problems, including sleeping much more or less than normal, are common. The likelihood of developing other emotional problems, including depression and anxiety disorders, is higher. As many as 20 percent of those diagnosed with depression, anxiety, or substance abuse also have ADHD.

The risk of substance use disorders for individuals with ADHD is twice that of the general population. According to several reports, between 15 and 25 percent of adults with substance use disorders have ADHD. In addition, individuals with ADHD start smoking at a younger age and have higher rates of smoking and drinking. (The use of stimulant medication to treat ADHD does not increase the risk of substance abuse.)

 The medications used for this disorder include stimulants (such as Ritalin), which improve behavior and cognition for about 70 percent of adolescents. Extended-release preparations (including a skin patch) are longer acting, so individuals do not have to take these medications as often as in the past. As discussed in Chapter 11, misuse of prescription stimulants by students without ADHD is a growing problem on college campuses. An estimated 10 percent of students reported using prescription stimulants at some point in their college years.[35] Their primary motivations were to stay awake or feel more energetic or to get high. ADHD medications do not have the same effects on individuals with the disorder.[36] Although many students take stimulants to improve performance, they generally get poorer grades, perhaps because they fall behind and then take stimulants in order to cram and catch up.

An alternative nonstimulant treatment is Strattera (atomoxetine), which treats ADHD and coexisting problems such as depression and anxiety. Its effects are more gradual, and it does not seem to have any known potential for abuse. Adverse effects include drowsiness, loss of appetite, nausea, vomiting, and headaches. Its long-term effects are not known.

 An estimated 1 percent of college students have an attention disorder that can have a significant impact on their academic performance and personal lives. Undergraduates with ADHD are at higher risk of becoming smokers, abusing alcohol and drugs, and having automobile accidents. The normal challenges of college—navigating the complexities of scheduling, planning courses, and honing study skills—may be especially daunting.

Psychological therapies have not been studied extensively in adolescents and young adults with ADHD. However, if you have ADHD, check with your student health or counseling center to see if any special services are available. College health services may provide support, but health insurance coverage for ADHD treatment is limited and costly.

Schizophrenia

Schizophrenia, one of the most debilitating mental disorders, profoundly impairs an individual's sense of reality. As the National Institute of Mental Health (NIMH) puts it, schizophrenia, which is characterized by abnormalities in brain structure and chemistry, destroys "the inner unity of the mind" and weakens "the will and drive that constitute our essential character." It affects every aspect of psychological functioning, including the ways in which people think, feel, view themselves, and relate to others.

The symptoms of schizophrenia include:

- **Hallucinations.**
- **Delusions.**
- **Inability to think** in a logical manner.
- **Talking** in rambling or incoherent ways.
- **Making odd or purposeless movements** or not moving at all.
- **Repeating others' words** or mimicking their gestures.
- **Showing few, if any, feelings;** responding with inappropriate emotions.
- **Lacking will or motivation** to complete a task or accomplish something.
- **Functioning at a much lower level** than in the past at work, in interpersonal relations, or in taking care of themselves.

Individuals with schizophrenia may hear, see, or feel things that do not exist—a voice telling them to jump from a bridge, a statue crying tears of blood, a spaceship beaming a light upon them. Frightened and vulnerable, they may devote all their energy to warding off the demons within. Unable to take care of themselves, they may look messy and disheveled. They often move in unusual ways, such as rocking or pacing, or repeat certain gestures again and again. They may believe that someone or something, such as the devil, is putting thoughts into their heads or controlling their actions. Some think they are reincarnations of Christ or Napoleon. About a third attempt to take their own lives, often in response to a command they hear inside their heads.

attention-deficit/hyperactivity disorder (ADHD) A spectrum of difficulties in controlling motion and sustaining attention, including hyperactivity, impulsivity, and distractibility.

schizophrenia A general term for a group of mental disorders with characteristic psychotic symptoms, such as delusions, hallucinations, and disordered thought patterns during the active phase of the illness, and a duration of at least six months.

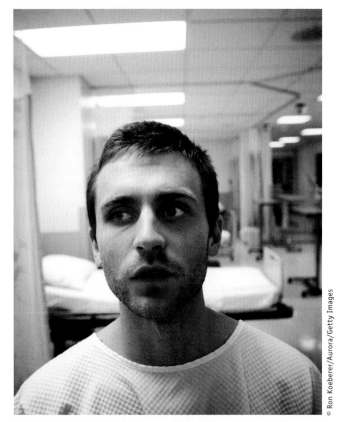

Individuals with schizophrenia, which often develops in young adulthood, may hear, see, or feel things that do not exist.

Researchers have identified early markers of schizophrenia, including impaired social skills, intellectual ability, and capacity for organization.

Schizophrenia is one of the leading causes of disability among young adults. The mean age for schizophrenia to develop is 21.4 years for men and 26.8 years for women. Although symptoms do not occur until then, they are almost certainly the result of a failure in brain development that occurs very early in life. The underlying defect is probably present before birth. Schizophrenia has a strong genetic basis and is not the result of upbringing, social conditions, or traumatic experiences.

For the vast majority of individuals with schizophrenia, antipsychotic drugs are the foundation of treatment. Newer agents are more effective in making most people with schizophrenia feel more comfortable and in control of themselves, help organize chaotic thinking, and reduce or eliminate delusions or hallucinations, allowing fuller participation in normal activities.[37]

Suicide

Suicide is not in itself a psychiatric disorder, but it is often the tragic consequence of emotional and psychological problems. Every year 30,000 Americans—among them many young people who seem to have "everything to live for"—commit suicide. An estimated 752,000 attempt to take their own lives; there may be 4.5 million suicide "survivors" in the United States.

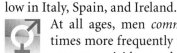 The suicide rate for African American and Caucasian men peaks between ages 20 and 40. It rises again after age 65 among white men and after age 75 among blacks. In general, whites are at highest risk for suicide, followed by Native Americans, African Americans, Hispanic Americans, and Asian Americans. Internationally, suicide rates are highest in Germany, Scandinavia, Eastern Europe, and Japan, average in the United States, Canada, and Great Britain, and low in Italy, Spain, and Ireland.

At all ages, men *commit* suicide three to four times more frequently than women, but women *attempt* suicide much more often than men (Table 4.2). Elderly men are ten times more likely to take their own lives than elderly women.[38]

Suicide in the Young

Although rates have declined in the last decade, suicide remains the third-leading cause of death among children and adolescents 10 to 19 years old in the United States. An estimated 500,000 U.S. teens attempt suicide every year. About 1,500 die.[39]

 Suicide is the second-leading cause of death among students at American colleges and universities. Although many people believe that suicide rates are increasing, the suicide rate for young adults has been stable or declining since 1976. Among college-aged women, the rate is the lowest it has been in the last 100 years. More young men than women take their own lives, but the suicide rate for college-aged men has declined 20 percent in the past ten years.[40] The suicide rate among college students is about 6.5 per 100,000, half the rate of the U.S. population in general.[41] (See Reality Check.)

One-half of the adolescents who take their own lives suffer from major depression. "In psychological interviews after a teen suicide, we see that the warning signs were there," notes child psychiatrist Madelyn Gould, M.D., of Columbia University, "but no one realized the underlying problem was depression."[42]

Table 4-2 Suicide Risk

	Who attempts suicide?	Who completes suicide?
Sex	Female	Male
Age	Under 35	Under 20 or over 60
Means	Less deadly, such as wrist slashing	More deadly, such as a gun
Circumstances	High chance of rescue	Low chance of rescue

© Ron Koeberer/Aurora/Getty Images

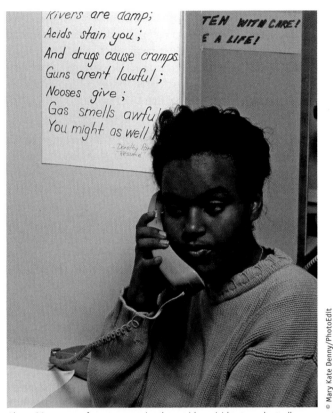

Kivers are damp;
Acids stain you;
And drugs cause cramps.
Guns aren't lawful;
Nooses give;
Gas smells awful
You might as well

—Dorothy Parker
"Résumé"

TEN WITH CARE!
E A LIFE!

About 20 percent of teenagers seriously consider suicide; a much smaller number actually attempt to take their own lives. Talking to a counselor at a suicide hot line may help a young person deal with feelings of despondency.

REALITYCHECK

- *How many college students felt things were hopeless at least once in the last year?* _____
- *How many felt so depressed it was difficult to function?* _____
- *How many seriously considered committing suicide?* _____
- *How many attempted suicide?* _____

Answers on next page.

cide. Among young people, early recognition and treatment for depressive disorders and alcohol and drug use could save thousands of lives each year.

Factors That Lead to Suicide

Researchers have looked for explanations for suicide by studying everything from phases of the moon to seasons (suicides peak in the spring and early summer) to birth order in the family. They have found no conclusive answers. A constellation of influences—mental disorders, personality traits, biologic and genetic vulnerability, medical illness, and psychosocial stressors—may combine in ways that lower an individual's threshold of vulnerability. The risk of suicide is higher in people who live in cities, are single, have a low income, or are unemployed. No one factor in itself may ever explain fully why a person chooses death.

Mental Disorders More than 95 percent of those who commit suicide have a mental disorder. Two in particular—depression and alcoholism—account for two-thirds of all suicides. Suicide also is a risk for those with other disorders, including schizophrenia, posttraumatic stress disorder, and personality disorders.

Antidepressant Medications As the FDA has warned, antidepressants can increase the risk of suicidal thoughts and attempts. Recent studies have confirmed an increase in suicide attempts in some individuals, including adolescents, during the first four weeks of treatment, especially the first nine days, with various antidepressants, including Prozac and Paxil.[45] Because depression itself increases the danger of suicide, psychiatrists contend that the benefits of treatment outweigh the risk but call for increased monitoring for increased agitation or suicidal thoughts.

Substance Abuse Many of those who commit suicide drink beforehand, and their use of alcohol may lower their inhibitions. Since alcohol itself is a depressant, it can intensify the despondency suicidal individuals are already feeling. Alcoholics who attempt suicide often have other risk factors, including major depression, poor social support, serious medical illness, and unemploy-

Native American communities have especially high rates of suicide among both young men and women. Young African American men, historically at low suicide risk, are narrowing the gap with their white peers, while suicide by Hispanic young men has declined. The lowest rates are for Asian Pacific males and African American females.[43]

Firearms and suffocation (mainly by hanging) are the most common methods of suicide among young people. In recent years, deaths with firearms have decreased, in part because of laws restricting access to guns by youngsters. However, deaths by hanging have increased, particularly among younger teens.[44]

Researchers also have identified factors that protect young people from suicide. Number one for both boys and girls was feeling connected to their parents and family. For girls, emotional well-being was also protective; grade point average was an additional protective factor for boys. High parental expectations for their child's school achievement, more people living in the household, and religiosity were protective for some of the boys, but not for the girls. Availability of counseling services at school and parental presence at key times during the day were protective for some of the girls, but not for the boys.

Suicide is not inevitable. Appropriate treatment can help as many as 70 to 80 percent of those at risk for sui-

ment. Drugs of abuse also can alter thinking and lower inhibitions against suicide.

Hopelessness   The sense of utter hopelessness and helplessness may be the most common contributing factor in suicide. When hope dies, individuals view every experience in negative terms and come to expect the worst possible outcomes for their problems. Given this way of thinking, suicide often seems a reasonable response to a life seen as not worth living. Optimism, on the other hand, correlates with fewer thoughts of suicide by college students.[46]

Family History   One of every four people who attempt suicide has a family member who also tried to commit suicide. While a family history of suicide is not in itself considered a predictor of suicide, two mental disorders that can lead to suicide—depression and bipolar disorder (manic depression)—do run in families.

Physical Illness   People who commit suicide are likely to be ill or to believe that they are. About 5 percent actually have a serious physical disorder, such as AIDS or cancer. While suicide may seem to be a decision rationally arrived at in persons with serious or fatal illness, this may not be the case. Depression, not uncommon in such instances, can warp judgment. When the depression is treated, the person may no longer have suicidal intentions.

Brain Chemistry   Investigators have found abnormalities in the brain chemistry of individuals who complete suicide, especially low levels of a metabolite of the neurotransmitter serotonin. There are indications that individuals with a deficiency in this substance may have as much as a ten times greater risk of committing suicide than those with higher levels.

Access to Guns   For individuals already facing a combination of predisposing factors, access to a means of committing suicide, particularly to guns, can add to the

Your Life Change Coach

Preventing Suicide

At some point thoughts of ending it all—the disappointments, problems, bad feelings—may cross your mind. It is not uncommon to fantasize about how such an act would make others, particularly those who have rejected or hurt you, feel. But persistent, specific ideas about suicide are not healthy or normal.

In the most recent ACHA survey, 91 percent of undergraduates said they had never seriously considered suicide in the previous year. About 7 percent reported having such thoughts one to four times; 1 percent said they had considered suicide five to eight times or nine times or more. One percent attempted suicide.[49]

Suicide is not inevitable. If the idea of ending your life persists or intensifies, respond as you would to other warnings of potential threats to your health: by getting the help you need.

If you are thinking about suicide . . .

- **Talk to a mental health professional.** If you have a therapist, call immediately. If not, call a suicide hot line.

- **Find someone you can trust and talk honestly about what you're feeling.** If you suffer from depression or another mental disorder, educate trusted friends or relatives about your condition so they are prepared if called upon to help.

- **Write down your more uplifting thoughts.** Even if you are despondent, you can help yourself by taking the time to retrieve some more positive thoughts or memories. A simple record of your hopes for the future and the people you value in your life can remind you of why your own life is worth continuing.

risk. Unlike other methods of suicide, guns almost always work. Suicide rates among children, women, and men of all ages are higher in states where more households have guns. Although only 5 percent of suicide attempts involve firearms, more than 90 percent of these attempts are fatal. By comparison, 75 percent of all suicide attempts involve drugs and result in death less than 3 percent of the time.[47] States with stricter gun-control laws have much lower rates of suicide than states with more lenient laws. Health professionals are urging parents whose children undergo psychological treatment or assessment to remove all weapons from their homes and to make sure their youngsters do not have access to potentially lethal medications or to alcohol.

Other Factors   Individuals who kill themselves often have gone through more major life crises—job changes, births, financial reversals, divorce, retirement—in the previous six months, compared with others. Long-standing, intense conflict with family members or other important people may add to the danger. In some cases, suicide may be an act of revenge that offers the person a sense of control—however temporary or illusory. For example, some may feel that, by rejecting life, they are rejecting a partner or parent who abandoned or betrayed them.

Among college students, dissatisfaction and unease with their bodies can be a source of psychological pain that increases their risk of depression and suicide.[48]

Overcoming Problems of the Mind

Mental illness costs our society an estimated $150 billion a year in lost work time and productivity, employee turnover, disability payments, and death. Yet many Americans do not have access to mental health services, nor do they have insurance for such services. Despite the fact that treatments for mental disorders have a higher success rate than those for many other diseases, employers often restrict mental health benefits. HMOs and health insurance plans are much more likely to limit psychotherapy visits and psychiatric hospitalizations than treatments for medical illnesses.

Even when cost is not a barrier, many people do not seek treatment because they see psychological problems as a sign of weakness rather than illness. They also may not realize that scientifically proven therapies can bring relief, often in a matter of weeks or months.

- **Avoid drugs and alcohol.** Most suicides are the results of sudden, uncontrolled impulses, and drugs and alcohol can make it harder to resist these destructive urges.

- **Go to the hospital.** Hospitalization can sometimes be the best way to protect your health and safety.

If someone you know may be thinking about suicide . . .

- **Encourage your friend to talk**. Ask concerned questions. Listen attentively. Show that you take the person's feelings seriously and truly care.

- **Don't offer trite reassurances.** Don't list reasons to go on living, try to analyze the person's motives, or try to shock or challenge him or her.

- **Suggest solutions or alternatives to problems.** Make plans. Encourage positive action, such as getting away for a while to gain a better perspective on a problem.

- **Don't be afraid to ask whether your friend has considered suicide.** The opportunity to talk about thoughts of suicide may be an enormous relief and—contrary to a long-standing myth—will not fix the idea of suicide more firmly in a person's mind.

- **Don't think that people who talk about killing themselves never carry out their threat.** Most individuals who commit suicide give definite indications of their intent to die.

- **Watch out for behavioral clues.** If your friend begins to behave unpredictably or suddenly emerges from a severe depression into a calm, settled state of mind, these could signal increased danger of suicide. Don't leave your friend alone. Call a suicide hotline, or get in touch with a mental health professional.

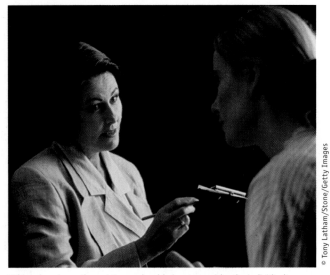

© Tony Latham/Stone/Getty Images

When choosing a therapist, you should always consider the individual's education, title, and qualifications. Also important are qualities such as compassion and caring.

Where To Turn for Help

As a student, your best contact for identifying local services may be your health education instructor or department. The health instructors can tell you about general and mental health counseling available on campus, school-based support groups, community-based programs, and special emergency services. On campus, you can also turn to the student health services or the office of the dean of student services or student affairs. (See the "Help Yourself" lab in *IPC*.) **IPC**

Within the community, you may be able to get help through the city or county health department and neighborhood health centers. Local hospitals often have special clinics and services; and there are usually local branches of national service organizations, such as United Way or Alcoholics Anonymous, other 12-step programs, and various support groups. You can call the psychiatric or psychological association in your city or state for the names of licensed professionals. (Check the telephone directory for listings.) Your primary physician may also be able to help.

The telephone book and the Internet are also good resources for special programs, found either by the nature of the service, by the name of the neighborhood or city, or by the name of the sponsoring group. In some places, the city's name may precede a listing: the New York City Suicide Hot Line, for instance. In addition to suicide-prevention programs, look for crisis intervention, violence prevention, and child-abuse prevention programs; drug-treatment information; shelters for battered women; senior citizen centers; and self-help and counseling services. Many services have special hot lines for coping with emergencies. Others provide information as well as counseling over the phone.

Types of Therapists

Only professionally trained individuals who have met state licensing requirements are certified as psychiatrists, psychologists, or social workers. Before selecting any of these mental health professionals, be sure to check the person's background and credentials.

Psychiatrists are licensed medical doctors (M.D.) who complete medical school; a year-long internship; and a three-year residency that provides training in various forms of psychotherapy, psychopharmacology, and both outpatient and inpatient treatment of mental disorders. They can prescribe medications and make medical decisions. *Board-certified* psychiatrists have passed oral and written examinations following completion of residency training.

Psychologists complete a graduate program (including clinical training and internships) in human psychology but do not study medicine and cannot prescribe medication. They must be licensed in most states in order to practice independently.

Certified social workers or **licensed clinical social workers (LCSWs)** usually complete a two-year graduate program and have specialized training in helping people with mental problems in addition to conventional social work.

Psychiatric nurses have nursing degrees and have passed a state examination. They usually have special training and experience in mental health care, although no specialty licensing or certification is required.

Marriage and family therapists, licensed in some but not all states, usually have a graduate degree, often in psychology, and at least two years of supervised clinical training in dealing with relationship problems.

Other therapists include pastoral counselors, members of the clergy who offer psychological counseling; hypnotherapists, who use hypnosis for problems such as smoking and obesity; stress-management counselors, who teach relaxation methods; and alcohol and drug counselors, who help individuals with substance abuse problems. Anyone can use these terms to describe themselves professionally, and there are no licensing requirements.

Types of Therapy

The term **psychotherapy** refers to any type of counseling based on the exchange of words in the context of the unique relationship that develops between a mental health professional and a person seeking help. The process of talking and listening can lead to new insight, relief from distressing psychological symptoms, changes in unhealthy or maladaptive behaviors, and more effective ways of dealing with the world.

Most mental health professionals today are trained in a variety of psychotherapeutic techniques and tailor their approach to the problem, personality, and needs of each person seeking their help. Because skilled therapists may combine different techniques in the course of therapy, the lines between the various approaches often blur.

Because insurance companies and health-care plans often limit the duration of psychotherapy, many mental health professionals are adopting a *time-limited* format in order to make the most of every session, regardless of the length of treatment. Brief or short-term psychotherapy typically focuses on a central theme, problem, or topic and may continue for several weeks to several months. The individuals most likely to benefit are those who are interested in solving immediate problems rather than changing their characters, who can think in psychological terms, and who are motivated to change.

Psychodynamic Psychotherapy

For the most part, today's mental health professionals base their assessment of individuals on a **psychodynamic** understanding that takes into account the role of early experiences and unconscious influences in *actively* shaping behavior. (This is the *dynamic* in psychodynamic.) Psychodynamic treatments work toward the goal of providing greater insight into problems and bringing about behavioral change. Therapy may be brief, consisting of 12 to 25 sessions, or may continue for several years. According to current thinking, psychotherapy can actually rewire the network of neurons within the brain in ways that ease distress and improve functioning in many areas of daily life.

Cognitive-Behavioral Therapy (CBT)

Cognitive-behavioral therapy (CBT) focuses on inappropriate or inaccurate thoughts or beliefs to help individuals break out of a distorted way of thinking. The techniques of **cognitive therapy** include identification of an individual's beliefs and attitudes, recognition of negative thought patterns, and education in alternative ways of thinking. Individuals with major depression or anxiety disorders are most likely to benefit, usually in 15 to 25 sessions. However, many of the positive messages used in cognitive therapy can help anyone improve a bad mood or negative outlook.

Behavioral therapy strives to substitute healthier ways of behaving for maladaptive patterns used in the past. Its premise is that distressing psychological symptoms, like all behaviors, are learned responses that can be modified or unlearned. Some therapists believe that changing behavior also changes how people think and feel. As they put it, "Change the behavior, and the feelings will follow." Behavioral therapies work best for disorders characterized by specific, abnormal patterns of acting—such as alcohol and drug abuse, anxiety disorders, and phobias—and for individuals who want to change bad habits.

Interpersonal Therapy (IPT)

Interpersonal therapy (IPT), originally developed for research into the treatment of major depression, focuses on relationships in order to help individuals deal with unrecognized feelings and needs and improve their communication skills. IPT does not deal with the psychological origins of symptoms but rather concentrates on current problems of getting along with others. The supportive, empathic relationship that is developed with the therapist, who takes an even more active role than in psychodynamic psychotherapy, is the most crucial component of this therapy. The emphasis is on the here and now and on interpersonal—rather than intrapsychic—issues. Individuals with major depression, chronic difficulties developing relationships, chronic mild depression, or bulimia (see Chapter 7 on eating disorders) are most likely to benefit. IPT usually consists of 12 to 16 sessions.

Other Approaches

Solution-focused therapy, originally developed as a short-term psychotherapy technique, accentuates the positive rather than focusing on problems and their causes. Guided by a therapist, a client thinks about hopes

psychiatrist Licensed medical doctor with additional training in psychotherapy, psychopharmacology, and treatment of mental disorders.

psychologist Mental health-care professional who has completed doctoral or graduate program in psychology and is trained in psychotherapeutic techniques, but who is not medically trained and does not prescribe medications.

certified social worker or licensed clinical social worker (LCSW) A person who has completed a two-year graduate program in counseling people with mental problems.

psychiatric nurse A nurse with special training and experience in mental health care.

marriage and family therapist A psychiatrist, psychologist, or social worker who specializes in marriage and family counseling.

psychotherapy Treatment designed to produce a response by psychological rather than physical means, such as suggestion, persuasion, reassurance, and support.

psychodynamic Interpreting behaviors in terms of early experiences and unconscious influences.

cognitive therapy A technique used to identify an individual's beliefs and attitudes, recognize negative thought patterns, and educate in alternative ways of thinking.

behavioral therapy A technique that emphasizes application of the principles of learning to substitute desirable responses and behavior patterns for undesirable ones.

interpersonal therapy (IPT) A technique used to develop communication skills and relationships.

solution-focused therapy A technique that accentuates the positive and focuses on goals and implementation of alternatives.

YOUR STRATEGIES FOR PREVENTION *Before Taking a Psychiatric Drug*

Before taking any psychoactive drug (one that affects the brain), talk to a qualified health professional. Here are some points to raise:

- What can this medication do for me? What specific symptoms will it relieve? Are there other possible benefits?

- When will I notice a difference? How long does it take for the medicine to have an effect?

- Are there any risks? What about side effects? Do I have to take it before or after eating? Will it affect my ability to study, work, drive, or operate machinery?

- Is there a risk of increased aggression or suicide? What should I do if I start thinking about taking my own life or of harming others?

- How will I be able to tell if the medication is working? What are the odds that it will help me?

- How long will I have to take medication? Is there any danger that I'll become addicted?

- What if it doesn't help?

- Is there an herbal or natural alternative? If so, has it been studied? What do you know about its possible risks and side effects?

and achievements and pays attention to goals rather than obstacles and strengths rather than weaknesses. Instead of making diagnoses or analyzing the past, solution-focused therapists encourage clients to recognize and implement alternatives so that they can successfully make changes in their lives.

Behavioral activation is a technique that helps depressed people do what they tend to avoid. Since depressed people often withdraw from routine activities and the demands of daily life, they have fewer positive experiences and receive fewer rewards. Over time they become more depressed. In behavioral activation, patients find out and record what gives them a sense of accomplishment, then do these things. With the therapist's help, they direct their attention to the immediate experience of their senses to avoid pessimism and gloomy rumination. In one study of people with major depression, behavioral activation was as effective as treatment with antidepressants.

Options for Treatment

Psychiatric Drugs

Medications that alter brain chemistry and relieve psychiatric symptoms have brought great hope and help to millions of people. Thanks to the recent development of a new generation of more precise and effective **psychiatric drugs,** success rates for treating many common and disabling disorders—depression, panic disorder, schizophrenia, and others—have soared. Often used in conjunction with psychotherapy, sometimes used as the primary treatment, these medications have revolutionized mental health care.

At some point in their lives, about half of all Americans will take a psychiatric drug. The reason may be depression, anxiety, a sleep difficulty, an eating disorder, alcohol or drug dependence, impaired memory, or another disorder that disrupts the intricate chemistry of the brain.

Psychiatric drugs are now among the most widely prescribed drugs in the United States. Serotonin-boosting medications (SSRIs) have become the drugs of choice in treating depression. They also are effective in treating obsessive compulsive disorder, panic disorder, social phobia, posttraumatic stress disorder, premenstrual dysphoric disorder, and generalized anxiety disorder. In patients who don't respond, psychiatrists may add another drug to boost the efficacy of the treatment.

 According to various studies, 5 to 7 percent of college students take antidepressant medications. Direct-to-consumer advertisements for antidepressant drugs can influence students' perceptions of what is wrong with them. In one study, college women were more likely to rate themselves as having mild-to-moderate depression as a result of reading pharmaceutical company information for popular antidepressants. The researchers cautioned that students should try alternative treatments for mild depression, including simple changes such as reduced class load, increased exercise, and more sleep, before starting medication.[50] (See Your Strategies for Prevention: "Before Taking a Psychiatric Drug.")

Alternative Mind-Mood Products

People with serious mental illnesses, including depression and bipolar disorder, often use at least one alternative health-care practice, such as yoga or meditation. In a recent survey of women with depression, about half (54 percent) reported trying herbs, vitamins, and manual therapies such as massage and acupressure.[51] Some "natural" products, such as herbs and enzymes, claim to have psychological effects. However, they have not undergone rigorous scientific testing.

St. John's wort has been used to treat anxiety and depression in Europe for many years. Data from clinical

---

behavioral activation A technique in which depressed people discover and do the things that give them a sense of accomplishment.

psychiatric drugs Medications that regulate a person's mental, emotional, and physical functions to facilitate normal functioning.

studies in the United States do not support the efficacy of St. John's wort for moderate to severe depression. In teo carefully controlled studies, the herb did not prove more effective than a placebo. However, more than two dozen studies have found that St. John's wort was similar in efficacy to standard antidepressants. Side effects include dizziness, abdominal pain and bloating, constipation, nausea, fatigue, and dry mouth. St. John's wort should not be taken in combination with other prescription antidepressants. St. John's wort can lower the efficacy of oral contraceptives and increase the risk of an unwanted pregnancy.

Learn It : Live It

Surviving and Thriving

Like physical health, psychological well-being is not a fixed state of being, but a process. The way you live every day affects how you feel about yourself and your world. Here are some basic guidelines that you can rely on to make the most of the process of living:

- **Accept yourself.** As a human being, you are, by definition, imperfect. Come to terms with the fact that you are a worthwhile person despite your mistakes.
- **Respect yourself.** Recognize your abilities and talents. Acknowledge your competence and achievements, and take pride in them.

- **Trust yourself.** Learn to listen to the voice within you, and let your intuition be your guide.
- **Love yourself.** Be happy to spend time by yourself. Learn to appreciate your own company and to be glad you're you.
- **Stretch yourself.** Be willing to change and grow, to try something new and dare to be vulnerable.
- **Look at challenges as opportunities for personal growth.** "Every problem brings the possibility of a widening of consciousness," psychologist Carl Jung once noted. Put his words to the test.
- **Think of not only where but also who you want to be a decade from now.** The goals you set, the decisions you make, the values you adopt now will determine how you feel about yourself and your life in the future.

SELFSURVEY : *Recognizing Depression*

Depression comes in different forms, just like other illnesses such as heart disease. Not everyone with a depressive disorder experiences every symptom. The number and severity of symptoms may vary among individuals and also over time.

Read through the following list, and check all the descriptions that apply.

- ❏ I am often restless and irritable.
- ❏ I am having irregular sleep patterns—either too much or not enough.
- ❏ I don't enjoy hobbies, my friends, family or leisure activities any more.
- ❏ I am having trouble managing my diabetes, hypertension, or other chronic illness.
- ❏ I have nagging aches and pains that do not get better no matter what I do.
- ❏ Specifically, I often experience:
  - ❏ Digestive problems
  - ❏ Headache or backache
  - ❏ Vague aches and pains like joint or muscle pains
  - ❏ Chest pains
  - ❏ Dizziness
- ❏ I have trouble concentrating or making simple decisions.

- ❏ Others have commented on my mood or attitude lately.
- ❏ My weight has changed a considerable amount.
- ❏ I have had several of the symptoms I checked above for more than two weeks.
- ❏ I feel that my functioning in my everyday life (work, family, friends) is suffering because of these problems.
- ❏ I have a family history of depression.
- ❏ I have thought about suicide.*

Checking several items on this list does not mean that you have a depressive disorder because many conditions can cause similar symptoms. However, you should take this list with you to discuss with your health care provider or mental health therapist. Even though it can be difficult to talk about certain things, your health care provider is knowledgeable, trained, and committed to helping you.

If you can't think of what to say, try these conversation starters:
"I just don't feel like myself lately."
"My friend (parent, roommate, spouse) thinks I might be depressed."
"I haven't been sleeping well lately."
"Everything seems harder than before."
"Nothing's fun anymore."

If you are diagnosed with depression, remember that it is a common and highly treatable illness with medical causes. Your habits or personality did not cause your depression, and you do not have to face it alone.

*University of Michigan Depression Center, 800-475-MICH, www.med.umich.edu/depression

Your Health Action Plan for Getting Help for a Psychological Problem

Sometimes we all need outside help from a trained, licensed professional to work through personal problems. Here is what you need to know if you are experiencing psychological difficulties.

Consider Therapy if You . . .

- Feel an overwhelming and prolonged sense of helplessness and sadness, which does not lift despite your efforts and help from family and friends.
- Find it difficult to carry out everyday activities such as homework, and your academic performance is suffering.
- Worry excessively, expect the worst, or are constantly on edge.
- Are finding it hard to resist or are engaging in behaviors that are harmful to you or others, such as drinking too much alcohol, abusing drugs, or becoming aggressive or violent.
- Have persistent thoughts or fantasies of harming yourself or others.

Most people who have at least several sessions of psychotherapy are far better off than individuals with emotional difficulties who do not get treatment. According to the American Psychological Association, 50 percent of patients noticeably improve after eight sessions, while 75 percent of individuals in therapy improved by the end of six months.

Choosing a Therapist

Ask your physician or another health professional. Call your local or state psychological association. Consult your university or college department of psychology or health center. Contact your area community mental health center. Inquire at your church or synagogue.

- A good rapport with your psychotherapist is critical. Choose someone with whom you feel comfortable and at ease.

- Ask the following questions:
  - Are you licensed?
  - How long have you been practicing?
  - I have been feeling (anxious, tense, depressed, etc.), and I'm having problems (with school, relationships, eating, sleeping, etc.). What experience do you have helping people with these types of problems?
  - What are your areas of expertise—phobias? ADHD? depression?
  - What kinds of treatments do you use? Have they proved effective for dealing with my kind of problem or issue?
  - What are your fees? (Fees are usually based on a 45- minute to 50-minute session.) Do you have a sliding-scale fee policy?
  - How much therapy would you recommend?
  - What types of insurance do you accept?

Is Therapy Working?

As you begin therapy, establish clear goals with your therapist. Some goals require more time to reach than others. You and your therapist should decide at what point you might expect to begin to see progress.

As they begin therapy, some people may have difficulty discussing painful and troubling experiences. Feelings of relief or hope are positive signs indicating that you are starting to explore your thoughts and behaviors.

CENGAGENOW If you want to write your own goals for avoiding mood slumps or getting psychological help, go to the Wellness Journal at HealthNow at **academic.cengage.com/login.**

Making This Chapter Work for YOU

Review Questions

1. Neurons
   a. transmit information within the brain and throughout the body by means of electrical impulses and chemical messengers.
   b. are specialized support cells that travel through the spinal cord, carrying signals related to movement.
   c. are protein molecules designed to bind with neurotransmitters.
   d. cross a synapse before reuptake.

2. A mental disorder can be described as
   a. a condition associated with migraine headaches and narcolepsy.
   b. a condition that is usually caused by severe trauma to the brain.
   c. a behavioral or psychological disorder that impairs an individual's ability to conduct one or more important activities of daily life.
   d. a psychological disorder that is easily controlled with medication and a change in diet.

3. Depression
   a. is not likely to occur in young adults.
   b. is twice as common in women as men.
   c. has the same symptoms in men and women.
   d. is twice as common in Hispanics than African Americans.

4. Some characteristic symptoms of major depression are
   a. difficulty concentrating, lack of energy, and eating more than usual.
   b. exaggerated sense of euphoria and energy.
   c. palpitations, sweating, numbness, and tingling sensations.
   d. talking in rambling ways, inability to think in a logical manner, and delusions.

5. Which statement about depression treatment is true?
   a. The most effective treatment for depression in adolescents is a combination of antidepressant medication and cognitive-behavioral therapy.
   b. Antidepressants help about 90 percent of individuals feel better within four weeks.
   c. Weight training has helped lift depression in most individuals.
   d. With the right therapy, depression will not reoccur.

6. Which of the following statements about anxiety disorders is true?
   a. Anxiety disorders are the least prevalent type of mental illness.
   b. An individual suffering from a panic attack may mistake her symptoms for a heart attack.
   c. The primary symptom of obsessive-compulsive disorder is irrational, intense, and persistent fear of a specific object or situation.
   d. Generalized anxiety disorders respond to systematic desensitization behavior therapy.

7. Students with attention-deficit/hyperactivity disorder
   a. perform as well on standardized tests as students without ADHD.
   b. have an increased risk of substance use disorders.
   c. have a decreased risk of developing depression or anxiety disorders.
   d. constitute 10 percent of the student population.

8. A person may be at higher risk of committing suicide if
   a. he is taking blood pressure medication.
   b. he lives in a rural environment and is married.
   c. he has been diagnosed with hyperactivity disorder.
   d. he has lost his job because of alcoholism.

9. Which of these therapies focuses on recognizing negative thought patterns and changing those patterns?
   a. psychodynamic psychotherapy
   b. behavioral activation
   c. interpersonal therapy
   d. cognitive therapy

10. Which of the following statements is true?
    a. Individuals with phobias are most likely to benefit from psychiatric medications.
    b. Antidepressant medications now require a warning label about the increased risk of suicidal thoughts.
    c. Only children have attention disorders.
    d. Interpersonal therapy focuses on the role of early experiences and unconscious influences in shaping patterns of behavior, such as repeated failed relationships.

Answers to these questions can be found on page 583.

Critical Thinking

1. Jake, who took antidepressants to recover from depression in high school, began feeling the same troubling symptoms. A physician at the student health center prescribed the same medication that had helped him in the past, but this time Jake noticed the warning about an increased risk of suicide. He has had thoughts of killing himself, and he worries whether or not to start the medication. When he did some online research, he learned that the risk of suicide is greater if depression is untreated than it is with medication. How would you counsel Jake? How would you weigh the risks and benefits of taking an antidepressant? Do you know someone who might benefit from taking antidepressants but is afraid to take them because of the possible risk of suicide?

2. Ever since breaking up with her boyfriend last month, Nicole has been feeling down. She sleeps in whenever she can, and she's lost her appetite. When friends ask her to join them for a night out, she usually says no. Although she can't explain why, she doesn't enjoy the things she once did. Do you think Nicole is recovering from a bad breakup or experiencing something more serious? What would you advise her to do? Where would you turn if you were in similar circumstances? Would you hesitate to seek psychological help for fear that friends may think you're crazy? Would your opinion of a friend change if you found out that he or she was in therapy?

3. Research has indicated that many homeless men and women are in need of outpatient psychiatric care, often because they suffer from chronic mental illnesses or alcoholism. Yet government funding for the mentally ill is inadequate, and homelessness itself can make it difficult, if not impossible, for people to gain access to the care they need. How do you feel when you pass homeless individuals who seem disoriented or out of touch with reality? Who should take responsibility for their welfare? Should they be forced to undergo treatment at psychiatric institutions?

Media Menu

CENGAGENOW™ Go to the HealthNow website at **academic.cengage.com/login** that will:

- Help you evaluate your knowledge of the material.
- Allow you to take an exam-prep quiz.
- Provide a Personalized Learning Plan targeting resources that address areas you should study.
- Coach you through identifying target goals for behavioral change and creating and monitoring your personal change plan throughout the semester.

INTERNET CONNECTIONS

SAVE: Suicide Awareness Voices of Education
www.save.org
This site (formerly American Foundation for Suicide Prevention) offers research, facts, survivor support, and more.

National Institute of Mental Health
www.nimh.nih.gov
The National Institute of Mental Health is a federally sponsored organization that provides useful information on a

variety of mental health topics including current mental health research.

American Psychological Association

www.apa.org

The APA is the scientific and professional organization for psychology in the United States. Its website provides up-to-date information on psychological issues and disorders.

National Mental Health Association

www.nmha.org

This site features fact sheets on a variety of mental health topics, including depression screening, college initiative, substance abuse prevention, and information for families. Also available are current mental health articles, an e-mail newsletter, and a bookstore.

Key Terms

The terms listed are used and defined on the page indicated. Definitions are also found in the Glossary at the end of this book.

antidepressant   85
anxiety disorders   91
attention deficit/hyperactivity disorder (ADHD) 93
axon   83
axon terminal   83
behavioral activation   100
behavioral therapy   99
bipolar disorder   91
certified social worker or licensed clinical social worker 99
cognitive therapy   99
dendrites   83
depression   85
dysthymia   89
generalized anxiety disorder (GAD) 91
glia   83
interpersonal therapy (IPT) 99
major depression   89
marriage and family therapist 99
mental disorder   85
neuron   83
neuropsychiatry   83
neurotransmitters   83
nucleus   83
obsessive-compulsive disorder (OCD) 91
panic attack   91
panic disorder   91
phobia   91
psychiatric drugs   100
psychiatric nurse   99
psychiatrist   99
psychodynamic   99
psychologist   99
psychotherapy   99
receptors   83
reuptake   85
schizophrenia   93
solution-focused therapy 99
synapse   83

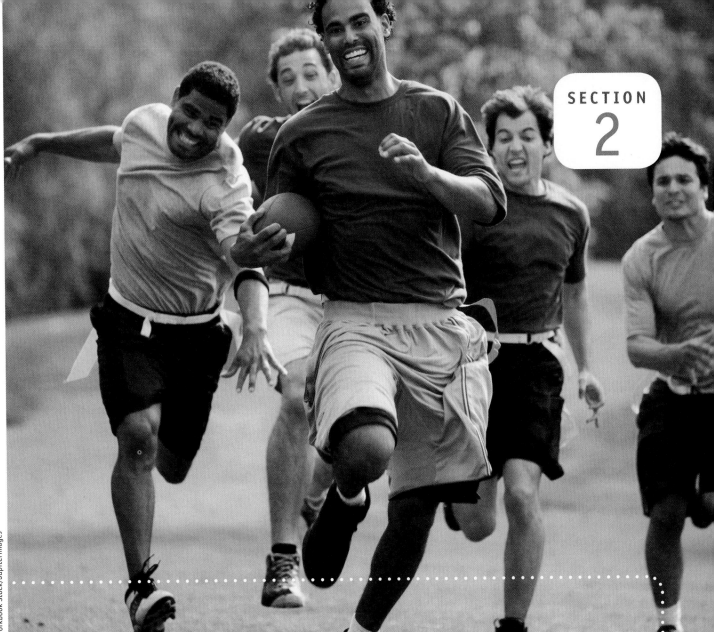

Healthy Lifestyles

You have enormous influence over your health and vitality. This section provides information about the tools you have at hand to become healthier and feel more energetic throughout your lifetime. By learning how to eat a balanced and varied diet, how to manage your weight, and how to become physically fit, you can get started on a lifelong journey of becoming all you can be. As you take better care of your body today, you'll build the foundation for feeling your best for many tomorrows to come.

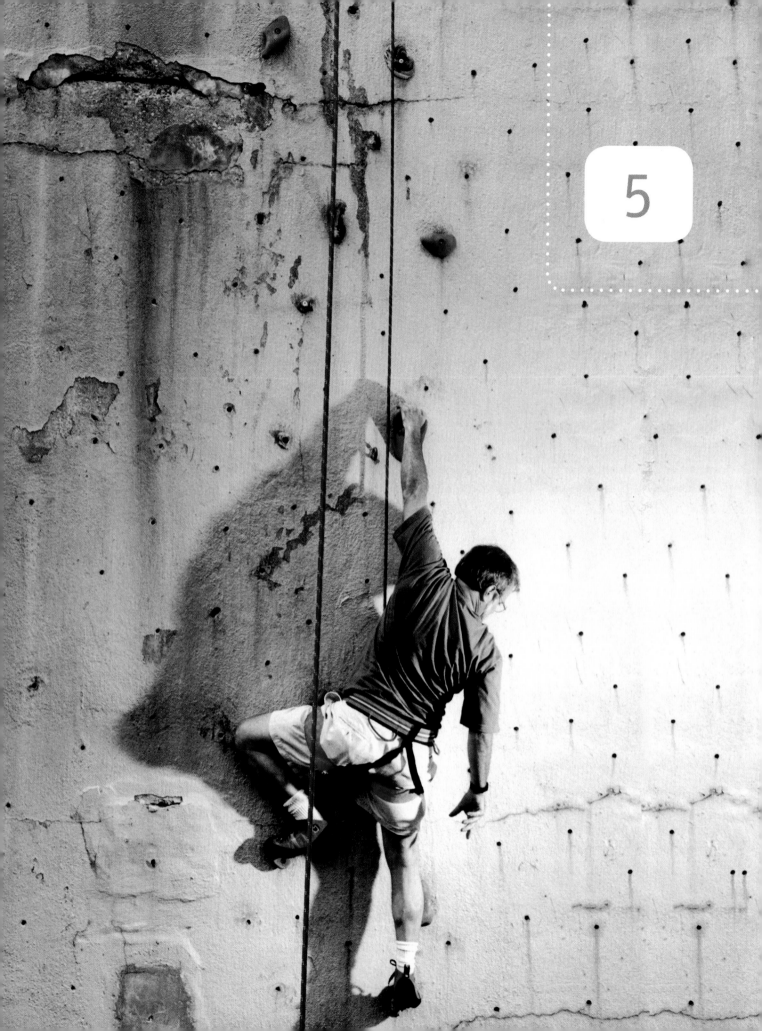

5

The Joy of Fitness

AS a boy, Derek never thought about doing anything special to stay physically fit. He loved sports so much that he spent every free moment on a softball field or basketball court. He could sprint faster, jump higher, and hit a ball harder than any of his friends. In high school Derek's life revolved around practices and games. He was a varsity athlete and a regional all-star.

Early in his first year in college, an injury sidelined Derek. Frustrated that he had to sit out the season, he gave up his rigorous training routine. As he became immersed in academics and other activities, Derek stopped going to the gym or working out on his own. Yet he continued to think of himself as an athlete in excellent physical condition. When Derek went home for spring break, he joined his younger brothers on a neighborhood basketball court. While he wasn't surprised that his long shots were off, Derek was amazed by how quickly he got winded. In fifteen minutes, he was panting for breath. "Getting old," one of his brothers joked. "Getting soft," the other teased.

Often the college years represent a turning point in physical fitness. Like Derek, many students, busy with classes and other commitments, devote less time to physical activity. About four in ten undergraduates do not participate in moderate or vigorous physical activity on a regular basis.[1]

The choices you make and the habits you develop now can affect how long and how well you'll live. As you'll see in this chapter, exercise yields immediate rewards: It boosts energy, improves mood, soothes stress, improves sleep, and makes you look and feel better. In the long term, physical activity slows many of the changes associated with chronological aging, such as loss of calcium and bone density, lowers the risk of serious chronic illnesses, and extends the lifespan.

This chapter can help you reap these rewards. It presents the latest activity recommendations, documents the benefits of exercise, describes types of exercise, and provides guidelines for getting into shape and exercising safely.

After studying the material in this chapter, you should be able to:

- **List** the five components of health-related fitness.
- **Describe** the health benefits of regular physical activity.
- **List** the different forms of cardiorespiratory activities and **describe** their potential health benefits and risks.
- **Explain** the benefits of a muscle training program and **describe** how to design a workout.
- **List** the potential health risks of strength-enhancing drugs and supplements.
- **Define** flexibility and describe the different types of stretching exercises.
- **Describe** the PRICE plan for handling an exercise injury.
- **Assess** yourself in the five components of health-related fitness, and **develop** a strategy to improve in at least two of them.

CENGAGENOW Log on to HealthNow at **academic.cengage.com/login** to find your Behavior Change Planner and to explore self-assessments, interactive tutorials, and practice quizzes.

You are designed to move. In ways far more complex than the fastest airplane or sleekest car, your body runs, stretches, bends, swims, climbs, glides, and strides—day after day, year after year, decade after decade. While mere machines break down from constant wear and tear, your body thrives on physical activity. The more you use your body, the stronger and healthier you can become.

What is Physical Fitness?

The simplest, most practical definition of **physical fitness** is the ability to respond to routine physical demands, with enough reserve energy to cope with a sudden challenge. You can consider yourself fit if you meet your daily energy needs; can handle unexpected extra demands; and are protecting yourself against potential health problems, such as heart disease. Fitness is important both for health and for athletic performance.

Health-Related Fitness

The five health-related components of physical fitness include aerobic or cardiorespiratory endurance, muscular strength, muscular endurance, flexibility, and body composition (the ratio of fat and lean body tissue).

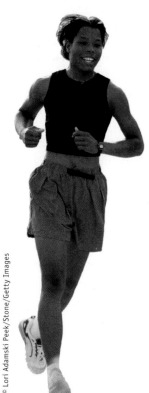

Fitness can enhance every dimension of your health—improving your mood and your mind as well as your body. Go for the joy!

Cardiorespiratory fitness refers to the ability of the heart to pump blood through the body efficiently. It is achieved through aerobic exercise—any activity, such as brisk walking or swimming, in which sufficient or excess oxygen is continually supplied to the body. In other words, aerobic exercise involves working out strenuously without pushing to the point of breathlessness.

Muscular strength refers to the force within muscles; it is measured by the absolute maximum weight that you can lift, push, or press in one effort. Strong muscles help keep the skeleton in proper alignment, improve posture, prevent back and leg aches, help in everyday lifting, and enhance athletic performance. Muscle mass increases along with strength, which makes for a healthier body composition and a higher metabolic rate.

Muscular endurance is the ability to perform repeated muscular effort; it is measured by counting how many times you can lift, push, or press a given weight. Important for posture, muscular endurance helps in everyday work as well as in athletics and sports.

Flexibility is the range of motion around specific joints—for example, the stretching you do to touch your toes or twist your torso. Flexibility depends on many factors: your age, gender, and posture; how muscular you are; and how much body fat you have. As children develop, their flexibility increases until adolescence. Then a gradual loss of joint mobility begins and continues throughout adult life. Both muscles and connective tissue, such as tendons and ligaments, shorten and become tighter if not consistently used through their full range of motion.

Body composition refers to the relative amounts of fat and lean tissue (bone, muscle, organs, water) in the body. As discussed in detail in Chapter 7, a high proportion of body fat has serious health implications, including increased incidence of heart disease, high blood pressure, diabetes, stroke, gallbladder problems, back and joint problems, and some forms of cancer.

Physical conditioning (or training) refers to the gradual building up of the body to enhance cardiorespiratory, or aerobic, fitness; muscular strength; muscular endurance; flexibility; and a healthy body composition.

Functional fitness, which is gaining greater emphasis among professional trainers, refers to the performance of activities of daily living. Exercises that mimic job tasks or everyday movements can improve an individual's balance, coordination, strength, and endurance.[2]

Athletic, or Performance-Related, Fitness

You may jog five miles, work out with weights, and start each day with a stretching routine. This doesn't qualify you for the soccer team. Most sports, such as softball, tennis, and basketball, require additional skills, including:

- **Agility,** the ability to change direction rapidly.

- **Balance,** or equilibrium, the ability to maintain a certain body position.

- **Coordination,** the ability to integrate the movement of body parts to produce smooth, fluid movements.

- **Power,** the product of force and speed.

- **Reaction time,** the time required to respond to a stimulus.

- **Speed,** or velocity, the ability to move rapidly.

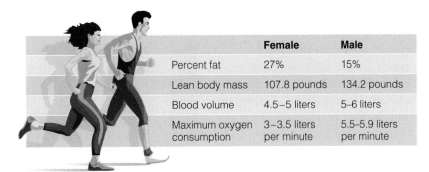

	Female	Male
Percent fat	27%	15%
Lean body mass	107.8 pounds	134.2 pounds
Blood volume	4.5–5 liters	5–6 liters
Maximum oxygen consumption	3–3.5 liters per minute	5.5–5.9 liters per minute

Figure 5.1 Physiological Differences Between Men and Women

While many amateur and professional athletes are in superb overall condition, you do not need athletic skills to keep your body operating at maximum capacity throughout life.

Fitness and the Dimensions of Health

The concept of fitness is evolving. Rather than focusing only on miles run or weight lifted, instructors, coaches, and consumers are pursuing a broader vision of total fitness that encompasses every dimension of health:

- **Physical.** As described later in this chapter, becoming fit reduces your risk of major diseases, increases energy and stamina, and may prolong your life.
- **Emotional.** Fitness lowers tension and anxiety, lifts depression, relieves stress, improves mood, and promotes a positive self-image.
- **Social.** Physical activities provide opportunities to meet new people and to work out with friends or family.
- **Intellectual.** Fit individuals report greater alertness, better concentration, more creativity, and improved personal health habits.
- **Occupational.** Fit employees miss fewer days of work, are more productive, and incur fewer medical costs.
- **Spiritual.** Fitness fosters appreciation for the relationship between body and mind and may lead to greater realization of your potential.
- **Environmental.** Fit individuals often become more aware of their need for healthy air and food and develop a deeper appreciation of the physical world.

Gender, Race, and Fitness

Men and women of all racial backgrounds benefit equally from fitness. However, there are some physiological differences between men and women, many of which are related to size.

 On average, men are 10 to 15 percent bigger than women, with roughly twice the percentage of muscle mass and half the percentage of body fat. They have more sweat glands and a greater maximum oxygen uptake. A man's bigger heart pumps more blood with each beat. His larger lungs take in 10 to 20 percent more oxygen (Figure 5.1). His longer legs cover more distance with each stride. If a man jogs along at 50 percent of his capacity, a woman has to push to 73 percent of hers to keep up.

 Women have a higher percentage of body fat than men, and more is distributed around the hips and thighs; men carry more body fat around the waist and stomach.

College-age men average 15 percent body fat; college-age women, 23 percent. On average, women have 11 percent more body fat and 8 percent less muscle mass than men.

The average woman has a smaller heart and blood volume than a man. Because women have a lower concentration of red blood cells, their bodies are less effective at transporting oxygen to their working muscles during exercise.

Even though training produces the same relative increases for both genders, a woman's maximum oxygen intake remains about 25 to 30 percent lower than that of an equally well-conditioned man. In elite athletes, the gender difference is smaller. Because the angle of the upper

physical fitness The ability to respond to routine physical demands, with enough reserve energy to cope with a sudden challenge.

cardiorespiratory fitness The ability of the heart and blood vessels to circulate blood through the body efficiently.

muscular strength Physical power; the maximum weight one can lift, push, or press in one effort.

muscular endurance The ability to withstand the stress of continued physical exertion.

flexibility The range of motion allowed by one's joints; determined by the length of muscles, tendons, and ligaments attached to the joints.

body composition The relative amounts of fat and lean tissue (bone, muscle, organs, water) in the body.

functional fitness The ability to perform real-life activities, such as lifting a heavy suitcase.

leg bone (femur) to the pelvis is greater in a woman, she is less efficient at running. Intense exercise provokes a rise in the stress hormone cortisol in men, but not women.[3]

In some endurance events, such as ultramarathon running and long-distance swimming, female anatomy and physiology may have some aerobic advantages. The longer a race—on land, water, or ice—the better women perform.

In absolute terms, men are 30 percent stronger, but gender differences in absolute strength do not apply to all muscle groups. Women have about 40 to 60 percent of the upper-body strength of men but 70 to 75 percent of the lower-body strength.

 Racial and ethnic backgrounds also influence fitness. Among women, physical fitness levels are similar between whites and blacks, but obesity is more common among African Americans. These findings suggest that if you are African American you may need to place even greater emphasis on improving your overall fitness to reduce your risk of heart disease.

The Inactivity Epidemic

One in four Americans reports no physical activity at all, according to the CDC. About half exercise occasionally, but not at the levels recommended by the National Center for Chronic Disease Prevention and Health Promotion. Fewer than one in four adults meets the levels of physical activity recommended by federal health officials.[4]

According to a national survey, about a third of adolescents and 14 percent of adults between ages 20 and 49 fall into the category of "low fitness" because they engage in little or no physical activity.[5] They are significantly more likely to develop diabetes, hypertension, and metabolic syndrome (discussed in Chapter 16) than those with higher fitness levels.

Many factors affect physical activity levels, including geographic location, gender, education, and income. According to the CDC, city-dwellers are more active than country folks, westerners more active than those in other regions. Men, people with higher education levels, and high-income earners work out more often.

How do Americans spend most of their leisure time? Watching television. We average more than 30 hours a week. Yet the more time spent in front of the TV, the greater the risk of obesity and related chronic diseases. Compared with other sedentary activities, such as reading, writing, or driving, watching TV lowers metabolic rate, so people burn fewer calories.

The Toll of Sedentary Living

Sedentary living claims some 250,000 lives, accounting for 10 percent of all deaths in America every year, and contributes to four of the six leading causes of death:

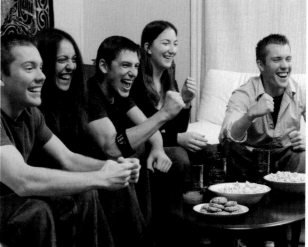

Watching football often replaces playing it when high school students go to college. Students exercise less with each succeeding year.

heart disease, cancer, stroke, and diabetes.[6] Inactivity doubles the risk of cardiorespiratory diseases, diabetes, and obesity and increases the risk of colon cancer, high blood pressure, osteoporosis, depression, and anxiety. As a risk factor for heart disease, physical inactivity ranks as high as elevated cholesterol, high blood pressure, or cigarette smoking.

Working Out on Campus: Student Bodies in Motion

 College students aren't necessarily more active or fit than the general population. (See "Reality Check" in this chapter.) Men are generally more active than women; Caucasians, Native Americans/Alaska Natives, and Native Hawaiians/Pacific Islanders are more active than other ethnic or racial groups. Full-time students and those without jobs exercise more than part-time or employed students. Undergraduates living on campus are more active than those living off campus; students living in fraternity or sorority housing engage in more exercise than those living in a house or an apartment. Single students report more days of vigorous workouts than married, divorced, or separated ones. How do you compare?[7]

As students progress from their first to fourth year of studies, they exercise less. The most drastic drop in physical activity occurs in the freshman year. In a recent study, physical fitness declined, and levels of total cholesterol, harmful LDL (low-density lipoprotein) cholesterol, and fasting glucose (blood sugar) levels increased over undergraduate's first 14-week school term.[8] (See Chapter 16 for a complete discussion of these risk factors for heart disease.)

Students are somewhat more active on exercise-friendly campuses that rank high in characteristics such as bike-

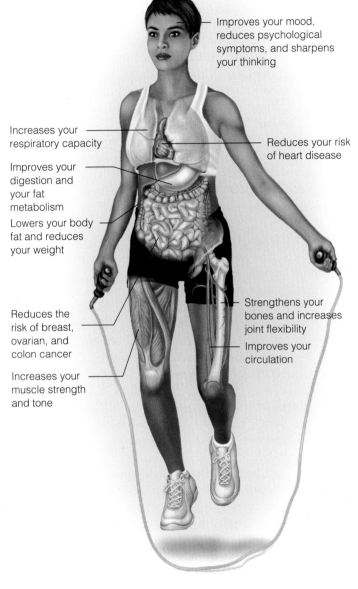

Improves your mood, reduces psychological symptoms, and sharpens your thinking

Increases your respiratory capacity

Improves your digestion and your fat metabolism

Lowers your body fat and reduces your weight

Reduces the risk of breast, ovarian, and colon cancer

Increases your muscle strength and tone

Reduces your risk of heart disease

Strengthens your bones and increases joint flexibility

Improves your circulation

Figure 5.2 The Benefits of Exercise

Regular physical activity enhances your overall physical and mental health and helps prevent disease.

know. In a survey, eight in ten undergraduates realized that physical activity can prevent heart disease and prevent and treat obesity. However, fewer than half knew that it maintains bone density and can help prevent diabetes.

As Figure 5.2 illustrates, exercise provides head-to-toe benefits. With regular activity, your heart muscles become stronger and pump blood more efficiently. Your heart rate and resting pulse slow down. Your blood pressure may drop slightly from its normal level.

Exercise thickens the bones and can slow the loss of calcium that normally occurs with age. Physical activity increases flexibility in the joints and improves digestion and elimination. It speeds up metabolism and builds lean body mass, so the body burns more calories and body fat decreases. It heightens sensitivity to insulin (a great benefit for diabetics) and may lower the risk of developing diabetes. In addition, exercise enhances clot-dissolving substances in the blood, helping to prevent strokes, heart attacks, and pulmonary embolisms (clots in the lungs), and it helps lower the risk of certain cancers. Regular exercise can actually extend your lifespan and sharpen your memory and mind.

Even your eyes benefit from physical activity. Individuals who exercise three or more times a week may reduce by 70 percent their risk of age-related macular degeneration, which destroys the sharp central vision needed for tasks such as reading and driving.[11]

Healthier Heart and Lungs

Regular physical activity makes blood less likely to clot and cause a stroke or heart attack. Sedentary people are about twice as likely to die of a heart attack as people who are physically active. Although rigorous exercise somewhat increases the risk of sudden cardiac death for men, regular physical activity lowers the overall danger, especially in women. (See Chapter 16 for a discussion of heart disease.)

Exercise also lowers levels of the indicators of increased risk of heart disease, such as high cholesterol and C-reactive protein, which are discussed in Chapter 16. Exercise itself, even without weight loss, may reduce the risk of developing

ability, an appealing neighborhood, perceived safety from traffic, and proximity to local shops.[9] However, even when campuses offer recreational facilities such as hiking trails and tennis courts, many students—particularly freshmen—are unaware of them.[10]

Physical Activity and Health

Why Exercise?

If exercise could be packed into a pill, it would be the single most widely prescribed and beneficial medicine in the nation. Why? Because nothing can do more to help your body function at its best—a fact that not all students

REALITYCHECK

PART II: *Just the Facts*

- **44** *percent of college students exercised—either vigorously for at least 20 minutes or moderately for at least 30 minutes—on three or more of the last seven days.*
- **48** *percent of students exercised to strengthen or tone their muscles at least two of the last seven days.*
- **55** *percent of students—44 percent of men and 63 percent of women—exercise to lose weight.*

Source: American College Health Association. "American College Health Association National College Health Assessment Spring 2006 Reference Group Data Report (Abridged)." *Journal of American College Health,* Vol. 55, No. 4, January–February 2007, pp. 195–206.

the prediabetic condition called metabolic syndrome, which if untreated can lead to type 2 diabetes and increase the risk of heart disease.

In addition to its effects on the heart, exercise makes the lungs more efficient. The lungs take in more oxygen, and their vital capacity (the maximum amount of air volume the lungs can take in and expel) increases, providing more energy for you to use.

Even in young men, physical fitness is associated with improvements in blood pressure and the makeup of blood fats, including cholesterol and triglycerides. Exercise, along with a healthy weight, keeps blood fats at healthy levels over time. Prolonged, sustained endurance training prevents the stiffening of the heart muscle once thought to be an inevitable consequence of aging.

Protection Against Cancer

Physical activity lowers the likelihood of getting some forms of cancer and, according to preliminary research, may lessen the risk of recurrence or a second cancer.[12] According to the American Institute for Cancer Research, physical activity may lower the risk of colon cancer by 40 to 50 percent, the risk of breast, endometrial, and lung cancers by 30 to 40 percent, and the risk of prostate cancer by 10 to 30 percent.

Among breast cancer survivors, the equivalent of walking three to five hours a week cuts the risk of recurrence in half, compared with those who exercise less than one hour per week. Women who exercised regularly in the year before a diagnosis of breast cancer have higher survival rates than sedentary women. Exercise also lowers the risk of recurrence in colon cancer, perhaps by lowering levels of substances such as insulin and insulin-like growth factor that drive the growth of cancer cells.[13]

Less Risk of Disease

Exercise may enhance immune function by reducing stress hormones like cortisol that can dampen resistance to disease. Women who walk briskly for 35 to 45 minutes five days a week experience half the number of sick days with cold symptoms as inactive women. While moderate exercise seems to bolster a person's immune system, heavy training may increase the risk of upper respiratory tract infections for endurance athletes.

An increase in physical activity can prevent type 2 diabetes even in those at high risk of developing the disease. In studies of high-risk individuals who exercised, took medication, or did nothing, those who became more active had the lowest incidence of diabetes.[14]

Brighter Mood

Exercise makes people feel good from the inside out. Exercise boosts mood, elevates self-esteem, increases energy, reduces anxiety, improves concentration and alertness, enables people to handle stress better, and may help ward off dementia.[15] During long workouts, some people experience what is called "runner's high," which may be the result of increased levels of mood-elevating brain chemicals called **endorphins.**

Better Mental Health and Functioning

Exercise is an effective—but underused—treatment for mild to moderate depression and may help in treating other mental disorders. Regular, moderate exercise, such as walking, running, or lifting weights, three times a week, has proved helpful for depression and anxiety disorders, including panic attacks. Exercise is as effective as medication in improving mood and also helps prevent relapse.

Lifelong fitness may protect the brain as we age. According to numerous long-term studies, physically fit adults perform better on cognitive tests than their less fit peers.[16] Improving cardiorespiratory fitness reduces the harmful effects of aging on brain structures as well as on memory and other functions.

Better Bones

By 2020, one in two Americans over age 50 may suffer from **osteoporosis**—a condition in which bones lose their mineral density and become susceptible to injury. Most are unaware that their bone health is in jeopardy. Four times as many men and almost three times as many women actually have osteoporosis than realize they do. (See Chapter 20 for more on osteoporosis and aging.)

 You may think that weak, brittle bones are a problem only for the elderly. However, 2 percent of college-age women have osteoporosis; another 15 percent have already sustained significant losses in bone density and are at high risk of osteoporosis.

Exercise during adolescence and young adulthood may prevent bone weakening and fractures in old age. Women who did not participate in high school sports are seven times more likely to have low bone density than those who did. The college women at greatest risk often are extremely skinny and maintain their low weights and slim looks by dieting and by avoiding exercise so as not to increase their muscle mass. Some eliminate dairy products, an important source of calcium, from their diets. Depo-Provera, a method of birth control that consists of hormone injections every three months, also is associated with low bone density, especially with long-term use. (See Chapter 10 on contraception.)

 What are the best exercises to boost bone density? According to a study of college women, high-impact aerobics, such as step exercising, "may offer the quickest route to building bone in young women." Resistance exercises such as squats, leg presses, and calf presses strengthened leg muscles but had no effect on bone density.[17] The American College of Sports Medicine recommends moderate-to-high-intensity weight-bearing activities to maintain bone mass in adults (Table 5.1).[18]

Lower Weight

For individuals on a diet, exercise provides extra benefits: A combination of dietary change and moderate- to high-level intensity exercise leads to greater weight loss than either alone. Dieters who work out lose more fat than lean muscle tissue, which improves their body composition.

 College-age men who start exercising lose abdominal fat, which poses the greatest risk to health. (See Chapter 7 for information on exercise and weight control.)

Table 5.1 Rx: Healthy Bones

Mode	Intensity	Frequency	Duration
Weight-bearing endurance activities, such as tennis and jogging; activities that involve jumping; and resistance exercise, such as weight lifting	Moderate to high	Weight-bearing activities, 3 to 5 times per week; resistance exercise, 2 or 3 times per week	30 to 60 minutes

Source: "Physical Activity and Bone Health." Position Stand, American College of Sports Medicine, www.acsm-/msse.org.

Sexuality

By improving physical endurance, muscle tone, blood flow, and body composition, exercise improves sexual functioning. Simply burning 200 extra calories a day can significantly lower the risk of erectile dysfunction in sedentary men. Exercise also may increase sexual drive, activity, and sexual satisfaction in people of all ages. In a recent study of about 400 students at a southeastern university, college students who exercise frequently and see themselves as physically fit rate themselves higher with regard to sexual performance and sexual desirability than those who exercise less and don't describe themselves as fit. All the men who exercised six to seven days per week rated their sexual desirability as above or much above average.[19]

In one recent study, physically fit men over age 55 reported higher levels of sexual desirability and better sexual performance than those who weren't in good shape. High fitness levels made women feel more sexually desirable but did not affect their sexual performance.[20]

Benefits for Students

Unlike middle-aged and older individuals, traditional-age college students cite improved fitness as the number-one advantage that exercise offers, followed by improved appearance and muscle tone. Undergraduates who recognize the benefits of exercise are more likely to be physically active than those who focus on barriers to working out.

Will exercise improve your grades? Not necessarily. A study at two Texas universities found that the fittest students didn't necessarily have higher GPAs. However, increasing their level of physical fitness did have a positive impact on the GPAs of the female students.

A More Active Old Age

Exercise slows the changes that are associated with advancing age: loss of lean muscle tissue, increase in body fat, and decrease in work capacity. In addition to lowering the risk of heart disease and stroke, exercise also helps older men and women retain the strength and mobility needed to live independently. Even in old age, exercise boosts strength and stamina, lessens time in wheelchairs, and improves outlook and sense of control.

Longer Life

People who exercise regularly enjoy 3.7 years of additional life expectancy when compared with sedentary

endorphins Mood-elevating, pain-killing chemicals produced by the brain.

osteoporosis A condition common in older people in which the bones become increasingly soft and porous, making them susceptible to injury.

individuals.[21] Formerly sedentary people, even the elderly, who begin to exercise live longer, on average, than those who remain inactive. However, for active people, light to moderate exercise won't do it—only vigorous exercise reduces the risk of dying of heart disease and of premature death from other causes.

New Exercise Guidelines

In 2007 the American College of Sports Medicine (ACSM) and the American Heart Association (AHA) updated the physical activity guidelines for Americans. For healthy adults under age 65, they recommend:

Moderately intense cardiorespiratory exercise
30 minutes a day, 5 days a week
or
Vigorously intense cardiorespiratory exercise
20 minutes a day, 3 days a week
and

8 to 10 strength-training exercises, with 8 to 12 repetitions of each exercise, twice a week.

According to the ACSM, moderate-intensity physical activity means working hard enough to raise your heart rate and break a sweat, yet still being able to carry on a conversation. The 30-minute recommendation is for the average healthy adult to maintain health and reduce the risk for chronic disease. To lose weight or maintain weight loss, 60 to 90 minutes of physical activity may be necessary.[27]

The new guidelines, based on more than a decade of research, clearly state the recommended aerobic activity should be in addition to the routine activities of daily life, such as house cleaning. However, vigorous activities, such as shoveling snow, do count as exercise. The new recommendations are a minimum requirement for maintaining good health. More exercise can produce more benefits. The recommendations for adults older than 65 include balance exercises if they are at risk of falling and developing a physical activity plan.[28]

Your Life Change Coach

Motivating Yourself to Move

Before you move a muscle, you need to be motivated. You may never even have thought about becoming more active. You may be thinking about getting into shape—someday. You may exercise, but not on a regular basis. Or you may have the best intentions but get too busy, stressed, or tired to work out. (See the "Excise Exercise Excuses" lab in *IPC*.) **IPC**

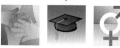

Gender and culture influence students' motivation to exercise and to enroll in fitness and wellness classes. Undergraduates in elective physical education classes cite having fun, staying active, and improving fitness as reasons for taking the courses.[22] College men say they choose fitness or wellness classes because they enjoy physical activity and want an opportunity to socialize.[23] Women consistently rank weight management as a greater incentive than men. In China, students report highly specific reasons for becoming more physically active,[24] while in Taiwan, the fittest students are most motivated to take more physical education courses.[25]

What would most motivate you to get moving? Take the Self-Survey at the end of this chapter to identify your readiness to become more active. Then try the following strategies to follow through:

• Work out with friends. If given a choice between exercising alone, with younger or older people, or with individuals their own age, most adults would rather exercise with others in their same age group.[26] Make regular dates to meet at the gym or a cardio class at the recreation center. Even if it's rainy and cold, you'll go if you know someone is waiting for you.

• Keep your athletic gear in a locker in the gym or in the trunk of your car so you can fit a workout into the breaks in your schedule. Build in time to walk or bike to class rather than take a bus or campus shuttle.

• Find a fun workout. Vary your usual activities with something new and challenging, like cardio kick-boxing, ice skating, or swing dancing.

• Sign up for a fitness class, such as spinning or step aerobics, so that exercise is built into your weekly schedule.

• Join a team—or root for one. College sports, whether competitive or informal, can help maintain fitness levels. So can cheerleading, which has become so physically demanding that college cheerleaders score as high in fitness levels as student athletes.

The Principles of Exercise

Your body is literally what you make of it. Superbly designed for multiple uses, it adjusts to meet physical demands. If you need to sprint for a bus, your heart will speed up and pump more blood. Beyond such immediate, short-term adaptations, physical training can produce long-term changes in heart rate, oxygen consumption, and muscle strength and endurance. Although there are limits on the maximum levels of physical fitness and performance that any individual can achieve, regular exercise can produce improvements in everyone's baseline wellness and fitness.

The following principles of exercise are fundamental to any physical activity plan:

Overload Principle

The **overload principle** requires a person exercising to provide a greater stress or demand on the body than it's usually accustomed to handling. For any muscle, including the heart, to get stronger, it must work against a greater-than-normal resistance or challenge. To continue to improve, you need further increases in the demands-but not too much too quickly. **Progressive overloading**—gradually

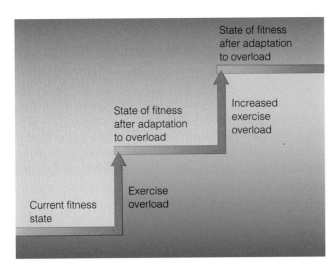

Figure 5.3 The Overload Principle

By increasing frequency, intensity, or duration, you will improve your level of fitness. Once your body adapts (becomes comfortable) to the demands, you can again apply the overload principle to achieve a higher level of fitness.

increasing physical challenges—provides the benefits of exercise without the risk of injuries (Figure 5.3).

Overloading is specific to each body part and to each component of fitness. Leg exercises develop only the lower limbs; arm exercises, only the upper limbs. This is why you need a comprehensive fitness plan that includes a variety of exercises to develop different parts of the body. If you play a particular sport, you also need training to develop sports-specific skills, such as a strong, efficient stroke in swimming.

FITT

Although low-intensity activity can enhance basic health, you need to work harder—that is, at a greater intensity—to improve fitness. Whatever exercise you do, there is a level, or threshold, at which fitness begins to improve; a target zone, where you can achieve maximum benefits; and an upper limit, at which potential risks outweigh any further benefits. The acronym **FITT** sums up the four dimensions of progressive overload: *frequency* (how often you exercise), *intensity* (how hard), *time* (how long), and *type* (specific activity).

Frequency

To attain and maintain physical fitness, you need to exercise regularly, but the recommended frequency varies with different types of exercise and with an individual's fitness goals. Health officials urge Americans to engage in moderate-intensity aerobic activity most days and in resistance and flexibility training two or three days a week.

Intensity

Exercise intensity varies with the type of exercise and with personal goals. To improve cardiorespiratory fitness, you need at a minimum to increase your heart rate to a target zone (the level that produces benefits). To develop muscular strength and endurance, you need to

overload principle Providing a greater stress or demand on the body than it is normally accustomed to handling.

progressive overloading Gradually increasing physical challenges once

the body adapts to the stress placed upon it to produce maximum benefits.

FITT A formula that describes the frequency, intensity, type, and length of time for physical activity.

increase the amount of weight you lift or the resistance you work against and/or the number of repetitions. For enhanced flexibility, you need to stretch muscles beyond their normal length.

Time (Duration)

The amount of time, or duration, of your workouts is also important, particularly for cardiorespiratory exercise. The American College of Sports Medicine recommends 30 to 45 minutes of aerobic exercise, preceded by 5 to 10 minutes of warm-up and followed by 5 to 10 minutes of stretching. However, experts have found similar health benefits from a single 30-minute session of moderate exercise as from several shorter sessions throughout the day. Duration and intensity are interlinked. If you're exercising at high intensity (biking or running at a brisk pace, for instance), you don't need to exercise as long as when you're working at lower intensity (walking or swimming at a moderate pace). For muscular strength and endurance and for flexibility, duration is defined by the number of sets or repetitions rather than total time.

Type (Specificity)

The **specificity principle** refers to the body's adaptation to a particular type of activity or amount of stress placed upon it. Jogging, for instance, trains the heart and lungs to work more efficiently and strengthens certain leg muscles. However, it does not build upper body strength or enhance flexibility.

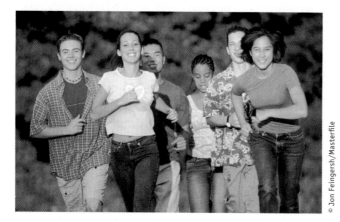

The goal of exercise isn't to become a competitive athlete but to improve your well-being and achieve your maximum fitness potential.

Reversibility Principle

The **reversibility principle** is the opposite of the overload principle. Just as the body adapts to greater physical demands, it also adjusts to lower levels. If you stop exercising, you can lose as much as 50 percent of your fitness improvements within two months. If you have to curtail your usual exercise routine because of a busy schedule, you can best maintain your fitness by keeping the inten-

sity constant and reducing frequency or duration. The principle of reversibility is aptly summed up by the phrase, "Use it or lose it."

How Much Exercise Is Enough?

The answer depends on your exercise goal: fitness or health. Both are related but not the same. Fit people, as epidemiological studies have shown, are healthy people with reduced risks of heart disease, hypertension, stroke, and diabetes and a lower mortality rate. Yet it is possible to get nearly all the health benefits of exercise without reaching high levels of fitness.[29]

Dozens of studies have shown dramatic benefits from moderate exercise. For example, gardening or walking at least one hour a week lowers the risk of sudden cardiac death. Walking for several hours a week lowers the risk of stroke, heart attack, and cardiac death. Even small amounts of physical exercise (approximately 75 minutes a week in a study of postmenopausal women of normal weight)[30] can improve fitness levels. But if a little exercise is good, more may be better.

While half an hour of exercise five days a week is good, working out more often and more intensely can yield more health dividends, including improved muscular strength and endurance. You may also need to exercise longer and harder to maintain a healthy weight and lose excess pounds. According to the Exercise Guidelines for Americans, individuals who've lost weight may need to exercise 60 to 90 minutes a day to keep off the pounds. Vigorous physical activity (such as jogging or spinning) burns calories more rapidly per unit of time than moderate activities like walking. It doesn't matter if your goal is to improve fitness or avoid fatness. The same strategy—regular physical activity—is the key to both.

Improving Cardiorespiratory Fitness

Cardiorespiratory endurance refers to the ability of the heart, lungs, and circulatory system to deliver oxygen to muscles working rhythmically over an extended period of time. Unlike muscular endurance (discussed later in this chapter), which is specific to individual muscles, cardiorespiratory endurance involves the entire body. **Aerobic exercise,** which improves cardiorespiratory endurance, can take many forms, but all involve working strenuously without pushing to the point of breathlessness. A person who builds up good aerobic capacity can maintain long periods of physical activity without great fatigue.

In **anaerobic exercise,** the amount of oxygen taken in by the body cannot meet the demands of the activity. This quickly creates an oxygen deficit that must be made up later. Anaerobic activities are high in intensity but short in duration, usually lasting only about ten seconds to two minutes. An example is sprinting the quarter-mile, which leaves even the best-trained athletes gasping for air. In *nonaerobic exercise*, such as bowling, softball, or doubles tennis, there is frequent rest between activities. Because the body can take in all the oxygen it needs, the heart and lungs don't get much of a workout.

Are You Working Hard Enough?

A variety of methods can indicate if you're exercising hard enough to condition your heart and lungs, but not overdoing it. Each of the following methods has both advantages and limitations. Fitness experts advise combining two methods—an objective one like target heart rate, for instance, and a subjective one like the talk test—to assess the intensity of your aerobic workouts.

Target Heart Rate

To use your pulse, or heart rate, as a guide, feel your pulse in the carotid artery in your neck. Slightly tilt your head back and to one side. Use your middle finger or forefinger, or both, to feel for your pulse. (Do not use your thumb; it has a beat of its own.) To determine your heart rate, count the number of pulses you feel for 10 seconds and multiply that number by six, or count for 30 seconds and multiply that number by two. Learn to recognize the pulsing of your heart when you're sitting or lying down. This is your **resting heart rate.**

Start taking your pulse during, or immediately after, exercise, when it's much more pronounced than when you're at rest. Three minutes after heavy exercise, take your pulse again. The closer that reading is to your resting heart rate, the better your condition. If it takes a long time for your pulse to recover and return to its resting level, your body's ability to handle physical stress is poor. As you continue working out, however, your pulse will return to normal much more quickly.

You don't want to push yourself to your maximum heart rate, yet you must exercise at about 60 to 85 percent of that maximum to get cardiorespiratory benefits from your training. This range is called your **target heart rate.** If you don't exercise intensely enough to raise your heart rate at least this high, your heart and lungs won't reap the most benefit from the workout. If you push too hard, and exercise at or near your absolute maximum heart rate, you run the risk of placing too great a burden on your heart. Figure 5.4 shows the target heart rate for various ages and activities. Find your age at the bottom of the figure and move up the grid to find your target heart rate for "aerobic workout."

You can also use the following steps to determine your maximum heart rate and target heart rate (in beats per minute):

1. Maximum heart rate: Subtract your age from 220. So if you are 20, your maximum heart rate is $220 - 20 = 200$ beats per minute.

2. Lower-limit target heart rate: Multiply your maximum heart rate by 0.6. So if you are 20, your lower-limit target heart rate is $200 \times 0.6 = 120$ beats per minute.

3. Upper-limit target heart rate. Multiply your maximum heart rate by 0.85. If you are 20, your upper-limit target heart range is $200 \times 0.85 = 170$.

Your target heart rate range is between your lower and upper limits.

According to the American College of Sports Medicine, for most people, exercising at the lower end of the target heart rate range for a long time is more beneficial than exercising at the higher end of the range for a short time. If your goal is losing weight, exercise at 60 to 70 percent of your maximum heart rate in order to burn fat calories. To improve aerobic endurance and strengthen your heart, work at 70 to 80 percent of your maximum heart rate. Competitive athletes may train at 80 to 100 percent of their maximum heart rate (Figure 5.4).

Rating of Perceived Exertion (RPE)

Another option besides heart rate for monitoring your exercise intensity is the **Rating of Perceived Exertion (RPE),** a self-assessment scale that rates symptoms of breathlessness and fatigue. You can use the RPE scale to describe your sensation of effort when exercising and gauge how hard you are working. The American College of Sports Medicine revised the original RPE scale to a range of 0 to 10 (Figure 5.5). Most exercisers should aim for a perceived exertion of "somewhat strong" or "strong," the equivalent of 4 or 5 on the RPE scale.

RPE is considered fairly reliable, but about 10 percent of the population tends to over- or underestimate their exertion. Your health or physical education instructor can help you learn to match what your body is feeling to the RPE scale. By paying attention to how you feel at different exercise intensities, you can learn how to challenge yourself without risking your safety.

---

specificity principle Each part of the body adapts to a particular type and amount of stress placed upon it.

reversibility principle The physical benefits of exercise are lost through disuse or inactivity.

aerobic exercise Physical activity in which sufficient or excess oxygen is continually supplied to the body.

anaerobic exercise Physical activity in which the body develops an oxygen deficit.

resting heart rate The number of heartbeats per minute during inactivity.

target heart rate Sixty to eighty-five percent of the maximum heart rate; the heart rate at which one derives maximum cardiovascular benefit from aerobic exercise.

Rating of Perceived Exertion (RPE) A self-assessment scale that rates symptoms of breathlessness and fatigue.

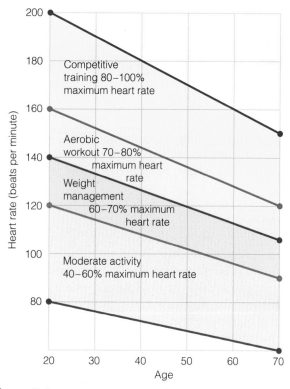

Figure 5.4 Target Heart Rates for Different Ages and Various Levels of Activity

Your maximum heart rate is 220 minus your age.

Rating of Perceived Exertion (RPE)	
0 Nothing at all	
0.5 Extremely weak (just noticeable)	
1 Very weak	
2 Weak (light)	
3 Moderate	
4 Somewhat strong	Correlate to target heart rate
5 Strong (heavy)	
6 —	
7 Very strong	
8 —	
9 —	
10 Extremely strong (almost maximum)	

Figure 5.5 Revised Scale for Rating of Perceived Exertion (RPE)

You can learn to rate your exertion based on this scale.

Source: Original scale from Borg, G. "Psychophysical Bases of Perceived Exertion." *Medicine and Science in Sports and Exercise*, Vol. 14, No. 5, 2003, pp. 377–381.

You can also experiment with other alternative ways for determining exercise intensity. One of the easiest follows.

"Talk Test"

During "aerobic" exercise you should be able to carry on a somewhat stilted conversation if you are indeed "with oxygen"—which is what the word "aerobic" means.

If you are gasping for air and unable to talk, you are most likely working at or beyond the anaerobic "without oxygen" threshold—a very, very, very hard intensity level at or beyond the high end of the aerobic zone.

If you can sing the entire Star Spangled Banner, you are probably not exerting much effort. If you can sing "Row Row Row Your Boat," but have to take a breath after every other word, you are probably working pretty hard—and just where you should be.

Designing an Aerobic Workout

Whatever activity you choose, your aerobic workout should consist of several stages: a warm-up, an aerobic activity, and a cool-down.

Warm-Up

Just as you don't get in your car and immediately gun your engine to 60 miles per hour, you shouldn't do the same with your body. You need to prepare your cardiorespiratory system for a workout, speed up the blood flow to your lungs, and increase the temperature and elasticity of your muscles and connective tissue to avoid injury.

After reviewing more than 350 scientific studies, the American College of Sports Medicine concluded that preparing for sports or exercise should involve a variety of activities and not be limited to stretching alone. They found little to no relationship between stretching and injuries or postexercise pain. A better option is a combination of warm-up, strength training, and balance exercises.

Aerobic Activity

The two key components of this part of your workout are intensity and duration. As described in the previous section, you can use your target heart rate range to make sure you are working at the proper intensity. The current recommendation is to keep moving for 30 to 60 minutes, either in one session or several briefer sessions, each lasting at least 10 minutes.

Cool-Down

After you've pushed your heart rate up to its target level and kept it there for a while, the worst thing you can do is slam on the brakes. If you come to a sudden stop, you put your heart at risk. When you stand or sit immediately after vigorous exercise, blood can pool in your legs. You need to keep moving at a slower pace to ensure an adequate supply of blood to your heart. Ideally, you should walk for 5 to 10 minutes at a comfortable pace before you end your workout session.

Your Long-Term Fitness Plan

One of the most common mistakes people make is to push too hard too fast. Often they end up injured or discouraged and quit entirely. If you are just starting an aerobic program, think of it as a series of phases: beginning, progression, and maintenance:

- **Beginning (4–6 weeks).** Start slow and low (in intensity). If you're walking, monitor your heart rate and aim for 55 percent of your maximum heart rate. Another good rule of thumb to make sure you're moving at the right pace: If you can sing as you walk, you're going too slow; if you can't talk, you're going too fast.

- **Progression (16–20 weeks).** Gradually increase the duration and/or intensity of your workouts. For instance, you might add 5 minutes every two weeks to your walking time. You also can gradually pick up your pace, using your target heart rate as your guide. Keep a log of your workouts so you can chart your progress until you reach your goal.

- **Maintenance (lifelong).** Once you've reached the stage of exercising for an hour every day, you may want to develop a repertoire of aerobic activities you enjoy. Combine or alternate activities to avoid monotony and keep up your enthusiasm (cross-training).

Aerobic Options

You have lots of choices for aerobic exercise, so experiment. Focus on one for a few weeks; alternate different activities on different days; try something new every month.

Stepping Out: Walk the Walk

More men and women are taking to their feet. Some are casualties of high-intensity sports and can no longer withstand the wear and tear of rigorous workouts. Others want to shape up, slim down, or ward off heart disease and other health problems. The good news for all is that walking is good exercise. Walking may reduce the risk of cardiorespiratory disease as much as vigorous activity does. Figure 5.6 shows good walking technique.

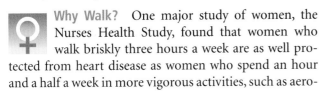 **Why Walk?** One major study of women, the Nurses Health Study, found that women who walk briskly three hours a week are as well protected from heart disease as women who spend an hour and a half a week in more vigorous activities, such as aero-

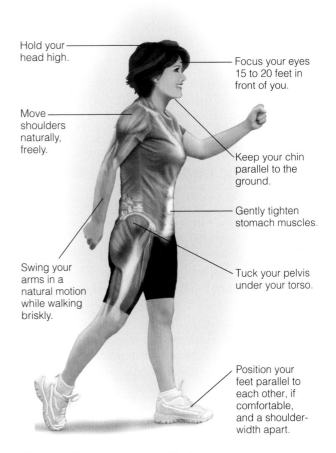

Figure 5.6 Good Walking Technique

bics or running. Women engaged in either form of exercise had a rate of heart attacks 30 to 40 percent lower than that of sedentary women.

Walking also protects men's hearts, whether they're healthy or have had heart problems. Men who regularly engage in light exercise, including walking, have a significantly lower risk of death than their sedentary counterparts.

Walking has proved to be one of the safest and most effective ways of preventing bone and joint disorders in obese individuals.

America on the Move How many steps do you walk every day? The typical adult averages about 5,310 steps; a child from 11,000 to 13,000. According to the American College of Sports Medicine, college students who used a pedometer to count their daily steps took an average of 7,700 steps per day. This falls short of the 10,000 steps recommended as part of the national "America on the Move" program.

How far is 10,000 steps? The average person's stride length is approximately 2.5 feet long. That means it takes just over 2,000 steps to walk 1 mile, and 10,000 steps is

YOUR STRATEGIES FOR CHANGE *The Right Way to Walk and Run*

Here are some guidelines for putting your best foot forward, whether you are walking or running:

- Take time to warm up.
- Maintain good posture. Keep your back straight, your head up, and your eyes looking straight ahead. Hold your arms slightly away from your body—your elbows should be bent slightly so that your forearms are almost parallel to the ground.

- Use the heel-to-toe method. The heel of your leading foot should touch the ground before the ball or toes of that foot do. Push off the ball of your foot, and bend your knee as you raise your heel. You should be able to feel the action in your calf muscles.
- Pump your arms back and forth. This burns more calories and gives you an upper-body workout as well.

- Do not walk or run on the balls of your feet. This produces soreness in the calves because the muscles must contract for a longer time. Avoid running on hard surfaces and making sudden stops and turns.
- End your walk or run with a cool-down period. Let your pace become more leisurely for the last 5 minutes.

close to 5 miles. Wearing a pedometer is an easy way to track your steps each day. Start by wearing the pedometer every day for one week. Put it on when you get up in the morning and wear it until bedtime. Record your daily steps in a log or diary. By the end of the week, you can calculate your average daily steps. To increase your steps, add 500 daily steps every week until you reach 10,000.

Why 10,000 steps? According to researchers' estimates, you take about 5,000 steps just to accomplish your daily tasks. Adding about 2,000 steps brings you to a level that can improve your health and wellness. Another 3,000 steps can help you lose excess pounds and prevent weight gain. People who walk at least 10,000 steps a day are more likely to have healthy weights. In addition, 10,000 steps generally translates into 30 minutes of activity, the minimum recommended by the U.S. Surgeon General.

Counting steps with a pedometer pays off. In one study, women who used a pedometer walked substantially more than those who simply tried to take a 30-minute brisk walk on most days.[31]

Treadmills are a good alternative to outdoor walks—and not just in bad weather. They keep you moving at a certain pace, they're easier on the knees, and they allow you to exercise in a climate-controlled, pollution-free environment—a definite plus for many city dwellers. Holding onto the handrails while walking on a treadmill reduces both heart rate and oxygen consumption, so you burn fewer calories. Experts advise slowing the pace if necessary so you can let go of the handrails while working out.

Jogging and Running

The difference between jogging and running is speed. You should be able to carry on a conversation with someone on a long jog or run; if you're too breathless to talk, you're pushing too hard.

If your goal is to enhance aerobic fitness, long, slow, distance running is best. If you want to improve your speed, try *interval training*—repeated hard runs over a certain distance, with intervals of relaxed jogging in between. Depending on what suits you and what your training goals are, you can vary the distance, duration, and number of fast runs, as well as the time and activity between them.

If you have been sedentary, it's best to launch a walking program before attempting to jog or run. Start by walking for 15 to 20 minutes three times a week at a comfortable pace. Continue at this same level until you no longer feel sore or unduly fatigued the day after exercising. Then increase your walking time to 20 to 25 minutes, speeding up your pace as well.

When you can handle a brisk 25-minute walk, alternate fast walking with slow jogging. Begin each session walking, and gradually increase the amount of time you spend jogging. If you feel breathless while jogging, slow down and walk. Continue to alternate in this manner until you can jog for 10 minutes without stopping. If you gradually increase your jogging time by 1 or 2 minutes with each workout, you'll slowly build up to 20 or 25 minutes per session. For optimal fitness, you should jog at least three times a week.

Be sure you're running right; see Your Strategies for Change "The Right Way to Walk and Run."

Other Aerobic Activities

Because variety is the spice of an active life, many people prefer different forms of aerobic exercise. All can provide many health benefits. Among the popular options:

- **Swimming.** For aerobic conditioning, you have to swim laps using the freestyle, butterfly, breaststroke, or backstroke. (The sidestroke is too easy.) You must also be a good enough swimmer to keep churning through the water for at least 20 minutes. Your heart will beat more slowly in water than on land, so your heart rate while swimming is not an accurate guide to exercise intensity. Try to keep up a steady pace that's fast enough to make you feel pleasantly tired, but not completely exhausted, by the time you get out of the pool.

- **Cycling.** Bicycling, indoors and out, can be an excellent cardiovascular conditioner, as well as an effective way to control weight—provided you aren't just along for the ride. If you coast down too

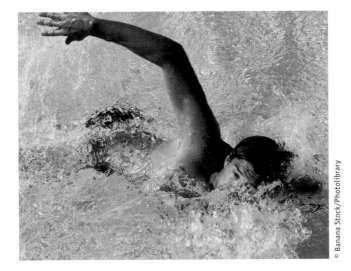
© Banana Stock/Photolibrary

Swimming laps for 20 minutes or longer at a steady pace is a good option for aerobic exercise.

many hills, you'll have to ride longer up hills or on level ground to get a good workout. An 18-speed bike can make pedaling too easy unless you choose gears carefully. To gain aerobic benefits, mountain bikers have to work hard enough to raise their heart rates to their target zone and keep up that intensity for at least 20 minutes.

- **Spinning™.** Spinning is a cardiovascular workout for the whole body that utilizes a special stationary bicycle. Led by an instructor, a group of bikers listens to music, and modifies their individual bike's resistance and their own pace according to the rhythm. An average spinning class lasts 45 minutes.

- **Cardio kick-boxing.** Also referred to as kick-boxing or boxing aerobics, this hybrid of boxing, martial arts, and aerobics offers an intense total-body workout. An hour of kick-boxing burns an average of 500 to 800 calories, compared to 300 to 400 calories in a typical step aerobics class.

- **Rowing.** Whether on water or a rowing machine, rowing provides excellent aerobic exercise as well as working the upper and lower body and toning the shoulders, back, arms, and legs. Correct rowing techniques are important to avoid back injury.

- **Skipping rope.** Essentially a form of stationary jogging with some extra arm action thrown in, skipping rope is excellent as both a heart conditioner and a way of losing weight. Always warm up before starting and cool down afterward.

- **Aerobic dancing.** This activity combines music with kicking, bending, and jumping. A typical class (you can also dance at home to a video or TV program) consists of stretching exercises and sit-ups, followed by aerobic dances and cool-down exer-

cises. "Soft," or low-impact, aerobic dancing doesn't put as much strain on the joints as "hard," or high-impact, routines.

- **Step training, or bench aerobics.** "Stepping" combines step, or bench, climbing with music and choreographed movements. Basic equipment consists of a bench 4 to 12 inches high. The fitter you are, the higher the bench—but the higher the bench, the greater the risk of knee injury.

- **Stair climbing.** You could run up the stairs in an office building or dormitory, but most people use stair-climbing machines available in home models and at gyms and health clubs.

- **Inline skating.** Inline skating can increase aerobic endurance and muscular strength and is less stressful on joints and bones than running or high-impact aerobics. Skaters can adjust the intensity of their workout by varying the terrain.

- **Tennis.** As with other sports, tennis can be an aerobic activity—depending on the number of players and their skill level. In general, a singles match requires more continuous exertion than playing doubles.

Building Muscular Fitness

Although aerobic workouts condition your insides (heart, blood vessels, and lungs), they don't exercise many of the muscles that shape your outsides and provide power when you need it. Strength workouts are important because they enable muscles to work more efficiently and reliably. Conditioned muscles function more smoothly and contract somewhat more vigorously and with less effort. With exercise, muscle tissue becomes firmer and can withstand much more strain—the result of toughening the sheath protecting the muscle and developing more connective tissue within it (Figure 5.7).

The two dimensions of muscular fitness are strength and endurance. Muscular strength is the maximal force that a muscle or group of muscles can generate for one movement. Muscular endurance is the capacity to sustain repeated muscle actions. Both are important. You need strength to hoist a shovelful of snow—and endurance so you can keep shoveling the entire driveway.

The latest research on fat-burning shows that the best way to reduce your body fat is to add muscle-strengthening exercise to your workouts. Muscle tissue is your very best calorie-burning tissue, and the more you have, the more calories you burn, even when you are resting. You don't have to become a serious body-builder. Using handheld weights (also called *free weights*) two or three times a week is enough. Just be sure you learn how to use them properly, because you can tear or strain muscles if you don't practice the proper weight-lifting

Strength workouts increase circulation

The heart's right half pumps oxygen-poor blood to capillary beds in lungs. There, O_2 diffuses into blood and CO_2 diffuses out. The oxygenated blood flows into the heart's left half where it is then pumped to capillary beds throughout the body.

Strength workouts build muscles

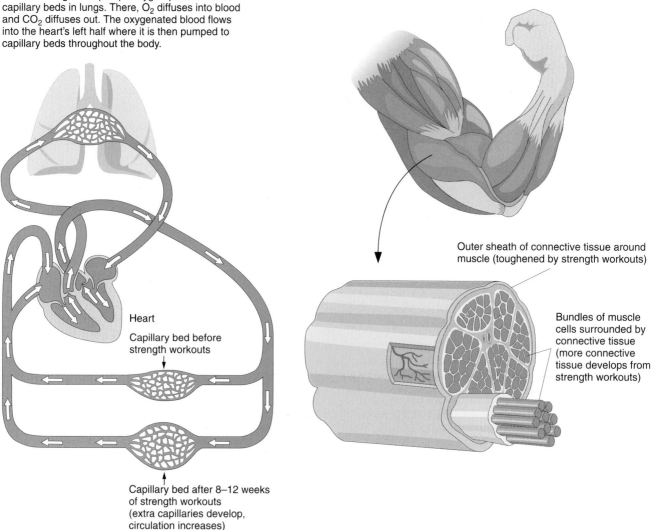

Heart
Capillary bed before strength workouts

Capillary bed after 8–12 weeks of strength workouts (extra capillaries develop, circulation increases)

Outer sheath of connective tissue around muscle (toughened by strength workouts)

Bundles of muscle cells surrounded by connective tissue (more connective tissue develops from strength workouts)

Figure 5.7 Benefits of Strength Training on the Body
Strength training increases blood circulation and oxygen supply to body tissues and develops muscles.

techniques. As more people have begun to lift weights, injuries have soared.

A balanced workout regimen of muscle building and aerobic exercise does more for you than just burn fat. It gives you more endurance by promoting better distribution of oxygen to your tissues and increasing the blood flow to your heart.

 Strength training has particular benefits for women: As numerous studies have documented, it makes their muscles stronger, their bodies leaner, and their bones more resistant to falls. In young women, it boosts self-esteem, body image, and emotional well-being. In middle-aged and older women, it enhances self-concept, boosts psychological health, and prevents weight gain.

Muscles at Work

Your muscles never stay the same. If you don't use them, they atrophy, weaken, or break down. If you use them rigorously and regularly, they grow stronger. The only way to develop muscles is by demanding more of them than you usually do. This is called **overloading.** (Remember the overload principle?) As you train, you have to gradually increase the number of repetitions or the amount of resistance and work the muscle to temporary fatigue. That's why it's important not to quit when your muscles start to tire. Progressive overload—steadily increasing the stress placed on the body—builds stronger muscles.

You need to exercise differently for strength than for endurance. *To develop strength,* do a few repetitions with

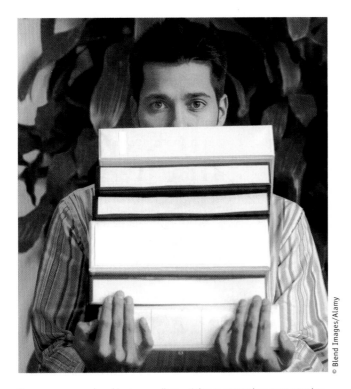

You can use everyday objects as well as weights to strengthen your muscles.

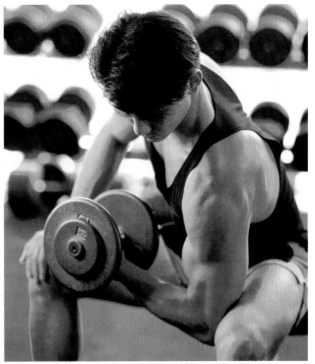

Various types of weight training, including free weights, build muscular strength and endurance.

heavy loads. As you increase the weight your muscles must move, you increase your strength. *To increase endurance,* you do many more repetitions with lighter loads. If your muscles are weak and you need to gain strength in your upper body, you may have to work for weeks to do a half-dozen regular push-ups. Then you can start building endurance by doing as many push-ups as you can before collapsing in exhaustion.

Muscles can do only two things: contract or relax. As they do so, skeletal muscles either pull on bones or stop pulling on bones. All exercise involves muscles pulling on bones across a joint. The movement that takes place depends on the structure of the joint and the position of the muscle attachments involved.

In an **isometric** contraction, the muscle applies force while maintaining an equal length. The muscle contracts and tries to shorten but cannot overcome the resistance. An example is pushing against an immovable object, like a wall, or tightening an abdominal muscle while sitting. The muscle contracts, but there is no movement. Push or pull against the immovable object, with each muscle contraction held for 5 to 8 seconds; repeat five to ten times daily.

An **isotonic** contraction involves movement, but the muscle tension remains the same. In an isotonic exercise, the muscle moves a moderate load several times, as in weight lifting or calisthenics. The best isotonic exercise for producing muscular strength involves high resistance and a low number of repetitions. On the other hand, you can develop the greatest flexibility, coordination, and endurance with isotonic exercises that incorporate lower resistance and frequent repetitions.

True **isokinetic** contraction is a constant speed contraction. Isokinetic exercises require special machines that provide resistance to overload muscles throughout the entire range of motion.

Designing a Muscle Workout

A workout with weights should exercise your body's primary muscle groups: the *deltoids* (shoulders), *pectorals* (chest), *triceps* and *biceps* (back and front of upper arms), *quadriceps* and *hamstrings* (front and back of thighs), *gluteus maximus* (buttocks), *trapezius* and *rhomboids* (back), and *abdomen* (Figure 5.8). Various machines and free-weight routines focus on each muscle group, but the

overloading Method of physical training involving increasing the number of repetitions or the amount of resistance gradually to work the muscle to temporary fatigue.

isometric Of the same length; exercise in which muscles increase their tension without shortening in length, such as when pushing an immovable object.

isotonic Having the same tension or tone; exercise requiring the -repetition of an action that creates tension, such as weight lifting or calisthenics.

isokinetic Having the same force; exercise with specialized equipment that provides resistance equal to the force applied by the user throughout the entire range of motion.

principle is always the same: Muscles contract as you raise and lower a weight, and you repeat the lift-and-lower routine until the muscle group is tired.

A weight-training program is made up of **reps** (the single performance, or **repetition,** of an exercise, such as lifting 50 pounds one time) and **sets** (a *set* number of repetitions of the same movement, such as a set of 20 push-ups). You should allow your breath to return to normal before moving on to each new set. Pushing yourself to the limit builds strength. Although the ideal number of sets in a resistance-training program remains controversial, recent evidence suggests that multiple sets lead to additional benefits in short- and long-term training in young and middle-aged adults.

Maintaining proper breathing during weight training is crucial. To breathe correctly, inhale when muscles are relaxed and exhale when you push or lift. Don't ever hold your breath, because oxygen flow helps prevent muscle fatigue and injury.

No one type of equipment—free weight or machine—has a clear advantage in terms of building fat-free body mass, enhancing strength and endurance, or improving a sport-specific skill. Each type offers benefits but also has drawbacks.

Free weights offer great versatility for strength training. With dumbbells, for example, you can perform a variety of exercises to work specific muscle groups, such as the chest and shoulders. (See Your Strategies for Prevention:

Figure 5.8 Primary Muscle Groups
Different exercises can strengthen and stretch different muscle groups.

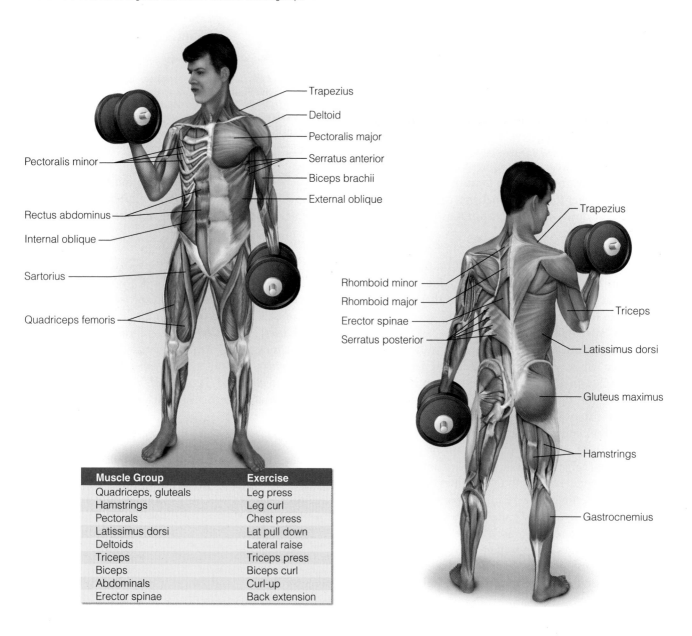

Muscle Group	Exercise
Quadriceps, gluteals	Leg press
Hamstrings	Leg curl
Pectorals	Chest press
Latissimus dorsi	Lat pull down
Deltoids	Lateral raise
Triceps	Triceps press
Biceps	Biceps curl
Abdominals	Curl-up
Erector spinae	Back extension

YOUR STRATEGIES FOR PREVENTION *How to Work with Free Weights*

If you plan to work with free weights, here are some guidelines for using them safely and effectively:

- Don't train alone—for safety's sake. Work with a partner so you can serve as spotters for each other and help motivate each other as well.
- Always warm up before weight training; also be sure to stretch after training.
- Breathe! Holding your breath during exertion can produce a dangerous rise in blood pressure.
- Begin with relatively light weights (50 percent of the maximum you can lift),

and increase the load slowly until you find the weight that will cause muscle failure at anywhere from eight to twelve repetitions. (Muscle failure is the point during a workout at which you can no longer perform or complete a repetition through the entire range of motion.)

- In the beginning, don't work at maximum intensity. Increase your level of exertion gradually over two to six weeks to allow your body to adapt to new stress without soreness.
- Always train your entire body, starting with the larger muscle groups. Don't focus only on specific areas, although

you may want to concentrate on your weakest muscles.

- Always use proper form. Unnecessary twisting, lurching, lunging, or arching can cause serious injury. Remember, quality matters more than quantity. One properly performed set of lifts can produce a greater increase in strength and muscle mass than many sets of improperly performed lifts.
- Work through the full range of motion. Be careful not to hyperextend or overextend.

POINT COUNTERPOINT *Sports Doping on Campus*

POINT

College athletes are among the groups most likely to use performance-enhancing drugs. To stop sports doping on campus, some suggest more rigorous drug testing and immediate suspension from a team if athletes test positive. However, school officials may not want to jeopardize the success of a team, since winning can affect a college's ability to attract talented athletes and to solicit contributions from alumni.

COUNTERPOINT

The penalties for use of performance-enhancing drugs should be steeper, including dismissal of coaches who turn a blind eye on

athletes' drug use. Rather than trying to win at any cost, schools should set and enforce a zero-tolerance standard for drug use in sports.

YOUR VIEW

Should college athletic departments focus on low-profile approaches to identifying and punishing students who test positive for performance-enhancing drug use? Do you think they should hold coaches and trainers who tolerate or endorse this practice responsible?

"How to Work with Free Weights.") Machines, in contrast, are much more limited; most allow only one exercise.

Strength-training machines have several advantages. They ensure correct movement for a lift, which helps protect against injury and prevent cheating when fatigue sets in. They isolate specific muscles, which is good for rehabilitating an injury or strengthening a specific body part. Because they offer high-tech options like varying resistance during the lifting motion, they can tax muscles in ways that a traditional barbell cannot.

Recovery

The American College of Sports Medicine recommends a minimum of eight to ten exercises involving the major muscle groups two to three days a week. Remember that your muscles need sufficient time to recover from a weight-training session. Never work a sore muscle, because soreness may indicate that too-heavy weights have caused tiny tears in the fibers. Allow no less than 48 hours, but no more than 96 hours, between training ses-

sions, so your body can recover from the work-out and you avoid overtraining. Workouts on consecutive days do more harm than good because the body can't recover that quickly. Strength training twice a week at greater intensity and for a longer duration can be as effective as working out three times a week. However, your muscles will begin to atrophy if you let more than three or four days pass without exercising them.

The use of drugs to boost muscle development has become a major problem, particularly among athletes (see Point/Counterpoint). The Savvy Consumer in this chapter discusses the risks and dangers.

rep (or repetition) In weight training, a single performance of a movement or exercise.

sets In weight training, the number of repetitions of the same movement or exercise.

▼ *Savvy* Consumer — What You Should Know About Performance-Boosting Drugs

Here's what we know—and don't know—about the most widely used performance boosters.

- **Anabolic steroids** are synthetic derivatives of the male hormone testosterone that promote the growth of skeletal muscle and increase lean body mass. Taking them to improve athletic performance is illegal.

  Anabolic steroids have been reported to increase lean muscle mass, strength, and ability to train longer and harder, but they pose serious health hazards, including liver tumors, jaundice (yellowish pigmentation of skin, tissues, and body fluids), fluid retention, high blood pressure, decreased immune function, and severe acne. Men may experience shrinking of the testicles, reduced sperm count, infertility, baldness, and development of breasts. Women may experience growth of facial hair, acne, changes in or cessation of the menstrual cycle, enlargement of the clitoris, and deepened voice. In women, these changes are irreversible. In men, side effects may be reversible once abuse stops. In adolescents, steroids may bring about a premature halt in skeletal maturation.

  Anabolic steroid abuse may lead to aggression and other psychiatric side effects. Many users report feeling good about themselves while on anabolic steroids, but researchers report that anabolic steroid abuse can cause wild mood swings including maniclike symptoms leading to "'roid rage," or violent, even homicidal, episodes. Researchers have reported that users may suffer from paranoid jealousy, extreme irritability, delusions, and impaired judgment stemming from feelings of invincibility. Stopping the drugs abruptly can lead to depression.

- **Androstenedione ("andro").** This testosterone precursor is normally produced by the adrenal glands and gonads. Manufacturers claim that androstenedione improves testosterone concentration, increases muscular strength and mass, helps reduce body fat, enhances mood, and improves sexual performance. Studies have shown that supplemental androstenedione doesn't increase testosterone and muscles don't get stronger with andro use. Andro has been classified as a controlled substance, making its use illegal.

- **Creatine.** This amino acid is made by the body and stored predominantly in skeletal muscle. Creatine serves as a reservoir to replenish adenosine triphosphate (ATP), a substance involved in energy production. Some studies show creatine may increase strength and endurance. Other effects on the body remain unknown.

  The Food and Drug Administration has warned consumers to consult a physician before taking creatine supplements. Creatine may cause dehydration and heat-related illnesses, reduced blood volume, and electrolyte imbalances. Some athletes drink quantities of water hoping to avoid such effects. However, many coaches forbid or discourage creatine use because its long-term effects remain unknown.

- **GBL (gamma butyrolactone).** This unapproved drug is being studied as a treatment for narcolepsy, a disabling sleep disorder. Nevertheless, it is marketed on the Internet and in some professional gyms as a muscle-builder and performance-enhancer.

  The Food and Drug Administration has warned consumers to avoid any products containing GBL, noting that they have been associated with at least one death and several incidents in which users became comatose or unconscious.

- **Ergogenic aids.** These are substances used to enhance energy and provide athletes with a competitive advantage. These include everyday substances. *Caffeine,* for instance, may boost alertness in some people but cause jitteriness in others. *Baking soda* (sodium bicarbonate) is believed to delay fatigue by neutralizing lactic acid in the muscles, but its potential drawbacks include explosive diarrhea, abdominal cramps, bloating, and nausea.

  Glycerol is a natural element derived from fats. Some sports-drink manufacturers are testing formulations that include glycerol, which they claim can lower heart rate and stave off exhaustion in marathon events. Glycerol-induced hyperhydration (holding too much water in the blood) can have a negative impact on performance, however, and may be hazardous to health.

Core Strength Conditioning

"Core strength," a popular trend in exercise and fitness, refers to the ability of the muscles to support your spine and keep your body stable and balanced. When you have good core stability, the muscles in your pelvis, lower back, hips, and abdomen work in harmony. This improves your posture, breathing, appearance, and performance in sports, while reducing your risk of muscle strain. When your core is weak, you become more susceptible to lower back pain and injury.

The major muscles of your core include the transverse abdominis, the deepest of the abdominal muscles; the external and internal obliques on the side and front of the abdomen around your waist; and the rectus abdominis, a long muscle that extends along the front of the abdomen.

YOUR STRATEGIES FOR PREVENTION *Watch out for "Pump Fiction"*

Shape up in seven days! Burn calories without breaking a sweat! A brand-new body in minutes a day!

Too good to be true? Absolutely. Advertisers promise no-sweat, no-effort ways to fitness with pills, potions, flab-melting belts, and thigh-slimming paddles. These claims amount to nothing more than what the American Council on Exercise calls "pump fiction." The benefits of fitness are real and well documented, but the only way to reap them is through regular exercise.

Here are some specific guidelines:

- **Be wary** of any program or product that promises "easy" or "effortless" results. Athletes in peak condition might use them without breaking a sweat. Chances are that you, like most people, won't.
- **Watch out for "spot" reducers.** You can't lose a "spare tire" or firm flabby thighs by targeting only that area of your body. You need to lose weight and tone your entire body.
- **Read the fine print.** Often it states that the results are based not just on the device but on dieting and exercise as well.

- **Don't believe testimonials** or celebrity endorsements. Slim, trim, smiling celebrities are paid well for their enthusiasm.
- **Be skeptical** of dramatic "before and after" photos. With today's technology, you never know if photos were doctored or if the results lasted.
- **Check the details** on warranties, guarantees, and return policies. The ads may promise a "30-day money-back guarantee" but fail to mention hefty shipping costs.

Strengthening all of your core muscles provides stability, improves balance, and protects you from injury.

Becoming More Flexible

Flexibility is the characteristic of body tissues that determines the **range of motion** achievable without injury at a joint or group of joints. There are two types of flexibility: static and dynamic. **Static flexibility**—the type most people think of as flexibility—refers to the ability to assume and maintain an extended position at one end point in a joint's range of motion. **Dynamic flexibility,** by comparison, involves movement. It is the ability to move a joint quickly and fluidly through its entire range of motion with little resistance. The static flexibility in the hip joint determines whether you can do a split; dynamic flexibility is what would enable you to perform a split leap.

Static flexibility depends on many factors, including the structure of a joint and the tightness of the muscles, tendons, and ligaments attached to it. Dynamic flexibility is influenced by static flexibility but also depends on additional factors, such as strength, coordination, and resistance to movement.

Genetics, age, gender, and body composition all influence how flexible you are. Girls and women tend to be more flexible than boys and men to a certain extent because of hormonal and anatomical differences. The way females and males use their muscles and the activities they engage in can also have an effect. Over time, the natural elasticity of muscles, tendons, and joints decreases in both genders, resulting in stiffness.

The Benefits of Flexibility

Just as cardiorespiratory fitness benefits the heart and lungs and muscular fitness builds endurance and strength, a stretching program produces unique benefits, including enhancement of the ability of the respiratory, circulatory, and neuromuscular systems to cope with the stress and demands of our high-pressure world (Figure 5.9). Among the other benefits of flexibility are:

- **Prevention of injuries.** Flexibility training stretches muscles and increases the elasticity of joints. Strong, flexible muscles resist stress better than weak or inflexible ones. Adding flexibility to a training program for sports such as soccer, football, or tennis can reduce the rate of injuries by as much as 75 percent. In one study of competitive runners, weekly stretching sessions significantly reduced the incidence of low-back pain.

- **Relief of muscle strain.** Muscles tighten as a result of stress or prolonged sitting. If you study or work in one position for several hours, you'll often feel stiffness in your back or neck. Stretching helps relieve this tension and enables you to work more effectively.

- **Relaxation.** Flexibility exercises are great stress-busters that reduce mental strain, slow the rate of breathing, and reduce blood pressure.

- **Relief of soreness after exercise.** Many people develop delayed-onset muscle soreness (DOMS) one or two days after they work out. This may be

anabolic steroids Drugs derived from testosterone and approved for medical use, but often used by athletes to increase their musculature and weight.

range of motion The fullest extent of possible movement in a particular joint.

static flexibility The ability to assume and maintain an extended position at one end point in a joint's range of motion.

dynamic flexibility The ability to move a joint quickly and fluidly through its entire range of motion with little resistance.

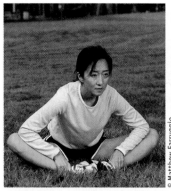

(a) Foot pull for the groin and thigh muscles

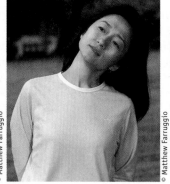

(b) Lateral head tilt

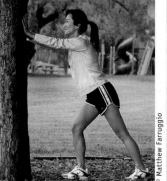

(c) Wall stretch for the Achilles tendon

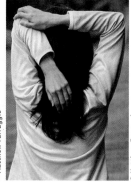

(d) Triceps stretch for the upper arm and shoulder

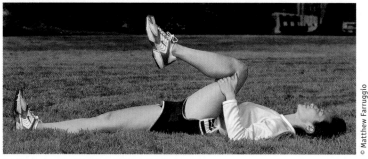

(e) Knee-chest pull for lower back muscles

Figure 5.9 Some Simple Stretching Exercises

(a) Sit on the ground and bend your legs so that the soles of your feet touch. Pull your feet closer as you press on your knees with your elbows. Hold for 10 seconds; repeat. **(b)** Gently tilt your head to each side. Repeat several times. **(c)** Stand 3 feet from a wall or post with your feet slightly apart. Keeping your heels on the ground, lean into the wall. Hold for 10 seconds; repeat. **(d)** Place your right hand behind your neck and grasp above the elbow with your left hand. Gently pull the elbow back. Repeat with the left elbow. **(e)** Lying on your back, clasp one knee and pull it toward your chest. Hold for 15–30 seconds; repeat with the other knee.

the result of damage to the muscle fibers and supporting connective tissue.

- **Improved posture.** Bad posture can create tight, stressed muscles. If you slump in your chair, for instance, the muscles in the front of your chest may tighten, causing those in the upper spine to overstretch and become loose.

Stretching

When you stretch a muscle, you are primarily stretching the connective tissue. The stretch must be intense enough to increase the length of the connective tissue without tearing it. (See Your Strategies for Prevention: "How to Avoid Stretching Injuries.")

Static stretching involves a gradual stretch held for a short time (10 to 30 seconds). A shorter stretch provides little benefit; a longer stretch does not provide additional benefits. Since a slow stretch provokes less of a reaction from the stretch receptors, the muscles can safely stretch farther than usual. Fitness experts most often recommend static stretching because it is both safe and effective. An example of such a stretch is letting your hands slowly slide down the front of your legs (keeping your knees in a soft, unlocked position) until you reach your toes and holding this final position for several seconds before slowly straightening up. You should feel a pull, but not pain, during this stretch.

In **passive stretching,** your own body, a partner, gravity, or a weight serves as an external force or resistance to

help your joints move through their range of motion. You can achieve a more intense stretch and a greater range of motion with passive stretching. There is a greater risk of injury, however, because the muscles themselves are not controlling the stretch.

Active stretching involves stretching a muscle by contracting the opposing muscle (the muscle on the opposite side of the limb). This method allows the muscle to be stretched farther with a low risk of injury.

Ballistic stretching is characterized by rapid bouncing movements, such as a series of up-and-down bobs as you try again and again to touch your toes with your hands. These bounces can stretch the muscle fibers too far, causing the muscle to contract rather than stretch. They also can tear ligaments and weaken or rupture tendons, the strong fibrous cords that connect muscles to bones. The heightened activity to stretch receptors caused by the rapid stretches can continue for some time, possibly causing injuries during any physical activities that follow. Because of its potential dangers, fitness experts generally recommend against ballistic stretching.

Stretching and Warming Up

Warming up means getting the heart beating, breaking a sweat, and readying the body for more vigorous activity. Stretching is a specific activity intended to elongate the muscles and keep joints limber, not simply a prelude to a game of tennis or a three-mile run. According to a review of recent studies, the value of stretching varies with different activities. While it does not prevent injuries from

YOUR STRATEGIES FOR PREVENTION *How to Avoid Stretching Injuries*

Before you begin, increase your body temperature by slowly marching or running in place. Sweat signals that you're ready to start stretching.

- Don't force body parts beyond their normal range of motion. Stretch to the point of tension, back off, and hold for ten seconds to a minute.
- Do a minimum of four repetitions of each stretch, with equal repetitions on each side.

- Don't hold your breath. Continue breathing slowly and rhythmically throughout your stretching routine.
- Don't attempt to stretch a weak or injured muscle.
- Start small. Work the muscles of the smaller joints in the arms and legs first and then work the larger joints like the shoulders and hips.
- Stretch individual muscles before you stretch a group of muscles, for instance,

the ankle, knee, and hip before a stretch that works all three.
- Don't make any quick, jerky movements while stretching. Stretches should be gentle and smooth.
- Certain positions can be harmful to the knees and lower back. In particular, avoid stretches that require deep knee bends or full squats, because they can harm your knees and lower back.

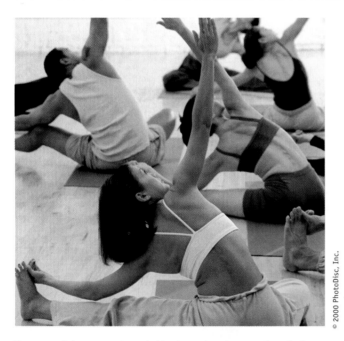

© 2000 PhotoDisc, Inc.

Yoga, one of the most ancient mind-body practices, has many benefits for people of all ages.

jogging, cycling, or swimming, stretching may be beneficial in sports, like soccer and football, that involve bouncing and jumping.

For aerobic activities, one of the best times to stretch is after an aerobic workout. Your muscles will be warm, more flexible, and less prone to injury. In addition, stretching after aerobic activity can help a fatigued muscle return to its normal resting length and possibly helps reduce delayed-onset muscle soreness.

Stretching and Athletic Performance

Conventional wisdom holds that stretching improves athletic performance, but a review of the research finds that this isn't necessarily so.[32] In some cases, active stretching can impede rather than improve performance in terms of muscle force and jumping height. Passive stretching prior to a sprint—a common practice—also has proved to reduce runners' speed. On the other hand,

regular stretching can improve athletic performance in a variety of sports.

Mind-Body Approaches

Yoga, Pilates, and t'ai chi, increasingly popular on campuses and throughout the country, can help reduce stress, enhance health and wellness, and improve physical fitness.

Yoga

One of the most ancient of mind-body practices, *yoga* comes from the Sanskrit word meaning "union." Traditionally associated with religion, yoga consists of various breathing and stretching exercises that unite all aspects of a person.

Once considered an exotic pursuit, yoga has gained acceptance as part of a comprehensive stress management and fitness program. Scientific studies have demonstrated its benefits, which include:

- **Improved flexibility,** which may offer protection from back pain and injuries.
- **Protection of joints** because yoga postures take joints through their full range of motion, providing a fresh supply of nutrients to joint cartilage.
- **Stronger, denser bones** from yoga's weight-bearing postures.
- **Enhanced circulation,** which also boosts the supply of oxygen throughout the body.

static stretching A gradual stretch held for a short time of 10 to 30 seconds.

passive stretching A stretching technique in which an external force or resistance (your body, a partner, gravity, or a weight) helps the joints move through their range of motion.

active stretching A technique that involves stretching a muscle by contracting the opposing muscle.

ballistic stretching Rapid bouncing movements.

> **YOUR STRATEGIES FOR PREVENTION** *How to Protect Your Back*
>
> Back pain is the most common health problem among college students, according to the National College Health Assessment. Here are some ways to prevent back problems now and in the future:
>
> - When standing, shift your weight from one foot to the other. If possible, place one foot on a stool, step, or railing 4 to 6 inches off the ground. Hold in your stomach, tilt your pelvis toward your back, and tuck in your buttocks to provide crucial support for the lower back.
>
> - Because sitting places more stress on the lower back than standing, try to get up from your seat at least once an hour to stretch or walk around. Whenever possible, sit in a straight chair with a firm back. Avoid slouching in overstuffed chairs or dangling your legs in midair. When driving, keep the seat forward so that your knees are raised to hip level; your right leg should not be fully extended. A small pillow or towel can help support your lower back.
>
> - Sleep on a flat, firm mattress. The best sleep position is on your side, with one or both knees bent at right angles to your torso. The pillow should keep your head in line with your body so that your neck isn't bent forward or to the side.
>
> - When lifting, bend at the knees, not from the waist. Get close to the load. Tighten your stomach muscles, but don't hold your breath. Let your leg muscles do the work.

- **Lower blood pressure.**
- **Lower levels of the stress hormone cortisol,** which (as discussed in Chapter 3) can affect the immune system, interfere with memory, and increase the risk of depression and osteoporosis.
- **Lower blood sugar in people with diabetes,** which reduces the risk of complications.
- **Reduced pain** in people with back problems, arthritis, carpal tunnel syndrome, fibromyalgia, and other chronic problems.

The best way to get started is to find a class that appeals to you and learn a few yoga moves and breathing techniques. Once you have mastered these, you can easily integrate yoga into your total fitness program.

The American College of Sports Medicine cautions that yoga should help, not hurt. To prevent injuries to your knees, back, neck, shoulders, wrists, or ankles, avoid forcing your body into difficult postures. Proper technique is essential to safety.

Pilates

Used by dancers for deep-body conditioning and injury rehabilitation, Pilates (pronounced Pilah-teez), was developed more than seven decades ago by German immigrant Joseph Pilates. Increasingly used to complement aerobics and weight training, Pilates exercises improve flexibility and joint mobility and strengthen the core by developing pelvic stability and abdominal control.

Pilates-trained instructors offer "mat" or "floor" classes that stress the stabilization and strengthening of the back and abdominal muscles. Fitness centers also may offer training on Pilates equipment, primarily a device called the Reformer, a wooden contraption with various cables, pulleys, springs, and sliding boards attached that is used for a series of progressive, range-of-motion exercises. Instructors typically work one on one or with small groups of two or three participants and tailor exercise sessions to individual flexibility and strength limitations. Unlike exercise techniques that emphasize numerous repetitions in a single direction, Pilates exercises involve very few, but extremely precise, repetitions in several planes of motion.

According to research from the American College of Sports Medicine, Pilates enhances flexibility and muscular endurance, particularly for intermediate and advanced practitioners, but its potential to increase cardiorespiratory fitness and reduce body weight is limited. The intensity of a Pilates workout increases from basic to intermediate to advanced levels, as does the number of calories burned. For intermediate practitioners, a 30-minute session burns 180 calories, with each additional quarter-hour burning another 90 calories. A single weekly session enhances flexibility but has little impact on body composition.

T'ai Chi

This ancient Chinese practice, designed to exercise body, mind, and spirit, gently works muscles, focuses concentration, and improves the flow of "qi" (often spelled "chi"), the vital life energy that sustains health. Popular with all ages, from children to seniors, t'ai chi is easy to learn and perform. Because of its focus on breathing and flowing gestures, t'ai chi is sometimes described as "meditation in motion."

Classes are available on campuses, in fitness centers, community centers, and some martial arts schools. Physicians may recommend t'ai chi for those with musculoskeletal disorders like arthritis to improve flexibility and build muscle strength gently and gradually. The American College of Sports Medicine reports that t'ai chi has proved effective in reducing falls in the elderly and those with balance disorders.

Keeping Your Back Healthy

The average person has an 80 percent chance of experiencing low-back pain in the course of a lifetime. Back pain strikes slightly more women than men and is most common between the ages of 20 and 55. You are at greater risk if you smoke or if you're overstressed, overweight, or out of shape. Back pain, which accounts for 40 percent of sickness absences, causes more lost workdays and costs the country more than any other malady. (See Your Strategies for Prevention: "How to Protect Your Back.")

Most severe back pain lasts only a few days, although less severe symptoms may persist for many months, and most patients have intermittent recurrences of back pain. More than 90 percent of individuals with back pain recover within three months.

Once bedrest was the primary treatment for back pain, but now doctors urge patients to avoid it. Even two to seven days of bedrest may provide little, if any, benefit. Acetaminophen (Tylenol) is the first-line therapy for pain relief. If it is not effective, doctors recommend nonsteroidal anti-inflammatory drugs, such as ibuprofen (Motrin or Advil). Muscle relaxants seem to be effective for a spasm in the lower back. The sooner that back patients return to normal activity, the less pain medication they require and the less long-term disability they suffer. Fewer than 1 percent of patients with chronic low-back pain benefit from surgery.

Body Composition

Body composition, the fifth component of fitness, can tell you a lot about risk for cardiorespiratory disease and diabetes.

A combination of regular exercise and good nutrition is the best way to maintain a healthy body composition. Aerobic exercise helps by burning calories and increasing metabolic rate (the rate at which the body uses calories) for several hours after a workout. Strength training increases the proportion of lean body tissue by building muscle mass, which also increases the metabolic rate.

Experts debate which measure of body composition—body mass index (BMI), waist circumference, or waist-to-hip ratio—is the best indicator of central or visceral obesity, which increases the risk of heart disease, metabolic syndrome, diabetes, and other illnesses.

Body Mass Index (BMI)

Body mass index (BMI), a ratio between weight and height, is a mathematical formula that correlates with body fat. You can determine your BMI from Figure 5.10. A healthy BMI ranges from 18.5 to 24.9.

A BMI of 25 or greater defines **overweight** and marks the point at which excess weight increases the risk of disease. If your BMI is between 25 and 29.9 (23.4 for Asians), your weight is undermining the quality of your life. You suffer more aches and pains. You find it harder to perform everyday tasks. You run a greater risk of serious health problems.

A BMI of 30 or greater defines **obesity** and marks the point at which excess weight increases the risk of death. If your BMI is between 30 and 34.9 (class 1 obesity), you face all the preceding dangers plus one more: dying. The risk of premature death increases even more if your BMI is between 35 and 39.9 (class 2 obesity). A BMI of 40 or higher indicates class 3 or severe obesity.

Doctors use BMI to determine whether a person is at risk for weight-related diseases like diabetes. However, using BMI as an assessment tool has limitations. Muscular individuals, including athletes and body builders, may be miscategorized as overweight or obese because they have greater lean muscle mass. BMI also does not reliably reflect body fat, an independent predictor of health risk, and is not useful for growing children, women who are pregnant or nursing, or the elderly. In addition, BMI, which was developed in Western nations, may not accurately indicate the risk of obesity-related diseases in Asian men and women.

Waist Circumference

Even if your scale shows that you haven't gained a lot of weight, your waist may widen—particularly if you've been under stress. Because of the physiological impact of stress hormones, fat accumulates around your midsection in times of tension and turmoil.

A widening waist or "apple" shape is a warning signal. In women, a wider waist correlates with high levels of harmful blood fats, such as LDL cholesterol and triglycerides.[33] In both sexes, abdominal fat, unlike fat in the thighs or hips, increases the risk of high blood pressure, type 2 diabetes, high cholesterol, and metabolic syndrome (a perilous combination of overweight, high blood pressure, and high levels of cholesterol and blood sugar, discussed in Chapter 16).

To measure your waist circumference, place a tape measure around your bare abdomen just above your hip bone. Be sure that the tape is snug but does not compress your skin. Relax, exhale, and measure.

When is a waist too wide? Various studies have produced different results, but the general guideline is that a waist measuring more than 35 inches in a woman or more than 40 inches in a man signals greater health risks. These waist circumferences indicate "central" obesity, which is characterized by fat deposited deep within the central abdominal area of the body. Such "visceral" fat is

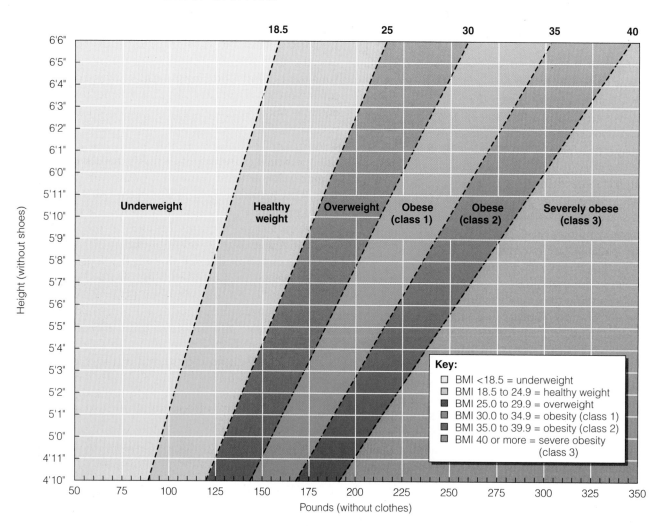

Figure 5.10 BMI Values Used to Assess Weight for Adults

more dangerous than "subcutaneous" fat just below the skin because it moves more readily into the bloodstream and directly raises levels of harmful cholesterol.

 Body composition varies with race and ethnicity. Asians, for instance, may be more likely and African Americans less likely to accumulate visceral fat than Caucasians.

Waist-to-Hip Ratio

Another way of determining your health risk is your **waist-to-hip ratio (WHR).** In addition to measuring your waist, measure your hips at the widest part. Divide your waist measurement by your hip measurement. For women, a ratio of 0.80 or less is considered safe; for men, the recommended ratio is 0.90 or less. For both men and women, a 1.0 or higher is considered "at risk" or in the danger zone for undesirable health consequences, such as heart disease and other ailments associated with being overweight.

Men of all ages are more prone to develop the "apple" shape characteristic of central obesity; women in their

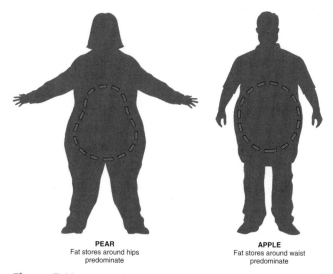

PEAR
Fat stores around hips predominate

APPLE
Fat stores around waist predominate

Figure 5.11 Pear-Shaped Versus Apple-Shaped Bodies

reproductive years are more likely to accumulate fat around the hips and thighs and acquire a pear shape (Figure 5.11).

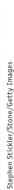

When men and women diet, men lose more visceral fat located around the abdominal area. This weight loss produces more cardiovascular benefits for men, including a decrease in triglycerides (fats circulating in the blood) and an increase in the "good" form of cholesterol, high-density lipoprotein (HDL).

Measuring Body Fat

Knowing your specific body composition can provide useful information about body fat and health. Ideal body fat percentages for men range from 7 to 25 percent and for women from 16 to 35 percent. Methods of assessing body composition range from skin calipers to more high-tech methods.

Skinfold Measurement
Skinfold measurement is determined using a caliper to measure the amount of skinfold. The usual sites include the chest, abdomen, and thigh for men, and the tricep, hip, and thigh for women. Various equations determine body fat percentage, including calculations that take into account age, gender, race, and other factors. This relatively simple and low-cost method requires considerable technical skill for an accurate reading.

Home Body Fat Analyzers
Handheld devices and stand-on monitors sold online and in specialty stores promise to make measuring your body fat percentage as easy as finding your weight. None has been extensively tested.

Laboratory Methods
- **Bioelectrical Impedance Analysis (BIA).** This noninvasive method is based on the principle that electrical current applied to the body meets greater resistance with different types of tissue. Lean tissue, which contains large amounts of water and electrolytes, is a good electrical conductor; fat, which does not, is a poor conductor. In theory, the easier the electrical conduction, the greater an individual's lean body mass.
- **Hydrostatic (underwater) weighing.** According to the Archimedes Principle, a body immersed in a fluid is buoyed by a force equal to the weight of the displaced fluid. Since muscle has a higher density than water and fat has a lower density, fat people tend to displace less water than lean people.
- **Dual-energy X-ray absorptiometry (DXA).** X rays are used to quantify the skeletal and soft tissue components of body mass. The test requires just 10 to 20 minutes, and radiation dosage is low (800 to 2,000 times lower than a typical chest X ray). Some researchers believe that DXA will supplant hydro-

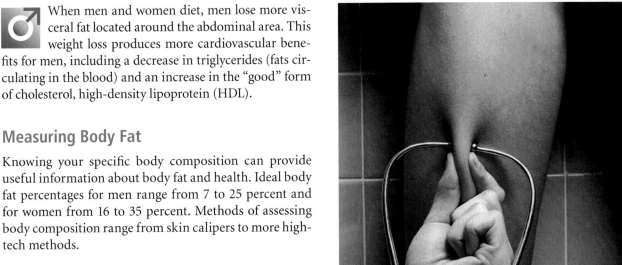

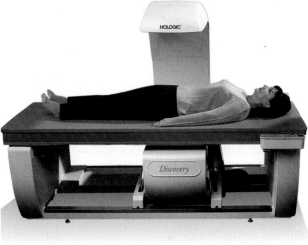

Skinfold measure accuracy depends on the technician's skill; laboratory methods such as DXA don't have that subjective component.

static testing as the standard for body composition assessment.
- **The Bod Pod®.** This large, egg-shaped fiberglass chamber uses an approach based on air displacement plethysmography, that is, the calculation of the relationship between pressure and volume to derive body volume.

body mass index (BMI) A mathematical formula that correlates with body fat; the ratio of weight to height squared.

overweight A condition of having a BMI between 25.0 and 29.9.

obesity The excessive accumulation of fat in the body; class 1 obesity is defined by a BMI between 30 and 34.9; class 2 obesity is defined by a BMI between 35 and 39.9; class 3, or severe obesity, is a BMI of 40 or higher.

waist-to-hip ratio (WHR) The proportion of one's waist circumference to one's hip circumference.

Evaluating Fitness Products and Programs

As fitness has become a major industry in the United States, consumers have been bombarded with pitches for products that promise to do everything from whittle a waistline to build up biceps. As always, you have to ask questions and do your own research—whether you're buying basic exercise aids or joining a health club. Beware of any promise that sounds too good to be true. And keep in mind that nothing matters more than your own commitment.

Exercise Equipment

Always try out equipment before buying it. If you decide to purchase a stationary bicycle, for instance, read all the product information. Ask someone in your physical education department or at a local gym for recommendations. Try out a bicycle at the gym. Make sure any equipment you purchase is safe and durable.

Athletic Shoes

Footwear has come a long way from the days of canvas sneakers. With so many new materials and high-tech options, choosing the right shoe for working out can be confusing. The best shoes aren't necessarily the most expensive but the ones that fit you best. Here are some basic guidelines:

- **Choose the right shoe for your sport.** If you're a walker or runner, you want maximum overall shock absorption for the foot, with extra cushioning in the heel and under the ball of the foot (the metatarsal area) to prevent pain, burning, and tenderness. If you also participate in other types of exercise, consider "cross-trainers," shoes that are flexible enough in the front for running but provide the side-to-side, or lateral, control you need for aerobics or tennis.

- **Check out the shoe.** A "slip-lasted" shoe, made by sewing together the upper like a moccasin and gluing it to the sole, is lightweight and flexible. A "board-lasted" shoe has a leather, nylon mesh, or canvas upper sewn to a cardboardlike material, which provides more support and control. A "combination-last" shoe offers the advantages of both and works well for a variety of foot types (Figure 5.12).

- **Shop late.** Try on shoes at the end of the day or after a workout, when your foot size is at its maximum (sometimes half a shoe size larger than in the morning). Wear socks similar to those you'll wear for workouts.

- **Give your toes room.** Allow a half-inch, or the width of your index finger, between the end of your longest toe and the tip of the shoe. Try on both shoes. If one foot is larger than the other, buy the larger size.

Figure 5.12   What to Look for When You Buy Running Shoes

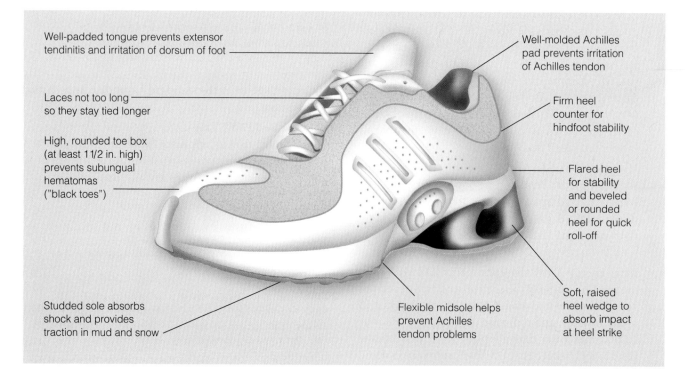

Well-padded tongue prevents extensor tendinitis and irritation of dorsum of foot

Laces not too long so they stay tied longer

High, rounded toe box (at least 1 1/2 in. high) prevents subungual hematomas ("black toes")

Studded sole absorbs shock and provides traction in mud and snow

Well-molded Achilles pad prevents irritation of Achilles tendon

Firm heel counter for hindfoot stability

Flared heel for stability and beveled or rounded heel for quick roll-off

Soft, raised heel wedge to absorb impact at heel strike

Flexible midsole helps prevent Achilles tendon problems

- **Check the width.** A shoe should be as wide as possible across the forefoot without allowing the heel to slip. Lace up the shoe completely and walk or jog a few steps to make sure the shoes are comfortable.
- **Replace shoes when they lose their cushioning.** After about 300 to 500 miles of running or 300 hours of aerobic activity, your shoes are no longer absorbing the pounding and jarring of your sport. Don't put yourself at increased risk of knee and ankle injuries.

Low-Cost Fitness Aids

Not all fitness equipment comes with a big price tag. Here are some affordable ways to expand and enhance a home workout:

- **Dumbbells.** You can purchase light weights to carry when walking and jogging to build and firm arm muscles. Training with heavier weights increases muscle strength and endurance, improves balance and body composition, and may reverse some bone loss. An adjustable dumbbell set allows you to add more weight as you build strength.
- **Stability balls.** A large inflatable rubber ball can be a fun, effective way of building core strength, improving posture, and increasing balance. When performing standard exercises like crunches and abdominal curls, the ball provides an additional challenge: maintaining a stable trunk throughout each exercise. You also can sit on the ball while working with hand weights to build core strength and balance. Introductory videos and DVDs are available for rental or purchase.
- **Resistance tubing.** Developed by physical therapists for rehabilitation after injuries, elastic bands and tubing come in different strengths, based on the thickness of the plastic. If you're a beginner, start with a thin band, particularly for the upper body. The lightweight, inexpensive, and easy-to-carry bands aren't particularly risky, but you should check for holes or worn spots, choose a smooth surface, maintain good posture, and perform the exercises in a slow, controlled manner.

Fitness Centers

Begin by checking out the recreational facilities on your own campus. Is there a gym, running track, pool, basketball court, athletic fields? Are they crowded at certain times? Are they convenient? Are classes in spinning or Pilates available?

If you decide to join a private gym or health club, find out exactly what facilities and programs it offers. The club should be located close to home, campus, or work and

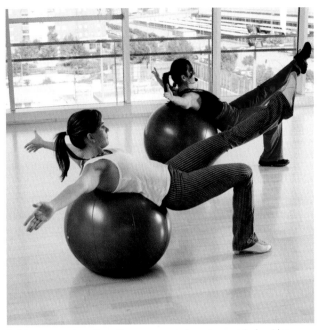

Build your core strength and improve your balance inexpensively with a stability ball. Maintaining appropriate air pressure is important—the exercise will become more difficult as air pressure increases.

© Polka Dot Images/Jupiterimages

should be open at convenient hours. Think about your schedule and when you'll have time to work out. Visit the club at the times you're most likely to use it.

A club should have facilities for a complete workout, including both aerobic and muscle workouts: exercycles, rowing machines, treadmills, stair-climbing machines, stationary bicycles, a running track, aerobics classes, a swimming pool, strength-training equipment, and, if it's what you're looking for, racquetball courts and a large gym for basketball and volleyball.

Find out whether all facilities are available to all members at all times. Some clubs reserve the pool for families only or kids' lessons at certain times. Ask if you can try out the club before joining. Find out what the membership includes. Will you end up paying extra for lockers, towels, classes, and the like? Are student discounts offered? Beware of long-term memberships; many clubs go out of business or change ownership often. Do the members seem to be significantly older or younger, or in much better or worse shape, than you are? You're more likely to work out regularly in a place, and with people, you like.

Sports Nutrition

In general, active people need the same basic nutrients as others and should follow the recommendations in Chapter 6. However, athletes in competitive sports—amateur as well as professional—may have increased energy requirements.

Contrary to a common misconception, athletes generally do not need more protein; the exception may be those engaged in intense strength training. Like most Americans, athletes typically consume more than the Recommended Daily Allowance for protein and do not need increased protein. A high-protein diet can be high in fat and low in the nutrients supplied by fruits, vegetables, and grains and can put a strain on the liver and kidneys. However, in a recent study of undergraduates, college men and women who engaged in vigorous exercise ate more fruits and vegetables than their less active classmates.[34]

Although complex carbohydrates are essential in an athlete's diet, fat also plays a role. Including the right types of fat in the daily diet can actually improve athletic performance—not just by providing calories, but by replenishing intramuscular fat stores (fat stored within the muscle and used to fuel extended exercise).

Not just *what* you eat but *when* you eat can affect your exercise performance. If you eat immediately prior to a workout, you may feel sluggish or develop nausea, cramping, or diarrhea. If you don't eat, you may feel weak, faint, or tired.

Time your meals so that you exercise three to four hours after a large meal and one to two hours after a small one. Most people can eat a snack right before exercise. After a workout, eat a meal containing both protein and carbohydrates within two hours to help your muscles recover and to replace fuel stores.

Water

Water, which we need more than any other nutrient, is even more important during exercise and exertion. Thirst, the body's way of telling you to replace lost fluids, is not a good way for athletes to monitor their fluid needs. Rather than waiting until you're already somewhat dehydrated, you should be fully hydrated when you begin your activity or exercise and, depending on the duration and intensity of your workout, continue to replace fluids both during and afterward.

The American College of Sports Medicine (ACSM) recommends fluid intake before, during, and after exercise to regulate body temperature and replace body fluids lost through sweating. The failure to replace fluids during exercise can lead to dehydration, which can cause muscle fatigue, loss of coordination, heat exhaustion, and an elevation of body-core temperature to dangerously high levels. To avoid this danger, the ACSM advises:

- **Consume a nutritionally balanced diet and drink adequate fluids** in the 24 hours before an exercise event.
- **Drink about 17 ounces of fluid** about two hours before.
- **During exercise, start drinking early** and at regular intervals to replace all the water lost through sweating (i.e., body weight loss).
- **Drink fluids with carbohydrates and/or electrolytes** for exercise lasting more than an hour. For

shorter periods, there is little evidence of differences between drinking a carbohydrate–electrolyte drink and plain water.[35]

Too much water during prolonged bouts of exercise, such as a marathon, can lead to *hyponatremia*, or water intoxication. This condition occurs when the body's sodium level falls below normal as a result of salt loss from sweat and dilution of sodium in the bloodstream by overdrinking. Symptoms of hyponatremia include nausea, vomiting, weakness, and in severe cases, seizures, coma, and death.

Sports Drinks

More than twenty "power" beverages compete for the $1 billion market of drinks for active people. As noted above, water best meets the fluid needs of most athletes, but you have other choices. According to a recent study, non-fat milk is more effective than even a soy protein beverage or sports drink such as Gatorade at burning fat and building lean muscle mass. Young men who consistently drank fat-free milk after resistance training gained 40 percent more muscle mass than those who consumed soy drinks, and 60 percent more than those consuming carbohydrate-based sport drinks.[36]

What you are actually consuming in a sports drink is a mixture of simple sugars, sodium, and other electrolytes. Sugars help maintain hydration and blood glucose and may be especially beneficial for strenuous endurance workouts that last longer than 45 minutes or during prolonged competitive games that demand repeated intermittent activity.

Most sports drinks contain about 7 percent carbohydrate (about half the sugar of ordinary soft drinks). Less than 6 percent may not enhance performance; more than 8 percent could cause abdominal cramping, nausea, and diarrhea.

Sodium and other electrolytes in sports drinks help replace those lost during physical activity. However, most exercisers do not have to replace minerals lost in sweat immediately. A meal eaten within several hours does so soon enough.

If you exercise to lose weight, sports drinks may be counterproductive since you take in 50 to 100 calories with every 8-ounce drink. Water, on the other hand, replenishes lost fluids without adding empty calories. (See Chapter 6 for a discussion of sodas and energy drinks.)

Dietary Supplements

Athletes and active individuals of all ages take dietary supplements, sometimes to ensure that they're getting the nutrients they need and sometimes to enhance their performance. Vitamin and mineral supplements, as discussed in Chapter 6, are safe when taken at recommended doses. Excess amounts can contribute to serious health problems. Vitamin supplements marketed for athletes are poorly regulated, and some may be adulterated with banned substances, such as ephedrine. Always look for the USP (United States Pharmacopeias) certification on the label when buying vitamins.

Athletes involved in heavy training may need more of several vitamins, such as thiamin, riboflavin, and B_6, which are involved in energy production. The best source, nutritionists advise, is vitamin-rich foods, such as fruits and vegetables.

Mineral deficiencies, such as too little iron in female athletes, can impair athletic performance. Women who exercise rigorously should undergo regular blood testing and, if needed, take iron supplements. In general, calcium, magnesium, iron, zinc, and copper supplements do not enhance sport performance in well-nourished athletes. Chromium, boron, and vanadium have been studied as possible performance boosters, but researchers have not reported any beneficial effects on body composition or muscular strength and endurance.

Energy Bars

Sold as snacks, meal substitutes, or performance enhancers, energy bars come in different forms. High-carbohydrate bars derive more than 70 percent of their calories from carbohydrates (such as corn syrup, grape and pear juice concentrate, oat bran, and brown rice) and are low in protein and fat. Another type gets 40 percent of its energy from carbohydrate, 30 percent from protein, and 30 percent from fat.

Little scientific research has studied the actual benefits of the various types of energy bars, including their effects on blood glucose levels and athletic performance. According to one nutritional analysis, high-carbohydrate energy bars are similar to candy bars in their impact on glucose—even though sugars composed 31 percent of the high-carbohydrate energy bar and 86 percent of the candy bar. In fact, the high-carbohydrate energy bar caused a more rapid peak in blood glucose followed by a sharper decline than did the candy bar. This effect may be desirable for athletes involved in short-duration events who want a quick increase in blood glucose.

Energy bars with a lower carbohydrate level produce a more moderate, sustained increase in blood glucose level, possibly because the protein and fat in a 40–30–30 bar diminish blood glucose response. These bars would be a better choice for athletes involved in endurance events. As an alternative, try fiber-rich whole foods, like nuts and fruit, that provide a steady release of energy.

Safe and Healthy Workouts

Whenever you work out, you don't want to risk becoming sore or injured. Starting slowly when you begin any new fitness activity is the smartest strategy. Keep a simple diary to record the time and duration of each workout. Get accustomed to an activity first and then begin to work harder or longer. In this way, you strengthen your musculoskeletal system so you're less likely to be injured, you lower the cardiorespiratory risk, and you build the exercise habit into your schedule.

To prevent exercise-related problems before they happen, use common sense and take appropriate precautions, including the following:

- **Get proper instruction** and, if necessary, advanced training from knowledgeable instructors.
- **Make sure you have good equipment** and keep it in good condition. Know how to check and do at least basic maintenance on the equipment yourself. Always check your equipment prior to each use (especially if you're renting it).
- **Always warm up before and cool down** after a workout.
- Rather than being sedentary all week and then training hard on weekends, **try to stay active throughout the week** and not overdo on weekends.
- **Use reasonable protective measures,** including wearing a helmet when cycling or skating.
- For some sports, such as boating, **always go with a buddy.**
- **Take each outing seriously**—even if you've dived into this river a hundred times before, even if you know this mountain like you know your own backyard. Avoid the unknown under adverse conditions (for example, hiking unfamiliar terrain during poor weather or kayaking a new river when water levels are unusually high or low) or when accompanied by a beginner whose skills may not be as strong as yours.
- **Never combine alcohol or drugs with any workout or sport.**

Temperature

Prevention is the wisest approach to heat and cold problems. (See Your Strategies for Prevention: "How to Cope with Climates.") And knowing what can go wrong is part of that preventive approach.

Heat Cramps

These muscle cramps are caused by profuse sweating and the consequent loss of electrolytes (salts). They occur most often during exercise in hot weather. Salty snacks and sports beverages like Gatorade can help, but be aware

YOUR STRATEGIES FOR PREVENTION *How to Cope with Climate*

Heeding Heat

- Increase your fluid intake during hot temperatures by two to four glasses of cool fluids each hour. Cold beverages can cause stomach cramps; alcoholic beverages can cause you to lose more fluid.
- Cool off with a cool shower or sponge bath.
- Move into an air-conditioned environment.
- Wear lightweight clothing.

- Check weather conditions. The National Weather Service has produced a Heat Index chart that can be accessed online at **www.crh.noaa.gov/pub/heat.php**.

Handling Cold

- Dress appropriately. Choose several layers of loose clothing made of wool, cotton, down, or synthetic down. Make sure your head, feet, and hands are well protected. A pair of cotton socks inside a pair of wool socks will keep your feet warm.

- Don't go out in the cold after drinking. Alcohol can make you more susceptible to cold and can impair your judgment and sense of time.
- When snowshoeing or cross-country skiing, always let a responsible person know where you're heading and when you expect to be back. Stick to marked trails.
- Carry a small emergency kit that includes waterproof matches, a compass, a map, high-energy food, and water.
- Don't eat snow; it could lower your body temperature.

that sports drinks can be very high in calories. Salt tablets usually aren't necessary except in cases of extreme sweating.

Heat Syndromes

More serious temperature-related conditions include heat exhaustion and heat stroke. These are most likely to occur when both temperature and humidity are high, because sweat does not evaporate as quickly, preventing the body from releasing heat quickly. Other conditions that limit the body's ability to regulate temperature are old age, fever, obesity, dehydration, heart disease, poor circulation, sunburn, and drug and alcohol use. Some medicines that increase the risk include allergy medicines (antihistamines), some cough and cold medicines, blood pressure and heart medicines, diet pills, laxatives, and psychiatric medications.

Heat Exhaustion   Heat exhaustion is a mild from of heat-related illness that can be caused by exercise or hot weather. The signs of heat exhaustion are heavy sweating, paleness, muscle cramps, tiredness, weakness, dizziness, headache, nausea or vomiting, and/or fainting. Your pulse rate or heart rate may be fast and weak, and your breathing fast and shallow.

If you think you may have heat exhaustion, get out of the heat quickly. Rest in a cool, shady place and drink plenty of water or other fluids. Do *not* drink alcohol, which can make heat exhaustion worse. If you do not feel better within 30 minutes, see your doctor. If left untreated, heat exhaustion may lead to a heat stroke.

Heat Stroke   A heat stroke can occur when the body temperature rises to 106 degrees Fahrenheit or higher within 10 to 15 minutes. A heat stroke is a medical emergency that can be fatal. The warning signs are extremely high temperature; red, hot, and dry skin; rapid, strong pulse; throbbing headache; dizziness; nausea; confusion or unconsciousness.

If you think someone might have heat stroke, you should take him or her to a cool, shady place quickly, and call a

doctor. Remove unnecessary clothing and bathe or spray the victim with cool water. People with heat stroke may seem confused. They may have seizures or go into a coma.

The incidence of heat stroke in urban areas of the United States during very warm periods is approximately 20 cases per 100,000 people, and heat stroke accounts for at least 240 deaths in the United States annually.

Protecting Yourself from the Cold

The tips of the toes, fingers, ears, nose, and chin and the cheeks are most vulnerable to exposure to high wind speeds and low temperatures, which can result in *frostnip*.

Because frostnip is painless, you may not even be aware that it is occurring. Watch for a sudden blanching or lightening of your skin. The best early treatment is warming the area by firm, steady pressure with a warm hand; blowing on it with hot breath; holding it against your body; or immersing it in warm (not hot) water. As the skin thaws, it becomes red and starts to tingle. Be careful to protect it from further damage. Don't rub the skin vigorously or with snow, as you could damage the tissue.

More severe is *frostbite*. There are two types of frostbite: *superficial* and *deep*. Superficial frostbite, the freezing of the skin and tissues just below the skin, is characterized by a waxy look and firmness of the skin, although the tissue below is soft. Initial treatment should be to slowly rewarm the area. As the area thaws, it will be numb and bluish or purple, and blisters may form. Cover the area with a dry, sterile dressing, and protect the skin from further exposure to cold. See a doctor for further treatment. Deep frostbite, the freezing of skin, muscle, and even bone, requires medical treatment. It usually involves the tissues of the hands and feet, which appear pale and feel frozen. Keep the victim dry and as warm as possible on the way to a medical facility. Cover the frostbitten area with a dry, sterile dressing.

The center of the body may gradually cool at temperatures above, as well as below, freezing—usually in wet, windy weather. When body temperature falls below 95 degrees Fahrenheit, the body is incapable of rewarming itself because of the breakdown of the internal system that regulates its temperature. This state is known as **hypothermia**. The first sign of hypothermia is severe shivering. Then the victim becomes uncoordinated, drowsy, listless, and confused and is unable to speak properly. Symptoms become more severe as body temperature continues to drop, and coma or death can result.

Hypothermia requires emergency medical treatment. Try to prevent any further heat loss. Move the victim to a warm place, cover him or her with blankets, remove wet clothing, and replace it with dry garments. If the victim is conscious, administer warm liquids, not alcohol.

Protect yourself in cold weather (or cold indoor gyms) by covering as much of your body as possible, but don't overdress. Wear one layer less than you would if you were outside but not exercising. Don't use warm-up clothes made of waterproof material, because they tend to trap heat and keep perspiration from evaporating. Make sure your clothes are loose enough to allow movement and exercise of the hands, feet, and other body parts, thereby maintaining proper circulation. Choose dark colors that absorb heat. And because 40 percent or more of your body heat is lost through your head and neck, wear a hat, turtleneck, or scarf. Make sure you cover your hands and feet as well; mittens provide more warmth and protection than gloves.

Types of Injuries

According to the American Physical Therapy Association, the most common exercise-related injury sites are the knees, feet, back, and shoulders, followed by the ankles and hips. **Acute injuries**—sprains, bruises, and pulled muscles—are the result of sudden trauma, such as a fall or collision. **Overuse injuries,** on the other hand, are the result of overdoing a repetitive activity, such as running. When one particular joint is overstressed—such as a tennis player's elbow or a swimmer's shoulder—tendinitis, an inflammation at the point where the tendon meets the bone, can develop. Other overuse injuries include muscle strains and aches and stress fractures, which are hairline breaks in a bone, usually in the leg or foot.

 Men and women may be vulnerable to different types of injuries. Studies of male and female college basketball and soccer players have shown that gender differences in the neuromuscular control of the knee places female athletes at higher risk for knee injuries. Balance training may reduce the risk.

Taking Care of Injuries

Sooner or later most active people suffer an injury. Although most are minor, they all require attention. Ignoring a problem or trying to push through the pain can lead to more serious complications.

PRICE

If you develop aches and pains beyond what you might expect from an activity, stop. Never push to the point of fatigue. If you do, you could end up with sprained or torn muscles. Figure 5.13 gives the PRICE prescription for coping with an exercise injury.

- **P**rotect the area with an elastic wrap, a sling, splint, cane, crutches, or an air cast.
- **R**est to promote tissue healing. Avoid activities that cause pain, swelling, or discomfort.
- **I**ce the area immediately, even if you're seeking medical help (don't put the ice pack directly on the skin). Repeat every two or three hours while you're awake for the first 48 to 72 hours. Cold reduces pain, swelling, and inflammation in injured muscles, joints, and connecting tissues and may slow bleeding if a tear has occurred.

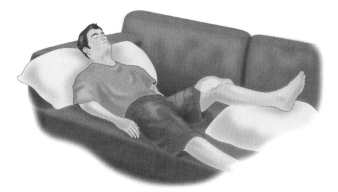

Figure 5.13 PRICE: How to Cope with an Exercise Injury

- **C**ompress the area with an elastic bandage until the swelling stops. Begin wrapping at the end farthest from your heart. Loosen the wrap if the pain increases, the area becomes numb, or swelling is occurring below the wrapped area.
- **E**levate the area above your heart, especially at night. Gravity helps reduce swelling by draining excess fluid.

After 48 hours, if the swelling is gone, you may apply warmth or gentle heat, which improves the blood flow and speeds healing.

hypothermia An abnormally low body temperature; if not treated appropriately, coma or death could result.

acute injuries Physical injuries, such as sprains, bruises, and pulled muscles, which result from sudden traumas, such as falls or collisions.

overuse injuries Physical injuries to joints or muscles, such as strains, fractures, and tendinitis, which result from overdoing a repetitive activity.

Overtraining

About half of all people who start an exercise program drop out within six months. One common reason is that they **overtrain,** pushing themselves to work too intensely too frequently. Signs of overdoing it include persistent muscle soreness, frequent injuries, unintended weight loss, nervousness, and an inability to relax. Overtraining for endurance sports like marathon running can damage the lungs and intensify asthma symptoms. You may find yourself unable to complete a normal workout or to recover after a normal workout.

If you develop any of the symptoms of overtraining, reduce or stop your workout sessions temporarily. Make gradual increases in the intensity of your workouts. Allow 24 to 48 hours for recovery between workouts. Make sure you get adequate rest. Check with a physical education instructor, coach, or trainer to make sure your exercise program fits your individual needs.

Exercise Addiction

Excessive exercise can become a form of addiction, and "exercise dependence" is not uncommon among young men and women. Although most physically active college students work out at healthy levels, some exercise to an extent that could signal dependence. In one study of 257 students at an East Coast university (none athletes in training or in season), about one in five exercised more than six hours a week and did so for reasons or in ways that appeared unhealthy. For example, they felt compelled to exercise even when ill or injured and felt guilty if they didn't work out.[37]

Learn It : Live It

Shaping Up

This chapter has given you the basic information you need to launch a fitness program. However, you're more likely to succeed if you create a plan and follow it. These basic steps can help you determine where you are now and how to get to where you want to be.

- **Evaluate your readiness for change.** Use this chapter's Self Survey to determine your stage of behavioral change. Don't expect to progress directly from one stage to another just once. Most people "recycle" several times before a change becomes permanent.

- **Consider your fitness goals.** Do you have an overall conditioning goal, such as losing weight? Or do you have a training goal, such as preparing for a 5K race or the tryouts for the volleyball team? Break down your goal into smaller "step" goals that lead you toward it.

- **Think through your personal preferences.** What are your physical strengths and weaknesses? Do you have good upper body strength but easily get winded? Do you have a stiff back? Do your allergies flare up when you exercise outdoors? By paying attention to your needs, likes, and dislikes, you can choose activities you enjoy—and are more likely to continue.

- **Schedule exercise into your daily routine.** If you can, block out a half-hour for working out at the beginning of the day, between classes, or in the evening. Write it into your schedule as if it were a class or doctor's appointment. If you can't find 30 minutes, look for two 15-minute or three 10-minute slots that you can use for "mini-workouts." Once you've worked out a schedule, write it down. A written plan encourages you to stay on track.

- **Assemble your gear.** Make sure you put your athletic shoes in your car or in the locker at the gym. Lay out the clothes you'll need to shoot hoops or play racquetball.

- **Start slowly.** If you are just beginning regular activity or exercise, begin at a low level. If you have an injury, disability, or chronic health problem, be sure you get medical clearance from a physician.

- **Progress gradually.** If you have not been physically active, begin by incorporating a few minutes of physical activity into each day, building up to 30 minutes or more of moderate-intensity activities. If you have been active but not as often or as intensely as recommended, become more consistent. Continue to increase the frequency, intensity, and duration of your workouts.

- **Take stock.** After a few months of leading a more active life, take stock. Think of how much more energy you have at the end of the day. Ask if you're feeling any less stressed, despite the push and pull of daily pressures. Focus on the unanticipated rewards of exercise. Savor the exhilaration of an autumn morning's walk; the thrill of feeling newly toughened muscles bend to your will; or the satisfaction of a long, smooth stretch after a stressful day. Enjoy the pure pleasure of living in the body you deserve.

overtrain   Working muscles too intensely or too frequently, resulting in persistent muscle soreness, injuries, unintended weight loss, nervousness, and an inability to relax.

SELFSURVEY : *Are You Ready to Become More Active?*

Physical Activity Stages of Change Questionnaire

For each of the following questions, please circle Yes or No. Please be sure to read the questions carefully.

Physical activity or exercise includes activities such as walking briskly, jogging, bicycling, swimming, or any other activity in which the exertion is at least as intense as these activities.

	NO	YES
1. I am currently physically active.	NO	YES
2. I intend to become more physically active in the next 6 months.	NO	YES

For activity to be regular, it must add up to a total of 30 minutes or more per day and be done at least 5 days per week. For example, you could take one 30-minute walk or take three 10-minute walks for a daily total of 30 minutes.

	NO	YES
3. I currently engage in regular physical activity.	NO	YES
4. I have been regularly physically active for the past 6 months.	NO	YES

Scoring Algorithm

	Question			
	1	2	3	4
Precontemplation	No	No		
Contemplation	No	Yes		
Preparation	Yes		No	
Action	Yes		Yes	No
Maintenance	Yes		Yes	Yes

Sources: Adapted from Marcus, Bess, and Beth Lewis. "Physical Activity and the Stages of Motivational Readiness for Change Model." *President's Council on Physical Fitness and Sports Research Digest,* Series 4, No. 1, March 2003, p. 1. Marcus, H., and L. J. Forsyth. *Motivating People to Be Physically Active.* Champaign, IL: Human Kinetics, 2003. Reprinted, by permission, from B. H. Marcus and L. H. Forsyth, 2003, *Motivating People to be Physically Active* (Champaign, IL: Human Kinetics), p. 21.

Your Health Action Plan for Physical Fitness

Once you know your stage of motivational readiness, you can employ the cognitive and behavioral strategies most likely to work for you now. As you progress through the stages of change, you can shift to other approaches. Here are some suggestions:

Precontemplation (not active and not thinking about becoming active)

- Use this course as an opportunity to learn about the benefits of physical activity, including better mood, lower stress, stronger bones, and a lower risk of cardiovascular disease.

- Set a small, reasonable goal that does not involve working up a sweat, such as looking up "exercise, benefits of" in the index of this book and reading the pages cited.

- List what you see as the cons of physical activity. For example, do you fear it would take time you need for your studies? Think of small changes that don't require time, for instance, standing rather than sitting when talking on the phone, doing stretches while watching television, or taking a quick walk down the hall or up the stairs while waiting for a friend or a class to begin.

- Identify barriers to physical activity, such as lack of money. Take advantage of your student status, and check out facilities, such as the swimming pool at the athletic center, or opportunities, such as an intramural soccer team, available to you free (or almost).

Contemplation (not active but thinking about becoming active)

- Think back to activities you found enjoyable in the past. You might consider inline skating to class or around campus, or plan a hike for a weekend or school break.

- Determine the types of activity you can realistically fit into your daily schedule. You might join friends for softball every Saturday, or sign up for an evening body-sculpting class.

- Visualize success. Focus on the person you want to become: How would you look? What would you do differently? Find an image—from a magazine advertisement, for example—and post it where you can see it often.

- Plan your rewards. Use a technique called shaping, which reinforces progress on the way to a goal. For instance, initially you might reward yourself once you engage in physical activity for 15 minutes a day. After a week, you get the reward only after 20 minutes a day. Over time you increase the number of days you are physically active as well as the number of minutes of activity per day.

- Reach out for support. Find a friend, family member, or classmate who is willing or able to provide support for being active. Or join an organized martial arts class or an informal team.

Preparation (active but not at recommended levels)

- Identify specific barriers that limit your activity. If your daily jogs are rained or snowed out, develop a list of indoor alternatives, such as walking stairs or working out to an exercise video.

- Set specific daily and weekly goals. Your daily goal might begin with 10 or 15 minutes of activity. Your weekly goal might be to try a new activity, such as spinning or a dance class.

- Divide physical activity over the course of the day with a 10 or 15 minute walk in the morning, another at lunch, and a third at the end of the day.

- Document your progress. You could use a monthly calendar to keep track of the number of days you've exercised as well as the length of each workout. Or you can keep a more detailed record, noting the types of exercise you do every day, the intensity you work at, the duration of each workout, and so forth.

Action and Maintenance (active at recommended levels for less than six months)

- Identify risk factors that might lead to relapse. If vacations or holiday breaks disrupt your routine, make a plan for alternative ways to remain active before you leave campus.
- Stress-proof your fitness program. In crunch times, you may feel you don't have time to spare for exercise. Multiple

10-minute walks during the day may be particularly useful both to keep up your fitness and to relieve stress buildup.

- Avoid boredom. Think through ways to vary your exercise routine. Take different routes on your walks. Invite different friends to join you. Alternate working with free weights and resistance machines at the gym.
- Set secondary goals. Once you've reached and maintained your goal for physical activity, set goals related to secondary benefits of exercise, for instance, losing weight or changing your body composition.

CENGAGENOW If you want to write your own goals for improved fitness, go to the Wellness Journal at HealthNow: **academic.cengage .com/login**

Making This Chapter Work
for YOU

Review Questions

1. Jessica takes a step aerobics class three times a week. Which component of physical fitness does her exercise routine emphasize?
   a. muscular strength and endurance
   b. flexibility
   c. cardiorespiratory fitness
   d. body composition

2. Which of the following statements is true?
   a. Inactivity does not affect health until middle age.
   b. Total fitness includes emotional and social dimensions of health besides the physical.
   c. Men and women have the same physiological capacities.
   d. Total fitness is one dimension of physical fitness.

3. The benefits of regular physical activity include
   a. decreased bone mass.
   b. lowered risk of shin splints.
   c. enhanced immune response.
   d. altered sleep patterns.

4. To motivate yourself to stick to an exercise program:
   a. Watch professional athletic competitions.
   b. Set a long-term goal, then break it down into short-term goals that can be achieved in a few months.
   c. Keep a detailed record of all the times that you avoided working out.
   d. Join an expensive health club so that you feel pressured to get your money's worth.

5. Michael started a walking program two weeks ago. Which of these workouts would you recommend to him for aerobic exercise?
   a. 5 minutes of brisk walking, 30 minutes of flexibility exercises, 5 minutes of brisk walking
   b. 5 minutes of stretching, 15 minutes of slow walking, 5 minutes of brisk walking, 15 minutes of slow walking

   c. 10 minutes of slow walking, 35 minutes of brisk walking, 5 minutes of slow walking
   d. 10 minutes of stretching, 45 minutes of brisk walking

6. For any muscle to get stronger, it must work against a greater-than-normal resistance. This is called the
   a. reversibility principle.
   b. overload principle.
   c. FITT principle.
   d. principle of compound interest.

7. A regular flexibility program provides which of the following benefits?
   a. stronger heart and lungs
   b. relief of muscle strain and soreness
   c. increased strength and endurance
   d. increased bone mass and leaner muscles

8. If you are a healthy weight,
   a. you are always hungry.
   b. your BMI is between 18.5 and 24.9.
   c. your waist measurement is 25 to 28 inches.
   d. your waist-to-hip ratio is greater than 1.0.

9. Which nutrient is the most important during exercise and exertion?
   a. water
   b. carbohydrates
   c. fat
   d. protein

10. Which of the following precautions could help to prevent a serious sports injury from occurring?
    a. Wear swimming goggles when doing laps to decrease the irritating effects of chlorine.
    b. Wear knee pads when cycling to prevent knee gashes if you fall off your bicycle.
    c. To eliminate persistent muscle soreness, increase the frequency and/or time period of your workout.
    d. Wear a helmet, wrist guards, and knee pads when inline skating to help prevent fractures and head injuries.

Answers to these questions can be found on page 583.

Critical Thinking

1. Allison knows that exercise is good for her health, but she figures she can keep her weight down by dieting and worry about her heart and health when she gets older. "I look good. I feel okay. Why should I bother exercising?" she asks. What would you reply?

2. College athletes have died unexpectedly from heart-related problems. The American Heart Association has identified guidelines to screen competitive athletes. Does your school follow these guidelines? If not, what precautions are taken to protect young athletes?

3. Your younger brother Andre is hoping to get a starting position on his high school football team. Practices began in July. You are aware that a couple of other players have suffered heat-related incidences, but according to Andre, these players just weren't tough enough. What can you do to help your brother protect his health?

4. Research is mixed on whether stretching can decrease delayed-onset muscle soreness. Do you think a placebo effect can occur in studies on exercise and training as it does in research on medications? Why or why not?

Media Menu

CENGAGENOW™ Go to the HealthNow website at **academic.cengage .com/login** that will:

- Help you evaluate your knowledge of the material.
- Allow you to take an exam-prep quiz.
- Provide a Personalized Learning Plan targeting resources that address areas you should study.
- Coach you through identifying target goals for behavioral change and creating and monitoring your personal change plan throughout the semester.

INTERNET CONNECTIONS

American Council on Exercise

www.acefitness.org

This website features information for the general public as well as for certified fitness trainers. The comprehensive site includes health and fitness news headlines, Fit Facts information sheets, a question and answer site, whole-body exercise workouts, daily fitness tips, discussion boards, newsletters, and information on ACE certification.

American Alliance for Health, Physical Education, Recreation and Dance

www.aahperd.org

This organization provides legislative advocacy for healthy lifestyles through high quality programs in health and physical education. The website features consumer news, career links, listing of graduate programs, research, and a link for the International Electronic Journal of Health Education.

Shape Up America

www.shapeup.org/fitness/index.php

At this site, you can perform a battery of physical fitness assessments, including activity level, strength, flexibility, and an aerobic fitness test. You get started by entering your weight, height, age, and gender and then take a quick screen test to assess your physical readiness for physical activity. Your final results in each area will be based on your personal data.

Start!

www.heart.org/presenter.jhtml?identifier=3041198

At this website sponsored by the American Heart Association, after a free registration you can access an interactive exercise diary where you can keep track of your own exercise progress. An information resource called MyStart! provides health and fitness resources.

Key Terms

The terms listed are used and defined on the page indicated. Definitions are also found in the Glossary at the end of this book.

active stretching 129
acute injuries 139
aerobic exercise 117
anabolic steroids 127
anaerobic exercise 117
ballistic stretching 129
body composition 109
body mass index (BMI) 133
cardiorespiratory fitness 109
dynamic flexibility 127
endorphins 113
FITT 115
flexibility 109
functional fitness 109
hypothermia 139
isokinetic 123
isometric 123
isotonic 123
muscular endurance 109
muscular strength 109
obesity 133
osteoporosis 113
overload principle 115
overloading 123
overtrain 140
overuse injuries 139
overweight 133
passive stretching 129
physical fitness 109
progressive overloading 115
range of motion 127
Rating of Perceived Exertion (RPE) 117
rep (or repetition) 125
resting heart rate 117
reversibility principle 117
sets 125
specificity principle 117
static flexibility 127
static stretching 129
target heart rate 117
waist-to-hip ratio 133

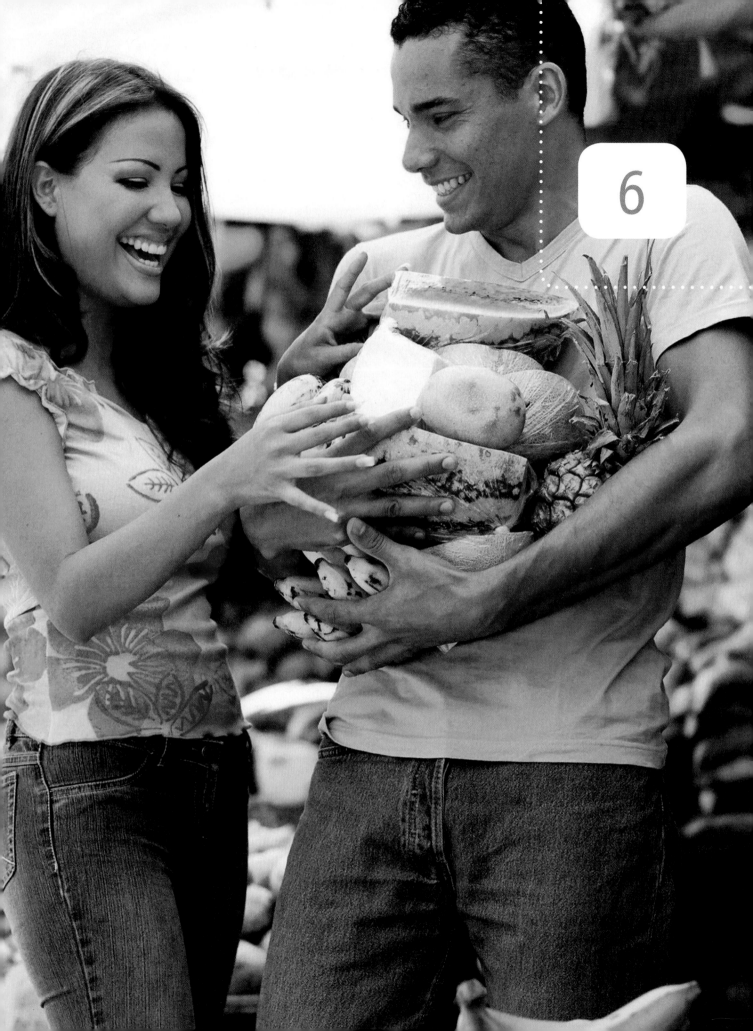

Personal Nutrition

THE freshmen on the fifth floor of a university dormitory decided to test a dubious premise: that man—and woman—can live on pizza alone. For a month, they vowed to eat nothing but pizza in all its savory varieties—mushroom, pepperoni, sausage, anchovies, extra cheese, thin crust, double crust. In less than a week, most cringed at the very sight of yet another cardboard delivery box. It wasn't just the boredom of having the same meal that got to them. Some felt bloated. Others had stomachaches. A few complained of headaches and fatigue. One was convinced she had scurvy, a vitamin deficiency disease caused by a lack of fruit and vegetables. None of them managed to stick with pizza for an entire month.

As these students discovered, we are indeed what we eat—and it shows in everything from our stamina and strength to the sheen in our hair and the glow in our cheeks. Eating well helps us live and feel well.

As demonstrated by the science of **nutrition,** the field that explores the connections between our bodies and the foods we eat, our daily diet affects how long and how well we live. Sensible eating can provide energy for our daily tasks, protect us from many chronic illnesses, and may even extend longevity. A high-quality diet also enhances day-to-day vitality, energy, and sense of well-being.

This chapter can help you make healthy food choices. It translates the latest scientific research into specific advice designed both to promote health and to prevent chronic disease. By learning more about nutrients, food groups, eating patterns, nutrition labels, and safety practices, you can nourish your body with foods that not only taste good but also are good for you. (See the "Mind Over Platter" lab in *IPC* to develop greater awareness and appreciation of the food you eat.) `IPC`

After studying the material in this chapter, you should be able to:

- **List** the basic nutrients necessary for a healthy body and **describe** their functions.
- **Describe** the key themes of the USDA MyPyramid Food Guidance System.
- **List** five specific nutrition guidelines of the MyPyramid system.
- **Explain** how to interpret the nutritional information provided on food labels.
- **List** the food safety hazards and **describe** prevention measures.
- **List** your nutrition pitfalls and **define** a strategy to avoid them.

© Ablestock/ Dynamic Graphics/ Jupiterimages

What You Need to Know About Nutrients

Every day your body needs certain **essential nutrients** that it cannot manufacture for itself. They provide energy, build and repair body tissues, and regulate body functions. The six classes of essential nutrients, which are discussed in this section, are water, protein, carbohydrates, fats, vitamins, and minerals (Table 6.1).

Water makes up about 60 percent of the body and is essential for health and survival. Besides water, we also need energy to live, and we receive our energy from the carbohydrates, proteins, and fats in the foods we eat. The digestive system (Figure 6.1) breaks down food into these **macronutrients.** They are the nutrients required by the human body in the greatest amounts. The amount of energy that can be derived from the macronutrients is measured in **calories.** There are 9 calories in every gram of fat and 4 calories in every gram of protein or carbohydrate. The other two essential nutrients—the vitamins and minerals—are called **micronutrients** because our bodies need them in only very small amounts.

Your need for macronutrients depends on how much energy you expend. Because fats, carbohydrates, and protein can all serve as sources of energy, they can, to some extent, substitute for one another in providing calories.

Adults, according to federal standards, should get 45 to 65 percent of calories from carbohydrates, 20 to 35 percent from fat, and 10 to 35 percent from protein. Children's fat intake should be slightly higher: 25 to 40 percent of their caloric intake.

To eat well without overeating, choose foods that are "nutrient-dense," that is, foods that provide the most nutritional value. For example, both a cup of nonfat milk and an ounce and a half of cheddar cheese provide about 300 mg of calcium, but the milk offers the same amount of calcium for half the calories. Foods that are extremely low in nutrient density—such as potato chips, candy, and soft drinks—deliver only calories. Fruits and vegetables are nutrient-dense foods that provide many health benefits. However, despite some claims, diets high in fruit and vegetables and low in fat have not proven to lower the risk of recurrence or death in women who have been treated for breast cancer.[1]

Calories

Calories are the measure of the amount of energy that can be derived from food. How many calories you need depends on your gender, age, body-frame size, weight, percentage of body fat, and your **basal metabolic rate (BMR)**—the number of calories needed to sustain your body at rest. Your activity level also affects your calorie

---

TABLE 6.1 The Essential Nutrients

	Sources	Functions
Water	Liquids, fruits, and vegetables	Carries nutrients and removes waste; dissolves amino acids, glucose, and minerals; cleans body by removing toxins; regulates body temperature
Proteins	Meat, poultry, fish, eggs, beans, nuts, cheese, tofu, vegetables, some fruits, pastas, breads, cereal, and rice	Help build new tissue to keep hair, skin, and eyesight healthy; build antibodies, enzymes, hormones, and other compounds; provide fuel for body
Carbohydrates	Grains, cereal, pasta, fruits and vegetables, nuts, milk, and sugars	Provide energy
Fats		
Saturated Fats	Red meat, dairy products, egg yolks, coconut and palm oils, shortening, stick margarine, baked goods	Provide energy; trigger production of cholesterol
Unsaturated Fats	Some fish; avocados; olive, canola, and peanut oils	Also provide energy, but trigger more "good" cholesterol production and less "bad" cholesterol production
Vitamins	Fruits, vegetables, grains, some meat and dairy products	Facilitate use of other nutrients; involved in regulating growth, maintaining tissue, and manufacturing blood cells, hormones, and other body components
Minerals	Many foods	Help build bones and teeth; aid in muscle function and nervous system activity; assist in various body functions including growth and energy production

© Gregg Adams/Stone/Getty Images

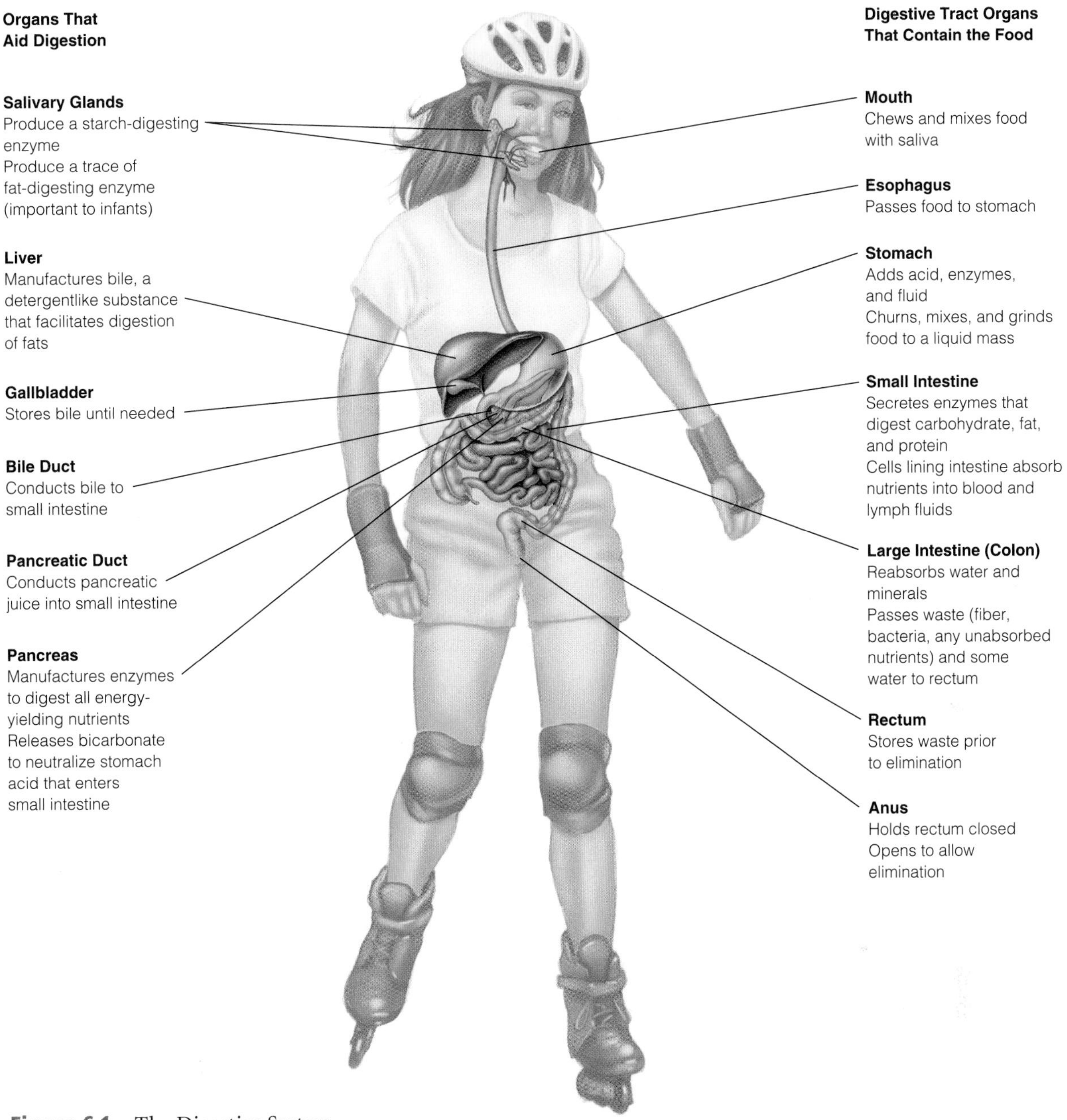

**Organs That
Aid Digestion**

**Digestive Tract Organs
That Contain the Food**

Salivary Glands
Produce a starch-digesting
enzyme
Produce a trace of
fat-digesting enzyme
(important to infants)

Liver
Manufactures bile, a
detergentlike substance
that facilitates digestion
of fats

Gallbladder
Stores bile until needed

Bile Duct
Conducts bile to
small intestine

Pancreatic Duct
Conducts pancreatic
juice into small intestine

Pancreas
Manufactures enzymes
to digest all energy-
yielding nutrients
Releases bicarbonate
to neutralize stomach
acid that enters
small intestine

Mouth
Chews and mixes food
with saliva

Esophagus
Passes food to stomach

Stomach
Adds acid, enzymes,
and fluid
Churns, mixes, and grinds
food to a liquid mass

Small Intestine
Secretes enzymes that
digest carbohydrate, fat,
and protein
Cells lining intestine absorb
nutrients into blood and
lymph fluids

Large Intestine (Colon)
Reabsorbs water and
minerals
Passes waste (fiber,
bacteria, any unabsorbed
nutrients) and some
water to rectum

Rectum
Stores waste prior
to elimination

Anus
Holds rectum closed
Opens to allow
elimination

Figure 6.1 The Digestive System
The organs of the digestive system break down food into nutrients that the body can use.

requirements. Regardless of whether you consume fat, protein, or carbohydrates, if you take in more calories than required to maintain your size and don't work them off in some sort of physical activity, your body will convert the excess to fat (see Chapter 7). On average, daily calorie needs are:

- Most women, some older adults, children ages two to six: 1,600
- Average adult: 2,000
- Most men, active women, teenage girls, older children: 2,200
- Active men, teenage boys: 2,800

nutrition The science devoted to the study of dietary needs for food and the effects of food on organisms.

essential nutrients Nutrients that the body cannot manufacture for itself and must obtain from food.

macronutrients Nutrients required by the human body in the greatest amounts, including water, carbohydrates, proteins, and fats.

calorie The amount of energy required to raise the temperature of

1 gram of water by 1 degree Celsius. In everyday usage related to the energy content of foods and the energy expended in activities, a calorie is actually the equivalent of a thousand such calories, or a kilocalorie.

micronutrients Vitamins and minerals needed by the body in very small amounts.

basal metabolic rate (BMR) The number of calories required to sustain the body at rest.

Water

Water, which makes up 85 percent of blood, 70 percent of muscles, and about 75 percent of the brain, performs many essential functions: It carries nutrients, maintains temperature, lubricates joints, helps with digestion, rids the body of waste through urine, and contributes to the production of sweat, which evaporates from the skin to cool the body. Research has correlated high fluid intake with a lower risk of kidney stones, colon cancer, and bladder cancer.

You lose about 64 to 80 ounces of water a day—the equivalent of eight to ten 8-ounce glasses—through perspiration, urination, bowel movements, and normal exhalation. You lose water more rapidly if you exercise, live in a dry climate or at a high altitude, drink a lot of caffeine or alcohol (which increase urination), skip a meal, or become ill. To assure adequate water intake, nutritionists advise drinking a minimum of 64 ounces, enough so that your urine is not dark in color. Healthy individuals can get adequate hydration from beverages other than plain water, including juice and soft drinks.

Protein

Critical for growth and repair, **proteins** form the basic framework for our muscles, bones, blood, hair, and fingernails. Supplying 4 calories per gram, they are made of combinations of 20 **amino acids,** 9 of which we must get from our diet because the human body cannot produce them. These are called *essential amino acids.*

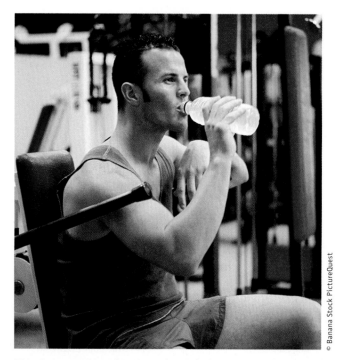

Water is an essential nutrient. Remember: Each day you must replace the amount you use.

© Banana Stock PictureQuest

Animal proteins—meat, fish, poultry, and dairy products—are **complete proteins** that provide the nine essential amino acids. Grains, dry beans, and nuts are **incomplete proteins** that may have relatively low levels of one or two essential amino acids but fairly high levels of others. Combining incomplete proteins, such as beans and rice, ensures that the body gets sufficient protein. The recommended level of daily protein intake is 0.8 gram per kilogram of body weight for adults.

Carbohydrates

Carbohydrates are organic compounds that provide our brains and bodies with *glucose,* their basic fuel. The major sources of carbohydrates are plants—including grains, vegetables, fruits, and beans—and milk. There are two types: *simple carbohydrates* (sugars) and *complex carbohydrates* (starches and fiber). All provide 4 calories per gram. Both adults and children should consume at least 130 grams of carbohydrates each day, the minimum needed to produce enough glucose for the brain to function.

Forms of Carbohydrates

Simple carbohydrates include *natural sugars,* such as the lactose in milk and the fructose in fruit, and *added sugars* that are found in candy, soft drinks, fruit drinks, pastries, and other sweets. Those whose diets are higher in added sugars typically have lower intakes of other essential nutrients.

Complex carbohydrates include grains, cereals, vegetables, beans, and nuts. Americans, however, get most of their complex carbohydrates from refined grains, which have been stripped of fiber and many nutrients.

Far more nutritious are whole grains, which are made up of all components of the grain: the *bran* (or fiber-rich outer layer), the *endosperm* (middle layer), and the *germ* (the nutrient-packed inner layer). Increasing whole-grain consumption has become a public health priority, and the 2005 Dietary Guidelines recommend that Americans increase their consumption of whole-grain foods.

Whole grains have proven effective in lowering the risk of diabetes and heart disease. In one recent seven-year study, individuals who consumed more fiber through cereal, bread, and other whole-grain products were less likely to develop diabetes than those who ate less fiber.[2] In an analysis of studies involving more than 285,000 people, those who consumed an average of 2.5 servings of whole grains each day had a significantly lower risk of cardiovascular disease than those who ate less than half a serving of grains. Yet only 8 percent of American adults consume three or more servings of whole grains; 42 percent eat no whole grains on a given day.[3]

Low-Carb Foods

The popularity of diets that restrict carbohydrate intake, such as the Atkins diet discussed in Chapter 7, prompted an explosion in products touted as "low-carb." You can get low-carb versions of everything from beer to bread. However, the Food and Drug Administration (FDA), which regulates health claims on food labels in the United States, hasn't defined what "low-carb" means. Words like "low-carb," "carb-wise," or "carb-free" are marketing terms created by manufacturers to sell their products.

Although many people may buy low-carb foods because they believe that they're healthier, that isn't necessarily the case. A low-carb nutrition bar, for instance, may be high in saturated fat and calories. Some low-carb food products cause digestive symptoms because food companies often replace the carbohydrates in a cookie or cracker with substances such as the sweetener sorbitol, which can cause diarrhea or stomach cramps.

Dieters often buy low-carb products in order to lose weight. According to proponents of low-carb diets, if carbohydrates raise blood sugar and insulin levels and cause weight gain, a decrease in carbs should result in lower blood sugar and insulin levels—and weight loss. With limited carbohydrates in the diet, the body would break down fat to provide needed energy.

Some people do lose weight when they switch to low-carb foods, but the reasons are probably that they consume fewer calories, lose water weight, and have decreased appetite because of a buildup of ketones (a by-product of fat metabolism) in the blood. As discussed in Chapter 7, a low-carb diet can lead to fairly rapid weight loss but is no easier to maintain over the long run than any other diet.

Glycemic Index and Glycemic Load

The glycemic index is a ranking of carbohydrates, gram for gram, based on their immediate effect on blood glucose (sugar) levels. Carbohydrates that break down quickly during digestion and trigger a fast, high glucose response have the highest glycemic index rating. Those that break down slowly, releasing glucose gradually into the bloodstream, have low glycemic index ratings. Potatoes, which raise blood sugar higher and faster than apples, for instance, earn a higher glycemic-index rating than apples. Glycemic index does not account for the amount of food you typically eat in a serving.

Glycemic load is a measure of how much a typical serving size of a particular food raises blood glucose. For example, the glycemic index of table sugar is high, but you use so little to sweeten your coffee or tea that its glycemic load is low.[4]

Some diets are based on the theory that high-glycemic-index foods raise blood sugar and insulin levels and cause weight gain, while low-glycemic-index foods lower your blood sugar and insulin levels so you'll lose weight. (See Chapter 7.)

Fiber

Dietary fiber is the nondigestible form of complex carbohydrates occurring naturally in plant foods, such as leaves, stems, skins, seeds, and hulls. **Functional fiber** consists of isolated, nondigestible carbohydrates that may be added to foods and that provide beneficial effects in humans. Total fiber is the sum of both.

The various forms of fiber enhance health in different ways: They slow the emptying of the stomach, which creates a feeling of fullness and aids weight control. They interfere with absorption of dietary fat and cholesterol, which lowers the risk of heart disease and stroke in both middle-aged and elderly individuals. In addition, fiber helps prevent constipation, diverticulosis (a painful inflammation of the bowel), and diabetes. The link between fiber and colon cancer is complex. Some studies have indicated that increased fiber intake reduces risk; others found no such correlation.

The Institute of Medicine has set recommendations for daily intake levels of total fiber (dietary plus functional fiber): 38 grams of total fiber for men and 25 grams for women. For men and women over 50 years of age, who consume less food, the recommendations are, respectively, 30 and 21 grams. The American Dietetic Association recommends 25 to 35 grams of dietary fiber a day, much more than the amount Americans typically consume.

Good fiber sources include wheat and corn bran (the outer layer); leafy greens; the skins of fruits and root vegetables; oats, beans, and barley; and the pulp, skin, and seeds of many fruits and vegetables, such as apples and strawberries (see Table 6.2). Because sudden increases in fiber can cause symptoms like bloating and gas, experts recommend gradually adding more fiber to your diet with an additional serving or two of vegetables, fruit, or whole-wheat bread.

---

proteins Organic compounds composed of amino acids; one of the essential nutrients.

amino acids Organic compounds containing nitrogen, carbon, hydrogen, and oxygen; the essential building blocks of proteins.

complete proteins Proteins that contain all the amino acids needed by the body for growth and maintenance.

incomplete proteins Proteins that lack one or more of the amino acids essential for protein synthesis.

carbohydrates Organic compounds, such as starches, sugars, and glycogen, that are composed of carbon, hydrogen, and oxygen, and are sources of bodily energy.

simple carbohydrates Sugars; like all carbohydrates, they provide the body with glucose.

complex carbohydrates Starches, including cereals, fruits, and vegetables.

dietary fiber The nondigestible form of carbohydrates found in plant foods, such as leaves, stems, skins, seeds, and hulls.

functional fiber Isolated, nondigestible carbohydrates with beneficial effects in humans.

TABLE 6.2 High-Fiber Foods

Grains

Whole-grain products provide about 1 to 2 grams (or more) of fiber per serving:
- 1 slice whole-wheat, pumpernickel, rye bread
- 1 oz ready-to-eat cereal (100% bran cereals contain 10 grams or more)
- ½ cup cooked barley, bulgur, grits, oatmeal

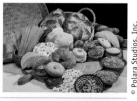

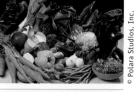

Vegetable

Most vegetables contain about 2 to 3 grams of fiber per serving:
- 1 cup raw bean sprouts
- ½ cup cooked broccoli, brussels sprouts, cabbage, carrots, cauliflower, collards, corn, eggplant, green beans, green peas, kale, mushrooms, okra, parsnips, potatoes, pumpkin, spinach, sweet potatoes, swiss chard, winter squash
- ½ cup chopped raw carrots, peppers

Fruit

Fresh, frozen, and dried fruits have about 2 grams of fiber per serving:
- 1 medium apple, banana, kiwi, nectarine, orange, pear
- ½ cup applesauce, blackberries, blueberries, raspberries, strawberries
- Fruit juices contain very little fiber

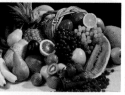

Legumes

Many legumes provide about 6 to 8 grams of fiber per serving:
- ½ cup cooked baked beans, black beans, black-eyed peas, kidney beans, navy beans, pinto beans

Some legumes provide about 5 grams of fiber per serving:
- ½ cup cooked garbanzo beans, great northern beans, lentils, lima beans, split peas

Fats

Fats carry the fat-soluble vitamins A, D, E, and K; aid in their absorption in the intestine; protect organs from injury; regulate body temperature; and play an important role in growth and development. They provide 9 calories per gram—more than twice the amount in carbohydrates or proteins.

Both high- and low-fat diets can be unhealthy. When people eat very low levels of fat and very high levels of carbohydrates, their levels of high-density lipoprotein, the so-called *good cholesterol*, decline. On the other hand, high-fat diets can lead to obesity and its related health dangers, discussed in Chapter 7.

saturated fats A chemical term indicating that a fat molecule contains as many hydrogen atoms as its carbon skeleton can hold. These fats are normally solid at room temperature.

unsaturated fats A chemical term indicating that a fat molecule contains fewer hydrogen atoms than its carbon skeleton can hold. These fats are normally liquid at room temperature.

trans fat Fat formed when liquid vegetable oils are processed to make table spreads or cooking fats; also found in dairy and beef products; considered to be especially dangerous dietary fats.

Forms of Fat

Saturated fats and **unsaturated fats** are distinguished by the type of fatty acids in their chemical structures. Unsaturated fats can be divided into monounsaturated or polyunsaturated, again depending on their chemical structure. All dietary fats are a mix of saturated and unsaturated fats but are predominantly one or the other. Unsaturated fats, like oils, are likely to be liquid at room temperature and saturated fats, like butter, are likely to be solid. In general, vegetable and fish oils are unsaturated, and animal fats are saturated. Table 6.3 lists the major sources of healthful monounsaturated and polyunsaturated fats.

Olive, soybean, canola, cottonseed, corn, and other vegetable oils are unsaturated fats. Olive oil is considered a good fat and one of the best vegetable oils for salads and cooking. Used for thousands of years, this staple of the Mediterranean diet, discussed later in this chapter, has been correlated with a lower incidence of heart disease, including strokes and heart attacks.

Fish oils are rich in omega-3 fatty acids, which make molecules such as prostaglandins that may enhance cardiovascular health. Long touted as "good" fats with numerous health benefits, omega-3 fatty acids may not live up to expectations. An extensive analysis of 89 studies on omega-3 fatty acids and their impact on cardiovascular disease, cancer, and stroke concluded that they

© Polara Studios, Inc.

© Polara Studios, Inc.

© Polara Studios, Inc.

© PhotoDisc Blue/Getty Images

do not improve health outcomes for the general population, although they do not cause harm or increase health risks.[5] Yet another large study yielded different findings, concluding that people who had higher intake of these fatty acids had lower death rates, primarily because of decreased heart attacks and strokes.[6]

Saturated fats can increase the risk of heart disease and should be avoided as much as possible. In response to consumer and health professionals' demand for less saturated fat in the food supply, many manufacturers switched to partially hydrogenated oils.

The process of hydrogenation creates unsaturated fatty acids called **trans fat.** They are found in some margarine products and most foods made with partially hydrogenated oils, such as baked goods and fried foods. Even though trans fats are unsaturated, they appear similar to saturated fats in terms of raising cholesterol levels. Epidemiological studies have suggested a possible link between cardiovascular disease risk and high intakes of trans fats, and researchers have concluded that they are, gram for gram, twice as damaging as saturated fat. There is no safe level for trans fats, which occur naturally in meats as well as in foods prepared with partially hydrogenated vegetable oils.

Some food manufacturers have reduced or eliminated trans fats in snacks and other products. Cities and communities across the country have banned trans fats in restaurants. Some campuses also have stopped using trans fats in their dining halls and food outlets.

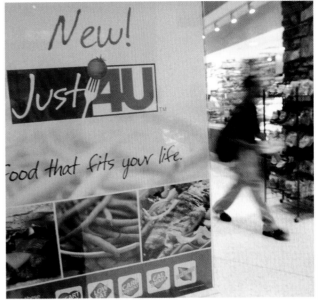

Many campus dining halls are providing nutritional information and healthier food options for students.

To cut down on both saturated and trans fats, choose soybean, canola, corn, olive, safflower, and sunflower oils, which are naturally free of trans fats and lower in saturated fats—see Table 6-3. Look for reduced-fat, low-fat, fat-free, and trans-fat-free versions of baked goods, snacks, and other processed foods. Some choices—such as butter versus margarine—are more difficult to make (see Figure 6.2).

TABLE 6.3   Major Sources of Various Fatty Acids

Healthful Fatty Acids

Monounsaturated	Polyunsaturated	Omega-3 Polyunsaturated
Avocado Oils (canola, olive, peanut, sesame) Nuts (almonds, cashews, filberts, hazelnuts, macadamia nuts, peanuts, pecans, pistachios) Olives Peanut butter Seeds (sesame)	Margarine (nonhydrogenated) Oils (corn, cottonseed, safflower, soybean) Nuts (pine nuts, walnuts) Mayonnaise Salad dressing Seeds (pumpkin, sunflower)	Fatty fish (herring, mackerel, salmon, tuna) Flaxseed Nuts (walnuts)

Unhealthful Fatty Acids

Saturated	Trans
Bacon Butter Chocolate Coconut Cream cheese Cream, half-and-half Lard Meat Milk and milk products (whole) Oils (coconut, palm, palm kernel) Shortening Sour cream	Fried foods (hydrogenated shortening) Margarine (hydrogenated or partially hydrogenated) Nondairy creamers Many fast foods Shortening Commercial baked goods (including doughnuts, cakes, cookies) Many snack foods (including microwave popcorn, chips, crackers)

Note: Keep in mind that foods contain a mixture of fatty acids.

Butter

Nutrition Facts

Serving Size 1 Tbsp (14g)
Servings per container about 32

Amount per serving

Calories 100 Calories from Fat 100

%Daily Value*

Total Fat 11g	17%
Saturated Fat 7g	37%
Trans Fat 0g	
Cholesterol 30mg	10%
Sodium 95mg	4%
Total Carbohydrate 0g	0%
Protein 0g	

Vitamin A 8%

Not a significant source of dietary fiber, sugars, vitamin C, calcium, and iron.

*Percent Daily Values are based on a 2,000 calorie diet.

INGREDIENTS: Cream, salt.

Margarine (stick)

Nutrition Facts

Serving Size 1 Tbsp (14g)
Servings per container about 32

Amount per serving

Calories 100 Calories from Fat 100

%Daily Value*

Total Fat 11g	17%
Saturated Fat 2g	11%
Trans Fat 2.5g	
Polyunsaturated Fat 3.5g	
Monounsaturated Fat 2.5g	
Cholesterol 0mg	0%
Sodium 105mg	4%
Total Carbohydrate 0g	0%
Protein 0g	

Vitamin A 10%

Not a significant source of dietary fiber, sugars, vitamin C, calcium, and iron.

*Percent Daily Values are based on a 2,000 calorie diet.

INGREDIENTS: Liquid soybean oil, partially hydrogenated soybean oil, water, buttermilk, salt, soy lecithin, sodium benzoate (as a preservative), vegetable mono and diglycerides, artificial flavor, vitamin A palmitate, colored with beta carotene (provitamin A).

Margarine (tub)

Nutrition Facts

Serving size 1 Tbsp (14g)
Servings per container about 32

Amount per serving

Calories 100 Calories from Fat 100

%Daily Value*

Total Fat 11g	17%
Saturated Fat 2.5g	13%
Trans Fat 2g	
Polyunsaturated Fat 4g	
Monounsaturated Fat 2.5g	
Cholesterol 0mg	0%
Sodium 80mg	3%
Total Carbohydrate 0g	0%
Protein 0g	

Vitamin A 10%

Not a significant source of dietary fiber, sugars, vitamin C, calcium, and iron.

*Percent Daily Values are based on a 2,000 calorie diet.

INGREDIENTS: Liquid soybean oil, partially hydrogenated soybean oil, buttermilk, water, butter (cream, salt), salt, soy lecithin, vegetable mono and diglycerides, sodium benzoate added as a preservative, artificial flavor, vitamin A palmitate, colored with beta carotene.

Margarine (liquid)

Nutrition Facts

Serving size 1 Tbsp (14g)
Servings per container about 24

Amount per serving

Calories 70 Calories from Fat 70

%Daily Value*

Total Fat 8g	13%
Saturated Fat 1.5g	7%
Trans Fat 0g	
Polyunsaturated Fat 4.5g	
Monounsaturated Fat 2g	
Cholesterol 0mg	0%
Sodium 110mg	8%
Total Carbohydrate 0g	0%
Protein 0g	

Vitamin A 10%

Not a significant source of dietary fiber, sugars, vitamin C, calcium, and iron.

*Percent Daily Values are based on a 2,000 calorie diet.

INGREDIENTS: Liquid soybean oil, water, salt, hydrogenated cottonseed oil, vegetable monoglycerides and soy lecithin (emulsifiers), potassium sorbate and sodium benzoate (to preserve freshness), artificial flavor, phosphoric acid (acidulant), colored with beta carotene (source of vitamin A), vitamin A palmitate.

Figure 6.2 Butter or Margarine?

Most of the fat in butter is saturated fat. Most of the fat in margarine is unsaturated, but the trans fats are twice as damaging as saturated fat. (If the list of ingredients includes hydrogenated oils, you know the food contains trans fat. The closer "partially hydrogenated oils" is to the beginning of the ingredients list, the more trans fats the product contains.)

Vitamins and Minerals

Vitamins, which help put proteins, fats, and carbohydrates to use, are essential to regulating growth, maintaining tissue, and releasing energy from foods. Together with the enzymes in the body, they help produce the right chemical reactions at the right times. They're also involved in the manufacture of blood cells, hormones, and other compounds.

The body produces some vitamins, such as vitamin D, which is manufactured in the skin after exposure to sunlight. Other vitamins must be ingested.

Vitamins A, D, E, and K are fat-soluble; they are absorbed through the intestinal membranes and stored in the body.

The B vitamins and vitamin C are water-soluble; they are absorbed directly into the blood and then used up or washed out of the body in urine and sweat. They must be replaced daily. Table 6.4 summarizes key information about the vitamins.

vitamins
Organic substances that are needed in very small amounts by the body and carry out a variety of functions in metabolism and nutrition.

antioxidant Substances that prevent the damaging effects of oxidation in cells.

minerals Naturally occurring inorganic substances, small amounts of some being essential in metabolism and nutrition.

Antioxidants are substances that prevent the harmful effects caused by oxidation within the body. They include vitamins C, E, and beta-carotene (a form of vitamin A), as well as compounds like carotenoids and flavonoids. All share a common enemy: renegade oxygen cells called free radicals released by normal metabolism as well as by pollution, smoking, radiation, and stress.

Diets high in antioxidant-rich fruits and vegetables have been linked with lower rates of esophageal, lung, colon, and stomach cancer. Nevertheless, scientific studies have not proved conclusively that any specific antioxidant, particularly in supplement form, can prevent cancer.

Carbon, oxygen, hydrogen, and nitrogen make up 96 percent of our body weight. The other 4 percent consists of **minerals** that help build bones and teeth, aid in muscle function, and help our nervous systems transmit messages. Every day we need about a tenth of a gram (100 milligrams) or more of the major minerals: sodium, potassium chloride, calcium, phosphorus, magnesium, and sulfur. We also need about a hundredth of a gram (10 milligrams) or less of each of the trace minerals: iron (although premenopausal

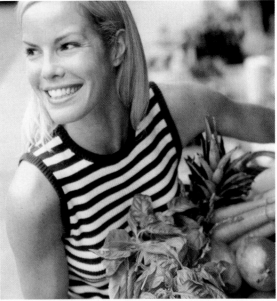

Vegetables and fruits are rich in antioxidants. By eating an orange at breakfast and half a carrot for lunch, you will get all the antioxidants you need for the day.

TABLE 6.4   Key Information About Vitamins

Fat-Soluble Vitamins   ADEK

Vitamin/Recommended Intake per Day	Significant Sources	Chief Functions	Signs of Severe, Prolonged Deficiency	Signs of Extreme Excess
Vitamin A Males 19–50: 900 μg Females 19–50: 700 μg	Fortified milk, cheese, cream, butter, fortified margarine, eggs, liver; spinach and other dark, leafy greens, broccoli, deep orange fruits (apricots, cantaloupes) and vegetables(carrots, sweet potatoes, pumpkins)	Antioxidant; needed for vision, health of cornea, epithelial cells, mucous membranes, skin health, bone and tooth growth, reproduction, immunity	Anemia, painful joints, cracks in teeth, tendency toward tooth decay, diarrhea, depression, frequent infections, night blindness, keratinization, corneal degeneration, rashes, kidney stones	Nosebleeds, bone pain, growth retardation, headaches, abdominal cramps and pain, vomiting, diarrhea, weight loss, overreactive immune system, blurred vision, fatigue, irritability, hair loss, dry skin
Vitamin D Males 19–50: 5 μg Females 19–50: 5 μg	Fortified milk or margarine, eggs, liver, sardines; exposure to sunlight	Mineralization of bones (promotes calcium and phosphorus absorption)	Abnormal growth, misshapen bones (bowing of legs), soft bones, joint pain, malformed teeth	Raised blood calcium, excessive thirst, headaches, irritability, loss of appetite, weakness, nausea, kidney stones, deposits in arteries
Vitamin E Males 19–50: 15 mg Females 19–50: 15 mg	Polyunsaturated plant oils (margarine, salad dressings, shortenings), green and leafy vegetables, wheat germ, whole-grain products, nuts, seeds	Antioxidant; needed for stabilization of cell membranes, regulation of oxidation reactions	Red blood cell breakage, anemia, muscle degeneration, difficulty walking, leg cramps	Augments the effects of anticlotting medication; general discomfort; blurred vision
Vitamin K Males 19–50: 120 μg Females 19–50: 90 μg	Green leafy vegetables, cabbage-type vegetables, soybeans, vegetable oils	Synthesis of blood-clotting proteins and proteins important in bone mineralization	Hemorrhage	Interference with anti-clotting medication; jaundice

Continued

TABLE 6.4 Key Information About Vitamins, *Continued*

Water-Soluble Vitamins

Vitamin/Recommended Intake per Day	Significant Sources	Chief Functions	Signs of Severe, Prolonged Deficiency	Signs of Extreme Excess
Vitamin B₆ Males 19–50: 1.3 mg Females 19–50: 1.3 mg	Meats, fish, poultry, liver, legumes, fruits, whole grains, potatoes, soy products	Part of a coenzyme used in amino acid and fatty acid metabolism, helps make red blood cells	Anemia, depression, abnormal brain wave pattern, convulsions, skin rashes	Impaired memory, irritability, headaches, numbness, damage to nerves, difficulty walking, loss of reflexes
Vitamin B₁₂ Males 19–50: 2.4 μg Females 19–50: 2.4 μg	Animal products (meat, fish, poultry, milk, cheese, eggs)	Part of a coenzyme used in new cell synthesis, helps maintain nerve cells	Anemia, nervous system degeneration progressing to paralysis, hypersensitivity	None known
Vitamin C Males 19–50: 90 mg Females 19–50: 75 mg	Citrus fruits, cabbage-type vegetables, dark green vegetables, cantaloupe, strawberries, peppers, lettuce, tomatoes, potatoes, papayas, mangoes	Antioxidant, collagen synthesis (strengthens blood vessel walls, forms scar tissue, matrix for bone growth), amino acid metabolism, strengthens resistance to infection, aids iron absorption	Anemia, pinpoint hemorrhages, frequent infections, bleeding gums, loosened teeth, muscle degeneration and pain, joint pain, blotchy bruises, failure of wounds to heal	Nausea, abdominal cramps, diarrhea, excessive urination, headache, fatigue, insomnia, rashes; deficiency symptoms may appear at first on withdrawal of high doses
Thiamin Males 19–50: 1.2 mg Females 19–50: 1.1 mg	Pork, ham, bacon, liver, whole grains, legumes, nuts; occurs in all nutritious foods in moderate amounts	Part of a coenzyme used in energy metabolism, supports normal appetite and nervous system function	Edema, enlarged heart, nervous/muscular system degeneration, difficulty walking, loss of reflexes, mental confusion	None reported
Riboflavin Males 19–50: 1.3 mg Females 19–50: 1.1 mg	Milk, yogurt, cottage cheese, meat, leafy green vegetables, whole-grain or enriched breads and cereals	Part of a coenzyme used in energy metabolism, supports normal vision and skin health	Cracks at corner of mouth, magenta tongue, hypersensitivity to light, reddening of cornea, skin rash	None reported
Niacin Males 19–50: 16 mg Females 19–50: 14 mg	Milk, eggs, meat, poultry, fish, whole-grain and enriched breads and cereals, nuts, and all protein-containing foods	Part of a coenzyme used in energy metabolism	Diarrhea, black smooth tongue, irritability, loss of appetite, weakness, dizziness, mental confusion, flaky skin rash on areas exposed to sun	Nausea, vomiting, painful flush and rash, sweating, liver damage
Folate Males 19–50: 400 μg Females 19–50: 400 μg	Leafy green vegetables, legumes, seeds, liver, enriched breads, cereal, pasta, and grains	Part of a coenzyme needed for new cell synthesis	Anemia, heartburn, frequent infections, smooth red tongue, depression, mental confusion	Masks vitamin B₁₂ deficiency
Panothenic acid Males 19–50: 5 mg Females 19–50: 5 mg	Widespread in foods	Part of a coenzyme used in energy metabolism	Vomiting, intestinal distress, insomnia, fatigue	Water retention (rare)
Biotin Males 19–50: 30 μg Females 19–50: 30 μg	Widespread in foods	Used in energy metabolism, fat synthesis, amino acid metabolism, and glycogen synthesis	Abnormal heart action, loss of appetite, nausea, depression, muscle pain, drying of facial skin	None reported

Source: Adapted from Sizer, Frances, and Ellie Whitney. *Nutrition: Concepts and Controversies,* 10th ed. Belmont, CA: Wadsworth, 2006.

women need more), zinc, selenium, molybdenum, iodine, copper, manganese, fluoride, and chromium. (See Table 6.5 for key information on minerals.)

Americans get adequate amounts of most nutrients. However, the 2005 Advisory Committee for Dietary Guidelines reported that intakes of several nutrients are low enough to be of concern.

- **For adults:** vitamins A, C, and E, calcium, magnesium, potassium, and fiber.

TABLE 6.5   Key Information About Minerals

Mineral	Significant Sources	Chief Functions	Signs of Severe, Prolonged Deficiency	Signs of Extreme Excess
Major Minerals				
Sodium	Salt, soy sauce, processed foods	Needed to maintain fluid balance and acid-base balance in body cells; critical to nerve impulse transmission	Mental apathy, poor appetite, muscle cramps	High blood pressure
Potassium	All whole foods: meats, milk, fruits, vegetables, grains, legumes	Needed to maintain fluid balance and acid-base balance in body cells; needed for muscle and nerve activity	Muscle weakness, mental confusion, paralysis	Irregular heartbeat, heart attack; muscular weakness
Chloride	Salt, soy sauce, processed foods	Aids in digestion; needed to maintain fluid balance and acid-base balance in body cells	Muscle cramps, apathy, poor appetite, growth failure in children	Vomiting
Calcium	Milk and milk products, oysters, small fish (with bones), tofu, greens, legumes	Component of bones and teeth, needed for muscle and nerve activity, blood clotting	Stunted growth in children, adult bone loss (osteoporosis)	Constipation; calcium deposits in kidneys, liver; decreased absorption of other minerals
Phosphorus	All animal tissues	Component of bones and teeth, energy formation, needed to maintain cell membranes	Loss of appetite, muscle weakness, impaired growth	Loss of calcium from bones
Magnesium	Nuts, legumes, whole grains, dark green vegetables, seafoods, chocolate, cocoa	Component of bones and teeth, nerve activity, energy and protein formation	Stunted growth in children, weakness, muscle spasms, personality changes	Diarrhea, dehydration, impaired nerve activity
Sulfur	All protein-containing foods	Component of certain amino acids; stabilizes protein shape	None known; protein deficiency would occur first	Depresses growth in animals
Trace Minerals				
Iron	Red meats, fish, poultry, shellfish, eggs, legumes, dried fruits	Aids in transport of oxygen, component of myoglobin, energy formation	Anemia, weakness, fatigue, pale appearance, reduced attention span, developmental delays in children	Vomiting, abdominal pain, blue coloration of skin, shock, heart failure, diabetes
Zinc	Protein-containing foods: fish, shellfish, poultry, grains, vegetables	Protein reproduction, component of insulin	Growth failure, delayed sexual maturation, slow wound healing	Nausea, vomiting, weakness, fatigue, metallic taste in mouth
Selenium	Meats and seafood, eggs, grains	Acts as an antioxidant in conjunction with vitamin E	Anemia, muscle pain and tenderness, heart failure	Hair and fingernail loss, weakness, liver damage, garlic or metallic breath
Molybdenum	Dried beans, grains, dark green vegetables, liver, milk and milk products	Aids in oxygen transfer from one molecule to another	Rapid heartbeat and breathing, nausea, vomiting, coma	Loss of copper from the body, joint pain, growth failure, anemia, gout
Iodine	Iodized salt, milk and milk products, seaweed, seafood, bread	Component of thyroid hormones that helps regulate energy production and growth	Goiter, cretinism in newborns (mental retardation, hearing loss, growth failure)	Pimples, goiter, decreased thyroid function
Copper	Organ meats, whole grains, nuts and seeds, seafood, drinking water	Component of enzymes involved in the body's utilization of iron and oxygen	Anemia, nerve and bone abnormalities in children, growth retardation	Vomiting, diarrhea, liver disease
Manganese	Whole grains, coffee, tea, dried beans, nuts	Formation of body fat and bone	Weight loss, rash, nausea and vomiting	Infertility in men, disruptions in the nervous system, muscle spasms

Continued

TABLE 6.5 Key Information About Minerals, *Continued*

Mineral	Significant Sources	Chief Functions	Signs of Severe, Prolonged Deficiency	Signs of Extreme Excess
Trace Minerals, continued				
Fluoride	Fluoridated water, foods, and beverages; tea; shrimp; crab	Component of bones and teeth (enamel)	Tooth decay and other dental diseases	Fluorosis, brittle bones, mottled teeth, nerve abnormalities
Chromium	Whole grains, liver, meat, beer, wine	Glucose utilization	Poor blood glucose control, weight loss	Kidney and skin damage

Source: Adapted from Brown, Judith E. *Nutrition Now*, 4th ed. Belmont, CA: Wadsworth, 2002; Sizer, Frances, and Ellie Whitney. *Nutrition: Concepts and Controversies*, 10th ed. Belmont, CA: Wadsworth, 2006.

- **For children:** vitamin E, calcium, magnesium, potassium, and fiber.

Are you getting enough of these nutrients?

Among the groups at highest risk of nutritional deficiencies are:

- **Teenage girls.**
- **Women of child-bearing age** (iron and folic acid).
- **Persons over age 50** (vitamin B$_{12}$).
- **The elderly, persons with dark skin,** and those who do not get adequate exposure to sunshine (vitamin D).[7]

Calcium

Calcium, the most abundant mineral in the body, builds strong bone tissue throughout life and plays a vital role in blood clotting and muscle and nerve functioning. Pregnant or nursing women need more calcium to meet the additional needs of their babies' bodies. Calcium may also help control high blood pressure, prevent colon cancer in adults, and promote weight loss. Adequate calcium and vitamin D intake during childhood, adolescence, and young adulthood is crucial to prevent *osteoporosis,* the bone-weakening disease that strikes one of every four women over the age of 60.

National health organizations are promoting greater calcium consumption among college students, particularly women, to increase bone density and safeguard against osteoporosis.

In both men and women, bone mass peaks between the ages of 25 and 35. Over the next 10 to 15 years, bone mass remains fairly stable. At about age 40, bone loss equivalent to 0.3 to 0.5 percent per year begins in both men and women. Women may experience greater bone loss, at a rate of 3 to 5 percent, at the time of menopause. This decline continues for approximately five to seven years and is the primary factor leading to postmenopausal osteoporosis.

The higher an individual's peak bone mass, the longer it takes for age- and menopause-related bone loss to increase the risk of fractures. Osteoporosis is less common in groups with higher peak bone mass—men versus women, blacks versus whites.

Calcium is a special concern for African Americans who, as a group, have a higher risk for high blood pressure and obesity than the rest of the population but, on average, consume less than one serving of dairy foods a day. In fact, more than 80 percent of African Americans fail to get their daily recommended amount of calcium.

Calcium and vitamin D supplements in healthy postmenopausal women provide a modest benefit in preserving bone mass and preventing hip fractures, but do not prevent other types of fractures or colorectal cancer, according to the results of a major clinical trial, part of the Women's Health Initiative, which studied more than 36,000 women over age 50.[8] Others have questioned the value of calcium supplementation in younger adults and children as well. A combination of regular exercise, dietary calcium, and vitamin D may be the best prescription for building and preserving strong bones.

Sodium

Sodium helps maintain proper fluid balance, regulates blood pressure, transmits muscle impulses, and relaxes muscles. Excess sodium isn't a problem for most healthy people, but for those who are sodium-sensitive—as many as 30 percent of the population—too much sodium contributes to high blood pressure.

The National Heart, Lung, and Blood Institute recommends less than 2.4 grams (2,400 milligrams) of sodium a day, the equivalent of about one teaspoon of table salt a day. For someone with high blood pressure, a daily intake of less than 1,500 mg of sodium is better for lowering blood pressure.

African Americans, who have higher rates of high blood pressure and diseases related to hypertension, such as stroke and kidney failure, tend to be more sensitive to salt. African Americans also have lower intakes of calcium and potassium—both of which can protect against heart disease.

Phytochemicals

Phytochemicals, compounds that exist naturally in plants, serve many functions, including helping a plant protect itself from bacteria and disease. Some phytochemicals such as solanine, an insect-repelling chemical found in the leaves and stalks of potato plants, are natural toxins, but many are beneficial to humans. Flavonoids, found in apples, strawberries, grapes, onions, green and black tea, and red wine, may decrease atherosclerotic plaque and DNA damage related to cancer development. Phytochemicals are associated with a reduced risk of heart disease, certain cancers, age-related macular degeneration, adult-onset diabetes, stroke, and other diseases.

Dietary Supplements

About two out of five Americans take a vitamin or mineral supplement regularly. Should you be among them? Or are you getting enough of the vitamins and minerals you need from your food? Despite intensive marketing of a host of supplements, large-scale studies have cast doubts on the benefits of many, especially antioxidants.

One recent analysis of research on more than 232,000 individuals found that vitamin E and other antioxidants provide no health benefits. Rather than reducing the likelihood of heart disease and cancer, they may even produce a small increase in the risk of death. Vitamin C has shown neither benefit nor risk.[9] Other studies have discredited lycopene, an antioxidant primarily found in tomatoes, a protective agent against prostate cancer in men.[10] Super-high doses of vitamin E also have not helped people with mild cognitive impairment, an early stage of Alzheimer's disease.[11]

High doses of vitamins carry potential risks. Certain antioxidants can interfere with the efficacy of cholesterol-lowering medications. High doses of vitamin E may increase the chances of earlier death. In cancer patients, those taking large doses had an increased risk of a new cancer.

In particular, the fat-soluble vitamins, primarily A and D, can build up in our bodies and cause serious complications, such as damage to the kidneys, liver, or bones. Large doses of water-soluble vitamins, including the B vitamins, may also be harmful. Excessive intake of vitamin B_6 (pyridoxine), often used to relieve premenstrual bloating, can cause neurological damage, such as numbness in the mouth and tingling in the hands. (An excessive amount in this case is 250 to 300 times the recommended dose.) High doses of vitamin C can produce stomachaches and diarrhea. Niacin, often taken in high doses to lower cholesterol, can cause jaundice, liver damage, and irregular heartbeats as well as severe, uncomfortable flushing of the skin.

If you do feel a need for vitamins, choose a multivitamin supplement that does not exceed the recommended doses listed in Tables 6.4 and 6.5. Another option for many people is to take herbal supplements, which are discussed in Chapter 17.

Using the MyPyramid Food Guidance System

Making healthy choices about what and how to eat isn't easy. However, the federal government is trying to help. In its most recent edition of *Nutrition and Your Health: Dietary Guidelines for Americans,* the U.S. Departments of Health and Human Services and of Agriculture provide science-based advice both to promote wellness and to reduce the risk of major chronic diseases. The MyPyramid Food Guidance System (Figure 6.3) translates the guidelines into a personalized, balanced, total diet.

The key themes of MyPyramid are:

- **Variety.** Eating foods from all food groups and subgroups.
- **Proportionality.** Eating more of some foods (fruits, vegetables, whole grains, fat-free or low-fat milk products) and less of others (foods high in saturated or trans fats, added sugars, cholesterol, salt, and alcohol). Critics of the new pyramid point out that the guidelines still do not take a hard enough line on the amount of refined starches or red meat in the American diet.
- **Moderation.** Choosing forms of foods that limit intake of saturated or trans fats, added sugars, cholesterol, salt, and alcohol.
- **Activity.** Being physically active every day.
- **Personalization.** To make the most of the new MyPyramid system, you need to go online to www.mypyramid.gov. By filling in your age, gender, and typical level of activity, you will be linked to one of twelve versions of the pyramid, ranging from 1,000 to 3,200 daily calories. You can print out your customized pyramid and use it as a dietary guide. Track what you eat for a week to see how it compares with the recommendations, and go back to the website for specific suggestions.

Critics of the new MyPyramid charge that it does not go far enough in urging Americans to cut back on harmful fats and simple carbohydrates and also lumps together various protein sources (red meat, poultry, fish, and beans)

phytochemicals Chemicals such as indoles, coumarins, and capsaicin, which exist naturally in plants and have disease-fighting properties.

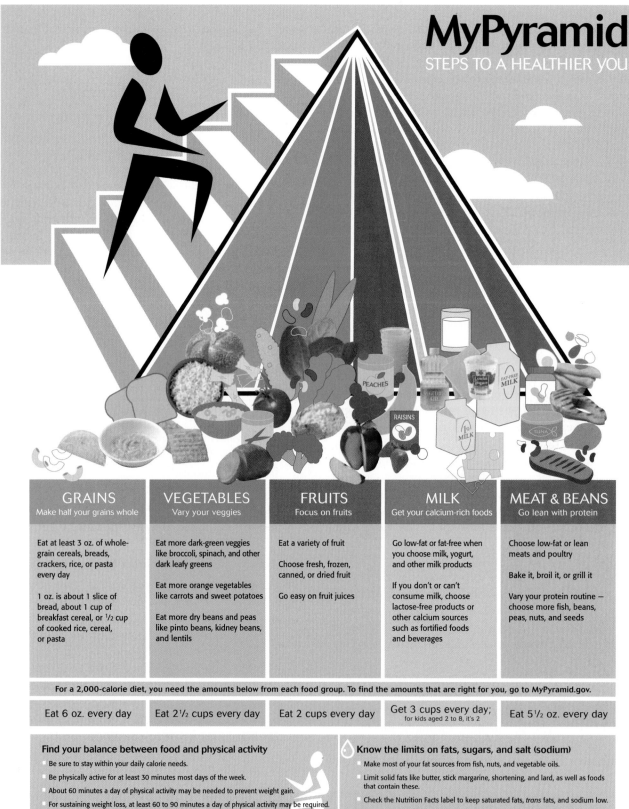

Figure 6.3 The MyPyramid Food Guidance System

as equally healthy.[12] However, national surveys show that a large majority of Americans have heard of the revised guidelines and had a generally positive reaction. About a third said they would change their habits, another third said they might change, and a third said they wouldn't alter their lifestyles.[13]

The following guidelines are based on the MyPyramid system.

Consume a Variety of Foods

The six colors on the MyPyramid graphic represent the five food groups—grains, vegetables, fruits, milk, and meat and beans—and oils. The greater the variety of colors and of foods you choose, the more likely you are to obtain the nutrients you need—see Figure 6.4. In general, the USDA recommends a diet that is high in fruits and vegetables, whole grains, and nonfat or low-fat milk products that provides amounts of nutrients (including potassium and fiber) that can help reduce the risk of chronic disease and is low in saturated fat, cholesterol, added sugars, trans fat, and sodium.

Manage Your Weight

As discussed in Chapter 7, you must expend as much energy (calories) as you take in to stay at the same weight. Among the best ways to balance this energy equation are limiting portion sizes (discussed later in this chapter), substituting nutrient-dense foods (such as raw vegetables or low-fat soups) for nutrient-poor foods (such as candy and cake), and limiting added sugars, solid fats, and alcoholic beverages.

Get Physical Every Day

As discussed in Chapter 5, regular physical activity helps maintain a healthy weight and reduces risk for several chronic diseases. While 30 minutes of moderate physical activity (such as walking at a pace of three or four miles an hour) on most days provides important benefits, exercising more often and more intensely yields additional health dividends. Many adults need up to 60 minutes of moderate to vigorous physical activity—the equivalent of 150 to 200 calories, depending on body size, daily to prevent unhealthy weight gain. Men and women who have lost weight may need 60 to 90 minutes to keep off excess pounds. Children and teenagers require at least 60 minutes of moderate physical activity every day.

Increase Foods from Certain Food Groups

 Fewer than a third of American adults eat the recommended amounts of fruits and vegetables. College-age young adults between ages 18 and

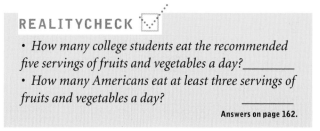

24 eat the fewest vegetables. Nearly four-fifths of this group don't put vegetables on their plates—or scrape them to the side if they do.[14] (See Reality Check.)

Greater consumption of fruits and vegetables (5 to 13 servings or 2½ to 6½ cups per day, depending on how many calories you burn) may reduce the risk of stroke, certain cancers, and type 2 diabetes (vegetables more so than fruit) as well as helping reach and maintain a healthy weight. The more fruits and vegetables men and women consume, the lower their levels of harmful low-density lipoprotein (LDL) cholesterol. Plant-based foods also reduce the risk of rectal cancer in both men and women. To increase the fruits and vegetables in your diet, fill half of your plate with them (see Figure 6.5).

Among the ways to increase your fruit and vegetable intake:

- **Toss fruit into a green salad** for extra flavor, variety, color, and crunch.
- **Start the day with a daily double:** a glass of juice and a banana or other fruit on cereal.
- **Buy pre-cut vegetables** for snacking or dipping (instead of chips).
- **Make or order sandwiches** with extra tomatoes or other vegetable toppings.

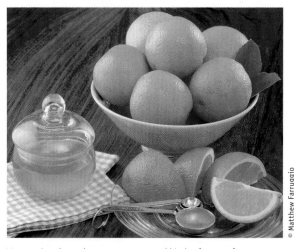

You receive about the same amount and kinds of sugars from an orange as from a tablespoon of honey, but the packaging makes a big nutrition difference.

Key:

● Foods generally high in nutrient density (choose most often)

△ Foods lower in nutrient density (limit selections)

FRUITS

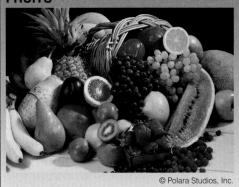

© Polara Studios, Inc.

Consume a variety of fruits and no more than one-third of the recommended intake as fruit juice.

These foods contribute folate, vitamin A, vitamin C, potassium, and fiber.

> **½ cup fruit is equivalent to ½ cup fresh, frozen, or canned fruit; 1 small fruit; ¼ cup dried fruit; ½ cup fruit juice.**

● Apples, apricots, avocados, bananas, blueberries, cantaloupe, cherries, grapefruit, grapes, guava, kiwi, mango, oranges, papaya, peaches, pears, pineapples, plums, raspberries, strawberries, watermelon; dried fruit (dates, figs, raisins); unsweetened juices.

△ Canned or frozen fruit in syrup; juices, punches, ades, and fruit drinks with added sugars; fried plantains.

VEGETABLES

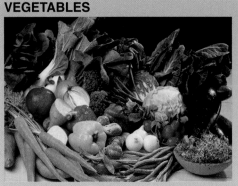

© Polara Studios, Inc.

Choose a variety of vegetables from all five subgroups several times a week.

These foods contribute folate, vitamin A, vitamin C, vitamin K, vitamin E, magnesium, potassium, and fiber.

> **½ cup vegetables is equivalent to ½ cup cut-up raw or cooked vegetables; ½ cup cooked legumes; ½ cup vegetable juice; 1 cup raw, leafy greens.**

● Dark green vegetables: Broccoli and leafy greens such as arugula, beet greens, bok choy, collard greens, kale, mustard greens, romaine lettuce, spinach, and turnip greens.

● Orange and deep yellow vegetables: Carrots, carrot juice, pumpkin, sweet potatoes, and winter squash (acorn, butternut).

● Legumes: Black beans, black-eyed peas, garbanzo beans (chickpeas), kidney beans, lentils, navy beans, pinto beans, soybeans and soy products such as tofu, and split peas.

● Starchy vegetables: Cassava, corn, green peas, hominy, lima beans, and potatoes.

● Other vegetables: Artichokes, asparagus, bamboo shoots, bean sprouts, beets, brussels sprouts, cabbages, cactus, cauliflower, celery, cucumbers, eggplant, green beans, iceberg lettuce, mushrooms, okra, onions, peppers, seaweed, snow peas, tomatoes, vegetable juices, zucchini.

△ Baked beans, candied sweet potatoes, coleslaw, French fries, potato salad, refried beans, scalloped potatoes, tempura vegetables.

GRAINS

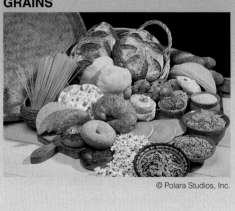

© Polara Studios, Inc.

Make at least half of the grain selections whole grains.

These foods contribute folate, niacin, riboflavin, thiamin, iron, magnesium, selenium, and fiber.

> **1 oz grains is equivalent to 1 slice bread; ½ cup cooked rice, pasta, or cereal; 1 oz dry pasta or rice; 1 cup ready-to-eat cereal; 3 cups popped popcorn.**

● Whole grains (amaranth, barley, brown rice, buckwheat, bulgur, millet, oats, quinoa, rye, wheat) and whole-grain, low-fat breads, cereals, crackers, and pastas; popcorn.

● Enriched bagels, breads, cereals, pastas (couscous, macaroni, spaghetti), pretzels, rice, rolls, tortillas.

△ Biscuits, cakes, cookies, cornbread, crackers, croissants, doughnuts, French toast, fried rice, granola, muffins, pancakes, pastries, pies, presweetened cereals, taco shells, waffles.

Figure 6.4   USDA Food Guide, 2005

MEAT, POULTRY, FISH, LEGUMES, EGGS, AND NUTS

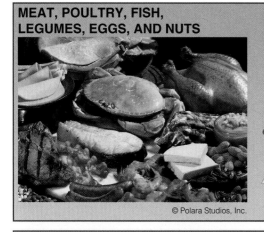

© Polara Studios, Inc.

Make lean or low-fat choices. Prepare them with little, or no, added fat.

Meat, poultry, fish, and eggs contribute protein, niacin, thiamin, vitamin B_6, vitamin B_{12}, iron, magnesium, potassium, and zinc; legumes and nuts are notable for their protein, folate, thiamin, vitamin E, iron, magnesium, potassium, zinc, and fiber.

> **1 oz meat is equivalent to 1 oz cooked lean meat, poultry, or fish; 1 egg; $\frac{1}{4}$ cup cooked legumes or tofu; 1 tbs peanut butter; $\frac{1}{2}$ oz nuts or seeds.**

● Poultry (no skin), fish, shellfish, legumes, eggs, lean meat (fat-trimmed beef, game, ham, lamb, pork); low-fat tofu, tempeh, peanut butter, nuts (almonds, filberts, peanuts, pistachios, walnuts) or seeds (flaxseeds, pumpkin seeds, sunflower seeds).

△ Bacon; baked beans; fried meat, fish, poultry, eggs, or tofu; refried beans; ground beef; hot dogs; luncheon meats; marbled steaks; poultry with skin; sausages; spare ribs.

MILK, YOGURT, AND CHEESE

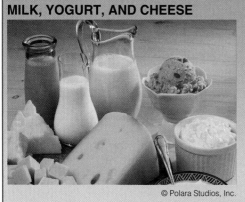

© Polara Studios, Inc.

Make fat-free or low-fat choices. Choose lactose-free products or other calcium-rich foods if you don't consume milk.

These foods contribute protein, riboflavin, vitamin B_{12}, calcium, magnesium, potassium, and, when fortified, vitamin A and vitamin D.

> **1 cup milk is equivalent to 1 cup fat-free milk or yogurt; $1\frac{1}{2}$ oz fat-free natural cheese; 2 oz fat-free processed cheese.**

● Fat-free milk and fat-free milk products such as buttermilk, cheeses, cottage cheese, yogurt; fat-free fortified soy milk.

△ 1% low-fat milk, 2% reduced-fat milk, and whole milk; low-fat, reduced-fat, and whole-milk products such as cheeses, cottage cheese, and yogurt; milk products with added sugars such as chocolate milk, custard, ice cream, ice milk, milk shakes, pudding, sherbet; fortified soy milk.

OILS

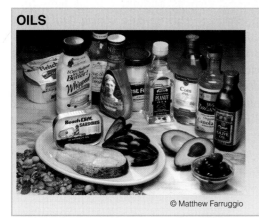

© Matthew Farruggio

Select the recommended amounts of oils from among these sources.

These foods contribute vitamin E and essential fatty acids, along with abundant kcalories.

> **1 tsp oil is equivalent to 1 tbs low-fat mayonnaise; 2 tbs light salad dressing; 1 tsp vegetable oil; 1 tsp soft margarine.**

● Liquid vegetable oils such as canola, corn, flaxseed, nut, olive, peanut, safflower, sesame, soybean, and sunflower oils; mayonnaise, oil-based salad dressing, soft *trans*-free margarine.

● Unsaturated oils that occur naturally in foods such as avocados, fatty fish, nuts, olives, seeds (flaxseeds, sesame seeds), and shellfish.

SOLID FATS AND ADDED SUGARS

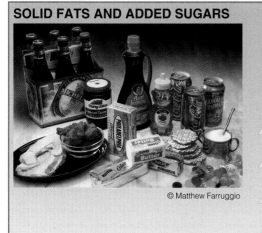

© Matthew Farruggio

Limit intakes of food and beverages with solid fats and added sugars.

Solid fats deliver saturated fat and *trans* fat, and intake should be kept low. Solid fats and added sugars contribute abundant kcalories but few nutrients, and intakes should not exceed the discretionary kcalorie allowance—kcalories to meet energy needs after all nutrient needs have been met with nutrient-dense foods. Alcohol also contributes abundant kcalories but few nutrients, and its kcalories are counted among discretionary kcalories.

△ Solid fats that occur in foods naturally such as milk fat and meat fat (see △ in previous lists).

△ Solid fats that are often added to foods such as butter, cream cheese, hard margarine, lard, sour cream, and shortening.

△ Added sugars such as brown sugar, candy, honey, jelly, molasses, soft drinks, sugar, and syrup.

△ Alcoholic beverages include beer, wine, and liquor.

Figure 6.4 USDA Food Guide, 2005, *Continued*

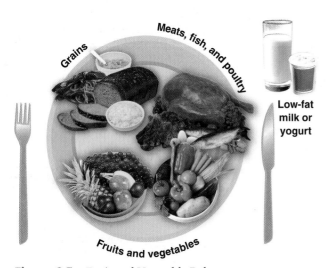

Figure 6.5 Fruit and Vegetable Balance
Fill half your plate with fruits and vegetables.

Consuming at least three servings (the equivalent of 3 ounces) of whole grains per day can reduce the risk of diabetes and coronary heart disease and maintain a healthy weight. To increase your intake of grains:

- **Check labels of rolls and bread,** and choose those with at least 2 to 3 grams of fiber per slice.
- **Add brown rice or barley** to soups.
- **Choose whole-grain,** ready-to-eat cereals.

To get more dairy products with less fat, try the following:

- **Substitute fat-free sour cream** or nonfat, plain yogurt for sour cream.
- **Add low-fat milk** instead of water to oatmeal and hot cereals.
- **Eat cereals with added calcium** and with milk.
- **Top salads or soups with low-fat shredded cheese.**

Be Finicky About Fats

Reducing saturated fat, trans fat, and cholesterol can lower harmful LDL cholesterol and your risk of heart disease. You should keep saturated fat below 10 percent of total calories, trans fat as low as possible, and cholesterol intake below 300 mg per day. Your total fat intake should make up no more than 20 to 35 percent of calories. For children ages 2 and 3, recommended minimum fat intake is 30 percent of calories; for those between ages 4 and 18, it is 25 percent.

To keep within these limits:

- **Restrict animal fats** (such as those in cheese, milk, butter, ice cream, and other full-fat dairy products, fatty meat, bacon, sausage, poultry skin and fat).
- **Cut back** on foods made with partially hydrogenated vegetable oils.
- **Limit your intake** of eggs and organ meats.

As noted earlier, some research has challenged the health benefits of omega-3 fats. However, foods containing these fats are generally healthful ones: oily fish (such as salmon or sardines), flaxseed, walnuts, and canola oils. You should continue to include them in your diet about two times a week. Choose safer fish varieties with lower mercury content, such as salmon, canned light tuna (rather than albacore), shrimp, and catfish. Do not eat swordfish, shark, large mackerel, and tilefish.

Omega-3 fatty acids are especially important for the proper development of the nervous system in the fetus. Omega-3s also play a role in nervous system development in young children. This poses a dilemma because while oily fish are a great source of omega-3s, they are also the ones highest in mercury and potentially other toxic substances such as dioxins. Pregnant and nursing women and children should limit their consumption of oily fish and always choose the safer varieties.

Choose Carbohydrates Wisely

Eating more fruits, vegetables, whole grains, and nonfat or low-fat milk and dairy products is a healthful way to get the carbohydrates you need. Fiber-rich choices—an apple rather than apple juice, for example—have the added benefit of promoting digestive health and reduce the risk of type 2 diabetes and heart disease.

The new guidelines do not include a specific message about sugar but caution against "added" sugars, those added to foods during processing or preparation or at the table. Carbohydrates (including sucrose, glucose, fructose, lactose, and starch) also can increase the risk of dental cavities. Drinking fluoridated water and/or using fluoride-containing dental hygiene products can protect your teeth.

To make sure your grains are whole, choose foods that name one of the following whole-grain ingredients first on the label's ingredient list: brown rice, bulgur, graham flour, oatmeal, whole-grain corn, whole oats, whole rye, whole wheat, wild rice. Foods labeled multi-grain, stone-ground, 100% wheat, cracked wheat, seven-grain, or bran are usually not whole-grain products.

Limit Salt

Reducing salt in your diet is one way to lower your blood pressure and reduce your risk of stroke, heart disease, and kidney disease. Another effective strategy is to eat more foods rich in potassium, which blunts the effects of salt on blood pressure, may decrease bone loss, and reduces the risk of kidney stones.

The USDA guidelines recommend less than 2,300 mg of sodium per day. Many people, including those with hypertension, African Americans, and older adults, should reduce their salt intake even more and increase potassium to at least 4,700 mg.

To reduce sodium intake:

- **Look for labels that say "low sodium."** They contain 140 mg or less of sodium per serving.
- **Learn to use spices and herbs rather than salt** to enhance the flavor of food.
- **Go easy on condiments** such as soy sauce, pickles, olives, ketchup, and mustard, which can add a lot of salt to your food.
- **Always check the amount of sodium** in processed foods, such as frozen dinners, packaged mixes, cereals, salad dressings, and sauces. The amount in different types and brands can vary widely.

If You Drink Alcoholic Beverages, Do So in Moderation

As discussed in Chapter 12, alcohol has different effects on health for different age groups. In middle-aged and older adults, one to two drinks a day seem to lower the risk of dying, primarily because moderate alcohol consumption protects against heart disease. Compared with nondrinkers, however, women who consume one alcoholic beverage per day appear to have a slightly higher risk of breast cancer. For younger people, alcohol provides little, if any, health benefits and increases the risk of traumatic injury and death. At any age, heavy drinking contributes to automotive accidents and deaths, assaults, liver disease, and other health problems.

MyPyramid includes a category for "discretionary calories," which can be used on fats, added sugar, alcohol, or more food from any food group. However, most people, especially those who are not physically active, "earn" very small discretionary calorie allowances, usually no more than 100 to 300 calories a day.[15]

Keep Food Safe to Eat

See page 173 for an in-depth discussion of food safety. The key steps you can take to ensure food safety and prevent a problem with foodborne illnesses are:

- **Thoroughly wash hands,** contact surfaces, and fruits and vegetables (but not meat and poultry).
- **Separate raw, cooked, and ready-to-eat foods** while shopping, preparing, or storing.
- **Cook foods to a safe temperature.**
- **Chill (refrigerate) perishable foods promptly.**

The Way We Eat

Just as there is no one perfect food, there is no one eating pattern that suits all people of all ages and backgrounds at all times. Your ethnic background and family makeup influenced the way you ate as a child. In college, you probably will find yourself eating in different—and not necessarily better—ways. Because the United States is so diverse, you also will have the opportunity to sample the cuisines of many cultures.

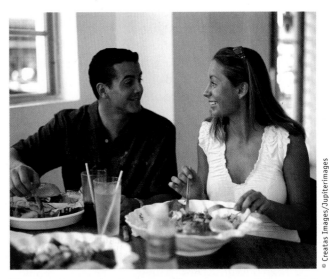

Why do most guys prefer a hamburger while many women will choose salad?

His Plate, Her Plate: Gender and Nutrition

Men and women do not need to eat different foods, but their nutritional needs are different. Because most men are bigger and taller than most women, they consume more calories. On average, a moderately active 125-pound woman needs 2,000 calories a day; a 175-pound man with a similar exercise pattern needs 2,800 calories. Eating more means it's easier for men to get the nutrients they need, even though many don't make the wisest food choices.

Are there "chick foods" and "guy foods"? According to psychological research, individuals who eat "feminine" foods (such as a bagel with cream cheese) are rated as more feminine and less masculine than those who choose a more "masculine" dish (such as flapjacks with syrup). Eating less and choosing "good" foods, such as fruit, oatmeal, and whole wheat bread, are seen as feminine behaviors, while preferring doughnuts, burgers, double-fudge ice cream sundaes, and other so-called "bad" foods qualifies as masculine.[16]

Women, particularly those who restrict their caloric intake or are chronically dieting, are more likely to develop specific deficiencies. Calcium is one example. Many teenage girls and young women under age 30 do not consume the recommended 800 to 1,200 milligrams of calcium daily and may be at increased risk of bone-weakening osteoporosis.

Many women also get too little iron. Even in adolescence, girls are more prone to iron deficiency than boys; some suffer memory and learning impairments as a result. In adult women, menstrual blood loss and poor eating habits can lead to low iron stores, which puts them at risk for anemia. According to U.S. Department of Agriculture research, most women consume only 60 percent of the recommended 18 milligrams of iron per day. (The recommendation for men is 8 milligrams.) Regular blood tests can monitor a woman's iron status.

Both genders should increase their fruit and vegetable intake to ensure that they are getting adequate amounts of vitamins and fiber in their daily diet.

Here are some gender-specific strategies for better nutrition:

 Men should cut back on fat and meat in their diets, two things they eat too much.

Women should increase their iron intake by eating meat (iron from animal sources is absorbed better than that from vegetable sources) or a combination of meat and vegetable iron sources together (for example, a meat and bean burrito). Those with iron deficiencies should consult a physician. Because large doses of iron can be toxic, iron supplements should be taken only with medical supervision.

Women should consume more calcium-rich foods, including low-fat and nonfat dairy products, leafy greens, and tofu. Women who cannot get adequate amounts of calcium from their daily diet should take calcium supplements. This is not advised for all men because of a possible connection between calcium and prostate cancer.

Women who could become pregnant should take a multivitamin with 400 micrograms of **folic acid**, which helps prevent neural tube defects such as spina bifida. Folic acid is also useful to men because it may cut the risk of heart disease, stroke, and colon cancer.

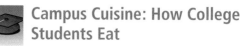

Campus Cuisine: How College Students Eat

Often on their own for the first time, college students typically change their usual eating patterns. In one recent survey, 59 percent of freshmen said their diet had changed since they began college. When they are making meal choices, the top two influences on students are price and convenience, with nutrition coming in third.

According to various national samples, many students do not consume adequate amounts of fruits and vegetables and consume too many fried and fast foods. In one study that followed students through their freshman and sophomore years, more than half remained in the precontemplation stage for adopting healthier eating behaviors throughout this time. Only 30 percent of the students consumed at least five fruits and vegetables daily; more than half reported eating high-fat fried or fast foods at least three times during the previous week.

Perhaps because they don't get five daily servings of fruit and vegetables, students also fall short in fiber intake. When 144 undergraduates at a four-year university completed three-day food intake reports, only 19 met the recommended 20 to 35 grams per day of dietary fiber: 13 percent of the women and 16 percent of the men.[17]

The same holds true for consumption of healthful omega-3 polyunsaturated fats, such as fish oils. In a recent study of 51 college-aged women, 84 percent failed to meet the recommended levels for adequate intake. Only the small percentage consuming higher-than-recommended levels for total fat intake met or exceeded the recommended amounts of beneficial fats.

Some colleges are doing their part to improve student nutrition. Many post nutritional information in dining halls; some have expanded their offerings to include more salads, fewer fried foods, and more ethnic dishes. On some campuses, students are taking the lead in demanding more healthful, fresher, and more varied dishes in their dining halls. (See the Point/Counterpoint feature.)

folic acid A form of folate used in vitamin supplements and fortified foods.

Fast Food: Nutrition on the Run

On any given day, about 25 percent of adults in the United States go to a fast-food restaurant. The typical American consumes three hamburgers and four orders of french fries every week. Not all fast foods are junk foods—that is, high in calories, sugar, salt, and fat and low in beneficial nutrients (Table 6.6). But while it's not all bad, fast food has definite disadvantages. A meal in a fast-food restaurant may cost twice as much as the same meal prepared at home and may provide half your daily calorie needs. The fat content of many items is extremely high. A Burger King Whopper with cheese contains 760 calories and 47 grams of fat, 16 grams from saturated fat. A McDonald's Sausage McMuffin with egg has 450 calories and 27 grams of fat, 10 grams from saturated fat. Many fast-food chains have switched from beef tallow or lard to unsaturated vegetable oils for frying, but the total fat content of the foods remains the same. For tips on choosing well in a fast-food restaurant, see Your Strategies for Prevention: "A Guide to Fast Foods."

You Are What You Drink

About 20 percent of the calories Americans over age 2 consume come from beverages, predominantly soft drinks and fruit drinks with added sugar.[18] The consumption of sugar-sweetened beverages has surged in recent decades. Calories from these drinks, which some call "liquid candy," account for half the rise in caloric intake by Americans since the 1970s.[19]

Serving sizes of drinks have morphed from big to superbig to gigantic. Some people sip several 32-ounce slurpies or 16-ounce lattes throughout the day, drinking in hundreds of calories that contribute few if any health benefits and that may increase the risk of obesity, heart disease, stroke, diabetes, cancer, and dementia.

Water—tap or bottled, sparkling or still, chilled or room temperature—is the medical experts' beverage of choice. But don't think that "fortified" or "enriched" water is better. There is no evidence that nutrients added to water confer any health benefits. Consumers who assume they're getting vitamins in their drinks may think they don't need to eat healthy foods and could end up short-changing themselves of vital nutrients.

Low-fat and skim milk (soy or cow) are other healthy alternatives. The calcium and vitamin D in milk help maintain bone density. Other essential nutrients in milk include magnesium, potassium, zinc, iron, vitamin A, riboflavin, folate, and protein. According to long-term research, milk drinkers are less likely to develop metabolic syndrome, the combination of coronary risk factors that includes high blood pressure and low levels of the beneficial form of cholesterol (see Chapter 14).

TABLE 6.6 Some Fast-Food Choices

	Calories	Fat (g)	% Calories from Fat	Protein (g)	Carb (g)	Fiber (g)
Arby's						
Martha's Vineyard Salad	276	8	25	26	24	4
Santa Fe Salad w/ Grilled Chicken	283	9	27	29	20	5
Burger King						
Tendergrill Chicken Sandwich w/o mayo	450	10	20	37	53	4
Big Fish Sandwich w/o tartar sauce	470	13	25	23	65	3
Veggie Burger w/o mayo	340	8	21	23	46	7
Tendergrill Chicken Garden Salad	240	9	34	33	8	4
Domino's 1 slice 12" Classic Hand-Tossed:						
with any veggies	220	7	28	9	32	1
with grilled chicken	235	8	30	11	32	1
Jack in the Box						
Chicken Fajita Pita	290	9	28	21	31	2
Asian Grilled Chicken Salad	160	2	10	22	18	5
Southwest Grilled Chicken Salad	320	12	34	31	27	7
KFC						
Original Recipe Chicken Breast w/o skin or breading	140	2	14	29	1	0
Honey BBQ Sandwich	280	3.5	11	22	40	3
Tender Roast Sandwich w/o sauce	300	4.5	13	37	28	2
KFC Snacker, Buffalo	260	8	27	15	31	1
Long John Silver's						
Baked Cod—1 piece	120	4.5	33	22	1	0
Buttered Lobster Bites—snack box	250	9	32	14	27	2
1 Corn Cobbette	90	3	28	3	14	3
McDonald's						
Hamburger	250	9	32	12	31	2
Premium Grilled Chicken Classic Sandwich	420	10	21	33	51	3
Ranch Snack Wrap w/ Grilled Chicken	270	10	33	18	26	1
Subway						
6" Ham	290	5	16	18	47	4
6" Roast Beef	290	5	16	19	45	4
6" Sweet Onion Teriyaki	370	5	12	26	59	5
Subway Club Wrap	310	8	23	22	40	3
Taco Bell						
Bean Burito	340	9	23	13	54	8
Fiesta Burrito—Chicken	350	10	26	18	47	3
Fiesta Burrito—Steak	340	11	29	15	47	3
Spicy Chicken Soft Taco	170	6	30	10	20	2
(Order "Fresco Style" to substitute cheese and sauce with Fiesta Salsa)						
Wendy's						
Jr. Hamburger	280	9	29	15	34	1
Ultimate Chicken Grill Sandwich	320	7	20	28	36	2
Large Chili	330	9	24	25	35	8

© Spencer Grant/PhotoEdit

Soft Drinks

Americans down an average of more than 600 soft drinks a year. In a recent review of 88 studies, researchers linked soft drinks with increased calorie intake, higher body weight, lower consumption of calcium and other nutrients, and greater risk of other medical problems, such as diabetes. In a long-term, large-scale study of women, those who consumed one or more soft drinks per day (less than the national average) were at twice the risk of developing diabetes as those who had less than one soft drink a month.[20] A single daily soft drink, either diet or regular, also increases the likelihood of metabolic syndrome.[21] Sweetened iced tea and many carbonated beverages can damage tooth enamel, especially when not consumed with food. Drinking regular and diet cola has been linked with the thinning of hip bones in women.

People who consume a lot of soft drinks generally take in more calories than others—and not just from the beverages. Instead of satisfying a sweet tooth, soft drinks seem to do the opposite. Although researchers cannot explain exactly why, soft drinks may increase hunger or decrease feelings of satiety or fullness. Even diet drinks made with artificial sweeteners may "condition" people to eat more sweets.

Energy Drinks

Coffee and tea, which both contain caffeine, are the classic "pick-me-up" beverages. As discussed in Chapter 11, regular coffee consumption may reduce the risk of several serious illnesses—including type 2 diabetes, colon cancer, and Parkinson's disease—and may protect against age-related memory and thinking defects. Studies of tea's benefits have produced mixed results, although some research suggests that tea may improve blood flow to the heart and help prevent kidney stones.

Consumption of energy drinks such as Red Bull and Rockstar has more than doubled in the last three years, particularly among young people.[22] The main ingredient in these drinks, including diet brands, is caffeine, sometimes in doses that can cause physical and psychological complications, including disrupted sleep, exaggerated stress response, heart palpitations, and increased risk of high blood pressure.[23]

Red Bull, for instance, contains nearly 80 mg of caffeine per can, about the same amount of caffeine as a cup of brewed coffee and twice the caffeine as a cup of tea. Other energy drinks contain several times this amount—see Table 6.7.

The drink formulations vary widely, and manufacturers make many different claims about their effects. Some brands contain fruit juices, teas, and dietary supplements such as ginseng and glucuronolactone. One can of Red Bull contains 1000 mg of taurine, a substance that plays an important role in muscle contraction (especially in the heart) and the nervous system. Some energy drinks contain guarana, a South American herbal caffeine source that could pose additional risks. We know very little about the effects of such combinations of ingredients, which may work synergistically with caffeine to boost its stimulant power.

The amount of caffeine in an energy drink isn't always indicated on the label, so it is difficult to gauge how much you are consuming. And unlike hot coffee and tea, which you sip slowly, you're more likely to drink large amounts of an energy drink quickly. This can be especially dangerous if you're exercising. The FDA, which recommends caffeine concentrations no higher than 68 mg per 12-ounce serving, soon may require warning labels on energy drinks. In a recent study at Northwestern University, 12 percent of patients calling a poison control center

TABLE 6.7	Energy Drinks: Caffeine in Cans and Cups	
Type of Drink	**Amount of Caffeine**
Regular Cola (12-oz can)	40 mg
Red Bull (8.3-oz can)	75 mg
Coffee (standard 8-oz cup)	95 mg
Monster (16-oz container)	140 mg
Rockstar (16-oz container)	240 mg

had caffeine overdoses, often from energy drinks. Their average age was 21.[24]

Millions of college students consume energy drinks for the jolt provided or because they believe the drinks enhance sports performance or sexual function. Yet health experts warn that these sugar- and caffeine-laded drinks pose serious health risks, including dehydration, accidents, and alcohol poisoning.

Particularly perilous is the combination of an energy drink like Red Bull with vodka, a cocktail called V-Bomb, Friday Flattener, or Raging Bull. In studies, college students drinking this concoction reported feeling less intoxicated than they actually were, with marked differences in their actual and perceived coordination and reaction times.[25] This increases their risk of accidents and of alcohol poisoning.

Dietary Diversity

Whatever your cultural heritage, you have probably sampled Chinese, Mexican, Indian, Italian, and Japanese foods. If you belong to any of these ethnic groups, you may eat these cuisines regularly. Each type of ethnic cooking has its own nutritional benefits and potential drawbacks.

Mediterranean Diet

Several years ago epidemiologists noticed something unexpected in the residents of regions along the Mediterranean Sea: a lower incidence of deaths from heart disease. Scientists have identified antioxidants in red wine and olive oil that may account for the beneficial effects on the heart of the Mediterranean diet, which features lots of fruits and vegetables, legumes, nuts, and grains. The Mediterranean diet also has beneficial effects on the lungs, reducing the risk of asthma[26] and progressive lung disease.[27] Meat is used mainly as a condiment rather than as a main course, and fish, yogurt, and low-fat feta cheese are the predominant animal foods. The diet is relatively high in fat, but the main source is olive oil, an unsaturated fat.

Ethnic Cuisines

The cuisine served in Mexico features rice, corn, and beans, which are low in fat and high in nutrients. However, the dishes Americans think of as Mexican are far less healthful. Burritos, especially when topped with cheese and sour cream, are very high in fat. Although guacamole has a high fat content, it contains mostly monounsaturated fatty acids, a better form of fat.

African American cuisine traces some of its roots to food preferences from west Africa (for example, peanuts, okra, and black-eyed peas), as well as to traditional American foods, such as fish, game, greens, and sweet potatoes. It uses many nutritious vegetables, such as collard greens and sweet potatoes, as well as legumes. However, some dishes include high-fat food products such as peanuts and pecans or involve frying, sometimes in saturated fat.

The mainland Chinese diet, which is plant-based, high in carbohydrates, and low in fats and animal protein, is considered one of the healthiest in the world. However, Chinese restaurants in the United States serve more meat and sauces than are generally eaten in China. According to laboratory tests of typical take-out dishes from Chinese restaurants, many have more fats and cholesterol than hamburger or egg dishes from fast-food outlets.

Traditional French cuisine, which includes rich, high-fat sauces and dishes, has never been considered healthful. Yet, nutritionists have been stumped to explain the so-called French paradox. Despite a diet high in saturated fats, the French have had one of the lowest rates of coronary artery disease in the world. The French diet increasingly resembles the American diet, but French portions tend to be one-third to one-half the size of American portions.

Many Indian dishes highlight healthful ingredients such as vegetables and legumes (beans and peas). However, many also use *ghee* (a form of butter) or coconut oil; both are rich in harmful saturated fats. The best advice in an Indian restaurant is to ask how each dish is prepared. Good choices include *daal* or *dal* (lentils), *karbi* or *karni* (chickpea soup), and *chapati* (tortilla-like bread).

The traditional Japanese diet is very low in fat, which may account for the low incidence of heart disease in Japan. Dietary staples include soybean products, fish, vegetables, noodles, and rice. A variety of fruits and vegetables are also included in many dishes. However, Japanese cuisine is high in salted, smoked, and pickled foods. Watch out for deep-fried dishes such as tempura and salty soups and sauces.

Table 6.8 summarizes some of the ethnic food choices by food group.

Vegetarian Diets

Not all vegetarians avoid all meats. Some, who call themselves *lacto-ovo-pesco-vegetarians*, eat dairy products, eggs, chicken, and fish but not red meat. **Lacto-vegetarians** eat dairy products as well as grains, fruits, and vegetables; **ovo-lacto-vegetarians** also eat eggs. Pure vegetarians, called **vegans**, eat only plant foods; often they take vitamin B_{12} supplements because that vitamin is normally found only in animal products. If they select their food with care, vegetarians can get sufficient amounts of protein, vitamin B_{12}, iron, and calcium without supplements.

TABLE 6.8   Ethnic Food Choices

	Grains	Vegetables	Fruits	Meats and Legumes	Milk
Asian	Rice, noodles, millet	Amaranth, baby corn, bamboo shoots, chayote, bok choy, mung bean sprouts, sugar peas, straw mushrooms, water chestnuts, kelp	Carambola, guava, kumquat, lychee, persimmon, melons, mandarin orange	Soybeans and soy products such as soy milk and tofu, squid, duck eggs, pork, poultry, fish and other seafood, peanuts, cashews	Usually excluded
Mediterranean	Pita pocket bread, pastas, rice, couscous, polenta, bulgur, focaccia, Italian bread	Eggplant, tomatoes, peppers, cucumbers, grape leaves	Olives, grapes, figs	Fish and other seafood, gyros, lamb, chicken, beef, port, sausage, lentils, fava beans	Ricotta, provolone, parmesan, feta, mozzarella, and goat cheeses; yogurt
Mexican	Tortillas (corn or flour), taco shells, rice	Chayote, corn, jicama, tomato salsa, cactus, cassava, tomatoes, yams, chilies	Guava, mango, papaya, avocado, plantain, bananas, oranges	Refried beans, fish, chicken, chorizo, beef, eggs	Cheese, custard

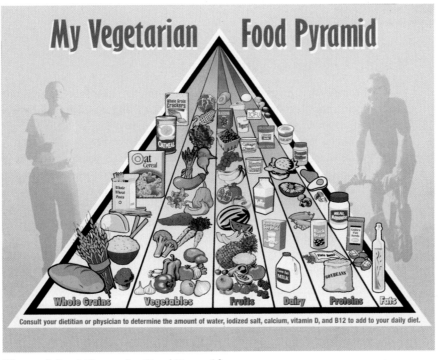

Figure 6.6 A Vegetarian Food Pyramid
Tips for planning a vegetarian diet can be found at MyPyramid.gov

Source: © GC Nutrition Council, 2006, adapted from USDA 2005 Dietary Guidelines and www.MyPyramid.gov. Copies can be ordered from 301-680-6717.

The key to getting sufficient protein from a vegetarian diet is understanding the concept of **complementary proteins.** Meat, poultry, fish, eggs, and dairy products are *complete proteins* that provide the nine essential amino acids—substances that the human body cannot produce itself. *Incomplete proteins,* such as legumes or nuts, may have relatively low levels of one or two essential amino acids but fairly high levels of others. By combining complementary protein sources, you can make sure that your body makes the most of the nonanimal proteins you eat. Many cultures rely heavily on complementary foods for protein. In Middle Eastern cooking, sesame seeds and chickpeas are a popular combination; in Latin American dishes, beans and rice, or beans and tortillas; in Chinese cuisine, soy and rice.

According to the 2005 Dietary Guidelines, vegetarians can best meet their nutrient needs by paying special attention to protein, iron, vitamin B_{12}, calcium, and vitamin D. Instead of a 6-ounce serving of meat, they can substitute one egg, 1.5 ounces of nuts, or two-thirds cup of legumes. Those who avoid milk because of its lactose content may obtain all the nutrients of milk by using lactose-reduced milk or eating other calcium-rich foods, such as broccoli, calcium-fortified orange juice, and fortified soy milk. Figure 6.6 shows a vegetarian food pyramid.

Vegetarian diets have proven health benefits. Studies show that vegetarians' cholesterol levels are low, and vegetarians are seldom overweight. As a result, they're less apt to be candidates for heart disease than those who consume large quantities of meat. Vegetarians also have lower incidences of breast, colon, and prostate cancer; high blood pressure; and osteoporosis.

Portions and Servings

Consumers often are confused by what a *serving* actually is, especially since many American restaurants have super-sized the amount of food they put on their customers' plates. The average bagel has doubled in size in the last ten to fifteen years. A standard fast-food serving of french fries is larger in the United States than in the United Kingdom.

A food-label *serving* is a specific amount of food that contains the quantity of nutrients described on the Nutrition Facts label. A *portion* is the amount of a specific food that an individual eats at one time. Portions can be

lacto-vegetarians People who eat dairy products as well as fruits and vegetables (but not meat, poultry, or fish).

ovo-lacto-vegetarians People who eat eggs, dairy products, and fruits and vegetables (but not meat, poultry, or fish).

vegans People who eat only plant foods.

complementary proteins Incomplete proteins that, when combined, provide all the amino acids essential for protein synthesis.

Taking Charge of What You Eat

You can't control what you don't know. Because of the Nutrition Labeling and Education Act, food manufacturers must provide information about fat, calories, and ingredients in large type on packaged food labels, and they must show how a food item fits into a daily diet of 2,000 calories. The law also restricts nutritional claims for terms such as *healthy, low-fat,* and *high-fiber.*

 At one university, almost two-thirds of the freshmen reported that they were aware of the nutrition labels posted in the dining commons. One-third used them to help make food choices. Female students were significantly more likely to base their food choices on the labels than the men. Students primarily checked overall good/balanced nutrition content of foods, calories, fat, saturated fat, and protein. Their top reason for checking labels: to be healthy now.[28]

In evaluating food labels and product claims, keep in mind that while individual foods vary in their nutritional value, what matters is your total diet. If you eat too much of any one food—regardless of what its label states—you may not be getting the variety and balance of nutrients that you need.

---

bigger or smaller than the servings on food labels. According to nutritionists, "marketplace portions"—the actual amounts served to customers—are two to eight times larger than the standard serving sizes defined by the USDA. In fast-food chains, today's portions are two to five times larger than the original sizes. As studies have shown, people presented with larger portions eat 30 to 50 percent more than they otherwise would.

If you are trying to balance your diet or control your weight, it's important to keep track of the size of your portions so that you do not exceed recommended servings. For instance, a 3-ounce serving of meat is about the size of a pack of playing cards—see Figure 6.7. If you eat a larger amount, count it as more than one serving. (See "Mind over Platter" in *IPC* for more on developing greater awareness of what and how you eat.) **IPC**

How to Read Nutrition Labels

As Figure 6.8 shows, the Nutrition Facts on food labels present a wealth of information—if you know what to look for. The label focuses on those nutrients most clearly associated with disease risk and health: total fat, saturated fat, cholesterol, sodium, total carbohydrate, dietary fiber, sugar, and protein.

- **Calories.** Calories are the measure of the amount of energy that can be derived from food. Science defines a *calorie* as the amount of energy required to raise the temperature of 1 gram of water by 1 degree Celsius. In the laboratory, the caloric content of food is measured in 1,000-calorie units called *kilocalories.* The calorie referred to in everyday usage is actually the equivalent of the laboratory kilocalorie.

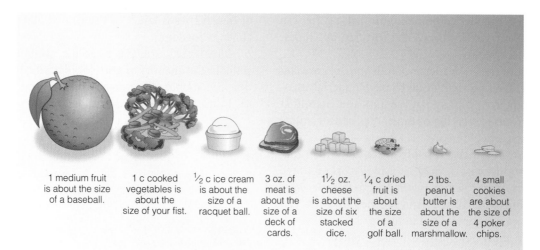

1 medium fruit is about the size of a baseball.

1 c cooked vegetables is about the size of your fist.

½ c ice cream is about the size of a racquet ball.

3 oz. of meat is about the size of a deck of cards.

1½ oz. cheese is about the size of six stacked dice.

¼ c dried fruit is about the size of a golf ball.

2 tbs. peanut butter is about the size of a marshmallow.

4 small cookies are about the size of 4 poker chips.

Figure 6.7 Understanding Nutrition Labels
Quick and Easy Estimates of Portion Sizes

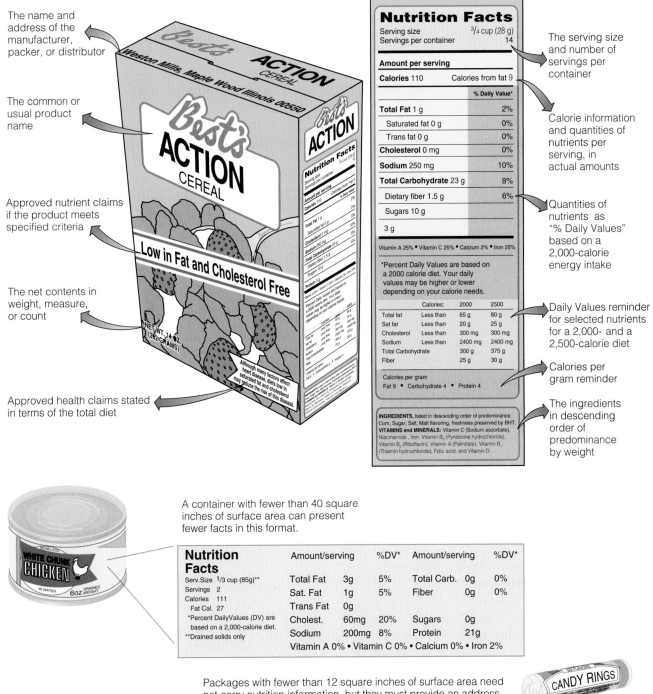

The name and address of the manufacturer, packer, or distributor

The common or usual product name

Approved nutrient claims if the product meets specified criteria

The net contents in weight, measure, or count

Approved health claims stated in terms of the total diet

The serving size and number of servings per container

Calorie information and quantities of nutrients per serving, in actual amounts

Quantities of nutrients as "% Daily Values" based on a 2,000-calorie energy intake

Daily Values reminder for selected nutrients for a 2,000- and a 2,500-calorie diet

Calories per gram reminder

The ingredients in descending order of predominance by weight

A container with fewer than 40 square inches of surface area can present fewer facts in this format.

Packages with fewer than 12 square inches of surface area need not carry nutrition information, but they must provide an address, phone number, or website for obtaining information.

Figure 6.8 Understanding Nutrition Labels
The Nutrition Facts label lists the essential nutrient content of packaged food as well as the amount of potentially harmful substances such as fat and sodium.

The Nutrition Facts label lists two numbers for calories: calories per serving and calories from fat per serving. This allows consumers to calculate how many calories they'll consume and to determine the percentage of fat in an item.

• **Serving size.** Rather than the tiny portions manufacturers sometimes used in the past to keep down the number of calories per serving, the new labels reflect more realistic portions. Serving sizes, which have been defined for approximately 150 food categories, must be the same for similar products (for example, different brands of potato chips) and for similar products within a category (for example, snack foods such as pretzels, potato chips, and popcorn). This makes it easier to compare the nutritional content of foods.

- **Daily Values (DVs).** DVs refer to the total amount of a nutrient that the average adult should aim to get or not exceed on a daily basis. The DVs for cholesterol, sodium, vitamins, and minerals are the same for all adults. The DVs for total fat, saturated fat, carbohydrate, fiber, and protein are based on a 2,000-calorie daily diet—the amount of food ingested by many American men and active women.

- **Percent Daily Values (%DVs).** The goal for a full day's diet is to select foods that together add up to 100 percent of the DVs. The %DVs show how a particular food's nutrient content fits into a 2,000-calorie diet. Individuals who consume (or should consume) fewer than 2,000 total calories a day have to lower their DVs for total fat, saturated fat, and carbohydrates. For example, if their caloric intake is 10 percent less than 2,000 calories, they would lower the DV by 10 percent. Similarly, those who consume more than 2,000 calories should adjust the DVs upward.

- **Calories per gram.** The bottom of the food label lists the number of calories per gram for fat, carbohydrates, and protein.

People zero in on different figures on the food label—for example, calories if they're watching their weight, specific ingredients if they have food allergies. Among the useful items to check are the following:

- **Calories from fat.** Get into the habit of calculating the percentage of fat calories in a food before buying or eating it.

- **Total fat.** Since the average person munches on 15 to 20 food items a day, it's easy to overload on fat. Saturated fat and trans fat numbers deserve special attention because of their link to several diseases.

- **Cholesterol.** Cholesterol is made by and contained in products of animal origin only. Many high-fat products, such as potato chips, contain 0 percent cholesterol because they're made from plants and are cooked in vegetable fats. However, if the vegetable fats are hydrogenated, the resulting trans fat is more harmful to the heart than cholesterol.

- **Sugars.** There is no Daily Value for sugars because health experts have yet to agree on a daily limit. The figure on the label includes naturally present sugars, such as lactose in milk and fructose in fruit, as well as those added to the food, such as table sugar, corn syrup, or dextrose.

- **Fiber.** A "high-fiber" food has 5 or more grams of fiber per serving. A "good" source of fiber provides at least 2.5 grams. "More" or "added" fiber means at least 2.5 grams more per serving than similar foods—10 percent more of the DV for fiber.

- **Calcium.** "High" equals 200 mg or more per serving. "Good" means at least 100 mg, while "more" indicates that the food contains at least 100 mg more calcium—10 percent more of the DV—than the item usually would have.

- **Sodium.** Most of us routinely get more sodium than we need. Read labels carefully to avoid excess sodium, which can be a health threat.

- **Vitamins.** A Daily Value of 10 percent of any vitamin makes a food a "good" source; 20 percent qualifies it as "high" in a certain vitamin.

Nutrition labeling for fresh produce, fish, meat, and poultry remains voluntary. Packages too small for a full-sized label must provide an address, phone number, or website so that consumers can obtain information from the manufacturer.

What Is Organic?

Foods certified as **organic** by the USDA must meet strict criteria, including:

- Processing or preservation only with substances approved by the USDA for organic foods.
- Processing without genetic modification or ionizing radiation.
- No use of most synthetic chemicals, such as pesticides, herbicides, or fertilizers.
- Fertilization without sewage sludge.
- Food-producing animals are grown without medication such as antibiotics or hormones, provided with living conditions similar to their natural habitat, and fed organic feed.

Are organic foods better for you? There has been limited research as to whether organic foods are nutritionally superior to conventional foods. Some studies have shown higher levels of specific nutrients, such as flavonoids, in organic produce, but no one knows if this translates into specific health benefits. However, you can avoid exposure to pesticides and other chemicals by opting for organic foods.

Functional Foods

As the American Dietetic Association has noted, all foods are functional at some physiological level. However, the term *functional* generally applies to a food specifically created to have health-promoting benefits. The International Food Information Council defines functional foods as those "that provide health benefits beyond basic nutrition."

Some manufacturers are adding biologically active components such as beta-carotene to food products and promoting them as functional foods. However, the amounts added are often too low to have any effect, and many such foods are high-sugared drinks and snack foods. More research is needed to evaluate their claims of health benefits.

Choosing Healthful Snacks

 Snacking has become more widespread on campuses, as in other places. College students snack primarily "to satisfy hunger"; the second-most common reason is "no time for meals." Other reasons for munching between meals: "for energy," "to be sociable," and "to relieve stress." One-third snack at 9:00 p.m. or later.

In response to consumer demands for smart snack choices, food manufacturers are offering "better-for-you" options that are lower in salt and sugar or free of trans fat and artificial colors. Some new snack items promoted as healthful options, such as sugar-free chocolate or organic potato chips, offer little nutritional value. Meat-based snacks, increasingly popular among young men, also can be high in fat and sodium. Read labels carefully, and be sure to check total calories and fat.

A best-for-you option is fruit, such as bananas, apples, or berries, rich in vitamins, low in calories, and packed with fiber. Other nutritious snacks include nuts, trail mix, granola bars, yogurt, sunflower seeds, soy nuts, and dried fruit (such as cranberries). If you enjoy fruit juice, buy 100 percent fruit juice without added sugar. Limit yourself to one serving of these calorie-rich beverages a day.

If you rely on snacks to keep you energized throughout the day, take time to plan in advance so you have choices other than the nearest vending machine. Try to prepare snacks from different food groups: low- or no-fat milk and a few graham crackers, for instance, or celery sticks with peanut butter and raisins. Save part of one meal—half of your breakfast bagel or lunch sandwich—to eat a few hours later. If you're trying to add fiber to your diet, eat high-fiber snacks, such as prunes, popcorn, or sunflower seeds.

Food Safety

Foodborne illnesses cause an estimated 76 million illnesses, 325,000 hospitalizations, and 5,000 deaths in the United States every year. Three organisms—*Salmonella*, *Listeria*, and *Toxoplasma*—are responsible for more than 75 percent of these deaths. Although most foodborne infections cause mild illness, severe infections and serious complications—including death—do occur.

Fight BAC!

To improve food safety awareness and practices, government and private agencies have developed the Fight Bac! campaign, which identifies four key culprits in foodborne illness:

- **Improper cooling.**
- **Improper hand washing.**
- **Inadequate cooking.**
- **Failure to avoid cross-contamination.**

Avoiding *E. coli* Infection

Eating unwashed produce, such as spinach or lettuce, or undercooked beef, especially hamburger, can increase your risk of infection with *Escherichia coli* (*E. coli*) bacteria. These bacteria, which live in the intestinal tract of healthy people and animals, are usually harmless. However, infection with the strain *E. coli* O157:H7 produces symptoms that can range from mild to life-threatening. This strain has made its way into hamburger in fast-food chains and into packaged spinach. *E. coli* can cause severe bloody diarrhea, kidney failure, and even death. Symptoms usually develop within 2 to 10 days and can include severe stomach cramps, vomiting, mild fever, and bloody diarrhea. Most people recover within 7 to 10 days. Others—especially older adults, children under the age of five, and those with weakened immune systems—may develop complications that lead to kidney failure.

The most common sources of *E. coli* infection are:

- **Contaminated food.** Although all beef can be contaminated, ground meat is a special concern because grinding combines meat from different animals and transfers bacteria from the meat's surface to its interior. Other sources of infection are raw milk, dry cured sausage, salami, alfalfa and clover sprouts, lettuce, unpasteurized apple juice and cider, and unwashed raw fruits and vegetables.
- **Contaminated water.** Drinking or inadvertently swallowing untreated water from lakes and streams can cause infection.
- **Person-to-person contact.** Family members of young children with the infection are especially likely to become sick themselves.

Proper handling and cooking of food can practically eliminate infection from meat. Especially if grilled, meat is likely to brown before it's completely cooked, so a meat thermometer should be used to ensure that meat is heated to at least 160°F at its thickest point. If a thermometer is not available, ground meat should be cooked until no pink shows in the center.

organic Term designating food produced with, or production based on the use of, fertilizers originating from plants or animals, without the use of pesticides or chemically formulated fertilizers.

Food Poisoning

Salmonella is a bacterium that contaminates many foods, particularly undercooked chicken, eggs, and sometimes processed meat. Eating contaminated food can result in salmonella poisoning, which causes diarrhea and vomiting. The Centers for Disease Control and Prevention (CDC) estimates 40,000 reported cases of salmonella poisoning a year; the actual number of cases could be anywhere from 400,000 to 4 million. The FDA has warned consumers about the dangers of unpasteurized orange juice because of the risk of salmonella contamination.

Another bacterium, *Campylobacter jejuni,* may cause even more stomach infections than salmonella. Found in water, milk, and some foods, campylobacter poisoning causes severe diarrhea and has been implicated in the growth of stomach ulcers.

Bacteria can also cause illness by producing toxins in food. *Staphylococcus aureus* is the most common culprit. When cooked foods are cross-contaminated with the bacteria from raw foods and not stored properly, staph infections can result, causing nausea and abdominal pain anywhere from thirty minutes to eight hours after ingestion.

Even many healthy foods can pose dangers. The FDA has urged consumers to avoid eating raw sprouts because of the risk of getting sick. Sprouts, particularly alfalfa and clover, can be contaminated by salmonella or *E. coli* bacteria. The FDA advises people to either cook sprouts before eating them or request that they be left off sandwiches and other food ordered in restaurants. Homegrown sprouts can also present a risk if they come from contaminated seeds.

An uncommon but sometimes fatal form of food poisoning is **botulism,** caused by the *Clostridium botulinum* organism. Improper home-canning procedures are the most common cause of this potentially fatal problem.

There have been several outbreaks of listeriosis, caused by the bacteria *listeria,* commonly found in deli meats, hot dogs, soft cheeses, raw meat, and unpasteurized milk. Although rare, listeriosis can be life-threatening. At greatest risk are pregnant women, infants, and those with weakened immune systems. You can reduce your risk by cooking meats and leftovers thoroughly and by washing everything that may come into contact with raw meat.

Pesticides

Plants and animals naturally produce compounds that act as pesticides to aid in their survival. The vast majority of the pesticides we consume are therefore natural, not added by farmers or food processors. *Commercial pesticides* save billions of dollars of valuable crops from pests, but they also may endanger human health and life. Fearful of potential risks in pesticides, many consumers are purchasing organic foods.

Food Allergies

As many as one in four Americans experience some adverse reaction to a particular food.[29] Food allergies are more common in children than adults.

Physicians disagree as to which foods are the most common triggers of food allergies. Cow's milk, eggs, seafood, wheat, soybeans, nuts, seeds, and chocolate have all been identified as culprits. The symptoms they provoke vary. One person might sneeze if exposed to an irritating food; another might vomit or develop diarrhea; others might suffer headaches, dizziness, hives, or a rapid heartbeat. Symptoms may not develop for up to 72 hours, making it hard to pinpoint which food was responsible.

If you suspect that you have a food allergy, see a physician with specialized training in allergy diagnosis. Medical opinion about the merits of many treatments for food allergies is divided. Once you've identified the culprit, the wisest and sometimes simplest course is to avoid it.

Nutritional Quackery

The American Dietetic Association describes nutritional quackery as a growing problem for unsuspecting consumers. Because so much nutritional nonsense is garbed in scientific-sounding terms, it can be hard to recognize bad advice when you get it. One basic rule: If the promises of a nutritional claim sound too good to be true, they probably are (see Savvy Consumer: "Spotting Nutrition Misinformation").

If you seek the advice of a nutrition consultant, carefully check his or her credentials and professional associa-

---

YOUR STRATEGIES FOR PREVENTION *How to Protect Yourself from Food Poisoning*

- Always wash your hands with liquid or clean bar soap before handling food. Rub your hands vigorously together for 10 to 15 seconds; the soap combined with the scrubbing action dislodges and removes germs.
- When preparing fresh fruits and vegetables, discard outer leaves, wash under

running water, and when possible, scrub with a clean brush or hands. Do not wash meat or poultry.

- To avoid the spread of bacteria to other foods, utensils, or surfaces, do not allow liquids to touch or drip onto other items. Wipe up all spills immediately.

- Clean out your refrigerator regularly. Throw out any leftovers stored for three or four days.

- To kill bacteria and viruses, sterilize wet kitchen sponges by putting them in a microwave for two minutes. Make sure they are completely wet to guard against the risk of fire.

ᵢ**Savvy**Consumer   Spotting Nutrition Misinformation

- Don't believe everything you read. A quick way to spot a bad nutrition self-help book is to look in the index for a diet to prevent or treat rheumatoid arthritis (none exists). If you find one, don't buy the book.

- Before you try any new nutritional approach, check with your doctor or a registered dietitian or call the American Dietetic Association's consumer hot line, (800)366–1655.

- Don't believe ads or advisers basing their nutritional recommendations on hair analysis, which is not accurate in detecting nutritional deficiencies.

- Be wary of anyone who recommends megadoses of vitamins or nutritional supplements, which can be dangerous. High doses of vitamin A, which some people take to clear up acne, can be toxic.

- Question personal testimonies about the powers of some magical pill or powder, and be wary of "scientific articles" in journals that aren't reviewed by health professionals.

- Be wary of any nutritional supplements sold in health stores or through health and body-building magazines. These products may contain ingredients that have not been tested and proven safe.

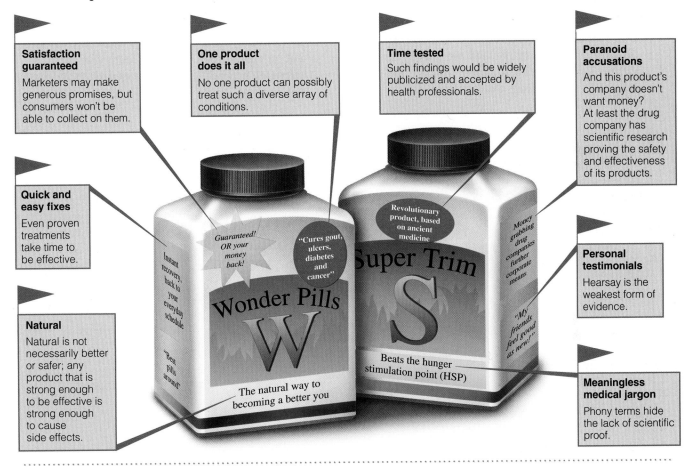

Satisfaction guaranteed
Marketers may make generous promises, but consumers won't be able to collect on them.

One product does it all
No one product can possibly treat such a diverse array of conditions.

Time tested
Such findings would be widely publicized and accepted by health professionals.

Paranoid accusations
And this product's company doesn't want money? At least the drug company has scientific research proving the safety and effectiveness of its products.

Quick and easy fixes
Even proven treatments take time to be effective.

Natural
Natural is not necessarily better or safer; any product that is strong enough to be effective is strong enough to cause side effects.

Personal testimonials
Hearsay is the weakest form of evidence.

Meaningless medical jargon
Phony terms hide the lack of scientific proof.

tions. Because licensing isn't required in all states, almost anyone can use the label "nutritionist," regardless of qualifications. Be wary of diplomas from obscure schools and organizations that allow anyone who pays dues to join. (One physician obtained a membership for his dog!) A registered dietitian (R.D.), who has a bachelor's degree and specialized training (including an internship) and who passed a certification examination, is usually a member of the American Dietetic Association (ADA), which sets the standard for quality in diets. A nutrition expert with an M.D. or Ph.D. generally belongs to the ADA, the American Institute of Nutrition, or the American Society of Clinical Nutrition; all have stringent membership requirements.

botulism Possibly fatal food poisoning caused by a type of bacterium that grows and produces its toxin in the absence of air and is found in improperly canned food.

Learn It ⋮ **Live It**

Making Healthful Food Choices

As nutritional knowledge expands and evolves, it's easy to be confused by changing advice on which foods to avoid and which to eat. But even though research may challenge or change thinking on a specific food, some basic principles always apply.

- **Eat breakfast.** Easy to prepare breakfasts include cold cereal with fruit and low-fat milk, whole-wheat toast with peanut butter, yogurt with fruit, or whole-grain waffles.

- **Don't eat too much of one thing.** Your body needs protein, carbohydrates, fat, and many different vitamins and minerals, such as vitamins C and A, iron, and calcium, from a variety of foods.

- **Eat more grains, fruits, and vegetables.** These foods give you carbohydrates for energy, plus vitamins, minerals, and fiber. Try breads such as whole-wheat, bagels, and pita. Spaghetti and oatmeal are also in the grain group.

- **Don't ban any food.** Fit in a higher-fat food, like pepperoni pizza, at dinner by choosing lower-fat foods at other meals. And don't forget about moderation. If two pieces of pizza fill you up, don't eat a third.

- **Make every calorie count.** Load up on nutrients, not on big portions. Choosing foods that are nutrient dense will help protect against disease and keep you healthy.

SELFSURVEY ⋮ *How Healthful Is Your Diet?*

STEP 1

Keep a food diary for a week, writing down everything you eat and drink for meals and snacks. Include the approximate amount eaten (for example, 1/2 cup, 1 large, 12-oz can, and so on).

	Mon	Tues	Wed	Thurs	Fri	Sat	Sun
Grains							
Vegetables							
Fruits							
Milk, yogurt, cheese							
Meat, poultry, dry beans, eggs, nuts							
Fats, oil, sweets, cheese							

STEP 2: Are You Getting Enough Vegetables, Fruits, and Grains?

How often do you eat:	Seldom/Never	1–2 times a week	3–5 times a week	Almost daily
At least three servings of vegetables a day?				
Starchy vegetables like potatoes, corn, or peas?				
Foods made with dry beans, lentils, or peas?				
Dark green or deep yellow vegetables (broccoli, spinach, collards, carrots, sweet potatoes, squash)?				
At least two servings of fruit a day?				

Citrus fruits and 100% fruit juices (oranges, grapefruit, tangerines)? _____

Whole fruit with skin or seeds (berries, apples, pears)? _____

At least six servings of breads, cereals, pasta, or rice a day? _____

The best answer for each is "almost daily." Use your food diary to see which foods you should be eating more often.

STEP 3: Are You Getting Too Much Fat?

How often do you eat:	Seldom/Never	1–2 times a week	3–5 times a week	Almost daily
Fried, deep-fat fried, or breaded food?				
Fatty meats, such as sausages, luncheon meat, fatty steaks or roasts?				
Whole milk, high-fat cheeses, ice cream?				
Pies, pastries, rich cakes?				
Rich cream sauces and gravies?				
Oily salad dressings or mayonnaise?				
Butter or margarine on vegetables, rolls, bread, or toast?				

Ideally, you should be eating these foods no more than one or two times a week. If your food diary indicates that you're eating them more frequently, your fat intake may well be too high.

STEP 4: Are You Getting Too Much Sodium?

How often do you eat:	Seldom/Never	1–2 times a week	3–5 times a week	Almost daily
Cured or processed meats, such as ham, sausage, frankfurters, or luncheon meats?				
Canned vegetables or frozen vegetables with sauce?				
Frozen TV dinners, entrees, or canned or dehydrated soups?				
Salted nuts, popcorn, pretzels, corn chips, or potato chips?				
Seasoning mixes or sauces containing salt?				
Processed cheese?				
Salt added to table foods before you taste them?				

Ideally, you should be eating these high-sodium items no more than one or two times a week. If your food diary indicates that you're eating them more frequently, your sodium intake may well be too high.

Your Health Action Plan for Better Nutrition

- **Eat five servings of fruits and vegetables per day.** For breakfast, have 100% fruit juice or add raisins, berries, or sliced fruit to cereal, pancakes, or waffles. For lunch, have vegetable soup or salad with your meal or pile vegetables on your sandwich. For dinner, choose vegetables that are green, orange (such as carrots or squash), and red (such as tomatoes or bell peppers).

- **Include three servings of whole-grain foods every day.** To identify whole-grain products, check the ingredient list. The first ingredient should be a whole grain, such as "whole-grain oats," "whole-grain wheat," or "whole wheat."

- **Consume a calcium-rich food at each meal.** Good options include low-fat and nonfat milk; cheese; or yogurt; tofu; broccoli; dried beans; spinach; and fortified soy milk.

- **Eat less meat.** Rather than making meat the heart of a meal, think of it as a flavoring ingredient.

- **Avoid high-fat fast foods.** Hot dogs, fried foods, packaged snack foods, and pastries are most likely to be laden with fat.

- **Check the numbers.** When buying prepared foods, choose items that contain no more than 3 grams of fat per 100 calories.

- **Think small.** A dinner-size serving of meat should be about the size of a deck of cards; half a cup is the size of a woman's fist; a pancake is the diameter of a CD.

- **Read labels carefully.** Remember that "cholesterol-free" doesn't necessarily mean fat-free. Avoid products that contain saturated coconut oil, palm oil, lard, or hydrogenated fats.

- **Switch to low-fat and nonfat dairy products.** Rather than buying whole-fat dairy products, choose skim milk, fat-free sour cream, and low- or nonfat yogurt.

- **The brighter the better.** When selecting fruits and vegetables, choose the most intense color. A bright orange carrot has more beta-carotene than a pale one. Dark green lettuce leaves have more vitamins than lighter ones. Orange sweet potatoes pack more vitamin A than yellow ones.

CENGAGENOW™ If you want to write your own goals for more nutritious choices, go to the Wellness Journal at HealthNow: **academic.cengage. com/login.**

Making This Chapter Work
for YOU

Review Questions

1. The classes of essential nutrients include which of the following?
   a. amino acids, antioxidants, fiber, and cholesterol
   b. proteins, calcium, calories, and folic acid
   c. carbohydrates, minerals, fat, and water
   d. iron, whole grains, fruits, and vegetables

2. Which type of fat is *not* considered a threat to heart health?
   a. omega-3 fatty acids
   b. trans fat
   c. triglycerides
   d. saturated fats

3. Antioxidants
   a. are nutrients important in the production of hemoglobin.
   b. are substances added to foods to make them more flavorful or physically appealing.
   c. are suspected triggers of food allergies.
   d. are substances that prevent the harmful effects of free radicals.

4. The MyPyramid system can be personalized to your age, gender, and activity level at www.MyPyramid.gov. Besides personalization, the MyPyramid system has these themes:
   a. variety, proportionality, moderation, and activity
   b. variety, bulimia, activity
   c. variety, moderation, activity, and food safety
   d. variety, moderation, activity, and correct food labeling

5. The MyPyramid system includes this recommendation:
   a. Make half your grains whole.
   b. Go lean with protein.
   c. Focus on fruits.
   d. All of the above.

6. The 2005 Dietary Guidelines for Americans include:
   a. Decrease intake of added sugars.
   b. Increase consumption of olive oil.
   c. Control calorie intake to manage body weight.
   d. Eat dessert no more than three days a week.

7. Food labels on packaged foods include all of the following *except*
   a. total weight of the package.
   b. total amount of nutrients contained in the food.
   c. the percent of nutrient Daily Values provided in the food.
   d. serving size.

8. Since Sam plays poker, it's been easy for him to remember that a recommended serving of 3 ounces of meat means a piece of meat about the size of
  a. one deck of cards.
  b. eight poker chips.
  c. two decks of cards.
  d. a roll of quarters.

9. Some vegetarians may
  a. include chicken and fish in their diets.
  b. avoid vitamin B$_{12}$ supplements if they eat only plant foods.
  c. eat only legumes or nuts because these provide complete proteins.
  d. have high cholesterol levels because of the saturated fats in fruits and vegetables.

10. Common causes of foodborne infections include which of the following?
  a. the influenza virus
  b. *Salmonella* and *E. coli* bacteria
  c. avian flu virus
  d. pesticides

Answers to these questions can be found on page 583.

Critical Thinking

1. Which alternative or ethnic diet do you think has the best tasting food? Which is the most healthy? Why?

2. Is it possible to meet nutritional requirements on a limited budget? Have you ever been in this situation? What would you recommend to someone who wanted to eat healthfully on $30 a week?

3. Consider the number of times a week you eat fast food. How much money would you have saved if you had eaten home-prepared meals? Which fast foods could you have selected that would have provided more nutritional value?

Media Menu

CENGAGENOW™Go to the HealthNow website at **academic.cengage.com/login** that will:
- Help you evaluate your knowledge of the material.
- Allow you to take an exam-prep quiz.
- Provide a Personalized Learning Plan targeting resources that address areas you should study.
- Coach you through identifying target goals for behavioral change and creating and monitoring your personal change plan throughout the semester.

Internet Connections

U.S. Food and Nutrition Information Center
www.nal.usda.gov/fnic/
This comprehensive governmental website features reports and scientific studies on a variety of nutrition information, including the 2005 USDA Dietary Guidelines, MyPyramid, dietary supplements, dietary assessment, food composition searchable databases, educational brochures, historical food guides, and a topics "A-Z" section.

USDA's MyPyramid
www.MyPyramid.gov
This interactive site features MyPyramid Plan, which gives you a personal eating plan, and MyPyramid Tracker, which offers a detailed assessment of your food intake and physical activity level.

Nutrient Analysis Tool
http://nat.crgq.com
This site, provided as a public service by the Food Science and Human Nutrition Department at the University of Illinois, features a free nutrient analysis interactive program that calculates the amount of calories, carbohydrates, protein, fat, vitamins, minerals, and fiber in the foods that make up your daily diet.

Cyberkitchen
www.nhlbisupport.com/chd1/Tipsheets/cyberkit.htm
This interactive site helps you discover how much you are really eating with an activity on comparing standard serving sizes versus real serving sizes. You also can provide personal information regarding your age, gender, height, weight, and activity level, and the Cyberkitchen will provide you with a healthy diet plan to meet your weight management goals. It's fun and educational.

Key Terms

The terms listed are used and defined on the page indicated.
Definitions are also found in the Glossary at the end of this book.

amino acids	149
antioxidants	152
basal metabolic rate (BMR)	147
botulism	175
calories	147
carbohydrates	149
complementary proteins	169
complete proteins	149
complex carbohydrates	149
dietary fiber	149
essential nutrients	147
folic acid	164
functional fiber	149
incomplete proteins	149
lacto-vegetarians	169
macronutrients	147
micronutrients	147
minerals	152
nutrition	147
organic	173
ovo-lacto-vegetarians	169
phytochemicals	157
proteins	149
saturated fats	150
simple carbohydrates	149
trans fat	150
unsaturated fats	150
vegans	169
vitamins	152

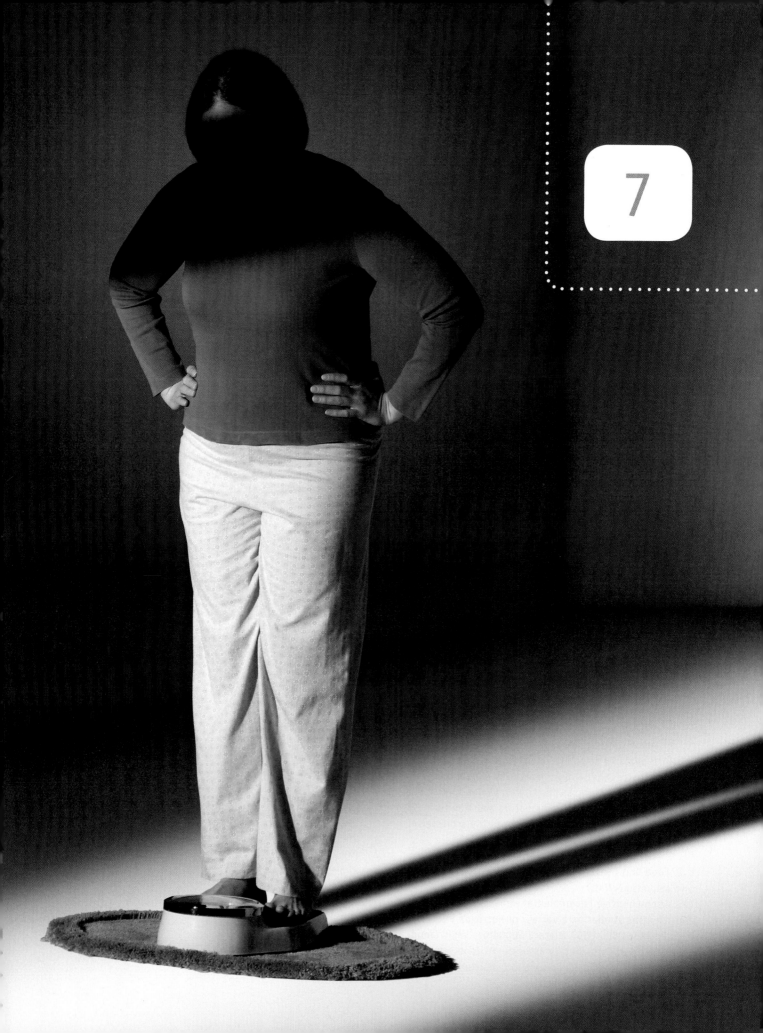

Taking Control of Your Weight

LINA'S mother called it "baby fat." "You'll outgrow it soon enough," she said. Yet Lina's cheeks grew chubbier and her waist wider every year. "Wait for your growth spurt," her mother reassured her. But Lina remained one of the shortest girls in her class—and, she was convinced, the roundest.

Lina went on her first diet in high school. For three days she ate nothing but carrot sticks, cottage cheese, and apples. Then she scarfed down two double cheeseburgers with fries and a chocolate shake. Her other attempts at dieting didn't last much longer. By graduation Lina was grateful to hide under the flowing black robe as she walked on stage to get her diploma.

When Lina heard about the "freshman 15," the extra pounds many students acquire during their first year at college, she groaned at the prospect of putting on more weight. In her Personal Health class, Lina set one primary goal: not to gain another pound. Rather than going on—and inevitably falling off—one diet after another, she developed a weight management plan that included healthful food choices and regular exercise. Armed with the information and tools provided in this chapter, Lina, for the first time in her life, took charge of her weight.

You can do the same. If you're already at a healthy weight, this chapter can ensure that you remain so in the future. If like two-thirds of Americans, you are overweight, you will find help in these pages. You can choose to lose.

Don't fool yourself into thinking that fat is only a cosmetic problem. Excess weight weakens hearts; raises blood pressure; clogs arteries; strains backs and joints; increases the risk of diabetes, stroke, and certain cancers; and steals years of productive life. The earlier the weight gain, the greater the danger it poses. Obesity at age 20 can cut 20 years off a person's life.

After studying the material in this chapter, you should be able to:

- **List** the factors besides genetics that have contributed to the global increase in overweight and obesity.
- **Define** overweight and obesity.
- **Identify** the main health risks of excess weight.
- **Assess** various approaches to weight loss.
- **Identify** and describe the symptoms and dangers associated with eating disorders.
- **Design** a personal plan for sensible weight management.

CENGAGENOW™ Log on to HealthNow at **academic.cengage.com/login** to find your Behavior Change Planner and to explore self-assessments, interactive tutorials, and practice quizzes.

This chapter explains how we grew so big, tells what obesity is and why excess pounds are dangerous, describes current approaches to weight loss, discusses diets that work (and some that don't), offers practical guidelines for exercise and behavioral approaches to losing weight, and examines unhealthy eating patterns and eating disorders. Regardless of your current weight, you will find insights and skills that you will need for healthy weight management throughout your life.

The Global Epidemic

An estimated 1.1 billion people around the world—seven in ten of the Dutch and Spanish, two in three Americans and Canadians, and one in two Britons, Germans, and Italians—are overweight or obese. In Europe, excess weight ranks as the most common childhood disorder. Since 1980, obesity rates have tripled in parts of Eastern Europe, the Middle East, China, and the Pacific Islands. In many poor countries, obesity is common among city dwellers, while people in rural areas remain underweight and malnourished.

The World Health Organization, in its first global diet, exercise, and health program to combat obesity, recommends that governments promote public knowledge about diet, exercise, and health; offer information that makes healthy choices easier for consumers to make; and require accurate, comprehensible food labels.[1] Although ultimately each individual decides what and how much to eat, policy makers agree that governments also must act to reverse the obesity epidemic.

Exposure to a Western lifestyle seems to bring out susceptibility to excess weight. Obesity is much more common among the Pima Indians of Arizona compared to Pimas living in Mexico, who have maintained a more traditional lifestyle, with more physical activity and a diet lower in fat and richer in complex carbohydrates. Native Hawaiians who follow a more traditional diet and lifestyle also have lower rates of obesity and cardiovascular disease.

Supersized Nation

Since 1980, the obesity rate has tripled for children and adolescents. The prevalence of obesity among men has increased significantly since 1999, rising to 31 percent. The rate of obesity among women has remained the same: 33 percent. About 3 percent of men and 7 percent of women are extremely obese. Men and women between ages 20 and 39 have the lowest rate of obesity: 29 percent. Among 40- to 59-year-olds, 37 percent are obese, as are 31 percent of those over age 60.[2] By some estimates, Americans are collectively more than 5 billion pounds overweight. Some 200 million men and women weigh more—often much more—than their recommended target weights.

Obesity rates vary by ethnic groups as well as by gender and age. About 30 percent of white Americans are obese, compared with 45 percent of African Americans and 37 percent of Mexican Americans. In some Native American communities, up to 70 percent of all adults are dangerously overweight. Differences in metabolic rates may be one factor.

Not all Americans are equally likely to be overweight or obese. As Figure 7.1 shows, the southern states have the highest concentration of obese residents. Mississippi is home to the county with the highest percentage of people with a body mass index (BMI) between 30 and 40. (BMI, as discussed in Chapter 5, is defined as the ratio between weight and height that correlates with percentage of body fat.)

Weight problems are starting earlier than ever. About one in four children between ages two and five is overweight or at risk of becoming overweight. Among those between ages six to eleven, the percentage rises to 37 percent. About one in three teenagers falls into this category.

How Did We Get So Fat?

A variety of factors, ranging from behavior to environment to genetics, played a role in the increase in overweight and obesity. They include:

1. **More calories.** Bombarded by nonstop commercials for taste treats, tempted by foods in every form to munch and crunch, in the last thirty years the average man has added 168 calories and the average woman 335 calories to their daily diets.[3] Many of these extra calories come from refined carbohydrates, which can raise levels of heart-damaging blood fats called triglycerides and increase the risk of diabetes as well as obesity. As discussed in Chapter 6, soft drinks account for half of the increase in caloric intake.[4]

2. **Bigger portions.** As Table 7.1 shows, the size of many popular restaurant and packaged foods has increased two to five times during the past 20 years. Some foods, like chocolate bars, have grown more than ten times since they were first introduced. Popular 64-ounce sodas can pack a whopping 800 calories. According to studies of appetite and satiety, people presented with larger portions eat up to 30 percent more than they otherwise would.

3. **Fast food.** Young adults who eat frequently at fast-food restaurants gain more weight and develop metabolic abnormalities that increase their risk of diabetes in early middle age. In a recent study,

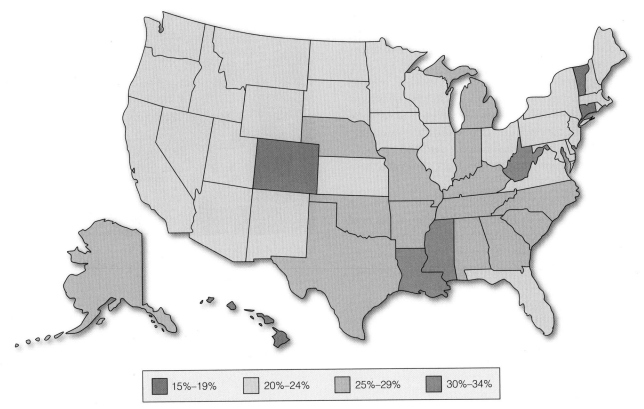

Figure 7.1 Obesity in the United States

This map shows the percentage of people in each state who are obese—they have a body mass index between 30 and 40.

Source: Data from National Center for Chronic Disease Prevention and Health Promotion, "At a Glance 2007," www.cdc.gov.nccdphp/publications/aag/dnpa.htm.

Legend: 15%–19% 20%–24% 25%–29% 30%–34%

TABLE 7.1 Supersized Portions

Food/Beverage	Original Size (year introduced)	Today (largest available)
Soda (Coca-Cola)	6.5 oz (1916)	34 oz
French fries (Burger King)	2.6 oz (1954)	6.9 oz
Hamburger (McDonald's); (beef only)	1.6 oz (1955)	8 oz
Nestle's Crunch	1.6 oz (1938)	5 oz
Budweiser (bottle)	7 oz (1976)	40 oz

Source: "Are Growing Portion Sizes Leading to Expanding Waistlines?" American Dietetic Association, www.eatright.org.

those who ate fast food at least twice a week gained an extra 10 pounds and had a twofold greater increase in insulin resistance, a risk factor for diabetes. The men in the study visited fast-food restaurants more often than the women; African Americans did so more frequently than whites.[5]

4. **Physical inactivity.** As Americans eat more, they exercise less. Experts estimate that most adults expend 200 to 300 fewer calories than people did 25 years ago. The most dramatic drop in physical activity often occurs during the college years.

5. **Passive entertainment.** Television is a culprit in an estimated 30 percent of new cases of obesity.

TV viewing may increase weight in several ways: It takes up time that otherwise might be spent in physical activities. It increases food intake since people tend to eat more while watching TV. And compared with sewing, reading, driving, or other relatively sedentary pursuits, watching television lowers metabolic rate so viewers burn fewer calories. The combination of watching television (at least two and one-half hours a day) and eating fast food more than twice a week can triple the risk of obesity.

6. **Modernization.** The growth of industry and technology has led to an abundance of food, less need for physical activity, urbanization, labor-saving devices, and a more sedentary lifestyle. Suburban sprawl directly contributes to obesity, according to research. People who live in neighborhoods where they must drive to get anywhere are significantly more likely to be obese than those who can easily walk to their destinations.

7. **Socioeconomics.** The less money you make, the more likely you are to be overweight. One in four adults below the poverty level is obese, compared with one in six in households earning $67,000 or more. Minorities are at even greater risk. One in three poor African Americans is obese.

8. **Prenatal factors.** A woman's weight before conception and weight gain during pregnancy influence her child's weight. A substantial number of children are prone to gaining weight because their mothers developed gestational diabetes during their pregnancies. Children born to obese women are more than twice as likely to be overweight by age four.

9. **Childhood development.** Today's children don't necessarily eat more food than in the past, but they eat more high-fat, high-calorie foods and they exercise much, much less. On days when they eat fast food, youngsters consume an average of 187 more calories per day. Fewer than half of grade schoolers participate in daily physical education classes. Many spend five hours or more a day in front of a computer or television screen.

10. **Genetics.** Scientists have identified a specific gene, found in one-sixth of people of European descent, that increases the risk of obesity by 30 percent or more.[6] It also may be that various genes contribute a small increase in risk or that rare abnormalities in many genes create a predisposition to weight gain and obesity.

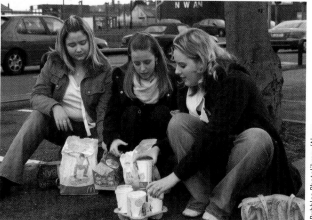

Round-the-clock snacking, fast-food restaurants on every corner, and hours in front of the TV have all contributed to the increase in overweight and obesity.

11. **Social networks.** Friends may have a significant effect on a person's risk of obesity. A 32-year detailed analysis of a large social network of 12,067 people, found that when one close friend became obese, the other's chances of doing the same increased by 171 percent. Among pairs of adult siblings, if one became obese, the chance that the other would become obese increased by 40 percent.[7] Researchers cannot fully explain why this happens. Perhaps one explanation is that friends alter each others' perception of fatness: When a close friend is obese, obesity seems normal and acceptable.[8]

12. **Emotional influences.** Obese people are neither more nor less psychologically troubled than others. Psychological problems, such as irritability, depression, and anxiety, are more likely to be the result of obesity than the cause. As discussed later in this chapter, emotions do play a role in weight problems. Just as some people reach for a drink or a drug when they're upset, others cope by overeating, bingeing, or purging.

Body Image

Throughout most of history, bigger was better. The great beauties of centuries past, as painted by such artistic masters as Rubens and Renoir, were soft and fleshy, with rounded bellies and dimpled thighs. Culture often shapes views of beauty and health.

Many developing countries still regard a full figure, rather than a thin one, as the ideal. Fattening huts, in which brides-to-be eat extra food to plump up before marriage, still exist in some African cultures. Among certain Native American tribes of the Southwest, if a girl is thin at puberty, a fat woman places her foot on the girl's back so she will magically gain weight and become more attractive.

Influenced by the media, many Americans are paying more attention to their body images than ever before—and at a younger age. In a study of high school girls, those who regularly read women's health and fitness magazines, which may present unrealistic physical ideals, were more likely to go on low-calorie diets, take pills to suppress their appetites, use laxatives, or force themselves to vomit after eating. Boys' body images also are influenced by media images depicting superstrong, highly muscular males.

 Being overweight for a long period of time has a cumulative negative impact on body image. In a study of 266 college women, those who described themselves as "always overweight" ranked much lower in current body self-esteem than those with more recent weight problems.

 College students of different ethnic and racial backgrounds, including Asians, express as much—and sometimes more—concern about their body shape and weight as whites. In a study of university students, African American and Caucasian men were similar in their ideals for body size and in their perceptions of their own shapes. As shown in Figure 7.2, both African American and white women perceived themselves as smaller than they actually were and desired an even smaller body size.

However, the African American women were more accepting of larger size.

Male and Female Body Image

 Although women generally report a more negative body image, many men are dissatisfied with their bodies but for different reasons. Often they want either to lose or gain weight or to add muscle and bulk. Women compare their appearance to others more frequently than men and worry more that others will think negatively about their looks. Yet appearance matters just as much to men, who are as likely as women to engage in efforts to improve their bodies.[9]

Women have long been bombarded by idealized images in the media of female bodies that bear little resemblance to the way most women look. Increasingly, more advertisements and men's magazines are featuring idealized male bodies. Sleek, strong, and sculpted, they do not resemble the bodies most men inhabit. The gap between reality and ideal is getting bigger for both genders.

When college men and women step on a scale or look in a mirror, they react in different ways. In a study of 525 undergraduates, the women failed to see themselves as underweight, even when they were, and perceived themselves as overweight, even when they were not. Many of the women who considered themselves normal weight nonetheless desired to be thinner. Men in the study generally saw themselves as under-

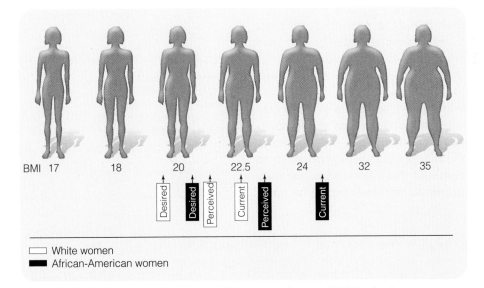

Figure 7.2 Body Dissatisfaction in African American and White Students
In a study of 630 undergraduates, both African American and white women perceived themselves to be smaller than they actually were—and wished to be even smaller. However, the white students saw themselves as and desired to be considerably smaller than did the African American women. Both African American and white men rated the silhouette depicting a BMI of 20 as the most desirable.

Source: "Body Dissatisfaction Among College Students." *Nutrition Research Newsletter*, Vol. 21, No. 3, March 2002, p. 9.

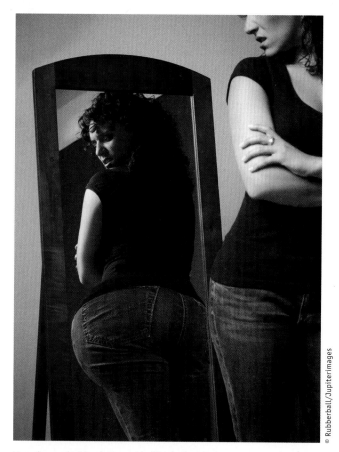

How do you decide what your ideal body size is?

weight, even when they were not. Most desired to be heavier, though not obese. Table 7.2 shows how students describe their own weight.

 The higher their body fat percentage, the more dissatisfied college women tend to be with their shape. Women at all-female schools are just as prone to distorted perceptions of body size and body dissatisfaction as those at coed institutions.[10]

The greater the discrepancy between a woman's current view of her body shape and the ideal she considers most attractive to men, the more likely she is to worry about how others will view her and to doubt her ability to make a desirable impression. Such "social physique anxiety" occurs often in women who feel they do not mea-

sure up to what they or others consider most desirable in terms of weight or appearance. Women with high BMIs and greater body-related anxiety may exercise to become thinner or more attractive. Those reporting the greatest distress because of body image are at highest risk of disordered eating or actual eating disorders (discussed later in this chapter). For tips on improving your body image, see Your Strategies for Change: "How to Boost Your Body Esteem."

Understanding Weight Problems

Weight problems don't develop overnight. Fat accumulates meal by meal, day by day, pound by pound. Ultimately, all weight problems are the result of a prolonged energy imbalance—of consuming too many calories and burning too few in daily activities.

How many calories you need depends on your gender, age, body-frame size, weight, percentage of body fat, and your *basal metabolic rate (BMR)*—the number of calories needed to sustain your body at rest. Your activity level also affects your calorie requirements. Regardless of whether you consume fat, protein, or carbohydrates, if you take in more calories than required to maintain your size and don't work them off in some sort of physical activity, your body will convert the excess to fat.

The average American consumes about one million calories a year. Given that number, what difference does an extra 100-calorie soda or 300-calorie brownie make?

TABLE 7.2 Students Weigh in on Weight

	Total	Women	Men
Percentage of Students Who Described Themselves as			
Very underweight	0.7%	0.4%	1.2%
Slightly underweight	10	7	14
About the right weight	53	53	53
Slightly overweight	33	35	28
Very overweight	4	5	3

Source: American College Health Association. "American College Health Association National College Health Assessment Spring 2006 Reference Group Data Report (Abridged)." *Journal of American College Health*, Vol. 55, No. 4, January–February 2007, pp. 195–206.

YOUR STRATEGIES FOR CHANGE *How to Boost Your Body Esteem*

Whatever your weight or shape, here are some ways to improve your body image:

- Start walking with more bounce in your step.
- Focus on the parts of your body you like. Take pride in your powerful shoulders or large eyes.

- Treat yourself with the respect you'd like to receive from others. Don't put yourself down or joke about your weight.
- Work with hand weights. As you build your muscles, your sense of strength and self-confidence also will grow.

- Don't put off special plans, such as learning to kayak or signing up for an exchange program, until you reach a certain magical weight: Do what you want to do *now*.
- Pull your shoulders back, suck in your stomach, and stand up straight. You'll look and feel better.

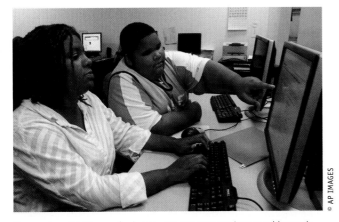

© AP IMAGES

If you gain weight in your freshman year, you may continue to add pounds as a sophomore.

YOUR STRATEGIES FOR PREVENTION *How to Hold the Line on College Weight Gain*

- **Plan meals.** Most campus cafeterias post the week's menus in advance. Plan which items you will eat before you see or smell high-fat dishes.
- **Don't linger.** If you use the cafeteria as a social gathering place, you may end up eating with two or three different groups of people. Set a time limit to eat—then leave.

- **Develop alternative behaviors.** People who eat when they are stressed or bored need substitute activities ready when they need them. Make a list of things you can do—shower, phone a friend, take a hike—when stress strikes.
- **Eat at "home."** If the dormitory has a small kitchen, cook some healthful dishes and invite friends to join you.

- **Take advantage of physical activity programs.** Many college students become less active during their years in college. Aim to maintain or increase the amount of exercise you did in high school. Join a biking club, take a salsa class, learn yoga, try tennis or raquetball.

A lot, because the extra calories that you don't burn every day accumulate, adding an average of 2 to 4 pounds to your weight every year.

Weight and the College Student

Obesity rates have increased most rapidly among 18- to 29-year-olds. About one in three college students may be overweight or obese. (See Reality Check.)

One in five college students has an unhealthy weight as well as at least one risk factor for metabolic disorder, an important cause of cardiovascular disease (discussed in Chapter 14).

As many students discover, it's easy to gain weight on campuses, which are typically crammed with vending machines, fast-food counters, and cafeterias serving up hearty meals. But the infamous *freshman 15,* the extra pounds acquired in the first year at college, seems to be a myth. Several studies have documented much lower weight gains, ranging from 2.45 to 7 pounds. In one recent study at a private school in the Northeast, males gained an average of 5.6 pounds and females 3.6 pounds in their freshman year. One in six freshmen gained 10 or more pounds. In another study at a public university in the Midwest, students gained an average of 7.8 pounds their freshman year. One in five piled on 15 or more pounds.[11]

Although students do put on the most weight in their first term of college, many continue to gain weight as sophomores. Among the suspected culprits in college weight gain are alcohol, socializing that involves eating, high-fat foods in dorm cafeterias, and less physical activity.

To avoid the freshman 15 and beyond, see Your Strategies for Prevention: "How to Hold the Line on College Weight Gain."

What Is a Healthy Weight?

Rather than relying on a range of ideal weights for various heights, as they did in the past, medical experts use various methods to assess body composition and weight. The best indicators of weight-related health risks are Body Mass Index (BMI); waist circumference (WC); and waist-to-hip ratio (WHR). (All are discussed in depth in Chapter 5.)

If you have a BMI higher than 25, you are **overweight** and at greater risk of health problems. If your BMI is between 30 and 34.9, you have class 1 **obesity.** If it is

overweight A condition of having a BMI between 25.0 and 29.9.

obesity The excessive accumulation of fat in the body; class 1 obesity is defined by a BMI between 30.0 and 34.9; class 2 obesity by a BMI between 35.0 and 39.9; class 3 or severe obesity by a BMI of 40 or higher.

between 35 and 39.9, you have class 2 obesity. Both indicate increased risk of dying of weight-related problems. A BMI over 40 signifies class 3 or severe obesity and poses the greatest threat to health and longevity.

If you're a young adult, even mild to moderate overweight poses a threat to your health because it puts you at risk for gaining even more weight—and for facing greater health risks. Obesity has been implicated as a culprit in rising rates of disability among younger Americans as well as a factor in chronic health problems. If you are older than a traditional-aged student, the risks to your health are more immediate.

Health Dangers of Excess Weight

The federal government has recognized obesity as a serious, potentially fatal disease. This designation cleared the way for insurance coverage for obesity treatments, rather than just for the medical problems it can cause. The effects of obesity on health are the equivalent of 20 years of aging. They include increased risk of cardiovascular disease, diabetes, and cancer, as well as rheumatoid arthritis, sleep apnea, gout, and liver disease (Figure 7.3). Being overweight or obese at age 25 increases your likelihood of difficulties in walking, balance, and rising from

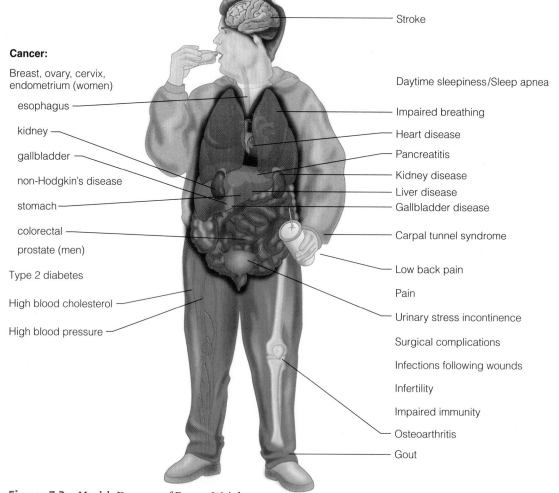

Figure 7.3 Health Dangers of Excess Weight

a chair.[12] Total medical costs, both direct and indirect, amount to more than $117 billion a year.

The Impact on the Body

The incidence of diabetes, gallstones, hypertension, heart disease, and colon cancer increases with the degree of overweight in both sexes. Those with BMIs of 35 or more are approximately 20 times more likely to develop diabetes. Overweight men and women are at least three times more likely to suffer knee injuries that require surgery to repair.

 Health risks may vary in different races, ethnic groups, and at-risk populations. Even relatively small amounts of excess fat—as little as 5 pounds—can add to the dangers in those already at risk for hypertension and diabetes. Obesity also causes alterations in various measures of immune function and increases the risk of kidney stones and disease. It may also affect the brain and contribute to cognitive problems and dementia.[13]

Overweight young adults have a 70 percent chance of becoming overweight or obese adults. They are two to three times more likely to have high total cholesterol levels and more than 43 times more likely to have cardiovascular disease risk factors such as elevated blood pressure. They also have a higher prevalence of type 2 diabetes.

Excess pounds affect people around the clock. Overweight and obese individuals sleep less than those with normal weights. (See Chapter 2 for a discussion of sleep.) The lost sleep could add to the risk of medical problems.

Major diseases linked to obesity include:

- **Type 2 diabetes.** More than 80 percent of people with type 2 diabetes are overweight. Although the reasons are not known, being overweight may make cells less efficient at using sugar from the blood. This then puts stress on the cells that produce insulin (a hormone that carries sugar from the blood to cells) and makes them gradually fail. You can lower your risk for developing type 2 diabetes by losing weight and increasing the amount of physical activity you do. If you have type 2 diabetes, losing weight and becoming more physically active can help you control your blood sugar levels and may allow you to reduce the amount of diabetes medication you take.

- **Heart disease and stroke.** People who are overweight are more likely to suffer from high blood pressure, high levels of triglycerides (blood fats) and harmful LDL cholesterol, and low levels of beneficial HDL cholesterol. In addition, people with more body fat have higher blood levels of substances that cause inflammation, which may

raise heart disease risk. Losing 5 to 15 percent of your weight can lower your chances for developing heart disease or having a stroke.

People who both smoke and are obese are at especially high risk of cardiovascular disease. Although some smokers have felt that they couldn't lose weight until they stopped smoking, researchers have found that weight loss among smokers is possible and beneficial, leading to a reduction in other risk factors, such as lower blood pressure and lower cholesterol.

- **Cancer.** Excess weight may account for 14 percent of all cancer deaths in men and 20 percent of those in women. Losing weight, researchers estimate, could prevent as many as one of every six cancer deaths. Excess weight has been linked to cancers of the colon and rectum, kidney, esophagus, and gallbladder; non-Hodgkin's lymphoma; multiple myeloma; and cancers of the pancreas and liver, the breast, uterus, cervix, and ovary (in women), and the stomach and prostate (in men).

Body size and higher BMI are linked with increased risk of breast cancer in premenopausal women and in postmenopausal women not using hormone replacement therapy.

Too much body fat can influence cancer in several ways: It increases the amount of estrogen in the blood, raising the risk of cancers of the female reproductive system. It raises the levels of insulin, which prompts the body to create a hormone that causes cells to multiply. Acid reflux, which can cause cancer of the esophagus, occurs more frequently in heavy men and women. Obesity also makes cancer harder to diagnose and treat.

The Impact on Life Expectancy

Obesity kills. Researchers attribute 112,000 to 280,000 deaths every year to excess weight.[14] Your weight in early adulthood and middle age can have an impact on how long and how well you live. Overweight and obesity after age 30 increase the risk of hospitalization and of dying from cardiovascular disease and diabetes later in life, even in individuals with no risk factors for heart disease (discussed in Chapter 14) and in those with just one risk factor.[15]

The Emotional Toll

In our calorie-conscious and thinness-obsessed society, obesity also affects quality of life, including sense of vitality and physical pain. Many see it as a psychological burden, a sign of failure, laziness, or inadequate willpower. Overweight men and women often blame themselves for becoming heavy and feel guilty and

POINT COUNTERPOINT *Whose Fault Is Fat?*

POINT

Many people assume that obesity occurs because of a failure of willpower. If they chose more healthful foods, didn't overeat, and exercised more, the 200 million overweight and obese Americans could take control of their weight. If they don't, they deserve to suffer the consequences, which include health problems, social prejudice, and discrimination on the job.

COUNTERPOINT

Society sets people up to get fat. The food industry spends $30 billion a year urging us to eat. Fast-food outlets peddle high-calorie treats on practically every street corner and in every shopping mall.

Changes in the social environment to make it easier to eat healthfully and exercise more are essential to solving America's weight problems.

YOUR VIEW

Who do you think is responsible for the widening of our waistlines? Do you see weight as a personal responsibility? Should society do more to prevent obesity and help the overweight lose excess pounds? What could your school do to prevent weight problems or help heavy students slim down?

---

depressed as a result. In fact, the psychological problems once considered the cause of obesity may be its consequence. (See the Point/Counterpoint feature.)

 Weight may affect risky sexual behaviors among college students. In a study of almost 1,000 undergraduates, sexually active women with the highest BMIs were more likely to have sex with a casual partner, to have multiple same-sex partners, and to recall being intoxicated at the time of their most recent sexual intercourse. There was no correlation between men's weight and their sexual behavior.[16]

If You're Too Thin: How to Gain Weight

Being underweight is not an uncommon problem, particularly among adolescent and young adult men as well as among those who diet excessively or suffer from an eating disorder (discussed later in this chapter). If you lose weight suddenly and don't know the reason, talk to a doctor. Rapid weight loss can be an early symptom of a health problem.

If you're trying to put on pounds, you need to do the opposite of dieters: Consume more calories than you burn. But as with losing weight, you should try to gain weight in healthy ways. Here are some suggestions:

- **Eat more of a variety of foods** rather than more high-fat, high-calorie foods. Get no more than 30 percent of your daily calories from fat. A higher percentage poses a threat to your heart and your health.
- **If your appetite is small, eat more frequently.** Try for five or six smaller meals rather than a big lunch and dinner.
- **Choose some calorie-rich foods,** such as dried fruits rather than fresh ones. Add nuts and cheese to salads and main dishes.

- **Drink juice** rather than regular or diet soda.
- **Try adding a commercial liquid meal** replacement as a snack.
- **Exercise regularly** to build up both appetite and muscle.

A Practical Guide to Weight Loss

More than half of college women and about a third of college men intend to lose weight. Readiness to change is the key to successful weight loss. However, individuals vary in their readiness to change their diets, increase their physical activity, and seek professional counseling. Take the Self Survey at the end of this chapter to determine your readiness to lose weight. (See the *IPC* lab "Thinking Thinner" for proven and practical strategies.) **IPC**

Why We Overeat

The answer lies not just in the belly but in the brain. Both **hunger,** the physiological drive to consume food, and **appetite,** the psychological desire to eat, influence and control our desire for food. Scientists have discovered appetite receptors within the brain that specifically respond to hunger messengers carried by hormones produced in the digestive tract (Figure 7.4).

Appetite usually begins with the fear of the unpleasant sensation of hunger. We learn to avoid hunger by eating a certain amount of food at certain times of the day, just as dogs in the laboratory learn to avoid electric shocks by jumping at the sound of a warning bell. But appetite is easily led into temptation. In one famous experiment, psychologists bought bags of high-calorie goodies—peanut butter, marshmallows, chocolate-chip cookies, and salami—for their test rats. The animals ate so much on this "supermarket diet" that they gained more weight than any laboratory rats ever had before. The snack-food diet that fattened up these rats was particularly high in

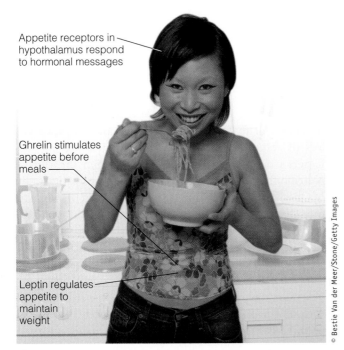

Appetite receptors in hypothalamus respond to hormonal messages

Ghrelin stimulates appetite before meals

Leptin regulates appetite to maintain weight

© Bestie Van der Meer/Stone/Getty Images

Figure 7.4 Hormones help regulate our appetites.

fats. Biologists speculate that creamy, buttery, or greasy foods may cause internal changes that increase appetite and, consequently, weight.

A hormone called leptin, produced by fat cells, sends signals to the brain that affect appetite. When leptin levels are normal, people eat just enough to maintain weight. When leptin is low, the brain responds as if fat stores had been depleted and slows down metabolism. This may be one reason why it is so difficult to lose weight by dieting alone.

Other hormones made in the stomach also influence how hungry we feel. One is ghrelin, a natural appetite stimulant. When given shots of ghrelin, people become very hungry and eat 30 percent more than they normally would. Ghrelin typically rises before meals and falls afterward. Dieters tend to have high levels of ghrelin, as if their bodies were trying to stimulate appetite so they regain lost fat.

We stop eating when we feel satisfied; this is called **satiety,** a feeling of fullness and relief from hunger. The neurotransmitter serotonin has been shown to produce feelings of satiety. In addition, several peptides, released from the digestive tract as we ingest food, may signal the brain to stop or restrict eating. However, it takes 20 minutes for the brain to register fullness.

Weight Loss Diets: What Works, What Doesn't

You've seen the ads. You've heard the hype. And like millions of others, you may have fallen for the pitch for the latest sure-to-lose diet. According to the ACHA–NCHA

survey, about 3 in 10 college students are dieting.[17] Do diets work? The answer is yes—and no. In the short term, people can and do lose weight on almost any diet. As recent research has confirmed, what matters is consuming fewer calories than you burn—whether by eating less (as in Weight Watchers), exercising more, or both.[18]

However, in the long run, dieting usually doesn't keep off excess pounds. Regardless of the diets they follow, people lose only about 5 percent of their initial weight after one year. Even in programs that provide intensive counseling by doctors, nurses, or dietitians, participants regain about half the weight they lost within three years. Five years after a successful diet, they typically have put on all the weight they lost.[19]

Low-Carb versus Low-Fat Diets

So which diet works best? None takes off and keeps off a lot of weight. However, most can lead to modest weight loss. In a one-year comparison of the Atkins (low-carbohydrate), Ornish (low-fat), Zone (balanced protein, carbohydrate and fat) and the LEARN program (low-fat, moderately high carbohydrate), overweight women steadily lost weight for the first six months on all of the diets. Those assigned to the Atkins

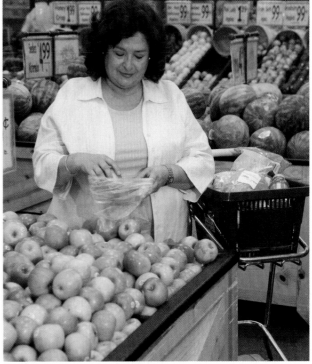

Healthful food choices are a first step toward a healthy weight.

© Jack Hollingsworth/Photodisc/Getty Images

hunger The physiological drive to consume food.

appetite A desire for food, stimulated by anticipated hunger, physiological changes within the brain and

body, the availability of food, and other environmental and psychological factors.

satiety A feeling of fullness after eating.

plan lost the most—an average of 14 pounds, compared with 6 to 8 pounds for the other three.

After six months, most of the women began to regain weight. At the end of the year, those in the Atkins groups were about 10 pounds lighter than when they had started, compared with 5.7 pounds for the LEARN group, 4.9 pounds for the Ornish group, and 3.5 pounds for the Zone group. However, few of the women stuck with their assigned diet. Those in the Atkins group took in almost triple the recommended carbohydrates, while those on the Ornish diet ate three times the fat. The other participants did the same.[20] Although many nutrition experts had warned that the Atkins diet, which advocates high intake of meat and cheese, might be hazardous to heart health, the women on the Atkins diet in this study had slightly better blood pressure and cholesterol readings than the others.[21]

The bottom line, according to weight experts, is that you can lose weight on any diet that helps you eat less. Finding strategies that help you balance the equation between calories-in and calories-used-up matters more than focusing on protein, carbohydrates, or fat.[22] (See Table 7.3 and Your Strategies for Change: "How to Design a Diet."

Low-Calorie and Very-Low-Calorie Diets

Over the course of a year the average adult man consumes about 900,000 calories, yet his weight may not rise or fall by more than a pound. Since a pound equals about 4,000 calories, just 11 calories a day—a mere potato chip—can throw off this equation.

Cutting back 500 to 1,000 calories a day typically leads to a loss of 1 to 2 pounds a week and an average weight loss of about 8 percent of body weight in six months. Expert groups, such as the American Society for Clinical Nutrition, the North American Association for the Study of Obesity, and the National Heart, Lung, and Blood Institute Obesity Education Initiative, recommend going no lower than 1,000 to 1,200 calories a day for women and 1,200 to 1,600 calories for men.

Very low-calorie diets, which provide fewer than 800 calories a day, lead to rapid weight loss but pose serious, potentially deadly health risks. Whenever people cut back drastically on calories, they immediately lose several pounds because of a loss of fluid. As soon as they return to a more normal way of eating, they regain this weight.

On a very low-calorie diet, as much as 50 percent of the weight you lose may be muscle (so you'll actually look flabbier). Because your heart is a muscle, it may become

---

TABLE 7.3 How the Three Most Popular Diets Compare

Atkins	Ornish	Weight Watchers
Premise With a diet high in protein and fat (meat, eggs, cheese) and low in carbohydrates (bread, pasta, cookies), the body burns fat instead of carbs.	**Premise** Reduce fats and simple carbohydrates like sugar and alcohol. Eat more fruits, vegetables, and complex carbohydrates.	**Premise** Nothing is forbidden. A point system assigns a value to portions of all sorts of foods to help track the number of calories taken in every day.
Promise Lose weight without hunger.	**Promise** Lose weight and prevent or reverse heart disease.	**Promise** Lose weight steadily with portion control and moderation.
Pitfall Can be hard to comply because so many foods are banned.	**Pitfall** Strictness makes it hard to stick with in the long run.	**Pitfall** Hunger.

YOUR STRATEGIES FOR CHANGE *How to Design a Diet*

There is no one perfect diet that will work for everyone who needs to lose weight. "Experiment with various methods for weight control," suggests Dr. Walter Willett of the Harvard School of Public Health. "Patients should focus on finding ways to eat that they can maintain indefinitely rather than seeking diets that promote rapid weight loss." In other words, design an eating plan that you can stick with for the rest of your life.

Whether you decide to focus on carbohydrates, fat, or calories, the following strategies can help you get to and maintain a healthy weight:

- Avoid "bad" fats, including trans-fatty acids and partially hydrogenated fats.
- Consume "good" fats, such as omega-3 fatty acids every day.
- Eat fewer "bad" carbohydrates, such as sugar and white flour.
- Eat more "good" carbs, including fruits, vegetables, legumes, and unrefined grains like whole-wheat flour and brown rice.

- Opt for quality over quantity. Eating a smaller amount of something delicious and nutritious can be far more satisfying than larger portions of junk foods.
- Exercise more. The key to balancing the equation between calories consumed and calories used is physical activity.
- Eliminate sweetened soft drinks and drink water instead.

so weak that it no longer can pump blood through your body. In addition, your blood pressure may plummet, causing dizziness, light-headedness, and fatigue. You may develop nausea and abdominal pain. You may lose hair. If you're a woman, your menstrual cycle may become irregular, or you may stop menstruating altogether. As you lose more water, you also lose essential vitamins, and your metabolism slows down. Even reaction time slows, and crash dieters may not be able to respond as quickly as usual.

Once you go off an extreme diet—as you inevitably must—your metabolism remains slow, even though you're no longer restricting your food intake. The human body appears to alter its energy use to compensate for weight loss. These metabolic changes may make it harder for people to maintain a reduced body weight after dieting.

Low-Glycemic-Load Diets

As discussed in Chapter 6, the glycemic index ranks carbohydrate-rich food based on their effect on blood sugar levels. Compared to high-glycemic foods such as white rice and French fries, low-glycemic foods, such as lentils, sweet potatoes, and apples produce more consistent blood glucose levels.

At least for those overweight individuals who secrete insulin at a higher rate, a low-glycemic-load diet may lead to greater weight loss than a low-fat one.[23] In an analysis of six studies in different nations, dieters who chose mainly low-glycemic foods lost more body fat and more pounds.[24] Because low-glycemic foods tend to be more filling, dieters may experience less hunger and find it easier to reduce total calories.

Avoiding Diet Traps

Whatever your eating style, there are only two effective strategies for losing weight: eating less and exercising more. Unfortunately, most people search for easier alternatives that almost invariably turn into dietary dead ends or unexpected dangers (see Savvy Consumer: "How to Spot a Dubious Diet"). Three common traps to avoid are diet pills, diet foods, and the yo-yo syndrome.

Over-the-Counter Diet Pills

An estimated 15 percent of adults—21 percent of women and 10 percent of men—have used weight-loss supplements. Women between ages 18 and 34 are the highest users.[25] In the 1920s, some women swallowed patented weight loss capsules that turned out to be tapeworm eggs. In the 1960s and 1970s, addictive amphetamines were common diet aids. In the 1990s, appetite suppressants known as fen-phen became popular but were taken off the market after being linked to heart valve problems.

In the last decade dieters tried ephedra products for weight loss, but a major study reported more than 16,000 adverse events associated with the use of ephedra-containing dietary supplements, including heart palpitations, tremors, and insomnia. The study also found little evidence that ephedra is effective in boosting physical activities and weight loss. The Food and Drug Administration has prohibited the sale of dietary supplements containing ephedra, because they present an unreasonable risk of illness or injury.

The weight loss prescription drug Orlistat is available as an over-the-counter weight loss pill called Alli. The drug, which blocks about a quarter of the fat consumed, works best with a low-fat diet. If dieters eat a meal made up of more than 15 fat grams, they can suffer nasty side effects, including flatulence, an urgent need to defecate, oily stools, and diarrhea.

Diet Foods

According to the Calorie Control Council, 90 percent of Americans choose some foods labeled "light." But even though these foods keep growing in popularity, Americans' weight keeps rising. There are several reasons: Many people think choosing a food that's lower in calories, fat-free, or light gives them a license to eat as much as they want. What they don't realize is that many foods that are low in fat are still high in sugar and calories. Refined carbohydrates, rapidly absorbed into the bloodstream, raise blood glucose levels. As they fall, appetite increases.

Diet products, including diet sodas and low-fat foods, are a very big business. Many people rely on meal replacements, usually shakes or snack bars, to lose or keep off weight. If used appropriately—as actual replacements rather than supplements to regular meals and snacks—they can be a useful strategy for weight loss. Yet people who use these products often gain weight because they think that they can afford to add high-calorie treats to their diets.

What about the artificial sweeteners and fake fats that appear in many diet products? Nutritionists caution to use them in moderation and not to substitute them for basic foods, such as grains, fruits, and vegetables. Foods made with fat substitutes may have fewer grams of fat, but they don't necessarily have significantly fewer calories. Many people who consume reduced-fat, fat-free, or sugar-free sodas, cookies, chips, and other snacks often cut back on more nutritious foods, such as fruits and vegetables. They also tend to eat more of the low- or no-fat foods so that their daily calorie intake either stays the same or actually increases.

The Yo-Yo Syndrome

On-and-off-again dieting, especially by means of very low-calorie diets (under 800 calories a day), can be self-defeating and dangerous. Some studies have shown that weight cycling may make it more difficult to lose weight or keep it off (Figure 7.5). Repeated cycles of rapid weight loss followed by weight gain may even change food preferences. Chronic crash dieters often come to prefer foods that combine sugar and fat, such as cake frosting.

To avoid the yo-yo syndrome and overcome its negative effects: Exercise. Researchers at the University of Pennsylvania found that when overweight women who also exercised went off a very low-calorie diet, their metabolism did not stay slow but bounced back to the appropriate level for their new, lower body weight. The reason may be exercise's ability to preserve muscle tissue. The more muscle tissue you have, the higher your metabolic rate.

If you've been losing (and regaining) the same 5 or 10 pounds for years, try the following suggestions for long-term success:

- **Set a danger zone.** Once you've reached your desired weight, don't let your weight climb more than 3 or 4 pounds higher. Take into account normal fluctuations, but watch out for an upward trend. Once you hit your upper weight limit, take action immediately rather than waiting until you gain 10 pounds.

- **Be patient.** Think of weight loss as a road trip. If you're going across town, you expect to get there in 20 minutes. If your destination is 400 miles away, you know it'll take longer. Give yourself the time you need to lose weight safely and steadily.

- **Try, try again.** Dieters don't usually keep weight off on their first attempt. The people who eventually succeed don't give up. Through trial and error, they find a plan that works for them.

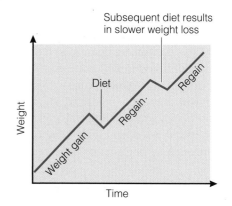

Figure 7.5 Weight-Cycling Effect of Repeated Dieting
Each round of dieting is typically followed by a rebound leading to a greater weight gain.

Physical Activity

Unplanned daily activity, such as fidgeting or pacing, can make a difference in preventing weight gain. Scientists use the acronym **NEAT**—for **nonexercise activity thermogenesis**—to describe such "nonvolitional" movement and have verified that it can be an effective way of burning calories. In a study of ten lean and ten mildly obese people—all self-confessed couch potatoes—the thinner ones sat an average of two hours less and moved and stood more often than the heavier individuals.[26] Small steps such as taking the stairs for a flight or two or parking farther away can make a difference.

Although physical activity and exercise can prevent weight gain and improve health, usually it does not lead to significant weight loss. However, when combined with diet, exercise ensures that you lose fat rather than muscle and

---

ˇSavvy Consumer   How to Spot a Dubious Diet

The National Council Against Health Fraud cautions dieters to watch for these warnings of dangerous or fraudulent programs.

- Promises of very rapid weight loss.
- Claims that the diet can eliminate "cellulite" (a term used to describe dimply fatty tissue on the arms and legs).
- "Counselors" who are really salespersons pushing a product or program.
- No mention of any risks associated with the diet.
- Unproven gimmicks, such as body wraps, starch blockers, hormones, diuretics, or "unique" pills or potions.
- No maintenance program.

If you hear about a new diet that promises to melt away fat, don't try it until you get answers to the following questions:

- Does it include a wide variety of nutritious foods?
- Does it provide at least 1,200 calories a day?
- Is it designed to reduce your weight by one-half to two pounds per week?
- Does it emphasize moderate portions?
- Does it use foods that are easy to find and prepare?
- Can you follow it wherever you eat—at home, work, restaurants, or parties?
- Is its cost reasonable?

If the answer to any of these questions is no, don't try the diet; then ask yourself one more question: Is losing weight worth losing your well-being?

helps keep off excess pounds. Moderate exercise, such as 30 to 60 minutes of daily physical activity, has proved effective in reducing the risk of heart disease and other health threats. Although there are no definitive data, experts generally agree that more exercise—an estimated 60 to 90 minutes daily of moderately intense activity—is necessary to prevent weight gain. Recommending such higher levels of activity to overweight men and women does indeed lead to more exercise—and more lasting weight loss.

Exercise has other benefits: It increases energy expenditure, builds up muscle tissue, burns off fat stores, and stimulates the immune system. Exercise also may reprogram metabolism so that more calories are burned during and after a workout.

An exercise program designed for both health benefits and weight loss should include both aerobic activity and resistance training. People who start and stick with an exercise program during or after a weight loss program are consistently more successful in keeping off most of the pounds they've shed.

Can a Person Be Fat and Fit?

Most people assume that fitness comes in only one size: small. That's not necessarily so. There is considerable controversy over how to define a healthy weight. But individuals of every size can improve their physical fitness.

In ten years of research on 25,000 men and 8,000 women, scientists at the Cooper Institute for Aerobics Research in Dallas, Texas, have found that heavier individuals can be just as healthy and physically fit as their leaner counterparts. In their studies, obese people who exercised moderately (30 minutes of daily walking at three or four miles per hour) had half the death rate of those who were slimmer but more sedentary. Low cardiorespiratory fitness, regardless of an individual's weight, is as great a risk factor for dying of heart disease or other causes such as diabetes, high blood pressure, and other well-recognized threats.

Nonetheless, fitness doesn't completely reverse the increased risks associated with excess weight. If you're obese, even a high level of physical activity does not protect you from premature death. And if you're sedentary, being thin does not cancel out the dangers of inactivity. In the long-term Nurses Health Study, which has followed more than 100,000 women for decades, women who were both obese and inactive were most likely to die. Those who were fit but fat and those who were thin but sedentary also had higher death rates than others.

The Psychology of Losing Weight

Diets change what you eat. Exercise changes body composition, stamina, and strength. But changing your food-related thoughts and behaviors can be the key to lasting weight loss. If you think that you can shed pounds, if you think that you can control what you put in your mouth, if you think that there is a form of exercise that you could enjoy, then you are on your way to reaching your weight loss goals. (See "Thinking Thinner" in *IPC*.) **IPC**

Maintaining Weight Loss

Surveys of people who lost significant amounts of weight and kept it off for several years show that most did so on their own—without medication, meal substitutes, or membership in an organized weight loss group. When a National Institutes of Health panel reviewed 48 separate weight loss trials, they found that participants lost about 8 percent of their body weight on average and kept it off.

Rather than focusing on why dieters fail, the creators of the National Weight Control Registry study the habits and lifestyles of those who've maintained a weight loss of at least 30 pounds for at least a year. The nearly 6,000 people in the registry have maintained their weight loss for almost six years.[27]

No one diet or commercial weight loss program helped all these formerly fat individuals. Many, through years of trial and error, eventually came up with a permanent exercise and eating program that worked for them. Despite the immense variety, their customized approaches share certain characteristics:

- **Personal responsibility for change.** Weight loss winners develop an internal locus of control. Rather than blaming others for their weight problem or relying on a doctor or trainer to fix it, they believe that the keys to a healthy weight lie within themselves.
- **Exercise.** Registry members report an hour of moderate physical activity almost every day. Their favorite exercise? Three in four say walking, followed by cycling, weight lifting, aerobics, running, and stair climbing. On average, they burn about 2,545 calories per week through physical activity.
- **Monitoring.** About 44 percent of registry members count calories, and almost all keep track of their food intake in some way, written or not.
- **Vigilance.** Rather than avoiding the scale or telling themselves their jeans shrunk in the wash, successful losers keep tabs on their weight and size. About a third check the scale every week. If the scale notches upward or their waistbands start to pinch, they take action.

nonexercise activity thermogenesis (NEAT) Nonvolitional movement that can be an effective way of burning calories.

Your Life Change Coach

Get a Grip on Emotional Eating

Occasionally all of us seek comfort at the tip of a spoon. However, many people use food as a way of coping with anger, frustration, stress, boredom, or fatigue. Whatever its motivation, emotional eating always involves eating for reasons other than physiological hunger. If you're not sure whether you do this, ask yourself the following questions:

- Do you eat when you're not hungry?
- Do you eat or continue eating even if the food doesn't taste good?
- Do you eat when you can't think of anything else to do?
- Do you eat when you're emotionally vulnerable—tired, frustrated, or worried?
- Do you eat after an argument or stressful situation to calm down?
- Do you eat as one of your favorite ways of enjoying yourself?
- Do you eat to reward yourself?
- Do you keep eating even after you're full?

If you answer yes to more than three of these, you're eating in response to what you feel, not what you need. Diets may work for you, but the extra weight will inevitably creep back unless you confront your hidden motives for overeating. Since neither emotions nor food ever go away, you have to learn to deal with both for as long as you live.

To get a grip on your emotional eating, try this three-step plan:

Step 1: Know Your Triggers

Whatever its specific motivation, emotional eating always involves eating for reasons other than physiological hunger. The key to getting it under control is awareness.

What are the feelings that set off an eating binge?

- **Anger?** Many people, especially women, swallow their anger by eating because they're afraid of what might happen if they express it.
- **Guilt?** Some people eat because they feel they're always falling short as children, partners, or parents.
- **Rebellion?** Eating may be the only way some people give themselves permission to take a break from being dutiful.

- **Breakfast.** Your mother probably told you that breakfast is the most important meal of the day, and 40 years of breakfast-related studies, as well as the experience of registry members, have proved her right. A morning meal improves concentration and problem-solving ability, boosts energy levels, and helps control weight. Regular breakfast skippers are four times more likely to be obese than those who eat a morning meal.

Treating Severe Obesity

The biggest Americans are getting bigger. The prevalence of severe or "morbid" obesity is increasing faster than obesity itself. The number of extremely obese adults—those at least 100 pounds overweight with BMIs over 40—has quadrupled in the last two decades from 1 in 200 to about 1 in every 50 men and women. The number with BMIs greater than 50 has jumped from 1 in 2,000 in the 1980s to 1 in 400.

 Extreme obesity poses extreme danger to health and survival and undermines quality of life. White women report more impairment than men or African American women, even when they have lower BMIs. Severe obesity also has a profound effect on every aspect of an adolescent's life.

Drug Therapy

Obesity medications are recommended only for patients with BMIs equal to or greater than 30 or those with a BMI equal to or greater than 27 with risk factors (like high blood pressure) that increase their risk of disease.

- **Deprivation?** At the end of a long day, a person may justify turning to food as a well-deserved reward, maybe the first nice thing done for herself or himself all day.

Did any of these possibilities hit home? If so, train yourself to take a step back and ask yourself a series of questions before you take a bite: Are you hungry? If not, what are you feeling? Stressed, tired, bored, anxious, sad, happy? Once you identify your true feeling, push deeper and ask why you feel this way. Try writing down your answers in a notebook. This is an even more effective way to help make sure that every bite you take is a conscious one.

Step 2: Put Your Body, Not Your Emotions, In Charge of What You Eat

To keep mind and body on an even keel, avoid getting so hungry and feeling so deprived that you become desperate and panicky. If you're facing an emotionally intense period—exam week or a visit from an ornery relative—plan your meals and snacks in advance and try, as much as you can, to stick with your program. Rather than swearing off sweets forever, work indulgences into your weekly routine. If you plan to have a brownie for dessert on Friday night, you can look forward to it all week and not waste calories on a candy bar that won't taste as good.

Step 3: Focus on Your Feelings

Let yourself feel how you're feeling without eating. Breathe deeply for a minute or two. Focus on the places in your body that feel tense. Rate the intensity of the emotion on a scale from ten (life or death) to one (truly trivial). Ask yourself: What's the worst-case scenario of feeling this way? Is food going to make it better in any way? Will it make it worse?

When you're tempted to eat but aren't hungry, write down the circumstances and try to discern the underlying reasons. If you eat cookies at night, ask, What does it get me? The answer might be that it relaxes you. Once you realize that the cookies are a means to an end, you can figure out something else you can do to get the same emotional benefits.

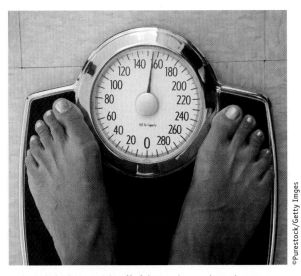

Vigilance helps keep weight off. If the number on the scale creeps upward, take action.

Researchers are experimenting with other medications, such as rimonabant and the epilepsy drug zonisamide, to enhance weight loss.[28] Currently, only two weight loss drugs are FDA approved.

Xenical (orlistat) (also available in a lower dose as the over-the-counter drug Alli) blocks fat absorption by the gut but also inhibits absorption of water and vitamins in some patients and may cause cramping and diarrhea. It produces a weight loss of 2 to 3 percent of initial weight beyond the weight lost by dieting over the course of a year.

Meridia (sibutramine) is in the same chemical class as amphetamines and works by suppressing appetite. It also may increase blood pressure, heart rate, or both. Other side effects include headache, insomnia, dry mouth, and constipation. Patients taking these drugs generally lose less than 10 percent of their body weight, and many regain weight after they stop treatment.

Obesity Surgery

Obesity, or bariatric, surgery is becoming the most popular weight loss approach for the estimated 15 million men and women who qualify as "morbidly obese" (100 or more pounds overweight) because of their increased health risks. This year as many as 200,000 Americans will undergo obesity surgery—four times the number who did so in 2000. Eight in ten are women. A growing number are teenagers, although adolescents make up less than 1 percent of patients having such procedures.[29] According to the Agency for Healthcare Research and Quality, three in four bariatric patients lose 50 to 75 percent of their excess weight within two years and keep it off.

As recent research has shown, bariatric surgery eliminates or improves diabetes, hypertension, sleep apnea, and high cholesterol in most patients. However, these

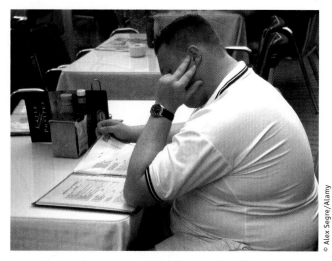

Severe obesity endangers a person's health and quality of life.

operations—particularly in the hands of poorly trained or inexperienced surgeons—pose serious risks, including potentially fatal leaks, infection, bleeding, hernias, and pneumonia. According to federal estimates, 4 in 10 patients suffer complications within six months. The mortality rate averages about two deaths in 1,000 operations. Long-term dangers—both physical and psychological—are unknown, particularly for adolescents. Even with excellent medical results, extreme weight loss creates drapes of excess skin that sag over the belly, buttocks, thighs, breasts, or upper arms.

The two most common types of procedures are:

- **Gastric bypass.** Surgeons create an egg-sized pouch with staples and reroute food around part of the upper intestine to block absorption of calories and nutrients. About 75 percent of bypass patients lose 50 to 75 percent of their excess weight within two years. For the "super obese," a more extensive procedure that bypasses most of the small intestine can lead to a loss of 80 percent of excess weight. However, the latter procedure carries the highest risks of complications, including serious vitamin and mineral deficiencies. Too little thiamine, for instance, can lead to a serious neurological condition called Wernicke encephalopathy.[30]

- **Banding.** In this newer, less risky procedure, surgeons slip an inflatable silicon band around the stomach; it can be tightened or loosened at a doctor's office without the need for further surgery. Patients lose about 40 to 55 percent of excess weight but may be more likely to regain lost pounds. The band also may slip or erode.

The individuals most likely to benefit from obesity surgery generally:

- Have a body mass index over 40.
- Have a BMI over 35 *and* a serious obesity-related problem, such as type 2 diabetes or severe sleep apnea (when breathing stops for brief periods during sleep).
- Have made repeated unsuccessful attempts to lose weight.
- Do not have any significant or untreated psychological problems.
- Are well-informed about the risks of the surgery.
- Recognize the need for lifestyle changes and daily vitamin and mineral supplements.

Unhealthy Eating Behaviors

Unhealthy eating behavior takes many forms, ranging from not eating enough to eating too much too quickly. Its roots are complex. In addition to media and external pressures, family history can play a role. Researchers have linked specific genes to some cases of anorexia nervosa and binge eating, but most believe that a variety of factors, including stress and culture, combine to cause disordered eating.

Sooner or later many people don't eat the way they should. They may skip meals, thereby increasing the likelihood that they'll end up with more body fat, a higher weight, and a higher blood cholesterol level. They may live on diet foods, but consume so much of them that they gain weight anyway. Some even engage in more extreme eating behavior: Dissatisfied with almost all aspects of their appearance, they continuously go on and off diets, eat compulsively, or binge on high-fat treats. Such behaviors can be warning signs of potentially serious eating disorders that should not be ignored.

Unhealthy Eating in College Students

 College students—particularly women, including varsity athletes—are at risk for unhealthy eating behaviors. While some college students have full-blown eating disorders, many others develop "partial syndromes" and experience symptoms that are not severe or numerous enough for a diagnosis of anorexia nervosa or bulimia nervosa. Distress over body image increases the risk of all forms of disordered eating in college women.

 In a survey at a large, public, rural university in the mid-Atlantic states, 17 percent of the women were struggling with disordered eating. Younger women (ages 18 to 21) were more likely than older students to have an eating disorder. In this study, eating disorders did not discriminate, equally affecting women of different races (white, Asian, African American, Native

American, and Hispanic), religions, athletic involvement, and living arrangements (on or off campus; with roommates, boyfriends, or family). Although the students viewed eating disorders as both mental and physical problems and felt that individual therapy would be most helpful, all said that they would first turn to a friend for help. Women in sororities are at slightly increased risk of an eating disorder compared with those in dormitories.

Extreme Dieting

Extreme dieters go beyond cutting back on calories or increasing physical activity. They become preoccupied with what they eat and weigh. Although their weight never falls below 85 percent of normal, their weight loss is severe enough to cause uncomfortable physical consequences, such as weakness and sensitivity to cold. Technically, these dieters do not have anorexia nervosa (discussed later in this chapter), but they are at increased risk for it.

Extreme dieters may think they know a great deal about nutrition, yet many of their beliefs about food and weight are misconceptions or myths. For instance, they may eat only protein because they believe complex carbohydrates, including fruits and whole-grain breads, are fattening.

Sometimes nutritional education alone can help change these eating patterns. However, many avid dieters who deny that they have a problem with food may need counseling (which they usually agree to only at their family's insistence) to correct dangerous eating behavior and prevent further complications.

Compulsive Overeating

People who eat compulsively cannot stop putting food in their mouths. They eat fast and they eat a lot. They eat even when they're full. They may eat around the clock rather than at set meal times, often in private because of embarrassment over how much they consume.

 Some mental health professionals describe compulsive eating as a food addiction that is much more likely to develop in women. According to Overeaters Anonymous (OA), an international 12-step program, many women who eat compulsively view food as a source of comfort against feelings of inner emptiness, low self-esteem, and fear of abandonment.

The following behaviors may signal a potential problem with compulsive overeating:

- **Turning to food** when depressed or lonely, when feeling rejected, or as a reward.
- **A history of failed diets** and anxiety when dieting.
- **Thinking about food** throughout the day.

- **Eating quickly** and without pleasure.
- **Continuing to eat** even when no longer hungry.
- **Frequently talking about food** or refusing to talk about food.
- **Fear of not being able to stop** eating after starting.

Recovery from compulsive eating can be challenging because people with this problem cannot give up entirely the substance they abuse. Like everyone else, they must eat. However, they can learn new eating habits and ways of dealing with underlying emotional problems. An OA survey found that most of its members joined to lose weight but later felt the most important effect was their improved emotional, mental, and physical health. As one woman put it, "I came for vanity but stayed for sanity."

Binge Eating

Binge eating—the rapid consumption of an abnormally large amount of food in a relatively short time—often occurs in compulsive eaters. The 25 million Americans with a binge-eating disorder typically eat a larger than ordinary amount of food during a relatively brief period, feel a lack of control over eating, and binge at least twice a week for at least a six-month period. During most of these episodes, binge eaters experience at least three of the following:

- **Eating much more rapidly** than usual.
- **Eating until they feel uncomfortably full.**
- **Eating large amounts of food** when not feeling physically hungry.
- **Eating large amounts of food** throughout the day with no planned mealtimes.
- **Eating alone** because they are embarrassed by how much they eat and by their eating habits.

Binge eaters may spend up to several hours eating, and consume 2,000 or more calories worth of food in a single binge—more than many people eat in a day. After such binges, they usually do not do anything to control weight, but simply get fatter. As their weight climbs, they become depressed, anxious, or troubled by other psychological symptoms to a much greater extent than others of comparable weight.

binge eating The rapid consumption of an abnormally large amount of food in a relatively short time.

Binge eating is probably the most common eating disorder. An estimated 8 to 19 percent of obese patients in weight loss programs are binge eaters.

If you occasionally go on eating binges, use the behavioral technique called *habit reversal,* and replace your bingeing with a competing behavior. For example, every time you're tempted to binge, immediately do something—text-message a friend, play solitaire, check your email—that keeps food out of your mouth.

If you binge twice a week or more for at least a six-month period, you may have binge-eating disorder, which can require professional help. Treatment usually consists of cognitive-behavioral therapy, either individually or in a group setting. As chronic binge eaters recognize their unhealthy behavior and confront the underlying issues, they usually are able to stop bingeing and resume normal eating patterns.

Eating Disorders

According to the American Psychiatric Association, patients with **eating disorders** display a broad range of symptoms that occur along a continuum between those of anorexia nervosa and those of bulimia nervosa.

 As many as 10 percent of teenage girls develop symptoms of or full-blown eating disorders. Among the factors that increase the risk are preoccupation with a thin body; social pressure; and childhood traits such as perfectionism and excessive cautiousness, which can reflect an obsessive-compulsive personality. Teenage girls who diet and have four specific risk factors—a high BMI, menarche (first menstruation) before sixth grade, extreme concern with weight or shape, and teasing by peers—are most likely to have an eating disorder.

The best known eating disorders are anorexia nervosa, which affects fewer than 1 percent of adolescent women, and bulimia nervosa, which strikes 2 to 3 percent. The American Psychiatric Association has developed practice guidelines for the treatment of patients with eating disorders, which include medical, psychological, and behavioral approaches. One of the most scientifically supported is cognitive-behavioral therapy.

Who Develops Eating Disorders?

Eating disorders affect an estimated 5 to 10 million women and 1 million men. Despite past evidence that eating disorders were primarily problems for white women, they are increasing among men and members of different ethnic and racial groups. Yet most college students believe mainly young white women develop eating disorders.[31]

 In the few studies of eating disorders in minority college students that have been completed, African American female undergraduates had a slightly lower prevalence of eating disorders than whites. Asian Americans reported fewer symptoms of eating disorders but more body dissatisfaction, concerns about shape, and more intense efforts to lose weight.

 In a survey of health-care professionals at the country's largest colleges and universities, 69 percent have professionals on staff who specialize in diagnosing and treating eating disorders. Of all the hurdles to helping students with eating disorders, 39 percent said denial is the biggest, while 24 percent felt it was unwillingness to seek treatment, and 20 percent blamed pressure from peers and the media to stay thin.

Eating disorders affect every aspect of college students' lives, including dating. Both men and women tend to avoid dating individuals with eating disorders, but men are far less accepting of obesity than women.

Male and female athletes are vulnerable to eating disorders, either because of the pressure to maintain ideal body weight or to achieve a weight that might enhance their performance. Many female athletes, particularly those participating in sports or activities that emphasize leanness (such as gymnastics, distance running, diving, figure skating, and classical ballet) have subclinical eating disorders that could undermine their nutritional status and energy levels. However, there is often little awareness or recognition of their disordered eating. To determine if you have this problem, see Your Strategies for Prevention: "Do You Have an Eating Disorder?"

If someone you know has an eating disorder, let your friend know you're concerned and that you care. Don't

---

YOUR STRATEGIES FOR PREVENTION *Do You Have an Eating Disorder?*

Physicians have developed a simple screening test for eating disorders, consisting of the following questions:

- Do you make yourself sick because you feel uncomfortably full?
- Do you worry you have lost control over how much you eat?

- Have you recently lost more than 14 pounds in a three-month period?
- Do you believe yourself to be fat when others say you are too thin?
- Would you say that food dominates your life?

Score one point for every "yes." A score of two or more is a likely indication of anorexia nervosa or bulimia nervosa.

Source: Miller, Karl. "Treatment Guideline for Eating Disorders." American Family Physician, Vol. 62, No. 1, July 1, 2000.

criticize or make fun of his or her eating habits. Encourage your friend to talk about other problems and feelings, and suggest that he or she talk to the school counselor or someone at the mental health center, the family doctor, or another trusted adult. Offer to go along if you think that will make a difference.

Anorexia Nervosa

Although *anorexia* means "loss of appetite," most individuals with **anorexia nervosa** are, in fact, hungry all the time. For them, food is an enemy—a threat to their sense of self, identity, and autonomy. In the distorted mirror of their mind's eye, they see themselves as fat or flabby even at a normal or below-normal body weight. Some simply feel fat; others think that they are thin in some places and too fat in others, such as the abdomen, buttocks, or thighs.

The characteristics of anorexia nervosa include:

- A refusal to maintain normal body weight (weight loss leading to body weight of less than 85 percent of that expected for age and height).
- An intense fear of gaining weight or becoming fat, even though underweight.
- A distorted body image so that the person feels fat even when emaciated.
- In women, the absence of at least three menstrual cycles.

The incidence of anorexia nervosa has increased in the last three decades in most developed countries. The peak ages for its onset are $14^1/_2$ and 18 years. According to the American Psychiatric Association's Work Group on Eating Disorders, cases are increasing among males, minorities, women of all ages, and possibly preteens. About 1 percent of American women develop anorexia.

In the *restricting* type of anorexia, individuals lose weight by avoiding any fatty foods, and by dieting, fasting, and exercising. Some start smoking as a way of controlling their weight. In the *binge-eating/purging* type, they engage in binge eating, purging (through self-induced vomiting, laxatives, diuretics, or enemas), or both. Obsessed with an intense fear of fatness, they may weigh themselves several times a day, measure various parts of their body, check mirrors to see if they look fat, and try on different items of clothing to see if they feel tight.

What Causes Anorexia Nervosa?

Many complex factors interact and contribute to this disorder, including biological, psychological, and social ones. Anorexia is more common among close relatives, particularly sisters, than it is in the general population. The relatives of anorexics also have a higher than expected frequency of depressive disorders.

Anorexia is associated with changes within the brain, including abnormalities in the stress-hormone cortisol, the neurotransmitters dopamine, serotonin, and norepinephrine—all of which influence appetite and satiety. Brain chemistry returns to normal after treatment and recovery.[32]

Anorexia also may be a response to a personal loss or a sign of a driven, perfectionist personality. Often young anorexics have above-average grades and an unwarranted fear of failure. Girls who develop anorexia often have little insight or awareness of their feelings, needs, and wants.

 In one study that followed 21 college women with eating disorders for six years, 11 got better during their postcollege years, while 10 continued to struggle with disordered eating. The major difference between the two groups revolved around issues of autonomy and relation. Those who could better negotiate the tension between being independent and relating to others had higher self-esteem, a more positive self-concept, and a healthier relationship with food.

About one-third of those with anorexia initially were mildly overweight and cut back on food just to lose a few pounds. Others had normal weights but began to diet to look more attractive or, in the case of male and female athletes and dancers, to gain a performance advantage. Sometimes illness, stress, or surgery triggers weight loss. Often the initial response to their weight loss—from parents, coaches, or friends—is positive. However, starvation seems to take on a life of its own, and anorexics cannot return to a healthy eating pattern. In time, they may place so much value on thinness that they cannot recognize the dangers to their health.

Health Dangers and Treatment

The medical consequences of anorexia nervosa are serious (Figure 7.6). Menstrual periods stop in women; testosterone levels decline in men. Adolescents with this disorder do not undergo normal sexual maturation, such as breast development, and may not reach their anticipated height. Even individuals who look and feel reasonably healthy may have subtle or hidden abnormalities, including heart irregularities and arrhythmias that can increase their risk of sudden death. Women who do not menstruate for six months or more may

eating disorders Bizarre, often dangerous patterns of food consumption, including anorexia nervosa and bulimia nervosa.

anorexia nervosa A psychological disorder in which refusal to eat and/or an extreme loss of appetite leads to malnutrition, severe weight loss, and possibly death.

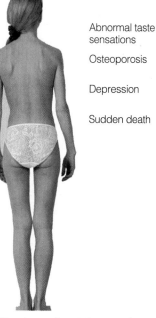

Loss of fat and muscle mass, including heart muscle

Increased sensitivity to cold

Irregular heartbeats

Bloating, constipation, abdominal pain

Amenorrhea (absence of menstruation)

Growth of fine, babylike hair over body

Abnormal taste sensations

Osteoporosis

Depression

Sudden death

© Amethyst/Custom Medical Stock Photo

Figure 7.6 Medical Complications of Weight Loss from Anorexia Nervosa

develop osteoporosis and suffer irreversible weakening and thinning of their bones as a result.

Even when they realize that they are jeopardizing their health, people with anorexia tend to fear that treatment will make them worse—that is, fatter. They need repeated reassurance that they will not become overweight and that they can and will find healthier ways of coping with life.

According to current practice guidelines, treatment of anorexia nervosa includes medical therapy (such as "refeeding" to overcome malnutrition) and behavioral, cognitive, psychodynamic, and family therapy. Antidepressant medication sometimes can help, particularly when there is a personal or family history of depression. Most people who get help do return to normal weight, but it can take a long time for their eating behaviors to become normal and for them to deal with troubling body image issues. Nutritional therapy is critical for a return to regular menstrual periods and an improvement in bone density.[33]

Bulimia Nervosa

Individuals with **bulimia nervosa** go on repeated eating binges and rapidly consume large amounts of food, usually sweets, stopping only because of severe abdominal pain or sleep, or because they are interrupted. Those with *purging* bulimia induce vomiting or take large doses of laxatives to relieve guilt and control their weight. In *nonpurging* bulimia, individuals use other means, such as fasting or excessive exercise, to compensate for binges.

The characteristics of bulimia nervosa include:

- Repeated binge eating.
- A feeling of lack of control over eating behavior.
- Regular reliance on self-induced vomiting, laxatives, or diuretics.
- Strict dieting or fasting, or vigorous exercise, to prevent weight gain.
- A minimum average of two bingeing episodes a week for at least three months.
- A preoccupation with body shape and weight.

An estimated 1 to 3 percent of adolescent and young American women develop bulimia. Some experiment with bingeing and purging for a few months and then stop when they change their social or living situation. Others develop longer-term bulimia. Among males, this disorder is about one-tenth as common. The average age for developing bulimia is 18.

What Causes Bulimia Nervosa?

Bulimia usually begins after a rigid diet that lasted from several weeks to a year or more. Strict dieting may affect brain chemistry in such a way as to disrupt the normal mechanisms for appetite and satiety. Semi-starvation eventually sets off a binge; bingeing leads to purging. Once dieters realize that vomiting reduces the anxiety triggered by gorging, they no longer fear overeating. When this happens, bingeing may become more frequent and severe until, in time, it becomes an all-purpose way of coping with stress. However, the driving force in this

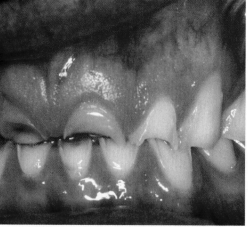

© Gill/Custom Medical Stock Photo

One of the health complications of purging is erosion and decay of dental enamel from the acid in vomit.

bulimia nervosa Episodic binge eating, often followed by forced vomiting or laxative abuse, and accompanied by a persistent preoccupation with body shape and weight.

disorder may not be the overeating but the vomiting or laxative use. If individuals felt they couldn't get rid of food, they might not overeat.

Obesity in adolescence may increase the likelihood of bulimia in adulthood. Extremely obese individuals may lose weight by vomiting and not want to stop because they fear regaining it. Sometimes bulimia develops after recovery from anorexia. Purging becomes an alternative way of staying thin.

As with anorexia, bulimia is associated with changes in brain chemistry, particularly low levels of the peptide cholescystokinin, which produces feelings of satiety. The cycle of bingeing and purging seems to wreak havoc on the biological controls that keep weight at a certain level.

Family conflicts, life stresses such as going away to school, and struggles with the transition to independent adulthood also may play a role. Bulimia also may be a symptom of depression. About 20 to 30 percent of those with this problem are chronically depressed; others have a history of depressive episodes. Bulimic individuals also are more likely to experience other problems, including anxiety disorders, substance abuse, and impulse disorders, such as shoplifting (kleptomania) and cutting themselves. A significant percentage of bulimics—from a quarter to a half,

by some estimates—may have been victims of incest, sexual molestation, or rape, but this correlation is controversial.

Bulimia may continue for many years, with binges alternating with periods of normal eating. Physiological consequences are cumulative. Often dentists are the first to detect bulimia because they notice damage to teeth and gums, including erosion of the enamel from the stomach acids in vomit (see photo). Repeated vomiting can lead to other complications as it robs the body of essential nutrients and fluids, causes dehydration and electrolyte imbalances, and impairs the ability of the heart and other muscles to function. Bulimia can trigger cardiac arrhythmias and, occasionally, sudden death.

Cognitive-behavioral therapy has proved more effective than other psychological approaches. Antidepressant medications that increase levels of the neurotransmitter serotonin can also help.

 Group therapy has proven effective in allowing university students with bulimia the opportunity to experience, express, and understand the emotions related to their disorder.[34] About 70 percent of those who complete treatment programs reduce their bingeing and purging, although flareups are common in times of stress.

Learn It | **Live It**

Managing Your Weight

No diet—high-protein, low-fat, or high-carbohydrate—can produce permanent weight loss. Successful weight management, the American Dietetic Association has concluded, "requires a lifelong commitment to healthful lifestyle behaviors emphasizing sustainable and enjoyable eating practices and daily physical activity." Studies have shown that successful dieters are highly motivated, monitor their food intake, increase their activity, set realistic goals, and receive social support from others. Another key to long-term success is tailoring any weight loss program to an individual's gender, lifestyle, and cultural, racial, and ethnic values.

Here are some practical guidelines.

- **Be realistic.** Trying to shrink to an impossibly low weight dooms you to defeat. Start off slowly and make steady progress. If your weight creeps up 5 pounds, go back to the basics of your program. Take into account normal fluctuations, but watch out for an upward trend. If you let your weight continue to creep up, it may not stop until you have a serious weight problem—again.

- **Recognize that there are no quick fixes.** Ultimately, quick-loss diets are very damaging physically and psychologically because when you stop dieting and put the pounds back on, you feel like a failure.

- **Note your progress.** Make a graph, with your initial weight as the base, to indicate your progress. View plateaus or occasional gains as temporary setbacks rather than disasters.

- **Adopt the 90 percent rule.** If you practice good eating habits 90 percent of the time, a few indiscretions won't make a difference. In effect, you should allow for occasional cheating, so that you don't have to feel guilty about it.

- **Look for joy and meaning beyond your food life.** Make your personal goals and your relationships your priorities, and treat food as the fuel that allows you to bring your best to both.

- **Try, try again.** Remember, dieters usually don't keep weight off on their first attempt. The people who eventually succeed try various methods until they find the plan that works for them.

SELFSURVEY : *Are You Ready to Lose Weight?*

As discussed in Chapter 1, people change the way they behave stage by stage and step by step. The same is true for changing behaviors related to weight. If you need to lose excess pounds, knowing your stage of readiness for change is a crucial first step. Here is a guide to identifying where you are right now.

If you are still in the *precontemplation* stage, you don't think of yourself as having a weight problem, even though others may. If you can't fit into some of your clothes, you blame the dry cleaners. Or you look around and think, "I'm no bigger than anyone else in this class." Unconsciously, you may feel helpless to do anything about your weight. So you deny or dismiss its importance.

In the *contemplation* stage, you would prefer not to have to change, but you can't avoid reality. Your coach or doctor may comment on your weight. You wince at the vacation photos of you in a swimsuit. You look in the mirror, try to suck in your stomach, and say, "I've got to do something about my weight."

In the *preparation* stage, you're gearing up by taking small but necessary steps. You may buy athletic shoes or check out several diet books from the library. Maybe you experiment with some minor changes, such as having fruit instead of cookies for an afternoon snack. Internally, you are getting accustomed to the idea of change.

In the *action* stage of change, you are deliberately working to lose weight. You no longer snack all evening long. You stick to a specific diet and track calories, carbs, or points. You hop on a treadmill or stationary bike for 30 minutes a day. Your resolve is strong, and you know you're on your way to a thinner, healthier you.

In the *maintenance* stage, you strengthen, enhance, and extend the changes you've made. Whether or not you have lost all the weight you want, you've made significant progress. As you continue to watch what you eat and to be physically active, you lock-in healthy new habits.

Where are you right now? Read each of the following statements and decide which best applies to you.

1. I never think about my weight.   Precontemplation Stage
2. I'm trying to zip up a pair of jeans and wondering when was the last time they fit.   Contemplation Stage
3. I'm downloading a food diary to keep track of what I eat.   Preparation Stage
4. I have been following a diet for three weeks and have started working out.   Action Stage
5. I have been sticking to a diet and engaging in regular physical activity for at least six months.   Maintenance Stage

Your Health Action Plan for Losing Weight

Here is a guide to strategies most likely to help you at your particular stage of readiness to change.

Precontemplation (not active and not thinking about becoming active)

- **Set a small, reasonable goal** that does not involve working up a sweat, such as standing rather than sitting when blow-drying your hair or doing squats while brushing your teeth.

- **Start paying attention** to what, when, where, and why you eat. Take note of the times you eat or continue eating even though you're not hungry.

- **List what you see** as the cons of physical activity. For example, do you fear it will take up too much time? Write down three activities you could do if you woke up half an hour earlier.

Contemplation (not active but thinking about becoming active)

- **Think back to activities** you found enjoyable in the past. Did you ever try inline skating? Play softball? Row? Ask friends if they can put you in touch with others with the same interest.

- **Start drinking more water.** Get used to the idea of ending every meal with water to wash away the taste of what you've eaten and signal that you've stopped putting food in your mouth.

- **Determine the types of activity** you can realistically fit into your daily schedule. If you have classes and work most of the day, sign up for an evening body-sculpting or spinning class.

- **Find an image of a slimmer body** you'd like to have—from a magazine advertisement, for example—and post it where you can see it often.

Preparation (active but not at recommended levels)

- **Record everything you put in your mouth.** List calories and carbs next to each entry. Also describe how you feel as you eat.

- **Set specific daily and weekly action-oriented goals.** Your daily goal might begin with 10 or 15 minutes of activity and increase by 5 minutes every week or two. Your weekly goal might be to try a new activity, such as kick-boxing or a dance class.

- **Document your progress.** You could use a monthly calendar to keep track of the number of days you've exercised as well as the length of each workout. Or you can keep a more detailed record, noting the types of exercise you do every day, the intensity you work at, the duration of each workout, and so forth.

Action and Maintenance (active at recommended levels for less than six months)

- **Find new comfort foods.** Good options include air-popped popcorn, chocolate fruit sundaes (fresh fruit with a spoonful of rich syrup), hot chocolate (with skim milk), and fudgsicles (creamy but low in calories).
- **Avoid boredom.** Think through ways to vary your exercise routine. Take different routes on your walks. Invite different friends to join you. Alternate working with free weights with resistance machines at the gym.

- **Try new athletic and sports skills.** Try snowshoeing, kayaking, rock climbing, dancing. Don't expect instant expertise. It usually takes four to six weeks to feel competent and get in the swing of a new activity.

Don't expect to progress through these stages just once. Most people "recycle" several times before a change becomes permanent. Whether you're moving forward or have temporarily fallen back, remember that change is a journey that happens step by step, meal by meal, day by day, stage by stage.

CENGAGENOW If you want to write your own goals for more nutritious choices, go to the Wellness Journal at HealthNow: **academic.cengage.com/login**.

Making This Chapter Work for YOU

Review Questions

1. Which of the following statements is true?
   a. Obesity is a problem only in industrialized countries.
   b. Obesity is a problem that starts in middle age.
   c. The southern states have the highest percentage of people who are obese.
   d. If you were heavy as child, you will always be obese.

2. People gain weight when
   a. their basal metabolic rate increases.
   b. they consume more calories than they use up in daily activity.
   c. they eat fast food more than two times a week.
   d. they watch two hours of television a day.

3. The health dangers of excess weight include all of the following *except*
   a. increased risk of type 2 diabetes, heart disease, and cancer.
   b. increased risk of impaired immunity.
   c. increased risk of auto accidents.
   d. increased risk of dying prematurely.

4. If you have gone online to check out weight reduction support groups in your area, which stage of readiness for weight behavior change are you in?
   a. precontemplation stage
   b. contemplation stage
   c. preparation stage
   d. action stage

5. Which of the following statements is *incorrect?*
   a. I can lose weight successfully on a low-carbohydrate diet.
   b. I can lose weight successfully on a low-fat diet.
   c. I can lose weight successfully on a low-calorie diet.
   d. I can lose weight successfully by working out once a week.

6. Successful weight management strategies include which of the following?
   a. Learn to distinguish between actual and emotional hunger.
   b. Ask friends for recommendations for methods that helped them to lose weight quickly.
   c. Practice good eating habits 50 percent of the time so that you can balance your cravings with healthy food.
   d. Look at celebrity photos and pick one for a model.

7. Which of the following statements is true?
   a. Very-low-calorie diets increase metabolism, which helps burn calories more quickly.
   b. An individual eating low-calorie or fat-free foods can increase the serving sizes.
   c. Low-carbohydrate diets have been shown safe over the short term but long-term studies have not been completed.
   d. Yo-yo dieting works best for long-term weight loss.

8. Which of the following eating behaviors may be a warning sign of a serious eating disorder?
   a. vegetarianism
   b. compulsive food washing
   c. binge eating
   d. weight gain during the first year of college

9. Individuals with anorexia nervosa
   a. believe they are overweight even if they are extremely thin.
   b. typically feel full all the time, which limits their food intake.
   c. usually look overweight, even though their body mass index is normal.
   d. have a reduced risk for heart-related abnormalities.

10. Bulimia nervosa
    a. is characterized by excessive sleeping followed by periods of insomnia.
    b. is found primarily in older women who are concerned with the aging process.
    c. is associated with the use of laxatives or excessive exercise to control weight.
    d. does not have serious health consequences.

    Answers to these questions can be found on page 583.

Critical Thinking

1. Visualize the body you would like to have—where did the image come from? From television, movies, magazines? Name five influences on your concept of your body image. Examine the validity of each influence. How much are you swayed by media presentations?

2. Do you think you have a weight problem? If so, what makes you think so? Is your perception based on your actual BMI measurement or on how you believe you look? If you found out that your BMI was within the ideal range, would that change your opinion about your body? Why or why not?

3. Suppose one of your roommates appears to have symptoms of an eating disorder. You have told him or her of your concerns, but your roommate has denied having a problem and brushed off your fears. What can you do to help this individual? Should you contact his or her parent? Why or why not?

Media Menu

CENGAGENOW Go to the HealthNow website at **academic.cengage.com/login** that will:
- Help you evaluate your knowledge of the material.
- Allow you to take an exam-prep quiz.
- Provide a Personalized Learning Plan targeting resources that address areas you should study.
- Coach you through identifying target goals for behavioral change and creating and monitoring your personal change plan throughout the semester.

Internet Connections

American Obesity Association

www.obesity.org

The American Obesity Association is the leading organization for advocacy and education on the nation's obesity epidemic. This comprehensive website features statistics on overweight and obesity in the United States, research articles, consumer protection links, prevention topics, library resources, fact sheets on a variety of weight management topics, and more.

Weight Control Information Network

http://win.niddk.nih.gov/index.htm

This government-sponsored website features a variety of publications in English and Spanish on nutrition, physical activity, and weight control for the general public and for health-care professionals. In addition, there are links for research, a newsletter, statistical data, and a bibliographic collection of journal articles on various aspects of weight management and obesity.

Something Fishy, A Website on Eating Disorders

www.something-fishy.org

This very comprehensive and popular site features the latest news on eating disorders, as well as links regarding signs to watch for, "Recovery: Reach Out," treatment finders, doctors and patients, cultural issues, and a support chat.

Key Terms

The terms listed are used and defined on the page indicated. Definitions are also found in the Glossary at the end of this book.

anorexia nervosa	201
appetite	191
binge eating	199
bulimia nervosa	202
eating disorders	201
hunger	191
NEAT (nonexercise activity thermogenesis)	195
obesity	187
overweight	187
satiety	191

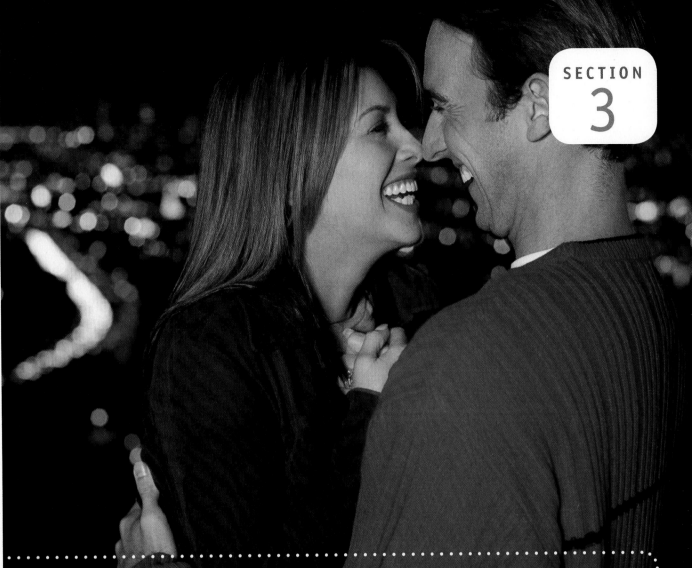

Responsible Sexuality

Our most special relationships are those that bring us closer to others—our friends, partners, spouses, parents, and children. Such intimacy is the most rewarding and often the most demanding of human involvements. The giving of ourselves to another—sharing thoughts, feelings, experiences, and sexual pleasure—touches the essence of what it means to be human. This section provides a comprehensive philosophical and practical view of relating to others. Each of the chapters focuses on the unique form of personal responsibility involved in every close relationship: a responsibility that looks beyond the self to those we care for and love.

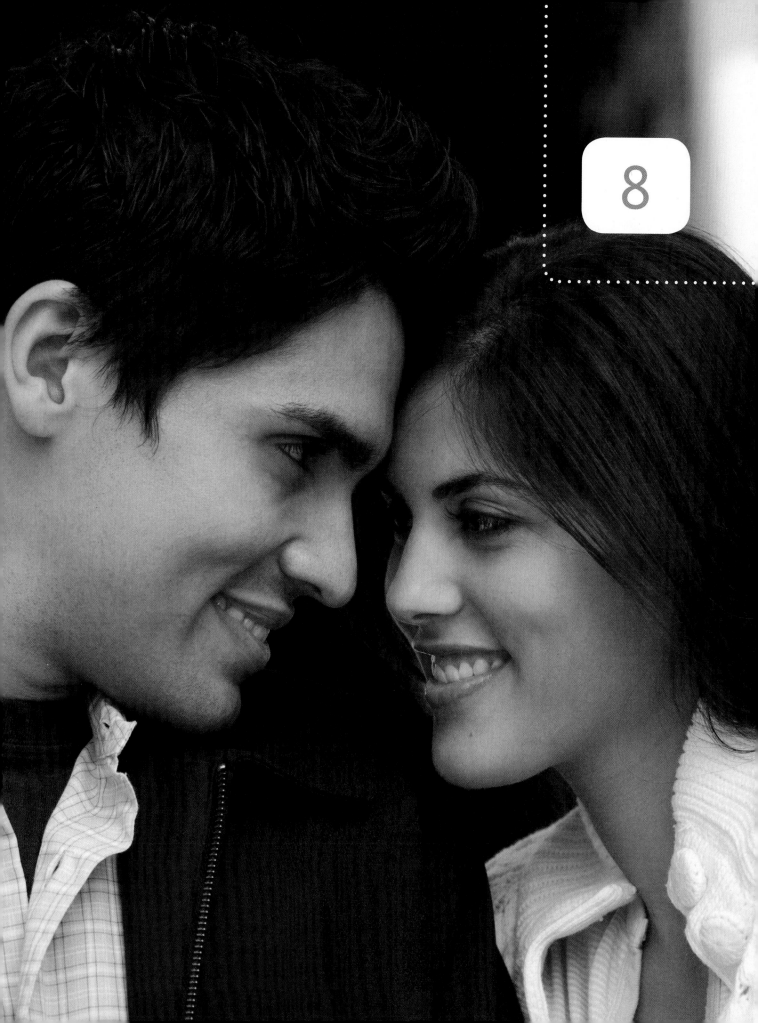

8

Communicating and Relating

OONA compares the people in her life to threads in a magnificent tapestry. Each brings different tones and textures that complement and contrast with others. Her earliest childhood memories are of loving circles of family and friends that she once thought revolved around only her. Now she sees that she is part of these concentric rings and that the friendship and support she offers others enrich all of their lives.

When she left for a college thousands of miles from her home, Oona worried about the people she was leaving behind and the strangers she would be living among. She wondered if she'd be welcomed or shunned, judged by her looks or her race, invited to join social groups or excluded from them. What she discovered was that the choice was largely hers. She could reach out to others, smile, and hope that others would smile in return, communicate clearly and honestly, strive to forge connections. Within months of her arrival, Oona was sure she had made friends she would keep forever.

Whether we are shy or outgoing, reserved or exuberant, we all crave human connection. As individuals and as part of society, we need to care about others and to know that others care about us, to feel for others and have others feel for us, to share what we know and to learn from what others know.

Sending clear messages through words, gestures, expressions, and behaviors is the essence of good communication. The more effectively we communicate, the more likely we are to create good relationships built on honesty, understanding, and mutual trust. Such relationships can infuse our lives with a richness no solitary pleasure can match.

This chapter discusses the social needs we all share, the ways some of us respond to those needs, healthy and unhealthy relationships, and the possibilities that exist for coming together from our solitude to warm ourselves in each other's glow.

After studying the material in this chapter, you should be able to:

- **Describe** the role verbal and nonverbal communication plays in forming and maintaining relationships and **discuss** gender differences in communication.

- **Define** friendship and **explain** how friendship grows.

- **Discuss** the behavior and emotional expectations for friendship, dating, and intimate relationships.

- **Identify** the behaviors that may result in dysfunctional relationships.

- **List** and **describe** the various living arrangements today's adults might choose.

- **Identify** the problems likely to affect long-term relationships and **explain** how they can be prevented.

- **Describe** at least two ways to improve one of your relationships.

CENGAGENOW™   Log on to HealthNow at **academic.cengage.com/login** to find your Behavior Change Planner and to explore self-assessments, interactive tutorials, and practice quizzes.

Your Social Health

Your relationships with your family, friends, coworkers, and loved ones may amaze, irritate, exhilarate, frustrate, and delight you. They also may affect your health. As noted in Chapter 1, your ability to communicate, to develop satisfying relationships, and to live in harmony with others is an important dimension of health and wellness.

Specific qualities in a relationship affect physical health, particularly *social support.* This term refers to the ways in which we provide information or assistance, show affection, comfort, and confide in others. As mounting evidence shows, people of all ages function best in socially supportive environments.

 This is particularly true of college students, who report more stress and more physical symptoms when they feel a lack of family support. More than any other component of social support, a sense of belonging may have the greatest impact on college students' health. In a study of undergraduates, belonging to a social network enhanced women's perceptions of their health and lowered the number of symptoms that men reported. Because college is a transition time, forming new attachments may be especially important—and beneficial to overall health.[1]

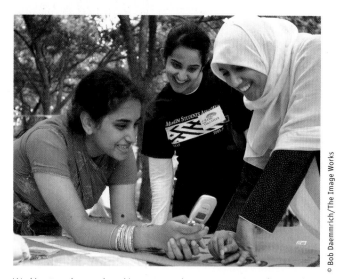

Working together on shared interests can be an opportunity to forge and strengthen friendships.

Personal Communications

Getting to know someone is one of life's greatest challenges and pleasures. When you find another person intriguing—as a friend, as a teacher, as a colleague, as a possible partner—you want to find out as much as you can about him or her and to share more and more information about yourself. Roommates may talk for endless hours. Friends may spend years getting to know each other. Partners in committed relationships may delight in learning new things about each other.

Communication stems from a desire to know and a decision to tell. The first step is learning how to listen. (See "Listen Up" lab in *IPC.*) **IPC** Then you mostly choose what information about yourself to disclose and what to keep private. But in opening up to others, you increase your own self-knowledge and understanding.

Communicating Feelings

A great deal of daily communication focuses on facts: on the who, what, where, when, and how. Information is easy to convey and comprehend. Emotions are not. Some people have great difficulty saying "I appreciate you" or "I care about you," even though they are genuinely appreciative and caring. Others find it hard to know what to say in response and how to accept such expressions of affection. Men and women vary in their communication styles.

Some people feel that relationships shouldn't require any effort, that there's no need to talk of responsibility between people who care about each other. Yet responsibility is implicit in our dealings with anyone or anything we value—and what can be more valuable than those with whom we share our lives? Friendships and other intimate relationships always demand an emotional investment, but the rewards they yield are great.

Sometimes people convey strong emotions with a kiss or a hug, a pat or a punch, but such actions aren't precise enough to communicate exact thoughts. Stalking out of a room and slamming the door may be clear signs of anger, but they don't explain what caused the anger or suggest what to do about it. You must learn how to communicate all feelings clearly and appropriately if you hope to become truly close to another person.

As two people build a relationship, they must sharpen their communication skills so that they can discuss all the issues they may confront. They must learn how to communicate anger as well as affection, hurt as well as joy—and they must listen as carefully as they speak.

Listening involves more than waiting for the other person to stop talking. Listening is an active process of trying to understand the other person's feelings and motivation. Effective listeners ask questions when they're not sure they understand the other person and prompt the other person to continue.

Nonverbal Communication

More than 90 percent of communication may be nonverbal. While we speak with our vocal cords, we communicate with our facial expressions, tone of voice, hands, shoulders, legs, torsos, posture. Body language is the

© Bob Daemmrich/The Image Works

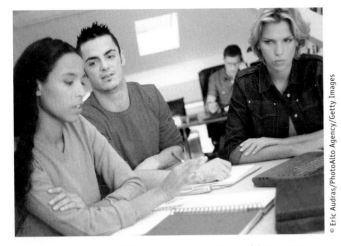

Body language and nonverbal expressions can send powerful messages about underlying tensions between people.

building block upon which more advanced verbal forms of communication rest.

Learning to interpret what people *don't* say can reveal more than what they *do* say. "Understanding nonverbal communication is probably the best tool there is for a good life of communicating, be it personally or professionally," says Marilyn Maple, an educator at the University of Florida. "It's one of the most practical skills you can develop. When you can consciously read what others are saying unconsciously, you can deal with issues before they become problems."[2]

 In a survey of undergraduates at a large southeastern university, those who saw themselves as "involved" daters were more concerned about nonverbal communication than "casual" daters. These individuals were more likely to "work hard" to ensure that their nonverbal behavior backed up the words they said—and to say their partners did the same. Regardless of their dating status, the female students valued nonverbal behavior more than men. They also engaged in more forms of nonverbal communication, such as looking their partners straight in the eye and nodding their heads as their partners spoke.

 Culture has a great deal of influence over body language. In some cultures, for example, establishing eye contact is considered hostile or challenging; in others, it conveys friendliness. A person's sense of personal space—the distance he or she feels most comfortable in keeping from others—varies in different societies.

How Men and Women Communicate

Gender differences in communication start early. By age one, boys make less eye contact than girls and pay more attention to moving objects like cars than to human faces. Both mothers and fathers talk less about feelings (except anger) to sons than daughters,

and boys' vocabularies include fewer "feeling" words. In the playground, if not at home, boys learn to choke back tears and show no fear. Their faces—once as openly emotional as girls—become less expressive as they move through the elementary years.

As adults, men use fewer words and talk, at least in public, as a means of putting themselves in a one-up situation—unlike women, who talk to draw others closer. Even with friends, men mainly swap information as they talk shop, sports, cars, computers. "Women talk to clear their heads, but men think before they talk," says psychiatrist Mark Goulston, author of *The 6 Secrets of a Lasting Relationship*. "If they didn't, they'd risk saying something stupid and being humiliated or offending another man and getting beaten up. They're safer not saying anything."[3]

In her insightful studies of language, linguist Deborah Tannen has noted that while men speak more often and for longer periods in public, women speak more in private, usually to build better connections to others. In public and private, women generally are better listeners, facilitating conversation by nodding, asking questions, and signaling interest by saying "uh-huh," or "yes." Men interrupt more, breaking in on another's monologue if they aren't getting the information they need. Women are more likely to wait for the speaker to finish. "There's more than one interpretation for why a woman is less likely to interrupt," says psychologist Judith Hall. "It could show that she's being submissive and not playing the aggressive role. But it also could mean that she is less of a social blunderer and is more adept at reading the other person's signals."[4]

In social interactions, two white women talking together look into each other's eyes far more often than two men; African American women are less likely to do so. When a man and a woman are together, the man gazes into the woman's eyes more often than he would a man's, while a woman makes eye contact less often than she would if she were with another woman—a nice exercise in reciprocity. "A man talking with a woman will act more like a woman, and a woman will act more like a man," observes Hall. "It's as if they're adjusting to accommodate each other's cultural norm."

In writing, women use more words overall, more words related to emotion (positive and negative), more idea words, more hearing, feeling, and sensing words, more causal words, such as *because,* and more modal words (*would, should, could*). Men use more numbers, more prepositions, and more articles, such as *an* and *the.*

Gender differences appear online. In general, women tend to write e-mails in much the same way that they talk, using words to build a connection with people. Men's e-mails are briefer and more utilitarian. In chat rooms and blogs, men are more likely to make strong assertions, disagree with others, and to use profanities and sarcasm. Women are more prone to posing questions, making suggestions, and including polite expressions. Communication researchers studying the differences between "he-mails" and "she-mails" have also found that people who are not generally verbally expressive—mainly men—often convey more feelings in e-mails than they do in face-to-face conversations.

Forming Relationships

We first learn how to relate in our families as children. Our relationships with parents and siblings change dramatically as we grow toward independence. Relationships between friends also change as they move or develop different interests; between lovers, as they come to know more about each other; between spouses, as they pass through life together; and between parents and children, as youngsters develop and mature. But throughout life, close relationships, tested and strengthened by time, allow us to explore the depths of our souls and the heights of our emotions. (See this chapter's Self Survey, "How Strong Are the Communication and Affection in Your Relationship?")

I, Myself, and Me

The way each of us perceives himself or herself affects all the ways we reach out and relate to others. If we feel unworthy of love, others may share that opinion. Self-esteem (discussed in Chapter 2) provides a positive foundation for our relationships with others. Self-esteem doesn't mean vanity or preoccupation with our own needs; rather, it is a genuine concern and respect for ourselves so that we remain true to our own feelings and beliefs. We can't know or love or accept others until we know and love and accept ourselves, however imperfect we may be.

 Partners with low self-esteem may feel responsible for a partner's unhappiness. In studies of college students, those who scored low on measures of self-esteem were far more likely to feel rejected or hostile if their partners seemed distraught. Regardless of the reason for the distress, insecure, self-doubting individuals may read nonexistent meaning into their partners' ambiguous cues. As a result, they may unwittingly sabotage their relationships. This misreading of cues occurs not just in dating couples, but among long-married partners who still fear that their spouses love them less than they actually do.

Friendship

Friendship has been described as "the most holy bond of society." Every culture has prized the ties of respect, tolerance, and loyalty that friendship builds and nurtures. An anonymous writer put it well:

A friend is one who knows you as you are,
Understands where you've been,
Accepts who you've become,
And still gently invites you to grow.

Friends can be a basic source of happiness, a connection to a larger world, a source of solace in times of trouble. Although we have different friends throughout life, often the friendships of adolescence and young adulthood are the closest we ever form. They ease the normal break from parents and the transition from childhood to independence.

In the past, many people believed that men and women couldn't become close friends without getting romantically involved. But as the genders have worked together and come to share more interests, this belief has changed. Yet unique obstacles arise in male-female friendships, such as distinguishing between friendship and romantic attraction and dealing with sexual tension. However, men and women who overcome such barriers and become friends benefit from their relationship—but in different ways. For men, a friendship with a woman offers support and nurturance. What they report liking most is talking and relating to women, something they don't do with their male buddies. Women view their friendships with men as more light-hearted and casual, with more joking and less fear of hurt feelings. They especially like getting insight into what guys really think.

Friendship transcends all boundaries of distance and differences and enhances feelings of warmth, trust, love, and affection between two people. It is a common denominator of human existence that cuts across major social categories: In every country, culture, and language, human beings make friends. Friendship is both a universal and a deeply satisfying experience.

"Wishing to be friends," Aristotle wrote, "is quick work, but friendship is a slowly opening fruit." The qualities that make a good friend include honesty, acceptance, dependability, empathy, and loyalty. To sustain a close friendship, both people must be able to see the other's perspective, anticipate each other's needs, and take each other's viewpoint into account. More than anything else, good friends are there when we need them. They see us at our worst but never lose sight of our best. They share our laughter and tears, our triumphs and tragedies.

Dating on Campus

 Dating isn't what it used to be. Many young people socialize in groups until a couple pairs off into a romantic relationship. Rather than the conventional dinner and a movie, college students may just get together to hang out. Is one person interested in something more? Is the other? Often it can take a while for couples to figure out if they are in fact dating.

By simplest definition, a date is any occasion during which two people share their time. Friends and lovers go on dates, so do complete strangers. Some men date other men; some women date other women. We don't expect to love, or even like, everyone we date. Yet the people you date reveal something about the sort of person you are.

With more people remaining single longer, the search for a good date has become more complex. Singles bars have become less popular; cafés, laundromats, health clubs, and bookstores have become more acceptable as places to meet new people. The Internet provides alternative ways to meet potential dates (see Savvy Consumer: "Dos and Don'ts of Online Dating").

Dating can do more than help you meet people. By dating, you can learn how to make conversation, get to know more about others as well as yourself, and share feelings, opinions, and interests. In adolescence and young adulthood, dating also provides an opportunity for exploring your sexual identity. Some people date for months and never share more than a good-night kiss. Others may fall into bed together before they fall in love or even "like."

Separating your emotional feelings about someone you're dating from your sexual desire is often difficult. The first step to making responsible sexual decisions is respecting your sexual values and those of your partner. If you care about the other person—not just his or her body—and the relationship you're creating, sex will be an important, but not the all-important, factor while you're dating.

Should You Stay Together?

You've met someone, gone out a few times, and enjoyed yourself. Is it infatuation, "like," or love? Should you keep seeing each other? Here are some positive indications of a relationship worth continuing:

- You feel at ease with your new partner.
- You feel good about your new partner when you're together and when you're not.
- Your partner is open with you about his or her life—past, present, and future.
- You can say no to each other without feeling guilty.
- You feel cared for, appreciated, and accepted as you are.
- Your partner really listens to what you have to say.

Following are some reasons to rethink your relationship:

- You don't feel comfortable together.
- You feel angry or let down when you're together or apart.
- Your partner is very secretive about his or her life.
- You feel your partner isn't attentive to you.
- You don't feel cared for and appreciated.

Hooking Up

Hooking up refers to a sexual encounter between two people who usually are not seriously dating and who may or may not know each other well. College students use the term to describe a variety of sexual interactions, including kissing, fondling, oral sex, and sexual intercourse. What makes hooking up unique is that the couple agrees there will be no commitment, no exclusivity, no feelings.

▼ Savvy Consumer   Dos and Don'ts of Online Dating

E-mail flirtations can be fun, but they also entail some risks, particularly if you decide to go off-line and meet in person. Here are some guidelines:

- Be careful of what you type. Anything you put on the Internet can end up almost anywhere. To avoid embarrassment, don't say anything you wouldn't want to see in newspaper print.
- Don't give out your address, telephone number, or any other identifying information. The people you meet online are strangers, and you should keep your guard up.
- Don't "date" on an office or university computer. You could end up supplying your professors, classmates, or coworkers with unintentional entertainment. Also, many organizations and institutions consider e-mail messages company property.
- Remember that you have no way of verifying if a correspondent is telling the truth about anything—sex, age, occupation, marital status. If your online partner seems insincere or strange in any way, stop corresponding.

- If you do decide to meet, make your first face-to-face encounter a double or group date and make it somewhere public, like a café or museum. Don't plan a full-day outing. Coffee or a drink in a crowded place makes the best transition from e-mails.
- Make sure you tell a friend or family member your plans and have your own way of getting home. It's also a good idea to schedule the first meeting in the afternoon or early in the evening rather than later at night.
- Don't let your expectations run wild. Finding Mr. or Ms. Right is no easier in cyberspace than anywhere else, so be realistic about where your relationship might lead.
- Don't rely on the Internet as your only method of meeting people. Continue to get out in the real world and meet potential dates the old-fashioned way: live and in-person.

Why do people hook up? According to a recent book on the subject, college students, focused on academic and career success, don't have time for a real relationship. But social commentators speculate that by not seeking a connection beyond the physical, young people may be shortchanging themselves of the richness of a caring, committed relationship. They also face a higher risk of sexually transmitted infections and of date rape (discussed in Chapter 18).[5]

 In an informal survey of college hookups, a sexuality instructor found that over 85 percent of students had engaged in a hookup. Ninety percent reporting having had a "really good" hookup for reasons that included good sex, no interruptions, or a resulting relationship. However, 78 percent reported a bad hookup experience because of bad sex, interruptions, or a partner wanting more out of the hookup than they did.[6]

Alcohol often plays a role in hooking up. Under its influence, individuals may engage in sexual activities, including unsafe sex, that they normally would avoid or with someone they usually would not choose. Most students surveyed believe that hooking up is more common than it may in fact be and that their peers—particularly men—are more comfortable with hooking up than they are.

Some young people also engage in sexual activities with friends with whom they are not romantically involved. Many "friends with benefits" may have had a sexual relationship in the past. Others have no expectation of any serious involvement.

Dysfunctional Relationships

Although they enrich and fulfill us in many ways, our relationships with friends, siblings, parents, or colleagues can also sabotage our health. Mental health professionals define a "toxic" relationship as one in which either person is made to feel worthless or incompetent.

Your Life Change Coach

Building Healthy Relationships

Healthy relationships are built on mutual respect, trust, and consideration. People who've grown up in dysfunctional families or who have had abusive relationships may not have a clear idea of what a healthy relationship is. Here are some of the characteristics to look and strive for:

- Emotional support and sensitivity.
- Mutual good will.
- Respectful asking rather than ordering.
- Encouragement.
- Being listened and responded to with courtesy.
- Acknowledgement and appreciation of your feelings.
- The right to express your own point of view.
- Freedom from accusations, blame, criticism, and judgment.
- Respect for your work and interests.
- No rage, outbursts of anger, or emotional or physical threats.
- Sincere apologies for comments or jokes you find offensive.

A healthy relationship requires empathy, the ability to appreciate what another person is experiencing. You may not agree with your roommate's political opinions or your sibling's wardrobe choices, yet you respect their rights to think and dress as the individuals they are.

In an intimate relationship, empathy becomes even more important. You can develop your capacity for empathy by pulling back periodically, particularly in moments of stress or conflict, and asking yourself: "What is my partner or spouse feeling right now? What does he or she need?" (See "Your Intimacy Quotient" in *IPC*.) **IPC**

Self-Disclosure in Relationships

A key element of relationships—whether friendships or romantic ones—is **self-disclosure,** that is, how much we reveal about ourselves to another person. What you share about yourself is a critical building block that affects the nature and quality of the bonds you establish with others. But both cultural and individual factors can influence self-disclosure.

Relationships that don't promote healthy communication, honesty, and intimacy are sometimes called **dysfunctional.** Individuals with addictive behaviors or dependence on drugs or alcohol (see Chapters 11 and 12), and the children or partners of such people, are especially likely to find themselves in such relationships, although they occur in all economic and social groups.

Often partners have magical, unrealistic expectations (e.g., they expect that a relationship with the right person will make their life okay), and one person uses the other almost as if he or she were a mood-altering drug. The partners may compulsively try to get the other to act the way they want. Both persons may not trust or may deceive each other. Often they isolate themselves from others, thus trapping themselves in a recurring cycle of pain.

"Physical symptoms, such as headaches, digestive troubles, tics, and inability to sleep well, can be signs of a destructive relationship," says sociologist Robert Billingham, professor of human development and family studies at Indiana University.[8] Yet, although one person may repeatedly attack, abandon, betray, badger, bully, criticize, deceive, dominate, or demean the other, the responsibility for changing the unhealthy dynamic belongs to both.

"The big question is, 'Do I want or have to keep this relationship going?'" says sociologist Jan Yager, author of *When Friendship Hurts.* "If yes, are you willing to invest time and energy to turn it around?"[9] (See Your Strategies for Change: "How to Cope with an Unhealthy Relationship."

Emotional Abuse

Abuse consists of any behavior that uses fear, humiliation, or verbal or physical assaults to control and subjugate another human being. Rather than being physical, emotional abuse often takes the form of constant berating, belittling, and criticism. Aggressive verbal abuse includes calling names, blaming, threatening, accusing, demeaning, and judging. Trivializing, minimizing, or

 In a study of American and Japanese college students, the Japanese undergraduates reported significantly less self-disclosure, whether in passionate love relationships, companionate love relationships, cross-sex friendships, or same-sex friendships. As previous studies have shown, Japanese people talk less about themselves than Americans do and may think that talking about their personal issues would hurt the feelings of people around them. On the other hand, Americans generally strive to express themselves.[7]

Yet both American and Japanese students disclosed more in romantic relationships than in friendships and more in same-sex than in cross-sex friendships. This might be because we talk about more topics with a romantic partner than with a friend. We also may have more in common with people of the same sex so we discuss more with them than with a friend of the other sex.

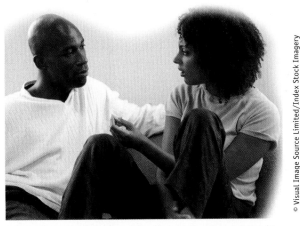

© Visual Image Source Limited/Index Stock Imagery

Talking about your feelings and listening intently move a relationship to a deeper and more meaningful level.

Assessing a Relationship

How do you know if you're in a healthy relationship? Ask yourself the following questions:

- **Do you have a clear sense of who you are,** what you believe and value, the goals you want? Such self-knowledge is critical for forming any mature relationship.
- **Do you feel that you can be yourself** when you're with this person? Do you feel good about yourself? Do you get—and give—compliments, support, and praise?
- **Do you share interests and values?** When you have things in common, you have a foundation to expand and build your relationship.
- **Do you respect the other person** and feel respected in return?
- **Do you have differences in values,** politics, religion, age, or race? Can you accept them?
- **Do you still feel like a unique, strong individual** within this relationship?

dysfunctional Characterized by negative and destructive patterns of behavior between partners or between parents and children.

self-disclosure Sharing personal information and experiences with another that he or she would not otherwise discover; self-disclosure involves risk and vulnerability.

YOUR STRATEGIES FOR CHANGE *How to Cope with an Unhealthy Relationship*

- **Start a dialogue.** Focus on communication, not confrontation. Start with a positive statement, for instance, saying what you really value in the relationship. Volunteer what you might do to make it better, and state what you need from the other person.

- **Distance yourself.** Take a vacation from a toxic friendship. Skip the family reunion or Thanksgiving dinner. When forced into proximity, be polite. If you refuse to engage—not arguing, not getting angry, not trying to make things better—toxic people give up trying to get under your skin.

- **Consult a professional.** A therapist or minister can help people recognize and change toxic behavior patterns. Changes you make in how you act and react may trigger changes in others.

- **Save yourself.** If you can never get what you need in a relationship, you may need to let it go. Nothing is worth compromising your mental or physical health.

---

denying what a person says or feels is a more subtle but equally destructive type of abuse. Even if done for the sake of "teaching" or "helping," emotional abuse wears away at self-confidence, sense of self-worth, and trust and belief in one's self. Because it is more than skin deep, emotional abuse can leave deeper, longer-lasting scars.

 In a recent survey of more than 1,500 never-married undergraduates, 25 percent reported that they had experienced at least two acts of physical abuse in a dating relationship. Far fewer (12 percent) believed that they had ever physically abused their current or most recent dating partner. The majority of students who abuse or are physically abused by a dating partner, the researchers concluded, may not identify themselves as being in an abusive relationship. This may be because of denial, ignorance, or acceptance of physical violence as a norm in a dating relationship.[10] (See Reality Check.)

No one wants to get into an abusive relationship, but often people who were emotionally abused in childhood find themselves in similar circumstances as adults. Dealing with an emotional abuser, regardless of how painful, may feel familiar or even comfortable. Individuals who think very little of themselves also may pick partners who treat them as badly as they believe they deserve.

Abusers also may have grown up with emotional abuse and view it as a way of coping with feelings of fear, hurt, powerlessness, or anger. They may seek partners who see themselves as helpless and who make them feel more powerful.

Among the signs of emotional abuse are:

- **Attempting to control various aspects of your life,** such as what you say or wear.

- **Frequently humiliating you** or making you feel badly about yourself.

- **Making you feel as if you are to blame** for what your partner does.

- **Wanting to know where you are** and whom you're with at all times.

- **Becoming jealous or angry** when you spend time with friends.

- **Threatening to harm you** if you break up.

- **Trying to coerce you** into unwanted sexual activity with statements such as, "If you loved me, you would. . ."

If you can never get what you need or if you're afraid, you need to get out of the relationship. Take whatever steps necessary to ensure your safety. Find a trusted adult who can help. Don't isolate yourself from family and friends. This is the time when you need their support and often the support of a counselor, minister, or doctor as well.

Codependency

Codependency has expanded its definition to include any maladaptive behaviors learned by family members in order to survive great emotional pain and stress, such as an addiction, chronic mental or physical illness, and abuse. Some therapists refer to codependency as a "relationship addiction" because codependent people often form or maintain relationships that are one-sided, emotionally destructive, or abusive. First identified in studies of the relationships in families of alcoholics, codependent behavior can occur in any dysfunctional family.

Codependent individuals, lacking in self-esteem, may develop compulsive behaviors, such as workaholism, or try to feel better by using alcohol or drugs. If they take on a martyr's role, they may sacrifice their own needs and dreams for the sake of helping a parent, child, or spouse. Although codependent people may initially relish being needed, in time they feel overwhelmed and trapped in the relationship, but cannot break away. They come to see themselves as victims and are attracted to that same role in friendships and romantic relationships.

Among the characteristics of codependency are:

- **An exaggerated sense of responsibility** for the actions of others.

- An attraction to people who need rescuing.
- Always trying to do more than one's share.
- Doing anything to cling to a relationship and avoid feeling abandoned.
- An extreme need for approval and recognition.
- A sense of guilt about asserting needs and desires.
- A compelling need to control others.
- Lack of trust in self and/or others.
- Fear of being alone.
- Difficulty identifying feelings.
- Rigidity/difficulty adjusting to change.
- Chronic anger.
- Lying/dishonesty.
- Poor communications.
- Difficulty making decisions.

Are You Codependent?

Check any of these statements that apply to you.

_____ I keep quiet to avoid arguments.

_____ I'm always worried about what other people think of me.

_____ One of my family members has an alcohol or drug problem.

_____ I have had relatives, friends, or partners who abused me verbally or physically.

_____ I always think that the opinions of others are more important than mine.

_____ I find it hard to adjust to changes at work or home.

_____ I feel hurt and rejected when someone close to me spends time with friends.

_____ I am uncomfortable expressing my true feelings.

_____ I feel inadequate and like a "bad person" when I make a mistake.

_____ I have difficulty accepting compliments or gifts.

_____ I think people in my life would fall apart without my constant efforts.

_____ I find it hard to talk to people in authority.

REALITYCHECK

- *How many students report being in an emotionally abusive relationship in the last year?* _____
- *What percentage of college men?* _____ *College women?* _____
- *How many have been in a physically abusive relationship?* _____

Answers on next page.

_____ I'm confused about who I am or where I'm going in my life.

_____ I have trouble saying "no" when asked for help and asking for help when I need it.

_____ I am trying to do so many things at once that I can't do any of them well.

If you identify with many of these statements, you may have been or are now in a codependent relationship. Learn as much as you can about it. Turn to the Internet, libraries, drug and alcohol abuse treatment centers, and mental health centers, which often offer educational materials and programs to the public. The more you understand codependency, the better you can cope with its effects.

Overcoming Codependency

Because the roots of codependency run so deep, people don't just "outgrow" this problem or magically find themselves in a healthy relationship. Treatment to resolve childhood hurts and deal with emotional issues may take the form of individual or group therapy, education, or programs such as Codependents Anonymous (www.codependents.org). The goal is to help individuals get in touch with long-buried feelings and build healthier family and relationship dynamics.

Enabling

Experts on the subject of addiction first identified traits of codependency in spouses of alcoholics, who followed a predictable pattern of behavior: While intensely trying to control the drinkers, the codependent mates would act in ways that allowed the drinkers to keep drinking. For example, if an alcoholic found it hard to get up in the morning, his wife would wake him up, pull him out of

codependency An emotional and psychological behavioral pattern in which the spouses, partners, parents, children, and friends of individuals with addictive behaviors allow or enable their loved ones to continue their self-destructive habits.

REALITYCHECK

PART II: *Just the Facts*

- **13** *percent of college students—***15** *percent of women and* **8** *percent of men—report being in an emotionally abusive relationship in the last year.*
- **2** *percent of college students have been in a physically abusive relationship.*

Source: American College Health Association. *American College Health Association National College Health Assessment Reference Group Executive Summary Fall 2006.* Baltimore: American College Health Association, 2007.

bed and into the shower, and drop him off at work. If he was late, she made excuses to his boss. The husband was the one with the substance-abuse problem, but without realizing it, his wife was enabling him to continue drinking. In fact, he might not have been able to keep up his habit without her unintentional cooperation.

The different styles or components of **enabling** include the following:

- **Shielding.** Codependents may cover up for abusers, preventing them from experiencing the full impact of the harmful consequences of their behavior—for example, by dropping off a paper or report so that the addicted person can avoid a missed deadline.

- **Controlling.** A codependent may try to control the significant other—for instance, by withholding sex or using sex as a reward for cutting down on an addictive behavior.

- **Taking over responsibilities.** The codependent may take over such household chores as shopping or running errands.

- **Rationalizing.** Codependents try to rationalize the person's addiction by telling themselves that a compulsive behavior pattern, like workaholism, is making the person more successful, or that drinking helps him or her relax.

- **Cooperating.** Sometimes codependents become involved in the person's compulsion, perhaps placing bets for a gambler or buying alcohol for a drinker.

- **Rescuing.** The codependent may become overprotective—for example, by allowing the user to use drugs at home to avoid the risk of an accident or arrest.

Codependency progresses just as an addiction does, and codependents excuse their own behavior with many of the same defense mechanisms used by addicts, such as rationalization ("I cut class so I could catch up on my reading, not to keep an eye on my partner") and denial ("He likes to gamble, but he never loses more than he

can afford"). In time, codependents lose sight of everything but their loved one. They feel that if they can only "fix" this person, everything will be fine.

Intimate Relationships

The term **intimacy**—the open, trusting sharing of close, confidential thoughts and feelings—comes from the Latin word for *within*. Intimacy doesn't happen at first sight, or in a day or a week or a number of weeks. Intimacy requires time and nurturing; it is a process of revealing rather than hiding, of wanting to know another and to be known by that other. Although intimacy doesn't require sex, an intimate relationship often includes a sexual relationship, heterosexual or homosexual.

All of our close relationships, whether they're with parents or friends, have a great deal in common. We feel we can count on these people in times of need. We feel that they understand us and we understand them. We give and receive loving emotional support. We care about their happiness and welfare. However, when we choose one person above all others, there is something even deeper and richer—something we call romantic love.

What Attracts Two People to Each Other?

What draws two people to each other and keeps them together: chemistry or fate, survival instincts or sexual longings? "Probably it's a host of different things," reports sociologist Edward Laumann, coauthor of *Sex in America,* a landmark survey conducted by the National Opinion Research Center at the University of Chicago.[11] "But what's remarkable is that most of us end up with partners much like ourselves—in age, race, ethnicity, socioeconomic class, education."

Why? "You've got to get close for sexual chemistry to occur," says Laumann. "Sparks may fly when you see someone across a crowded room, but you only see a preselected group of people—people enough like you to be in the same room in the first place. This makes sense because initiating a sexual relationship is very uncertain. We all have such trepidations about being too fat, too ugly, too undesirable. We try to lower the risk of rejection by looking for people more or less like us."

 Scientists have tried to analyze the combination of factors that attracts two people to each other. In several studies of college students, four predictors ranked as the most important reasons for attraction: warmth and kindness, desirable personality, something specific about the person, and reciprocal liking.

Do opposites attract, or do people find greater happiness with partners who are similar to them? One of the most comprehensive studies ever undertaken on these questions found no evidence that opposites attract. Most people, the researchers found, tend to marry those who are similar in attitudes, religion, and values. However, these similarities have little to do with having a happy marriage. What does matter are similarities in personality, such as being extroverted or conscientious. These take more time to recognize but have a greater impact on how a couple gets along over the long term.[12]

In his cross-cultural research, psychologist David Buss, author of *The Evolution of Desire*, found that men in 37 sample groups drawn from Africa, Asia, Europe, North and South America, Australia, and New Zealand rated youth and attractiveness as more important in a possible mate than did women. Women placed greater value on potential mates who were somewhat older, had good financial prospects, and were dependable and hardworking.[13]

Attractive women in different cultures, including the United States, use different mating strategies than less attractive ones, including more "attractiveness enhancement tactics" (such as wearing makeup), flirting with other men to make a date jealous, and acting possessively. Attractive women also may have more opportunities for "trial liaisons" in selecting long-term partners and for replacing a mate who fails to live up to expectations.

Infatuation

It is tempting to think of love as scenes from a movie script: blazing sunsets and misty nights, fiery glances and passionate embraces, consuming desire and happily-ever-after endings. However, movies only last for 2 hours; ideally, love lasts a lifetime. Infatuation falls somewhere in between.

Certainly, falling in love is an intense, dizzying experience. A person not only enters our life, but also takes possession. We are intrigued, flattered, captivated, delighted—but is this love or a love of loving?

At the time you're experiencing it, there is no difference between infatuation and lasting love. You feel the same giddy, wonderful way. However, if it's infatuation, it won't last. Infatuation refers only to falling in love. People genuinely in love with each other do more than fall: They start building a relationship together.

Infatuation also can be a disguise for something quite different: a strong sex drive, a fear of loneliness, loneliness itself, or a hunger for approval. Sometimes lovers in love with love may become infatuated with someone who doesn't even exist: the projection of their unmet needs for unconditional love.

The Science of Romantic Love

We like to think of this powerful force, this source of both danger and delight, as something that defies analy-

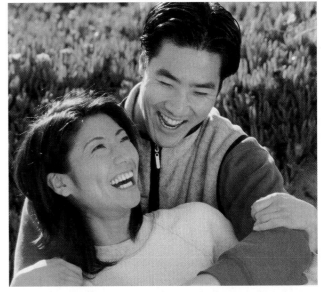

We tend to be attracted to people who are similar to ourselves in age, race, ethnicity, socioeconomic class, and education.

© Comstock/Jupiterimages

sis. However, scientists have provided new perspectives on its true nature.

A Psychological View

According to psychologist Robert Sternberg, love can be viewed as a triangle with three faces: passion, intimacy, and commitment (Figure 8.1). Each person brings his or her own triangle to a relationship. If they match well, their relationship is likely to be satisfying.

Sternberg also identified six types of love:

- **Liking,** the intimacy friends share.

- **Infatuation,** the passion that stems from physical and emotional attraction.

- **Romantic love,** a combination of intimacy and passion.

- **Companionate love,** a deep emotional bond in a relationship that may have had romantic components.

enabling To unwittingly contribute to a person's addictive or abusive behavior. Components of enabling include shielding or covering up for an abuser/addict; controlling them; taking over responsibilities; rational- izing addictive behavior; or cooperating with them.

intimacy A state of closeness between two people, characterized by the desire and ability to share one's innermost thoughts and feelings with each other either verbally or nonverbally.

- **Fatuous love,** a combination of passion and commitment in two people who lack a deep emotional intimacy.
- **Consummate love,** which combines passion, intimacy, and commitment over time.

An Anthropological View

When you first fall in love, you may be sure that no one else has ever known the same dizzying, wonderful feelings. Yet, while every romance may be unique, romantic love is anything but. Anthropologists have found evidence of romantic love between individuals in most of the cultures they have studied—it seems to be a human universal or, at the least, a near-universal.

Anthropologist Helen Fisher, author of *Anatomy of Love: The Natural History of Monogamy, Adultery and Divorce,* describes romantic love "as a very primitive, basic human emotion, as basic as fear, anger or joy." As she explains, it pulled men and women of prehistoric times into the sort of partnerships that were essential to child rearing. But after about four years—just "long enough to rear one child through infancy," says Fisher—romantic love seemed to wane, and primitive couples tended to break up and find new partners. This "four-year itch" may well have endured through the centuries, contends Fisher, who notes that divorce statistics from most of the 62 cultures she has studied still show a pattern of restlessness four years into a marriage.[14]

A Biochemical View

The heart is the organ we associate with love, but the brain may be where the action really is. According to research on neurotransmitters (the messenger chemicals within the brain), love sets off a chemical chain reaction that causes our skin to flush, our palms to sweat, and our lungs to breathe more deeply and rapidly. The "love chemicals" within the brain—dopamine, norepinephrine, and phenylethylamine (PEA)—have effects similar to those of amphetamines, stimulant drugs that intensify physiological reactions (see Chapter 11).

Infatuation may indeed be a natural high, but like other highs, this rush doesn't last—possibly because the body develops tolerance for love-induced chemicals, just as it does with amphetamines. However, as the initial lovers' high fades, other brain chemicals may come into play: the endorphins, morphinelike chemicals that can help produce feelings of well-being, security, and tranquility. These feel-good molecules may increase in partners who develop a deep attachment.

The hormone *oxytocin,* best known for its role in inducing labor during childbirth, seems particularly important in our ability to bond with others. By measuring blood levels of women as they recalled positive and negative relationships, researchers have found that women whose oxytocin levels rose when remembering a positive relationship reported having little difficulty setting appropriate boundaries, being alone, or trying too hard to please

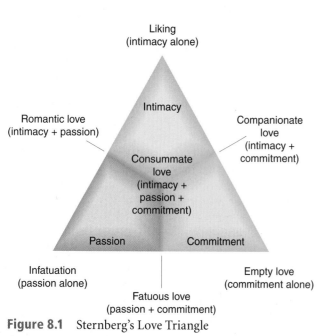

Figure 8.1 Sternberg's Love Triangle

The three components of love are intimacy, passion, and commitment. The various kinds of love are composed of different combinations of the three components.

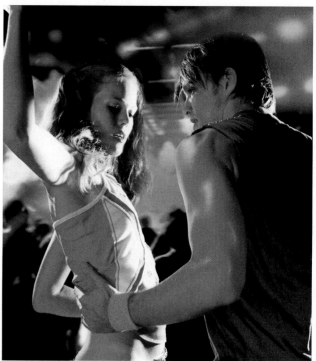

Can romantic love be just a matter of chemistry? Our neurotransmitters and hormones definitely play a role in sexual attraction.

© Daly and Newton/Stone/Getty Images

YOUR STRATEGIES FOR CHANGE *How to Deal with Rejection*

- Remind yourself of your own worth. You are no less attractive, intelligent, interesting, or lovable because someone ends a relationship with you.

- Accept the rejection as a statement of the other person's preference rather than trying to debate or defend yourself.

- Think of other people who value or have valued you, who accept and even see as appealing the same characteristics the rejecting person viewed as undesirable.

- Don't withdraw from others. Although you may not want to risk further rejection, it's worth the gamble to get

involved again. The only individuals who've never been rejected are those who've never reached out to connect with another.

others. Women whose oxytocin levels fell in response to remembering a negative emotional relationship reported greater anxiety in close relationships.

Mature Love

Social scientists have distinguished between *passionate love* (characterized by intense feelings of elation, sexual desire, and ecstasy) and *companionate love* (characterized by friendly affection and deep attachment). Often relationships begin with passionate love and evolve into a more companionate love. Sometimes the opposite happens and two people who know each other well discover that their friendship has "caught fire" and the sparks have flamed an unexpected passion.

Mature love is a complex combination of sexual excitement, tenderness, commitment, and—most of all—an over-riding passion that sets it apart from all other love relationships in one's life. This passion isn't simply a matter of orgasm but also entails a crossing of the psychological boundaries between oneself and one's lover. You feel as if you're becoming one with your partner while simultaneously retaining a sense of yourself.

When Love Ends

Breaking up is indeed hard to do. Sometimes two people grow apart gradually, and both of them realize that they must go their separate ways. More often, one person falls out of love first. It hurts to be rejected; it also hurts to inflict pain on someone who once meant a great deal to you. (See Your Strategies for Change: "How to Deal with Rejection.")

 In surveys, college students say it's more difficult to initiate a breakup than to be rejected. Those who decided to end a relationship report greater feelings of guilt, uncertainty, discomfort, and awkwardness than their girlfriends or boyfriends. However, students with high levels of jealousy are likely to feel a desire for vengeance that can lead to aggressive behavior.

Research suggests that people do not end their relationships because of the disappearance of love. Rather a sense of dissatisfaction or unhappiness develops, which may then cause love to stop growing. The fact that love does not dissipate completely may be why breakups are so painful. While the pain does ease over time, it can help both parties if they end their relationship in a way that shows kindness and respect. Your basic guideline should be to think of how you would like to be treated if someone were breaking up with you. Would it hurt more to find out from someone else? Would it be more painful if the person you cared for lied to you or deceived you, rather than admitted the truth? Saying "I don't feel the way I once did about you; I don't want to continue our relationship" is hard, but it's also honest and direct.

Living Arrangements

Today's adults have many choices to explore regarding how and with whom they might live: returning to one's primary family, staying single, living with one or more friends, living in a long-term relationship with a lover of the same or opposite sex, or getting married. Increasingly, men and women in their twenties and thirties are spending more time considering all their options before committing themselves to an exclusive relationship.

Transition into Adulthood

According to the U.S. Census Bureau, young adults between the ages of 18 and 24 are more likely to be living in their parents' homes than young people were in the 1970s. Some 18 million Americans between the ages of 18 and 34 are still living with their parents. Of those between ages 19 and 24, 66 percent (including college students) are living at home, compared to 50 percent in 1980.[15] Their reasons include the high cost of housing and the low incomes most men and women earn in their early twenties.

Sociologists debate the benefits and drawbacks of delaying traditional adult milestones, such as supporting one's self and getting one's own apartment. Trying different fields or jobs and waiting to commit may help young people make better long-term choices. Yet they also may be ducking responsibility for their own lives.

> **YOUR STRATEGIES FOR CHANGE** *How to Stay Single and Satisfied*
>
> - Fill your life with meaningful work, experiences, and people.
> - Build a network of supportive friends who care for and about you.
> - Be open to new experiences that can expand your feelings about yourself and your world.
> - Don't miss out on a special event because you don't have someone to accompany you: Go alone.
> - Enjoy your own company. Allow yourself to be amazed by your own witty or off-the-wall observations.
> - Volunteer to help others less fortunate, or become involved in church and social organizations.

Single Life

In young adulthood, single men outnumber single women; after age 40, however, there are more single women than single men. Perhaps because there are so many singles, more and more Americans are living alone. The number of women living alone has doubled since 1970 and has nearly tripled for men. Approximately one-quarter of the households in the nation are one-person homes.

Among Americans between 25 and 34 years old, about 35 percent (14 million) have never been married. Of African Americans in this age group, 53 percent have never been married. Being single no longer marks a transition phase between living with parents and living with a spouse, but is an accepted, appealing lifestyle for millions of men and women. (See Your Strategies for Change: "How to Stay Single and Satisfied.")

More women in the United States now live without a husband than with one (see Table 8.1). Younger women are marrying later and living with unmarried partners more often and for longer periods. After divorce, women are more likely to delay remarriage than men. And since women generally live longer than men, many spend the last years of their lives as widows. About 53 percent of men are married and live with their spouses. [16]

Cohabitation

Although couples have always shared homes in informal relationships without any official ties, "living together," or **cohabitation,** has become more common. Some 5 million couples are cohabiting in the United States; the vast majority are heterosexual; 40 percent have children.

The number of unmarried couples increased by nearly 1200 percent between 1960 and 2005 (Figure 8.2). About a quarter of unmarried women ages 25 to 39 are currently living with a partner; an additional quarter lived with a partner in the past. Couples live together before more than half of all marriages, a practice that was practically unknown 50 years ago. In addition, the proportion of cohabiting women between the ages of 20 and 50 has tripled in the last 50 years. [17]

 Asians and non-Hispanic white couples are the least likely to cohabit. A higher percentage of Native American, black, and Hispanic couples are unmarried. "Cohabiters" tend to have lower income and education levels. They also are younger—on average, some 12 years younger than married men and women.

According to the U.S. Census Bureau, unmarried couples tend to cluster in several zones in the United States, including the western states and the Northeast. In these regions, married couples flock to the suburbs, while unmarried couples, especially same-sex ones, are most likely to live in central cities. As more states and nations are increasing the legal obligations of all intimate partners, the lines between cohabitation and conventional marriage are blurring.

Cohabitation can be a prelude to marriage, an alternative to living alone, or an alternative to marriage. Does living together help couples to find out if they get along and avoid a bad marriage? That does not seem to be the case. About half of men and women living together get married within five years; 40 percent break up; 10 percent continue to cohabit for a longer period.

Committed Relationships

Even though men and women today may have more sexual partners than in the past, most still yearn for an intense, supportive, exclusive relationship, based on mutual commitment and enduring over time. In our society, most such relationships take the form of heterosexual marriages, but partners of the same sex or heterosexual

TABLE 8.1 Women Without Husbands

Percent of Women Who Do Not Live with a Spouse	
Asian	40%
Non-Hispanic white	45%
Hispanic	51%
African-American	70%

Source: U.S. Census Bureau

© Steve Murez/The Image Bank/Getty Images

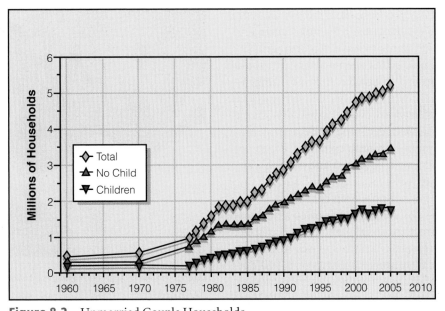

Figure 8.2   Unmarried Couple Households

The number of unmarried couples living together, both with and without children, has risen dramatically in the last fifty years.

Source: U.S. Census Bureau

partners who never marry also may sustain long-lasting, deeply committed relationships. These couples are much like married people: They make a home, handle daily chores, cope with problems, celebrate special occasions, plan for the future—all the while knowing that they are not alone, that they are part of a pair that adds up to far more than just the sum of two individual souls.

Domestic Partners

Committed couples, both heterosexual and homosexual, can register as domestic partners in certain areas. This may enable them to qualify for benefits such as health insurance. Employers may require that the couple has lived together for a specified period (generally, at least six months) and are responsible for each other's financial welfare. Recent court rulings have placed domestic partners on the same legal footing as married couples in dealings with businesses.

Long-Term Same-Sex Relationships

Contrary to the stereotype that same-sex relationships tend to be brief, researchers have studied couples who have been together for more than 20 years. Like heterosexual ("straight") couples, same-sex relationships progress through various stages. The first, blending, is a time of intense passion and romantic love. Gradually the couples move through nesting (starting a home together), to building trust and dependability, to merging assets, to establishing a strong sense of partnership.

Because there are no social norms for same-sex unions, researchers describe these relationships as more egalitarian. Each partner tends to be more self-reliant, and homosexual men and women tend to be more willing to communicate and experiment in terms of sexual behaviors.

Gay and lesbian relationships are comparable to straight relationships in many ways. But same-sex couples have to deal with every day ups-and-downs in a social context of isolation from family, workplace prejudice, and other social barriers. However, gay and lesbian couples are more upbeat in the face of conflict. Compared to straight couples, they use more affection and humor when they bring up a disagreement and remain more positive after a disagreement. They also display less belligerence, domineering, and fear with each other than straight couples do. When they argue, they are better able to soothe each other so they show fewer signs of physiological arousal, such as an elevated heart rate or sweaty palms, than heterosexual couples.

Marriage

Like everything which is not the involuntary result of fleeting emotion but the creation of time and will, any marriage, happy or unhappy, is infinitely more interesting and significant than any romance, however passionate.

W. H. Auden

cohabitation   Two people living together as a couple, without official ties such as marriage.

Contemporary marriage has been described as an institution that everyone on the outside wants to enter and everyone on the inside wants to leave. According to the U.S. Census Bureau, nine in ten people marry, but about half of first marriages end in divorce after an average of seven or eight years.

The proportion of married people, especially among younger age groups, has been declining for decades. Across North America and many European countries, the age of first marriage has risen, with both men and women waiting an extra three years before saying, "I do," and the rate of first marriages among men has been cut in half.[18]

 Not too long ago, marriage was often a business deal, a contract made by parents for economic or political reasons when the spouses-to-be were still very young. Today, in some countries, it is still culturally acceptable to arrange marriages in this manner. Even in America, certain ethnic groups, such as Asians who have recently immigrated to the United States, plan marriages for their children. In such arrangements, the marriage partners are likely to have similar values and expectations. However, the newlyweds also start out as strangers who may not even know whether they like—let alone love—each other. Sometimes arranged marriages do lead to loving unions; sometimes they trap both partners in loneliness and longing.

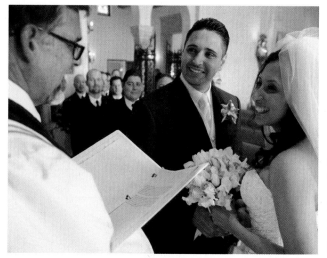

Marriage is a formal and legal, lifetime commitment to another person—and a great occasion for celebration!

Types of Marriage

Sociologists have categorized marriages as traditional or companion-oriented. In **traditional marriages,** the couples assume prescribed societal roles. In **companion-oriented marriages,** the partnership and its rewards—rather than the roles of fathering, mothering, and breadwinning—are primary. In addition, there are **romantic marriages,** in which sexual passion never seems to die, and **rescue marriages,** in which one partner suffered a traumatic childhood and sees marriage as a way of healing. About a fifth of all marriages belong to another category that has grown significantly in recent years: marriages of equally dependent spouses. Each partner in these unions earns between 40 and 59 percent of the total family income. According to research on these marriages, divorces are more common and occur more often at the wife's initiative. Researchers theorize that wives who are not economically dependent on their spouses may be more likely to leave an emotionally unfulfilling relationship. Regardless of type, a marriage can succeed if it fulfills basic tasks, such as providing a sense of intimacy and autonomy and providing a safe haven that is strong enough to absorb inevitable conflicts.

Preparing for Marriage

Most people say they marry for one far-from-simple reason: love. However, with more than half of all marriages ending in divorce, there's little doubt that modern marriages aren't made in heaven. Are some couples doomed to divorce even before they swap vows? Could counseling before a marriage increase its odds of success? According to recent research findings, the answer to both questions is yes.

There have been government attempts to set requirements for couples who want to marry. Some states, such as Arizona and Louisiana, have established "covenant" marriages in which engaged couples are required to get premarital counseling. Utah allows counties to require counseling before issuing marriage licenses to minors and people who have been divorced. Florida requires high school students to take marriage education classes.

YOUR STRATEGIES FOR PREVENTION *Think Twice About Getting Married If . . .*

- You or your partner are constantly asking the other such questions as, "Are you sure you love me?"
- You spend most of your time together disagreeing and quarreling.

- You're both still very young (under the age of 20).
- Your boyfriend or girlfriend has behaviors (such as nonstop talking), traits (such as bossiness), or problems (such as drinking too much) that really bother you and that

you're hoping will change after you're married.
- Your partner wants you to stop seeing your friends, quit a job you enjoy, or change your life in some other way that diminishes your overall satisfaction.

Finding Mr. or Ms. Right

Generally, men and women marry people from the geographical area they grew up in and from the same social background. Differences in religion and race can add to the pressures of marriage, but they also can enrich the relationship if they aren't viewed as obstacles. In our culturally diverse society, interracial and cross-cultural marriages are becoming more common and widely accepted, although the odds are much greater for partners of the same race to live together or marry.

 In a study of 75,000 couples who lived together and 480,000 married couples in the United States, researchers found that African Americans were 365 times more likely to marry a black than a nonblack spouse and 110 times more likely to cohabit with a black partner than someone of another racial group. Asians were 55 times more likely to marry another Asian and 17 times more likely to cohabit with another Asian. Hispanics were 12 times more likely to select a Hispanic spouse and nine times more likely to live with a Hispanic partner. Whites were about eight times more likely to marry another white person and five times more likely to cohabit with someone white rather than nonwhite.[19]

Some of the traits that appeal to us in a date become less important when we select a mate; others become key ingredients in the emotional cement holding two people together. According to psychologist Robert Sternberg of Yale University, the crucial ingredients for commitment are the following:

- **Shared values.**
- **A willingness to change in response to each other.**
- **A willingness to tolerate flaws.**
- **A match in religious beliefs.**
- **The ability to communicate effectively.**

The single best predictor of how satisfied one will be in a relationship, according to Sternberg, is not how one feels toward a lover, but the difference between how one would like the lover to feel and how the lover actually feels. Feeling that the partner you've chosen loves too little or too much is, as he puts it, "the best predictor of failure." For other predictors, see Your Strategies for Prevention: "Think Twice About Getting Married If . . ."[20]

Premarital Assessments

There are scientific ways of predicting marital happiness. Some premarital assessment inventories identify strengths and weaknesses in many aspects of a relationship: realistic expectations, personality issues, communication, conflict resolution, financial management, leisure activities, sex, children, family and friends, egalitarian roles, and religious orientation. Couples who become aware of potential conflicts by means of such inventories may be able to resolve them through professional counseling. In some cases, they may want to reconsider or postpone their wedding.

Other common predictors of marital discord, unhappiness, and separation are:

- **A high level of arousal during a discussion.**
- **Defensive behaviors** such as making excuses and denying responsibility for disagreements.
- **A wife's expressions of contempt.**
- **A husband's stonewalling** (showing no response when a wife expresses her concerns).

By looking for such behaviors, researchers have been able to predict with better than 90 percent accuracy whether a couple will separate within the first few years of marriage.

The Benefits of Marriage

Despite its problems, marriage endures because it is a fulfilling way for two people to live. As researchers have proved, saying "I do" can do wonders for your health. According to a CDC study of more than 127,000 adults, married people are healthier than those who are divorced, widowed, never-married, or live with a partner. The connection between marriage and health was strongest in the youngest group, aged 18 to 44.[21]

Married people are less likely to suffer from health conditions like back pain, headaches, and serious psychological distress. That is true for all ages, ethnicities, and levels of income and education. Married people are less likely to smoke, drink heavily, and be physically inactive.

Marriage does pose one health hazard: weight gain. Married men are more likely to be overweight or obese. Three in four married men aged 45 to 64 are overweight or obese. The slimmest groups are men and women who had never married.

Married men and women also have lower rates of most mental disorders than single or divorced individuals. Both husbands and wives live longer than single or divorced individuals. In one national survey, about 90 percent of husbands and wives survived until at least age 65, compared with only about 60 to 70 percent of divorced and never-

traditional marriage A marital relationship in which the roles of the partners are distinct; defined by gender-based cultural norms and expectations.

companion-oriented marriage A marital relationship in which the partners share interests, activities, and domestic responsibilities.

romantic marriage A marital relationship in which sexual passion never fades.

rescue marriage A marital relationship in which one partner has had a traumatic childhood and views marriage as a way of healing the past.

POINT COUNTERPOINT *Should Same-Sex Marriages Be Legal?*

POINT

Marriage "by definition" can only unite a man and a woman. Any attempt to extend it beyond heterosexuals would threaten and devalue the institution of marriage. Homosexual unions are abnormal, immoral, and unworthy of the law's protection.

COUNTERPOINT

All human beings should have the same fundamental rights. The fact that they were denied equality in the past does not justify continuing to treat lesbians and gays unfairly. Same-sex couples should have the same economic and civil rights guaranteed only in a legally recognized marriage such as heterosexual couples have.

YOUR VIEW

Should marriage be restricted to heterosexual couples? Should homosexual couples have the same recognition? Are committed relationships between gays or lesbians different or less deserving of legal protection than those between heterosexuals?

---

married men and women. Although there has not been much research on same-sex committed relationships, most experts believe that gay couples are likely to enjoy similar benefits, as long as they remain together and receive social support for doing so.

For years researchers thought that marriage was especially beneficial to men. Married men have lower rates of alcohol and drug abuse, depression, and risk-taking behavior than divorced men. They also earn more money—possibly because they have more incentive to do so. However, more recent research indicates that a happy marriage boosts mental health and well-being in both spouses.

Same-Sex Marriage

Same-sex marriage, also called gay or single-sex or gender-neutral marriage, refers to a governmentally, socially, or religiously recognized marriage in which two people of the same sex live together as a family. Several countries, including Canada, the Netherlands, Belgium, and Spain have legitimized same-sex marriages. The state of Massachusetts recognizes same-sex marriages. Several other states recognize domestic partnerships and civil unions that grant some of the legal and economic benefits of marriage.

Same-sex marriages have triggered intense controversy. (See Point/Counterpoint: "Should Same-Sex Marriages Be Legal?") Some oppose gay unions on religious and moral grounds. Others argue that marriage is a right based on procreation and designed to protect the children of a man and a woman. Advocates of gay marriage contend that the ban on same-gender unions discriminates against homosexuals and denies them the same civil rights and legal protection as heterosexual couples.[22]

Issues Couples Confront

No two people can live together in perfect harmony all the time. Some of the issues that crop up in any long-term relationship include expectations, money, sex, and careers.

Unrealistic Expectations Partners may think that their significant others should always be as attractive, charming, and tolerant as they were when they were dating. They may assume that their partners will always agree with them or will automatically see their point of view; or they may believe that their one true love will always be able to meet all their needs. Because no one could ever live up to such expectations, the partners are doomed to disappointment.

Togetherness does not necessarily guarantee happiness. According to one study of more than 2,000 couples, too much time together—particularly doing shopping and chores—may be bad for a marriage.

Money Money may make the business world go around, but it has the opposite effect on relationships: It knocks them off their tracks, brings them to a halt, twists them upside down. However, even though almost all couples quarrel about money, they rarely fight over how much they have. What matters more—whether they make $10,000 or $100,000 a year—is what money means to both part-

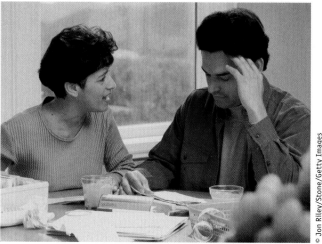

Fight fair. You can learn to argue effectively, without attacking others or damaging relationships.

© Jon Riley/Stone/Getty Images

ners. How does each person use money to meet emotional needs? Who decides how the money is spent? Who keeps track? Until they resolve these issues, couples may quarrel over money as long as they're together.

To avoid fighting over money, understand that having different money values or expectations doesn't make one of you right and the other wrong. Recognize the value of unpaid work. A partner who's finishing school or taking care of the children is making an important contribution to the family and its future. It also helps to go over your finances together so that you have a firm basis in reality for what you can and can't afford. Talk about the financial goals you hope to attain five years from now. Set priorities to meet them. Also, set aside money for each of you to spend without asking or answering to the other. Even a small amount can make each partner feel more independent.

Sex Like every other aspect of a relationship, sex evolves and changes over the course of marriage. The redhot sexual chemistry of the early stages of intimacy invariably cools down. Even so, the happiest couples have sex more often than unhappily married pairs do.

What matters most isn't quantity alone, but the quality of sexual activity and intimacy. Are both partners satisfied with their sexual relationship? Does one partner always initiate sex? Do the partners talk about their preferences and pleasures? Sexuality, like personality, is dynamic and changes throughout life. Do the partners acknowledge and adapt to these changes? Do they feel sufficiently at ease with each other to discuss anxieties about sex? The answers to these questions can determine how sexually gratifying a marriage is for both spouses.

Extramarital Affairs How faithful are American mates? The answer depends on the questions researchers ask and who they ask. In face-to-face interviews, University of Chicago researchers found that 25 percent of men and 15 percent of women had had affairs and that 94 percent of the married subjects had been monogamous in the last year. Another survey of Americans found that one out of six Americans had had an extramarital relationship—19 percent of the men and 15 percent of the women.[23]

High or low, numbers are little comfort when affairs do occur. A husband or wife who learns about a spouse's affair typically feels a devastating sense of betrayal as well as deep feelings of shame, fear of abandonment, depression, and anger. Two crucial questions determine whether a marriage can survive: Do the spouses still feel a serious commitment to each other? And do they love each other and want to remain together?

Two-Career Couples More than 75 percent of women with children work—a dramatic increase from the 1960s, when only 30 percent of mothers worked outside the home. Two careers can bring pressure to a relationship: Both individuals may come home tired and irritable;

both may have to spend a great deal of time on their jobs; both may have to travel or work on weekends. Two-career couples must be able to discuss their problems openly to resolve these pressures.

Couples pursuing individual careers sometimes face difficult choices. What happens, for example, if one of them is offered a promising job in another city? Does the spouse quit his or her job, pack up, and move? Some couples resolve such dilemmas by working in different cities and spending weekends together. Others try to alternate career and home priorities. However imperfect these arrangements may be, they work for some couples.

Conflict in Marriage

While all couples may wish to live happily and peacefully ever after, sooner or later, they argue. Years of research have shown that while conflict is inevitable, the key difference between happy and unhappy couples is the way they fight.

Happier couples interject positive interactions, like a joke or a smile, into their arguments. As long as the ratio of positive to negative interactions remains at least five to one, the relationship remains intact. By comparison, unhappy couples unfurl a barrage of negative words, gestures, criticisms, and hostility at their mates with hardly any positive interactions. Based on observations of couples in conflict, researchers have been able to predict which would divorce with 94 percent accuracy.[24]

Although many assume that women are more nurturing than men, research on married couples at the University of Toledo has found that husbands can be as emotionally sensitive and supportive as wives. However, their timing tends to be off.[25] "Men aren't oblivious," says researcher Lisa Neff, "but wives need to communicate their needs directly to their husbands."

Among the other suggestions therapists offer couples are:

- **Focus on friendship.** If a marriage is not built on a strong friendship, it may be difficult to stay connected over time.

- **Remember what you loved and admired in your partner in the first place.** Focusing on these qualities can foster a much more positive attitude toward him or her.

- **Show respect.** Your spouse deserves the same courtesy and civility that your colleagues do. Without respect, love cannot survive.

same-sex marriage Governmentally, socially, or religiously recognized marriage in which two people of the same sex live together as a family.

- **Compliment what your partner does right.** Noticing the positive can change how both of you feel about each other.

- **Forgive one another.** When your partner hurts your feelings but then reaches out, don't reject his or her attempts to make things better.

Saving Marriages

Fewer than two-thirds of couples—65 percent of husbands and 60 percent of wives—say they are "very happy" in their marriages. Each year, hundreds of thousands of couples go into counseling in an effort to make their unions happier. Among the approaches currently in use are marriage education and various forms of couples therapy.

Marriage education consists of workshops that teach couples practical skills so they get along better. Some studies indicate that graduates of these programs have a lower divorce rate than unhappy couples who do not enroll in them.

Couples therapy, also called marriage counseling or marriage therapy, uses a variety of psychological techniques to help couples understand and overcome their conflicts. These include:

- **Behavioral marital therapy,** which teaches partners to communicate better and to improve their conflict resolution skills.

- **Emotionally focused therapy,** which helps couples identify and break free of destructive emotional cycles.

- **Insight-oriented marital therapy,** which combines behavioral therapy with techniques for understanding negative behaviors, such as power struggles, within the relationship.

Divorce

According to the most recent U.S. Census Bureau data, 2,230,000 marriages occur every year. The marriage rate now stands at 7.5 per 1,000 Americans. The divorce rate is almost 50 percent: 3.6 per 1,000 Americans.[26] Your risk of divorce depends on many factors. Simply having some college education improves your odds of a happy marriage. Other factors that do the same are an income higher than $50,000, marrying at age 25 or older, not having a baby during the first seven months after the wedding, coming from an intact family, and having some religious affiliation.

 Race also influences marriage and divorce rates. African American couples are more likely to break up than white couples, and black divorcées are less likely to marry again. Researchers have found that African Americans place an equally high value on marriage. However, there is a smaller "marriageable pool" of black men for a variety of reasons, including a higher mortality rate.

Children whose parents divorced are less likely to marry and to stay married. However, their adult relationships aren't doomed to fail. "Divorce isn't in the genes," says child psychologist Judith Wallerstein, who has studied divorced families for thirty years. "Divorce is an avoidable human error."

Family Ties

Children have become the exception rather than the rule in American households. A century ago most households contained children under age 18. In 1960, slightly fewer than half did. In 2000, fewer than a third of households included children, and this figure is expected to drop to 28 percent by 2010 (Figure 8.3).

Attitudes also have changed. While many traditionally viewed having children as the primary purpose for getting married, nearly 70 percent of Americans now cite another reason. When young adults—ages 18 to 34—react to the statement, "Those who want children should get married," only about half of men and even fewer women agree.

Fertility has declined in the United States since 1960. At that time, the average woman had about three and one-

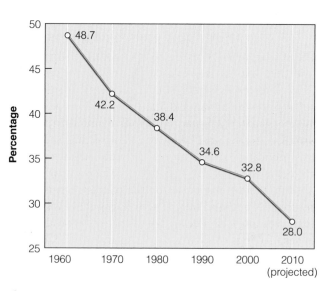

Figure 8.3 Percentage of Households with a Child or Children Under Age 18 (United States)

Source: Poponoe, David, and Barbara Dafoe Whitehead. *The State of Our Union: The Social Health of Marriage in America in 2005.* Copyright 2005 by the National Marriage Project at Rutgers University. Reprinted by permission of the National Marriage Project. http://marriage.rutgers.edu.

half children over the course of her life. Today's woman has an average of about two children, which is lower than the "replacement level" of 2.1 children per woman. This is the level at which the population would be replaced by births alone. In most European and several Asian countries, fertility has dropped even lower.

Diversity Within Families

Families have become as diverse as the American population and reflect different traditions, beliefs, and values. Within African American families, for instance, traditional gender roles are often reversed, with women serving as head of the household, a kinship bond uniting several households, and a strong religious commitment or orientation. In Chinese American families, both spouses may work and see themselves as breadwinners, but the wife may not have an equal role in decision making. In Hispanic families, wives and mothers are acknowledged and respected as healers and dispensers of wisdom. At the same time, they are expected to defer to their husbands, who see themselves as the strong, protective, dominant head of the family. As time passes and families from different cultures become more integrated into American life, traditional gender roles and decision-making patterns often change, particularly among the youngest family members.

American families are diverse in other ways. *Multigenerational families,* with children, parents, and grandparents, make up 3.7 percent of households. They occur most often in areas where new immigrants live with relatives, where housing shortages or high costs force families to double up their living arrangements, or where high rates of out-of-wedlock childbearing force unwed mothers to live with their children in their parents' home.

Three of every ten households consist of **blended families,** formed when one or both of the partners bring children from a previous union. In the future, social scientists predict, American families will become even more diverse, or pluralistic. But as norms or expectations about the configurations of families have changed, values or ideas about the intents and purposes of families have not. American families of every type still support each other and strive toward values such as commitment and caring.

Working Parents

The traditional family with a breadwinner and a homemaker has been replaced by what some call "the juggler family." Two working parents or an unmarried working parent head 70 percent of American families with chil-

dren. As a result, American parents have fewer hours to spend with their children. Women, balancing multiple roles as parents, spouses, caregivers, and employees often give their own personal needs the lowest priority.

The Family and Work Institute of New York calculates that American husbands put in 75 percent as much time as wives on workday chores—a dramatic rise from 30 percent in 1977. In actual clocktime, the gender difference in domestic "scutwork" amounts to just 45 minutes a day.

Plenty of sociologists—and lots of weary women still doing the lioness's share of chores—doubt whether all men in all income groups are doing as much. However, the trend toward greater husbandly involvement is real—and likely to continue.

Single Parents

About 35 percent of births—up from 5 percent a half-century ago—occur outside of marriage.[27] About 28 percent of all children under age 18 live with just one parent, the majority with their mothers. The number of families headed by single mothers has increased 25 percent since 1990, to more than 7.5 million households.

The new breed of single mother doesn't fit the old stereotype of an unwed, minority teenager. The median age for unmarried mothers is the late 20s; the fastest growing group is white women. She may be divorced or unmarried. Forty percent live with men who may be the fathers of one or more of their children.

Single fathers head over two million households. The typical single father is 38 years old. One in 9 is under age 25; and 1 in 70 is 60 or older. About 5 of every 6 (83 percent) of the nation's single fathers are white. African Americans and Hispanics together constitute about 13 percent.

Median family income for one-parent families is significantly lower than the median for two-parent families. Twenty percent are poor, compared with 9 percent of two-parent families. Half live in rental housing, compared with one-quarter of two-parent families.

family A group of people united by marriage, blood, or adoption; residing in the same household; maintaining a common culture; and interacting with one another on the basis of their roles within the group.

blended family A family formed when one or both of the partners bring children from a previous union to the new marriage.

Learn It : Live It

Creating Better Relationships

We are born social. From our first days of life, we reach out to others, struggle to express ourselves, strive to forge connections. The fabric of our lives becomes richer as family and friends weave through it the threads of their experiences. No solitary pleasure can match the gifts that we gain by reaching out and connecting with others.

As with other significant endeavors, good relationships require work—through hard times, despite conflicts, over months and years and decades. As you strive to improve the ties that bind you to others, keep in mind the characteristics of a good relationship. They can serve as the goals you strive to attain:

- **Trust.** Partners are able to confide in each other openly, knowing their confidences will be respected.
- **Togetherness.** In a healthy relationship, two people create a sense of both intimacy and autonomy. They enjoy each other's company but also pursue solitary interests.
- **Expressiveness.** Partners in healthy relationships say what they feel, need, and desire.

- **Staying power.** People in committed relationships keep their bond strong through tough times by proving that they will be there for each other.
- **Security.** Because a good relationship is strong enough to absorb conflict and anger, partners know they can express their feelings honestly. They also are willing to risk vulnerability for the sake of becoming closer.
- **Laughter.** Humor keeps things in perspective—always crucial in any sort of ongoing relationship or enterprise.
- **Support.** Partners in good relationships continually offer each other encouragement, comfort, and acceptance.
- **Physical affection.** Sexual desire may fluctuate or diminish over the years, but partners in loving, long-term relationships usually retain some physical connection.
- **Personal growth.** In the best relationships, partners are committed to bringing out the best in each other and have the other's best interests at heart.
- **Respect.** Caring partners are aware of each other's boundaries, need for personal space, and vulnerabilities. They do not take each other or their relationship for granted.

SELFSURVEY : *How Strong Are the Communication and Affection in Your Relationship?*

Effective, caring communication and loving affection markedly enhance a couple's relationship. The following self-test may help you to assess the degree of good communication, love, and respect in your intimate relationship. If you agree or mostly agree with a statement, answer yes. If you disagree or mostly disagree, answer no. You may wish to have your partner respond to this assessment as well. If so, mark your answers on a separate sheet.

	Yes	No
1. My partner seeks out my opinion.	Yes	No
2. My partner cares about my feelings.	Yes	No
3. I don't feel ignored very often.	Yes	No
4. We touch each other a lot.	Yes	No
5. We listen to each other.	Yes	No
6. We respect each other's ideas.	Yes	No
7. We are affectionate toward one another.	Yes	No
8. I feel my partner takes good care of me.	Yes	No
9. What I say counts.	Yes	No
10. I am important in our decisions.	Yes	No
11. There's lots of love in our relationship.	Yes	No
12. We are genuinely interested in one another.	Yes	No
13. I love spending time with my partner.	Yes	No
14. We are very good friends.	Yes	No

15. Even during rough times, we can be empathetic.	Yes	No
16. My partner is considerate of my viewpoint.	Yes	No
17. My partner finds me physically attractive.	Yes	No
18. My partner expresses warmth toward me.	Yes	No
19. I feel included in my partner's life.	Yes	No
20. My partner admires me.	Yes	No

Scoring:

A preponderance of yes answers indicates that you enjoy a strong relationship characterized by good communication and loving affection. If you answered yes to fewer than seven items, it is likely that you are not feeling loved and respected and that the communication in your relationship is decidedly lacking.

Source: John Gottman, *Why Marriages Succeed or Fail*. New York: Simon & Schuster, 1994.

Your Health Action Plan For Improving Your Relationships

Being in a relationship should be an opportunity for fun, personal growth, and mutual support, never an excuse for hurting or controlling someone else. The following guidelines can help keep a relationship healthy:

- **Recognize that both people in the relationship have the right to be accepted** as they are, to be treated with respect, to feel safe, to ask for what they want, to say no without feeling guilty, to express themselves, to give and receive affection, and to make some mistakes and be forgiven.

- **Remember that no one in a relationship has the right to force the other to do anything,** to tell the other where or when to speak up or go out, to humiliate the other in public or private, to isolate the other from friends and family, to read personal material without permission, to pressure the other to give up goals or interests, or to abuse the other person verbally or physically.

- **Be willing to open up.** The more you share, the deeper the bond between you and your friend will become.

- **Be sensitive to your friend's or partner's feelings.** Keep in mind that, like you, he or she has unique needs, desires, and dreams.

- **Express appreciation.** Be generous with your compliments. Let your friends and family know you recognize their kindnesses.

- **Know that people will disappoint you from time to time.** We are only human. Accept your loved ones as they are. Admitting their faults need not reduce your respect for them.

- **Talk about your relationship.** If you have any gripes or frustrations, air them.

CENGAGENOW If you want to write your own goals for enhanced relationship, go to the Wellness Journal at HealthNow: **academic.cengage.com/login**

Making This Chapter Work
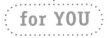
for YOU

Review Questions

1. In friendships and other intimate relationships, which of the following is *not* true?
   a. Friends can communicate feelings as well as facts.
   b. Listening is just as important as talking.
   c. Emotional investment is required but the rewards are great.
   d. There is no need to pay attention to nonverbal communication.

2. Which of the following scenarios demonstrates what might be considered gender differences in verbal and nonverbal communication styles?
   a. While Alyssa and Peter are discussing their vacation plans, Alyssa is gazing at the television and Peter is looking at Alyssa.
   b. Good friends Eva and Julia see each other for the first time after Christmas break and greet each other with a nod and a quick "Hi."
   c. New bank manager Alejandro tells the staff that they should consider him "the team coach and the keeper of the playbook."
   d. During an argument, Tony complains to Nicki, "I don't appreciate your crude jokes and constant swearing."

3. Romantic love
   a. is associated with the depletion of the hormone oxytocin.
   b. is an emotional phenomenon between humans that has its roots in prehistoric times and occurs in almost all cultures.
   c. can only occur between people who share interests and goals.
   d. always results in a committed long-term relationship.

4. The characteristics of a good relationship include which of the following?
   a. trust
   b. financial stability
   c. identical interests
   d. physical attractiveness

5. Which of these is an example of self-disclosure?
   a. Steve tells his friend Twana that he would really like to change jobs sometime in the next year.
   b. Mike and Nicole talk about which cars they prefer.
   c. Maria mentions to Carrie that she and her brother don't get along so he won't be at the picnic.
   d. Angela lets her boyfriend Paul know that she used to be bulimic.

6. Which of the following is more likely a sign of a dysfunctional relationship?
   a. The partners have frequent disagreements about money.
   b. One partner makes all the decisions for the couple and the other partner.
   c. Each partner has a demanding career.
   d. One partner is much older than the other partner.

7. Partners in successful marital relationships
   a. are generally from the same social and ethnic background.
   b. usually lived together before marrying.
   c. were usually very young at the time of their marriage.
   d. have premarital agreements.

8. Married people
   a. have sex less frequently than unmarried partners.
   b. are more likely to become alcoholics and drug users.
   c. typically have at least one extramarital affair during their marriage.
   d. live longer than single or divorced individuals.

9. Some disagreement is part of every relationship. Here's a good communication method when arguing:
   a. Ignore the subject of the disagreement.
   b. Make fun of your partner's point of view.
   c. Keep your partner's good qualities in mind.
   d. Vent about every misunderstanding over the past two years.

10. Which of the following statements is *false*?
    a. College education increases your chances of a happy marriage.
    b. African American couples are more likely to divorce than white couples.
    c. Children whose parents divorced are more likely to stay married.
    d. The divorce rate is lower now than it was in 1980.

Answers to these questions can be found on page 583.

Critical Thinking

1. Reread the section on Personal Communication in this chapter, and think about your own communication skills. How does your communication style compare to the patterns for your gender? Do your personal experiences support or contradict the research results?

2. While our society has become more tolerant, marriages between people of different religious and racial groups still face special pressures. What issues might arise if a Christian marries a Jew or Muslim? What about the issues facing partners of different races? How could these issues be resolved? What are your own feelings about mixed marriages? Would you date someone of a different religion or race? Why or why not?

3. What are your personal criteria for a successful relationship? Develop a brief list of factors you consider important, and support your choices with examples or experiences from your own life.

Chapter 8 • COMMUNICATING AND RELATING 233

Media Menu

INTERNET CONNECTIONS

Go Ask Alice

www.goaskalice.columbia.edu

Sponsored by the health education and wellness program of the Columbia University Health Service, this site features educators' answers to questions on a wide variety of topics, including those related to relationships and marriage and family.

Family and relationship articles from the APA

www.apahelpcenter.org/articles/topic.php?id=2

The American Psychological Association provides a wealth of articles and information on sustaining healthy relationships.

Parenting and Families—information from the University of Minnesota's Children, Youth, and Family Consortium

www.cyfc.umn.edu/family/index.html

This site offers research, programs, publications, and information on all types of parenting, relationships, and family issues.

Key Terms

The terms listed are used and defined on the page indicated. Definitions are also found in the Glossary at the end of this book.

blended families 229
codependency 217
cohabitation 223
companion-oriented marriages 225
dysfunctional 215
enabling 219
family 229
intimacy 219
rescue marriages 225
romantic marriages 225
same-sex marriages 227
self-disclosure 215
traditional marriages 225

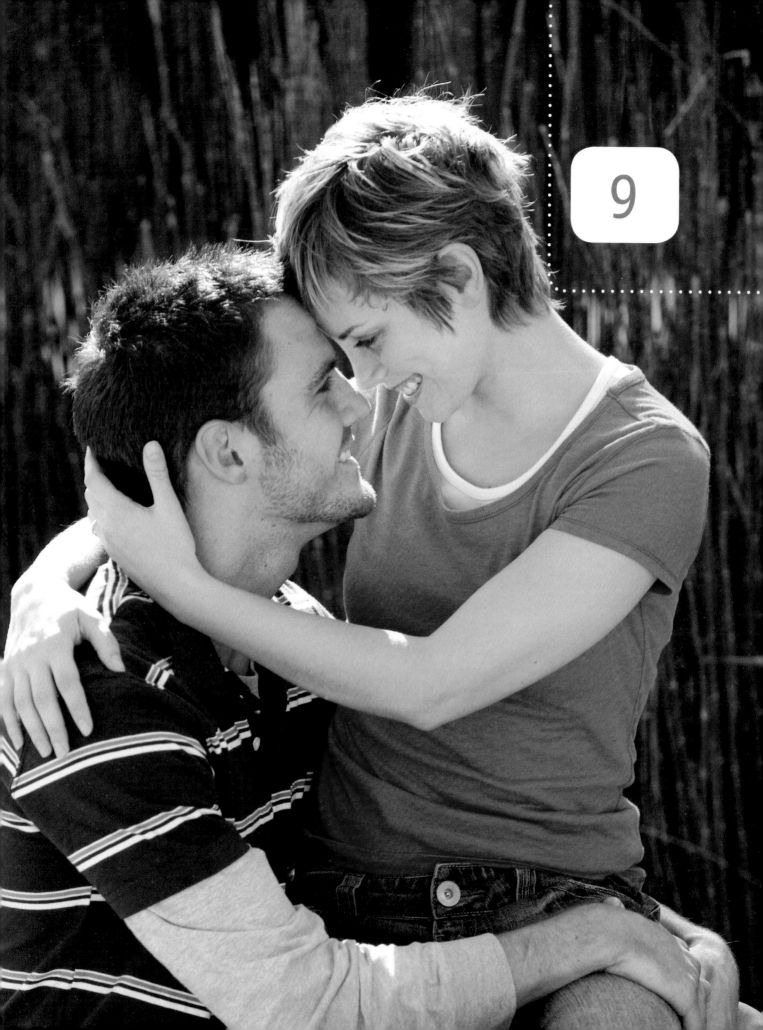

Personal Sexuality

CHARLES, several years older than the typical college freshman, usually doesn't think much about the age difference—until the conversation turns to sex. He understands his younger classmates' seemingly endless fascination with sex, but his perspective is different. As a teenager, he had plunged recklessly into dangerous territory of every type. Sex—casual and sometimes unprotected—was one of them. Looking back, he feels lucky that he didn't, as he puts it, "end up a statistic." But he still regrets the irresponsible ways he acted.

At 28 Charles is a veteran of military service, a married man, and an expectant father. His enjoyment of sex hasn't faded—in many ways, it's deepened and become more gratifying. He now realizes that there is no such thing as casual sex, that sexual choices have consequences and effects on one's own life and on other people. These are the lessons he hopes someday to pass on to his own children.

As Charles learned with time and experience, you are ultimately responsible for your sexual health and behavior. You make decisions that affect how you express your sexuality, how you respond sexually, and how you give and get sexual pleasure. Yet most sexual activity involves another person. Therefore, your decisions about sex—more so than those you make about nutrition, drugs, or exercise—have important effects on other people. Recognizing this fact is the key to responsible sexuality.

Sexual responsibility means learning about your body, your partner's body, your sexual development and preferences, and the health risks associated with sexual activity. This chapter is an introduction to your sexual self and an exploration of sexual issues in today's world. It provides the information and insight you can use in making decisions and choosing behaviors that are responsible for all concerned.

After studying the material in this chapter, you should be able to:

- **Explain** the roles of hormones in sexual development.
- **Describe** the male and female reproductive systems and the functions of the individual structures of each system.
- **Describe** conditions or issues unique to women's and men's sexual health.
- **Define** sexual health and list behaviors that can contribute to sexually healthy relationships.
- **Define** sexual orientation and **give examples** of sexual diversity.
- **List** the range of sexual behaviors practiced by adults.
- **Describe** the phases of sexual response.
- **List** the common sexual concerns of men and women.
- **Evaluate** your ability to communicate about sex with a potential partner.

CENGAGENOW Log on to HealthNow at **academic.cengage.com/login** to find your Behavior Change Planner and to explore self-assessments, interactive tutorials, and practice quizzes.

Human **sexuality**—the quality of being sexual—is as rich, varied, and complex as life itself. Along with our **sex,** or biological maleness or femaleness, it is an integral part of who we are, how we see ourselves, and how we relate to others. Of all of our involvements with others, sexual **intimacy,** or physical closeness, can be the most rewarding. But while sexual expression and experience can provide intense joy, they also can involve great emotional turmoil.

Sexuality and the Dimensions of Health

Our sexuality both affects and is affected by the various dimensions of health. Responsible sexuality and high-level **sexual health** contribute to the fullest possible functioning of body, mind, spirit, and social relationships. In turn, other aspects of health enhance our sexuality. Here are some examples:

- **Physical.** As described in Chapter 15, safer sex practices reduce the risk of sexually transmitted infections that can threaten sexual health, physical health, and even survival. When our bodies are healthy and well, we feel better about how we look and move—which enhances both self-esteem and healthy sexuality.

- **Emotional.** By acknowledging and respecting the intimacy of a sexual relationship, responsible sexuality builds trust and commitment. When our emotional health is high, we can better understand and cope with the complex feelings related to being sexual.

- **Social.** From dating to mating, we express and fulfill our sexual identities in the context of families, friends, and society as a whole. Having strong friendships, intimate relationships, and caring partnerships enables us to explore our sexuality in safe and healthy ways.

- **Intellectual.** Our most fulfilling relationships involve a meeting of minds as well as bodies. High-level intellectual health enables us to acquire and understand sexual information, analyze it critically, and make healthy sexual decisions.

- **Spiritual.** At its deepest, most fulfilling level, sexuality uplifts the soul by allowing us to connect to something greater than oneself. Individuals who have developed their spirituality bring to their most intimate relationships an awareness and appreciation that lifts them beyond the physical.

- **Environmental.** Responsible sexuality makes people more aware of the impact of their decisions on others. Protecting yourself from sexual threats and creating a supportive environment in which to study and work are crucial to high-level health and to healthy sexuality.

Becoming Male or Female

Physiological maleness or femaleness, or biological sex, is indicated by the sex chromosomes, hormonal balance, and genital anatomy. **Gender** refers to the psychological and sociological, as well as the physical, aspects of being male or female. You are born with a certain *sexual identity* based on your sexual anatomy and appearance; you, your parents, and society mold your *gender identity*.

Are You an X or a Y?

Biologically, few absolute differences separate the sexes: Males alone can make sperm and contribute the chromosome that causes embryos to develop as males; females alone are born with sex cells (eggs, or ova), menstruate, give birth, and breast-feed babies. But the process of becoming male or female is a long and complex one.

In the beginning, all human embryos have undifferentiated sex organs. Only after several weeks do the sex organs differentiate, becoming either male or female *gonads* (testes or ovaries), the structures that produce the future reproductive cells of an individual. This initial differentiation process depends on genetic instructions in the form of the sex chromosomes, referred to as X and Y. If a Y (or male) chromosome is present in the embryo, about seven weeks after conception, it signals the sex organs to develop into testes. If a Y chromosome isn't present, an embryo begins developing ovaries in the eighth week. From this point on, the sex hormones produced by the gonads, not the chromosomes, play the crucial role in making a male or female.

How Hormones Work

In Greek, *hormone* means "set into motion"—and that's exactly what our **hormones** do. These chemical messengers, produced by various organs in the body, including the sex organs, and carried to target structures by the bloodstream, arouse cells and organs to specific activities and influence the way we look, feel, develop, and behave.

The group of organs that produce hormones is referred to as the **endocrine system.** Except for the sex organs, males and females have identical endocrine systems. Directing the endocrine system is the *hypothalamus,* a pea-sized section of the brain. The pituitary gland, directly beneath the hypothalamus, turns the various glands on and off in response to messages from it.

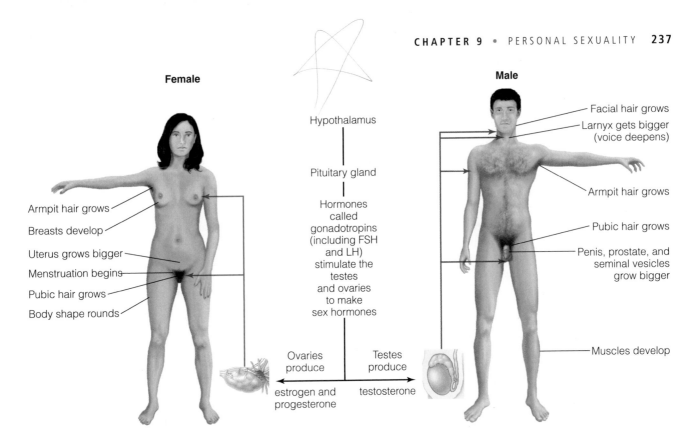

Figure 9.1 Puberty

The body's endocrine system produces hormones that trigger body changes, including growth spurts, in boys and girls.

The ovaries produce the sex hormones most crucial to women, **estrogen** and **progesterone.** The primary sex hormone in men is **testosterone,** which is produced by the testes and the adrenal glands. However, both men and women have small amounts of the hormones of the opposite sex. Estrogen, in fact, is crucial to male fertility and gives sperm what researchers describe as their "reproductive punch."

The sex hormones begin their work early in an embryo's development. As soon as the testes are formed, they start releasing testosterone, which stimulates the development of other structures, such as the penis. The absence of testosterone in an embryo causes female genitals to form. (If the testes of a genetic male don't produce testosterone, the fetus will develop female genitals. Similarly, if a genetic female is exposed to excessive testosterone, the fetus will have ovaries but will also develop male genitals.)

As puberty begins, the pituitary gland initiates the changes that transform boys into men and girls into women (Figure 9.1). When a boy is about 14 years old and a girl about 12, their brains stimulate the hypothalamus to secrete a hormone called *gonadotropin-releasing hormone (GnRH).* This substance causes the pituitary gland to release hormones called **gonadotropins.** These, in turn, stimulate the gonads to make sex hormones.

The gonadotropins are *follicle-stimulating hormone (FSH)* and *luteinizing hormone (LH).* In girls, these hormones travel to the ovary and stimulate the production of estrogen. As estrogen increases, a girl's **secondary sex characteristics**

develop. Her breasts become fuller, her external genitals enlarge, and fat is deposited on her hips and buttocks. Estrogen keeps her hair thick and skin smooth. She begins menstruating because she has begun ovulating, the process that prepares her body to conceive and carry a baby.

sexuality The behaviors, instincts, and attitudes associated with being sexual.

sex Maleness or femaleness, resulting from genetic, structural, and functional factors.

intimacy A state of closeness between two people, characterized by the desire and ability to share one's innermost thoughts and feelings with each other either verbally or nonverbally.

sexual health The integration of the physical, emotional, intellectual, social, and spiritual aspects of sexual being in ways that are positively enriching and that enhance personality, communication, and love.

gender Maleness or femaleness, as determined by a combination of anatomical and physiological factors, psychological factors, and learned behaviors.

hormone Substance released in the blood that regulates specific bodily functions.

endocrine system The group of ductless glands that produce hormones and secrete them directly into the blood for transport to target organs.

estrogen The female sex hormone that stimulates female secondary sex characteristics.

progesterone The female sex hormone that stimulates the uterus, preparing it for the arrival of a fertilized egg.

testosterone The male sex hormone that stimulates male secondary sex characteristics.

gonadotropins Gonad-stimulating hormones produced by the pituitary gland.

secondary sex characteristics Physical changes associated with maleness or femaleness, induced by the sex hormones.

This process seems to be beginning earlier than in the past. "By eight, 15 percent of white girls and 48 percent of African American girls show signs of sexual development," says Marcia Herman-Giddens, Ph.D., of the University of North Carolina at Chapel Hill, who analyzed 17,077 growth charts from pediatricians around the country. In her study, the mean ages for breast development were 8.87 years for African American girls and 9.96 years for white girls. African American girls reach **menarche**—the term for first menstruation—at a mean age of 12.16 years; white girls, at 12.88 years. By comparison, a hundred years ago girls didn't reach menarche until the relatively ripe age of fifteen.[1]

Improved nutrition and good health seem to be the primary factors. Girls today are bigger, taller, better fed, more sedentary, and have a higher percentage of body fat (one of the triggers of sexual maturation). They also grow up amid a host of environmental influences that may further speed development.

Cultural influences affect a girl's response to menarche. In a cross-cultural study of college students, the most common emotions expressed by American women at menarche were embarrassment, pride, and anxiety. Malaysian women cited fear, embarrassment, and worry. Lithuanian women described themselves as happy or scared, while Sudanese women cited fear, anxiety, embarrassment, and anger. On the positive side, the Lithuanian women reported feeling more valuable and believing they had entered the world of women. American girls worried about whether they could still play sports but felt superior to friends who had not reached menarche and became eager to learn about sex. Malaysians described feeling wise, respected, and mature. Sudanese women felt more beautiful and aware that they could now have children.

In boys, the gonadotropins stimulate the testes to produce testosterone, which triggers the development of male secondary sex characteristics. Their voices deepen, hair grows on their faces and bodies, their penises become thicker and longer, and their muscles become stronger.

The sex hormones released during puberty change the growth pattern of childhood, so that a boy or girl may now spurt up 4 to 6 inches in a single year. The skeleton matures very rapidly until, at the end of puberty (usually around age 18), the growth centers at the ends of the bones close off. Estrogen causes girls' bones to stop growing at an earlier age than boys' bones.

Sexual and Gender Identity

It's a boy! It's a girl! These statements confer an instant identity on a newborn. However, in recent years, researchers have challenged such either/or distinctions as male or female, masculine or feminine, heterosexual or homosexual. Although most people have the biological characteristics of a male or a female, some possess some degree of both male and female reproductive structures. They are referred to as intersexual.

The continuum for gender identity ranges from extreme stereotypical masculine notions to extreme stereotypical feminine behaviors. Different cultures vary in defining what is masculine or feminine. Individuals who consider themselves androgynous choose not to conform to sexual stereotypes. **Androgyny** includes those who are "positively androgynous," combining positive attributes linked with both sexes, for example, feminine compassion and masculine independence and individuals who are "negatively androgynous" and might show less desirable characteristics of each gender, such as feminine dependency and masculine assertiveness. (Transgenderism is discussed on page 123.)

Women's Sexual Health

Only recently has medical research devoted major scientific investigations to issues in women's health. Until about a decade ago, the National Institutes of Health routinely excluded women from experimental studies because of concerns about menstrual cycles and pregnancy. In clinical settings, women are more likely to have their symptoms dismissed as psychological and not to be referred to a specialist than are men with identical complaints. Some physicians are suggesting the creation of a new medical specialty (distinct from obstetrics and gynecology) that would be devoted to women's health.

Female Sexual Anatomy

As illustrated in Figure 9.2a, the **mons pubis** is the rounded, fleshy area over the junction of the pubic bones. The folds of skin that form the outer lips of a woman's genital area are called the **labia majora.** They cover soft flaps of skin (inner lips) called the **labia minora.** The inner lips join at the top to form a hood over the **clitoris,** a small elongated erectile organ, and the most sensitive spot in the entire female genital area. Below the clitoris is the **urethral opening,** the outer opening of the thin tube that carries urine from the bladder. Below that is a larger

---

menarche The onset of menstruation at puberty.

androgyny The expression of both masculine and feminine traits.

mons pubis The rounded, fleshy area over the junction of the female pubic bones.

labia majora The fleshy outer folds that border the female genital area.

labia minora The fleshy inner folds that border the female genital area.

clitoris A small erectile structure on the female, corresponding to the penis on the male.

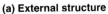

(a) External structure

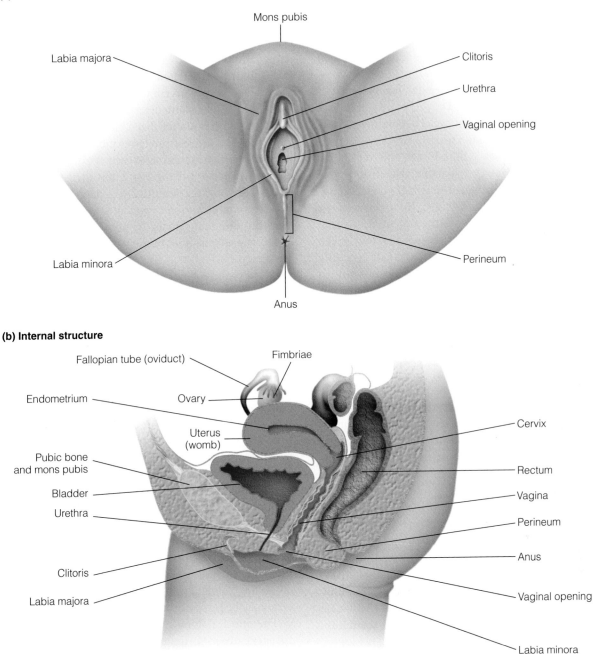

Mons pubis

Labia majora

Clitoris

Urethra

Vaginal opening

Perineum

Labia minora

Anus

(b) Internal structure

Fallopian tube (oviduct)

Fimbriae

Endometrium

Ovary

Uterus (womb)

Cervix

Pubic bone and mons pubis

Rectum

Bladder

Vagina

Urethra

Perineum

Anus

Clitoris

Vaginal opening

Labia majora

Labia minora

Figure 9.2   The Female Sex Organs and Reproductive Structures

opening, the mouth of the **vagina,** the canal that leads to the primary internal organs of reproduction. The **perineum** is the area between the vagina and the anus (the opening to the rectum and large intestine).

At the back of the vagina is the **cervix,** the opening to the womb, or **uterus** (see Figure 9.2b). The uterine walls are lined by a layer of tissue called the **endometrium.** The **ovaries,** about the size and shape of almonds, are located on either

urethral opening   The outer opening of the thin tube that carries urine from the bladder.

vagina   The canal leading from the exterior opening in the female genital area to the uterus.

perineum   The area between the anus and vagina in the female and between the anus and scrotum in the male.

cervix   The narrow, lower end of the uterus that opens into the vagina.

uterus   The female organ that houses the developing fetus until birth.

endometrium   The mucous membrane lining the uterus.

ovary   The female sex organ that produces egg cells, estrogen, and progesterone.

side of the uterus and contain egg cells called **ova** (singular, **ovum**). Extending outward and back from the upper uterus are the **fallopian tubes,** the canals that transport ova from the ovaries to the uterus. When an egg is released from an ovary, the fingerlike ends of the adjacent fallopian tube "catch" the egg and direct it into the tube.

 Discharge and changes in odor normally occur in a healthy vagina. They typically fluctuate through the menstrual cycle, depending on hormone level. In the past, many women practiced douching, the introduction of a liquid into the vagina, to cleanse the vagina. However, particularly if done frequently, douching may increase the risk of pelvic inflammatory disease (discussed in Chapter 16) and ectopic or out-of-uterus pregnancy. Despite the potential dangers, according to data from a southern university, four in ten female students had douched in the past; half currently douche. African American women were encouraged to douche by their mothers; white women were more influenced by television advertisements. When advised to stop douching by a doctor or nurse, most students do so.

The Menstrual Cycle

Scientists have discovered that the menstrual cycle actually begins in the brain with the production of gonadotropin-releasing hormone (GnRH). Each month a surge of GnRH sets into motion the sequence of steps that lead to ovulation, the potential for conception, and if conception doesn't occur, menstruation. The hypothalamus monitors hormone levels in the blood and sends messages to the pituitary gland to release follicle-stimulating hormone (FSH) and luteinizing hormone (LH).

As shown in Figure 9.3, in the ovaries, these hormones stimulate the growth of a few of the immature eggs, or ova, stored in follicles in every woman's body. Usually, only one ovum matures completely during each monthly cycle. As it does, it increases its production of the female sex hormone estrogen, which in turn triggers the release of a larger surge of LH.

At midcycle, the increased LH hormone levels trigger **ovulation,** the release of the egg cell, or ovum, from the follicle. Estrogen levels drop, and the remaining cells of the follicle then enlarge, change character, and form the **corpus luteum,** or yellow body. In the second half of the menstrual cycle, the corpus luteum secretes estrogen and larger amounts of progesterone. The endometrium (uterine lining) is stimulated by progesterone to thicken and become more engorged with blood in preparation for nourishing an implanted, fertilized ovum.

If the ovum is not fertilized, the corpus luteum disintegrates. As the level of progesterone drops, **menstruation** occurs; the uterine lining is shed during the course of a menstrual period. If the egg is fertilized and pregnancy occurs, the cells that eventually develop into the placenta secrete *human chorionic gonadotropin (HCG)*, a messenger hormone that signals the pituitary not to start a new cycle. The corpus luteum then steps up its production of progesterone.

Many women experience physical or psychological changes, or both, during their monthly cycles. Usually the changes are minor, but more serious problems can occur. (See Your Strategies for Prevention: "How to Reduce Premenstrual Problems.")

Premenstrual Syndrome

Women with **premenstrual syndrome (PMS)** experience bodily discomfort and emotional distress for up to two weeks, from ovulation until the onset of menstruation. Up to 75 percent of menstruating women report one or more premenstrual symptoms; 3 to 9 percent experience disabling, incapacitating symptoms.

Once dismissed as a psychological problem, PMS has been recognized as a very real physiological disorder that may be caused by a hormonal deficiency; abnormal levels of thyroid hormone; an imbalance of estrogen and progesterone; or social and environmental factors, particularly stress. Recent studies indicate that PMS may originate in the brain. Changes in brain receptors during the ovarian cycle may be responsible.

The most common symptoms of PMS are mood changes, anxiety, irritability, difficulty concentrating, forgetfulness, impaired judgment, tearfulness, digestive symptoms (diarrhea, bloating, constipation), hot flashes, palpitations, dizziness, headache, fatigue, changes in appetite, cravings (usually for sweets or salt), water retention, breast tenderness, and insomnia. For a diagnosis to be made, women—using a self-rating symptom scale or calendar—must report troubling premenstrual symptoms in the period before menstruation in at least two successive menstrual cycles.

Treatments for PMS depend on specific symptoms. Diuretics (drugs that speed up fluid elimination) can relieve water retention and bloating. Relaxation techniques have led to a 60 percent reduction in anxiety symptoms. Sleep deprivation, or the use of bright light to adjust a woman's circadian or daily rhythm, also has proven

ovum (plural, **ova**) The female gamete (egg cell).

fallopian tubes The pair of channels that transport ova from the ovaries to the uterus; the usual site of fertilization.

ovulation The release of a mature ovum from an ovary approximately 14 days prior to the onset of menstruation.

corpus luteum A yellowish mass of tissue that is formed, immediately after ovulation, from the remaining cells of the follicle; it secretes estrogen and progesterone for the remainder of the menstrual cycle.

menstruation Discharge of blood from the vagina as a result of the shedding of the uterine lining at the end of the menstrual cycle.

premenstrual syndrome (PMS) A disorder that causes physical discomfort and psychological distress prior to a woman's menstrual period.

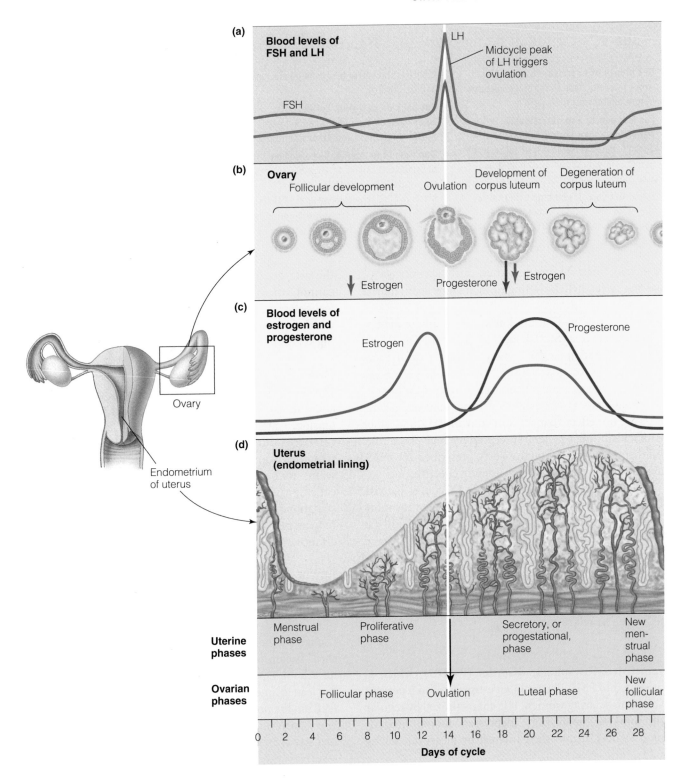

Figure 9.3 Menstrual Cycle

(a) In response to the hypothalamus, the pituitary gland releases the gonadotropins FSH and LH. Levels of FSH and LH stimulate the cycle (and in turn are affected by production of estrogen and progesterone).

(b) FSH does what its name says—it stimulates follicle development in the ovary. The follicle matures and ruptures, releasing an ovum (egg) into the fallopian tube.

(c) The follicle produces estrogen, and the corpus luteum produces estrogen and progesterone. The high level of estrogen at the middle of the cycle produces a surge of LH, which triggers ovulation.

(d) Estrogen and progesterone stimulate the endometrium, which becomes thicker and prepares to receive an implanted, fertilized egg.

If a fertilized egg is deposited in the uterus, pregnancy begins. If the egg is not fertilized, progesterone production decreases, and the endometrium is shed (menstruation). At this point, both estrogen and progesterone levels have dropped, so the pituitary responds by producing FSH, and the cycle begins again.

YOUR STRATEGIES FOR PREVENTION *How to Reduce Premenstrual Problems*

- **Get plenty of exercise.** Physically fit women usually have fewer problems both before and during their periods.

- **Eat frequently and nutritiously.** In the week before your period, your body doesn't regulate the levels of sugar, or glucose, in your blood as well as it usually does.

- **Swear off salt.** If you stop using salt at the table and while cooking, you may gain less weight premenstrually, feel less bloated, and suffer less from headaches and irritability.

- **Cut back on caffeine.** Coffee, colas, diet colas, chocolate, and tea can increase breast tenderness and other symptoms.

- **Don't drink or smoke.** Some women become so sensitive to alcohol's effects before their periods that a glass of wine hits with the impact of several stiff drinks. Nicotine worsens low blood sugar problems.

- **Watch out for sweets.** Premenstrual cravings for sweets are common, but try to resist. Sugar may pick you up, but later you'll feel worse than before.

- **Add more low-fat dairy products to your diet.** They can lower your risk of problems.

---

beneficial. Behavioral approaches, such as exercise or charting cycles, help by letting women know when they're vulnerable.

Low doses of medications known as *selective serotonin-reuptake inhibitors* (SSRIs), such as fluoxetine (marketed as Prozac, Sarafem, and in generic forms) provide relief for symptoms such as tension, depression, irritability, and mood swings, even when taken only during the premenstrual phase rather than daily throughout the month. SSRIs are not effective in all women with PMS, and other factors, including a genetic susceptibility, may play a role. Oral contraceptives, though widely prescribed for PMS, have not been shown to be consistently effective.

A diet rich in calcium and vitamin D reduces the risk of PMS. In recent studies that followed women for more than ten years, those whose daily diet included low-fat milk, yogurt, and other good calcium sources lowered their likelihood of PMS symptoms.[2] Other treatments with some reported success include calcium supplements; vitamins; exercise; less caffeine, alcohol, salt and sugar; acupuncture; and stress management techniques such as meditation or relaxation training.

Premenstrual Dysphoric Disorder

Premenstrual dysphoric disorder (PMDD), which is not related to PMS, occurs in an estimated 3 to 5 percent of all menstruating women. It is characterized by regular symptoms of depression (depressed mood, anxiety, mood swings, diminished interest or pleasure) during the last week of the menstrual cycle. Women with PMDD cannot function as usual at work, school, or home. They feel better a few days after menstruation begins. SSRIs, which are used to treat PMS, also are effective in relieving symptoms of PMDD.

Menstrual Cramps

Dysmenorrhea is the medical name for the discomforts—abdominal cramps and pain, back and leg pain, diarrhea, tension, water retention, fatigue, and depression—that can occur during menstruation. About half of all menstruating women suffer from dysmenorrhea. The cause seems to be an overproduction of bodily substances called prostaglandins, which typically rise during menstruation. Medications that inhibit prostaglandins can reduce menstrual pain, and exercise can also relieve cramps.

Amenorrhea

Women may stop menstruating—a condition called **amenorrhea**—for a variety of reasons, including a hormonal disorder, drastic weight loss, strenuous exercise, or change in the environment. "Boarding-school amenorrhea" is common among young women who leave home for school. Distance running and strenuous exercise also can lead to amenorrhea. The reason may be a drop in body fat from the normal range of 18 to 22 percent to a range of 9 to 12 percent. To be considered amenorrheic, a woman's menstrual cycle is typically absent for three or more consecutive months. Prolonged amenorrhea can have serious health consequences, including a loss of bone density that may lead to stress fractures or osteoporosis.

Scientists have developed chemical mimics, or analogues, of GnRH—usually administered by nasal spray—that trigger ovulation in women who don't ovulate or menstruate normally.

Toxic Shock Syndrome

This rare, potentially deadly bacterial infection primarily strikes menstruating women under the age of 30 who

---

premenstrual dysphoric disorder (PMDD) A disorder that causes symptoms of psychological depression during the last week of the menstrual cycle.

dysmenorrhea Painful menstruation.

amenorrhea The absence or suppression of menstruation.

toxic shock syndrome (TSS) A disease characterized by fever, vomiting, diarrhea, and often shock, caused by a bacterium that releases toxic waste products into the bloodstream.

penis The male organ of sex and urination.

scrotum The external sac or pouch that holds the testes.

testes (singular, **testis**) The male sex organs that produce sperm and testosterone.

A. External structure

B. Internal structure

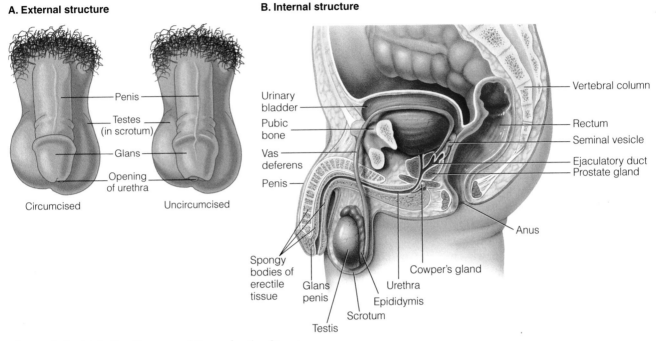

Figure 9.4 Male Sex Organs and Reproductive Structures

use tampons. Both *Staphylococcus aureus* and group A *Streptococcus pyogenes* can produce **toxic shock syndrome (TSS).** Symptoms include a high fever; a rash that leads to peeling of the skin on the fingers, toes, palms, and soles; dizziness; dangerously low blood pressure; and abnormalities in several organ systems (the digestive tract and the kidneys) and in the muscles and blood. Treatment usually consists of antibiotics and intense supportive care; intravenous administration of immunoglobulins that attack the toxins produced by these bacteria also may be beneficial.

Men's Sexual Health

Because the male reproductive system is simpler in many ways than the female, it's often ignored—especially by healthy young men. However, men should make regular self-exams (including checking their penises and testes, as described in Chapter 16) part of their routine.

Male Sexual Anatomy

The visible parts of the male sexual anatomy are the **penis** and the **scrotum,** the pouch that contains the **testes** (Figure 9.4). The testes manufacture testosterone, the hormone that stimulates the development of a male's secondary sex characteristics, and **sperm,** the male reproductive cells. Immature sperm are stored in the **epididymis,** a collection of coiled tubes adjacent to each testis.

The penis contains three hollow cylinders loosely covered with skin. The two major cylinders, the *corpora cavernosa,* extend side by side through the length of the penis. The third cylinder, the *corpus spongiosum,* surrounds the **urethra,** the channel for both seminal fluid and urine; see Figure 9.4.

When hanging down loosely, the average penis is about 3 3/4 inches long. During erection, its internal cylinders fill with so much blood that they become rigid, and the penis stretches to an average length of 6 1/4 inches. About 90 percent of all men have erect penises measuring between 5 and 7 inches in length. There is no relation, however, between penis size and female sexual satisfaction: A woman's vagina naturally adjusts during intercourse to the size of her partner's penis.

Inside the body are several structures involved in the production of seminal fluid, or **semen,** the liquid in which sperm cells are carried out of the body during ejaculation. The **vas deferens** are two tubes that carry sperm from the epididymis into the urethra. The **seminal vesicles,** which make some of the seminal fluid, join with the vas

sperm The male gamete produced by the testes and transported outside the body through ejaculation.

epididymis That portion of the male duct system in which sperm mature.

urethra The canal through which urine from the bladder leaves the body; in the male, also serves as the channel for seminal fluid.

semen The viscous whitish fluid that is the complete male ejaculate; a combination of sperm and secretions from the prostate gland, seminal vesicles, and other glands.

vas deferens Two tubes that carry sperm from the epididymis into the urethra.

seminal vesicles Glands in the male reproductive system that produce the major portion of the fluid of semen.

deferens to form the **ejaculatory ducts.** The **prostate gland** produces some of the seminal fluid, which it secretes into the urethra during ejaculation. The **Cowper's glands** are two pea-sized structures on either side of the urethra (just below where it emerges from the prostate gland) and connected to it via tiny ducts. When a man is sexually aroused, the Cowper's glands often secrete a fluid that appears as a droplet at the tip of the penis. This fluid is not semen, although it occasionally contains sperm.

Circumcision

In its natural state, the tip of the penis is covered by a fold of skin called the *foreskin.* About 60 percent of baby boys in the United States undergo **circumcision,** the surgical removal of the foreskin.

An estimated 1.2 million newborn males are circumcised in the United States annually for reasons that vary from religious traditions to preventive health measures. Until the last half century, scientific evidence to support or repudiate routine circumcision was limited. Large, carefully controlled studies in sub-Saharan Africa have shown that circumcision significantly reduces a man's risk of acquiring HIV through heterosexual intercourse. It is still not known whether circumcision also lowers the risk in men who have sex with men.[3] Male circumcision may help to prevent the spread of HIV in part because the cells on the foreskin of the penis are more susceptible to HIV infection. Circumcision does not protect against herpes, syphilis, or gonorrhea, suggesting a biological rather than a behavioral explanation for the protective effect of circumcision against HIV.

Boys who are not circumcised are four times as likely to develop urinary tract infections in their first year; however, such infections develop in only 1 percent of circumcised boys. Uncircumcised men are three times as likely to develop penile cancer, but the absolute risk is low. (Only about nine in every million American men ever gets cancer of the penis.)

Your Life Change Coach

Making Responsible Sexual Decisions

Sexual decision making always takes place within the context of an individual's values and perceptions of right and wrong behavior. Making sexually responsible decisions means considering all the possible consequences of sexual behavior for both yourself and your partner. It must always take into account, not just personal preferences and desires, but the very real risks of unwanted pregnancy, sexually transmitted infections (STIs), and long-term medical consequences (such as impaired fertility). You also must consider the emotional consequences of a sexual relationship— not just for yourself but also for your partner. (See "Your Intimacy Quotient" in *IPC.*) **IPC**

Talking About Sex

Prior to any sexual activity that involves a risk of sexually transmitted infection or pregnancy, both partners should talk about their prior sexual histories (including number of partners and exposure to STIs) and other high-risk behavior, such as the use of injection drugs. They should also discuss the issue of birth control and which methods might be best for them to use. If you know someone well enough to consider having sex with that person, you should be able to talk about such sensitive subjects. If a potential partner is unwilling to talk or hedges on crucial questions, you shouldn't be engaging in sex.

Styles of communicating vary among white Americans, African Americans, Hispanic Americans, and Asian Americans. While white and African Americans may openly discuss sex with partners, Hispanic-American couples generally do not discuss their sexual relationship. Asian Americans also are less inclined to discuss sex and to value nonverbal, indirect, and intuitive communication over explicit verbal interaction.[4]

Here are some questions to consider as you think and talk about the significance of becoming sexually intimate with a partner:

- **What role do we want relationships and sex to have in our life at this time?**
- **What are my values and my potential partner's values as they pertain to sexual relationships?** Does each of us believe that intercourse should be reserved for a permanent partnership or committed relationship?
- **Will a decision to engage in sex enhance my positive feelings about myself or my partner?** Does either of us have questions about sexual orientation or the kinds of people we are attracted to?

- **Do I and my partner both want to have sex?** Is my partner pressuring me in any way? Am I pressuring my partner? Am I making this decision for myself or my partner?
- **Have my partner and I discussed our sexual histories and risk factors?** Have I spoken honestly about any STIs I've had in the past? Am I sure that neither my partner nor I have a sexually transmitted infection?
- **Have we taken precautions against unwanted pregnancy and STIs?**

Talking about sex means talking about values, trust, commitment, and responsibility.

Saying No to Sex

Whether couples are on a first date or have been married for years, each partner always has the right not to have sex. Unfortunately, "no" sometimes seems to mean different things to men and women.

The following strategies can help you assert yourself when saying no to sex:

- **First of all, recognize** your own values and feelings. If you believe that sex is something to be shared only by people who've already become close in other ways, be true to that belief.
- **Be direct.** Look the person in the eyes, keep your head up, and speak clearly and firmly.
- **Just say no.** Make it clear you're rejecting the offer, not the person. You don't owe anyone an explanation for what you want, but if you want to expand on your reasons, you might say, "I enjoy your company, and I'd like to do something together, but no," or "Thank you. I appreciate your interest, but no."
- **If you're still at a loss for words,** try these responses: "I like you a lot, but I'm not ready to have sex." "You're a great person, but sex isn't something I do to prove I like someone." "I'd like to wait until I'm married to have sex."
- **If you're feeling pressured,** let your date know that you're uncomfortable. Be simple and direct. Watch out for emotional blackmail. If your date says, "If you really like me, you'd want to make love," point out that if he or she really likes you, he or she wouldn't try to force you to do something you don't want to do.
- **If you're a woman, monitor your sexual signals.** Men impute more sexual meaning to gestures (such as casual touching) that women perceive as friendly and innocent.
- **Communicate your feelings** to your date sooner rather than later. It's far easier to say, "I don't want to go to your apartment" than to fight off unwelcome advances once you're there.
- **Remember that if saying no to sex** puts an end to a relationship, it wasn't much of a relationship in the first place.

Creating a Sexually Healthy Relationship

A sexually healthy relationship, as defined by the Sexuality Information and Education Council of the United States (SIECUS), is based on shared values and has five characteristics: It is consensual, nonexploitative, honest, mutually pleasurable, and protected against unintended pregnancy and sexually transmitted infections. All individuals also have sexual rights, which include the right to the information, education, skills, support, and services they need to make responsible decisions about their sexuality consistent with their own values, as well as the right to express their sexual orientation without violence or discrimination.

Communication is vital in a sexually healthy relationship, even though these discussions can be awkward. Yet if you have a need or a problem that relates to your partner, it is your responsibility to bring it up. Choose an appropriate time and place for an intimate discussion. In a new relationship, talking in a public place, such as a park bench or a quiet table at a coffee house, can seem safer. If you're in an established relationship, choose a time when you can give each other complete attention and a setting in which you can both relax.

ejaculatory duct The canal connecting the seminal vesicles and vas deferens.

prostate gland A structure surrounding the male urethra that produces a secretion that helps liquefy the semen from the testes.

Cowper's gland Two small glands that discharge into the male urethra; also called bulbourethral glands.

circumcision The surgical removal of the foreskin of the penis.

Here are some specific suggestions that can help:

- **Ask open-ended questions** that encourage a dialogue, for instance, "How do you feel about . . . ?" or "What are your thoughts about . . . ?"
- **Listen actively** rather than passively when your partner speaks. Show that you're paying attention by nodding, smiling, and leaning forward. Paraphrase what he or she says to show you understand it fully. (See the "Listen Up" lab in *IPC*.) **IPC**
- **Use "I" statements,** such as "I really enjoy making love, but I'm so tired right now that I won't be a responsive partner. Why don't we get the kids to bed early tomorrow so we can enjoy ourselves a little earlier?"
- **Speak up** if something hurts during sex. Be specific.
- **If you would like to try something different, say so.** Practice saying the words first if they embarrass you. If your partner feels uncomfortable, don't force the issue, but do try talking it through.
- **If you want to request changes** or tackle a touchy topic, start with positive statements. Let your partner know how much you enjoy having sex, and then express your desire to enjoy lovemaking more often or in different ways.
- **Encourage small changes.** If you want your partner to be less inhibited, start slowly, perhaps by suggesting sex in a different room or place.

The drawbacks of circumcision include the risk of complications (which tend to be uncommon and minor) and pain. The AAP recommends that when circumcision is performed, analgesic creams or anesthetic shots be used to minimize discomfort. There is little consensus on what impact the presence or absence of a foreskin has on sexual functioning or satisfaction.

Responsible Sexuality

The World Health Organization defines sexual health as "the integration of the physical, emotional, intellectual, and social aspects of sexual being in ways that are positively enriching, and that enhance personality, communication, and love. . . . Every person has a right to receive sexual information and to consider sexual relationships for pleasure as well as for procreation."

Sexuality education is a lifelong process. Your own knowledge about sex may not be as extensive as you might assume. Most people grow up with a lot of myths and misconceptions about sex. (See this chapter's Self-Survey: "How Much Do You Know About Sex?"). Rather than relying on what peers say or what you've always thought was true, find out the facts. This textbook is a good place to start. The student health center and the library can provide additional materials on sexual identity, orientation, behavior, and health, as well as on options for reducing your risk of acquiring sexually transmitted infections (discussed in Chapter 16) or becoming pregnant.

Sexual Behavior

From birth to death, we are sexual beings. Our sexual identities, needs, likes, and dislikes emerge in adolescence and become clearer as we enter adulthood, but we con-

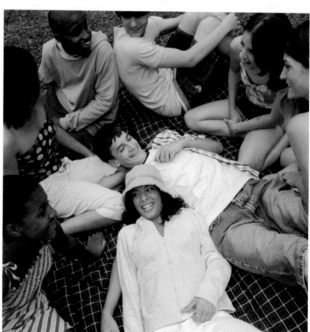

During adolescence, teens explore different social and intimate relationships as they begin to develop a sexual identity.

© Stephen Mallon/Photonica/Getty Images

tinue to change and evolve throughout our lives. In men, sexual interest is most intense at age 18; in women, it reaches a peak in the 30s. Although age brings changes in sexual responsiveness, we never outgrow our sexuality.

Adolescent Sexuality

Early in adolescence, sexual curiosity explodes, and sexual exploration—both alone and with a partner—takes on new meaning and intensity. Sexual education programs can make a difference by helping young people become sexually responsible, enabling them to form satisfying relationships, helping them assess their own attitudes toward sex, and giving them information on sexuality. Good programs can clarify values and enhance communication.

It's not unusual for teenage boys to experience frequent erections during the day and night, including **nocturnal emissions,** or wet dreams, during which ejaculation occurs. **Masturbation** (discussed later in this chapter) is the primary form of sexual expression for many teenagers, especially boys. Self-stimulation helps teens learn about their bodies and their sexual potential and serves as an outlet for sexual tension. By the end of adolescence, the majority of teens have masturbated to orgasm.

Other common sexual activities during adolescence include kissing and petting—erotic physical contact that may include holding, touching, manual stimulation of the genitals, and oral sex. As many as 25 percent of teens experience some same-sex attractions. Although many experiment with heterosexual and homosexual sexual experiences, adolescent sexual behavior does not always foretell sexual orientation. Young people, who often feel confused about their sexual identity, may engage in sexual activity with members of the same or the other sex as a way of testing how they really feel.

Teen Sexual Behaviors

For the first time since the federal government started keeping statistics in the early 1970s, fewer American teenagers are becoming sexually active. According to the CDC, the percentage of high school students who had intercourse dropped from 54.1 to 45.6 percent. The U.S. teenage birth rate has fallen to the lowest levels ever recorded: about 40 births per 1,000, down from a peak of almost 62 births per 1,000 in 1991. One-fourth of the drop is from delaying sex; three-fourths from increased use of contraceptives.[5]

According to a national survey of 1,800 teenagers and young adults sponsored by the Kaiser Family Foundation, young people are more concerned about sex and sexual health than any other health issue in their lives. Most—but especially males—report peer pressure to have sex. Three in five respondents described putting off sex as a "nice idea," but something nobody does. One in five reported initial sexual intercourse by age 15. Sexually experienced young teens were far more likely than virgins to engage in other risky behaviors, such as smoking, drinking, and using drugs. Almost a third said they had "done more sexually" because of alcohol or drug use.[6]

One in six young adults and adolescents regard unprotected sex as "not that big a deal." Males are twice as likely as females to feel this way. Pregnancy remains a real concern among young people. Seven in ten college-age young adults have or have had a partner who had a pregnancy test. Nearly two in five reported that they or a partner have been pregnant.[7]

REALITYCHECK

- *How many students say they have not had vaginal intercourse?* _____
- *How many students report having vaginal intercourse in the past 30 days?* _____
- *How many students say they have never had oral sex?* _____

Answers on next page.

In recent years the popular media have called attention to a rise in casual oral sex among teenagers. In the great majority of cases, girls perform fellatio, rather than boys performing cunnilingus. Some researchers initially thought the increasing incidence of oral sex represented a greater comfort level in talking about sexual issues. However, as studies have confirmed, oral sex has become more widespread among both teens who have already engaged in vaginal intercourse and those who have not. Many young people view oral sex as less risky than intercourse, and few report using barrier protection, such as condoms, during oral sex.[8]

Sex on Campus

Sexual behavior on campus has changed dramatically in the last 25 years. Surveys conducted in the United States and in Canada since 1980 reveal a steady increase in the number of students who have had intercourse and an increase in safer sex practices among sexually active students. Today's undergraduates are more likely to question potential partners about their past, use condoms with a new partner, and maintain fairly long-term monogamous relationships.

College students see sexual activity as normal behavior for their peer group. When researchers at Pennsylvania State University conducted focus groups with undergraduates, most agreed that the majority of college students (80 to 90 percent, in their estimate) are sexually active and that alcohol and drug use make sexual activity more likely.

College students tend to overestimate how much sex their peers are having. In a study at a large university in the Northeast, the mean number of sexual partners the students reported was 2.6, but they believed that the typical student had had 4.8 partners in the previous year.[9] (See Reality Check.)

College students who binge drink or participate in drinking games, which often involve physical skills (such

nocturnal emissions Ejaculations while dreaming; wet dreams.

masturbation Manual (or nonmanual) self-stimulation of the genitals, often resulting in orgasm.

as bouncing a coin into a glass) or word play, increase their odds of sexually risky behavior. Both men and women report being taken advantage of sexually, including someone having sex with them when they were too drunk to give consent, after such games.

Annual spring breaks provide what researchers describe as "ideal conditions for the potentially lethal interaction between alcohol, drugs, and sexual risk-taking." Students typically engage in binge drinking, illicit drug use, and unsafe sexual practices. The likelihood of casual sex depends on several factors, including peer influences, prior experiences with casual sex, alcohol consumption prior to sex, and impulsivity.

 As with other aspects of health, cultural, religious, and personal values affect students' sexual behaviors. Researchers raised concern about young Latina women, who have the highest teen birth rate in the United States (twice the national rate) and are at greater risk of sexually transmitted infections. Although Latinas represent about 10 percent of women over age 21, they account for 20 percent of female AIDS cases. Among college students and other populations, Latinas are more likely to engage in unprotected intercourse than women from other ethnic groups. Sexually active Latina college students also are less likely to use condoms than their peers from other ethnic groups.[11]

Acculturation—the process of adaptation that occurs when immigrants enter a new country—also affects sexual behavior. As Latina immigrants become more acculturated in the United States, some aspects of their sexual behavior become more Americanized; for instance, they become more likely to engage in nonmarital sexual activity and to have multiple partners. In a study of Cuban American college women, older, less religious, and U.S.-born Latinas were more likely to be sexually active and to engage in risky sexual behavior than other Latinas.[11]

The Sex Life of American Adults

The scientific study of Americans' sexual behavior began in 1938, when Alfred Kinsey, Ph.D., a professor of biol-

ogy at the University of Indiana, and his colleagues asked 5,300 white men and 5,940 white women about their sexual practices. In his landmark studies—*Sexual Behavior in the Human Male,* published in 1948, and *Sexual Behavior in the Human Female,* published in 1953—Kinsey reported that 73 percent of men and 20 percent of women had premarital intercourse by age 20, and 37 percent of men and 17 percent of women had some homosexual experience in their lifetime.

The Janus Report on Sexual Behavior, published in 1993, was based on a survey of 2,765 individuals across the United States. A larger survey, conducted by researchers at the University of Chicago, was based on face-to-face interviews with 3,432 Americans, aged 18 to 59. It became the basis for two books published in 1994: *Sex in America,* aimed at a lay audience, and *The Social Organization of Sexuality,* a more scholarly work. Since then, the researcher's General Social Survey (GSS) database on sexual activity has grown to nearly 10,000 respondents.

The average American adult reports having sex about once a week. However, 1 in 5 Americans has been celibate for at least a year, and 1 in 20 engages in sex at least every other day. Men report more sexual frequency than women—not because men are more boastful about their prowess, the researchers contend, but because the sample of women includes many widows and older women without partners. Among married people, the frequency reports of husbands and wives (not in the same couples) are within one episode per year—58.6 for married men and 57.9 for married women. If other differences between men and women are statistically controlled (such as sexual preference, age, and educational attainment), married women actually report a slightly higher frequency than men.

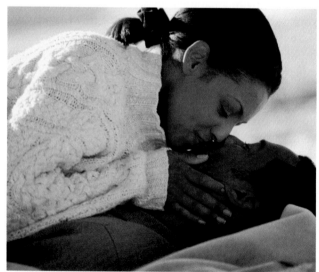

In a loving, committed relationship, sex serves as an intimate form of communication.

Sexual frequency peaks among those with some college education, then decreases among four-year college graduates, and declines even further among those with professional degrees. Americans who have attended graduate school are the least sexually active educational group in the population. These respondents may be more honest than others in reporting sexual activity, or they may be more precise in their definition of what counts as sex.

Does sex make people happier or healthier? Researchers have concluded that the more sex a person has, the more likely he or she is to report having a happy life and a happy marriage. This connection is stronger among women than men. A second and more important predictor of sexual frequency is the feeling that one's life is exciting rather than routine or dull. "Being excited by life is most strongly associated with being happier," the researchers noted. "It seems that increased sexual activity is one of the many benefits of having a positive attitude."

Why People Have Sex

The reasons people engage in sex long seemed so obvious that scientists didn't bother to investigate them. They assumed that heterosexuals had sex primarily to reproduce, experience sexual pleasure, and relieve sexual tension.

 In the most extensive study of why humans have sex, researchers identified 237 motivations. The study sample included 1,549 undergraduates ranging in age from 16 to 42.[12] The reasons people gave fell into nine categories:

- Pure attraction to the other person in general.
- Experiencing physical pleasure.
- Expressing love.
- Feeling desired by the other.
- Escalating the depth of a relationship.
- Curiosity or seeking new adventures.
- Marking a special occasion for celebration.
- Mere opportunity.
- Sex "just happening" due to seemingly uncontrollable circumstances.

The responses of men and women were generally similar. (see Table 9.1). However, men were significantly more likely to report having sex for reasons of opportunity and experience—for instance, because a person "was available" or wanting "to increase the number of partners I experienced." Women were more likely to endorse certain emotional motivations, such as, "I wanted to express my love for the person," or "I realized I was in love." Men also endorsed more reasons related to pure physical pleasure, such as wanting to have sex because it felt good or because they were "horny."

TABLE 9.1 Top 10 Reasons Why Men and Women Have Sex

	Women	Men
1.	I was attracted to the person.	I was attracted to the person.
2.	I wanted to experience the physical pleasure.	It feels good.
3.	It feels good.	I wanted to experience the physical pleasure.
4.	I wanted to show my affection to the person.	It's fun.
5.	I wanted to express my love for the person.	I wanted to show my affection to the person.
6.	I was sexually aroused and wanted the release.	I was sexually aroused and wanted the release.
7.	I was "horny."	I was "horny."
8.	It's fun.	I wanted to express my love for the person.
9.	I realized I was in love.	I wanted to achieve an orgasm.
10.	I was "in the heat of the moment."	I wanted to please my partner.

Source: Meston, Cindy and David Buss. "Why Humans Have Sex." *Archives of Sexual Behavior*, Vol. 36, August 2007, pp. 477–507.

© Marili Forastieri/ Digital Vision/ Getty Images

Sexual Diversity

Human beings are diverse in all ways—including sexual preferences and practices. Physiological, psychological, and social factors determine whether we are attracted to members of the same sex or the other sex. This attraction is our **sexual orientation.** Sigmund Freud argued that we all start off **bisexual,** or attracted to both sexes. But by the time we reach adulthood, most males prefer female sexual partners, and most females prefer male partners. **Heterosexual** is the term used for individuals whose primary orientation is toward members of the other sex. In virtually all cultures, some men and women are **homosexuals,** preferring partners of their own sex.

In our society, we tend to view heterosexuality and homosexuality as very different. In reality, these orientations are opposite ends of a spectrum. Sex researcher Alfred Kinsey devised a seven-point continuum representing sexual orientation in American society. At one end of the continuum are those exclusively attracted to members of the other sex; at the opposite end are

sexual orientation The direction of an individual's sexual interest, either to members of the opposite sex or to members of the same sex.

bisexual Sexually oriented toward both sexes.

heterosexual Primary sexual orientation toward members of the other sex.

homosexual Primary sexual orientation toward members of the same sex.

people exclusively attracted to members of the same sex. In between are varying degrees of homosexual, bisexual, and heterosexual orientation.

According to Kinsey's original data, 4 percent of men and 2 percent of women are exclusively homosexual. More recent studies have found lower numbers. For instance, in the University of Chicago's national survey, 2.8 percent of men and 1.4 percent of women defined themselves as homosexual. However, when asked if they'd had sex with a person of the same gender since age 18, about 5 percent of men and 4 percent of women said yes. When asked if they found members of the same gender sexually attractive, 6 percent of men and 5.5 percent of women said yes.

Most lesbian and bisexual women report that their first sexual experience occurred with a man (at the median age of 18) and that sex with a woman followed a few years later (at median age 21).

Heterosexuality

Heterosexuallity, the most common sexual orientation, refers to sexual or romantic attraction between opposite sexes. The adjective *heterosexual* describes intimate relationships and/or sexual relations between a man and a woman. The term *straight* is used predominantly for self-identified heterosexuals of either sex. In his landmark research in the 1940s, Alfred Kinsey reported that while many men and women were exclusively heterosexual, a significant number (37 percent of men and 13 percent of women) had at least one adult sexual experience with a member of the same sex.

Bisexuality

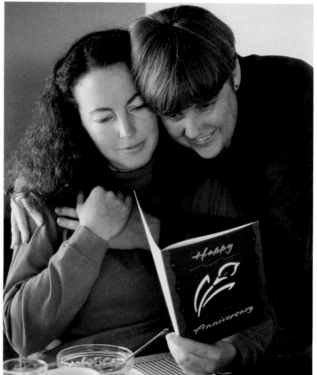 Bisexuality—sexual attraction to both males and females—can develop at any point in one's life. In some cultures, bisexual activity is considered part of normal sexual experimentation. Among the Sabmia Highlanders in Papua New Guinea, for instance, boys perform oral sex on one another as part of the rites of passage into manhood.

Some people identify themselves as bisexual even if they don't behave bisexually. Some are *serial* bisexuals— that is, they are sexually involved with same-sex partners for a while and then with partners of the other sex, or vice versa. An estimated 7 to 9 million men, about twice the number thought to be exclusively homosexual, could be described as bisexual during some extended period of their lives. The largest group are married, rarely have sexual relations with women other than their wives, and have secret sexual involvements with men.

Fear of HIV infection has sparked great concern about bisexuality, particularly among heterosexual women who worry about becoming involved with a bisexual man. About 20 to 30 percent of women with AIDS were infected by bisexual partners, and health officials fear that bisexual men who hide their homosexual affairs could transmit HIV to many more women.

Homosexuality

Homosexuality—social, emotional, and sexual attraction to members of the same sex—exists in almost all cultures. Men and women homosexuals are commonly referred to as *gays;* women homosexuals are also called *lesbians.*

Homosexuality threatens and upsets many people, perhaps because homosexuals are viewed as different, or perhaps because no one understands why some people are heterosexual and others homosexual. *Homophobia* has led to an increase in *gay bashing* (attacking homosexuals) in many communities, including college campuses. Some blame the emergence of AIDS as a societal danger. However, researchers have found that fear of AIDS has not created new hostility but has simply given bigots an excuse to act out their hatred.

Different ethnic groups respond to homosexuality in different ways. To a greater extent than white homosexuals, gays and lesbians from ethnic groups tend to stay in the closet longer rather than risk alienation from their families and communities. Often they feel forced to choose between their gay and their ethnic identities.

Close-couple homosexual relationships are similar to stable heterosexual relationships.

In general, the African American community has stronger negative views of homosexuals than whites, possibly because of the influence of strong fundamentalist Christian beliefs. Stigma may contribute to a phenomenon called "the Down Low" or DL, which refers to African American men who publicly present themselves as heterosexuals while secretly having sex with other men. This practice, which is neither new nor limited to African American men, can increase the risk of HIV infection in unsuspecting female partners.[13] Hispanic culture, with its emphasis on machismo, also has a very negative view of male homosexuality. Asian cultures, which tend to view an individual as a representative of his or her family, tend to view open declarations of sexual orientation as shaming the family and challenging their reputation and future.

Roots of Homosexuality

Most mental health experts agree that nobody knows what causes a person's sexual orientation. Research has discredited theories tracing homosexuality to troubled childhoods or abnormal psychological development. Sexual orientation probably emerges from a complex interaction that includes biological and environmental factors.

Homosexuality on Campus

In a study of almost 700 heterosexual students at six small liberal arts colleges, attitudes toward homosexuals and homosexuality varied, depending on students' membership in fraternities or sororities, sex role attitudes, religion and religiosity, and contact with and knowledge of gays, lesbians, and bisexuals. The students most likely to be accepting were those who were women, had less traditional sex-role attitudes, were less religious, attended colleges that did not have Greek social clubs, and had gay, lesbian, and/or bisexual friends.

A survey of colleges and universities found great variation in the resources available to gay, lesbian, and bisexual students. Most (71 percent) have a student organization; 32 percent provide a paid staff member to deal with the students' needs and issues; 40 percent provide a support identification program; 36 percent offered at least one course on gay, lesbian, and bisexual issues.

Transgenderism and Transsexuality

The term **transgender** is used as an umbrella term to describe people who have gender identities, expressions, or behaviors not traditionally associated with their birth sex. Male-to-female transgenders have been assigned a male gender at birth, but identify their gender as female. Female-to-male people were assigned a female gender at birth, but identify their gender as male.

Transgender individuals may be happy with the biological sex in which they are born but enjoy dressing up and behaving like the other sex. Most do so for psychological and social pleasure rather than sexual gratification.

Transsexuals feel trapped in the body of the wrong gender—a condition called *gender dysphoria*. In general, more men than women have this experience. Transsexualism is now viewed as a disorder that can be treated with sexual reassignment surgery. However, this intervention, which requires long psychological counseling, hormonel treatments, and complicated operations, remains controversial. Some studies report healthy postoperative functioning, while others note that many male and female transsexuals do not escape their psychological misery.[14]

Transgender individuals face varied health risks, including unprotected sex, sexually transmitted diseases, and HIV infection. Violence, including rape, sexual abuse, physical abuse, and suicide, is a major public health issue. In one study the majority of the transgender individuals reported being afraid for their life or physical safety at some point during their lives.[15]

Sexual Activity

Part of learning about your own sexuality is having a clear understanding of human sexual behaviors. Understanding frees us from fear and anxiety so that we can accept ourselves and others as the natural sexual beings we all are.

Celibacy

A celibate person does not engage in sexual activity. Complete **celibacy** means that the person doesn't masturbate (stimulate himself or herself sexually) or engage in sexual activity with a partner. In partial celibacy, the person masturbates but doesn't have sexual contact with others. Many people decide to be celibate at certain times of their lives. Some don't have sex because of concerns about pregnancy or STIs; others haven't found a partner for a permanent, monogamous relationship. Many simply have other priorities, such as finishing school or starting a career, and realize that sex outside of a committed relationship is a threat to their physical and psychological well-being.

---

transgender Having a gender identity opposite one's biological sex.

celibacy Abstention from sexual activity; can be partial or complete, permanent or temporary.

abstinence Voluntary refrainment from sexual intercourse.

POINT COUNTERPOINT *Advocating for Abstinence*

POINT

Campus abstinence clubs are gaining in popularity at Ivy League schools and other colleges around the country. They sponsor parties, lectures, and discussion panels that encourage abstinence. By publicly committing themselves to a chaste lifestyle, their members are presenting an alternative to casual "hookups" between two people who make no commitment to each other.

COUNTERPOINT

Sexual choices are private and personal. If students organized clubs to promote hookups and casual sex, there would be immediate protests. Rightly so, but neither should campus abstinence clubs be allowed. Consenting adults have the right to choose not to have sex, but not the right to impose their moral values and judgments on others.

YOUR VIEW

Do students have the right to proclaim and defend their personal values in a club setting? Do you think abstinence clubs are a reaction to the anything-goes sexual culture on many campuses? Are these clubs trying to impose a certain standard of behavior on others? What do you think of the students who join such groups? Are you or would you become a member?

Abstinence

The CDC defines **abstinence** as "refraining from sexual activities which involve vaginal, anal, and oral intercourse." The definition of abstinence remains a subject of debate and controversy, with some emphasizing positive choices and others avoidance of specific behaviors. In reality, abstinence means different things to different people, cultures, and religious groups.

Increasing numbers of adolescents and young adults are choosing to remain virgins and abstain from sexual intercourse until they enter a permanent, committed, monogamous relationship. About 2.5 million teens have taken pledges to abstain from sex. (See Point-Counterpoint: "Advocating for Abstinence.")

Many people who were sexually active in the past also are choosing abstinence because the risk of medical complications associated with STIs increases with the number of sexual partners a person has. Practicing abstinence is the safest, healthiest option for many. However, there is confusion about what it means to abstain, and individuals who think they are abstaining may still be engaging in behaviors that put them at risk for HIV and STIs. (See Chapter 10 for more on abstinence as a form of birth control.)

Why abstain? Among the reasons students give are:

- **Remaining a virgin until** you meet someone you love and see as a life partner.
- **Being true to your religious and moral values.**
- **Getting to know a partner better.**
- **If you're heterosexual, to avoid pregnancy.**
- **To be sure you're safe from sexually transmitted infections.**

Abstinence education programs, which received federal support and became widespread in American schools, have had little, if any, impact on teen sexual behavior. In a five-year study of adolescents, the same percentage—49 percent—of teens did not have sex, regardless of whether or not they'd had abstinence education. Scientists have found no difference in age of first intercourse for students who had graduated from abstinence programs and those who had not.[16]

Fantasy

The mind is the most powerful sex organ in the body, and erotic mental images can be sexually stimulating. Sexual fantasies can accompany sexual activity or be pleasurable in themselves. Fantasies lived out via the Internet are becoming more common but may also be harmful to psychological health (see the Savvy Consumer feature).

Fantasies generally enhance sexual arousal, reduce anxiety, and boost sexual desire. They're also a way to anticipate and rehearse new sexual experiences, as well as to bolster a person's self-image and feelings of desirability.

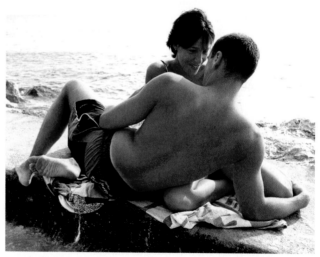

The magic of touch. Thrilling, soothing, stimulating—touch is a powerful way to communicate affection and sexual pleasure.

X-Rated Websites

Sex is the number-one word searched for online. About 15 percent of Americans logging onto the Internet visit sexually oriented sites. Men are the largest consumers of sexually explicit material and outnumber women by a ratio of six to one. However, while men look for visual erotica, women are more likely to visit chat rooms, which offer more interactions. Most people who check out sex sites on the Internet do not suffer any negative impact, but psychologists warn of some potential risks, including the following:

• *Dependence.* Individuals who spend 11 hours or more a week online in sexual pursuits show signs of psychological distress and admit that their behavior interferes with some areas of their lives.

• *Interference with work and study.* While most individuals use their home computers when surfing the Internet for sex-related sites, one in ten has used a school computer. Some universities have strict policies barring such practices and may take punitive actions against employees who violate the rules.

• *Sexual compulsivity.* A small but significant number of users are at risk of a serious problem as a result of their heavy Internet use.

• *Dishonesty.* Most Internet surfers admit that they occasionally "pretend" about their age on the Internet. Most keep secret how much time they spend on sexual pursuits in cyberspace.

Part of what makes fantasies exciting is that they provide an opportunity for expressing forbidden desires, such as sex with a different partner or with a past lover.

Men and women have different types of sexy thoughts, with men's fantasies containing more explicit genital images and culminating in sexual acts more quickly than women's. In women's fantasies, emotional feelings play a greater role, and there is more kissing and caressing rather than genital contact. For many women, fantasy helps in reaching orgasm during intercourse; a loss of fantasy often is a sign of low sexual desire.

Masturbation

Not everybody masturbates, but most people do. Kinsey estimated that 7 out of 10 women and 19 out of 20 men masturbate (and admit they do). Their reason is simple: It feels good. Masturbation produces the same physical responses as sexual activity with a partner and can be an enjoyable form of sexual release.

Masturbation has been described as immature; unsocial; tiring; frustrating; and a cause of hairy palms, warts, blemishes, and blindness. None of these myths is true. Sex educators recommend masturbation to adolescents as a means of releasing tension and becoming familiar with their sexual organs. Throughout adulthood, masturbation often is the primary sexual activity of individuals not involved in a sexual relationship and can be particularly useful when illness, absence, divorce, or death deprives a person of a partner. In the University of Chicago survey, about 25 percent of men and 9 percent of women said they masturbate at least once a week.

 White men and women have a higher incidence of masturbation than African American men and women. Latina women have the lowest rate of masturbation, compared with Latino men, white men and women, and African American men and women. Individuals with a higher level of education are more likely to masturbate than those with less schooling, and people living with sexual partners masturbate more than those who live alone.

Nonpenetrative Sexual Activity (Outercourse)

Various pleasurable behaviors can lead to orgasm with little risk of pregnancy or sexually transmitted disease. The options for "outercourse" include kissing, hugging, and touching but do not involve genital-to-genital, mouth-to-genital, or insertive anal sexual contact.

A kiss is a universal sign of affection. A kiss can be just a kiss—a quick press of the lips—or it can lead to much more. Usually kissing is the first sexual activity that couples engage in, and even after years of sexual experimentation and sharing, it remains an enduring pleasure for partners.

Touching is a silent form of communication between friends and lovers. Although a touch to any part of the body can be thrilling, some areas, such as the breasts and genitals, are especially sensitive. Stimulating these **erogenous** regions can lead to orgasm in both men and women. Though such forms of stimulation often accompany intercourse, more couples are gaining an appreciation of these activities as primary sources of sexual fulfillment—and as safer alternatives to intercourse.

Intercourse

Vaginal **intercourse,** or coitus, refers to the penetration of the vagina by the penis (Figure 9.5). This is the preferred form of sexual intimacy for most heterosexual couples, who may use a wide variety of positions. The

erogenous   Sexually sensitive.

intercourse   Sexual stimulation by means of entry of the penis into the vagina; coitus.

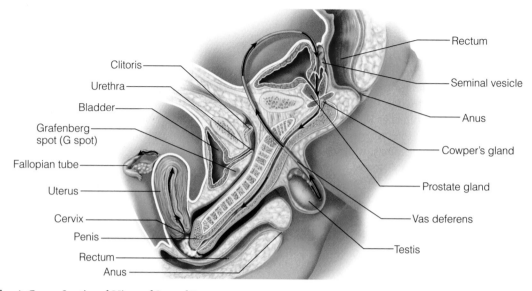

Figure 9.5 A Cross-Sectional View of Sexual Intercourse

Sperm are formed in each of the testes and stored in the epididymis. When a man ejaculates, sperm traveling in semen travel up the vas deferens. (The prostate gland and seminal vesicles contribute components of the semen.) The semen is expelled from the penis through the urethra and deposited in the vagina, near the cervix. During sexual excitement and orgasm in a woman, the upper end of the vagina enlarges and the uterus elevates. After orgasm, these organs return to their normal states, and the cervix descends into the pool of semen.

most familiar position for intercourse in our society is the so-called missionary position, with the man on top, facing the woman. An alternative is the woman on top, either lying down or sitting upright. Other positions include lying side by side (either face to face or with the man behind the woman, his penis entering her vagina from the rear); lying with the man on top of the woman in a rear-entry position; and kneeling or standing (again, in either a face-to-face or rear-entry position). Many couples move into several different positions for intercourse during a single episode of lovemaking; others may have a personal favorite or may choose different positions at different times.

Sexual activity, including intercourse, is possible throughout a woman's menstrual cycle. However, some women prefer to avoid sex while menstruating because of uncomfortable physical symptoms, such as cramps, or concern about bleeding or messiness. Others use a diaphragm or cervical cap (see Chapter 10) to hold back menstrual flow. Since different cultures have different views on intercourse during a woman's period, partners should discuss their own feelings and try to respect each other's views. If they choose not to have intercourse, there are other gratifying forms of sexual activity.

Vaginal intercourse, like other forms of sexual activity involving an exchange of bodily fluids, carries a risk of sexually transmitted infections, including HIV infection. In many other parts of the world, in fact, heterosexual intercourse is the most common means of HIV transmission (see Chapter 16).

Oral Sex

Our mouths and genitals give us some of our most intense pleasures. Though it might seem logical to combine the two, some people are very uncomfortable with it. Some people consider oral–genital sex a perversion; it is against the law in some states and a sin in some religions. However, others find it normal and acceptable. (The same comments apply to anal sex as well—see the next section.)

The formal terms for oral sex are **cunnilingus,** which refers to oral stimulation of the woman's genitals, and **fellatio,** oral stimulation of the man's genitals. For many couples, oral sex is a regular part of their lovemaking. For others, it's an occasional experiment. Oral sex with a partner carrying a sexually transmitted infection, such as herpes or HIV infection, can lead to infection, so a condom should be used (with cunnilingus, a condom cut in half to lay flat can be used).

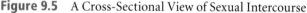 Different groups of the population have diverse views of oral sex. In one survey, more African American than white men reported never having performed or received oral sex.

Anal Stimulation and Intercourse

Because the anus has many nerve endings, it can produce intense erotic responses. Stimulation of the anus by the fingers or mouth can be a source of sexual arousal; anal intercourse involves penile penetration of the anus. An estimated 25 percent of adults have experienced anal intercourse at least once. However, anal sex involves important health risks, such as damage to sensitive rectal tissues and the transmission of various intestinal infections, hepatitis, and STIs, including HIV.

Cultural Variations

While the biological mechanisms underlying human sexual arousal and response are essentially universal, the particular sexual stimuli or behaviors that people find arousing are greatly influenced by cultural conditioning. For example, in Western societies, where the emphasis during sexual activity tends to be heavily weighted toward achieving orgasm, genitally focused activities are frequently defined as optimally arousing. In contrast, devotees to Eastern Tantric traditions (where spirituality is interwoven with sexuality) often achieve optimal pleasure by emphasizing the sensual and spiritual aspects of shared intimacy rather than orgasmic release.

Kissing on the mouth, a universal source of sexual arousal in Western society, may be rare or absent in many other parts of the world. Certain North American Eskimo people and inhabitants of the Trobriand Islands would rather rub noses than lips, and among the Thonga of South Africa, kissing is viewed as odious behavior. The Hindu people of India are also disinclined to kiss because they believe such contact symbolically contaminates the act of sexual intercourse. One survey of 190 societies found that mouth kissing was acknowledged in only 21 societies and practiced as a prelude or accompaniment to coitus in only 13.

Oral sex (both cunnilingus and fellatio) is a common source of sexual arousal among island societies of the South Pacific, in industrialized nations of Asia, and in much of the Western world. In contrast, in Africa (with the exception of northern regions), such practices are likely to be viewed as unnatural or disgusting behavior.

Foreplay in general, whether it be oral sex, sensual touching, or passionate kissing, is subject to wide cultural variation. In some societies, most notably those with Eastern traditions, couples may strive to prolong intense states of sexual arousal for several hours. While varied patterns of foreplay are common in Western cultures, these activities often are of short duration as lovers move rapidly toward the "main event" of coitus. In still other societies, foreplay is either sharply curtailed or absent altogether. For example, the Lepcha farmers of the southeastern Himalayas limit foreplay to men briefly caressing their partners' breasts, and among the Irish inhabitants of Inis Beag, precoital sexual activity is reported to be limited to mouth kissing and rough fondling of the woman's lower body by her partner.

Sexual Response

Sexuality involves every part of you: mind and body, muscles and skin, glands and genitals. The pioneers in finding out exactly how human beings respond to sex were William Masters and Virginia Johnson, who first studied more than 800 individuals in their laboratory in the 1950s. They discovered that sexual response is a well-ordered sequence of events, so predictable it could be divided into four phases: excitement, plateau, orgasm, and resolution (Figure 9.6). In real life, individuals don't necessarily follow this well-ordered pattern. But the responses for both sexes are remarkably similar. And sexual response always follows the same sequence, whatever the means of stimulation.

Excitement

Stimulation is the first step: a touch, a look, a fantasy. In men, sexual stimuli set off a rush of blood to the genitals, filling the blood vessels in the penis. Because these vessels are wrapped in a thick sheath of tissue, the penis becomes erect. The testes lift.

Women respond to stimulation with vaginal lubrication within 10 to 20 seconds of exposure to sexual stimuli. The clitoris becomes larger, as do the vaginal lips (the labia), the nipples, and later the breasts. The vagina lengthens, and its inner two-thirds increase in size. The uterus lifts, further increasing the free space in the vagina.

Plateau

During this stage, the changes begun in the excitement stage continue and intensify. The penis further increases in both length and diameter. The outer one-third of the vagina swells. During intercourse, the vaginal muscles grasp the penis to increase stimulation for both partners. The upper two-thirds of the vagina become wider as the uterus moves up; eventually its diameter is 2 1/2 to 3 inches.

Orgasm

Men and women have remarkably similar **orgasm** experiences. Both men and women typically have 3 to 12 pelvic muscle contractions approximately four-fifths of a

cunnilingus Sexual stimulation of a woman's genitals by means of oral manipulation.

fellatio Sexual stimulation of a man's genitals by means of oral manipulation.

orgasm A series of contractions of the pelvic muscles occurring at the peak of sexual arousal.

ejaculation The expulsion of semen from the penis.

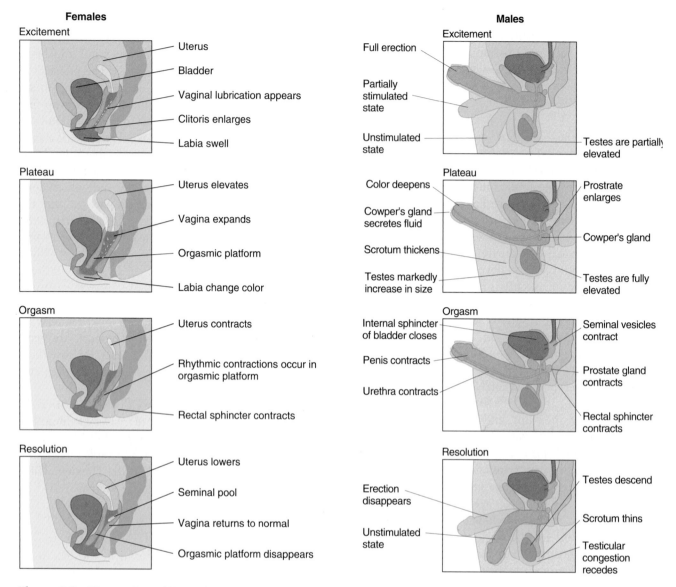

Females

Excitement
- Uterus
- Bladder
- Vaginal lubrication appears
- Clitoris enlarges
- Labia swell

Plateau
- Uterus elevates
- Vagina expands
- Orgasmic platform
- Labia change color

Orgasm
- Uterus contracts
- Rhythmic contractions occur in orgasmic platform
- Rectal sphincter contracts

Resolution
- Uterus lowers
- Seminal pool
- Vagina returns to normal
- Orgasmic platform disappears

Males

Excitement
- Full erection
- Partially stimulated state
- Unstimulated state
- Testes are partially elevated

Plateau
- Color deepens
- Cowper's gland secretes fluid
- Scrotum thickens
- Testes markedly increase in size
- Prostrate enlarges
- Cowper's gland
- Testes are fully elevated

Orgasm
- Internal sphincter of bladder closes
- Penis contracts
- Urethra contracts
- Seminal vesicles contract
- Prostate gland contracts
- Rectal sphincter contracts

Resolution
- Erection disappears
- Unstimulated state
- Testes descend
- Scrotum thins
- Testicular congestion recedes

Figure 9.6 Human Sexual Response
The four stages of sexual response are excitement, plateau, orgasm, and resolution.

second apart and lasting up to 60 seconds. Both undergo contractions and spasms of other muscles, as well as increases in breathing and pulse rates, and blood pressure. Both can sometimes have orgasms simply from kisses, stimulation of the breasts or other parts of the body, or fantasy alone.

The process of **ejaculation** (the discharge of semen by a male) requires two separate events. First, the vas deferens, the seminal vesicles, the prostate, and the upper portion of the urethra contract. The man perceives these subtle contractions deep in his pelvis just before the point of no return—which therapists refer to as the point of "ejaculatory inevitability." Then, seconds later, muscle contractions force semen out of the penis via the urethra.

Female orgasms follow several patterns. Some women experience a series of mini-orgasms—a response some-

times described as "skimming." Another pattern consists of rapid excitement and plateau stages, followed by a prolonged orgasm. This is the most frequent response to stimulation by a vibrator.

Female orgasms are primarily triggered by stimulating the clitoris. When stimulation reaches an adequate level, the vagina responds by contracting. Although it sometimes seems that vaginal stimulation alone can set off an orgasm, the clitoris is usually involved—at least indirectly during full penile penetration.

Some researchers have identified what they call the *Grafenberg* (or G) *spot* (or area) just behind the front wall of the vagina, between the cervix and the back of the public bone (see Figure 9.5). When this region is stimulated, women report various sensations, including slight discomfort, a brief feeling that they need to urinate, and increasing pleasure. Continued stimulation may result in an orgasm of great intensity, accompanied by ejaculation of fluid from the urethra. However, other researchers have failed to confirm the existence and importance of the G spot, and sex therapists disagree about its significance for a woman's sexual satisfaction.

Resolution

The sexual organs of men and women return to their normal, nonexcited state during this final phase of sexual response. Heightened skin color quickly fades after orgasm, and the heart rate, blood pressure, and breathing rate soon return to normal. The clitoris also resumes its normal position and appearance very shortly thereafter, whereas the penis may remain somewhat erect for up to 30 minutes.

After orgasm, men typically enter a **refractory period,** during which they are incapable of another orgasm. The duration of this period varies from minutes to days, depending on age and the frequency of previous sexual activity. If either partner doesn't have an orgasm after becoming highly aroused, resolution may be much slower and may be accompanied by a sense of discomfort.

Other Models of Sexual Response

Since Masters and Johnson's pioneering work, other researchers have challenged and expanded their theories. Some argue that their model neglects the importance of desire in sexual response and that the plateau stage is virtually indistinguishable from excitement. Others note that arousal may come before desire, particularly for women who may not have spontaneous feelings of sexual desire.

As many experts have concluded, physiology alone can never explain the complexity of human sexual response. Desire, arousal, pleasure, and satisfaction are highly subjective. Positive feelings like trust and happiness enhance them. Negative emotions like anger and anxiety can undermine them. For women, sexual satisfaction cannot be defined, as it typically is for men, by whether or not they achieved orgasm.

Sexual Concerns

Many sexual concerns stem from myths and misinformation. There is no truth, for instance, behind these misconceptions: men are always capable of erection, sex always involves intercourse, partners should experience simultaneous orgasms, or people who truly love each other always have satisfying sex lives.

Cultural and childhood influences can affect our attitudes toward sex. Even though America's traditionally puritanical values have eased, our society continues to convey mixed messages about sex. Some children, repeatedly warned of the evils of sex, never accept the sexual dimensions of their identity. Others—especially young boys—may be exposed to macho attitudes toward sex and feel a need to prove their virility. Young girls may feel confused by media messages that encourage them to look and act provocatively and a double standard that blames them for leading boys on. In addition, virtually everyone has individual worries. A woman may feel self-conscious about the shape of her breasts; a man may worry about the size of his penis; both partners may fear not pleasing the other.

The concept of sexual normalcy differs greatly in different times, cultures, or racial and ethnic groups. In certain times and places, only sex between a husband and wife has been deemed normal. In other circumstances, "normal" has been applied to any sexual behavior—alone or with others—that does not harm others or produce great anxiety and guilt. The following are some of the most common contemporary sexual concerns.

Safer Sex

Having sex is never completely safe; the only 100 percent risk-free sexual choice is abstinence. By choosing not to be sexually active with a partner, you can safeguard your physical health, your fertility, and your future.

For men and women who are sexually active, a mutually faithful sexual relationship with just one healthy partner is the safest option. For those not in such relationships, safer-sex practices are essential for reducing risks. See Chapter 16 and "The Seduction of Safer Sex" lab in *IPC* for a complete discussion of safer sex. **IPC**

Sexual Dysfunction

SIECUS defines **sexual dysfunction** as the inability to react emotionally and/or physically to sexual stimulation in a way expected of the average healthy person or according to one's own standards. Sexual dysfunctions, which have a wide range of psychological and physiological origins, can affect different stages in the sexual response cycle. They are not all-or-nothing problems but vary considerably in how severe they are and how frequently they occur. In as many as one-third of people with sexual problems, the partner also has a sexual dysfunction.

refractory period The period of time following orgasm during which the male cannot experience another orgasm.

sexual dysfunction The inability to react emotionally and/or physically to sexual stimulation in a way expected of the average healthy person or according to one's own standards.

Most men and women at one time or another experience some sort of sexual difficulty, but they tend to develop different types. Men are more likely to seek and receive treatment for sexual problems. Nevertheless, they find them very difficult to talk about and may delay or avoid seeking help. In women, the most common sexual dysfunction is loss of desire for sexual activity.

Erectile Dysfunction (ED)

An NIH consensus conference has defined **erectile dysfunction** (**ED,** also referred to as *impotence*) as the consistent inability to maintain a penile erection sufficient for adequate sexual relations. Virtually all men are occasionally unable to achieve or maintain an erection because of fatigue, stress, alcohol, or drug use, but the incidence of erectile disorders increases with age.

Erectile dysfunction affects an estimated 18 million men—about 18 percent of those over age 20—in the United States. Only 5 percent of men between ages 20 and 40 report ED, which becomes more prevalent with age and illness. Almost 90 percent of men with ED have at least one risk factor for cardiovascular disease, including hypertension or diabetes.[17]

Psychological factors, such as anxiety about performance, may cause erectile dysfunction. But in as many as 80 percent of cases, the problem has physical origins. Diabetes and reactions to drugs—including an estimated 200 prescription medications—are the most frequent organic causes. Even cigarettes can create erection problems for men sensitive to nicotine.

Preventing Erectile Dysfunction "The way a man lives can affect the way he loves." This was the conclusion of the Harvard's Health Professionals Follow-up Study, which found that healthy habits directly affect a man's risk of ED. Here are their key findings:

- **Smoking.** Men who smoke are twice as likely to develop ED. than nonsmokers.
- **Exercise.** Men who exercise for 30 minutes a day are less likely to develop erectile dysfunction than sedentary men.
- **Obesity.** Overweight men are more likely to have ED. even after age, diabetes, exercise, and other risk factors are taken into account. For example, a man with a 42-inch waist is 50 percent more likely to be impotent than a man with a 32-inch waist.
- **Alcohol.** The effects of alcohol are complex: A man who averages one to two drinks a day is less likely to have erectile dysfunction than a nondrinker, but a man who drinks more will increase his risk of sexual dysfunction.
- **Cycling.** Sitting on a bicycle for a long time puts pressure on the perineum, the area between the genitals and anus. This pressure can harm nerves and temporarily block blood flow, causing tingling or numbness in the penis and eventually leading to ED. To prevent this problem:
  - Wear padded biking shorts.
  - Raise the handlebars so you sit relatively upright, which shifts pressure from the perineum to the buttocks.
  - Use a wide, well-padded or gel-filled seat rather than a narrow one. Position the seat so you don't have to extend your legs fully at the bottom of your pedal stroke. Don't tilt the seat upward.
  - Shift position and take regular breaks during long rides.
  - If you feel tingling or numbness in the penis, stop riding for a week or two.[18]

Lifestyle therapy has promise for erectile dysfunction, but men have to make changes early enough to prevent irreversible changes in the arteries and nerves required for normal sexual function.

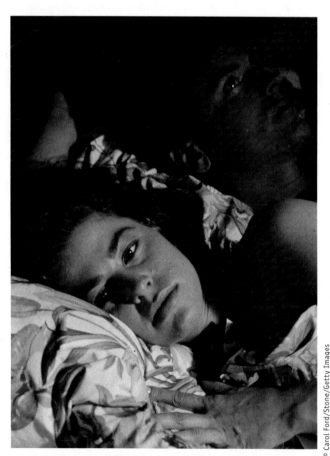

Sexual problems can be difficult for partners to talk about, but lack of communication can create tension and anxiety.

© Carol Ford/Stone/Getty Images

Treating Erectile Dysfunction   Men with erectile dysfunction can get help. If medication for a chronic medical problem is the culprit, a change in treatment may work. Treating underlying diseases, such as diabetes, may also help restore erectile function.

Millions of men have used the "erection pills": Viagra, Levitra, and Cialis. The three ED medications have similar success rates. In all, about 70 percent of men respond to the drugs but the rates vary according to what is responsible for ED. About half of men with diabetes respond well, while 90 percent of those without an underlying disease benefit.

Because of their effects on the arteries, men with cardiovascular disease should try ED pills only with their doctors' supervision, and some cannot use them under any circumstances. The FDA has warned doctors that some erectile dysfunction drugs, including Viagra, Cialis, and Levitra, could cause vision loss. The FDA is uncertain whether the drugs are directly to blame, or if the problems were caused by high blood pressure or diabetes. Other side effects include headache, facial flushing, nasal congestion, indigestion, and diarrhea.

Men can purchase ED drugs on the Internet, but they are taking a risk in using them without a legitimate medical evaluation. Other men turn to herbal remedies. The FDA warns that "all-natural" supplements may actually contain prescription-strength levels of Viagra that could be life-threatening for men with heart disease.

Erection drugs are not aphrodisiacs, but they can improve the erectile response to erotic stimulation. They correct impotence but do not enhance sexual performance.

Orgasm Problems in Men

About 20 percent of men complain of **premature ejaculation,** which is defined as ejaculating within 30 to 90 seconds of inserting the penis into the vagina, or after 10 to 15 thrusts. Another definition is that a premature ejaculator cannot control or delay his ejaculation long enough to satisfy a responsive partner at least half the time. By this definition, a man may be premature with some women but not with others.

To delay orgasm, men may try to think of baseball or other sports, but this just makes sex boring. Others may masturbate before intercourse, hoping to take advantage of the refractory period, during which they cannot ejaculate again. Others may bite their lips or dig their nails into their palms—although usually this just results in premature ejaculators with bloody lips and scarred palms. Topical anesthetics used to prevent climax dull pleasurable sensations for the woman as well as for the man.

Researchers are studying several medications, including clomipramine, SSRIs, and Viagra, in the treatment of premature ejaculation. The combination of medication and psychological and behavioral counseling seems most effective.

Men can learn to control their ejaculation by concentrating on their sexual responses, rather than by trying to distract themselves or ignore their reactions. Some men find that they have greater control by lying on their backs with their partner on top, by relaxing during intercourse, and by communicating with their partner about when to stop or slow down movements.

Other techniques for delaying ejaculation include *stop-start,* in which a man learns to sense the feelings that precede ejaculation and stop his movements before the point of ejaculatory inevitability, allowing his arousal to subside slightly before restarting sexual activity. In the *squeeze technique,* a man's partner applies strong pressure with the thumb on the frenum (the thin strip of skin that connects the glans to the shaft on the underside of the penis) and the second and third fingers on the top side of the penis, one above and one below the corona (rim of penile glans), until the man loses the urge to ejaculate.

Female Sexual Dysfunction

The American Foundation for Urological Disease classifies female sexual dysfunction into four categories: sexual desire disorders, arousal disorders, orgasmic disorders, and sexual pain disorders. How common are these problems? That's hard to estimate. Some sex therapists have speculated that as many as 43 percent of American women may have some form of sexual dysfunction.

Many health professionals remain dubious about the "medicalization" of various patterns of female sexual response. Scientists at the Kinsey Institute for Research in Sex, Gender, and Reproduction, for instance, caution that a pill, whatever its nature, may not be the solution to many women's sexual concerns. In women, psychology often is as or even more important than physiology, and effective therapy must address psychological problems in a sexual relationship as well as social constraints and inhibitions.

Some forms of female sexual dysfunction do respond to various therapies. These include **dyspareunia,** or pain during intercourse, and **vaginismus,** an extreme form of painful intercourse in which involuntary contractions of the muscles of the outer third of the vagina are so intense that they totally or partially close the vaginal opening. This

---

erectile dysfunction (ED)   The consistents inability to maintain a penile erection sufficient for adequate sexual relations.

premature ejaculation   A sexual difficulty in which a man ejaculates so rapidly that his partner's satisfaction is impaired.

dyspareunia   A sexual difficulty in which a woman experiences pain during sexual intercourse.

vaginismus   A sexual difficulty in which a woman experiences painful spasms of the vagina during sexual intercourse.

problem often derives from a fear of being penetrated. Relaxation techniques, such as Kegel exercises (alternately tightening and relaxing the muscles of the pelvic floor), or the use of fingers or dilators to gradually open the vagina, can make penetration easier.

The female orgasm has long been a controversial sexual topic. According to recent estimates, about 90 percent of sexually active women have experienced orgasm, but only a much smaller percentage achieve orgasm through intercourse alone. Even fewer reach orgasm if intercourse isn't accompanied by direct stimulation of the clitoris. Is intercourse without orgasm a sexual problem? The best answer is that it is a problem if a woman wants to experience orgasm during intercourse but doesn't.

Many counseling programs urge women who have never had orgasms to masturbate. They are then encouraged to share with their partners what they've learned, communicating with words or gestures what is most pleasing to them. Some women want more than a single orgasm during intercourse. Partners can help by varying positions and experimenting with sexual techniques. However, in sexual response, more is not necessarily better, and the couple should keep in mind that no one else is counting.

Sex Therapy

Modern sex therapy, pioneered by Masters and Johnson in the 1960s, views sex as a natural, healthy behavior that enhances a couple's relationship. Their approach emphasizes education, communication, reduction of performance anxiety, and sexual exercises that enhance sexual intimacy.

Today most sex therapists, working either alone or with a partner, have modified Masters and Johnson's approach. Most see couples once a week for eight to ten weeks; the focus of therapy is on correcting dysfunctional behavior, not exploring underlying psychodynamics.

Contrary to common misconceptions, sex therapy does not involve conducting sexual activity in front of therapists. The therapist may review psychological and physiological aspects of sexual functioning and evaluate the couple's sexual attitudes and ability to communicate. The core of the program is the couple's "homework"—a series of exercises, carried out in private, that enhances their sensory awareness and improves nonverbal communication. These techniques have proved effective for couples regardless of their age or general health.

You and your partner should consider consulting a sex therapist if any of the following is true for you:

- **Sex is painful** or physically uncomfortable.
- **You're having sex less** and less frequently.
- **You have a general fear** of, or revulsion toward, sex.
- **Your sexual pleasure is declining.**

- **Your sexual desire is diminishing.**
- **Your sexual problems are increasing** in frequency or persisting for longer periods.

Drugs and Sex

Many recreational drugs, such as alcohol and marijuana, are believed to enhance sexual performance. However, none of the popular drugs touted as *aphrodisiacs*—including amphetamines, barbiturates, cantharides ("Spanish fly"), cocaine, LSD and other psychedelics, marijuana, amyl nitrite ("poppers"), and L-dopa (a medication used to treat Parkinson's disease)—is truly a sexual stimulant. In fact, these drugs often interfere with normal sexual response. Researchers are studying one drug that may truly enhance sexual performance: yohimbine hydrochloride, which is derived from the sap of the tropical yohimbe tree that grows in West Africa.

Because many psychiatric problems can lower sexual desire and affect sexual functioning, medications appropriate to the specific disorders can help. In addition, psychiatric drugs may be used as part of therapy. Drugs such as certain antidepressants may be used to prolong sexual response in conditions such as premature ejaculation.

Medications can also cause sexual difficulty. In men, drugs that are used to treat high blood pressure, anxiety, allergies, depression, muscle spasms, obesity, ulcers, irritable colon, and prostate cancer can cause impotence, breast enlargement, testicular swelling, priapism (persistent erection), loss of sexual desire, inability to ejaculate, and reduced sperm count. In women, they can diminish sexual desire, inhibit or delay orgasm, and cause breast swelling or secretions.

Atypical Behavior

Although sexual desire and response are universal, some individuals develop sexual appetites or engage in activities that are not typical sexual behaviors.

Sexual Addiction

Some men and women can get relief from their feelings of restlessness and worthlessness only through sex (either masturbation or with a partner). Once the sexual high ends, however, they're overwhelmed by the same negative feelings and driven, once more, to have sex.

Some therapists describe this problem as sexual addiction; others, as sexual compulsion. Professionals continue to debate exactly what this controversial condition is, how to diagnose it, and how to overcome it. However, most agree that for some people, sex is more than a normal pleasure: It is an overwhelming need that must be met, even at the cost of their careers and marriages.

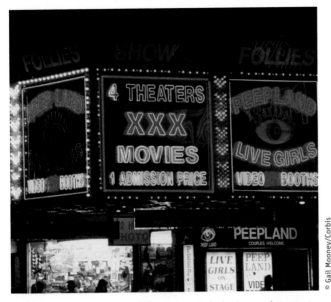

© Gail Mooney/Corbis

Sex sells. Topless bars and strip clubs are among the businesses that cater to those who enjoy sexual stimulation outside a loving relationship.

Sex addicts can be heterosexual or homosexual, male or female. Their behaviors include masturbation, phone sex, reading or viewing pornography, attending strip shows, having affairs, engaging in anonymous sex with strangers or prostitutes, exhibitionism, voyeurism, child molestation, incest, and rape. Many were physically and emotionally abused as children or have family members who abuse drugs or alcohol. They typically feel a loss of control and a compulsion for sexual activity, and they continue their unhealthy (and sometimes illegal) sexual behavior despite the dangers, including the risk of contracting STIs.

With help, sex addicts can deal with the shame that both triggers and follows sexual activity. Professional therapy may begin with a month of complete sexual abstinence, to break the cycle of compulsive sexual behavior. Several organizations, such as Sexaholics Anonymous and Sexual Addicts Anonymous, offer support from people who share the same problem.

Sexual Deviations

Sexual deviations listed by the American Psychiatric Association include the following:

- **Fetishism:** Obtaining sexual pleasure from an inanimate object or an asexual part of the body, such as the foot.
- **Transvestitism:** Becoming sexually aroused by wearing the clothing of the opposite sex.

- **Exhibitionism:** Exposing one's genitals to an unwilling observer.
- **Voyeurism:** Obtaining sexual gratification by observing people undressing or involved in sexual activity.
- **Sadism:** Becoming sexually aroused by inflicting physical or psychological pain.
- **Masochism:** Obtaining sexual gratification by suffering physical or psychological pain.

Another, increasingly common sexual variation, hypoxyphilia, involves attempts to enhance the pleasure of orgasm by reducing oxygen intake. Individuals who do so by tying a noose around the neck have accidentally killed themselves.

Psychiatrists distinguish between passive sexual deviancy, which doesn't involve actual contact with another, and aggressive deviancy. Most voyeurs and obscene phone callers don't seek physical contact with the objects of their sexual desire. These behaviors are performed predominantly, but not exclusively, by males.

The Business of Sex

Sex, without affection and individuality, becomes a product to be packaged, marketed, traded, bought, and sold. Two of the billion-dollar industries that treat sex as a commodity are prostitution and pornography.

Prostitution, described as the world's oldest profession, is a nationwide industry grossing more than $1 billion annually. In every state except Nevada (and in all but a few counties there), prostitution is illegal. Besides the threat of jail and fines, prostitutes and their clients face another danger: sexually transmitted infections, including HIV infection and hepatitis B.

Pornography is a multimedia industry—books, magazines, movies, the Internet, phone lines, and computer games are available to those who find sexually explicit material entertaining or exciting. Most laws against pornography are based on the assumption that such materials can set off uncontrollable, dangerous sexual urges, ranging from promiscuity to sexual violence. Research indicates that exposure to scenes of rape or other forms of sexual violence against women, or to scenes of degradation of women, does lead to tolerance of these hostile and brutal acts.

Learn It : **Live It**

Being Sexually Responsible

We remain sexual beings throughout life. At different ages and stages, sexuality can take on different meanings. As you forge relationships and explore your sexuality, you may encounter difficult situations and unfamiliar feelings. But sex is never just about hormones and body parts. People describe the brain as the sexiest of our organs. Using your brain to make responsible sexual decisions leads to both a smarter and a more fulfilling sex life.

- **Communicate openly.** If you or your partner cannot talk openly and honestly about your sexual histories and contraception, you should avoid having sex. For the sake of protecting your sexual health, you have to be willing to ask—and answer—questions that may seem embarrassing.

- **Share responsibility in a sexual relationship.** Both partners should be involved in protecting themselves and each other from STIs and, if heterosexual, unwanted pregnancy.

- **Respect sexual privacy.** Revealing sexual activities violates the trust between two partners. Bragging about a sexual conquest demeans everyone involved.

- **Do not sexually harass others.** Pinches, pats, sexual comments or jokes, and suggestive gestures are offensive and disrespectful.

- **Be considerate.** A public display of sexual affection can be extremely embarrassing to others. Roommates, in particular, should be sensitive and discrete in their sexual behavior.

- **Be prepared.** If there's any possibility that you may be engaging in sex, be sure you have the means to protect yourself against unwanted pregnancy and sexually transmitted infections.

- **In sexual situations, always think ahead.** For the sake of safety, think about potential dangers—parking in an isolated area, going into a bedroom with someone you hardly know, and the like—and options to protect yourself.

- **Be aware of your own and your partner's alcohol and drug intake.** The use of such substances impairs judgment and reduces the ability to say no. While under their influence, you may engage in sexual behavior you'll later regret.

- **Be sure sexual activity is consensual.** Coercion can take many forms: physical, emotional, and verbal. All cause psychological damage and undermine trust and respect. At any point in a relationship, whether the couple is dating or married, either individual has the right to say no.

Source: Adapted from Hatcher, Robert, et al. *Sexual Etiquette 101 and More.* Atlanta, GA: Emory University School of Medicine, 2002.

SELFSURVEY : *How Much Do You Know About Sex?*

Mark each of the following statements True or False:
1. Men and women have completely different sex hormones.
2. Premenstrual syndrome (PMS) is primarily a psychological problem.
3. Circumcision diminishes a man's sexual pleasure.
4. Sexual orientation may have a biological basis.
5. Masturbation is a sign of emotional immaturity.
6. Only homosexual men engage in anal intercourse.
7. Despite their awareness of AIDS, many college students do not practice safe sex.
8. After age 60, lovemaking is mainly a fond memory, not a regular pleasure of daily living.
9. Doctors advise against having intercourse during a woman's menstrual period.
10. Only men ejaculate.
11. It is possible to be infected with HIV during a single sexual encounter.
12. Impotence is always a sign of emotional or sexual problems in a relationship.

Answers:

1. False. Men and women have the same hormones, but in different amounts.
2. False. PMS has been recognized as a physiological disorder that may be caused by a hormonal deficiency, abnormal levels of thyroid hormone, or social and environmental factors, such as stress.
3. False. Sex therapists have not been able to document differences in sensitivity to stimulation between circumcised and uncircumcised men.
4. True. Researchers documented structural differences in the brains of homosexual men and women.
5. False. Throughout a person's life, masturbation can be a form of sexual release and pleasure.
6. False. As many as one in every four married couples under age 35 have reported that they occasionally engage in anal intercourse.
7. True. In one recent study, more than a third of college students had engaged in vaginal or anal intercourse at least once in the previous year without using effective protection from conception or sexually transmitted infections (STIs).
8. False. More than a third of American married men and women older than 60 make love at least once a week, as do 10 percent of those older than 70.
9. False. There's no medical reason to avoid intercourse during a woman's menstrual period.
10. False. Some researchers say that stimulation of the Grafenberg spot in a woman's vagina may lead to a release of fluid from her urethra during orgasm.
11. True. Although the risk increases with repeated sexual contact with an infected partner, an individual can contract HIV during a single sexual encounter.
12. False. Many erection difficulties have physical causes.

Your Action Plan for Responsible Sexuality

Your score on the Self Survey may indicate that you know a lot more—or less—about sex than you thought you did. Part of sexual responsibility is being informed about sexuality, including reproductive anatomy, sexual orientation, the range of sexual behaviors, and ways of protecting yourself from sexually transmitted diseases.

The Sexuality Information and Education Council of the United States (SIECUS) has worked with nongovernmental organizations around the world to develop a consensus about the life behaviors of a sexually healthy and responsible adult. These include:

- Appreciating one's own body.
- Seeking information about reproduction as needed.
- Affirming that sexual development may or may not include reproduction or genital sexual experience.
- Interacting with both genders in respectful and appropriate ways.
- Affirming one's own sexual orientation and respecting the sexual orientation of others.
- Expressing love and intimacy in appropriate ways.
- Developing and maintaining meaningful relationships.
- Avoiding exploitative or manipulative relationships.
- Making informed choices about family options and lifestyles.
- Enjoying and expressing one's sexuality throughout life.
- Expressing one's sexuality in ways congruent with one's values.
- Discriminating between life-enhancing sexual behaviors and those that are harmful to oneself and/or others.
- Expressing one's sexuality while respecting the rights of others.

- Seeking new information to enhance one's sexuality.
- Using contraception effectively to avoid unintended pregnancy.
- Preventing sexual abuse.
- Seeking early prenatal care.
- Avoiding contracting or transmitting a sexually transmitted infection, including HIV.
- Practicing health-promoting behaviors, such as regular checkups, breast and testicular self-exam, and early identification of potential problems.
- Demonstrating tolerance for people with different sexual values and lifestyles.
- Exercising democratic responsibility to influence legislation dealing with sexual issues.
- Assessing the impact of family, cultural, religious, media, and societal messages on one's thoughts, feelings, values, and behaviors related to sexuality.
- Promoting the rights of all people to accurate sexuality information.
- Avoiding behaviors that exhibit prejudice and bigotry.
- Rejecting stereotypes about the sexuality of diverse populations.

CENGAGENOW If you want to write your own goals for responsible sexual behavior, go to the Wellness Journal at HealthNow: **academic .cengage.com/login.**

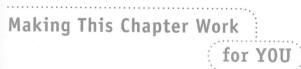

Making This Chapter Work for YOU

Review Questions

1. The hormones that influence the early development of sexual organs
   a. are released by the ovaries in the female and the testes in the male.
   b. begin to work soon after conception during the embryo's development.
   c. begin to work during puberty, when they stimulate the development of secondary male and female sex characteristics.
   d. determine one's biological sex.

2. Which of the following statements about the menstrual cycle is true?
   a. The pituitary gland releases estrogen and progesterone.
   b. Ovulation occurs at the end of the menstrual cycle.
   c. Premenstrual syndrome is a physiological disorder that usually results in amenorrhea.
   d. The endometrium becomes thicker during the cycle and is shed during menstruation.

3. Which statement about male anatomy is *incorrect?*
   a. The testes manufacture testosterone and sperm.
   b. Sperm cells are carried in the liquid semen.
   c. Cowper's glands secrete semen.
   d. Circumcision is the surgical removal of the foreskin of the penis.

4. Which of the following behaviors is most likely to be a characteristic of sexually healthy and responsible adults?
   a. engages in frequent sexual encounters with many partners
   b. avoids the use of condoms in order to heighten sexual enjoyment for both partners
   c. uses alcohol sparingly and only to help loosen the inhibitions of a resistant partner
   d. engages in sex that is unquestionably consensual

5. Which of the following statements is true about sexual orientation?
   a. Most individuals who identify themselves as bisexual are really homosexual.
   b. Homosexuality is caused by a poor family environment.
   c. Homosexual behavior is found only in affluent and well-educated cultures.
   d. The African American, Hispanic, and Asian cultures tend to be less accepting of homosexuality than the white community.

6. According to the Centers for Disease Control, abstinence is defined as
   a. refraining from all sexual behaviors that result in arousal.
   b. refraining from all sexual activities that involve vaginal, anal, and oral intercourse.
   c. having sexual intercourse with only one partner exclusively.
   d. refraining from drinking alcohol before sexual activity.

7. Which statement about sexual activity is *not* true?
   a. College students consider sexual activity normal for their peer group.
   b. The frequency of sexual activity is highest among those with some college education.
   c. Men and women have sex for generally similar reasons.
   d. Masters and Johnson discovered five stages in human sexual response.

8. Which of the following statements about erectile dysfunction (ED) is *false?*
   a. ED is usually caused by physical factors.
   b. A popular treatment for ED is Viagra.
   c. ED is usually caused by psychological factors.
   d. Men who are heavy smokers are at risk for developing ED.

9. Women may experience which of the following problems during intercourse?
   a. vaginismus
   b. excitement
   c. vaginal expansion
   d. amenorrhea

10. Atypical sexual behaviors include which of the following?
    a. masochism
    b. sexual desire
    c. masturbation
    d. celibacy

Answers to these questions can be found on page 583.

Critical Thinking

1. Tad has told his girlfriend, Kylie, that he has never taken any sexual risks. But when she suggested that they get tested for STIs, he became furious and refused. Now Kylie says she doesn't know what to believe. Could Tad be telling the truth, or is he hiding something? If he is telling the truth, why is Tad so upset? Kylie doesn't want to take any risks, but she doesn't want to lose him either. What would you advise her to say or do? What would you advise Tad to say or do?

2. Sex education is always a controversial topic. In SIECUS national surveys, nine in ten parents believe it is important to have sex education as part of the curriculum. Other parents feel that boys and girls should learn about sex and sexual values in the home. Did you have "sex ed" in junior high or high school? What do you think about such classes—and why?

3. Do you think it is okay to read or look at pornographic books, magazines, websites, and videos? Why or why not?

Media Menu

CENGAGENOW™ Go to the HealthNow website at **academic.cengage .com/login** that will:

- Help you evaluate your knowledge of the material.
- Allow you to take an exam-prep quiz.
- Provide a Personalized Learning Plan targeting resources that address areas you should study.
- Coach you through identifying target goals for behavioral change and creating and monitoring your personal change plan throughout the semester.

INTERNET CONNECTIONS

The Sexuality Information and Education Council of the United States (SIECUS)

www.siecus.org

This website is sponsored by SIECUS, a national nonprofit organization that promotes comprehensive education about sexuality and advocates the right of all individuals of all sexual orientations to make responsible sexual choices. The site features a library of fact sheets and articles on a variety of sexuality topics and STIs designed for educators, adults, teens, parents, media, international audiences, and religious organizations.

Human Rights Campaign

www.hrc.org

The Human Rights Campaign is America's largest gay, lesbian, bisexual, and transgender civil rights organization. Its website features up-to-date information on issues related to gay rights and suggests courses of action to change government policies.

Go Ask Alice

www.goaskalice.columbia.edu/

Sponsored by the health education and wellness program of the Columbia University Health Service, this site features educators' answers to questions on a wide variety of topics of concern to young people, including those related to sexual orientation and healthy sexuality.

Key Terms

The terms listed are used and defined on the page indicated. Definitions are also found in the Glossary at the end of this book.

abstinence 251
amenorrhea 242
androgyny 238
bisexual 249
celibacy 251
cervix 239
circumcision 245
clitoris 238
corpus luteum 240
Cowper's glands 245
cunnilingus 255
dysmenorrhea 242
dyspareunia 259
ejaculation 255

ejaculatory ducts 245
endocrine system 237
endometrium 239
epididymis 243
erectile dysfunction (ED) 259
erogenous 253
estrogen 237
fallopian tubes 240
fellatio 255
gender 237
gonadotropins 237
heterosexual 249
homosexual 249
hormones 237
intercourse 253
intimacy 237
labia majora 238
labia minora 238
masturbation 247
menarche 238
menstruation 240
mons pubis 238
nocturnal emissions 247
orgasm 255
ovaries 239
ovulation 240
ovum (ova) 240
penis 242
perineum 239
premature ejaculation 259
premenstrual dysphoric disorder (PMDD) 242
premenstrual syndrome (PMS) 240
progesterone 237
prostate gland 245
refractory period 257
scrotum 242
secondary sex characteristics 237
semen 243
seminal vesicles 243
sex 237
sexual dysfunction 257
sexual health 237
sexual orientation 249
sexuality 237
sperm 243
testes 242
testosterone 237
toxic shock syndrome (TSS) 242
transgender 251
urethra 243
urethral opening 239
uterus 239
vagina 239
vaginismus 259
vas deferens 243

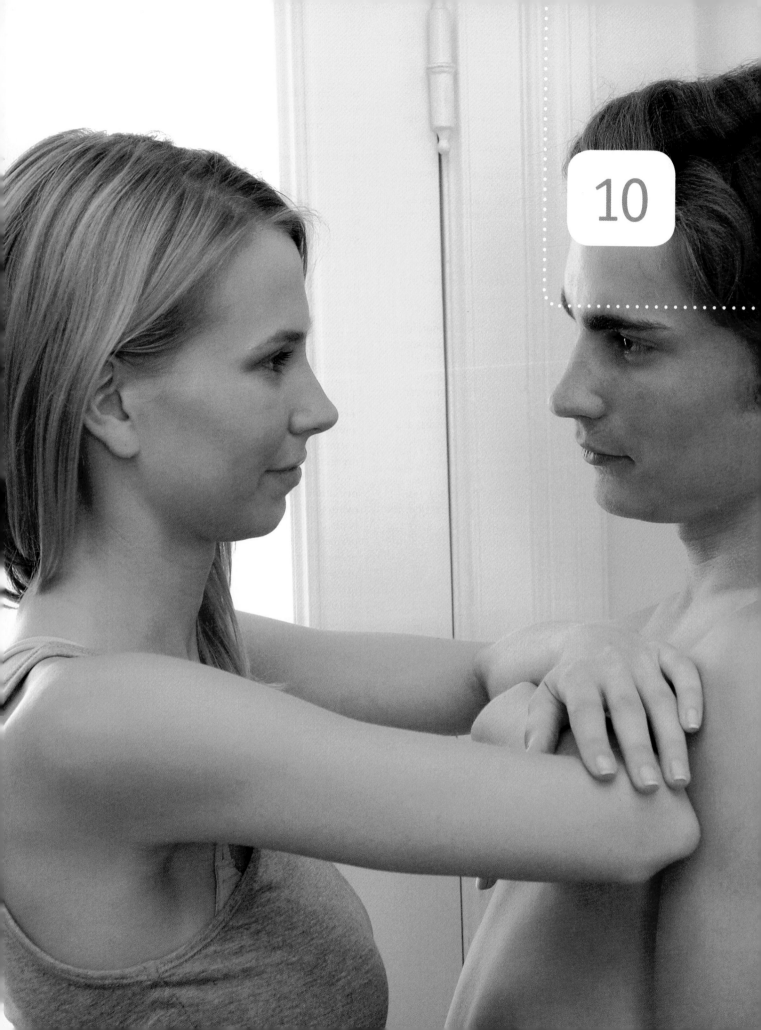

Reproductive Choices

JESS and Sara, juniors at the same community college, can't remember a time when abortion was illegal, when AIDS wasn't a deadly threat, and when safe sex wasn't a concern of every sexually active individual. Yet even though they were aware of the risks and the realities involved, neither used contraception during every single sexual encounter. Then one of Jess's partners had a pregnancy scare. He decided never again to engage in unprotected sex. Sara had a different reality check: At her regular physical, she learned that she had contracted chlamydia, the most common sexually transmitted infection in the United States.

When Jess and Sara started dating, both of them felt that something was special about their relationship. Despite their mutual attraction, they decided to take every step toward intimacy slowly. Both considered and talked about their personal priorities and concerns. Even though it was awkward, they also discussed their own sexual histories and underwent tests for STIs. Looking toward a continuing committed relationship, they decided on not one but two forms of contraception: the birth control pill and a condom. In the future, they realized that they might switch to other forms of birth control—and might well consider different options, including both marriage and parenthood.

As human beings, we have a unique power: the ability to choose to conceive or not to conceive. No other species on Earth can separate sexual activity and pleasure from reproduction. However, simply not wanting to get pregnant is never enough to prevent conception, nor is wanting to have a child always enough to get pregnant. Both desires require individual decisions and actions. (See the lab "To Have or Have Not" in *IPC*.) **IPC**

This chapter provides information on conception, birth control, abortion, infertility, adoption, and the processes by which a new human life develops and enters the world.

After studying the material in this chapter, you should be able to:

- **Describe** the process of human conception.

- **List** the major options available for contraception, and **identify** the advantages and disadvantages of each.

- **Describe** the commonly used abortion methods.

- **Discuss** the physiological effects of pregnancy on a woman and describe fetal development.

- **Give examples** of prenatal care measures.

- **Describe** the three stages of labor and the birth process.

- **Identify** the options available to infertile couples wanting children.

- If contraception is one of your reproductive choices for the next three years, **name** the methods you will likely use and why.

CENGAGENOW™ Log on to HealthNow at **academic.cengage.com/login** to find your Behavior Change Planner and to explore self-assessments, interactive tutorials, and practice quizzes.

Anyone who engages in vaginal intercourse must be willing to accept the consequences of that activity—the possibility of pregnancy and responsibility for the child who might be conceived—or take action to avoid those consequences. Although many people are concerned about the risks associated with contraception, using birth control is safer and healthier than not using it. According to the Population Reference Bureau, the use of contraceptives, including oral contraceptives, saves millions of lives each year.

Conception

The equation for making a baby is quite simple: One sperm plus one egg equals one fertilized egg, which can develop into an infant. But the processes that affect or permit **conception** are quite complicated. The creation of sperm, or **spermatogenesis,** starts in the male at puberty, and the production of sperm is regulated by hormones. Sperm cells form in the seminiferous tubules of the testes and are passed into the epididymis, where they are stored until ejaculation; a single male ejaculation may contain 500 million sperm. Each sperm released into the vagina during intercourse moves on its own, propelling itself toward its target, an ovum.

To reach its goal, the sperm must move through the acidic secretions of the vagina, enter the uterus, travel up the fallopian tube containing the ovum, then fuse with the nucleus of the egg (**fertilization**). Just about every sperm produced by a man in his lifetime fails to accomplish its mission.

There are far fewer human egg cells than there are sperm cells. Each woman is born with her lifetime supply of ova, and between 300 and 500 eggs eventually mature and leave her ovaries during ovulation. As discussed in Chapter 9, every month, one or the other of the woman's ovaries releases an ovum to the nearby fallopian tube. It travels through the fallopian tube until it reaches the uterus, a journey that takes three to four days. An unfertilized egg lives for about 24 to 36 hours, disintegrates, and during menstruation is expelled along with the uterine lining.

Even if a sperm, which can survive in the female reproductive tract for two to five days, meets a ripe egg in a fallopian tube, its success is not assured. A mature ovum releases the chemical allurin, which attracts the sperm. A sperm is able to penetrate the ovum's outer membrane because of a protein called fertilin. The egg then pulls the sperm inside toward its nucleus (Figure 10.1). The fertilized egg travels down the fallopian tube, dividing to form a tiny clump of cells called a **zygote.** When it reaches the uterus, about a week after fertilization, it burrows into the endometrium, the lining of the uterus. This process is called **implantation.**

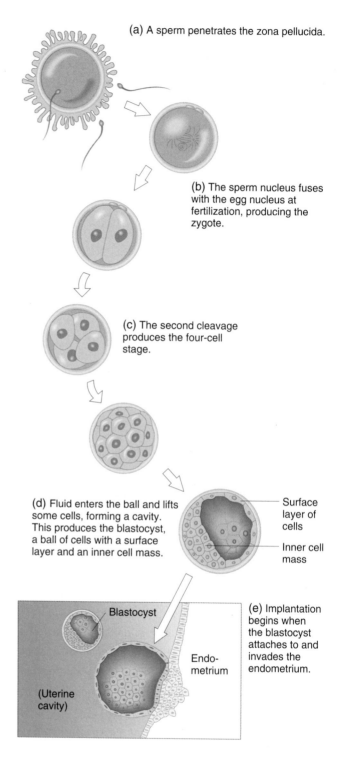

(a) A sperm penetrates the zona pellucida.

(b) The sperm nucleus fuses with the egg nucleus at fertilization, producing the zygote.

(c) The second cleavage produces the four-cell stage.

(d) Fluid enters the ball and lifts some cells, forming a cavity. This produces the blastocyst, a ball of cells with a surface layer and an inner cell mass.

Surface layer of cells

Inner cell mass

Blastocyst

(Uterine cavity)

Endo-metrium

(e) Implantation begins when the blastocyst attaches to and invades the endometrium.

Figure 10.1 Fertilization

(a) The efforts of hundreds of sperm may allow one to penetrate the ovum's corona radiata, an outer layer of cells, and then the zona pellucida, a thick inner membrane. (b) The nuclei of the sperm and the egg cells merge, and the male and female chromosomes in the nuclei come together, forming a zygote. (c) The zygote divides into two cells, then four cells, and so on. (d) As fluid enters the ball, cells form a ball of cells called a blastocyst. (e) The blastocyst implants itself in the endometrium.

Conception can be prevented by **contraception.** Some contraceptive methods prevent ovulation or implantation, and others block the sperm from reaching the egg. Some methods are temporary; others permanently alter one's fertility.

Birth Control Basics

Most sexually active women use some form of birth control. According to the Centers for Disease Control and Prevention, more than 98 percent of women between the ages of 15 and 44 who have ever had intercourse have used at least one contraceptive method. Most of the women not using any form of contraception are pregnant, trying to get pregnant, unable to conceive, or not having intercourse. (See Reality Check.)

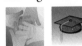 The use of contraception has declined in recent years, particularly among poor women. As a result, they are more likely to get pregnant unintentionally and to have abortions. An estimated 11 percent of sexually active women, including white, Hispanic, and African American women who are not trying to get pregnant do not use birth control, up from 7 percent in 1994. The rate of unintended births also has risen. About half of the three million pregnancies that occur every year in the United States are unintended. Half of these are carried to term. About 14,000 women who continue their pregnancies put the children up for adoption; 1.3 million women have

REALITYCHECK

• *How many students used birth control the last time they had vaginal intercourse?* _____
• *How many students used condoms last time they had vaginal intercourse?* _____
• *How many sexually active students reported using (or reported their partner using) emergency contraception within the last 12 months?* _____

Answers on next page.

abortions.[1] Among sexually active students, 2 percent of women and 2 percent of men report having become pregnant or having gotten someone pregnant unintentionally in the past year.[2]

If you are engaging in sexual activity that could lead to conception, you have to be realistic about your situation. This means assuming full responsibility for your reproductive ability, whether you're a man or a woman. The more you know about contraception, the more likely you are to use birth control.

You also have to recognize the risks associated with various methods of contraception. If you're a woman, the risks are chiefly yours. Various methods of birth control have side effects, but pregnancy and childbirth account for much higher rates of medical complications and deaths than any contraceptive. Although most women never experience any serious complications, it's important to be aware of the potential for long-term risks. Risks that are acceptable to others may not be acceptable to you.

Your Life Change Coach

Choosing a Birth Control Method

When it comes to deciding which form of birth control to use, there's no one "right" decision. Good decisions are based on sound information. You should consult a physician or family-planning counselor if you have questions or want to know how certain methods might affect existing or familial medical conditions, such as high blood pressure or diabetes.

Table 10.1 presents your contraceptive choices. As the table indicates, contraception doesn't always work. When you evaluate any contraceptive, always consider its effectiveness (the likelihood that it will indeed prevent pregnancy). The **failure rate** refers to the number of pregnancies that occur per year for every 100 women using a particular method of birth control.

The reliability of contraceptives in actual, real-life use is much lower than those reported in national surveys or clinical trials. In general, failure rates are highest among cohabiting and other unmarried women, very poor families, African American and Hispanic women, adolescents, and women in their twenties.

Some couples use withdrawal or **coitus interruptus**, removal of the penis from the vagina before ejaculation, to prevent pregnancy, even though this is not a reliable form of birth control. About half the men who have tried coitus interruptus find it unsatisfactory, either

conception The merging of a sperm and an ovum.

spermatogenesis The process by which sperm cells are produced.

fertilization The fusion of sperm and egg nucleus.

zygote A fertilized egg.

implantation The embedding of the fertilized ovum in the uterine lining.

contraception The prevention of conception; birth control.

failure rate The number of pregnancies that occur per year for every 100 women using a particular method of birth control.

coitus interruptus The removal of the penis from the vagina before ejaculation.

PART II: *Just the Facts*

- **96** *percent of students said they used birth control the last time they had vaginal intercourse.*
- **54** *percent of students used condoms the last time they had vaginal intercourse.*
- **11** *percent of sexually active students reported using (or reported their partner using) emergency contraception within the last 12 months.*

Source: American College Health Association. *American College Health Association National College Health Assessment Reference Group Executive Summary Fall 2006.* Baltimore: American College Health Association, 2007.

because they don't know when they're going to ejaculate or because they can't withdraw quickly enough. Also, the Cowper's glands, two pea-sized structures located on each side of the urethra, often produce a fluid that appears as drops at the tip of the penis any time from arousal and erection to orgasm. This fluid can contain active sperm and, in infected men, human immunodeficiency virus (HIV).

Many unintentional pregnancies are the result of contraceptive failure, either from problems with the drug or device itself or from improper use. Partners can lower the risk of unwanted pregnancy by using backup methods—that is, more than one form of contraception simultaneously. Emergency or after-intercourse contraception (discussed later in this chapter) could prevent as many as 1.7 million unwanted pregnancies each year.

 Even college students aware of the risks associated with unprotected sexual intercourse often do not practice safe-sex behaviors. There are many reasons, ranging from the influence of sex and alcohol to embarrassment about buying condoms. Generally, the ability to talk about a desire to use condoms has been found to be associated with a greater use of condoms.

The bottom line is that it takes two people to conceive a baby, and two people should be involved in deciding not to conceive a baby. In the process, they can also enhance their skills in communication, critical thinking, and negotiating. (See "Listen Up" in *IPC*.) **IPC** (See Your Strategies for Prevention: "How to Choose a Contraceptive.")

Table 10.1 Overview of Contraceptive Options

Method	Failure Rate	Frequency of Use	Protection against STIs	Cost
None	85%	—	No	None
Spermicide	20–50%	Each time	No	$0.35 to 12
Withdrawal	27%	Each time	No	None
Periodic abstinence	20%	Each month	No	None
Sponge*	14–28%	Each time	No	$2.50 to $3 a sponge
Cervical cap* (FemCap) (women who have not had children)	23–24% (possibly higher in women who have had children)	Each time	No	$70 or more for cap; $50 to $200 for fitting
Diaphragm*	16%	Each time	No	$30 to $50 plus fitting
Female condom	21%	Each time	Yes	$2 to $3 each
Male condom	15% (5% when used with spermicide)	Each time	Yes	$0.50 to $2 each
Progestin-only pill	8%	Taken daily	No	$30 to $35 per month
Injection	3%	Injection every 12 weeks	No	$60 to $75 per shot plus exam
The pill (combination)	1–8%	Taken daily	No	$20 to $50 per cycle plus annual exam
Contraceptive patch	1–2%	Applied weekly	No	$30 to $40 per month
NuvaRing	1–2%	Inserted every 4 weeks	No	$43 per month
Seasonale	1–2%	Taken daily for 3 months	No	$160 to $200 for 91 pills
Copper-containing IUD	<1%	Inserted every 10 years	No	$200 to $400
Mirena	0.1%	Inserted every 5 years	No	$300 to $400 every 5 years
Female sterilization	<1%	Done once	No	$2,500 to $4,000
Male sterilization	<1%	Done once	No	$250 to $1,000
Emergency contraception		After unprotected intercourse		$8 to $25 for Plan B

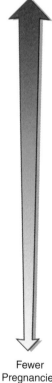

More Pregnancies

Fewer Pregnancies

STI, sexually transmitted infection; IUD, intrauterine device. *Used with spermicide. Source: Food and Drug Administration, www.fda.gov., www.mayoclinic.com

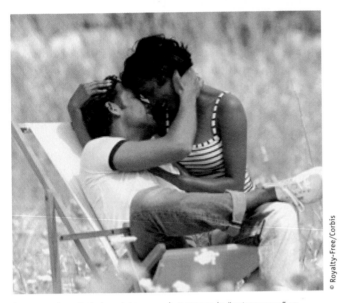

© Royalty-Free/Corbis

Some couples refrain from intercource but engage in "outercourse," or intimacy that includes kissing and hugging.

Abstinence and Nonpenetrative Sexual Activity

The contraceptive methods discussed in this chapter are designed to prevent pregnancy as a consequence of vaginal intercourse. Couples who choose abstinence make a very different decision—to abstain from vaginal intercourse and forms of nonpenetrative sexual activity that could result in conception (any in which ejaculation occurs near the vaginal opening).

For many individuals, abstinence represents a deliberate choice regarding their bodies, minds, spirits, and sexuality. People choose abstinence for various reasons, including waiting until they are ready for a sexual relationship or until they find the "right" partner, respecting religious or moral values, enjoying friendships without sexual involvement, recovering from a breakup, or preventing pregnancy and sexually transmitted infection (see Chapter 16).

Practicing abstinence is the only form of birth control that is 100 percent effective and risk-free. It is also an important, increasingly valued lifestyle choice. A growing number of individuals, including some who have been sexually active in the past, are choosing abstinence until they establish a relationship with a long-term partner.

Abstinence offers special health benefits for women. Those who abstain until their twenties and engage in sex with fewer partners during their lifetime are less likely to get sexually transmitted infections, to suffer infertility, or to develop cervical cancer. However, some people find it difficult to abstain for long periods of time. There also is a risk that people will abruptly end their abstinence without being prepared to protect themselves against pregnancy or infection.

Individuals who choose abstinence from vaginal intercourse often engage in activities sometimes called *outercourse,* such as kissing, hugging, sensual touching, and mutual masturbation. Outercourse is nearly 100 percent effective as a contraceptive measure, but pregnancy is possible if there is genital contact. If the man ejaculates near the vaginal opening, sperm can swim up into the vagina and fallopian tubes to fertilize an egg. Outercourse also may lower the risk of contracting sexually transmitted infections. It is an effective form of safe sex as long as no body fluids are exchanged.

Some couples routinely restrict themselves to outercourse; others temporarily choose such sexual activities when it is inadvisable for them to have vaginal intercourse, for example, after childbirth. Other benefits: Outercourse has no medical or hormonal side effects; it may prolong sex play and enhance orgasm, and it can be used when no other birth control methods are available.

Barrier Contraceptives

Table 10.2 presents the contraceptives by type and how accessible they are. We start with the barriers. As their name implies, **barrier contraceptives** block the meeting of egg and sperm by means of a physical barrier (condom, sponge, diaphragm, cervical cap, or FemCap) or a chemical one (vaginal spermicide in jellies, foams, creams, suppositories, or film).

barrier contraceptives Birth control devices that block the meeting of egg and sperm, either by physical barriers, such as condoms, diaphragms, or cervical caps, or by chemical barriers, such as spermicide, or both.

Nonprescription Barriers

The nonprescription barrier contraceptives include the male and female condom, the contraceptive sponge, and vaginal spermicides. Condoms provide some protection against HIV infection and other STIs; spermicides, sponges, and films do not.

Male Condom

The male **condom** covers the erect penis and catches the ejaculate, thus preventing sperm from entering the woman's reproductive tract (Figure 10.2). Most are made of thin surgical latex or sheep membrane; a new type is made of polyurethane, which is thinner, stronger, more heat sensitive, and more comfortable than latex. In a study of 901 couples over six months, the polyurethane condom was not as effective as the latex condom for pregnancy prevention. Experts now advise against use of condoms with nonoxynol-9 which may increase rather than lower the risk of sexual infections (see discussion in Chapter 16).

Although the theoretical effectiveness rate for condoms is 97 percent, the actual rate is only 80 to 85 percent. The condom can be torn during the manufacturing process or during its use; testing by the manufacturer may not be as strenuous as it could or should be. Careless removal can also decrease the effectiveness of condoms. However, the major reason that condoms have such a low actual effectiveness rate is that couples don't use them each and every time they have sex. Users who have little experience with condoms—who are young, single, or childless, or who engage in risky behaviors—are more likely to have condoms break.

 Condoms are second only to the pill in popularity among college-age adults. About half (54 percent) of sexually active students report using condoms the last time they had vaginal intercourse. However, only 17 percent of students say they always used condoms during vaginal intercourse during the previous 30 days; 20 percent said they never used them.[3] Nearly one-third of students in one survey reported discomfort, such as a too-tight fit or loss of pleasurable sensation. These students were less likely to use condoms correctly and more likely to report condom breakage. Larger-sized condoms and/or vaginal lubricants can eliminate many complaints of discomfort.[4]

College men also may try to avoid condom use because of concern about erectile dysfunction (ED), the inability to maintain a penile erection sufficient for sexual relations. In an anonymous survey of 234 sexually active males between the ages of 18 to 25 on three university campuses, 25 percent reported ED with condom use. These men were much more inconsistent in their use of condoms than other students. Six percent of all the students surveyed had taken ED medications, such as Viagra. Almost two-thirds mixed these medications with alcohol and drugs, such as ecstasy or methamphetamine.[5]

Female Condom

The female condom, made of polyurethane, consists of two rings and a polyurethane sheath, and is inserted into the vagina with a tamponlike applicator (Figure 10.3). Once in place, the device loosely lines the walls of the vagina. Internally, a thickened rubber ring keeps it anchored near the cervix. Externally, another rubber ring, 2 inches in diameter, rests on the labia and resists slippage.

TABLE 10.2 Contraceptive Options: Types and Accessibility

Type	Accessibility
Barrier Contraceptives	
Male condom	Over-the-counter
Female condom	Over-the-counter
Sponge	Over-the-counter
Spermicide	Over-the-counter
Diaphragm	Requires fitting by physician
Cervical cap	Prescription required
FemCap	Prescription required
Hormonal Contraceptives	
Oral contraceptives	
Combination pills	Prescription required
Progestin-only pills	Prescription required
Extended-use pills	Prescription required
The Patch	Prescription required
The NuvaRing	Prescription required
Contraceptive injections Requires injection every 12 weeks (Depo-Provera)	Prescription required
Contraceptive implants	Requires insertion by physician
Intrauterine Contraceptive	Requires insertion by physician
Fertility Awareness and Periodic Abstinence	Requires woman to chart her menstrual cycle, estimate ovulation, and abstain from vaginal intercourse during ovulation
Emergency Contraception	Over-the-counter if over 18. Prescription required if 17 or younger
Sterilization	
Men—vasectomy	Outpatient procedure
Women—tubal ligation	Outpatient procedure

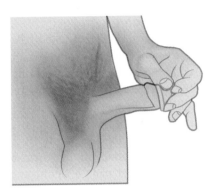

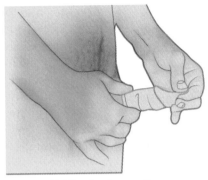

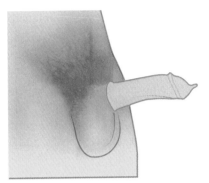

Pinch or twist the tip of the condom, leaving one-half inch at the tip to catch the semen.

Holding the tip, unroll the condom.

Unroll the condom until it reaches the pubic hairs.

Figure 10.2 Male Condom
Condoms effectively reduce the risk of pregnancy as well as STIs if used consistently and correctly.

 Although not widely used in the West, the female condom is gaining acceptance in Africa, Asia, and Latin America. Properly used, it is believed to be as good or better than the male condom for preventing infections, including HIV, because it is stronger and covers a slightly larger area. Female condoms may be more prone to slipping and other mechanical problems but are as effective as male condoms in blocking semen.[6] The efficacy of female condoms does increase with a woman's experience in using them.

How They Work

Male Condoms   Most physicians recommend prelubricated, spermicide-treated, American-made latex or polyurethane condoms, not membrane condoms ("natural" or "sheepskin"). Before using a condom, check the expiration date and make sure it's soft and pliable. If it's yellow or sticky, throw it out. Don't check for leaks by blowing up a condom before using it; you may weaken or tear it.

The condom should be put on at the beginning of sexual activity, before genital contact occurs. There should be a little space left at the top of the condom to catch the semen (Figure 10.2). Any vaginal lubricant should be water-based. Petroleum-based creams or jellies (such as Vaseline, baby oil, massage oil, vegetable oils, or oil-based hand lotions) can deteriorate the latex. After ejaculation, the condom should be held firmly against the penis so that it doesn't slip off or leak during withdrawal. Couples engaging in anal intercourse should use a water-based lubricant as well as a condom, but should never assume the condom will provide 100 percent protection from HIV infection or other STIs.

Female Condoms   As illustrated in Figure 10.3, a woman removes the condom and applicator from the wrapper and inserts the condom slowly by gently pushing the applicator toward the small of the back. When properly inserted, the outer ring should rest on the folds of skin around the vaginal opening, and the inner ring (the closed end) should fit against the cervix.

The female condom can be washed and reused several times and still meet the standards set by the FDA, according to the study conducted in South Africa in which a sample of women washed, dried, and relubricated female condoms up to seven times.

Advantages

- Effective when used correctly.
- Lower a woman's risk of pelvic inflammatory disease (PID) and may protect against some urinary tract and genital infections.
- No side effects, unless you're allergic to latex.
- No prescription required.
- Inexpensive.
- The female condom gives women more control in reducing their risk of pregnancy and STIs and does not require a prescription or medical appointment.

Disadvantages

- Requires consistent and diligent use.
- Not 100 percent effective in preventing pregnancy or STIs.
- Risk of manufacturing defects, such as pin-size holes, and breaking or slipping off during intercourse.

condom   A latex sheath worn over the penis during sexual acts to prevent conception and/or the transmission of disease; the female condom lines the walls of the vagina.

- May inhibit sexual spontaneity.
- Users or partners may complain about odor, lubrication (too much or too little), feel, taste, difficulty opening the packages, and disposal.
- Some men dislike reduced penile sensitivity or cannot sustain an erection while putting on a condom.
- Some women complain that the female condom is difficult to use, squeaks, and looks odd.

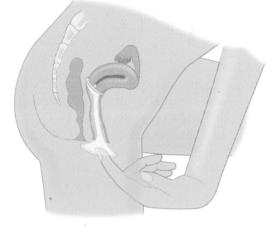

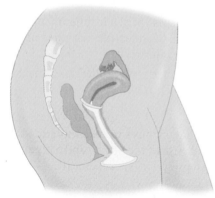

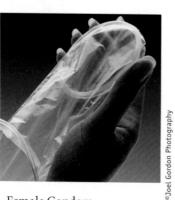

©Joel Gordon Photography

Figure 10.3 Female Condom

No spermicide is used with the female condom. Like the male condom, this method does not require a prescription.

Do Men and Women Use Condoms for Different Reasons?

The genders have very different motives both for engaging in sex and for using condoms. In focus groups, young women say they engage in sexual relations because of a desire for physical intimacy and a committed relationship. They generally report having sex only with men they care for and deeply trust and expect that these men would be honest and forthright about their sexual history. This trust plays a significant role in their decision whether to insist on condom use.

In contrast, few young men say relationships are an important dimension of their sexual involvements. Their primary motivation is a desire for physical and sexual satisfaction. Most say they are not interested in commitment and view emotional expectations as a complication of becoming sexually involved with a woman. Young men also admit to making judgments about types of girls. To them, young women they didn't care about were "sluts" with whom they used a condom for their own protection.

Which partner determines whether a couple uses a condom? The answer is often the women—if they choose to do so. Regardless of race or ethnicity, many young women are adamant in demanding that their partners use condoms—and many young men say they would not challenge such a demand out of fear of losing the opportunity for sex. Men often expect potential partners to want to use condoms and describe themselves as "suspicious" of women who do not.

Both sexes name two primary reasons for using condoms: preventing pregnancy and protecting against sexually transmitted infections. Young women see an unwanted pregnancy as an occurrence that would be disruptive, expensive, and could "ruin" their lives and their parents' lives. Young men see condom use as a way of protecting themselves against emotional entanglements and paternity issues.

Contraceptive Sponge

The Today Sponge, which is made of soft polyurethane foam laced with spermicide was sold as an over-the-counter contraceptive in the United States from 1983 to 1995, when it was withdrawn because of contamination problems at the manufacturing plant. It has returned to stores several times.

How It Works

The contraceptive sponge acts as a barrier by blocking the entrance to the uterus and absorbing and deactivating sperm. Prior to inserting it in the vagina, moisten the sponge with water to activate the spermicide. Then fold it in half and insert deep into the vagina. Check to make sure it is covering the cervix. Intercourse can occur

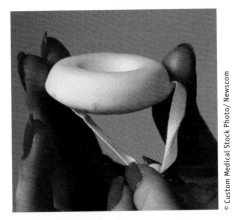

The contraceptive sponge prevents sperm from entering the uterus and is available without a prescription.

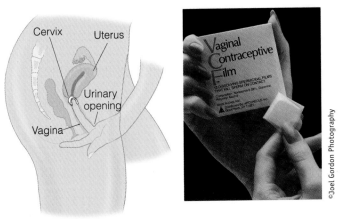

Figure 10.4 Vaginal Contraceptive Film
The effectiveness of this thin film, laced with spermicide, is similar to other spermicides and greatest when used with a condom.

immediately or at any time during the next 24 hours. However, the sponge must remain in place for six hours after intercourse. To remove, gently pull the cloth loop or the tabs on the outside.

Advantages

- Easy to use.
- Can be inserted up to 24 hours before intercourse.
- Effective immediately if used correctly.
- No effect on fertility.

Disadvantages

- May be difficult to remove.
- May be less effective in women who have had children.
- No reliable protection against STIs.
- Requires advance planning to place the sponge.
- Side effects include vaginal irritation and allergic reactions.
- Should not be used during menstruation.

Vaginal Spermicides

The various forms of **vaginal spermicide** include chemical foams, creams, jellies, vaginal suppositories, gels, and film. Some creams and jellies are made for use with a diaphragm; others can be used alone. Several vaginal suppositories claim high effectiveness, but no American studies have confirmed these claims. In general, failure rates for vaginal suppositories are as high as 10 to 25 percent.

One widely used spermicide, nonoxynol-9, has proven to be less effective than once believed. It does not protect against many STIs, including chlamydia and gonorrhea.

Nonoxynol-9 also may increase the risk of infection with human papillomavirus (HPV).[7] The CDC has concluded that it is ineffective against HIV, and the World Health Organization describes it as only "moderately effective" for pregnancy prevention.

Vaginal contraceptive film, a thin two-inch square film laced with spermicide, is folded and inserted into the vagina, where it dissolves into a stay-in-place gel (see Figure 10.4). VCF, which can be used by people allergic to foams and jellies, is as effective as most spermicides and almost 100 percent effective when paired with a condom.

Although more effective methods of birth control now provide good alternatives to spermicides, they remain popular as a means of lowering the risk of STIs.

How They Work

Spermicides consist of a chemical that kills sperm and potential pathogens and an inert base, such as jelly, cream, foam, or film, that holds the spermicide close to the cervix. The jelly, cream, or foam spermicide is inserted into the vagina with an applicator or finger. Vaginal suppositories take about 20 minutes to dissolve and cover the vaginal walls. Follow package directions precisely.

You must apply additional spermicide or insert another VCF film before each additional intercourse. After sex, women should shower rather than bathe to prevent the spermicide from being rinsed out of the vagina, and they should not douche for at least six hours.

vaginal spermicide A substance that kills or neutralizes sperm, inserted into the vagina in the form of a foam, cream, jelly, suppository, or film.

vaginal contraceptive film (VCF) A small dissolvable sheet saturated with spermicide that can be inserted into the vagina and placed over the cervix.

Advantages

- Easy to use.
- Effective if used with another form of contraception, such as condoms.
- Reduces the risk of some vaginal infections, PID, and STIs.
- No effect on fertility.

Disadvantages

- Insertion interrupts sexual spontaneity.
- May cause irritation.
- Some people cannot use foams or jellies because of an allergic reaction.
- Some users complain that spermicides are messy or interfere with oral-genital contact.
- Spermicidal suppositories that do not dissolve completely can feel gritty.

Prescription Barriers

The prescription barrier contraceptives are used by women: the diaphragm, cervical cap, and FemCap. They are placed in the vagina with a spermicide. They do not protect against HIV infection and most STIs.

Diaphragm

The **diaphragm** is a bowl-like rubber cup with a flexible rim that is inserted into the vagina to cover the cervix and prevent the passage of sperm into the uterus during sexual intercourse (Figure 10.5). When used with a spermicide, the diaphragm is both a physical and a chemical barrier to sperm. The effectiveness of the diaphragm in preventing pregnancy depends on strong motivation (to use it faithfully) and a precise understanding of its use. If diaphragms with spermicide are used consistently and carefully, they can be 95 to 98 percent effective. Without a spermicide, the diaphragm is not effective.

Cervical Cap

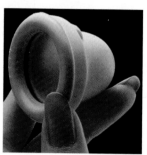

©Joel Gordon Photography

Like the diaphragm, the **cervical cap** combined with spermicide serves as both a chemical and physical barrier blocking the path of the sperm to the uterus. The rubber or plastic cap is smaller and thicker than a diaphragm. It resembles a large thimble that fits snugly around the cervix and may work better for some women. It is about as effective as a diaphragm (95 to 98 percent).

FemCap

The FemCap is a nonhormonal, latex-free barrier contraceptive that works with a spermicide (Figure 10.6). The FemCap, designed to conform to the anatomy of the cervix and vagina, comes in three sizes. The smallest usually best suits women who have never been pregnant; the medium size, for women who have been pregnant but have not had a vaginal delivery; the largest, for those who have delivered a full-term baby vaginally.

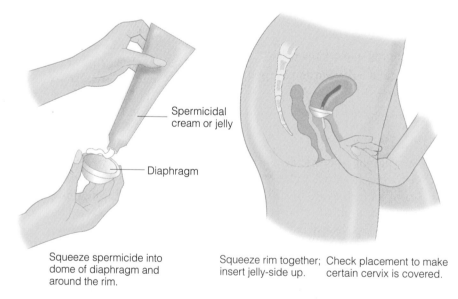

Spermicidal cream or jelly

Diaphragm

Squeeze spermicide into dome of diaphragm and around the rim.

Squeeze rim together; insert jelly-side up.

Check placement to make certain cervix is covered.

Figure 10.5 Diaphragm

When used correctly and consistently and with a spermicide, the diaphragm is effective in preventing pregnancy. It must be fitted by a health-care professional.

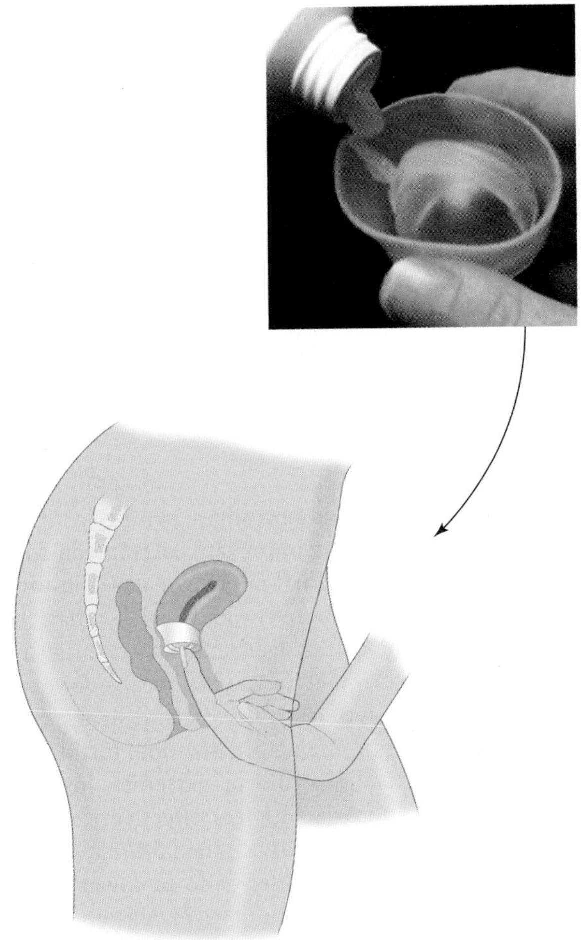

Cervical Cap   Like the diaphragm, the cervical cap is fitted by a qualified health-care professional. For use, the woman fills it one-third to two-thirds full with spermicide and inserts it by holding its edges together and sliding it into the vagina. The cup is then pressed onto the cervix. (Most women find it easiest to do so while squatting or in an upright sitting position.) The cap can be inserted up to 6 hours prior to intercourse and should not be removed for at least 6 hours afterward. It can be left in place up to 24 hours. Pulling on one side of the rim breaks the suction and allows easy removal. Oil-based lubricants should not be used with the cap because they can deteriorate the latex.

FemCap   A prescription is required to purchase FemCap, and the woman selects the appropriate size. Apply spermicide to the bowl of the FemCap (which goes over the cervix), to the outer brim, and to the groove that will face into the vagina. Insert the squeezed, flattened cap into the vagina with the bowl facing upward. The FemCap must be pushed all the way in to cover the cervix completely and left in place at least six hours after intercourse.

Advantages

- Relatively inexpensive.
- Don't interrupt sexual activity; can be inserted hours ahead of time.
- Usually not felt by either partner.
- Can easily be carried in pocket or purse.
- No hormones or side effects.
- Cervical caps are an alternative for women who cannot use diaphragms or find them too messy.

Disadvantages

- Less effective than hormonal contraceptives.
- Available by prescription only.
- Require advance planning or interruption of sexual activity to position the device before intercourse.
- May slip out of place during intercourse.
- May be uncomfortable for some women and their partners.
- Spermicidal foams, creams, and jellies may be messy, cause irritation, and detract from oral–genital sex.

Courtesy of FemCap, Inc., and Alfred Shihata, MD

Figure 10.6   FemCap

The FemCap must be used with spermicide and correctly positioned to cover the cervix completely.

Source: Reproduced with permission from FemCap, Inc., and Alfred Shihata, M.D.

How They Work

Diaphragm   Diaphragms are fitted and prescribed by a qualified health-care professional in diameter sizes ranging from 2 to 4 inches (50 to 105 millimeters). The diaphragm's main function is to serve as a container for a spermicidal (sperm-killing) foam or jelly, which is available at pharmacies without a prescription. A diaphragm should remain in the vagina for at least six hours after intercourse to ensure that all sperm are killed. If intercourse occurs again during this period, additional spermicide must be inserted with an applicator tube.

The key to proper use of the diaphragm is having it available. A sexually active woman should keep it in the most accessible place—her purse, bedroom, bathroom. Before every use, a diaphragm should be checked for tiny leaks (hold up to the light or place water in the dome). A health-care provider should check its fit and condition every year when the woman has her annual Pap smear. Oil-based lubricants will deteriorate the latex of the diaphragm and should not be used with one.

diaphragm   A bowl-like rubber cup with a flexible rim that is inserted into the vagina to cover the cervix and prevent the passage of sperm into the uterus during sexual intercourse; used with a spermicidal foam or jelly, it serves as both a chemical and a physical barrier to sperm.

cervical cap   A thimble-sized rubber or plastic cap that is inserted into the vagina to fit over the cervix and prevent the passage of sperm into the uterus during sexual intercourse; used with a spermicidal foam or jelly, it serves as both a chemical and a physical barrier to sperm.

- Some diaphragm users report bladder discomfort, urethral irritation, or recurrent cystitis.
- Some cap users find it difficult to insert and remove and uncomfortable to wear.

Hormonal Contraceptives

In recent years, birth control methods made with synthetic hormones have become available in a variety of forms. Oral contraceptives have been available for decades, and the birth control pill is one of the most well-researched medications. Other options for hormonal birth control include a skin patch, a vaginal ring, and a quarterly injection. All are extremely effective when used consistently and conscientiously.

Hormonal contraceptives do not protect against HIV infection and other STIs, so condoms and spermicides should also be used if you need protection against infections.

Oral Contraceptives

The pill—the popular term for **oral contraceptives**—is the method of birth control preferred by unmarried women and by those under age 30, including college students (Table 10.3). Women 18 to 24 years old are most likely to choose oral contraceptives. In use for 40 years, the pill is one of the most researched, tested, and carefully followed medications in medical history—and one of the most controversial.

Although many women incorrectly think that the risks of the pill are greater than those of pregnancy and childbirth, long-term studies show that oral contraceptive use does not increase mortality rates. Combination oral contraceptives significantly reduce the risk of ovarian

TABLE 10.3 Contraception on Campus

Method	Percentage of Students Who Used It During Last Intercourse
Birth control pills	38%
Condoms (male or female)	37
Withdrawal	14
Fertility awareness	3
Spermicide	3
Depo-Provera	2
Diaphragm/cervical cap/sponge	.5
Norplant	.2

Source: American College Health Association. "American College Health Association National College Health Assessment Spring 2006 Reference Group Data Report (Abridged)." *Journal of American College Health,* Vol. 55, No. 4, January–February 2007, pp. 195–206.

and endometrial cancer and produce no increase in breast cancer, diabetes, multiple sclerosis, rheumatoid arthritis, and liver disease.

Although research is limited, the use of common antibiotics, including many prescribed for dental procedures or skin conditions, may lower the effectiveness of oral contraceptives, particularly low-dose birth control pills. Always ask a dentist or doctor who prescribes an antibiotic about its potential effect on your oral contraceptive, and check with your gynecologist or primary physician about using an additional nonhormonal means of contraception (such as a condom) to ensure protection against an unwanted pregnancy.

Combination Pills

These pills consist of two hormones, synthetic estrogen and progestin, which play important roles in controlling ovulation and the menstrual cycle. The doses in today's oral contraceptives are much lower—less than one-fourth the amount of estrogen and one-twentieth the progestin in the original pill. This means fewer side effects and lower risk of heart disease and stroke. Stroke risk among women taking newer, low-dose formulations of oral contraceptive pills may be extremely low. However, these pills appear to be less effective than those approved decades ago, with twice the failure rate of previous products. The reason seems to be lower doses of hormones that stop ovulation. The FDA is considering higher standards for these drugs.[8]

Monophasic pills release a constant dose of estrogen and progestin throughout a woman's menstrual cycle. **Multiphasic pills** mimic normal hormonal fluctuations of the natural menstrual cycle by providing different levels of estrogen and progesterone at different times of the month. Multiphasic pills reduce total hormonal dose and side effects. Both monophasic and multiphasic pills block the release of hormones that would stimulate the process leading to ovulation. They also thicken and alter the cervical mucus, making it more hostile to sperm, and they make implantation of a fertilized egg in the uterine lining more difficult.

One combination pill, Yasmin, contains a unique progestin that works like a mild diuretic and prevents fluid retention. Researchers have found that it lessens symptoms of premenstrual problems. Women who are taking potassium supplements, daily anti-inflammatory drugs, or heparin, a blood-thinner, should not take Yasmin because of potentially dangerous drug interactions. Other pills offer different benefits, such as clearer skin and reduced facial hair.

Progestin-Only Pills

Progestin-only **"minipills"** contain only a small amount of progestin and no estrogen. They work somewhat differently than combination pills. Women taking

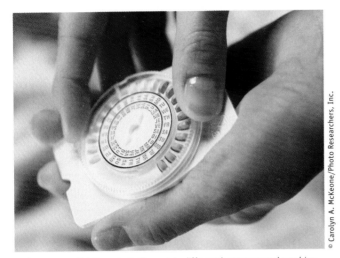

Various types of birth control pills contain different hormones and combinations of hormones.

© Carolyn A. McKeone/Photo Researchers, Inc.

progestin-only pills probably ovulate, at least occasionally. In those cycles, the pills prevent pregnancy by thickening cervical mucus, making it hard for sperm to penetrate, and by interfering with implantation of a fertilized egg.

The risk of heart disease and stroke is lower with progestin-only pills than with any combination pill. For this reason, they are a good choice for women over age 35 and others who cannot take estrogen-containing pills because of high blood pressure, diabetes, or clotting disorders. Because they do not affect the quality or quantity of breast milk, progestin-only pills often are recommended for nursing mothers, and they are recommended for smokers. Because progestin can affect mood and worsen the symptoms of depression, progestin-only pills are not recommended for women with a history of depression. Anti-seizure medications, such as Dilantin, which accelerate liver metabolism, may make the minipill less effective.

Users of progestin-only pills have to be conscientious about taking these pills, not just every day, but at the same time every day. If you take a progestin-only pill three or more hours later than usual, use a back-up method of contraception, such as a condom, for two days after you resume taking the pill.

How They Work

The pill usually comes in 28-day packets: 21 of the pills contain the hormones, and 7 are "blanks," included so that the woman can take a pill every day, even during her menstrual period. If a woman forgets to take one pill, she should take it as soon as she remembers. However, if she forgets during the first week of her cycle or misses more than one pill, she should rely on another form of birth control until her next menstrual period.

Even if you experience no discomfort or side effects while on the pill, see a physician at least once a year for an examination, which should include a blood pressure test, a pelvic, and a breast exam. Notify your doctor at once if you develop severe abdominal pain, chest pain, coughing, shortness of breath, pain or tenderness in the calf or thigh, severe headaches, dizziness, faintness, muscle weakness or numbness, speech disturbance, blurred vision, a sensation of flashing lights, a breast lump, severe depression, or yellowing of your skin.

Generally, when a woman stops taking the pill, her menstrual cycle resumes the next month, but it may be irregular for the next couple of months. However, 2 to 4 percent of pill users experience prolonged delays. Women who become pregnant during the first or second cycle after discontinuing use of the pill may be at greater risk of miscarriage; they also are more likely to conceive twins.

Advantages

- Extremely effective when taken consistently.
- Convenient.
- Moderately priced.
- Do not interrupt sexual activity.
- Reversible within three months of stopping the pill.
- Reduce the risk of benign breast lumps, ovarian cysts, iron-deficiency anemia, pelvic inflammatory disease, endometrial and ovarian cancer.
- May relieve painful menstruation.

Disadvantages

- Require a prescription.
- Increased risk of cardiovascular problems, primarily for women over age 35 who smoke and those with high blood pressure or other health problems.
- Side effects vary with different brands but include spotting between periods, weight gain or loss, nausea and vomiting, breast tenderness, and decreased sex drive.
- Must be taken at the same time every day (especially critical with low-dose estrogen and progestin-only pills).
- No protection against STIs.

oral contraceptives Preparations of synthetic hormones that inhibit ovulation; also referred to as birth control pills or simply the pill.

monophasic pills An oral contraceptive that releases synthetic estrogen and progestin at constant levels throughout the menstrual cycle.

multiphasic pill An oral contraceptive that releases different levels of estrogen and progestin to mimic the hormonal fluctuations of the natural menstrual cycle.

minipill, progestin-only pill An oral contraceptive containing a small amount of progestin and no estrogen, which prevents contraception by making the mucus in the cervix so thick that sperm cannot enter the uterus.

Savvy Consumer   How to Evaluate the Risks of Contraceptives

For individuals with certain medical conditions, specific types of birth control can pose a health risk. To be safe, follow these guidelines:

- **High blood pressure** (180/110 mmHg or higher): Avoid birth control pills or injections containing estrogen, which may increase your risk of a heart attack or stroke.

- **Episodes of depression:** Avoid products that contain progestin, such as Depo-Provera, contraceptive implants, and the minipill. In some women with depression, progestin may worsen depressive symptoms. Also, check with your doctor if you are taking an antidepressant medication; it may affect or be affected by oral contraceptives and you may require a different dose.

- **Seizure disorder:** Avoid low-dose birth control pills. Some antiseizure medications, such as Dilantin, accelerate liver metabolism of all substances, including oral contraceptives, and make them less effective.

- **Ectopic pregnancy:** Avoid IUDs. Although IUDs do not cause ectopic pregnancies, if your fallopian tubes have been scarred by a previous ectopic gestation, you're more likely to have another ectopic if you use an IUD.

- **Hepatitis:** Avoid birth control pills or injections containing estrogen, which is metabolized in the liver—an organ damaged by hepatitis.

- Must use a secondary form of birth control for the initial seven days of use.

Before Using Oral Contraceptives   Before starting on the pill, you should undergo a thorough physical examination that includes the following tests:

- Routine blood pressure test.
- Pelvic exam, including a Pap smear.
- Breast exam.
- Blood test.
- Urine sample.

Let your doctor know about any personal or family incidence of high blood pressure or heart disease, diabetes, liver dysfunction, hepatitis, unusual menstrual history, severe depression, sickle-cell anemia, cancer of the breast, ovaries, or uterus, high cholesterol levels, or migraine headaches. (See Savvy Consumer: "How to Evaluate the Risks of Contraceptives.")

Extended-Use Pills

For years physicians have prescribed prolonged use of birth control pills to lessen the number of menstrual cycles for women with asthma, migraines, rashes, or other conditions that flare up during their periods. Eliminating periods eliminates symptoms, and having fewer cycles also may lower a woman's long-term risk of ovarian cancer. However, some women are wary of long-term hormone use or consider a lack of menstrual cycles unnatural.

Seasonale®

Seasonale® is a prescription form of oral contraception that prevents pregnancy as effectively as other birth control pills but produces only four menstrual periods a year.

How It Works

Unlike traditional birth control pills, women take "active" pills continuously for three months or 84 days. During this time, Seasonale® prevents the uterine lining from thickening enough to produce a full menstrual period. Every three months, a woman takes one week of inactive pills to produce a "pill period," which may be lighter than a regular period.

The chance of getting pregnant ranges from 5 percent with typical use to 1 percent with perfect use. For maximum effectiveness, each pill should be taken at the same time of day.

Advantages

- Fewer periods
- Tri-monthly periods are usually lighter, with less blood flow.

Disadvantages

- Similar to those of other oral contraceptives in terms of health risks, costs, and side effects. Cigarette smoking increases these risks.
- No protection from STIs.
- More spotting and breakthrough bleeding than with a 28-day pill.
- Determining pregnancy is difficult without a monthly period.

Lybrel, the "No-Period" Pill

Lybrel, described as a continuous contraceptive, works the same way as other combination hormonal birth control pills. However, women take the "365-day" pill every single day without interruption.

How It Works

Like other oral contraceptives, Lybrel stops the body's monthly preparation for pregnancy by lowering the production of hormones that make pregnancy possible. However, it does not include the "week-off" of placebo pills that lead to vaginal bleeding. Most women resume menstruation within 90 days of stopping Lybrel.

Medical experts see no long-term risk in doing away with regular monthly periods. A two-year study of more than 2,400 women showed no increased risk of endometrial cancer in those taking Lybrel.[9] However, the long-term safety of menstrual suppression is unknown.

Advantages

- No menstrual periods, cramps, or other symptoms.
- No need to stop taking pills or switch to dummy pills for a week.
- Relief from menstruation-linked conditions such as endometriosis and menstrual migraine.

Disadvantages

- Spotting, which generally tapers off over the first year of use.
- Health risks similar to those of other combination pills.
- Determining pregnancy is difficult without a monthly period.
- Some women feel that eliminating periods is unnatural.

The Patch (Ortho Evra)

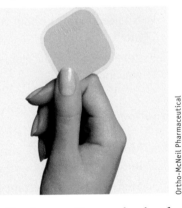

Ortho-McNeil Pharmaceutical

The Ortho Evra birth control patch, the first transdermal (through the skin) contraceptive, works like a combination pill but looks like a band-aid. Embedded in its adhesive layer are two hormones, a low-dose estrogen and a progestin. It prevents pregnancy by delivering continuous levels of estrogen and progestin through the skin directly into the bloodstream so women are exposed to higher overall levels of estrogen, which may increase their risk of blood clots.[10] The patch is waterproof and stays on in the shower, swimming pools, or hot tubs.

How It Works

A woman applies the $1^3/_4$ inch square to her back, upper arm, lower abdomen, or buttocks and changes it every seven days for three weeks. During the patch-free week, she experiences menstrual bleeding. A user should check every day to make sure the patch is still in place. If you don't replace a detached patch within 24 hours, use a backup method of contraception until your next period.

Advantages

- Good alternative for women who can't remember, don't like, or have problems swallowing daily pills.
- Highly effective when used correctly.
- Does not interrupt sexual activity.
- Fewer side effects, such as nausea, breakthrough bleeding, and mood swings, than pills.
- Fertility returns quickly after you stop using it.

Disadvantages

- Must apply a new patch every week.
- Requires a prescription.
- No protection against STIs.
- Increased risk of blood clots, heart attack, and stroke, particularly for women who smoke or have certain health conditions. The risk of dying or suffering a survivable blood clot while using the patch is estimated to be about three times higher than while using birth control pills.[11]
- Less effective in women who weigh more than 198 pounds.
- Some women report breast tenderness, headaches, upper respiratory infections, or self-consciousness wearing the patch.
- Contact lens wearers may experience vision changes.
- Five percent of women report that at least one patch slipped off; 2 percent report skin irritation.
- Must use another form of birth control for the initial seven days of use.

The NuvaRing

The silver-dollar-sized NuvaRing, a 2-inch ring made of flexible, transparent plastic, slowly emits the same hormones as oral contraceptives through the vaginal tissues (Figure 10.7). Smaller than the smallest diaphragm, it contains less estrogen than any pill. As effective as the pill, it provides a steady dose of hormones and causes fewer side effects.

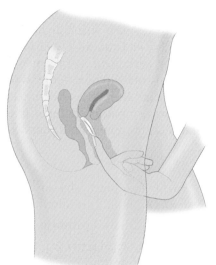

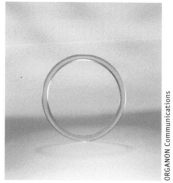

ORGANON Communications

Figure 10.7 NuvaRing

The NuvaRing releases estrogen and progestin, preventing ovulation. The exact position of NuvaRing in the vagina is not critical.

How It Works

Unlike a diaphragm, the NuvaRing does not have to be exactly positioned within the vagina or used with a spermicide. The flexible, plastic 2-inch ring compresses so a woman can easily insert it. Each ring stays in place for three weeks, then is removed for the fourth week of the menstrual cycle.

If a NuvaRing pops out (uncommon but possible), it should be washed, dried, and replaced within three hours. If a longer time passes, users should rely on a backup form of birth control until the ring has been reinserted for a week and the medications have risen to protective levels again.

Advantages

- Under medical supervision, may be safer than birth control pills for women with mild hypertension or diabetes.
- Less likelihood of pill-related side effects, such as nausea, mood swings, spotting, and cramping.
- No need to remember a daily pill or weekly patch.
- Fertility returns quickly when ring is removed.

Disadvantages

- Some women do not feel comfortable placing and removing something inside their vaginas.
- Possible side effects include vaginal discharge, irritation, and infection.
- Cannot use oil-based vaginal medications for yeast infections while ring is in place.
- No protection against STIs.

Contraceptive Injections

A hormonal contraceptive is available in the form of "shots" or injections. Depo-Provera, which contains only progestin, must be given every 12 weeks. Contraceptive injections provide no protection against HIV and other STIs.

How It Works

One injection of Depo-Provera, a synthetic version of the natural hormone progesterone, provides three months of contraceptive protection. This long-acting hormonal contraceptive raises levels of progesterone, thereby simulating pregnancy. The pituitary gland doesn't produce FSH and LH, which normally cause egg ripening and release. The endometrial lining of the uterus thins, preventing implantation of a fertilized egg.

Advantages

- Because it contains only progestin, it is safe for women who cannot take combination birth control pills.
- No risk of user error.
- No worry about buying, storing, or using contraceptives.
- No need to think about contraception for three months at a time.
- Possible protection against endometrial and ovarian cancer.

Disadvantages

- Must visit a doctor or clinic every three months for injection.
- Menstrual cycles become irregular or cease.
- Potential side effects include decreased libido, depression, headaches, dizziness, frequent urination, and allergic reactions.
- Increased weight gain, especially for obese women and teenage girls.[12]
- No protection against STIs.

- According to recent NIH study, appears to triple risk of acquiring chlamydia and gonorrhea compared to women not using a hormonal contraceptive. Scientists do not know the reason for this increased risk.
- Delayed return of fertility.
- Long-term use may significantly reduce bone density.

Contraceptive Implants

Hormonal implants, placed under the skin, deliver a constant low dose of progestin. They work primarily by suppressing ovulation, but they also thicken the cervical mucus (which inhibits sperm migration), inhibit the development and growth of the uterine lining, and limit secretion of progesterone during the second, or luteal, half of the menstrual cycle.

Norplant, consisting of six thin silicone rubber capsules containing a synthetic form of progestin, was the first such implant available in the United States. Approximately 9 million women used this method before it was taken off the market for reasons unrelated to its efficacy. Women with Norplant implants, who include many adolescents and young adults, should consult their doctors. They can safely leave the rods in place for the entire five-year period of contraceptive protection. However, they should discuss all options, including removal of the Norplant rods and switching to an alternative form of contraception.

A newer generation of implants may provide the benefits of long-term pregnancy protection with fewer complications. Implanon, a single Silastic rod that is simpler to insert and remove than Norplant, provides at least three years of contraception. Available in Europe and Australia, it uses a different type of progestin than Norplant and may cause fewer side effects like weight gain or acne. It has been approved but is not yet widely available in the United States.

Intrauterine Contraceptives

An **intrauterine device (IUD)** is a small piece of molded plastic, with a nylon string attached, that is inserted into the uterus through the cervix. It prevents pregnancy by interfering with implantation. Once widely used, IUDs became less popular after most brands were removed from the market because of serious complications such as pelvic infection and infertility.

Mirena

A new option is the Mirena intrauterine system, which consists of a T-shaped device inserted in the uterus by a physician, that releases a continuous low dose of progestin and provides five years of protection from pregnancy. Used in Europe, Asia, and Latin America for years, it is 99 percent effective.

Mirena is increasingly being used, not just for contraception, but as an alternative to hysterectomy for extremely heavy menstrual bleeding and as a treatment for problems such as iron-deficiency anemia.

How It Works

A physician must insert the Mirena in a woman's uterus. In a five-year clinical trial, about 5 in every 100 women reported that the Mirena had slipped out of the uterus. Users should check for the string that extends from the device through the vagina at least once a month.

Advantages

- Highly effective at preventing pregnancy.
- No need to think about contraception for five years.
- Allows sexual spontaneity; neither partner can feel it.
- Starts working immediately.
- New mothers can breast-feed while using it.
- Periods become shorter and lighter or stop altogether.
- Low incidence of side effects.
- Can be removed at any time.

Disadvantages

- Spotting or breakthrough bleeding in first three to six months.
- No protection against STIs.
- Potential side effects include acne, headaches, nausea, breast tenderness, mood changes.
- Increased risk of benign ovarian cysts.
- May take up to a year for fertility to return after discontinuation.

Fertility Awareness Methods

Awareness of a woman's cyclic fertility can help in both contraception and conception. The different methods of birth control based on a woman's menstrual cycle are

intrauterine device (IUD) A device inserted into the uterus through the cervix to prevent pregnancy by interfering with implantation.

sometimes referred to as *natural family planning* or *fertility awareness methods.* They include the calendar method, the basal-body-temperature method, and the cervical mucus method. New fertility monitors that use saliva to determine time of ovulation can improve the accuracy of these methods.

Women's menstrual cycles vary greatly. To use one of the fertility awareness methods, a woman must know and understand her cycle. She should track her cycle for at least eight months—marking day one (the day bleeding begins) on a calendar and counting the length of each cycle. Figure 10.8 shows the days in a 28-day cycle when abstinence or other contraceptive methods would be necessary.

How It Works

The calendar method, often called the **rhythm method,** is based on counting the woman's safe days based on her individual menstrual cycle. The basal-body-temperature method determines the safe days based on the woman's *Basal body temperature,* which rises after ovulation. The cervical mucus method, also called the *ovulation method,* is based on observation of changes in the consistency of the woman's vaginal mucus throughout her menstrual cycle. The period of maximum fertility occurs when the mucus is smooth and slippery.

Advantages

- No expense.
- No side effects.
- No need for a prescription, medical visit, or fittings.
- Nothing to insert, swallow, or check.
- No effect on fertility.
- Complies with the teachings of the Roman Catholic Church.

Disadvantages

- Less reliable than other forms of birth control.
- Couples must abstain from vaginal intercourse eight to eleven days a month or use some form of contraception.
- Conscientious planning and scheduling is essential.
- May not work for women with irregular menstrual cycles.
- Some women find the mucus or temperature methods difficult to use.

Emergency Contraception

Emergency contraception (EC) is the use of a method of contraception to prevent unintended pregnancy after

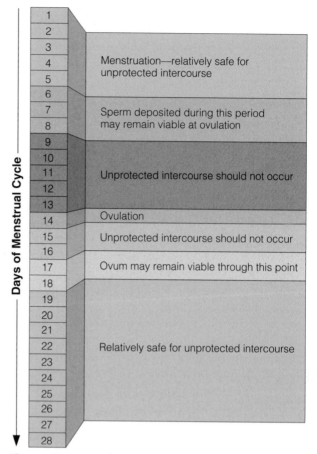

Figure 10.8 Safe and Unsafe Days

Events in the menstrual cycle determine the relatively safe days for unprotected intercourse.

unprotected intercourse or the failure of another form of contraception, such as a condom breaking or slipping off. If emergency contraception were more widely used, it would result in 800,000 fewer abortions and 1.7 million fewer unintended pregnancies.[13] EC has proved extremely safe in almost all women, as confirmed by numerous health organizations, including the World Health Organization and American College of Obstetricians and Gynecologists.

Combination estrogen-progestin pills, progestin-only pills, and the copper-bearing intrauterine device (IUD) have been used as methods of emergency contraception for decades. The progestin-only pills, referred to as Plan B, have proved more effective with fewer side effects than the combination pills. Plan B morning-after pills are available without a prescription for anyone over age 18; a prescription is required for anyone 17 or younger. Plan B, which should be taken without five days (120 hours) of unprotected sex, can reduce the risk of pregnancy up to 89 percent.[14]

Most women can safely use ECPs, even if they cannot use birth control pills as their regular method of birth control. (Although ECPs use the same hormones as birth control pills, not all brands of birth control pills can be used for emergency contraception.) Some women may experience spotting or a full menstrual period a few days after taking ECPs, depending on where they were in their cycle when they began therapy. Most women have their next period at the expected time.

The easier availability of EC has not yet resulted in a decrease in unintended pregnancies because many women, particularly foreign-born Hispanic women, women with incomes below the poverty level, and women who did not complete high school, are unaware of this option.[15]

 Among sexually active college women, 11 percent report having used emergency contraception in the past year.[16] According to a national survey of colleges and universities, slightly more than half of student health centers offer emergency contraception.[17] The primary reasons for not dispensing EC are religious affiliation, insufficient staff, and lack of funding. None of the two-year colleges surveyed provide EC. More public institutions, rural schools, four-year institutions, and schools with enrollments smaller than 15,000 are offering EC than in the past.

How It Works

Emergency contraception pills (ECPs) stop pregnancy in the same way as other hormonal contraceptives: They delay or inhibit ovulation, inhibit fertilization, or block implantation of a fertilized egg, depending on a woman's phase of the menstrual cycle. They have no effect once a pregnancy has been established.

Sterilization

The most popular method of birth control among married couples in the United States is **sterilization** (surgery to end a person's reproductive capability). Each year an estimated 1 million men and women in the United States undergo sterilization procedures. Fewer than 25 percent ever seek reversal.

Male Sterilization

In men, the cutting of the vas deferens, the tube that carries sperm from one of the testes into the urethra for ejaculation, is called **vasectomy.** During the 15- or 20-minute office procedure, done under a local anesthetic, the doctor makes small incisions in the scrotum, lifts up each vas deferens, cuts them, and ties off the ends to block the flow of sperm (Figure 10.9). Sperm continue to form, but they are broken down and absorbed by the body.

The man usually experiences some local pain, swelling, and discoloration for about a week after the procedure. More serious complications, including the formation of a blood clot in the scrotum (which usually disappears with-

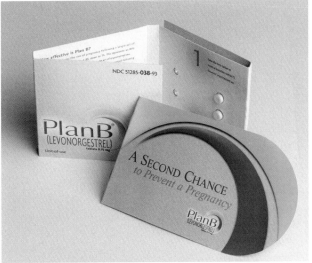

Emergency contraception can prevent unintended pregnancy after unprotected intercource or another form of contraception fails.

out treatment), infection, and an inflammatory reaction, occur in a small percentage of cases.

Sometimes men want to reverse their vasectomies, usually because they want to have children with a new spouse. Although anyone who chooses to have a vasectomy should consider it permanent, surgical reversal (*vasovasostomy*) is sometimes successful. New microsurgical techniques have led to annual pregnancy rates for the wives of men having undergone vasovasostomies of about 50 percent, depending on such factors as the doctor's expertise and the time elapsed since the vasectomy.

Female Sterilization

Eleven million U.S. women ages 15 to 44 rely on tubal sterilization for contraception. An estimated 750,000 tubal sterilization procedures are performed each year in the United States. The average age of sterilization is about 30. Female sterilization procedures modify the fallopian tubes, which each month normally carry an egg from the ovaries to the uterus. The two terms used to describe female sterilization are **tubal ligation** (the cutting or tying of the fallopian tubes) and **tubal occlusion** (the blocking of the tubes). The tubes may be cut or sealed

rhythm method   A birth control method in which sexual intercourse is avoided during those days of the menstrual cycle in which fertilization is most likely to occur.

emergency contraception (EC)   Types of oral contraceptive pills, usually taken within 72 hours after intercourse, that can prevent pregnancy.

sterilization   A surgical procedure to end a person's reproductive capability.

vasectomy   A surgical sterilization procedure in which each vas deferens is cut and tied shut to stop the passage of sperm to the urethra for ejaculation.

tubal ligation   The suturing or tying shut of the fallopian tubes to prevent pregnancy.

tubal occlusion   The blocking of the fallopian tubes to prevent pregnancy.

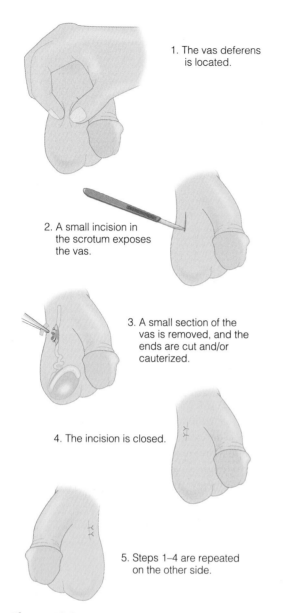

1. The vas deferens is located.

2. A small incision in the scrotum exposes the vas.

3. A small section of the vas is removed, and the ends are cut and/or cauterized.

4. The incision is closed.

5. Steps 1–4 are repeated on the other side.

Figure 10.9 Male Sterilization, or Vasectomy

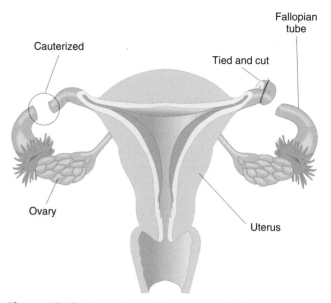

Figure 10.10 Female Sterilization, or Tubal Ligation

with thread, a clamp, or a clip, or by electrical coagulation to prevent the passage of eggs from the ovaries (Figure 10.10). They also can be blocked with bands of silicone.

One of the common methods of tubal ligation or occlusion uses **laparoscopy,** commonly called *belly-button* or *band-aid surgery.* This procedure is done on an outpatient basis and takes 15 to 30 minutes. A lighted tube called a *laparoscope* is inserted through a half-inch incision made right below the navel, giving the doctor a view of the fallopian tubes. Using surgical instruments that may be inserted through the laparoscope or through other tiny incisions, the doctor then cuts or seals the tubes, most commonly by electrical coagulation.

The cumulative failure rate of tubal sterilization is about 1.85 percent during a 10-year period. Complications include problems with anesthesia, hemorrhage, organ damage, and mortality.

Essure is a relatively new method for permanent sterilization that involves placement of small, flexible microcoils into the fallopian tubes via the vagina by a physician. Unlike other methods, it does not require the risks of general anesthesia and surgery. The procedure itself does not require incisions and takes an average of about 35 minutes. Recovery occurs quickly. In clinical trials, about 90 percent of women returned to work within 24 hours. For the first three months after insertion, women should use another form of contraception. An X-ray called a hystero-salpingogram must confirm that the inserts are correctly placed and the fallopian tubes are completely blocked.

Like traditional forms of tubal ligation, Essure cannot be reversed. It is recommended only for women who definitely do not want more children and especially for those with medical and health problems (such as diabetes, heart disease, or obesity) that make surgery and anesthesia more dangerous. There is a risk that the microinserts may not be placed correctly at the first attempt (this occurred in 14 percent of women in one study). Because the procedure is new, long-term data on the effectiveness of Essure are not yet available.

Advantages of Sterilization

- Offers permanent protection against unwanted pregnancy.
- No effect on sex drive in men or women. Many couples report greater sexual activity and pleasure because they no longer have to worry about pregnancy or deal with contraceptives.
- Vasectomy and tubal ligation are performed as outpatient procedures, with a quick recovery time.
- Use of Essure requires no incision, so there's less discomfort and very rapid recovery. Essure may be an option for women with chronic health conditions, such as obesity, diabetes, or heart disease.

Disadvantages of Sterilization

- All procedures should be considered permanent and used only if both partners are certain they want no more children.
- No protection against STIs.
- Must use another form of birth control for first three months.
- Many long-term risks remain unknown, but there is no evidence of any link between vasectomy and prostate cancer.

Abortion

More than half of unintended pregnancies end in induced abortions. In the United States one in three women under age 45 has had an abortion. Women between ages 18 and 24 account for 45 percent of abortions; minors under age 18, for 7 percent. Abortion rates vary greatly around the world. The U.S. abortion rate, which has declined, still remains higher than that of many Western countries, including Canada, Great Britain, the Netherlands, and Sweden. Although there is no one single or simple explanation for this difference, researchers focus on America's high rate of unintended pregnancies. In many nations with fewer unwanted pregnancies and lower abortion rates, contraceptives are generally easier and cheaper to obtain, and early sex education strongly emphasizes their importance.

No woman in any country ever chooses to be in a situation where she has to consider abortion. But if faced with an unwanted pregnancy, many women consider *elective abortion* as an option.

After rising steadily through the 1970s, the number of legal abortions leveled off in the 1980s and declined in the 1990s. As fewer Americans have used contraception, the decline in abortion rates has halted. Although women of all backgrounds have abortions, abortion in the United States is most likely to occur among single women, racial or ethnic minorities, low-income women, and women who have had at least one child.

Claims that abortion increases the risk of breast cancer, based on retrospective studies that are less accurate because they rely on individuals' recall, have proved false. Research has found no correlation between the termination of a pregnancy, whether induced or spontaneous, and increased risk of breast cancer.[18]

Thinking Through the Options

A woman faced with an unwanted pregnancy—often alone, unwed, and desperate—can find it extremely difficult to decide what to do. The political debate over the right to life almost always is secondary to practical and emotional matters, such as the quality of her relationship with the baby's father, their capacity to provide for the child, the impact on any children she already has, and other important life issues.

Giving up her child for adoption is an option for women who do not feel abortion is right for them. Because the number of would-be adoptive parents greatly exceeds the number of available newborns, some women considering adoption may feel pressured by offers of money from couples eager to adopt. Others, particularly minority women, may feel cultural pressures to keep a child—regardless of their age, economic situation, or ability to care for an infant. Advocates of adoption reform are pressing for mandatory counseling for all pregnant women considering adoption (available now in agency-arranged, but not private, adoptions) and for extending the period of time during which a new mother can change her mind about giving up her child for adoption.

Medical Abortion

The term **medical abortion** describes the use of drugs, also called *abortifacients,* to terminate a pregnancy. In 2000, the abortion pill mifepristone (Mifeprex), formerly known as RU-486, became available for use in the United States. Mifepristone, which is 97 percent effective in inducing abortion, blocks progesterone, the hormone that prepares the uterine lining for pregnancy. Two days after taking this compound, a woman takes a prostaglandin to increase uterine contractions. The uterine lining is expelled along with the fertilized egg (Figure 10.11).

Women have compared the discomfort of this experience to severe menstrual cramps. Common side effects include excessive bleeding, nausea, fatigue, abdominal pain, and dizziness. About 1 woman in 100 requires a blood transfusion. The FDA has warned doctors about rare but deadly bloodstream infections in women using mifepristone. The rate of infection is about 1 in 100,000 uses, comparable to infection risks with surgical abortions and childbirth.

Although condemned by right-to-life advocates, abortion medications may in time lower the public profile of pregnancy termination. They are not painless, cheap, or equally available to all, but they do offer women a chance

laparoscopy A surgical sterilization procedure in which the fallopian tubes are observed, with a laparoscope inserted through a small incision, and then cut or blocked

medical abortion Method of ending a pregnancy within nine weeks of conception using hormonal medications that cause expulsion of the fertilized egg.

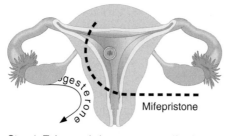

Step 1. Taken early in pregnancy, mifepristone blocks the action of progesterone and makes the body react as if it weren't pregnant.

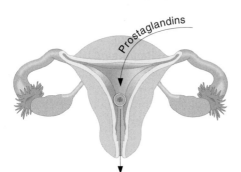

Step 2. Prostaglandins, taken two days later, cause the uterus to contract and the cervix to soften and dilate. As a result, the fertilized egg is expelled in 97 percent of cases.

Figure 10.11   Medical Abortion

Mifepristone works by blocking the action of progesterone, a hormone produced by the ovaries that is necessary for the implantation and development of a fertilized egg.

to carry through on their personal choice in greater privacy and safety.

Medical abortion does not require anesthesia and can be performed very early in pregnancy. However, women experience more cramping and bleeding during medical abortion than during surgical abortion, and bleeding lasts for a longer period.

Other Abortion Methods

About half of all abortions (54 percent) are performed within the first 8 weeks of pregnancy. Only about 1 percent of abortions occur after 20 weeks. Medically, first-trimester abortion is less risky than childbirth. However, the likelihood of complications increases when abortions are performed in the second trimester (the second three-month period) of pregnancy.

The majority of abortions performed in the United States today are surgical. **Suction curettage,** usually done from 7 to 13 weeks after the last menstrual period, involves the gradual dilation (opening) of the cervix, often by inserting into the cervix one or more sticks of *laminaria* (a sterilized seaweed that absorbs moisture and expands, thus gradually stretching the cervix). Some women feel pressure

or cramping with the laminaria in place. Occasionally, the laminaria itself starts to bring on a miscarriage.

At the time of abortion, the laminaria is removed, and dilators are used to further enlarge the cervical opening, if needed. The physician inserts a suction tip into the cervix, and the uterine contents are drawn out via a vacuum system (Figure 10.12). A *curette* (a spoon-shaped surgical instrument used for scraping) is used to check for complete removal of the contents of the uterus. With suction curettage, the risks of complication are low. Major complications, such as perforation of the uterus, occur in fewer than 1 in 100 cases.

For early second-trimester abortions, physicians generally use a technique called **dilation and evacuation (D and E)**, in which they open the cervix and use medical instruments to remove the fetus from the uterus. D and E procedures are performed under local or general anesthesia.

To induce abortion from week 16 to week 20, prostaglandins (natural substances found in most body tissues) are administered as vaginal suppositories or injected into the amniotic sac by inserting a needle through the abdominal wall. They induce uterine contractions, and the fetus and placenta are expelled within 24 hours. Injecting saline or urea solutions into the amniotic sac also can terminate the pregnancy by triggering contractions that expel the fetus and placenta. Sometimes vaginal suppositories or drugs that help the uterus contract are used. Complications from abortion techniques that induce labor include nausea, vomiting, diarrhea, tearing of the cervix, excessive bleeding, and possible shock and death.

The Psychological Impact of Abortion

Many assume that abortion must be psychologically devastating, that women who abort a fetus sooner or later develop what some have termed *postabortion trauma syndrome.* In her studies at the University of Chicago, psychiatrist Nada Stotland found that there is no such thing. The primary emotion of women who have just had an abortion, she discovered, is relief. Although many women also express feelings of sadness or guilt, their anxiety levels eventually drop until they are lower than they were immediately before the abortion.

Nonetheless, although psychologists consider the mental health risks minimal compared to those of bearing an unwanted child, this does not mean women who have abortions never have regrets. But a feeling—even one as painful as loss, sadness, or guilt—is not a syndrome, and a woman's responses to abortion often change with passing days, weeks, months, or years. Anniversaries—of conception, of the date a woman found out she was pregnant, of the abortion, of the delivery date—can trigger memories and a sense of loss, but most women deal with these and move on with their lives.

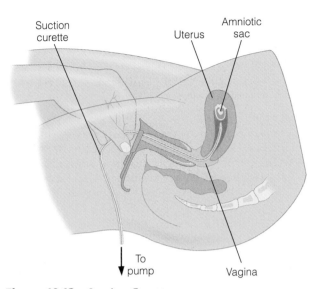

Figure 10.12 Suction Curettage

The contents of the uterus are extracted through the cervix with a vacuum apparatus.

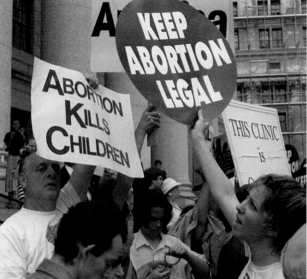

The controversy over abortion has resulted in countless demonstrations and encounters between pro-choice and pro-life supporters.

The best predictor of psychological well-being after abortion is a woman's emotional well-being prior to pregnancy. At highest risk are women who have had a psychiatric illness, such as an anxiety disorder or clinical depression, prior to an abortion, and those whose abortions occurred among complicated circumstances (such as a rape, or coercion by parents or a partner). The vast majority of women manage to put the abortion into perspective as one of many life events.

The Politics of Abortion

Abortion is one of the most controversial political, religious, and ethical issues of our time. The issues of when life begins, a woman's right to choose, and an unborn child's right to survival are among the most divisive Americans face. Abortions were legal in the United States until the 1860s. For decades after that, women who decided to terminate unwanted pregnancies did so by attempting to abort on their own or by obtaining illegal abortions—often performed by untrained individuals using unsanitary and unsafe procedures. In the late 1960s, some states changed their laws to make abortions legal. In 1973, the U.S. Supreme Court, following a 1970 ruling on the case of *Roe v. Wade* by the New York Supreme Court, said that an abortion in the first trimester of pregnancy was a decision between a woman and her physician and was protected by privacy laws. The Court further ruled that abortion during the second trimester could be performed on the basis of health risks and that abortion during the final trimester could be performed only for the sake of the mother's health.

The debate over abortion continues to stir passionate emotions, with pro-life supporters arguing that life begins at conception and that abortion is therefore immoral, and pro-choice advocates countering that an individual woman should have the right to make decisions about her body and health. The controversy over abortion has at times become violent: Physicians who perform abortions have been shot and killed; abortion clinics have been bombed, wounding and killing patients and staff members. Although the majority of Americans continue to support abortion, many feel that it should be more restricted and difficult to obtain.

In 2007 the Supreme Court upheld a federal law, passed in 2003, banning "partial-birth" abortions, a late-term procedure involving the removal of a fetus from the uterus and the collapsing of its skull. Pro-life groups hailed this ruling as a step toward the overthrow of *Roe v. Wade*. More than 40 years after this landmark ruling, the controversy over abortion and the conflict between pro-lifers and pro-choicers remains intense. (See Point/Counterpoint.)

A Cross-Cultural Perspective

 More than one in four pregnancies worldwide ends in abortion. Of the estimated 46 million global abortions, an estimated 20 million are illegal and lead to the death of about 70,000 women.

suction curettage A procedure in which the contents of the uterus are removed by means of suction and scraping.

dilation and evacuation (D and E) A medical procedure in which the contents of the uterus are removed through the use of instruments.

POINT COUNTERPOINT *Pro-Life or Pro-Choice?*

POINT

Life, from the moment of conception, is sacred, and no one has the right to end it. The laws permitting abortion in this country should be overturned. Because abortion is morally wrong, women should be counseled toward other options, such as adoption.

COUNTERPOINT

A woman's body is her own, and she alone has the right to choose whether to carry a pregnancy to term. Rather than forcing women

to jeopardize their own lives to resorting to illegal abortions, the government should guarantee safe, legal abortions to women who choose to terminate a pregnancy.

YOUR VIEW

Where do you stand on one of the most heated controversies of our time? Do you see abortion as a moral or a political issue? How do you feel about those with opposing views? Why do you think that the issue of abortion ignites such intense and emotional debate?

More than 50 countries now allow abortion up to at least the 12th week of pregnancy. Some, such as Great Britain, permit it up to 24 weeks; others have no time limit. In recent years abortion has become more restrictive in terms of limits on timing, grounds, or methods in the United States, Russia, Hungary and Poland. Nicaragua and El Salvador have banned the practice outright. Romania has the world's highest abortion rate; three in four pregnancies are terminated. In the United States, Australia, Canada, Great Britain, and most of Western Europe, around 15–25 percent of pregnancies end in abortion.[19]

Childfree by Choice

More women and men are deliberately choosing to remain "childfree." According to the limited data available, single childfree women tend to be better educated, more cosmopolitan, less religious, and more professional than those in the general population. In general, childfree women are high achievers, often in demanding careers, who describe their work as exciting and satisfying. Childfree couples are predominantly urban, well-educated, and upper middle class, with egalitarian and long-running marriages.

Their reasons for not having children are diverse: a desire to maintain their freedom, more time with their partners, career ambitions, concern about overpopulation and the fate of Earth. Some women cite the hostile work environment for mothers and the inadequacy of day care. Others say they're disillusioned with the have-it-all hopes of baby boomers and believe in a have-most-of-it philosophy.

Pregnancy

In the last half century, pregnancy rates have generally declined. The average age of mothers in the United States has risen, but about 70 percent of babies are still born to women in their twenties. Mothers are now averaging about two children each.

The number of never-married, college-educated, career women who are becoming single parents has risen dramatically. They want children—with or without an ongoing relationship with a man—and may feel that, because of their age, they can't delay getting pregnant any longer.

Preconception Care

The time *before* a child is conceived can be crucial in assuring that an infant is born healthy, full-size, and full-term. Women who smoke, drink alcohol, take drugs, eat poorly, are too thin or too heavy, suffer from unrecognized infections or illnesses, or are exposed to toxins at work or home may start pregnancy with one or more strikes against them and their unborn babies. The best chance for lowering the infant mortality rate and preventing birth defects is before pregnancy. **Preconception care**—the enhancement of a woman's health and well-being prior to conception in order to ensure a healthy pregnancy and baby—includes risk assessment (evaluation of medical, genetic, and lifestyle risks), health promotion (such as teaching good nutrition), and interventions to reduce risk (such as treatment of infections and other diseases, and assistance in quitting smoking or drug use).

For tips on *post*conception care, see Your Strategies for Prevention: "A Mother-to-Be's Guide to a Healthy Pregnancy."

Home Pregnancy Tests

The sooner a woman realizes she is pregnant, the more she can do to take care of herself and her child. Home pregnancy tests detect the presence of human chorionic gonadotropin (hCG), which is secreted as the fertilized egg implants in the uterus. If the concentration of hCG is high enough, a woman will test positive for pregnancy. If the test is done too early, the result will be a false negative. A follow-up test a week later can usually confirm a pregnancy. Although home pregnancy tests are 85 to 95

YOUR STRATEGIES FOR PREVENTION *A Mother-to-Be's Guide to a Healthy Pregnancy*

- The American College of Obstetricians and Gynecologists (ACOG) recommends consuming about 300 more calories a day than before pregnancy and concentrating on eating the right foods, not on watching your weight. Never diet during pregnancy. Don't restrict salt intake either, unless specifically directed to by your doctor.

- Drink six to eight glasses of liquids each day, including water, fruit and vegetable juices, and milk.

- Don't exercise strenuously for more than 15 minutes, ACOG advises. Avoid vigorous exercise in hot, humid weather. Never let your body temperature rise above 100°F or your heart rate climb above 140 beats per minute.

- Stretch and flex carefully because the joints and connective tissue soften and loosen during pregnancy. After the fourth month of pregnancy, don't do any exercises while lying on your back, as this could impair blood flow to the placenta.

- Walk, swim, and jog in moderation; play tennis only if you played before pregnancy. Ski only if you're experienced, and stick to low altitudes and safe slopes. Do not water-ski, surf, or ride a horse.

---

percent accurate, medical laboratory tests provide definitive confirmation of a pregnancy.

How a Woman's Body Changes During Pregnancy

The 40 weeks of pregnancy transform a woman's body. At the beginning of pregnancy, the woman's uterus becomes slightly larger, and the cervix becomes softer and bluish due to increased blood flow. Progesterone and estrogen trigger changes in the milk glands and ducts in the breasts, which increase in size and feel somewhat tender. The pressure of the growing uterus against the bladder causes a more frequent need to urinate. As the pregnancy progresses, the woman's skin stretches as her body shape changes, her center of gravity changes as her abdomen protrudes, and her internal organs shift as the baby grows (Figure 10.13). Pregnancy is typically divided into three-month periods called trimesters.

How a Baby Grows

Silently and invisibly, over a nine-month period, a fertilized egg develops into a human being. When the zygote reaches the uterus, it's still smaller than the head of a pin. Once nestled into the spongy uterine lining, it becomes an **embryo.** The embryo takes on an elongated shape, rounded at one end. A sac called the **amnion** envelops it (see photo on page 133). As water and other small molecules cross the amniotic membrane, the embryo floats freely in the absorbed fluid, cushioned from shocks and bumps. At nine weeks the embryo is called a **fetus.**

A special organ, the **placenta,** forms. Attached to the embryo by the umbilical cord, it supplies the growing baby with fluid and nutrients from the maternal bloodstream and carries waste back to the mother's body for disposal (Figure 10.14).

Complications of Pregnancy

In about 10 to 15 percent of all pregnancies, there is increased risk of some problem, such as a baby's failure to grow normally. *Perinatology,* or maternal-fetal medicine, focuses on the special needs of high-risk mothers and their unborn babies. Perinatal centers, with state-of-the-art equipment and 24-hour staffs of specialists in this field, have been set up around the country. Several of the most frequent potential complications of pregnancy are discussed next.

Ectopic Pregnancy

Any woman who is of childbearing age, has had intercourse, and feels abdominal pain with no reasonable cause may have an **ectopic pregnancy.** In this type of pregnancy, the fertilized egg remains in the fallopian tube instead of traveling to the uterus. Ectopic, or tubal, pregnancies have increased dramatically in recent years, now accounting for 2 percent of all reported pregnancies. STIs, particularly chlamydia infections (discussed in Chapter 16), have become a major cause of ectopic pregnancy. Other risk factors include previous pelvic surgery, particularly involving the fallopian tubes; pelvic inflammatory disease; infertility; and use of an IUD.

---

preconception care   Health care to prepare for pregnancy.

embryo   An organism in its early stage of development; in humans, the embryonic period lasts from the second to the eighth week of pregnancy.

amnion   The innermost membrane of the sac enclosing the embryo or fetus.

fetus   The human organism developing in the uterus from the ninth week until birth.

placenta   An organ that develops after implantation and to which the embryo attaches, via the umbilical cord, for nourishment and waste removal.

ectopic pregnancy   A pregnancy in which the fertilized egg has implanted itself outside the uterine cavity, usually in the fallopian tube.

miscarriage   A pregnancy that terminates before the twentieth week of gestation; also called spontaneous abortion.

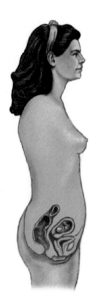

First Trimester

Increased urination because of hormonal
  changes and the pressure of the enlarging
  uterus on the bladder.
Enlarged breasts as milk glands develop.
Darkening of the nipples and the area around them.
Nausea or vomiting, particularly in the morning,
  may occur.
Fatigue.
Increased vaginal secretions.
Pinching of the sciatic nerve, which runs from
  the buttocks down through the back of the legs,
  may occur as the pelvic bones widen and begin
  to separate.

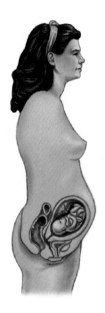

Second Trimester

Thickening of the waist as the
  uterus grows.
Weight gain.
Increase in total blood volume.
Slight increase in size and change
  in position of the heart.
Darkening of the pigment around
  the nipple and from the navel to the pubic region.
Darkening of the face.
Increased salivation and perspiration.
Secretion of colostrum from the breasts.

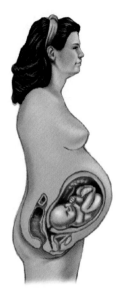

Third Trimester

Increased urination because of
  pressure from the uterus.
Tightening of the uterine muscles
  (called Braxton-Hicks
  contractions).
Shortness of breath because of
  increased pressure by the uterus
  on the lungs and diaphragm.
Interrupted sleep because of the
  baby's movements or the need to urinate.
Descending ("dropping") of the baby's
  head into the pelvis about two to
  four weeks before birth.
Navel pushed out.

Figure 10.13   Physiological Changes of Pregnancy

Miscarriage

About 10 to 20 percent of pregnancies end in **miscarriage,** or spontaneous abortion, before the 20th week of gestation. Major genetic disorders may be responsible for 33 to 50 percent of pregnancy losses. The most common cause is an abnormal number of chromosomes. About 0.5 to 1 percent of women suffer three or more miscarriages, possibly because of genetic, anatomic, hormonal, infectious, or autoimmune factors. An estimated 70 to 90 percent of women who miscarry eventually become pregnant again.

Infections

The infectious disease most clearly linked to birth defects is **rubella** (German measles). All women should be vaccinated against this disease at least three months prior to conception, to protect themselves and any children they may bear. (See Chapter 15 for more on immunization.) The most common prenatal infection today is *cytomegalovirus.* This infection produces mild flulike symptoms in adults but can cause brain damage, retardation, liver disease, cerebral palsy, hearing problems, and other malformations in unborn babies.

STIs, such as syphilis, gonorrhea, and genital herpes, can be particularly dangerous during pregnancy if not recognized and treated. If a woman has a herpes outbreak around the date her baby is due, her physician will deliver the baby by caesarean section to prevent infecting the baby. HIV infection endangers both a pregnant woman and her unborn baby, and all pregnant women and new mothers should be aware of the HIV epidemic, the risks to them and their babies, and the availability of anonymous testing.

Genetic Disorders

In some sense, each of us is a carrier of a genetic problem. Every individual has an estimated four to six defective genes, but the chances of passing them on to a child are slim. Almost all are recessive, which means they are "masked" by a more influential dominant gene. The likelihood of a child inheriting the same faulty recessive gene from both parents is remote—unless the parents are so closely related that they have very similar genetic makeup.

The child of a parent with an abnormal dominant gene has a 50 percent likelihood of inheriting it. The most common of such defects are minor, such as the growth of an

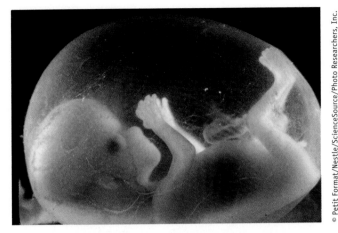

Embryo within the amnion.

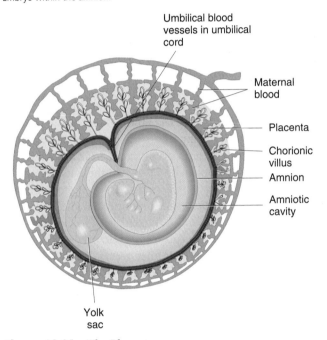

Umbilical blood
vessels in umbilical
cord

Maternal
blood

Placenta

Chorionic
villus

Amnion

Amniotic
cavity

Yolk
sac

Figure 10.14 The Placenta

The placenta supplies the growing embryo with fluid and nutrients from the maternal bloodstream and carries waste back for disposal.

extra finger or toe. However, some single-gene defects can be fatal. Huntington's chorea, for example, is a degenerative disease that in the past was usually not diagnosed until midlife.

Genetic tests can identify "carriers" of abnormal recessive genes for diseases such as sickle-cell anemia (the most common genetic disorder among African Americans), beta-thalassemia (found in families of Mediterranean origin), and Tay-Sachs (found in Jews of Eastern European origin). Two carriers of the same abnormal recessive genes can pass such problems on to their children.

The American College of Obstetricians and Gynecologists recommends a blood test for biochemical markers and ultrasound to screen for chromosomal abnormalities for all women in their first trimester. More invasive techniques, such as chorionic villus sampling (CVS) and second-trimester amniocentesis, can provide a precise diagnosis but carry a small risk for pregnancy loss.[20]

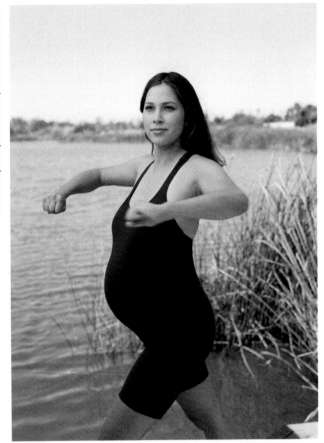

Most pregnant women benefit from regular moderate exercise

Premature Labor

Approximately 10 percent of all babies are born too soon (before the 37th week of pregnancy). According to researchers, prematurity is the main underlying cause of stillbirth and infant deaths within the first few weeks after birth. Bed rest, close monitoring, and, if necessary, medications for at-risk women can buy more time in the womb for their babies. But women must recognize the warning signs of **premature labor**—dull, low backache; a feeling of tightness or pressure on the lower abdomen; and intestinal cramps, sometimes with diarrhea. Low-birthweight premature babies face the highest risks, but comprehensive, enriched programs can reduce developmental and health problems.

rubella   An infectious disease that may cause birth defects if contracted by a pregnant woman; also called German measles.

premature labor   Labor that occurs after the twentieth week but before the thirty-seventh week of pregnancy.

Childbirth

A generation ago, delivering a baby was something a doctor did in a hospital. Today parents can choose from many birthing options, including a birth attendant, who can be a physician or a nurse-midwife, and a birthing center, hospital, or home birth.

Preparing for Childbirth

The most widespread method of childbirth preparation is the **Lamaze method** (*psychoprophylaxis*). Fernand Lamaze, a French doctor, instructed women to respond to labor contractions with prelearned, controlled breathing techniques. As the intensity of each contraction increases, the laboring woman concentrates on increasing her breathing rate in a prescribed way. Her partner coaches her during each contraction and helps her cope with discomfort.

Women who attend prenatal classes are less likely to undergo Caesarean deliveries and more likely to breast feed. They also tend to have fewer complications and require fewer medications. However, painkillers or anesthesia are always an option if labor is longer or more painful than expected. The lower body can be numbed with an *epidural block,* which involves injecting an anesthetic into the membrane around the spinal cord, or a *spinal block,* in which the injection goes directly into the spinal canal. General anesthesia is usually used only for emergency caesarean births.

Labor and Delivery

There are three stages of **labor.** The first starts with *effacement* (thinning) and *dilation* (opening up) of the cervix. Effacement is measured in percentages, and dilation in centimeters or finger-widths. Around this time, the amniotic sac of fluids usually breaks, a sign that the woman should call her doctor or midwife.

The first contractions of the early, or *latent,* phase of labor are usually not uncomfortable; they last 15 to 30 seconds, occur every 15 to 30 minutes, and gradually increase in intensity and frequency. The most difficult contractions come after the cervix is dilated to about 8 centimeters, as the woman feels greater pressure from the fetus. The first stage ends when the cervix is completely dilated to a diameter of 10 centimeters (or five finger-widths) and the baby is ready to come down the birth canal (Figure 10.15). For women having their first baby, this first stage of labor averages 12 to 13 hours. Women having another child often experience shorter first-stage labor.

When the cervix is completely dilated, the second stage of labor occurs, during which the baby moves into the vagina, or birth canal, and out of the mother's body. As

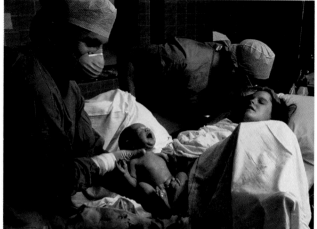

© SIU/Peter Arnold, Inc.

Today's fathers are active participants at the birth of their children.

this stage begins, women who have gone through childbirth preparation training often feel a sense of relief from the acute pain of the transition phase and at the prospect of giving birth.

This second stage can take up to an hour or more. Strong contractions may last 60 to 90 seconds and occur every two to three minutes. As the baby's head descends, the mother feels an urge to push. By bearing down, she helps the baby complete its passage to the outside.

As the baby's head appears, or *crowns,* the doctor may perform an *episiotomy*—an incision from the lower end of the vagina toward the anus to enlarge the vaginal opening. The purpose of the episiotomy is to prevent the baby's head from causing an irregular tear in the vagina, but routine episiotomies have been criticized as unnecessary. Women may be able to avoid this procedure by trying different birthing positions or having an attendant massage the perineal tissue.

Usually the baby's head emerges first, then its shoulders, then its body. With each contraction, a new part is born. However, the baby can be in a more difficult position, facing up rather than down, or with the feet or buttocks first (a *breech birth*), and a cesarean birth may then be necessary.

In the third stage of labor, the uterus contracts firmly after the birth of the baby and, usually within five minutes, the placenta separates from the uterine wall. The woman may bear down to help expel the placenta, or the doctor may exert gentle external pressure. If an episiotomy has been performed, the doctor sews up the incision. To help the uterus contract and return to its normal size, it may be massaged manually, or the baby may be put to the mother's breast to stimulate contraction of the uterus.

Caesarean Birth

In a **caesarean delivery** (also referred to as a *caesarean section*), the doctor lifts the baby out of the woman's

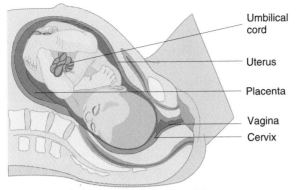

Umbilical cord
Uterus
Placenta
Vagina
Cervix

(a) The cervix is partially dilated, and the baby's head enters the birth canal.

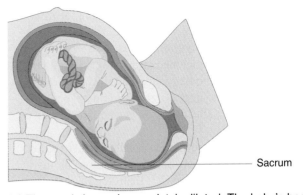

Sacrum

(b) The cervix is nearly completely dilated. The baby's head rotates so that it can move through the birth canal.

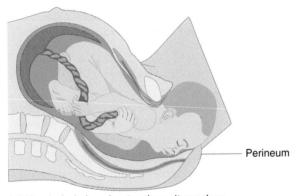

Perineum

(c) The baby's head extends as it reaches the vaginal opening, and the head and the rest of the body pass through the birth canal.

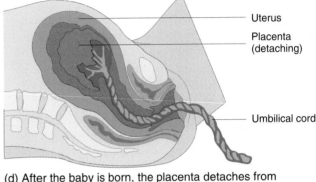

Uterus
Placenta (detaching)
Umbilical cord

(d) After the baby is born, the placenta detaches from the uterus and is expelled from the woman's body.

Figure 10.15 Birth

body through an incision made in the lower abdomen and uterus. The most common reason for caesarean birth is *failure to progress,* a vague term indicating that labor has gone on too long and may put the baby or mother at risk. Other reasons include the baby's position (if feet or buttocks are first) and signs that the fetus is in danger.

Thirty years ago, only 5 percent of babies born in America were delivered by caesarean birth; the current rate is 22.6 percent, substantially higher than in most other industrialized countries. About 36 percent of caesarean sections are performed because the woman has had a previous caesarean birth. However, four of every five women who have had caesarean births can have successful vaginal deliveries in subsequent pregnancies.

Caesarean birth involves abdominal surgery, so many women feel more physical discomfort after a caesarean than a vaginal birth, including nausea, pain, and abdominal gas. Women who have had a caesarean section must refrain from strenuous activity, such as heavy lifting, for several weeks.

Infertility

The World Health Organization defines **infertility** as the failure to conceive after one year of unprotected intercourse. Infertility affects one in seven couples. Women between ages 35 and 44 are about twice as likely to have fertility problems as women ages 30 to 34.

Infertility is a problem of the couple, not of the individual man or woman. In 40 percent of cases, infertility is caused by female problems, in 40 percent by male problems, in 10 percent by a combination of male and female problems, and in 10 percent by unexplained causes. A

Lamaze method A method of childbirth preparation taught to expectant parents to help the woman cope with the discomfort of labor; combines breathing and psychological techniques.

labor The process leading up to birth: effacement and dilation of the cervix; the movement of the baby into and through the birth canal, accompanied by strong contractions; and contraction of the uterus and expulsion of the placenta after the birth.

caesarean delivery The surgical procedure in which an infant is delivered through an incision made in the abdominal wall and uterus.

infertility The inability to conceive a child.

thorough diagnostic workup can reveal a cause for infertility in 90 percent of cases.

In women, the most common causes of subfertility or infertility are age, abnormal menstrual patterns, suppression of ovulation, and blocked fallopian tubes. A woman's fertility peaks between ages 20 and 30 and then drops quickly: by 20 percent after 30, by 50 percent after 35, and by 95 percent after 40.

Male subfertility or infertility is usually linked to either the quantity or the quality of sperm, which may be inactive, misshapen, or insufficient (less than 20 million sperm per milliliter of semen in an ejaculation of 3 to 5 milliliters). Sometimes the problem is hormonal or a blockage of a sperm duct. Some men suffer from the inability to ejaculate normally, or from retrograde ejaculation, in which some of the semen travels in the wrong direction, back into the body of the male.

Infertility can have an enormous emotional impact. Many women long to experience pregnancy and childbirth and feel great loss if they cannot conceive. Women in their thirties and forties fear that their biological clock is running out of time. Men may be confused and surprised by the intensity of their partner's emotions.

Options for Infertile Couples

The treatment of infertility has become a $2 billion a year enterprise in the United States. The odds of successful pregnancy range from 30 to 70 percent, depending on the specific cause of infertility. One result of successful infertility treatments has been a boom in multiple births, including quintuplets and sextuplets. Multiple births are associated with greater risk, both to the babies—including prematurity, low birthweight, neonatal death, and lifelong disability—and to the mothers, including caesarean section and hemorrhage.

Artificial Insemination

Since the 1960s, **artificial insemination**—the introduction of viable sperm into the vagina by artificial means—has led to an estimated 250,000 births in the United States, primarily in couples in which the husband was infertile. Some states do not recognize such children as legitimate; others do, but only if the woman's husband gave consent for the insemination.

Assisted Reproductive Technology

Approximately 1 percent of the babies born in the United States every year are conceived through assisted repro-

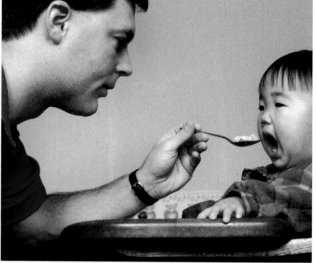

© Mike Greenlar/The Image Works

Adoption matches would-be parents yearning for youngsters to love with infants or children who need loving homes.

ductive technology (ART).[21] More than 35,000 babies are born each year as a result of ART.

The most common ART procedure is *in vitro fertilization (IVF)*, which removes the ova from a woman's ovary and places the woman's egg and her mate's sperm in a laboratory dish for fertilization. If the fertilized egg cell shows signs of development, within several days it is returned to the woman's uterus, the egg cell implants itself in the lining of the uterus, and the pregnancy continues as normal.

One of the most common complications of ART is multiple births. More than half of ART-conceived twins and more than 95 percent of ART triplets are born prematurely or have low birthweights. Born too soon or too small, they face greater risks of short- and long-term complications.[22]

Adoption

Men and women who cannot conceive children biologically can still become parents. **Adoption** matches would-be parents yearning for youngsters to love with infants or children who need loving. Couples interested in adoption can work with either public agencies or private counselors who contact obstetricians directly. Or they can contact organizations that arrange adoptions of children in need from other countries.

There are no reliable statistics on the annual number of adoptions in the United States, but census records indicate there are currently 1.5 million adopted children in the United States. Each year some 50,000 U.S. children become available for adoption—far fewer than the number of would-be parents looking for youngsters to adopt. By some estimates, only 1 in 30 couples receive a child—and they spend about two years and as much as $100,000 on the adoption process.

artificial insemination The introduction of viable sperm into the vagina by artificial means for the purpose of inducing conception.

adoption The legal process for becoming the parent to a child of other biological parents.

Learn It : Live It

Protecting Your Reproductive Health

The decisions you make about birth control can affect your reproductive health—and your partner's. Here are guidelines that can help prevent pregnancy and protect your reproductive well-being.

- **Abstain.** The only 100 percent safe and effective way to avoid unwanted pregnancy is not to engage in heterosexual intercourse.

- **Limit sexual activity to outercourse or oral sex.** You can engage in many sexual activities—kissing, hugging, touching, massage, oral–genital sex— without risking pregnancy.

- **Talk about birth control with any potential sex partner.** If you are considering sexual intimacy with a person, you should feel comfortable enough to talk about contraception.

- **Know what doesn't work—and don't rely on it.** There are many misconceptions about ways to avoid getting pregnant, such as having sex in a standing position or during menstruation. Only the methods described in this chapter are reliable forms of birth control.

- **Talk with a health-care professional.** A great deal of information and advice is available—in writing, from family planning counselors, from physicians on the Internet. Check it out.

- **Choose a contraceptive method that matches your personal habits and preferences.** If you can't remember to take a pill every day, oral contraceptives aren't for you. If you're constantly forgetting where you put things, a diaphragm might not be a good choice.

- **Consider long-term implications.** Since you may well wish to have children in the future, find out about the reversibility of various methods and possible effects on future fertility.

- **Resist having sex without contraceptive protection "just this once."** It only takes once—even the very first time—to get pregnant. Be wary of drugs and alcohol. They can impair your judgment and make you less conscientious about using birth control— or using it properly.

- **Use backup methods.** If there's a possibility that a contraceptive method might not offer adequate protection (for instance, if it's been almost three months since your last injection of Depo-Provera), use an additional form of birth control.

- **Inform yourself about emergency contraception.** Just in case a condom breaks or a diaphragm slips, find out about the availability of forms of after-intercourse contraception.

SELFSURVEY : *Which Contraceptive Method Is Best for You?*

Answer yes or no to each statement as it applies to you and, if appropriate, your partner.
1. You have high blood pressure or cardiovascular disease.
2. You smoke cigarettes.
3. You have a new sexual partner.
4. An unwanted pregnancy would be devastating to you.
5. You have a good memory.
6. You or your partner have multiple sexual partners.
7. You prefer a method with little or no bother.
8. You have heavy, crampy periods.
9. You need protection against STIs.
10. You are concerned about endometrial and ovarian cancer.
11. You are forgetful.
12. You need a method right away.
13. You're comfortable touching your own and your partner's genitals.
14. You have a cooperative partner.
15. You like a little extra vaginal lubrication.
16. You have sex at unpredictable times and places.
17. You are in a monogamous relationship and have at least one child.

Scoring:
Recommendations are based on Yes answers to the following numbered statements:

The combination pill: 4, 5, 6, 8, 10, 16
The progestin-only pill: 1, 2, 5, 7, 16
The patch: 4, 7, 8, 11, 16
The NuvaRing: 4, 7, 8, 11, 13, 16
Condoms: 1, 2, 3, 6, 9, 12, 13, 14
Depo-Provera: 1, 2, 4, 7, 11, 16
Diaphragm, cervical cap, or FemCap: 1, 2, 13, 14
Mirena IUD: 1, 2, 7, 8, 11, 13, 16, 17
Spermicides: 1, 2, 12, 13, 14, 15
Sponge: 1, 2, 12, 13

Your Health Action Plan For Choosing a Contraceptive

Your responses may indicate that there's more than one appropriate method of birth control for you. Remember that you may choose different types of birth control at different stages of your life, or switch contraceptives for various reasons. You and your partner should always consider and discuss these factors:

- **Effectiveness.** Keep in mind that your own conscientiousness will play an important role. If you forget to take your daily pill, or if you decide not to use a condom "just this once," you'll increase the odds of pregnancy by interfering with effective birth control.

- **Suitability.** If you don't have sex very often, a contraceptive with many risks and side effects, such as the pill, may be wrong for you. If you have many sexual partners and are at risk of contracting a sexually transmitted infection, a condom may provide protection against pregnancy and infection, especially if used with a diaphragm or cervical cap.

- **Side effects.** Some complications related to contraceptives are serious health threats. Be sure to ask questions and gather as much information as possible about what side effects to expect.

- **Safety.** The risks of certain contraceptives, such as the pill, may be too great to allow their use if, for example, you have high blood pressure. Be honest in describing your medical history to your physician.

- **Future fertility.** Some women don't return to regular menstrual cycles for six months to a year after discontinuing oral contraceptives. This possibility may or may not be important to you now, but you should try to look ahead.

- **Cost.** The only free contraceptive methods are abstinence and rhythm methods. If you're on a tight budget, you might consider the relative costs of a year's prescription of oral contraceptives compared to a year's supply of condoms or spermicidal foam or jelly. You should also think about the long-term costs and consequences.

- **Reduced risk of sexually transmitted infections.** Some forms of contraception, in particular barrier contraceptives and spermicides, help reduce the risk of transmission of some STIs. However, none provides complete protection.

CENGAGENOW™ If you want to write your own goals for safe and effective contraception, go to the Wellness HealthNow Journal: **academic .cengage.com/login**

Making This Chapter Work
for YOU

Review Questions

1. Conception occurs
   a. when a fertilized egg implants in the lining of the uterus.
   b. when sperm is blocked from reaching the egg.
   c. when a sperm fertilizes the egg.
   d. after the uterine lining is discharged during the menstrual cycle.

2. Factors to consider when choosing a contraceptive method include all of the following *except*
   a. cost.
   b. failure rate.
   c. effectiveness in preventing sexually transmitted infections.
   d. preferred sexual position.

3. When used correctly, which is the most effective non-hormonal contraceptive method?
   a. male condom
   b. female condom
   c. spermicide
   d. diaphragm

4. Which of the following contraceptive choices offers the best protection against STIs?
   a. condom alone
   b. condom plus spermicide
   c. abstinence
   d. withdrawal plus spermicide

5. Which statement about prescription contraceptives is *not* true?
    a. Prescription contraceptives do not offer protection against STIs.
    b. Some prescription contraceptives contain estrogen and progestin, and some contain only progestin.
    c. The contraceptive ring must be changed every week.
    d. IUDs prevent pregnancy by preventing or interfering with implantation.

6. Which of the following statements is true about sterilization?
    a. In women, the most frequently performed sterilization technique is Essure.
    b. Many couples experience an increase in sexual encounters after sterilization.
    c. Vasectomies are easily reversed with surgery.
    d. Sterilization is recommended for single men and women who are unsure about whether they want children.

7. Which statement about abortion is *false?*
    a. The abortion rate in the United States started declining in the 1990s.
    b. The U.S. abortion rate is higher than the rate in Canada and England.
    c. Most women are traumatized by an abortion.
    d. Mifepristone is 97 percent effective in inducing abortion.

8. In the third trimester of pregnancy,
    a. the woman experiences shortness of breath as the enlarged uterus presses on the lungs and diaphragm.
    b. the embryo is now called a fetus.
    c. the woman should begin regular prenatal checkups.
    d. the woman should increase her activity level to ensure that she is fit for childbirth.

9. During childbirth,
    a. breech birth can be prevented by practicing the Lamaze method.
    b. the cervix thins and dilates so that the baby can exit the uterus.
    c. the intensity of contractions decreases during the second stage of labor.
    d. the placenta is expelled immediately before the baby's head appears.

10. Which of the following statements is true about infertility?
    a. Infertility is most often caused by female problems.
    b. In men, infertility is usually caused by a combination of excess sperm production and an ejaculation problem.

c. In vitro fertilization involves introducing sperm into the vagina with a long needle.
d. In some cases of infertility, no cause can be demonstrated.

Answers to these questions can be found on page 583.

Critical Thinking

1. After reading about the various methods of contraception, which do you think would be most effective for you? What factors enter into your decision (convenience, risks, effectiveness, etc.)?

2. If you are sexually active, how do you start the conversation about contraception with a potential partner? What do you say and do if your partner is not ready for sex? What would you do if you do not have condoms with you to prevent sexually transmitted infection and do not have another form of birth control, such as a diaphragm?

3. Suppose that you and your partner were told that your only chance of having a child is by using fertility drugs. After taking the drugs, you and your partner are informed that there are seven fetuses. Would you carry them all to term? What if you knew that the chances of them all surviving were very slim and that eliminating some of them would improve the odds for the others? What ethical issues do cases like this raise?

Media Menu

CENGAGENOW™ Go to the HealthNow website at **academic.cengage .com/login** that will:
- Help you evaluate your knowledge of the material.
- Allow you to take an exam-prep quiz.
- Provide a Personalized Learning Plan targeting resources that address areas you should study.
- Coach you through identifying target goals for behavioral change and creating and monitoring your personal change plan throughout the semester.

INTERNET CONNECTIONS

Guttmacher Institute
www.guttmacher.org
This site offers excellent resources on teen pregnancy rates and sexual health for teens and young adults, including discussions on contraceptives versus abstinence.

Association of Reproductive Health Professionals
www.arhp.org
ARHP calls their website "the ultimate resource offering comprehensive information and education on all reproductive health topics to healthcare professionals, policymakers, the media, and the public."

National Abortion Rights Action League

www.naral.org

The website of this national organization provides information on the politics of the pro-choice movement.

National Right to Life Committee

www.nrlc.org

The website of this national organization provides information on the politics of the pro-life movement.

Planned Parenthood

www.plannedparenthood.org

The website for the Planned Parenthood Federation of America offers a wealth of information on sexual and reproductive health, reproductive choices, methods of contraception, and reproductive policy.

Key Terms

The terms listed are used and defined on the page indicated. Definitions are also found in the Glossary at the end of this book.

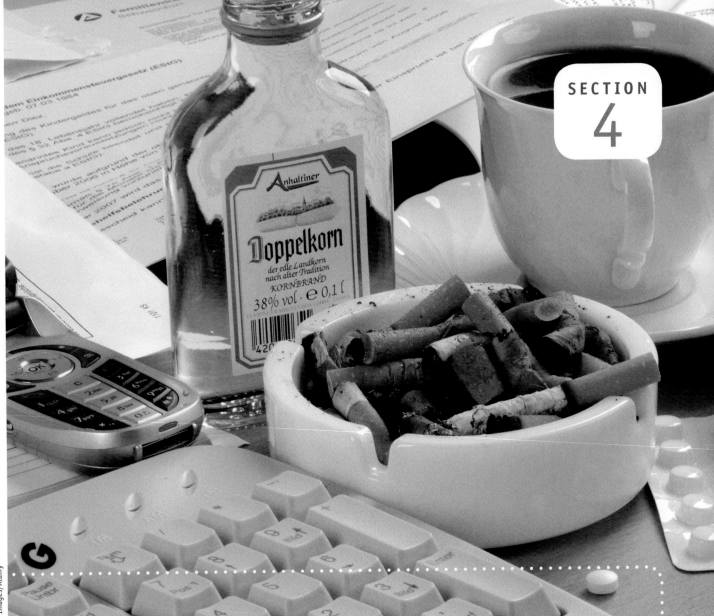

©Arco Images/Alamy

Avoiding Health Risks

You may constantly hear messages encouraging you to take risks with your health—to try drugs, to have another drink, to smoke cigarettes. We have another message for: Don't go there! You have nothing to gain and everything to lose when you let an addiction run your life. You also live with the consequences of others' drug abuse, alcoholism, and smoking. That's why it's important to know about potentially harmful habits—even if you never rely on drugs to pick you up or bring you down, never drink to excess, and never smoke. This section provides information you can use to avoid or overcome habits that jeopardize or destroy your health, happiness, and life.

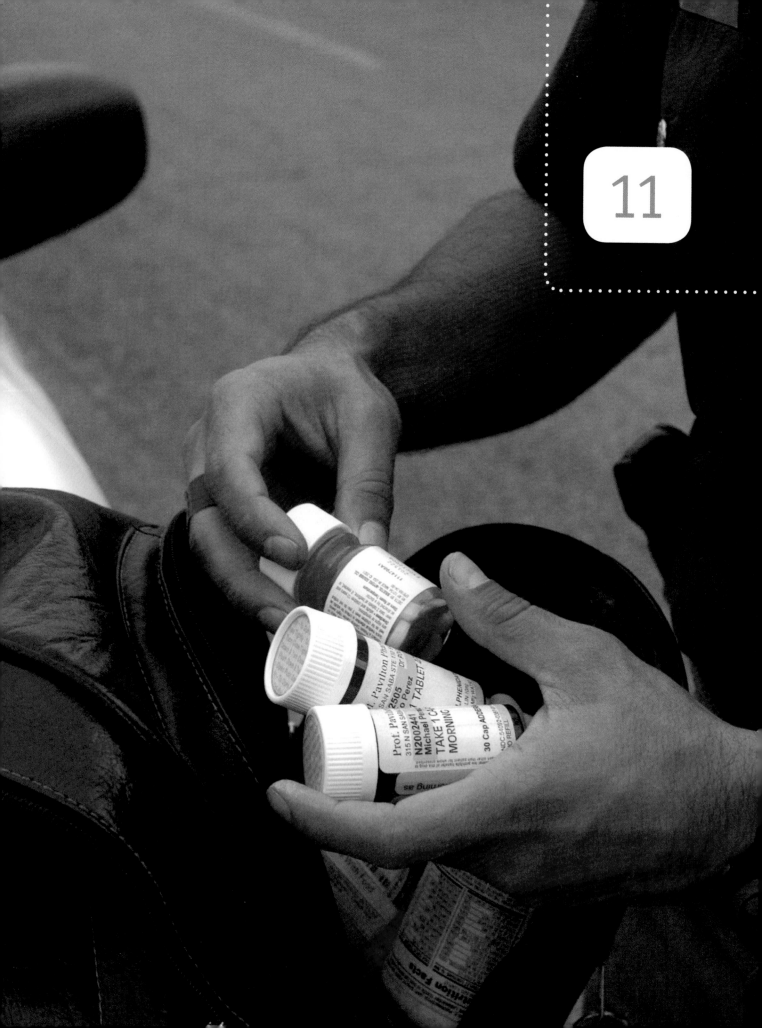

Avoiding Addictive Behaviors and Drug Abuse

TYLER had too many papers to write and too little time to finish them. One of the guys in his fraternity suggested a prescription stimulant a friend took for an attention deficit disorder. The jolt felt like just what Tyler needed. During midterms Tyler bought another prescription stimulant from a classmate. As finals approached, he started hoarding stimulants from several people. He popped the final ones to rev up for the last-bash of the school year parties. Without realizing it, Tyler put himself at risk for drug-related problems— physical, psychological, and legal.

People who try drugs don't think they'll ever lose control. Even regular users believe they are smart enough, strong enough, lucky enough not to get caught or hooked. But with continued use, drugs produce changes in an individual's body, brain, and behavior. In time the need for a drug can outweigh everything else a person values and holds dearest.

Globally the production, trafficking, and production of illegal drugs has stabilized.[1] Over the last five years, illegal drug use has declined by more than 20 percent among middle- and high-school students.[2] However, abuse of prescription drugs is skyrocketing and will soon exceed illegal drug use worldwide.[3]

On college campuses, abuse of both illegal and prescription drugs is a major health problem. Student abuse of prescription drugs, including painkillers, stimulants, and tranquilizers, has exploded in the last 15 years. The proportion of students smoking marijuana daily has doubled since the early 1990s. Almost one in four full-time students meets the medical criteria for substance abuse or dependence, two-and-a-half times the proportion for the rest of the population.[4]

The impact of drug taking in college ranges from short-term consequences, such as academic difficulties, to long-term physical and psychological problems.

After studying the material in this chapter, you should be able to:

- **Name** some of the risk factors for problem gambling.
- **Describe** the different types of drug actions and factors affecting individuals' response to drugs.
- **Give examples** of appropriate and inappropriate use of over-the-counter and prescription medications.
- **Identify** the types of drug dependence, and discuss the factors affecting drug dependence.
- **Describe** the effects and health risks of common drugs of abuse.
- **Describe** the treatment methods available for individuals seeking help for drug dependence.
- **Review** your drug history (legal and illegal) and **assess** the health risks you chose to take.

CENGAGENOW™   Log on to HealthNow at **academic.cengage.com/login** to find your Behavior Change Planner and to explore self-assessments, interactive tutorials, and practice quizzes.

Its toll also includes more than 1,700 deaths, 700,000 assaults, and almost 100,000 sexual attacks and rapes.[5] But knowing the risks isn't enough to keep many students from heading down the dead end road of addiction.

Going beyond warnings, this chapter provides information and insights into why students use and abuse drugs, how addictions start, the nature and effect of drugs, and the most commonly used, misused, and abused drugs. It also offers practical strategies for preventing, recognizing the signs of, and seeking help for drug-related problems.

Addictive Behaviors and the Dimensions of Health

Substance abuse and other self-destructive behaviors, such as gambling or compulsive eating, can affect every dimension of health. Yet often individuals are unaware of the harmful effects of their unhealthy choices:

- **Physical health.** As shown in this and the following chapters, the abuse of alcohol, tobacco, and drugs takes a toll on every organ system in the body, increasing the likelihood of disease, disability, and premature death.

- **Psychological health.** Sometimes people begin abusing substances or engaging in addictive behavior as a way of "self-medicating" symptoms of anxiety or depression. However, alcohol or drugs provide only temporary relief. As abuse continues, shame and guilt increase, and coping with daily stressors becomes more difficult. Depression and anxiety are as likely to be the consequences as the causes of substance abuse.

- **Spiritual health.** Addictive behavior blocks the pursuit of meaning and inner fulfillment. As they rely more and more on a chemical or behavioral escape, individuals lose their sense of self and of connection with others and with a higher power.

- **Social health.** Addictive behavior strains and, in time, severs the ties that bind an individual to family, friends, colleagues, and classmates. The primary relationship in the life of alcoholics or addicts is with a behavior or a drug. They withdraw from others and become increasingly isolated.

- **Intellectual health.** The brain is one of the targets of alcohol and drugs. Under their influence, logic and reasoning break down. Impulses become more difficult to control. Judgment falters. Certain substances, such as ecstasy, can lead to permanent changes in brain chemistry.

- **Environmental health.** The use of some substances, such as tobacco, directly harms the environment. Abusers of alcohol and drugs also pose indirect threats to others because their behavior can lead to injury and damage.

See the "Don't Go There" lab in *IPC*. **IPC**

Gambling

Although gambling is illegal for anyone under 18 to 21 years of age, depending on individual state law, underage gambling is a significant and growing problem across the country. In a survey of almost 1,000 university students, a majority had gambled—60 percent of the 18-year-olds, 73 percent of the 19-year-olds, 86 percent of the 20-year-olds, and 93 percent of those over 21 years of age—had gambled at least once in a casino.[6]

 College students who gamble do so for fun or excitement, to socialize, to win money, or to "just have something to do"—reasons similar to those for adults who gamble. Simply having access to casino machines, ongoing card games, or Internet gambling sites increases the likelihood that students will gamble.

Although most people who gamble limit the time and money they spend, some cross the line and lose control of their gambling "habit." The term *problem gambling* refers to all individuals with gambling-related problems, including mild or occasional ones. To determine whether you are such an individual, see Your Strategies for Change: "Do You Have a Gambling Problem?" Pathological or compulsive gambling is defined as "persistent and recur-

---

YOUR STRATEGIES FOR CHANGE *Do You Have a Gambling Problem?*

- Have you ever felt that your gambling or betting was out of control?

- Have you ever gotten into a fight with your family or friends because of gambling or betting?

- Have you ever felt that you lost too much money in gambling or betting?

- Have you ever felt the need to bet more and more money?

- Have you ever had to lie to people important to you about how much you gamble?

Even a single yes answer may indicate a problem. Go online or check with a counselor on campus to find resources, such as a local chapter of Gamblers Anonymous.

rent maladaptive behavior." Researchers now view problem or pathological gambling as an addiction that runs in families. Individuals predisposed to gambling because of their family history are more likely to develop a problem if they are regularly exposed to gambling. Alcoholism and drug abuse often occur along with gambling, leading to chaotic lives and dysfunctional relationships.

Risk Factors for Problem Gambling

Among young people (ages 16 to 25) the following behaviors indicate increased risk of problem gambling:

- Being male.
- Gambling at an early age (as young as age eight).
- A big win earlier in one's gambling career.
- Consistently chasing losses (betting more to recover money already lost).
- Gambling alone.
- Feeling depressed before gambling.
- Feeling excited and aroused during gambling.
- Behaving irrationally during gambling.
- Poor grades at school.
- Other addictive behaviors (smoking, drinking alcohol, illegal drug use).
- Lower socioeconomic class.
- Parents with a gambling or other addiction problem.
- A history of delinquency or stealing money to fund gambling.
- Skipping class to go gambling.

Pathological Gamblers

Adult pathological gamblers are more likely to be male, single, nonwhite, and less educated. Women start gambling later than men, but they progress more rapidly to pathological gambling. Genetics and exposure to gambling in childhood are significant influences. More than half of pathological gamblers report at least one first-degree relative with symptoms consistent with gambling problems.

Gamblers typically progress through various stages. In the winning phase, they feel empowered by their winnings and success. Next comes the losing phase, during which gamblers try to win back their losses. This is followed by the desperation phase, during which a gambler may resort to illegal activity, including stealing, to continue gambling. Some gamblers experience a fourth phase, the giving-up phase, where they desperately try to stay afloat in a game even though they realize they can't win.

As many as three-fourths of adult pathological gamblers suffer from depression. They also are at higher risk of other mood or anxiety disorders, such as panic disor-

REALITYCHECK
- *How many college students binge-drink and/or abuse prescription or illegal drugs?* _____
- *How many college students meet the medical criteria for substance abuse and dependence?* _____

Answers on next page.

der, phobias, obsessive-compulsive disorder, generalized anxiety, or post-traumatic stress disorder. An estimated 20 percent suffer from attention-deficit/hyperactivity disorder (ADHD). Even more—30 to 50 percent of pathological gamblers—abuse drugs or alcohol.

No standard or proven treatment exists for pathological gambling, but inpatient treatment centers, self-help groups, cognitive-behavioral psychotherapy, and addiction-based psychotherapy can help.

Drug Use on Campus

Drugs are a fact of life on almost every college campus. *Wasting the Best and the Brightest: Substance Abuse at America's Colleges and Universities* is a recent study by the National Center on Addiction and Substance Abuse at Columbia University. This report found that 3.8 million full-time undergraduates binge-drink (see Chapter 12 for a definition and discussion) and/or abuse illegal or prescription drugs. (See Reality Check.)

Although 9 in 10 college students do not abuse drugs, the percentage of those who do has soared. For instance, the proportion who abuse prescription painkillers like Percocet, Vicodin, and OxyContin increased by 343 percent—from .7 percent to 3 percent—from 1993 to 2005. During the same time period, the percentage of students using illicit drugs other than marijuana, such as cocaine and Ecstasy, increased by 52 percent, from 5 to 8 percent.

The biggest barrier to getting "the high out of higher education," as one health expert puts it,[7] is the public perception that substance abuse on campus is a normal, rite of passage for fun-loving students. In fact, substance abuse is neither normal nor fun. As research has conclusively shown, substance abuse is linked to poor academic performance, depression, anxiety, suicide, property damage, vandalism, fights, serious medical problems, and death.

Why Students *Do* Use Drugs

Various factors influence which students use drugs, including the following:

- **Genetics and family history.** Some college students inherit a genetic or biological predisposition to

REALITYCHECK

PART II: *Just the Facts*

- *Almost half (**49** percent) of college students binge-drink and/or abuse prescription or illegal drugs.*
- ***23** percent of college students meet the medical criteria for substance abuse and dependence.*

Source: *Wasting the Best and the Brightest: Substance Abuse at America's Colleges and Universities.* New York: National Center on Addiction and Substance Abuse at Columbia University, March 2007.

substance abuse. Research, which has focused almost exclusively on alcohol, has identified gene variations that affect the way certain students react to alcohol (for instance, with alcohol-induced headaches and more severe hangovers). Also, the risk for problem drinking and alcohol abuse is higher among children of substance abusers.

- **Parental attitudes and behavior.** In a survey of 2,000 students, 70 percent said that their parents' concerns or expectations influenced whether or how much they drink, smoke, or use drugs. Students also tend to imitate their parents' behavior in terms of substance use. Those who perceive that their parents approve of their drinking, for instance, are more likely to report a drinking-related problem, such as memory loss or missing class. More than one in five underage students report acquiring alcohol from their parents or relatives.[8]

- **Substance use in high school.** Many students start abusing drugs or alcohol well before getting to college. Only 8 percent of undergraduate marijuana users and even fewer cocaine users began their use in college. Students who used Ecstasy in high school are more than seven times likelier to report college use.[9]

- **Positive expectations.** Many students expect a drug to make them feel less stressed or anxious, more relaxed or confident, less shy or inhibited. Among students who use illicit drugs, 46 percent say they do so to relieve stress. (See Figure 11.1.) Others self-medicate, taking drugs to relieve depression or anxiety. Some abuse prescription medications, such as Adderall and Ritalin, because they think these drugs will energize them to study longer or perform better. Even when drugs don't live up to students' expectations, they may continue taking them for some short-term relief or because they have become addicted and cannot stop.

- **Mental health problems.** Students with feelings of hopelessness, sadness, depression, and anxiety as well as those with clinical mental disorders have higher rates of prescription drug abuse and illegal drug use. Students diagnosed with depression in the past school year have higher rates of marijuana, cocaine, alcohol, and tobacco use. Suicidal feelings also have been linked with substance abuse.[10]

- **Social influences.** More than 9 in 10 students who use illegal drugs were introduced to the habit

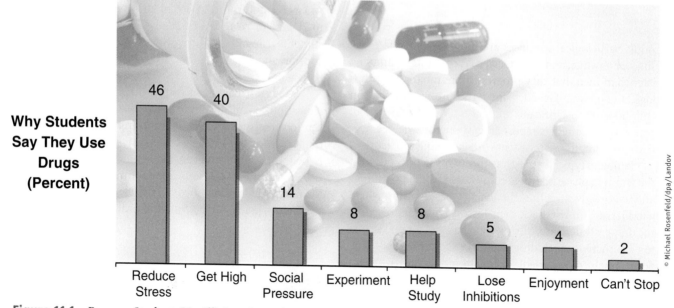

Why Students Say They Use Drugs (Percent)

Reduce Stress: 46
Get High: 40
Social Pressure: 14
Experiment: 8
Help Study: 8
Lose Inhibitions: 5
Enjoyment: 4
Can't Stop: 2

© Michael Rosenfeld/dpa/Landov

Figure 11.1 Reasons Students Use Illicit or Prescription Drugs

Source: *Wasting the Best and the Brightest: Substance Abuse at America's Colleges and Universities.* New York: National Center on Addiction and Substance Abuse at Columbia University, March 2007.

through friends; most use drugs with friends. Undergraduates who describe parties as "very important" to their lifestyle are almost three times as likely to use marijuana as those who don't consider parties very important. Sorority and fraternity members, who tend to socialize more often, are likelier to abuse prescription stimulants, but students who live off campus have higher rates of marijuana and cocaine use. Students tend to overestimate how many of their peers use drugs. Such misperceptions may affect their decisions about drugs.[11]

- **Alcohol use.** Often individuals engage in more than one risk behavior. College students, researchers have found that those who report binge drinking are much more likely than other students to report current or past use of marijuana, cocaine, or other illegal drugs.

- **Race/ethnicity.** In general, white students have higher levels of alcohol and drug use than do African American students. In a comparison of African American students at predominantly white and predominantly black colleges, those at historically black colleges had lower rates of alcohol and drug use than did either white or African American students at white schools. The reason, according to the researchers, may be that these colleges provide a greater sense of self-esteem, which helps prevent alcohol and drug use.

- **Sexual identity.** Gay, lesbian, and bisexual teens may rely on alcohol and marijuana to lessen social anxiety and boost self-confidence when they first come out. However, once they become more involved in the gay community, many are less likely to do so. Nonetheless, self-identified lesbian women are significantly more likely than heterosexual women to use marijuana, Ecstasy, and other drugs. Gay and bisexual men are significantly less likely than heterosexual men to drink heavily but more likely to use drugs.

Why Students *Don't* Use Drugs

The majority of undergraduates do not use illegal drugs or abuse prescription drugs. What keeps them drug-free? Here are some important factors:

- **Spirituality and religion.** The greater a student's religiosity—a term that encompasses hours spent in prayer, attendance at religious services, and reading spiritual materials—the less likely the student is to use alcohol, illegal drugs, or tobacco. Researchers have noted a drop in students' religiosity during college, along with an increase in their alcohol and marijuana use.

- **Academic engagement.** Substance abuse is much less common among students who actively participate in classes and feel connected with the subject matter. However, many students report never working closely with a faculty member, never being inspired by an educational experience, or never having an educational or extra-curricular experience that motivates them to make an active contribution to a greater goal.[12]

- **Athletics.** Although male and female college athletes drink at higher rates than nonathletes, they are less likely to use illegal drugs. One exception is the use of anabolic steroids (discussed in Chapter 5), which college athletes use more than other students.[13]

Understanding Drugs and Their Effects

A **drug** is a chemical substance that affects the way you feel and function. In some circumstances, taking a drug can help the body heal or relieve physical and mental distress. In other circumstances, taking a drug can distort reality, undermine well-being, and threaten survival. No drug is completely safe; all drugs have multiple effects that vary greatly in different people at different times. Knowing how drugs affect the brain, body, and behavior is crucial to understanding their impact and making responsible decisions about their use.

Drug misuse is the taking of a drug for a purpose or by a person other than that for which/whom it was medically intended. Borrowing a friend's prescription for penicillin when your throat feels scratchy is an example of drug misuse. The World Health Organization defines **drug abuse** as excessive drug use that's inconsistent with accepted medical practice. Taking prescription painkillers to get high is an example of drug abuse.

Risks are involved with all forms of drug use. Even medications that help cure illnesses or soothe symptoms have side effects and can be misused. Some substances that millions of people use every day, such as caffeine, pose some health risks. Others—like the most commonly used drugs in our society, alcohol and tobacco—can lead to potentially life-threatening problems. With some illicit drugs, any form of use can be dangerous.

drug Any substance, other than food, that affects bodily functions and structures when taken into the body.

drug misuse The use of a drug for a purpose (or person) other than that for which it was medically intended.

drug abuse The excessive use of a drug in a manner inconsistent with accepted medical practice.

Your Life Change Coach

Developing Positive Addictions

When you're anxious, bored, restless, or confused, when drugs seem all too appealing as a "quick fix," there are real solutions, "positive addictions" that can help you solve your problems without creating new and bigger ones. A positive addiction—whether it is exercising, mountain-climbing, or listening to music—can produce very real "highs." But there's a crucial difference between this sort of stimulation and drug dependency: one is real, the other is chemical. With one, you're in control; with the other, drugs are.

Here are some examples:

- **If you feel a need for physical relaxation,** if you want more energy or distraction from physical discomforts, you can turn to athletics, exercise (including walking and hiking), dance, or outdoor hobbies.

- **If you want to stimulate your senses,** enhance sexual stimulation, or magnify the sensations of sight, sound, and touch, train yourself to be more sensitive to nature and beauty. Take time to appreciate the sensations you experience when you're walking in the woods or embracing a person you love. Through activities like sailing or sky-diving, you can literally fill up your senses without relying on chemicals.

- **If you have psychological troubles,** if you're anxious or depressed, if you feel inhibited or uptight, if you don't know how to solve complex personal problems and want relief from emotional pain, turn to people who can offer lasting help: in some cases, friends; in others, professional counselors or support groups.

Many factors determine the effects a drug has on an individual. These include how the drug enters the body, the dosage, the drug action, and the presence of other drugs in the body—as well as the physical and psychological makeup of the person taking the drug and the setting in which the drug is used.

Routes of Administration

Drugs can enter the body in a number of ways (Figure 11.2). The most common way of taking a drug is by swallowing a tablet, capsule, or liquid. However, drugs taken orally don't reach the bloodstream as quickly as drugs introduced into the body by other means. A drug taken orally may not have any effect for 30 minutes or more.

Drugs can enter the body through the lungs either by inhaling smoke, for example, from marijuana, or by inhaling gases, aerosol sprays, or fumes from solvents or other compounds that evaporate quickly. Young users of such inhalants, discussed later in this chapter, often soak a rag with fluid and press it over their nose. Or they may place inhalants in a plastic bag, put the bag over their nose and mouth, and take deep breaths—a practice called *huffing* and one that can produce serious, even fatal consequences.

Drugs can also be injected with a syringe subcutaneously (beneath the skin), intramuscularly (into muscle tissue, which is richly supplied with blood vessels), or intravenously (directly into a vein). **Intravenous** (IV) injection gets the drug into the bloodstream immediately (within seconds in most cases); **intramuscular** injection, moderately fast (within a few minutes); and **subcutaneous** injection, more slowly (within ten minutes).

Injecting drugs is extremely dangerous because many diseases, including hepatitis and infection with human immune deficiency virus (HIV), can be transmitted by sharing contaminated needles. Injection-drug users who are HIV-positive are a major source of transmission of HIV among heterosexuals (see Chapter 16).

Dosage and Toxicity

The effects of any drug depend on the amount an individual takes. Increasing the dose usually intensifies the effects produced by smaller doses. Also, the kind of effect may change at different dose levels. For example, low doses of barbiturates may relieve anxiety, while higher doses can induce sleep, loss of sensation, even coma and death.

The dosage level at which a drug becomes poisonous to the body, causing either temporary or permanent damage, is called its **toxicity.** In most cases, drugs are eventually broken down in the liver by special body chemicals called *detoxification enzymes.*

Individual Differences

Each person responds differently to different drugs, depending on circumstances or setting. The enzymes in the body reduce the levels of drugs in the bloodstream;

- **If you want peer acceptance,** if you'd like to overcome your shyness, if you want to communicate and relate more effectively, you can join expertly managed sensitivity or encounter groups, enroll in confidence-building seminars, seek counseling, or volunteer in programs in which you can assist others and not focus only on your self-consciousness.

- **If you want to escape mental boredom,** gain new understanding of the world around you, study better, experiment with your levels of awareness, or indulge your intellectual curiosity, challenge your mind through reading, classes, creative games, discussion groups, memory training, or travel.

- **If you want to enhance your creativity** or your appreciation of the arts, pursue training in music, art, singing, gardening, or writing. Sign up for a nongraded course in art history or music appreciation. Attend more concerts, ballets, museum shows.

- **If you want to promote political or social change,** defy the establishment, change drug legislation, or gain power, you can volunteer in political campaigns, work on nonpartisan projects, or join lobbying and political action groups.

- **If you want to find meaning in life,** understand the nature of the universe, or expand your personal awareness, explore various philosophical theories through classes, seminars, and discussion groups. Study different religious orientations, including mysticism, try yoga and meditation, or try prayer.

- **If you're looking for kicks,** adventure, danger, and excitement, sign up for a wilderness survival course. Take up an adventurous sport, like hang gliding or rock climbing. Set a challenging professional or personal goal and direct your energies to meeting it.

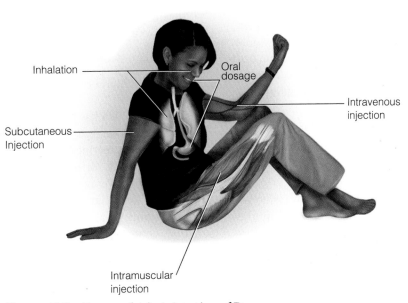

Figure 11.2   Routes of Administration of Drugs

because there can be 80 variants of each enzyme, every person's body may react differently.

Often drugs intensify the emotional state a person is in. If you're feeling depressed, a drug may make you feel more depressed. A generalized physical problem, such as having the flu, may make your body more vulnerable to the effects of a drug. Genetic differences among individuals also may account for varying reactions.

Personality and psychological attitude also play a role in drug effects. Each user's *mind-set*—his or her expectations or preconceptions about using the drug—affects the experience. Someone who takes a "club drug" (discussed further later in this chapter) to feel more "connected" may feel more sociable simply because that's what he or she expects.

intraveneous   Into a vein.
intramuscular   Into or within a muscle.
subcutaneous   Under the skin.

toxicity   Poisonousness; the dosage level at which a drug becomes poisonous to the body, causing either temporary or permanent damage.

Setting

The setting for drug use also influences its effects. Passing around a marijuana joint at a friend's is not a healthy or safe behavior, but the experience of going to a crack house is very different—and entails greater dangers.

Types of Action

A drug can act *locally,* as novocaine does to deaden pain in a tooth; *generally,* throughout a body system, as barbiturates do on the central nervous system; or *selectively,* as a drug does when it has a greater effect on one specific organ or system than on others, such as a spinal anesthetic. A drug that accumulates in the body because it's taken in faster than it can be metabolized and excreted is called *cumulative;* alcohol is such a drug.

Interaction with Other Drugs or Alcohol

A drug can interact with other drugs in four different ways:

- An **additive** interaction is one in which the resulting effect is equal to the sum of the effects of the different drugs used.

- A **synergistic** interaction is one in which the total effect of the two drugs taken together is greater than the sum of the effects the two drugs would have had if taken by themselves on separate occasions. Mixing barbiturates and alcohol, for example, has up to four times the depressant effect than either drug has alone.

- A drug can be **potentiating**—that is, one drug can increase the effect of another. Alcohol, for instance, can increase the drowsiness caused by antihistamines (antiallergy medications).

- Drugs can interact in an **antagonistic** fashion—that is, one drug can neutralize or block another drug with opposite effects. Tranquilizers, for example, may counter some of the nervousness and anxiety produced by cocaine.

The danger of mixing alcohol with other drugs cannot be emphasized too strongly. Alcohol and marijuana intensify each other's effects, making driving and many other activities extremely dangerous. Some people who have mixed sedatives or tranquilizers with alcohol never regained consciousness.

Men, Women, and Drugs

 Beginning at a very early age, males and females show different patterns in drug use. Men generally encounter more opportunities to use drugs than women, but given an opportunity to use drugs for the first time, both genders are equally likely to do so and to progress from initial use to dependence. Vulnerability to some drugs varies with gender. Both are equally likely to become addicted to or dependent on cocaine, heroin, hallucinogens, tobacco, and inhalants. Women are more likely than men to become addicted to or dependent on sedatives and drugs designed to treat anxiety or sleeplessness and less likely than men to abuse alcohol and marijuana.

Males and females may differ in their biological responses to drugs. In studies of animals given the opportunity to self-administer intravenous doses of cocaine or heroin, females began self-administration sooner than males and administered larger amounts of the drugs. Male and female long-term cocaine users showed similar impairment in tests of concentration, memory, and academic achievement following sustained abstinence, even though women in the study had substantially greater exposure to cocaine. Female cocaine users also were less likely than men to exhibit abnormalities of blood flow in the brain's frontal lobes. These findings suggest a gender-related mechanism that may protect women from some of the damage cocaine inflicts on the brain. However, women are more vulnerable to poor nutrition and below-average weight, depression, physical abuse, and if pregnant, preterm labor or early delivery.

Caffeine and Its Effects

Caffeine, which has been drunk, chewed, and swallowed since the Stone Age, is the most widely used **psychoactive** (mind-affecting) drug in the world. Eighty percent of Americans drink coffee, our principal caffeine source—an average of 3.5 cups a day. Coffee contains 100 to 150 milligrams of caffeine per cup; tea, 40 to 100 milligrams; cola, about 45 milligrams. Most medications that contain caffeine are one-third to one-half the strength of a cup of coffee. However, some, such as Excedrin, are very high in caffeine (Table 11.1).

TABLE 11.1 Caffeine Counts

Substance (typical serving)	Caffeine (milligrams)
No Doz, one pill	200
Coffee (drip), one 5-ounce cup	130
Excedrin, two pills	130
Espresso, one 2-ounce cup	100
Energy drink (Red Bull), one can	80
Instant coffee, one 5-ounce cup	74
Coca-Cola, 12 ounces	46
Tea, one 5-ounce cup	40
Dark chocolate, 1 ounce	20
Milk chocolate, 1 ounce	6
Cocoa, 5 ounces	4
Decaffeinated coffee, one 5-ounce cup	3

As a stimulant, caffeine relieves drowsiness, helps in the performance of repetitive tasks, and improves the capacity for work. Caffeine improves performance and endurance during prolonged, exhaustive exercise and to a lesser degree, enhances short-term, high-intensity athletic performance. Additional benefits include improved concentration, reduced fatigue, and sharpened alertness.

You'll stay more alert, particularly if you are fighting sleep deprivation, if you spread your coffee consumption over the course of the day. For instance, rather than drinking two 8-ounce cups in the morning, try consuming smaller servings of an ounce or two during the course of the day.

In recent decades, some 19,000 studies have examined caffeine's impact on health. Their conclusion: For most people, caffeine poses few serious health risks—and may convey a surprising range of benefits. Coffee may reduce the risk of type 2 diabetes, Parkinson's disease, colon cancer, liver cirrhosis, and gallstones. There is also some evidence that coffee may relieve migraines, boost mood, and even prevent cavities. Despite these positive findings, doctors still advice pregnant women, heart patients, and those at risk for osteoporosis to limit or avoid coffee. And too much caffeine, particularly in high-powered energy drinks (discussed in Chapter 5), can be dangerous for everyone.

You can overdose on caffeine and develop symptoms such as restlessness, nervousness, excitement, insomnia, flushed face, increased urination, digestive complaints, muscle twitching, rambling thoughts and speech, rapid heart rate or arrhythmias, periods of inexhaustibility, and physical restlessness. Some people develop these symptoms after as little as 250 milligrams of caffeine a day; others, only with much larger doses. Higher doses may produce ringing in the ears or flashes of light, grand mal seizures, and potentially fatal respiratory failure.

Caffeine withdrawal for those dependent on this substance can cause headaches and other neurological symptoms. Those who must cut back should taper off gradually. One approach is to mix regular and decaffeinated coffee, gradually decreasing the quantity of the former.

Medications

As many as half of all patients take the wrong medications, in the wrong doses, at the wrong times, or in the wrong ways. Every year these inadvertent errors lead to an estimated 125,000 deaths and more than $8.5 billion in hospital costs.[14] Mistakes occur among people of all ages, both genders, and every race, occupation, level of education, and personality type. Their number-one cause: not understanding directions (see Savvy Consumer: "How to Avoid Medication Mistakes").

Doctors occasionally make errors when it comes to prescription drugs. The most frequent are over- or under-dosing, omitting information from prescriptions, ordering the wrong dosage form (a pill instead of a liquid, for example), and not recognizing a patient's allergy to a drug.

Over-the-Counter Drugs

More than half a million health products—remedies for everything from bad breath to bunions—are readily available without a doctor's prescription. This doesn't mean that they're necessarily safe or effective. Indeed, many widely used **over-the-counter (OTC) drugs** pose unsuspected hazards.

Federal regulators have issued warnings for many popular painkillers, including over-the-counter pills like Advil (ibuprophen) and Aleve (naproxin). Their labels cite risks to the heart, stomach, and skin. Tylenol (acetaminophen) and aspirin are generally considered safe for people with temporary pain like headaches and muscle aches. However, aspirin can cause stomach irritation and bleeding. Tylenol and other products containing acetaminophen account for 40 to 50 percent of all acute cases of liver failure, many the result of unintentional overdose. Doctors caution against taking more than eight Tylenol Extra Strength pills (which contain 500 mg per tablet) in a 24-hour period.[15]

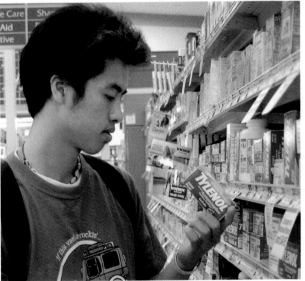

© Geri Engberg Photography

Practically all of these packages carry warnings to consumers. Read them before using an over-the-counter drug.

additive Characterized by a combined effect that is equal to the sum of the individual effects.

synergistic Characterized by a combined effect that is greater than the sum of the individual effects.

potentiating Making more effective or powerful.

antagonistic Opposing or counteracting.

psychoactive Mind-affecting.

over-the-counter (OTC) drugs Medications that can be obtained legally without a prescription from a medical professional.

Like other drugs, OTC medications can be used improperly, often simply because of a lack of education about proper use. Among those most often misused are the following:

- **Nasal sprays.** Nasal sprays relieve congestion by shrinking blood vessels in the nose. If they are used too often or for too many days in a row, the blood vessels widen instead of contracting, and the surrounding tissues become swollen, causing more congestion. To make the vessels shrink again, many people use more spray more often. The result can be permanent damage to nasal membranes, bleeding, infection, and partial or complete loss of smell.

- **Laxatives.** Believing that they must have one bowel movement a day (a common misconception), many people rely on laxatives. Brands that contain phenolphthalein irritate the lining of the intestines and cause muscles to contract or tighten, often making constipation worse rather than better. Bulk laxatives are less dangerous, but regular use is not advised. A high-fiber diet and more exercise are safer and more effective remedies for constipation.

- **Eye drops.** Eye drops make the blood vessels of the eye contract. However, as in the case of nasal sprays, with overuse (several times a day for several weeks), the blood vessels expand, making the eye look redder than before.

- **Sleep aids.** Although OTC sleeping pills are widely used, there has been little research on their use and possible risks. A national consensus panel on insomnia concluded that they are not effective and cause side effects such as morning-after grogginess.[16] Medications like Tylenol PM and Excedrin PM combine a pain reliever with a sleep-inducing antihistamine, the same ingredient that people take for hay fever or cold symptoms. Although they make people drowsy, they can leave you feeling groggy the next day, and they dry out the nose and mouth.

- **Cough syrup.** Many of the "active" ingredients in over-the-counter cough preparations may be ineffective. Chugging cough syrup (also called *roboing*, after the OTC medication Robitussin) is a growing problem, in part because young people think of dextromethorphan (DXM), a common ingredient

Savvy Consumer How to Avoid Medication Mistakes

- Whenever you get a prescription, be sure to find out from your doctor and pharmacist the name of the drug, what it's supposed to do, and how and when to take it and for how long. Are there foods, drinks, other medications, or activities you should avoid while taking the medication?

- Ask if the drug causes any side effects and what you should do if any occur.

- Keep a record of all your medicines, listing both their brand and generic (chemical) names and the reason you are taking them, and update it regularly. Give a copy of this list to every physician and every pharmacy providing health-care services.

- Inform your doctors of any over-the-counter drugs, vitamins, and herbal products you use regularly. Popular herbal supplements like gingko bilboa and common over-the-counter drugs like aspirin can interact with many prescription drugs to cause serious problems, such as excessive bleeding.

- Always turn on the lights when you take your medication. Familiarize yourself with the imprint on each tablet or capsule so you can recognize each pill. If a refill looks different, check with your pharmacist or doctor before taking it.

- Don't crush or chew a medicine without checking with your doctor or pharmacist first. Some medications are

designed for gradual release rather than all at once and could be harmful if absorbed too quickly.

- Don't use a kitchen spoon to dispense liquid medications. Household teaspoons can hold between 3 and 7 milliliters; a prescription "teaspoon" means 5 milliliters. Either measure the dose in the cup or dropper that came with the medicine or ask the pharmacist for a measuring device.

- Never take someone else's medications. They could interact with your medications or the dose may be different.

- Always check labels for warnings on interactions with alcohol and instructions on whether or not to take before, with, or after meals.

- Don't take medicine with grapefruit juice, which can interact with more than 200 medications, including cholesterol-lowering statins, sleeping pills, and anti-anxiety agents.

- Plan ahead to make sure you have adequate amounts of the medications you need.

- Don't leave medicines in a car for prolonged periods. Temperature extremes, along with moisture, light, and oxygen, can affect the potency of many medications.

- Use cues, such as the alarm on your cell phone or Palm Pilot or Post-it notes, to remind you to take your medication on schedule.

in cough medicine, as a "poor man's version" of the popular drug Ecstasy.

Prescription Drugs

 In a recent study of about 9,000 undergraduates at a large midwestern university, 57 percent reported that they had used prescription drugs for medical reasons at some point in their lives. The most widely used ones were pain medications, sedative or anxiety medications, sleeping medications, and stimulant medications. College women used more pain, anxiety, and sleeping pills; college men used more medically prescribed stimulants.[17]

Nonadherence

Many prescribed medications aren't taken the way they should be; millions simply aren't taken at all. As many as 70 percent of adults have trouble understanding dosage information and 30 percent can't read standard labels, according to the FDA, which has called for larger, clearer drug labeling. The dangers of nonadherence (not properly taking prescription drugs) include recurrent infections, serious medical complications, and emergency hospital treatment. The drugs most likely to be taken incorrectly are those that treat problems with no obvious symptoms (such as high blood pressure), require complex dosage schedules, treat psychiatric disorders, or have unpleasant side effects.

The most common reason that college students fail to take medicines as directed is forgetting. Others are concerned about cost, or they stop when they feel better. Students' underlying health beliefs, such as a conviction that taking medicine reflects weakness, can affect their compliance.[18]

Physical Side Effects

Most medications, taken correctly, cause only minor complications. However, no drug is entirely without side effects for all individuals taking it. Serious complications that may occur include heart failure, heart attack, seizures, kidney and liver failure, severe blood disorders, birth defects, blindness, memory problems, and allergic reactions.

Allergic reactions to drugs are common. The drugs that most often provoke allergic responses are penicillin and other antibiotics (drugs used to treat infection). Aspirin, sulfa drugs, barbiturates, anticonvulsants, insulin, and local anesthetics can also provoke allergic responses.

Psychological Side Effects

Dozens of drugs—both over-the-counter and prescription—can cause changes in the way people think, feel, and behave. Unfortunately, neither patients nor their physicians usually connect such symptoms with medications.

Doctors may not even mention potential mental and emotional problems because they don't want to scare patients away from what otherwise may be a very effective treatment. What you don't know about a drug's effects on your mind *can* hurt you.

Among the medications most likely to cause psychiatric side effects are drugs for high blood pressure, heart disease, asthma, epilepsy, arthritis, Parkinson's disease, anxiety, insomnia, and depression. Some drugs—such as the powerful hormones called *corticosteroids,* used for asthma, autoimmune diseases, and cancer—can cause different psychiatric symptoms, depending on dosage and other factors. The older you are, the sicker you are, and the more medications you're taking, the greater your risk of developing some psychiatric side effects.

Drug Interactions

OTC and prescription drugs can interact in a variety of ways. For example, mixing some cold medications with tranquilizers can cause drowsiness and coordination problems, thus making driving dangerous. Moreover, what you eat or drink can impair or completely wipe out the effectiveness of drugs or lead to unexpected effects on the body. For instance, aspirin takes five to ten times as long to be absorbed when taken with food or shortly after a meal than when taken on an empty stomach. If tetracyclines encounter calcium in the stomach, they bind together and cancel each other out.

To avoid potentially dangerous interactions, check the label(s) for any instructions on how or when to take a medication, such as "with a meal." If the directions say that you should take a drug on an empty stomach, take it at least one hour before eating or two or three hours after eating. Don't drink a hot beverage with a medication; the temperature may interfere with the effectiveness of the drug.

Whenever you take a drug, be especially careful of your intake of alcohol, which can change the rate of metabolism and the effects of many different drugs. Because it dilates the blood vessels, alcohol can add to the dizziness sometimes caused by drugs for high blood pressure, angina, or depression. Also, its irritating effects on the stomach can worsen stomach upset from aspirin, ibuprofen, and other anti-inflammatory drugs.

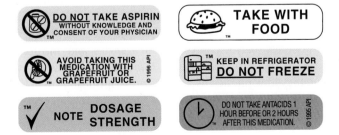

Check the labels on prescription medications.

Generic Drugs

The **generic** name is the chemical name for a drug. A specific drug may appear on the pharmacist's shelf under a variety of brand names, which may cost more than twice the generic equivalent. About 75 percent of all prescriptions specify a brand name, but pharmacists may—and in some states must—switch to a generic drug unless the doctor specifically tells them not to. Prescriptions filled with generic drugs cost 20 to 85 percent less than their brand-name counterparts.

Generic drugs have the same active ingredients as brand-name prescriptions, but their fillers and binders, which can affect the absorption of a drug, may be different. For some serious illnesses, the generics may not be as effective; some experts recommend sticking with brand names for heart medications, psychiatric drugs, and anticonvulsant drugs (for epilepsy and other seizure disorders).

To determine whether you should buy the generic version of a drug, ask your physician whether it matters if you get a brand-name or generic drug. If it does, ask which brand name is best. Also, find out if switching to a generic or from one generic to another might harm your condition in any way.

Buying Drugs Online

Millions of people in the United States purchase prescription medications online. Although some websites fill only faxed prescriptions from medical doctors, others ignore or sidestep traditional regulations and safeguards. Cyberspace distributors often ship pills across state lines without requiring a physical examination by a medical doctor. Instead, a "cyberdoc," who may or may not be qualified or up-to-date in a given specialty, reviews information submitted by a "patient." International pharmacies sometimes sell drugs that are not available or approved in the United States. And patients themselves use bulletin boards and other online resources to sell unused or unwanted medications to each other.

Many individuals turn to the Internet for "lifestyle" drugs such as pills for erectile dysfunction, weight control, and smoking cessation. Customers like the convenience and anonymity of buying drugs online. Although many assume drugs cost less on the Internet, shipping costs tend to drive prices up to the same amount or more than the price at a pharmacy.

The dangers of unregulated distribution of medications have alarmed government agencies and medical groups. The American Medical Association has declared it unethical for physicians to write prescriptions for people they've never met. The National Association of Boards of Pharmacy has developed a seal of approval to help customers determine which sites are legitimate. The FDA and other federal agencies, such as the Federal Trade Commission, which regulates advertising, are trying to find ways to impose some controls.

Consumers have to be wary. Ordering a drug like Accutane, an acne treatment, online may seem harmless. However, without close monitoring by a physician, you could develop complications, such as a bad reaction that aggravates hepatitis or inflames the pancreas. Quality control is another concern. Counterfeit drugs, increasingly sold online, may do little, if any, good and could be harmful. Cyberspace pharmacies provide no information on how the drug was stored or whether its expiration date has passed. In addition, since importing medications without a prescription is against the law, you could find yourself in legal trouble.

Prescription Drug Abuse

The abuse of prescription medications is becoming more widespread than illicit drug use around the world. In the United States, only marijuana is more widely abused.[19] The three most commonly abused classes of prescription drugs are:

- **Opioids.** Most often prescribed to treat pain. Examples include codeine, oxycodone (OxyContin and Percocet), and morphine (Kadian and Avinza).
- **Central nervous system (CNS) depressants.** Used to treat anxiety and sleep disorders. Examples include barbiturates (Mebaral and Nembutal) and benzodiazepines (Valium and Xanax).
- **Stimulants.** prescribed to treat the sleep disorder narcolepsy, attention-deficit/hyperactivity disorder (ADHD), and obesity. Examples include dextroamphetamine (Dexedrine and Adderall) and methylphenidate (Ritalin and Concerta).[20]

Table 11.2 presents the commonly abused prescription drugs and summarizes the dangers associated with them. While illegal drug use has dropped among teenagers, prescription drug use has increased. Nearly 1 in 10 high school seniors abused a prescription drug in the previous year.[21] Students in 8th, 10th, and 12th grade reported using cold or cough medicines containing dextromethorphan to get high.[22]

Soaring abuse of prescription drugs has led to a surge in counterfeit medications. Many end up in less developed countries, where 25 to 50 percent of medicines sold on the black market may be counterfeit.[23] Growing amounts of prescription drugs, including counterfeits, are sold online.

Although many assume that prescription medicines, which help so many sick people, are safer than illegal drugs, they can be more potent and pose a higher over-

TABLE 11.2 Abused Prescription Drugs

Pain killers—Opioids
Derivative or synthetic versions of opium, like heroin.

Such as: OxyContin, Codeine, Percodan, Fentanyl, Vicodin (hydrocodone), Methadone, Morphine, Percocet, Demoral.

How taken: Ingested orally as a tablet or capsule or liquid form; crushed and snorted; or cooked so it can be injected intravenously.

Occasional use: At first you may feel indifferent to physical or emotional pain, nauseated, and a little drowsy. You may be constipated later. If you take too much (overdose), your breathing may slow down and you could die.

Sustained use over time: Painkillers are highly addictive and tolerance can increase over time.

Most dangerous when used with: Alcohol, antihistamines, barbiturates, benzodiazepines.

Antianxiety Drugs—Benzodiazepines

Such as: Xanax, Valium, Librium, Klonopin, Ativan.

How taken: Orally; or crushed and snorted.

Occasional use: You may feel calm and sleepy, with less tension, anxiety, or panic. This feeling will diminish over time as the body builds a tolerance to the substance.

Sustained use over time: Potential for addiction. Withdrawal can be lengthy, painful, and cause seizures, and should be medically supervised.

Most dangerous when used with: Alcohol, pain medications, some over-the-counter cold and allergy medications.

"Study Drugs"—Stimulants

Such as: Ritalin, Concerta, Adderall, Focalin, Dexedrine.

How taken: As a tablet; crushed and snorted; or liquefied so it can be injected intravenously. Some people opt for inserting the drug anally (plugging).

Occasional use: You may feel alert, focused, and awake. These drugs can make blood pressure and heart rate go up. They can also suppress appetite and cause sleep problems.

Sustained use over time: High potential for addiction, paranoia, and sleep deprivation, which can cause psychotic episodes (like amphetamine psychosis). Also can cause insomnia, digestive problems, and erratic weight change.

Most dangerous when used with: Over-the-counter medications, including cold medications containing decongestants; antidepressants, unless supervised by a physician; some asthma medications.

Over the Counter Drugs—OTCs
This category includes a wide variety of substances. The similarity is that they are all cheap, widely available, and legal without a prescription.

Such as: Dextromethorphan (Coricidin Cough and Cold, Robitussin DM, Drixoral), caffeine pills, Sudafed, diet pills, vitamin supplements, herbal remedies.

How taken: Cough medicines containing DXM are taken orally as a liquid or in capsules, in as much as 10–30 times the recommended dose.

Occasional use: You may feel euphoric or disconnected. You may experience heart palpitations, dizziness, blackouts, insomnia, delusions, or seizures, and even coma or death from respiratory distress or heat stroke.

Sustained use over time: Commonly causes nausea, stomach cramps, or other unpleasant gastrointestinal effects that may persist for days after use. At risk for liver, kidney, lung, pancreas, and/or brain damage. Also can cause users to pee blood. Addiction is possible.

Most dangerous when used with: Cold medicines that contain acetaminophen (like Tylenol), chlorpheniramine maleate, MAO inhibitors and other antidepressants, unless supervised by a physician.

Antidepressants
Includes selective serotonin reuptake inhibitors (SSRIs), MAO inhibitors, Tricyclics.

Such as: Prozac, Zoloft, Celexa, Paxil, Wellbutrin.

How taken: Orally, with the substance building up in the body over time, so one dose does not have immediate effects.

Occasional use: You may not feel much. Most antidepressants take days or weeks to kick in.

Sustained use over time: If you take (unprescribed) antidepressants for long enough to feel the effects, you are in jeopardy of unbalancing the chemicals in your brain and causing emotional disturbances and risk of withdrawal symptoms. The bigger risk actually is for the person whose medication you are taking, who is being deprived of the medication they may need to function optimally.

Most dangerous when used with: Alcohol. Use of any drug will detract from the efficacy of most antidepressants.

Source: Adapted from wwww.factsontap.org/factsontap/wrong_prescription/types.htm.

dose risk than illicit drugs. The number of emergency room visits stemming from prescription drug abuse and the number of related deaths have spiked in recent years. Counterfeits add to the dangers.

generic Refers to products without trade names that are equivalent to other products protected by trademark registration.

Prescription Drug Abuse on Campus

 The abuse of prescription medications on college campuses has increased in the last 15 years. As many as one in five college students misuses or abuses a prescription medication every year. The rates of illicit use of prescribed drugs are higher than for the use of cocaine, Ecstasy, inhalants, LSD, other psychedelics, crystal methamphetamine, heroin, GHB, or Ketamine. Only marijuana use is more widespread on campus.

 College men have higher rates of prescription drug abuse than women. White and Hispanic undergraduates are significantly more likely to abuse medications than African American and Asian students. Many students taking prescription drugs for medical purposes report being approached by classmates seeking drugs. Undergraduates who misuse or abuse prescription medications are much more likely to report heavy binge drinking and use of illicit drugs.

Students who abuse prescription drugs may use both stimulants and painkillers. However, most students choose these agents for different reasons. Students who abuse stimulants say they do so to help improve performance at school, to increase alertness, or to enjoy partying more. A much smaller number take stimulants to lose weight or prevent weight gain. Students who abuse prescription painkillers say they do so to relax or get high, although some report taking the drugs to help with depression and anxiety or for chronic pain.[24]

Prescription Stimulants

The most widely abused prescription drugs are stimulant medications such as Ritalin. Although proper medical use of this agent appears safe, misuse or abuse of any stimulant medication can be dangerous, even deadly. When taken in high doses, either orally or nasally, the risk of addiction increases. Physical side effects include cardiorespiratory complications, increased blood pressure, and headache. High doses can trigger panic attacks, aggressive behavior, and suicidal or homicidal impulses. Overdoses can kill.

 In a recent survey at a northeastern university, 16 percent of students—about equal numbers of men and women—reported misuse or abuse of stimulants. About half used the drugs two or three times a year; a third took them two or three times a month. Most swallowed pills, but a high percentage reported snorting the drug. The majority expressed little concern about the potential negative effects of stimulants.[25]

Prescription Painkillers

 Abuse of prescription painkillers, such as Oxy-Contin and Vicodin, is also widespread on campuses. In a survey of more than 10,000 students attending 119 colleges, 12 percent of undergraduates reported lifetime use of a prescription painkiller for nonmedical reasons; 7 percent did so in the previous year. Students who are members of fraternities and sororities, enrolled at more competitive schools, earning lower grade point averages, and engaging in substance use and other risky behaviors are more likely to abuse these drugs.[26]

Substance Use Disorders

People have been using psychoactive chemicals for centuries. Citizens of ancient Mesopotamia and Egypt used opium. More than 3,000 years ago, Hindus included cannabis products in religious ceremonies. For centuries the Inca in South America have chewed the leaves of the coca bush. Yet while drugs existed in most societies, their use was usually limited to small groups. Today millions of people regularly turn to drugs to pick them up, bring them down, alter perceptions, or ease psychological pain.

The word **addiction**, as used by the general population, refers to the compulsive use of a substance, loss of control, negative consequences, and denial. Mental health professionals describe drug-related problems in terms of *dependence* and *abuse*.

Dependence

Individuals may develop **psychological dependence** and feel a strong craving for a drug because it produces pleasurable feelings or relieves stress and anxiety. **Physical dependence** occurs when a person develops *tolerance* to the effects of a drug and needs larger and larger doses to achieve intoxication or another desired effect. Individuals who are physically dependent and have a high tolerance to a drug may take amounts many times those that would produce intoxication or an overdose in someone who was not a regular user.

Men and women with a substance dependence disorder may use a drug to avoid or relieve withdrawal symptoms, or they may consume larger amounts of a drug or use it over a longer period than they'd originally intended. They may repeatedly try to cut down or control drug use without success; spend a great deal of time obtaining or using drugs or recovering from their effects; give up or reduce important social, occupational, or recreational activities because of their drug use; or continue to use a drug despite knowledge that the drug is likely to cause or worsen a persistent or recurring physical or psychological problem.

Specific symptoms of dependence vary with particular drugs. Some drugs, such as marijuana, hallucinogens, and phencyclidine, do not cause withdrawal symptoms. The degree of dependence also varies. In mild cases, a person may function normally most of the time. In severe cases, the person's entire life may revolve around obtaining, using, and recuperating from the effects of a drug.

Individuals with drug dependence become intoxicated or high on a regular basis—whether every day, every weekend, or several binges a year. They may try repeatedly to stop using a drug and yet fail, even though they realize their drug use is interfering with their health, family life, relationships, and work.

Abuse

Some drug users do not develop the symptoms of tolerance and withdrawal that characterize dependence, yet they use drugs in ways that clearly have a harmful effect on them. These individuals are diagnosed as having a *psychoactive substance abuse disorder.* They continue to use drugs despite their awareness of persistent or repeated social, occupational, psychological, or physical problems related to drug use, or they use drugs in dangerous ways or situations (before driving, for instance).

Intoxication and Withdrawal

Intoxication refers to maladaptive behavioral, psychological, and physiologic changes that occur as a result of substance use. **Withdrawal** is the development of symptoms that cause significant psychological and physical distress when an individual reduces or stops drug use. (Intoxication and withdrawal from specific drugs are discussed later in this chapter.)

Polyabuse

Most users prefer a certain type of drug but also use several others; this behavior is called **polyabuse.** The average user who enters treatment is on five different drugs. The more drugs anyone uses, the greater the chance of side effects, complications, and possibly life-threatening interactions.

Coexisting Conditions

Mental disorders and substance abuse disorders have a great deal of overlap.[27] Many individuals with substance abuse disorders also have another psychiatric disorder, such as depression. Individuals with such *dual diagnoses* require careful evaluation and appropriate treatment for the complete range of complex and chronic difficulties they face. However, they can benefit from participation in 12-step groups, like Double Trouble in Recovery, that provide treatment for both.

Causes of Drug Dependence and Abuse

No one fully understands why some people develop drug dependence or abuse disorders, whereas others, who may experiment briefly with drugs, do not. Inherited body chemistry, genetic factors, and sensitivity to drugs may make some individuals more susceptible. These disorders may stem from many complex causes.

The Biology of Dependence

Scientists now view drug dependence as a brain disease triggered by frequent use of drugs that change the biochemistry and anatomy of neurons and alter the way they work. A major breakthrough in understanding dependence has been the discovery that certain mood-altering substances and experiences—a puff of marijuana, a slug of whiskey, a snort of cocaine, a big win at blackjack—trigger a rise in a brain chemical called *dopamine,* which is associated with feelings of satisfaction and euphoria. This brain chemical or neurotransmitter is one of the crucial messengers that links nerve cells in the brain and its level rises during any pleasurable experience, whether it be a loving hug or a taste of chocolate.

The mechanism governing the rise in dopamine levels is not the same for all drugs. Figure 11.3 shows the one for cocaine. Normally, after dopamine is released from the axon terminal of a neuron and activates dopamine receptors on the adjacent neuron, the dopamine is then transported back to its original neuron by "uptake pumps." Cocaine binds to the uptake pumps and prevents them from transporting dopamine back into the neuron terminal. So more dopamine builds up in the synapse and is free to activate more dopamine receptors.

Addictive drugs have such a powerful impact on dopamine and its receptors that they change the pathways within the brain's pleasure centers. Various psychoactive chemicals create a craving for more of the same. According to this hypothesis, addicts do not specifically yearn for heroin, cocaine, or nicotine but for the rush of dopamine that these drugs produce. Some individuals, born with low levels of dopamine, may be particularly susceptible to this craving and thus to addiction.

addiction A behavioral pattern characterized by compulsion, loss of control, and continued repetition of a behavior or activity in spite of adverse consequences.

psychological dependence The emotional or mental attachment to the use of a drug.

physical dependence The physiological attachment to, and need for, a drug.

intoxication Maladaptive behavioral, psychological, and physiologic changes that occur as a result of substance abuse.

withdrawal Development of symptoms that cause significant psychological and physical distress when an individual reduces or stops drug use.

polyabuse The misuse or abuse of more than one drug.

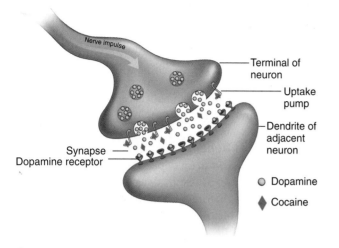

Figure 11.3 Dopamine Levels for Cocaine
Within the synapses between adjacent neurons, cocaine binds to the dopamine uptake pumps and thus allows the neurotransmitter dopamine to build up in the synapse and bind to more dopamine receptors.

The Psychology of Vulnerability

Although scientists do not believe there is an addictive personality, certain individuals are at greater risk of drug dependence because of psychological factors, including difficulty controlling impulses, a lack of values that might constrain drug use (whether based in religion, family, or society), low self-esteem, feelings of powerlessness, and depression. The one psychological trait most often linked with drug use is denial. Young people in particular are absolutely convinced that they will never lose control or suffer in any way as a result of drug use.

Many diagnosed drug users have at least one mental disorder, particularly depression or anxiety. Disorders that emerge in adolescence, such as bipolar disorder, may increase the risk of substance abuse. Many people with psychiatric disorders abuse drugs. Individuals may self-administer drugs to treat psychiatric symptoms; for example, they may take sedating drugs to suppress a panic attack.

Early Influences

Teen drug abuse has declined in the last decade, but some teens remain more vulnerable. Young people from lower socioeconomic backgrounds are more likely to use drugs than their more affluent peers, possibly because of economic disadvantage; family instability; a lack of realistic, rewarding alternatives and role models; and increased hopelessness.

 Those whose companions are substance abusers are far more likely to use drugs. Peer pressure to use drugs can be a powerful factor for adolescents, although having a drug-using roommate does not increase the odds that a college student will use drugs.[28] The likelihood of drug abuse is also related to family instability, parental rejection, and divorce.

Parents' own attitudes and drug-use history affect their children's likelihood of using marijuana, according to the Substance Abuse and Mental Health Services Administration. Parents who perceive little risk associated with marijuana use have children with similar attitudes, and the children of parents who used marijuana are more likely to try the drug than children whose parents never used the drug. For help in staying away from drugs, see Your Strategies for Prevention: "How to Say No to Drugs."

Drugs and Driving

About one in three adult drivers ages 21 to 25 have driven under the influence of alcohol or drugs during the past year, according to the Substance Abuse and Mental Health Services Administration. Older drivers are less likely than younger drivers to drive while under the influence of alcohol or illicit drugs. Among those ages 26 to 34, 24 percent drove while under the influence of alcohol or illicit drugs in the past year, as did 19 percent of those ages 35 to 49.[29]

Different drugs affect driving ability in different ways. Here are the facts from the National Institute on Drug Abuse:

- **Alcohol affects perception, coordination, and judgment,** and increases the sedative effects of tranquilizers and barbiturates.

- **Marijuana affects a wide range of driving skills—** including the ability to track (stay in the lane) through curves, brake quickly, and maintain speed and a safe distance between cars—and slows thinking and reflexes. Normal driving skills remain

---

YOUR STRATEGIES FOR PREVENTION *How to Say No to Drugs*

If people offer you a drug, here are some ways to say no.

- Let them know you're not interested. Change the subject. If the pressure seems threatening, just walk away.

- Have something else to do: "No, I'm going for a walk now."

- Be prepared for different types of pressure. If your friends tease you, tease them back.

- Keep it simple. "No, thanks," "No," or "No way" all get the point across.

- Hang out with people who won't offer you drugs.

impaired for four to six hours after smoking a single joint.

- **Sedatives, sedative-hypnotics, and antianxiety agents slow reaction time** and interfere with hand–eye coordination and judgment; the greatest impairment is in the first hour after taking the drug. The effects depend on the particular drug: some build up in the body and can impair driving skills the morning after use; others make drivers very sleepy and therefore incapable of driving safely.

- **Amphetamines, after repeated use, impair coordination.** They can also make a driver more edgy and less coordinated and thus more likely to be involved in an accident.

- **Hallucinogens distort judgment** and reality and cause confusion and panic, thus making driving extremely dangerous.

Common Drugs of Abuse

Table 11.3 describes the common drugs of abuse within these categories: cannabis, "club drugs," stimulants, depressants, hallucinogens, and inhalants.

Cannabis

Marijuana (pot) and **hashish** (hash)—the most widely used illegal drugs—are derived from the cannabis plant. The major psychoactive ingredient in both is *THC (delta-9-tetrahydrocannabinol)*. Marijuana is the most widely abused substance, with more than 150 million people reporting they've used it at least once in the last year. Some 12 million Americans use cannabis; more than 1 million cannot control this use.

Teens and young adults who use marijuana are more likely to develop serious mental health problems. According to the National Survey on Drug Use and Health, among individuals age 18 years or older, those who first used marijuana before age 12 were twice as likely to have a serious mental illness as those who first used marijuana at age 18 or older.[30]

Researchers have documented an association between frequent marijuana use and increased anxiety and depression in young adults, regardless of whether they use other illicit drugs.[31] Marijuana also increases the risk for psychotic symptoms, with greater use leading to greater risk.[32]

 Marijuana use is generally less pervasive than binge drinking (see Chapter 12) on most campuses, although at some schools as many as a third of students report smoking pot. Students who used marijuana in high school are more likely to do so in college. Roommates have very little impact on drug use. Men who have not used marijuana before college seem, if anything, turned off rather than turned on by roommates who have smoked pot. Peers have no clear impact on women's marijuana use.

Different types of marijuana have different percentages of THC. Because of careful cultivation, the strength of today's marijuana is much greater than that used in the 1970s. Today a marijuana joint contains 150 mg of THC, compared to 10 mg in the 1960s. Usually, marijuana is smoked in a joint (hand-rolled cigarette) or pipe; it may also be eaten as an ingredient in other foods (as when baked in brownies), though with a less predictable effect.

Marijuana has shown some medical benefits, including boosting appetite in patients who are HIV-positive or undergoing chemotherapy, alleviating cancer and neck pain, reducing pressure on the eyeball in glaucoma patients, and helping people with spasticity (extreme muscle tension) due to multiple sclerosis or injuries.

A growing number of states have passed voter referenda (or legislative actions) making marijuana to smoke available for a variety of medical conditions upon a doctor's recommendation. However, the FDA, after a comprehensive investigation, concluded that "no sound scientific studies supported medical use of marijuana for treatment in the United States, and no animal or human data supported the safety or efficacy of marijuana for general

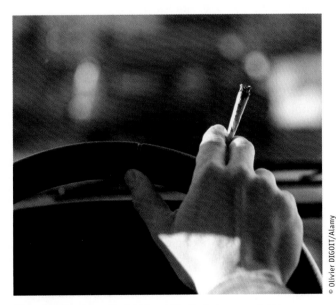

© Olivier DIGOIT/Alamy

All psychoactive drugs affect driving ability. For instance, marijuana decreases the ability to stay in the lane through curves and to brake quickly, and it slows thinking and reflexes.

marijuana   The drug derived from the cannabis plant, containing the psychoactive ingredient THC, which causes a mild sense of euphoria when inhaled or eaten.

hashish   A concentrated form of a drug, derived from the cannabis plant, containing the psychoactive ingredient TCH, which causes a sense of euphoria when inhaled or eaten.

TABLE 11.3 Commonly Abused Drugs

Drug	Street Names	How It's Used	Intoxication Effects/Potential Health Consequences
Cannabis			
Marijuana	Pot, grass, reefer, weed, blunt, dope, ganja, grass, herb, joints, Mary Jane, sinsemilla, skunk	Smoked, swallowed	Euphoria, slowed thinking and reaction time, confusion, impaired balance and coordination/Cough, frequent respiratory infections; impaired memory and learning; increased heart rate, anxiety; panic attacks; tolerance, addiction
Club Drugs			
MDMA	Ecstasy, E, Eve, X, XTC, clarity, lover's speed, peace, STP	Swallowed	Mild hallucinogenic effects, increased tactile sensitivity, empathic feelings/Impaired memory and learning, hyperthermia, cardiac toxicity, renal failure, liver toxicity
GHB	G, Georgia home boy, grievous bodily harm, liquid ecstasy	Swallowed	Reduced anxiety, feeling of well-being, lowered inhibitions, slowed pulse and breathing, lowered blood pressure, poor concentration/Fatigue; confusion; impaired coordination, memory, judgment; addiction, drowsiness, nausea/vomiting, headache, loss of consciousness, loss of reflexes, seizures, coma, death
Ketamine	Cat, Valiums, K, Special-K, vitamin K	Injected, snorted, smoked	Increased heart rate and blood pressure, impaired motor function/Memory loss; numbness; nausea/vomiting; at high doses, delirium, depression, respiratory depression, and arrest
Nitrites	Poppers	Inhaled	Stimulation, loss of inhibition; headache; nausea/vomiting; slurred speech; loss of motor coordination; wheezing/Unconsciousness, cramps, weight loss, muscle weakness, depression, memory impairment, damage to cardiovascular and nervous systems, sudden death
Stimulants			Increased heart rate, blood pressure, metabolism; feelings of exhilaration, energy, increased mental alertness/Rapid or irregular heart beat; reduced appetite, weight loss, heart failure, nervousness, insomnia
Amphetamine	Bennies, black beauties, crosses, hearts, LA turnaround, speed, truck drivers, uppers	Injected, swallowed, smoked, snorted	In addition to preceding: Rapid breathing/Tremor, loss of coordination; irritability, anxiousness, restlessness, delirium, panic, paranoia, impulsive behavior, aggressiveness, tolerance, addiction, psychosis
Methamphetamine	Chalk, crank, crystal, fire, glass, go fast, ice, meth, speed	Injected, swallowed, smoked, snorted	In addition to preceding: Aggression, violence, psychotic behavior/Memory loss, cardiac and neurological damage; impaired memory and learning, tolerance, addiction
Cocaine	Blow, bump, C, candy, Charlie, coke, crack, flake, rock, snow, toot	Injected, smoked, snorted	In addition to preceding: Increased temperature/Chest pain, respiratory failure, nausea, abdominal pain, strokes, seizures, headaches, malnutrition, panic attacks

continued

medical use." FDA-approved medications are available as treatment alternatives for many of the proposed uses of smoked marijuana, such as relief of nausea and vomiting induced by chemotherapy. Synthetic versions of the active ingredient in marijuana, developed for medical use, act on the brain like the THC in smoked marijuana but eliminate the need to inhale harmful smoke.

How Users Feel

The circumstances in which marijuana is smoked, the communal aspects of its use, and the user's experience all can affect the way a marijuana-induced high feels.

In low to moderate doses, marijuana typically creates a mild sense of euphoria, a sense of slowed time (five minutes may feel like an hour), a dreamy sort of self-absorption, and some impairment in thinking and communicating. Users report heightened sensations of color, sound, and other stimuli, relaxation, and increased confidence. The sense of being stoned peaks within half an hour and usually lasts about three hours. Even when alterations in perception seem slight, it is not safe to drive a car for as long as four to six hours after smoking a single joint.

Some users—particularly those smoking marijuana for the first time or taking a high dose in an unpleasant or unfamiliar setting—experience acute anxiety, which may be accompanied by a panicky fear of losing control. They may believe that their companions are ridiculing or threatening them and experience a panic attack, a state of intense terror.

TABLE 11.3 Commonly Abused Drugs, *Continued*

Drug	Street Names	How It's Used	Intoxication Effects/Potential Health Consequences
Depressants			Reduced anxiety; feeling of well-being; lowered inhibitions; slowed pulse and breathing; lowered blood pressure; poor concentration/Fatigue; confusion; impaired coordination, memory, judgment; addiction; respiratory depression and arrest, death
Benzodiazepines	Candy, downers, sleeping pills, tranks	Swallowed, injected	In addition to preceding: Sedation, drowsiness/Dizziness
Rohypnol	Forget-me pill, Mexican Valium, R2, Roche, roofies, roofinol, rope, rophies	Swallowed, snorted	Visual and gastrointestinal disturbances, urinary retention, memory loss for the time under the drug's effects
Barbiturates	Barbs, reds, red birds, phennies, tooies, yellows, yellow jackets	Injected, swallowed	In addition to preceding: Sedation, drowsiness/Depression, unusual excitement, fever, irritability, poor judgment, slurred speech, dizziness, life-threatening withdrawal
Opioids			Pain relief, euphoria, drowsiness/Nausea, constipation, confusion, sedation, respiratory depression and arrest, tolerance, addiction, unconsciousness, coma, death
Heroin	Brown sugar, dope, H, horse, junk, skag, skunk, smack, white horse	injected, smoked, snorted	
Morphine	Miss Emma, monkey, white stuff	Injected, swallowed, smoked	
Codeine	Captain Cody, Cody, schoolboy	Injected, swallowed	
OxyContin	Oxy, OC, Killer	Swallowed, snorted, injected	
Vicodin	Vike, Watson-387	Swallowed	
Hallucinogens			Altered states of perception and feeling/Nausea; persisting perception disorder (flashbacks)
LSD	Acid, blotter, boomers, cubes, microdot, yellow sunshines	Swallowed, absorbed through mouth tissues	In addition to preceding: Increased body temperature, heart-rate, blood pressure; loss of appetite, sleeplessness, numbness, weakness, tremors, persistent mental disorders
PCP	Angel dust, boat, hog, love boat, peace pill	Injected, swallowed, smoked	Impaired motor function, possible decrease in blood pressure and heart rate, panic, aggression, violence/Memory loss; numbness, nausea/vomiting, loss of appetite, depression
Inhalants			
Solvents (paint thinners, gasoline, glues) Gases (butane, propane, aerosol propellants, nitrous oxide)		Inhaled through nose or mouth	Stimulation, loss of inhibition; headache; nausea/vomiting; slurred speech, loss of motor coordination; wheezing/Unconsciousness, cramps, weight loss, muscle weakness, depression, memory impairment, damage to cardiovascular and nervous systems, sudden death

Source: National Institute on Drug Abuse, www.nida.nih.gov/DrugPages/DrugsofAbuse.html

The immediate physical effects of marijuana include increased pulse rate, bloodshot eyes, dry mouth and throat, slowed reaction times, impaired motor skills, increased appetite, and diminished short-term memory (Figure 11.4). High doses reduce the ability to perceive and to react; all the reactions experienced with low doses are intensified, leading to sensory distortion and, in the case of hashish, vivid hallucinations and LSD-like, psychedelic reactions. The drug remains in the body's fat cells 50 hours or more after use, so people may experience psychoactive effects for several days after use. Drug tests may produce positive results for days or weeks after last use.

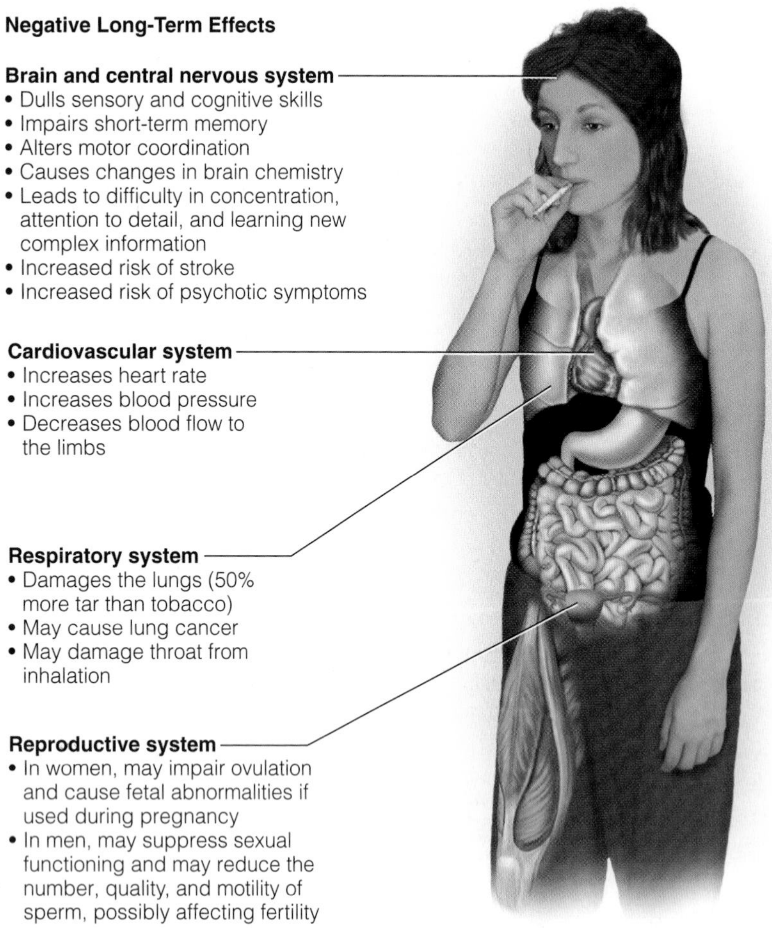

Negative Long-Term Effects

Brain and central nervous system
- Dulls sensory and cognitive skills
- Impairs short-term memory
- Alters motor coordination
- Causes changes in brain chemistry
- Leads to difficulty in concentration, attention to detail, and learning new complex information
- Increased risk of stroke
- Increased risk of psychotic symptoms

Cardiovascular system
- Increases heart rate
- Increases blood pressure
- Decreases blood flow to the limbs

Respiratory system
- Damages the lungs (50% more tar than tobacco)
- May cause lung cancer
- May damage throat from inhalation

Reproductive system
- In women, may impair ovulation and cause fetal abnormalities if used during pregnancy
- In men, may suppress sexual functioning and may reduce the number, quality, and motility of sperm, possibly affecting fertility

Figure 11.4 Impact of Marijuana
Marijuana has negative long-term effects on many systems of the body.

Risks

Marijuana produces a range of effects in different bodily systems, such as depression, diminished immune responses, and impaired fertility in men. Other risks include damage to the brain, lungs, and heart and to babies born to mothers who use marijuana during pregnancy or while nursing (see Figure 11.4).

Brain THC produces changes in the brain that affect learning, memory, and the way the brain integrates sensory experiences with emotions and motivations. Short-term effects include problems with memory and learning; distorted perceptions; difficulty thinking and problem solving; loss of coordination; increased anxiety; and panic attacks. Long-term use produces changes in the brain similar to those seen with other major drugs of abuse. Long-term heavy users of marijuana perform significantly worse on tests of verbal fluency, memory, and coordination than short-term users or nonusers, even after abstaining from pot for more than 24 hours.[33]

Over time, continued heavy marijuana use can interfere with students' ability to learn and perform well in school and in challenging careers. Marijuana contributes significantly to accidental death and injury among adolescents, especially through motor vehicle crashes.

Lungs Smoking cannabis may cause similar effects to smoking tobacco, with many of them appearing at a younger age. They include chronic bronchitis, emphysema, and other lung disorders and increased risk of heart attacks and sudden death. The amount of tar inhaled by marijuana smokers and the level of carbon monoxide absorbed are three to five times greater than among tobacco smokers. The reasons may be that marijuana users inhale more deeply, hold the smoke in the lungs longer, and do not use filters. Smoking a single joint can be as damaging to the lungs as smoking five tobacco cigarettes. Someone who smokes five joints a week may take in as many cancer-causing chemicals as a person who smokes a pack of cigarettes a day.

Heart Otherwise healthy people have suffered heart attacks shortly after smoking marijuana. Experiments have also linked marijuana use to elevated blood pressure and decreased oxygen supply to the heart muscle. The risk of heart attack triples within an hour of smoking pot. Smoking marijuana while shooting cocaine can potentially cause deadly increases in heart rate and blood pressure.

Pregnancy   Babies born to mothers who use marijuana during pregnancy are smaller than those born to mothers who did not use the drug, and the babies are more likely to develop health problems. A nursing mother who uses marijuana passes some of the THC to the baby in her breast milk. This may impair the infant's motor development (control of muscle movement).

Withdrawal

Marijuana users can develop a compulsive, often uncontrollable craving for the drug. More than 120,000 people enter treatment every year for marijuana addiction. In addition, animal studies suggest that marijuana causes physical dependence. Stopping after long-term marijuana use can produce *marijuana withdrawal syndrome,* which is characterized by insomnia, restlessness, loss of appetite, and irritability. People who smoke marijuana daily for many years may become aggressive after they stop using it and may relapse to prevent aggression and other symptoms.

Club Drugs (Designer Drugs)

The National Institute on Drug Abuse identifies a variety of drugs—alcohol, LSD (acid), MDMA (Ecstasy), GHB, GBL, ketamine (Special-K), fentanyl, Rohypnol, and nitrites—as **"club drugs."** They first became popular among teens and young adults at nightclubs, bars, or raves and trances—night-long dances often held in warehouses or other unusual settings. Their use by teenagers has been dropping in recent years.

Young people may take club drugs to relax, energize, and enhance their social interactions, but a large number

also experience negative consequences. As many as three in four report side effects such as profuse sweating, hot and cold flashes, tingling or numbness, blurred vision, trouble sleeping, hallucinations, depression, confusion, anxiety, irritability, paranoia, and loss of libido (sex drive). Some also experience difficulty with their usual daily activities and financial and work troubles.

Ecstasy

Ecstasy (E, XTC, X, hug, beans, love drug) is the most common street name for methylenedioxymethamphetamine (MDMA), a synthetic compound with both stimulant and mildly hallucinogenic properties.

 According to various studies, students who take Ecstasy were more likely to use marijuana, binge-drink, smoke cigarettes, have multiple sexual partners, spend more time socializing with friends and less time studying, and consider parties important and religion as less important. However, researchers who compared students who used Ecstasy and other illicit drugs with those who used only marijuana have concluded that undergraduates who use Ecstasy may be a subgroup of marijuana users who tend to engage in many risk-taking behaviors. Ecstasy users also think that their peers smoke more marijuana and use more Ecstasy than they actually do.

How Users Feel   Although it can be smoked, inhaled (snorted), or injected, Ecstasy is almost always taken as a pill or tablet. Its effects begin in 45 minutes and last for two to four hours.

MDMA belongs to a family of drugs called *enactogens,* which literally means "touching within." As a mood elevator, it produces a relaxed, euphoric state but does not produce hallucinations. Users of Ecstasy often say they feel at peace with themselves and a sense of connectedness with others. In some settings, they reveal intimate details of their lives (which they may later regret); in other settings, they join in collective rejoicing. Like hallucinogenic drugs, MDMA can enhance sensory experience, but it rarely causes visual distortions, sudden mood changes, or psychotic reactions. Regular users may experience depression and anxiety the week after taking MDMA.

Risks   Ecstasy poses risks similar to those of cocaine and amphetamines. These include psychological difficulties (confusion, depression, sleep problems, drug craving, severe anxiety, and paranoia) and physical symptoms (muscle tension, involuntary teeth clenching, nausea, blurred vision, rapid eye movement, faintness, chills,

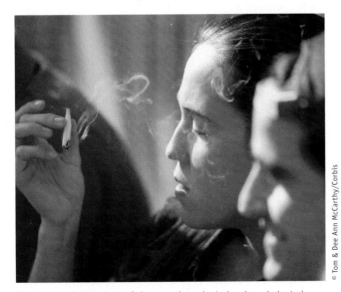

Marijuana and other drugs of abuse produce physical and psychological effects that can have a long-term impact on health.

© Tom & Dee Ann McCarthy/Corbis

club drugs   Illegally manufactured psychoactive drugs that have dangerous physical and psychological effects.

Ecstasy (MDMA)   A synthetic compound, also known as methylenedioxymethamphetamine, that is similar in structure to methamphetamine and has both stimulant and hallucinogenic effects.

sweating, and increases in heart rate and blood pressure that pose a special risk for people with circulatory or heart disease).

Ecstasy can produce nausea, vomiting, and dizziness. When combined with extended physical exertion like dancing, club drugs can lead to hyperthermia (severe overheating), severe dehydration, serious increases in blood pressure, stroke, and heart attack. Without sufficient water, dancers at raves may suffer dehydration and heat stroke, which can be fatal. Individuals with high blood pressure, heart trouble, or liver or kidney disease are in the greatest danger. Several deaths have occurred in teens who suffered brain damage by drinking large amounts of water to counteract the raised body temperature induced by the drug.

MDMA has been implicated in some cases of acute hepatitis, which can lead to liver failure. Even after liver transplantation, the mortality rate for individuals with this condition is 50 percent. Another danger comes from the practice of taking SSRIs (see Chapter 4), which modulate the mood-altering brain chemical serotonin, before Ecstasy. This can cause jaw clenching, nausea, tremors, and in extreme cases, potentially fatal elevations in body temperature.

Although not a sexual stimulant (if anything, MDMA has the opposite effect), Ecstasy fosters strong feelings of intimacy that may lead to risky sexual behavior. The psychological effects of Ecstasy become less intriguing with repeated use, and the physical side effects become more uncomfortable. Ecstasy poses risks to a developing fetus, including a greater likelihood of heart and skeletal abnormalities and long-term learning and memory impairments in children born to women who used MDMA during pregnancy.

Because Ecstasy is *neurotoxic* (damaging to brain cells), it depletes the brain of serotonin, a messenger chemical involved with mood, sleep, and appetite, and can lead to depression, anxiety, and impaired thinking and memory. Even short-term use of Ecstasy can have long-term neurological consequences that may affect memory and the brain's ability to perform complex thought processes.

According to brain-imaging studies, users, although as mentally alert as nonusers, fared far worse on measures of memory, learning, and general intelligence. The more frequently they took Ecstasy, the worse they did, probably because Ecstasy alters neuronal function in a brain structure called the hippocampus, which helps create short-term memory. The effect on memory persists for years after discontinuing use.

GHB and GBL

Once sold in health food stores for its muscle-building and alleged fat-burning properties, **gammahydroxybutyrate (GHB,** G, Georgia home boy) was banned because of its effects on the brain and nervous system. The main ingredient is **GBL (gamma butyrolactone),** an industrial solvent often used to strip floors, which converts into GHB once ingested. GHB acts as a sedative while producing feelings of euphoria and heightened sexuality. Because of its amnesic properties, GHB has been used as a "date rape" drug, similar to Rohypnol. Alcohol intensifies its effects.

Large doses can cause someone to pass out in 15 minutes and fall into a coma within half an hour. Other side effects include nausea, amnesia, hallucinations, decreased heart rate, convulsions, and sometimes blackouts. Longterm use at high doses can lead to a withdrawal reaction: rapid heartbeat, tremor, insomnia, anxiety, and occasionally hallucinations that last a few days to a week.

GHB is addictive. Users who attempt to quit may experience significant withdrawal symptoms, including anxiety, tremors, and insomnia. Most symptoms decrease within one to two weeks of cessation, but severe psychological effects can last for weeks to months.

Ketamine

Ketamine—called K, Special-K, and Vitamin K—is an anesthetic used by veterinarians. When cooked, dried, and ground into powder for snorting, ketamine blocks chemical messengers in the brain that carry sensory input. As a result, the brain fills the void with hallucinations. Users may report an "out-of-body" experience with distorted perceptions of time and space. The effects typically begin within 30 minutes and last for approximately two hours.

Ketamine has become common in club and rave scenes and has been used as a date rape drug. It can cause anxiety, agitation, paranoia, and vomiting. Higher doses can cause lethal breathing impairments, stroke, and heart attack. Repeated ketamine use can be addictive and even a single use can occasionally produce audiovisual "flashbacks," similar to those described by phencyclidine (PCP) users, and long-term memory loss.

Nitrites

Nitrites (amyl, butyl, and isobutyl nitrite) are clear, amber-colored liquids that have had a history of abuse for more than three decades, especially in gay and bisexual men. Popular in dance clubs, they are used recreationally for a high feeling, a slowed sense of time, a carefree sense of well-being, and intensified sexual experiences.

Sold in small glass ampules containing individual doses, nitrites are usually inhaled and rapidly absorbed into the bloodstream. Users feel their physiological and psychological impact in seconds. Acute adverse effects include headache, dizziness, a drop in blood pressure, changes in heart rate, increased pressure within the eye, and skin flushing. Some individuals develop respiratory irritation and cough, sneezing, or difficulty breathing. Chronic use can lead to crusty skin lesions and chemical burns around the nose, mouth, and lips.

Herbal Ecstasy

Herbal ecstasy, also known as herbal bliss, cloud 9, and herbal X, is a mixture of stimulants such as ephedrine, pseudoephedrine, and caffeine. Sold in tablet or capsule form as a "natural" and safe alternative to Ecstasy, its ingredients vary greatly. Herbal ecstasy can have dangerous and unpleasant side effects, including stroke, heart attack, and a disfiguring skin condition.

Stimulants

Central nervous system **stimulants** are drugs that increase activity in some portion of the brain or spinal cord. Some stimulants increase motor activity and enhance mental alertness, and some combat mental fatigue. Amphetamine, methamphetamine, caffeine, cocaine, and khat are stimulants. Stimulant medications are used to treat conditions such as ADHD.

Amphetamine

Amphetamines trigger the release of epinephrine (adrenaline), which stimulates the central nervous system. They were once widely prescribed for weight control because they suppress appetite, but they have emerged as a global danger. Amphetamines are sold under a variety of names: amphetamine (brand name Benzedrine, streetname bennies), dextroamphetamine (Dexedrine, dex), methamphetamine (Methedrine, meth, speed, crank), and Desoxyn (copilots). Related *uppers* include the prescription drugs methylphenidate (Ritalin), pemoline (Cylert), and phenmetrazine (Preludin). Amphetamines are available in tablet or capsule form.

How Users Feel Amphetamines produce a state of hyper-alertness and energy. Users feel confident in their ability to think clearly and to perform any task exceptionally well—although amphetamines do not, in fact, significantly boost performance or thinking. Higher doses make users feel *wired:* talkative, excited, restless, irritable, anxious, moody.

If taken intravenously, amphetamines produce a characteristic rush of elation and confidence, as well as adverse effects, including confusion, rambling or incoherent speech, anxiety, headache, and palpitations. Individuals may become paranoid; be convinced they are having profound thoughts; feel increased sexual interest; and experience unusual perceptions, such as ringing in the ears, a sensation of insects crawling on their skin, or hearing their name called. Methamphetamine users may feel high and sleepy or may hallucinate and lose contact with reality.

Risks Dependence on amphetamines can develop with episodic or daily use. Bingeing—taking high doses over a period of several days—can lead to an extremely intense and unpleasant *crash,* characterized by a craving

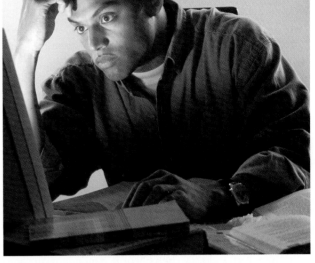

Some college students try stimulants to stay alert while cramming for exams, but these medications do not improve academic performance and cause harmful side effects.

for the drug, shakiness, irritability, anxiety, and depression. Two or more days are required for recuperation.

Amphetamine intoxication may cause the following symptoms:

- **Feelings of grandiosity,** anxiety, tension, hypervigilance, anger, social hypersensitivity, fighting, jitteriness or agitation, paranoia, and impaired judgment in social or occupational functioning.

- **Increased heart rate,** dilated pupils, elevated blood pressure, perspiration or chills, and nausea or vomiting.

- **Less frequent effects such as speeding up** or slowing down of physical movement; muscular weakness; impaired breathing, chest pain, heart arrhythmia; confusion, seizures, impaired movements or muscle tone; or even coma.

GHB (gamma hydroxybutyrate) A brain messenger chemical that stimulates the release of human growth hormone; commonly abused for its high and its alleged ability to trim fat and build muscles. Also known as "blue nitro" or the "date rape drug."

GBL (gamma butyrolactone) The main ingredient in gamma hydroxybutyrate (GHB), also known as the "date rape drug"; once ingested, GBL converts to GHB and can cause the ingestor to lose consciousness.

stimulant An agent, such as a drug, that temporarily relieves drowsiness, helps in the performance of repetitive tasks, and improves capacity for work.

amphetamine Any of a class of stimulants that trigger the release of epinephrine, which stimulates the central nervous system; users experience a state of hyper-alertness and energy, followed by a crash as the drug wears off.

- **In high doses, a rapid or irregular heartbeat,** tremors, loss of coordination, and collapse.

The long-term effects of amphetamine abuse include malnutrition, skin disorders, ulcers, insomnia, depression, vitamin deficiencies, and in some cases, brain damage that results in speech and thought disturbances. Sexual dysfunction and impaired concentration or memory also may occur.

Withdrawal

Withdrawal When the immediate effects of amphetamines wear off, users experience a *crash* and become shaky, irritable, anxious, and depressed. Amphetamine withdrawal usually persists for more than 24 hours after cessation of prolonged, heavy use. Its characteristic features include fatigue, disturbing dreams, much more or less than usual sleep, increased appetite, and speeding up or slowing down of physical movements. Those who are unable to sleep despite their exhaustion often take sedative-hypnotics (discussed later in this chapter) to help them rest and may then become dependent on them in addition to amphetamines. Symptoms usually reach a peak in two to four days, although depression and irritability may persist for months. Suicide is a major risk.

Methamphetamine

Methamphetamine, an addictive stimulant that is less expensive and possibly more addictive than cocaine or heroin, has become America's leading drug problem. More than 12 million Americans have tried methamphetamine, and 1.5 million are regular users, according to federal estimates.

Methamphetamine is chemically related to amphetamine, but its effects on the central nervous system are greater. Made in illegal laboratories, street methamphetamine is referred to by many names, such as speed, meth, and chalk. Methamphetamine hydrochloride, clear chunky crystals resembling ice that can be inhaled by smoking, is called ice, crystal, glass, and tina. Methamphetamine can be snorted, smoked, or injected.

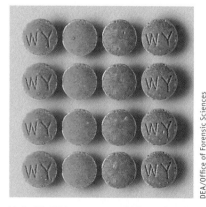

DEA/Office of Forensic Sciences

Ya-ba/Thai Tabs are a powerful form of methamphetamine that tastes sweet like candy.

How Users Feel Methamphetamine causes the release of large amounts of dopamine, which creates a sensation of euphoria, increased self-esteem, and alertness. Users also report a marked increase in sexual appetite, which often leads to risky sexual behaviors while under the drug's influence.

Smoking or intravenous injection leads to an intense, pleasurable sensation, called a rush or flash, that lasts only a few minutes. Oral or intranasal use produces a high but not a rush. Users may become addicted quickly, using more methamphetamine more and more frequently. Despair and suicidal thinking can develop when the stimulant effect wears off.

Risks Even small amounts of methamphetamine can increase wakefulness and physical activity, depress appetite, and raise body temperature. Other effects on the central nervous system include irritability, insomnia, confusion, tremors, convulsions, anxiety, paranoia, and aggressiveness.

Methamphetamine increases heart rate and blood pressure and can cause irreversible damage to blood vessels in the brain, producing strokes. Other effects of methamphetamine include respiratory problems, irregular heartbeat, and extreme loss of appetite and weight. During intoxication, the body (and probably brain) temperature rises, sometimes resulting in convulsions. High fevers or collapse of the circulatory system can cause death.

Common psychiatric symptoms are insomnia, irritability, and aggressive behavior. The drug causes intellectual impairment, anxiety, and depression. Chronic users become disorganized and unable to cope with everyday problems. The risk of developing psychotic symptoms—hallucinations and delusions—is very high. They may persist for months or years after use stops.[34]

Another side effect is called meth mouth. In short periods of time, sometimes just months, teeth can turn a grayish-brown, twist, begin to fall out, and take on a peculiar texture. This may be the result of methamphetamine's effects on the metabolic system, plus the huge quantities of sugary soft drinks that users consume for the dry mouth caused by the drug.[35]

Meth users engage in more sex, more carelessly. Meth has become popular among gay and bisexual men, and it has been linked to an increase in unsafe sex practices. Methamphetamine use and needle sharing has been linked to a spike in HIV and hepatitis C infections in gay communities.

Methamphetamine causes abnormalities in brain regions associated with selective attention and in those associated with memory. The brain may recover somewhat after months of abstinence, but problems often remain. Former methamphetamine addicts may suffer from chronic apathy and anhedonia (inability to experience pleasure) for years.

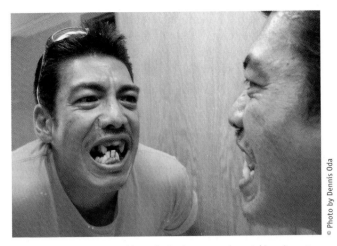

© Photo by Dennis Oda

In addition to respiratory problems, brain damage, and mental impairment, methamphetamine damages teeth. This is how "meth mouth" looks.

The Toll on Society   Law enforcement officials consider methamphetamine their biggest drug problem. Meth-related arrests have soared. Meth addicts are pouring into prisons and recovery centers at an ever-increasing rate. "Meth babies" are crowding the foster-care system. Meth-making operations have been uncovered in all 50 states, with the greatest number in Missouri. Production releases poisonous gases and results in toxic waste that is often dumped down household drains, in a backyard, or at a roadside. The cost of cleaning up the environment is a growing problem for many communities.

Over-the-counter cold medicines (ephedrine and pseudoephedrine) are commonly used in meth production, which is one reason for federal and state restrictions on their sale. As drug stores and retailers have placed nonprescription cold pills behind the pharmacy counter, meth manufacturing has moved into Mexico, where labs produce hundreds of pounds of meth a year and smuggle it into the United States.

Withdrawal   Methamphetamine addiction is difficult to treat. As with cocaine, coming off methamphetamine causes intense distress, so users often seek out the drug to relieve their pain. Treatment usually requires the intervention of the patient's family as well as a substance abuse specialist team experienced in treating methamphetamine addiction. Standard substance abuse treatment methods such as education, behavior therapy, individual and family counseling, and support groups may be effective for some. Methamphetamine abusers often use other illicit drugs as well, a problem that can be addressed as part of a comprehensive program.

Cocaine

Cocaine (coke, snow, lady) is a white crystalline powder extracted from the leaves of the South American coca plant. Usually mixed with various sugars and local anesthetics like lidocaine and procaine, cocaine powder is generally inhaled. When sniffed or snorted, cocaine anesthetizes the nerve endings in the nose and relaxes the lung's bronchial muscles.

Cocaine can be dissolved in water and injected intravenously. The drug is rapidly metabolized by the liver, so the high is relatively brief, typically lasting only about 20 minutes. This means that users will commonly inject the drug repeatedly, increasing the risk of infection and damage to their veins.

Cocaine alkaloid, or *freebase*, is obtained by removing the hydrochloride salt from cocaine powder. *Freebasing* is smoking the fumes of the alkaloid form of cocaine. *Crack*, pharmacologically identical to freebase, is a cheap, easy-to-use, widely available, smokeable, and potent form of cocaine named for the popping sound it makes when burned. Because it is absorbed rapidly into the bloodstream and large doses reach the brain very quickly, it is particularly dangerous. However, its low price and easy availability have made it a common drug of abuse in poor urban areas.

How Users Feel   A powerful stimulant to the central nervous system, cocaine targets several chemical sites in the brain, producing feelings of soaring well-being and boundless energy. Users feel they have enormous physical and mental ability, yet are also restless and anxious. After a brief period of euphoria, users slump into a depression. They often go on cocaine binges, lasting from a few hours to several days, and consume large quantities of cocaine.

With crack, dependence develops quickly. As soon as crack users come down from one high, they want more crack. Whereas heroin addicts may shoot up several times a day, crack addicts need another hit within minutes. Thus, a crack habit can quickly become more expensive than heroin addiction.

Risks   Cocaine dependence is an easy habit to acquire. With repeated use, the brain becomes tolerant of the drug's stimulant effects, and users must take more of it to get high. Those who smoke or inject cocaine can develop dependence within weeks. Those who sniff cocaine may not become dependent on the drug for months or years. It is thought that 5 to 20 percent of all coke users—a group as large as the estimated total number of heroin addicts—are dependent on the drug.

The physical effects of acute cocaine intoxication include dilated pupils, elevated or lowered blood pressure, perspiration or chills, nausea or vomiting, speeding up or slowing down of physical activity, muscular weakness, impaired breathing, chest pain, and impaired movements or muscle tone. Prolonged cocaine snorting can result

cocaine A white crystalline powder extracted from the leaves of the coca plant that stimulates the central nervous system and produces a brief period of euphoria followed by a depression.

in ulceration of the mucous membrane of the nose and damage to the nasal septum (the membrane between the nostrils) severe enough to cause it to collapse.

Although some users initially try cocaine as a sexual stimulant, it does not enhance sexual performance. At low doses, it may delay orgasm and cause heightened sensory awareness, but men who use cocaine regularly have problems maintaining erections and ejaculating. They also tend to have low sperm counts, less active sperm, and more abnormal sperm than nonusers. Both male and female chronic cocaine users tend to lose interest in sex and have difficulty reaching orgasm.

Cocaine use can cause blood vessels in the brain to clamp shut and can trigger a stroke, bleeding in the brain, and potentially fatal brain seizures. Cocaine users can also develop psychiatric or neurological complications (Figure 11.5). Repeated or high doses of cocaine can lead to impaired judgment, hyperactivity, nonstop babbling, feelings of suspicion and paranoia, and violent behavior. The brain never learns to tolerate cocaine's negative effects; users may become incoherent and paranoid and may experience unusual sensations, such as ringing in their ears, feeling insects crawling on the skin, or hearing their name called.

Cocaine can damage the liver and cause lung damage in freebasers. Smoking crack causes bronchitis as well as lung damage and may promote the transmission of HIV through burned and bleeding lips. Some smokers have died of respiratory complications, such as pulmonary edema (the buildup of fluid in the lungs).

Cocaine causes the heart rate to speed up and blood pressure to rise suddenly. Its use is associated with many cardiac complications, including arrhythmia (disruption of heart rhythm), angina (chest pain), and acute myocardial infarction (heart attack).

The combination of alcohol and cocaine is particularly lethal. The liver combines the two agents and manufactures cocaethylene, which intensifies cocaine's euphoric effects, while possibly increasing the risk of sudden death. Cocaine users who inject the drug and share needles put themselves at risk for another potentially lethal problem: HIV infection.

Cocaine is dangerous for pregnant women and their babies, causing miscarriages, developmental disorders, and life-threatening complications during birth. Cocaine can reduce the fetal oxygen supply, possibly interfering with the development of the fetus's nervous system.

Withdrawal When addicted individuals stop using cocaine, they often become depressed. This may lead to further cocaine use to alleviate depression. Other symptoms of cocaine withdrawal include fatigue, vivid and disturbing dreams, excessive or too little sleep, irritability, increased appetite, and physical slowing down or speeding up. This initial crash may last one to three days

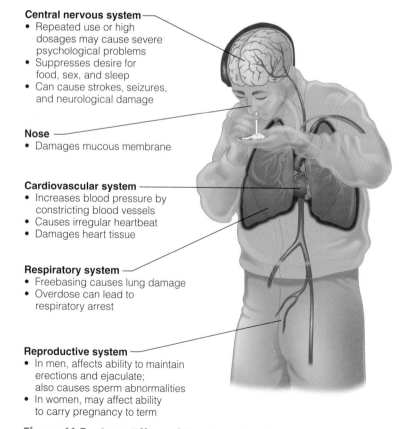

Central nervous system
• Repeated use or high dosages may cause severe psychological problems
• Suppresses desire for food, sex, and sleep
• Can cause strokes, seizures, and neurological damage

Nose
• Damages mucous membrane

Cardiovascular system
• Increases blood pressure by constricting blood vessels
• Causes irregular heartbeat
• Damages heart tissue

Respiratory system
• Freebasing causes lung damage
• Overdose can lead to respiratory arrest

Reproductive system
• In men, affects ability to maintain erections and ejaculate; also causes sperm abnormalities
• In women, may affect ability to carry pregnancy to term

Figure 11.5 Some Effects of Cocaine on the Body

after cutting down or stopping the heavy use of cocaine. Some individuals become violent, paranoid, and suicidal.

Symptoms usually reach a peak in two to four days, although depression, anxiety, irritability, lack of pleasure in usual activities, and low-level cravings may continue for weeks. As memories of the crash fade, the desire for cocaine intensifies. For many weeks after stopping, individuals may feel an intense craving for the drug.

Despite years of research, there is no drug approved in the United States for treating cocaine dependence. Some cocaine abusers fare better with cognitive-behavioral therapy (discussed in Chapter 4); others, with 12-step programs.

Khat (Kat, Catha, Chat, Abyssinian Tea)

For centuries people in East Africa and the Arabian peninsula consumed the fresh young leaves of the *Catha edulis* shrub in ways similar to our drinking coffee. Its active ingredients are two controlled substances, cathinone and cathine. Chewing alleviates fatigue and reduces appetite. Compulsive use may result in manic behavior, grandiose illusions, paranoia, and hallucinations.

Depressants

Depressants depress the central nervous system, reduce activity, and induce relaxation, drowsiness, or sleep. They include the benzodiazepines and the barbiturates, the opioids, and alcohol.

Benzodiazepines and Barbiturates

These depressants are the sedative-hypnotics, also known as anxiolytic or antianxiety drugs. The **benzodiazepines**—the most widely used drugs in this category—are commonly prescribed for tension, muscular strain, sleep problems, anxiety, panic attacks, anesthesia, and in the treatment of alcohol withdrawal. They include such drugs as *chlordiazepoxide* (Librium), *diazepam* (Valium), *oxazepam* (Serax), *lorazepam* (Ativan), *flurazepam* (Dalmane), and *alprazolam* (Xanax). They differ widely in their mechanism of action, absorption rate, and metabolism, but all produce similar intoxication and withdrawal symptoms.

Rohypnol, a trade name for flunitrazepam, is one of the benzodiazepines that has been of particular concern for the last few years because of its abuse in date rape. When mixed with alcohol, Rohypnol can incapacitate victims and prevent them from resisting sexual assault. It produces "anterograde amnesia," which means individuals may not remember events they experienced while under the effects of the drug. Rohypnol may be lethal when mixed with alcohol or other depressants.

Benzodiazepine sleeping pills have largely replaced the **barbiturates,** which were used medically in the past for inducing relaxation and sleep, relieving tension, and treating epileptic seizures. These drugs are usually taken

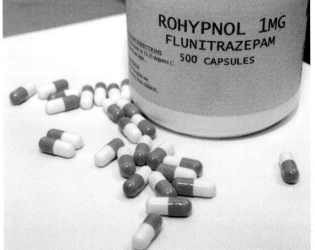

Because Rohypnol is colorless, tasteless, and odorless, it can be added to beverages without your knowledge.

by mouth in tablet, capsule, or liquid form. When used as a general anesthetic, they are administered intravenously.

How Users Feel   Low doses of these drugs may reduce or relieve tension, but increasing doses can cause a loosening of sexual or aggressive inhibitions. Individuals using this class of drugs may experience rapid mood changes, impaired judgment, and impaired social or occupational functioning.

Risks   All sedative-hypnotic drugs can produce physical and psychological dependence within two to four weeks. A complication specific to sedatives is *cross-tolerance* (cross-addiction), which occurs when users develop tolerance for one sedative or become dependent on it and develop tolerance for other sedatives as well.

Intoxication with these drugs can produce changes in mood or behavior, such as inappropriate sexual or aggressive acts, mood swings, and impaired judgment. Physical signs include slurred speech, poor coordination, unsteady gait, involuntary eye movements, impaired attention or memory, and stupor or coma.

Taken in combination with alcohol, these drugs have a synergistic effect that can be dangerous or even lethal. For example, an individual's driving ability, already impaired by alcohol, will be made even worse, increasing the risk of an accident. Alcohol in combination with sedative-hypnotics

---

benzodiazepines Antianxiety drugs that depress the central nervous system, reduce activity, and induce relaxation, drowsiness, or sleep; often prescribed to relieve tension, muscular strain, sleep problems, anxiety, and panic attacks; also used as an anesthetic and in the treatment of alcohol withdrawal.

barbiturates Antianxiety drugs that depress the central nervous system, reduce activity, and induce relaxation, drowsiness, or sleep; often prescribed to relieve tension and treat epileptic seizures or as a general anesthetic.

leads to respiratory depression and may result in respiratory arrest and death. Regular users of any of these drugs who become physically dependent should not try to cut down or quit on their own. If they try to quit suddenly, they run the risk of seizures, coma, and death.

Withdrawal   Withdrawal from sedative-hypnotic drugs may range from relatively mild discomfort to a severe syndrome with grand mal seizures, depending on the degree of dependence. Withdrawal symptoms include malaise or weakness, sweating, rapid pulse, coarse tremors (of the hands, tongue, or eyelids), insomnia, nausea or vomiting, temporary hallucinations or illusions, physical restlessness, anxiety or irritability, and grand mal seizures. Withdrawal may begin within two to three days after stopping drug use, and symptoms may persist for many weeks.

Opioids

The **opioids** include *opium* and its derivatives (*morphine, codeine,* and *heroin*) and synthetic drugs that have similar sleep-inducing and pain-relieving properties. The opioids come from a resin taken from the seedpod of the Asian poppy. Synthetic opioids, such as *meperidine* (Demerol), *methadone,* and *propoxyphene* (Darvon), are synthesized in a chemical laboratory. Whether natural or synthetic, these drugs are powerful *narcotics,* or painkillers.

Heroin (also known as horse, junk, smack, or downtown), the most widely abused opioid, is illegal in this country. In other nations it is used as a potent painkiller for conditions such as terminal cancer. There are an estimated 600,000 heroin addicts in the United States, with men outnumbering women addicts by three to one. Among people aged 18 to 25, the percentage of heroin users who inject the drug has doubled in the last decade. While the number of young heroin users in major cities has dropped by 50 percent, their numbers almost tripled in suburban and rural areas.

Heroin users typically inject the drug into their veins. However, individuals who experiment with recreational

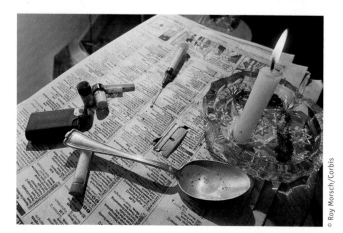

Opioid drugs, made from the Asian poppy, come in both legal and illegal forms. All are highly addictive.

drugs often prefer *skin-popping* (subcutaneous injection) rather than *mainlining* (intravenous injection); they also may snort heroin as a powder or dissolve it and inhale the vapors. To try to avoid addiction, some users begin by *chipping,* taking small or intermittent doses. Regardless of the method of administration, tolerance can develop rapidly.

Morphine, used as a painkiller and anesthetic, acts primarily on the central nervous system, eyes, and digestive tract. By producing mental clouding, drowsiness, and euphoria, it does not decrease the physical sensation of pain as much as it alters a person's awareness of the pain; in effect, he or she no longer cares about it.

Prescription Opioids

Two semisynthetic derivatives of morphine are *hydromorphone* (trade name Dilaudid, street name little D), with two to eight times the painkilling effect of morphine, and *oxycodone* (OxyContin, Percocet, Percodan, perkies), similar to codeine but more potent. The synthetic narcotic *meperidine* (Demerol, demies) is now probably second only to morphine for use in relieving pain. It is also used by addicts as a substitute for morphine or heroin.

Codeine, a weaker painkiller than morphine, is an ingredient in liquid products prescribed for relieving coughs and in tablet and injectable form for relieving pain. The synthetic narcotic *propoxyphene* (Darvon), a somewhat less potent painkiller than codeine, is no more effective than aspirin in usual doses. It has been one of the most widely prescribed drugs for headaches, dental pain, and menstrual cramps. At higher doses, Darvon produces a euphoric high, which may lead to misuse.

Like other addictions, a prescription drug "habit" is a treatable brain disease. Recovery usually requires carefully supervised detoxification, appropriate medications (similar to those used for opioid dependence), behavioral therapy, and ongoing support.

How Users Feel   All opioids relax the user. When injected, they can produce an immediate *rush* (high) that lasts 10 to 30 minutes. For two to six hours thereafter, users may feel indifferent, lethargic, and drowsy; they may slur their words and have problems paying attention, remembering, and going about their normal routine. The primary attractions of heroin are the euphoria and pain relief it produces. However, some people experience very unpleasant feelings, such as anxiety and fear. Other effects include a sensation of warmth or heaviness, dry mouth, facial flushing, and nausea and vomiting (particularly in first-time users).

Risks   Addiction is common. Almost all regular users of opioids rapidly develop drug dependence, which can lead to lethargy, weight loss, loss of sex drive, and the continual effort to avoid withdrawal symptoms through repeated drug administration. In addition, they experience anxiety, insomnia, restlessness, and craving for the drug. Users continue taking opioids as much to avoid the discomfort of withdrawal, a classic sign of opioid addiction, as to experience pleasure.

Physical symptoms include constricted pupils (although pupils may dilate from a severe overdose), drowsiness, slurred speech, and impaired attention or memory. Morphine affects blood pressure, heart rate, and blood circulation in the brain. Both morphine and heroin slow down the respiratory system; overdoses can cause fatal respiratory arrest.

Over time, users who inject opioids may develop infections of the heart lining and valves, skin abscesses, and lung congestion. Infections from unsterile solutions, syringes, and shared needles can lead to hepatitis, tetanus, liver disease, and HIV. Depression is common and may be both an antecedent and a risk factor for needle sharing.

Opioid abuse during pregnancy can cause miscarriage, stillbirth, or low birth weight. Babies born to addicted mothers experience withdrawal symptoms after birth.

Withdrawal   If a regular user stops taking an opioid, withdrawal begins within 6 to 12 hours. The intensity of the symptoms depends on the degree of the addiction; they may grow stronger for 24 to 72 hours and gradually subside over a period of 7 to 14 days, though some symptoms, such as insomnia, may persist for several months. Individuals may develop craving for an opioid, irritability, nausea or vomiting, muscle aches, runny nose or eyes, dilated pupils, sweating, diarrhea, yawning, fever, and insomnia. Opioid withdrawal usually is not life-threatening.

Hallucinogens

The drugs known as **hallucinogens** produce vivid and unusual changes in thought, feeling, and perception. Hallucinogens do not produce dependence in the same way as cocaine or heroin. Individuals who have an unpleasant experience after trying a hallucinogen may stop using the drug completely without suffering withdrawal symptoms. Others continue regular or occasional use because they enjoy the effects.

LSD and Mescaline
LSD (*lysergic acid diethylamide*, acid) was initially developed as a tool to explore mental illness. It became popular in the 1960s and resurfaced among teenagers in the 1990s. LSD is taken orally, either blotted onto pieces of paper that are held in the mouth or chewed along with another substance, such as a sugar cube. Peyote (whose active ingredient is *mescaline*) is another hallucinogen, but it is much less commonly used in this country.

Phencyclidine (PCP)
PCP (**phencyclidine,** brand name Sernyl; street names angel dust, peace pill, lovely, and green) is an illicit drug manufactured as a tablet, capsule, liquid, flake, spray, or crystal-like white powder that can be swallowed, smoked, sniffed, or injected. Sometimes it is sprinkled on crack, marijuana, tobacco, or parsley, and smoked. A fine-powdered form of PCP can be snorted or injected.

PCP use peaked in the 1970s, but it remains a popular drug of abuse in both inner-city ghettos and suburban high schools. Users often think that the PCP they take together with another illegal psychoactive substance, such as amphetamines, coke, or hallucinogens, is responsible for the highs they feel, so they seek it out specifically.

How Users Feel   The effects of PCP are utterly unpredictable. It may trigger violent behavior or irreversible psychosis the first time it is used, or the twentieth time, or never. In low doses, PCP produces changes—from hallucinations or euphoria to feelings of emptiness or numbness—similar to those produced by other psychoactive drugs. Higher doses may produce a stupor that lasts several days, increased heart rate and blood pressure, skin flushing, sweating, dizziness, and numbness.

Risks   Some people experience repetitive motor movements (such as facial grimacing), hallucinations, and paranoia. Suicide is a definite risk. Intoxication typically lasts four to six hours, but some effects can linger for several days. Delirium may occur within 24 hours of taking PCP or after recovery from an overdose and can last as much as a week.

Inhalants

Inhalants or *deleriants* are chemicals that produce vapors with psychoactive effects. The most commonly abused inhalants are solvents, aerosols, model-airplane glue, cleaning fluids, and petroleum products like kerosene and butane. Some anesthetics and nitrous oxide (laughing gas) are also abused.

Young people who have been treated for mental health problems, have a history of foster care, or already abuse other drugs have an increased risk of abusing or becoming dependent on inhalants. In addition, adolescents who first begin using inhalants at an early age are more likely to become dependent on them. Approximately 11 percent of adolescents nationwide report having used inhalants in their lifetime. Teens with inhalant use disorders report coexisting multiple drug abuse and dependence, mental health treatment, and delinquent behaviors.[36]

opioids   Drugs that have sleep-inducing and pain-relieving properties, including opium and its derivatives and nonopioid, synthetic drugs.

hallucinogen   A drug that causes hallucinations.

PCP (phencyclidine)   A synthetic psychoactive substance that produces effects similar to other psychoactive drugs when swallowed, smoked, sniffed, or injected, but also may trigger unpredictable behavioral changes.

inhalants   Substances that produce vapors having psychoactive effects when sniffed.

How Users Feel Inhalants very rapidly reach the lungs, bloodstream, and other parts of the body. At low doses, users may feel slightly stimulated; at higher doses, they may feel less inhibited. Intoxication often occurs within five minutes and can last more than an hour. Inhalant users do not report the intense rush associated with other drugs; nor do they experience the perceptual changes associated with LSD. However, inhalants interfere with thinking and impulse control, so users may act in dangerous or destructive ways.

Often there are visible external signs of use: a rash around the nose and mouth; breath odors; residue on face, hands, and clothing; redness, swelling, and tearing of the eyes; and irritation of throat, lungs, and nose that leads to coughing and gagging. Nausea and headache also may occur.

Risks Regular use of inhalants leads to tolerance, so the sniffer needs more and more to attain the desired effects. Younger children who use inhalants several times a week may develop dependence. Older users who become dependent may use the drugs many times a day.

Although some young people believe inhalants are safe, this is far from true. Inhalation of butane from cigarette lighters displaces oxygen in the lungs, causing suffocation. Users also can suffocate while covering their heads with a plastic bag to inhale the substance or from inhaling vomit into their lungs while high. The effects of inhalants are unpredictable, and even a single episode can trigger asphyxiation or cardiac arrhythmia, leading to disability or death. Abusers also can develop difficulties with memory and abstract reasoning, problems with coordination, and uncontrollable movements of the extremities.

Treating Substance Dependence and Abuse

An estimated 6.1 million Americans are in need of drug treatment, but the majority—some 5 million—never get treatment.[37] (See "Point/Counterpoint: Treat or Punish?")

for different perspectives on treatment vs. criminal prosecution.) The most difficult step for a drug user is to admit that he or she *is* in fact an addict. If drug abusers are not forced to deal with their problem through some unexpected trauma, such as being fired or going bankrupt, those who care—family, friends, coworkers, doctors—may have to confront them and insist that they do something about their addiction. Often this *intervention* can be the turning point for addicts and their families. Treatment has proved equally successful for young people and for older adults.

Some universities offer interventions for students who violate college substance abuse policies. *Motivational interviewing,* a brief intervention in which counselors express empathy to support personal change, has proved effective in reducing alcohol and drug consumption.[38]

Treatment may take place in an outpatient setting, a residential facility, or a hospital. Increasingly, treatment thereafter is tailored to address coexisting or dual diagnoses. A personal treatment plan may consist of individual psychotherapy, marital and family therapy, medication, and behavior therapy. Once an individual has made the decision to seek help for substance abuse, the first step usually is detoxification, which involves clearing the drug from the body.

Controlled and supervised withdrawal within a medical or psychiatric hospital may be recommended if an individual has not been able to stop using drugs as an outpatient or in a residential treatment program. Detoxification is most likely to be complicated in a polysubstance abuser, who may require close monitoring and treatment of potentially fatal withdrawal symptoms. Other reasons for inpatient treatment include lack of psychosocial support for maintaining abstinence and the absence of a drug-free living environment. Restrictions on insurance coverage may limit the number of days of inpatient care. Increasingly, once individuals complete detoxification, they continue treatment in residential programs or as outpatients.

Anti-addiction medications that target neurotransmitters in the brain are becoming safer and more effec-

---

POINT COUNTERPOINT *Treat or Punish?*

POINT

Substance abuse is a disorder that should be treated rather than punished. Some states have set up programs that send people arrested for possession of illegal drugs into treatment programs rather than jails. If they commit crimes, such as robbery, these men and women face prosecution for these offenses, but not for drug use.

COUNTERPOINT

Drug users are breaking the law. Not punishing them sends a message of approval for their behavior. Like other criminals, drug users should have to face the consequences of their behavior.

YOUR VIEW

What do you think is the best way of dealing with drug addiction? Do you see it as a medical problem needing treatment or a crime that should be punished? Do you know any students on your campus with serious drug problems that could get them in trouble with the law? What do you think would be the appropriate method of dealing with their drug use?

tive. With treatment, substance abusers are less prone to relapse. If they do return to drug use, their relapses tend to be shorter and less frequent.[39]

The aim of chemical dependence treatment is to help individuals establish and maintain their recovery from alcohol and drugs of abuse. Recovery is a dynamic process of personal growth and healing in which the drug user makes the transition from a lifestyle of active substance use to a drug-free lifestyle.

Whatever their setting, chemical dependence treatment programs initially involve some period of intensive treatment followed by one or two years of continuing aftercare. Most freestanding programs (those not affiliated with a hospital) follow what is known as the *Minnesota model,* a treatment approach developed at Hazelden Recovery Center in Center City, Minnesota, more than 30 years ago. Its key principles include a focus on drug use as the primary problem, not as a symptom of underlying emotional problems; a multidisciplinary approach that addresses the physical, emotional, spiritual, family, and social aspects of the individual; a supportive community; and a goal of abstinence and health.

12-Step Programs

Since its founding in 1935, Alcoholics Anonymous (AA)—the oldest, largest, and most successful self-help program in the world—has spawned a worldwide movement. As many as 200 different recovery programs are based on the spiritual **12-step program** of AA. Participation in 12-step programs for drug abusers, such as Substance Anonymous, Narcotics Anonymous, and Cocaine Anonymous, is of fundamental importance in promoting and maintaining long-term abstinence.

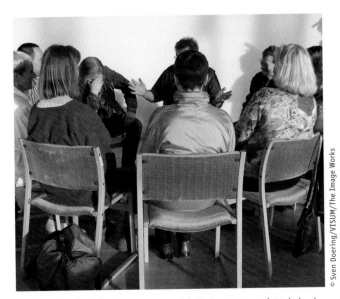

Based on the Alcoholics Anonymous model, 12-step programs have helped many people overcome addiction. The one requirement for membership is a desire to end a pattern of addictive behavior.

The basic precept of 12-step programs is that members have been powerless when it comes to controlling their addictive behavior on their own. These programs don't recruit members. The desire to stop must come from the individual, who can call the number of a 12-step program, listed in the telephone book, and find out when and where the next nearby meeting will be held. A representative may offer to send someone to the caller's house to talk about the problem and to escort him or her to the next meeting.

Meetings of various 12-step programs are held daily in almost every city in the country. (Some chapters, whose members often include the disabled or those in remote areas, meet via Internet chat rooms or electronic bulletin boards.) There are no dues or fees for membership. Many individuals belong to several programs because they have several problems, such as alcoholism, substance abuse, and pathological gambling. All have only one requirement for membership: a desire to stop an addictive behavior.

To get the most out of a 12-step program:

- Try out different groups until you find one you like and in which you feel comfortable.

- Once you find a group in which you feel comfortable, go back several times (some recommend a minimum of six meetings) before making a final decision on whether to continue.

- Keep an open mind. Listen to other people's stories and ask yourself if you've had similar feelings or experiences.

- Accept whatever feels right to you and ignore the rest. One common saying in 12-step programs is, "Take what you like and leave the rest."

Relapse Prevention

The most common clinical course for substance abuse disorders involves a pattern of multiple relapses over the course of a lifespan. It is important for individuals with these problems and their families to recognize this fact. (See Your Strategies for Prevention: "Relapse-Prevention Planning.") When relapses do occur, they should be viewed as neither a mark of defeat nor evidence of moral weakness. While painful, they do not erase the progress that has been achieved and ultimately may strengthen self-understanding. They can serve as reminders of potential pitfalls to avoid in the future.

One key to preventing relapse is learning to avoid obvious cues and associations that can set off intense cravings.

12-step programs Self-help group programs based on the principles of Alcoholics Anonymous

This means staying away from the people and places linked with past drug use. Some therapists use conditioning techniques to give former users some sense of control over their urge to use the drug. The theory behind this approach, which is called *extinction* of conditioned behavior, is that with repeated exposure—for example, to videotapes of dealers selling crack cocaine—the arousal and craving will diminish. While this technique by itself cannot ward off relapses, it does seem to enhance the overall effectiveness of other therapies.

Another important lesson that therapists emphasize is that every lapse does not have to lead to a full-blown relapse. Users can turn to the skills acquired in treatment—calling people for support or going to meetings—to avoid a major relapse. Ultimately, users must learn much more than how to avoid temptation; they must examine their entire view of the world and learn new ways to live in it without turning to drugs. This is the underlying goal of the recovery process.

Learn It : Live It

Choosing an Addiction-Free Lifestyle

People with substance abuse disorders and addictive behaviors lose control of their choices and their lives. Their compulsion to gamble or to use a drug seems irresistible. You, in contrast, have a choice. You can create a life and a lifestyle with no need and no room for reliance on a substance or a self-destructive behavior. Here are some ways to go about it:

- **Set goals for yourself.** Think about who you want to become, what you'd like to do, the future you wish for yourself. Focus on what it will take—years of education, perhaps, or specialized training—to achieve these goals. Understand that drugs can only get in the way and diminish your potential.

- **Participate in drug-free activities.** If you're bored or unfocused, drugs may appeal to you simply as something to do. Take charge of your time. Play a sport. Work out at the gym. Join a club. Volunteer. Start a blog.

- **Educate yourself.** Much of the information that young people hear from friends, particularly drug-using friends, is wrong. Drugs that are used as medicines are not safe for recreational use. The fact that many people at a rave are having fun doesn't mean that some aren't endangering their brains and their lives by taking club drugs. Get the facts for yourself from sites such as those on page 337.

- **Choose friends with a future.** The world of drug users shrinks. Nothing matters more than the next hit, the next high, the next fix. Losing all sense of tomorrow, they focus on getting through the day with the help of drugs. Are these the people you want to spend time with? Choose friends who can broaden your world with new ideas, ambitious plans, and great dreams for tomorrow.

SELFSURVEY : *Do You Have a Substance Use Disorder?*

Check the statements that apply to you.

- Use more of an illegal drug or a prescription medication or use a drug for a longer period of time than you desire or intend. _____

- Try, repeatedly and unsuccessfully, to cut down or control drug use. _____

- Spend a great deal of time doing whatever is necessary in order to get drugs, taking them, or recovering from their use. _____

- Be so high or feel so bad after drug use that you often cannot work or fulfill other responsibilities. _____

- Give up or cut back on important social, work, or recreational activities because of drug use. _____

- Continue to use drugs even though you realize that they are causing or worsening physical or mental problems. _____

- Use a lot more of a drug in order to achieve a "high" or desired effect or feel fewer such effects than in the past. _____

- Use drugs in dangerous ways or situations. _____

- Have repeated drug-related legal problems, such as arrests for possession. _____

- Continue to use drugs, even though the drug causes or worsens social or personal problems, such as arguments with a spouse. _____

- Develop hand tremors or other withdrawal symptoms if you cut down or stop drug use. _____

- Take drugs to relieve or avoid withdrawal symptoms. _____

The more blanks that you (or someone close to you) checks, the more reason you have to be concerned about drug use. The most difficult step for anyone with a substance use disorder is to admit that he or she has a problem. Sometimes a drug-related crisis, such as being arrested or fired, forces individuals to acknowledge the impact of drugs. If not, those who care—family, friends, boss, physician—may have to confront them and insist that they do something about it. This confrontation, planned beforehand, is called an *intervention* and can be the turning point for drug users and their families.

Your Health Action Plan for Recognizing Substance Abuse

How can you tell if a friend or loved one has a substance use disorder? Look for the following warning signs:

- **An abrupt change in attitude.** Individuals may lose interest in activities they once enjoyed or in being with friends they once valued.

- **Mood swings.** Drug users may often seem withdrawn or "out of it," or they may display unusual temper flareups.

- **A decline in performance.** Students may start skipping classes, stop studying, or not complete assignments; their grades may plummet.

- **Increased sensitivity.** Individuals may react intensely to any criticism or become easily frustrated or angered.

- **Secrecy.** Drug users may make furtive telephone calls or demand greater privacy concerning their personal possessions or their whereabouts.

- **Physical changes.** Individuals using drugs may change their pattern of sleep, spending more time in bed or sleeping at odd hours. They also may change their eating habits and lose weight.

- **Money problems.** Drug users may constantly borrow money, seem short of cash, or begin stealing.

- **Changes in appearance.** As they become more involved with drugs, users often lose regard for their personal appearance and look disheveled.

- **Defiance of restrictions.** Individuals may ignore or deliberately refuse to comply with deadlines, curfews, or other regulations.

- **Changes in relationships.** Drug users may quarrel more frequently with family members or old friends and develop strong allegiances with new acquaintances, including other drug users.

CENGAGENOW™ If you want to write your own goals for avoiding drug misuse, go to the Wellness Journal at HealthNow: **academic.cengage. com/login.**

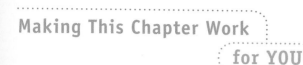

Making This Chapter Work for YOU

Review Questions

1. Which of the following statements about drugs is *false?*
   a. Toxicity is the dosage level of a prescription.
   b. Drugs can be injected into the body intravenously, intramuscularly, or subcutaneously.
   c. Drug misuse is the taking of a drug for a purpose other than that for which it was medically intended.
   d. An individual's response to a drug can be affected by the setting in which the drug is used.

2. To help ensure that an over-the-counter or prescription drug is safe and effective:
   a. take smaller dosages than indicated in the instructions.
   b. test your response to the drug by borrowing a similar medication from a friend.
   c. ask your doctor or pharmacist about possible interactions with other medications.
   d. buy all of your medications online.

3. Prescription drug abuse on college campuses
   a. is not a problem.
   b. is higher among college women than college men.
   c. is more widespread than the use of marijuana.
   d. is more widespread than the use of Ecstasy, cocaine, and meth.

4. Individuals with substance use disorders
   a. are usually not physically dependent on their drug of choice.
   b. have a compulsion to use one or more addictive substances.
   c. require less and less of the preferred drug to achieve the desired effect.
   d. suffer withdrawal symptoms when they use the drug regularly.

5. Amphetamine is very similar to which of the following in its effects on the central nervous system?
   a. marijuana
   b. heroin
   c. cocaine
   d. alcohol

6. Which of the following statements about marijuana is *false?*
   a. People who have used marijuana may experience psychoactive effects for several days after use.
   b. Marijuana has shown some effectiveness in treating chemotherapy-related nausea.
   c. Unlike long-term use of alcohol, regular use of marijuana does not have any long-lasting health consequences.
   d. Depending on the amount of marijuana used, its effects can range from a mild sense of euphoria to extreme panic.

7. Cocaine dependence can result in all of the following *except*
   a. stroke.
   b. paranoia and violent behavior.
   c. heart failure.
   d. enhanced sexual performance.

8. Which of the following statements about club drugs is true?
   a. Club drugs can produce many unwanted effects, including hallucinations and paranoia.
   b. Most club drugs do not pose the same health dangers as "hard" drugs such as heroin.
   c. MDMA is the street name for ecstasy.
   d. When combined with extended physical exertion, club drugs can lead to hypothermia (lowered body temperature).

9. The opioids
   a. are not addictive if used in a prescription form such as codeine or Demerol.
   b. produce an immediate but short-lasting high and feeling of euphoria.
   c. include morphine, which is typically used for cough suppression.
   d. are illegal in the United States, although they are allowed in other countries to help control severe pain.

10. Which of the following statements about drug dependence treatment is *false?*
    a. Chemical dependence treatment programs usually involve medications to alleviate withdrawal symptoms.
    b. Detoxification is usually the first step in a drug treatment program.
    c. Relapses are not uncommon for a person who has undergone drug treatment.
    d. The 12-step recovery program associated with Alcoholics Anonymous has been shown to be ineffective with individuals with drug dependence disorders.

Answers to these questions can be found on page 583.

Critical Thinking

1. Suppose that a close friend is using amphetamines to keep her energy levels high so that she can continue to attend school full-time and hold down a job to pay her school expenses. You fear that she is developing a substance abuse disorder. What can you do to help her realize the dangers of her behavior? What resources are available at your school or in your community to help her deal with both her drug problem and her financial needs?

2. Television ads market prescription drugs direct to consumers. Do you think the ads change the social perception of drug use? Do you think many consumers ask their doctors about these medications? Have you ever done so?

3. Some Web enthusiasts oppose any kind of government regulations on the Internet. Do you agree or disagree? How would you address the problems associated with distributing drugs online, including the sale of counterfeit drugs?

Media Menu

CENGAGENOW™ Go to the HealthNow website at **academic.cengage .com/login** that will:

- Help you evaluate your knowledge of the material.
- Allow you to take an exam-prep quiz.
- Provide a Personalized Learning Plan targeting resources that address areas you should study.
- Coach you through identifying target goals for behavioral change and creating and monitoring your personal change plan throughout the semester.

Internet Connections

National Institute on Drug Abuse

www.nida.nih.gov

This government site—a virtual clearinghouse of information for students, parents, teachers, researchers, and health professionals—features current treatment and research, as well as a comprehensive database on common drugs of abuse. The science of drug abuse and addictions is discussed with a focus on the major illegal drugs in use, with additional resources on drug testing, treatment research, and trends/statistics.

Partnership for a Drug-Free America

www.drugfree.org

This site features current resources and photographs on a wide spectrum of drugs, including performance-enhancing drugs, club drugs, and commonly abused prescription drugs.

The drug guide even allows you to search for a drug using its slang name.

Club Drugs

www.clubdrugs.org

This site is a service of the National Institute on Drug Abuse to provide information on club drugs.

Phoenix House

www.factsontap.org

Facts on Tap is one of the programs of Phoenix House, the largest nonprofit alcohol and drug abuse treatment and prevention facility in the United States.

Key Terms

The terms listed are used and defined on the page indicated. Definitions are also found in the Glossary at the end of this book.

addiction	317	
additive	311	
amphetamines	325	
antagonistic	311	
barbiturates	329	
benzodiazepines	329	
club drugs	323	
cocaine	327	
drug	307	
drug abuse	307	
drug misuse	307	
Ecstasy (MDMA)	323	
GBL (gamma butyrolactone)		325
GHB (gamma hydroxybutyrate)		325
generic	315	
hallucinogens	331	
hashish	319	
inhalants	331	
intoxication	317	
intramuscular	309	
intravenous	309	
marijuana	319	
opioids	331	
over-the-counter (OTC) drugs	311	
PCP (phencyclidine)	331	
physical dependence	317	
polyabuse	317	
potentiating	311	
psychoactive	311	
psychological dependence	317	
stimulant	325	
subcutaneous	309	
synergistic	311	
toxicity	309	
12-step program	333	
withdrawal	317	

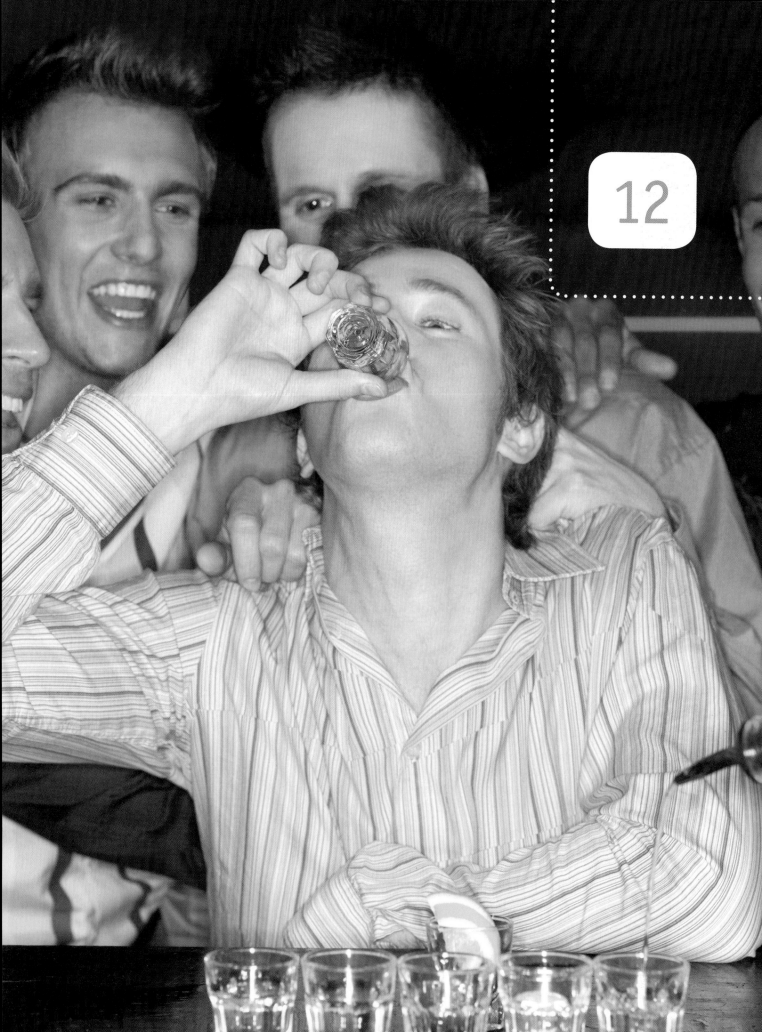

Alcohol Use, Misuse, and Abuse

IT was just another Friday night at the frat house. The drinking started early and usually didn't stop until dawn. One of the brothers, a popular easygoing guy named Ryan—not usually much of a drinker—was celebrating a big birthday: his twenty-first. Egged on by the hooting crowd, Ryan bolted down one drink after another, after another, after another.

By the time Ryan reached 12 drinks, he was slurring his words. As he kept chugging drinks, his face looked flushed; he started sweating heavily. When Ryan lurched to his feet, he swayed unsteadily for a few moments and then collapsed. At first everyone laughed. Then two of his buddies tried to revive him. They couldn't.

"He's not breathing!" one of them shouted. Someone called 911, and paramedics rushed Ryan to the nearest hospital. His blood-alcohol concentration was several times above the legal limit. Despite intensive efforts by the medical team, nothing helped. Ryan's twenty-first birthday was his last.

As Ryan's tragic death shows, alcohol, when not used responsibly, can take an enormous toll. Alcohol is the most widely used drug in the United States. No medical conditions, other than heart disease, cause more disability and premature death than alcohol-related problems. No mental or medical disorders touch the lives of more families. No other form of disability costs individuals, employers, and the government more for treatment, injuries, reduced worker productivity, and property damage. The costs in emotional pain and in lost and shattered lives because of irresponsible drinking are beyond measure.

This chapter provides information about alcohol: its impact on the body, brain, behavior, and society; patterns of drinking; drinking on campus; binge drinking; and the recognition, understanding, and treatment of drinking problems and of alcoholism.

After studying the material in this chapter, you should be able to:

- **Describe** the impact of alcohol misuse among college students, and **define** binge drinking.

- **Define** a standard drink.

- **Describe** the factors affecting a drinker's response to alcohol consumption.

- **Describe** the symptoms of alcohol poisoning and state what you should do if someone exhibits any of the symptoms.

- **List** the effects of alcohol on the body systems.

- **Define** alcohol abuse, dependence, and alcoholism, and **list** their symptoms.

- **List** the negative consequences to individuals, and to our society, from alcohol abuse.

- **Explain** the common treatment methods for alcoholism.

- **Evaluate** your drinking habits and **list** any health risks you are taking.

CENGAGENOW™ Log on to HealthNow at **academic.cengage.com/login** to find your Behavior Change Planner and to explore self-assessments, interactive tutorials, and practice quizzes.

Drinking in America

Many Americans drink alcohol; most do not misuse or abuse it. According to the most recent statistics available from the National Institute on Alcohol Abuse and Alcoholism, two-thirds of American adults use alcohol, although they vary in how much and how often they drink.

Whites are more likely to be daily or near-daily drinkers than nonwhites. Men tend to drink more and more often than women. In general the rates of women who drink have not changed much in the last twenty years. However, the drinking behavior of women in their twenties has changed in two seemingly contradictory ways: More young women don't drink at all, and more of the women who do consume alcohol drink to intoxication.[1]

The median age of first alcohol use is 15. Drinking typically increases in the late teens, peaks in the early 20s, and decreases as people age. The median age of onset for alcohol-use disorders is 19 to 20.

Choosing Not to Drink

More Americans are choosing not to drink, and alcohol consumption is at its lowest level in decades. About a third of adults over age 21 report not using alcohol in the last year.[2] According to the National College Health Assessment, 17 percent of undergraduates have never used alcohol. Among those who have tried alcohol, 13 percent did not have a drink in the previous month.[3]

With fewer people drinking alcohol, nonalcoholic beverages have grown in popularity. They appeal to drivers, boaters, individuals with health problems that could worsen with alcohol, those who are older and can't tolerate alcohol, anyone taking medicines that interact with alcohol (including antibiotics, antidepressants, and muscle relaxers), and everyone interested in limiting alcohol intake. Under federal law, these drinks can contain some alcohol but a much smaller amount than regular beer or wine. Nonalcoholic beers and wines on the market also are lower in calories than alcoholic varieties.

Certain people should not drink at all. These include:

- Anyone younger than age 21. Underage drinking (discussed later in this chapter) poses many medical, behavioral, and legal dangers.
- Anyone who plans to drive, operate motorized equipment, or engage in other activities that require alertness and skill (including sports and recreational activities).
- Women who are pregnant or trying to become pregnant.

- Individuals taking certain over-the-counter or prescription medications. (See the Savvy Consumer in this chapter.)
- People with medical conditions that can be made worse by drinking.
- Recovering alcoholics.

Why People Drink

The most common reason people drink alcohol is to relax. Because it depresses the central nervous system, alcohol can make people feel less tense. Some psychologists theorize that men engage in *confirmatory drinking;* that is, they drink to reinforce the image of masculinity associated with alcohol consumption. Both genders may engage in *compensatory drinking,* consuming alcohol to heighten their sense of masculinity or femininity.

Here are some other reasons why men and women, drink:

- **Social ease.** When people use alcohol, they may seem bolder, wittier, sexier. At the same time, they become more relaxed and seem to enjoy each other's company more. Because alcohol lowers inhibitions, some people see it as a prelude to seduction.
- **Role models.** Athletes, some of the biggest celebrities in our country, have a long history of appearing in commercials for alcohol. Many advertisements feature glamorous men and women holding or sipping alcoholic beverages.
- **Advertising.** Brewers and beer distributors spend multimillions of dollars every year promoting the message: If you want to have fun, have a drink. Young people may be especially responsive to such sales pitches.
- **Relationship issues.** Single, separated, or divorced men and women drink more and more often than married ones.

Individuals with drinking problems often turn to alcohol for other reasons, including:

- **Psychological factors.** Both men and women may drink to compensate for feelings of inadequacy. Yet women who tend to ruminate or mull over bad feelings may find that alcohol increases this tendency and makes them feel more distressed.
- **Self-medication.** More so than men, some women feel it's permissible to use alcohol as if it were a medicine. As long as they're taking it for a reason, it seems acceptable to them.

- **Childhood traumas.** Female alcoholics often report that they were physically or sexually abused as children or suffered great distress because of poverty or a parent's death.
- **Depression.** Women are more likely than men to be depressed prior to drinking and to suffer from both depression and a drinking problem at the same time.
- **Inherited susceptibility.** In both women and men, genetics accounts for 50 to 60 percent of a person's vulnerability to a serious drinking problem. Simply attending college gives young people with a genetic predisposition to alcoholism an extra boost toward heavy drinking.[4]

Safe and Unsafe Drinking

Many drugs, including nicotine, are toxic in any amount. Alcohol is different. In limited quantities, alcohol does not threaten a person's health and may even be beneficial for prevention of heart disease in middle-aged men and women.

Many people describe themselves as "light" or "moderate" drinkers. However, these are not scientific terms. It is more precise to think in terms of the amount of alcohol that seems safe for most people. The federal government's Dietary Guidelines for Americans recommend no more than one drink a day for women and no more than two drinks a day for men (Figure 12.1). The American Heart Association (AHA) advises that alcohol account for no more than 15 percent of the total calories consumed by an individual every day, up to an absolute maximum of 1.75 ounces of alcohol a day—the equivalent of three beers, two mixed drinks, or three and a half glasses of wine.

The dangers of alcohol increase along with the amount you drink. Heavy drinking destroys the liver, weakens the heart, elevates blood pressure, damages the brain, and increases the risk of cancer. Individuals who drink heavily have a higher mortality rate than those who have two or fewer drinks a day. However, the boundary between safe and dangerous drinking isn't the same for everyone. For some people, the upper limit of safety is zero: Once they start, they can't stop.

Unsafe drinking can take many forms, but one of the most dangerous is episodic heavy drinking or **binge drinking**. A binge consists of having five or more drinks in a single sitting for a man or four drinks in a single sitting for a woman. Although this definition is widely used, some criticize it for overlooking body weight and the length of time over which drinking occurs—both factors that influence the effects of alcohol consumption.[5] It also does not take into account alcohol tolerance, metabolism, and medications.

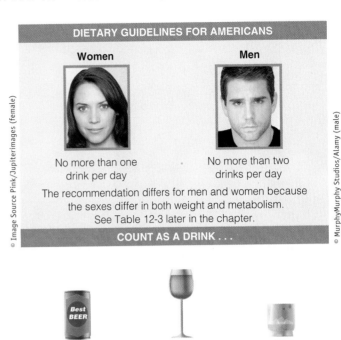

Figure 12.1 Recommendations from Dietary Guidelines for Americans
The recommendation differs for men and women because the sexes differ in both weight and metabolism. See Table 12.3 later in the chapter.
Source: National Council on Alcoholism and Drug Dependence, www.ncadd.org/facts/health.html.

By any measure, drinking multiple drinks at a single setting is common—and hazardous. Binges account for about half of the alcohol consumed by adults—and 90 percent of alcohol drunk by underage young people. They lead to half of alcohol-related deaths and a wide range of serious health and social problems, including motor vehicle accidents, injuries from falls, drowning, hypothermia, and burns; heart attacks; suicide; violence to others; unplanned pregnancy; and sexually transmitted infection. There is a strong link between binge drinking and violence, including murders, assaults, robberies, and sexual offenses.

Among high school students who drink, 60 percent report binge drinking, as do about 40 percent of college students. Among adults, about 29 percent of current drinkers report having engaged in a binge in the last months. While the prevalence of binge drinking has remained relatively constant over recent years, the

binge drinking For a man, having five or more alcoholic drinks at a single sitting; for a woman, having four drinks or more at a single sitting.

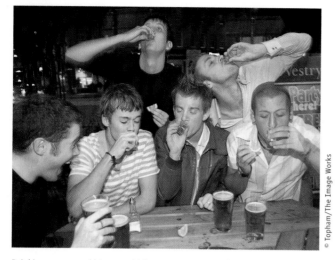

Drinking games and binges, which are common on college campuses, are dangerous in themselves and increase the likelihood of other risky behaviors, such as driving while intoxicated.

TABLE 12.1	Number of Drinks Students Had the Last Time They Drank
Number of Drinks	Percentage of Students
1	11%
2–3	34%
4–5	27%
6–10	22%
11 or more	4%

Source: *Wasting the Best and the Brightest: Substance Abuse at America's Colleges and Universities.* New York: National Center on Addiction and Substance Abuse at Columbia University, March 2007.

number of binge-drinking episodes by adults has increased 29 percent—up to 1.5 billion.

Binge drinking among women ages 18 to 44 may endanger not only a woman's health but that of her unborn child. Binge drinking during pregnancy doubles the risk of mental retardation and delinquent behavior in children.

Drinking on Campus

Young adults are the most frequent users of alcohol in the United States, and college students consume more alcohol more often and more dangerously than nonstudents the same age. Many health experts consider the use and abuse of alcohol as the primary health concern for college students.

In a National Center on Addiction and Substance Abuse survey conducted at Columbia University, about two-thirds of undergraduates reported having a drink within the last 30 days. About 60 percent drank one to five days in the month. On the days that they drank, 45 percent consumed fewer than three drinks. (See Table 12.1 on how much students drink.) Compared to the amount of drinking they did in high school, 64 percent said they drink more in college.[6]

College men drink more, more often, and more intensely than women. Caucasians drink more than African or Asian Americans. Fraternity and sorority members and athletes also use more alcohol more often than other students. (See Reality Check.) The students who drink the least are those attending two-year institutions, religious schools, commuter schools, and historically black colleges and universities.

Why Students *Don't* Drink

According to the National College Health Assessment, 17 percent of students report never using alcohol. Students who don't drink give various reasons for their choice, including not having access to alcohol, parental or peer pressure, being underage, costs, religious reasons, and not liking the taste.[7]

African American students are more likely than white undergraduates to abstain and to report never having had an alcoholic drink or not having a drink in the past 30 days. They also drink less frequently and consume fewer drinks per occasion than whites. Black undergraduates experience fewer negative consequences of drinking and more regularly use strategies to prevent problem drinking, such as eating before drinking and keeping track of how many drinks they consume.

Why Students *Do* Drink

Most college students drink for the same reasons undergraduates have always turned to alcohol: Away from home, often for the first time, many are excited by and apprehensive about their newfound independence. When new pressures seem overwhelming, when they feel awkward or insecure, when they just want to let loose and have a good time, they reach for a drink.

In the National Center on Addiction and Substance Abuse survey, the most common reason students gave for drinking was to relax or reduce stress, followed by enjoyment of the taste of alcohol and socializing. One in ten students said getting drunk was the most important reason for their drinking. (See Figure 12.2.) Most students say their drinking patterns have no relation to their schoolwork. They are most likely to drink on Fridays and Saturdays.[8]

Among other motives for student drinking are:

- **Positive expectations.** College students drink because they believe alcohol will make them feel better—more at ease, less stressed, more sociable, less self-conscious. The behaviors most commonly reported by students when they drink reflect these expectations: flirting, dancing, telling jokes, and laughing harder or more frequently.[9]

- **Coping.** Students turn to alcohol to cope with everyday problems and personal issues. Those with symptoms of depression who lack skills to cope with daily problems, particularly males, are more likely to drink than others.[10]

- **Social norms.** Social norms, discussed in Chapter 1, have proved among the best predictors of alcohol consumption. The more alcohol students believe their peers are drinking, the more they drink.[11] Students generally overestimate how much and how often their classmates drink.[12] However, those with high social anxiety (discussed in Chapter 4) drink more than less socially anxious students even when both groups believe the same social norms about campus drinking.[13]

- **First-year transition.** Some students who drank less in high school than classmates who weren't headed for college start drinking, and drinking heavily, in college—often during their first six weeks on campus. Students who engaged in binge drinking and other dangerous behaviors in high school also are at risk for heavy drinking in college.[14]

- **Drinking culture on campus.** At large colleges and universities where most of the students live on campus, students' social lives, at least on weekends, may revolve around parties, athletic games, and drinking. Colleges and universities in the Northeast, those with a strong Greek system, and those where athletics predominate have higher drinking rates than others. Historically, black universities and colleges have the lowest drinking rates.

- **Living arrangements.** Drinking rates are highest among students living in fraternity and sorority houses, followed by those in on-campus housing (dormitories, residence halls) and off-campus

apartments or houses. Students living at home with their families drink the least.

- **Celebrations.** Students turning 21 average 7.4 drinks on their birthdays—fewer than the 10.6 drinks college students assume their peers have, but still a dangerous amount of alcohol. Tailgating parties, big game rallies, Halloween bonfires, and other events fueled by "fun" also become occasions for drinking. Students have more drinks on the days of a semifinal or championship game—and on the Monday after a victory.[15] The most notorious celebratory drinking occurs during Spring break. (See Point/Counterpoint.)

- **Participation in sports.** College athletes drink more often and more heavily than nonathletes. They may be at greater risk because many are younger than 21, belong to Greek organizations, have lower GPAs, or spend more time socializing than other students.[16] Individual sports also matter. Male hockey and female soccer players drink the most; male basketball players and cross-country or track athletes of both sexes, the least.[17] Female athletes may drink more than other college women because they are following the male athletic model of taking the lead, not just on the field, but also at the party or bar.[18]

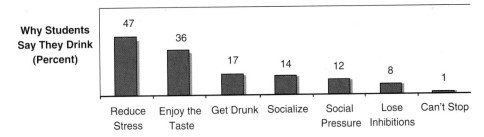

Figure 12.2 Why Students Drink

Source: *Wasting the Best and the Brightest: Substance Abuse at America's Colleges and Universities.* New York: National Center on Addiction and Substance Abuse at Columbia University, March 2007.

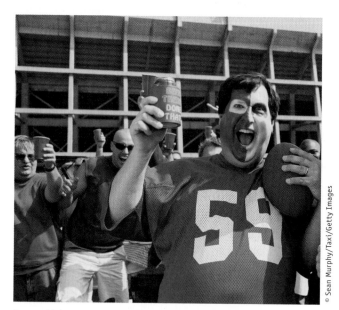

Do you drink at sports events? Why or why not?

© Sean Murphy/Taxi/Getty Images

- **Parental Approval.** Students who believe that their parents approve of drinking are more likely to drink and to report a drinking-related problem. This relationship is even stronger in younger students and those who perceive that their mothers approve of drinking.

High-Risk Student Drinking

 Binge drinking is the leading cause of preventable death among undergraduates and the most serious threat to their intellectual, physical, and psychological development. In spite of great efforts across U.S. college campuses to decrease binge drinking, the national average—two out of five students—remained steady for 20 years.

Colleges vary widely in their binge-drinking rates—from 1 percent to more than 70 percent. The federal government has set a goal of cutting the current binge-drinking rate of 40 percent among college students in half as a goal for Healthy People 2010. How does your campus compare?

Frequent binge drinkers account for almost 70 percent of all alcohol consumed by college students. Students in four-year colleges are more likely to binge than those in two-year colleges.

 Binge drinkers are most likely to be white, fraternity and sorority members, under 24 years of age, involved in athletics, and frequent socializers. White males binge-drink the most; African American women, the least. Students who study a great deal or are involved in community service or the arts are less likely to binge-drink.

Binge drinking has jumped from one in four women to almost one in three: Women who report binge-drinking are more likely to have greater weight concerns than those who did not binge.

POINT COUNTERPOINT *Is Spring Break Broken?*

POINT

No Mom. No Dad. No rules. Nothing to do but party. Spring break has long been an anything-goes celebration, but often it turns into what medical experts describe as a "dangerous binge fest." Many students drink until they pass out. Alcohol poisoning, fights, and accidents are frequent. Young men and women under the influence are at risk for blackouts, sexual assaults, and sexually transmitted infections. The promoters of Spring break trips have gone too far and are endangering the health and lives of college students. Colleges should eliminate this time off.

COUNTERPOINT

Spring break doesn't have to be a time for students to go wild. Rather than eliminating the time off, colleges and student groups should develop alternative experiences for undergraduates. An increasing number of students spend the break on community service projects, such as building houses for Habitat for Humanity or teaching reading in underserved areas.

YOUR VIEW

Should colleges eliminate Spring Break? Or should they encourage students to devote their time to more useful and less dangerous pursuits? Does your school have a Spring break? How do you plan to spend it?

Unplanned sexual activities, date rape, and sexual assault are 150 percent more likely among women who drink than among those who do not. Sophomore, junior, and senior women are much less likely to engage in heavy episodic drinking than freshmen women.

Surveys consistently show that students who engage in binge drinking, particularly those who do so more than once a week, experience a far higher rate of problems than other students. Frequent binge drinkers are likely to miss classes, vandalize property, drive after drinking, and abuse other substances, including nicotine, marijuana, cocaine, and LSD.

Why Students Binge-Drink

Young people who came from, socialized within, or were exposed to "wet" environments—settings in which alcohol is cheap and accessible and drinking is prevalent—are more likely to engage in binge drinking. Students who report drinking at least once a month during their final year of high school are over three times more likely to binge-drink in college than those who drank less frequently in high school.

The factors that most influence students to binge-drink are:

- **Low price** for alcohol. Beer, which is cheap and easy to obtain, is the beverage of choice among binge drinkers.
- **Easy access to alcohol.** In one study, the density of alcohol outlets (such as bars) near campus affected the drinking of students.
- **Attending a school** or living in a residence with many binge drinkers.
- **Belief** that close friends were likely to binge.
- **Drinking games**—such as beer pong or drinking whenever a certain phrase is mentioned in a song or on a TV program—can result in high levels of intoxication in a short period of time. Such games are particularly likely to increase drinking by student athletes.[19]
- **Parents who drank** or did not disapprove of their children drinking.
- **Recreational drinking** before age 16.

Some educators view bingeing as a product of the college environment. More students binge-drink at the beginning of the school year and then cut back as the semester progresses and academic demands increase. Binge drinking also peaks following exam times, during home football weekends, and during Spring break. Many new students engage in binge drinking for the first time very soon after they arrive on campus. Binges become less common in their subsequent years at school and almost always end with education. Real life, one educator notes, is "a strong disincentive" to this type of drinking.

Underage Drinking on Campus

Each year, approximately 5,000 young people under the age of 21 die as a result of underage drinking. This figure includes about 1,900 deaths from motor vehicle crashes, 1,600 as a result of homicides, 300 from suicide, as well as hundreds from other injuries such as falls, burns, and drownings. Students under age 21 drink less often than older students, but tend to drink more heavily and to experience more negative alcohol-related consequences. More underage students report drinking "to get drunk" and drinking at binge levels when they consumed alcohol.

Underage college students are most likely to drink if they can easily obtain cheap alcohol, especially beer. They tend to drink in private settings, such as dorms and fraternity parties, and to experience such drinking-related consequences as doing something they regretted, forgetting where they were or what they did, causing property damage, getting into trouble with police, and being hurt or injured. The drinking behavior of underage students also depends on their living arrangements. Those in controlled settings, such as their parents' home or a substance-free dorm, are less likely to binge-drink. Students living in fraternities or sororities were most likely to binge-drink, regardless of age.

Students under age 21 in states with tough laws against underage drinking are less likely to drink than those in states with fewer restrictions.

Why Students Stop Drinking

Only 1 percent of students ages 18 to 24 receive treatment for alcohol or drug abuse.[20] Nonetheless, as many as 22 percent of alcohol-abusing college students "spontaneously" reduce their drinking as they progress through college. Unlike older adults, who often hit bottom before they change their drinking behaviors, many college students go through a gradual process of reduced drinking. Researchers refer to this behavioral change as early cessation, natural reduction, natural recovery, or spontaneous recovery.[21]

Even though most are underage, freshmen drink more—and often more recklessly—than upperclassmen. The reason may be their fervent, even desperate desire to fit in and feel connected. Unsure of their social skills, anxious about being accepted, they rely on alcohol to make them feel more at ease. Because freshmen seem more susceptible to external influences, perceived drinking norms on campus may have a greater impact on them than on older students.

Why do students say they stop heavy drinking? One common response: "It was just getting old." Some describe more specific reasons why alcohol lost its appeal, including vomiting, urinating in hallways, being physically fondled, sexual assault, violence, accidents, injuries, unprotected intercourse, and emergency room visits. Alcohol-induced blackouts scare many students, especially women, into cutting back, at least temporarily. Vicarious experiences, such as a roommate's arrest for driving under the influence or a sorority sister's date rape, also have a powerful impact.

Students often change their lifestyles during college. They may move out of a dorm or Greek house. As they choose majors, they may meet different friends and form relationships that don't revolve around drinking. Looking toward graduate school and finding a job, many focus more on grades. And as research has shown, students who believe that dedicated studying and high GPAs will enhance their future employment opportunities, economic rewards, and respect from other students are less likely to engage in excessive alcohol consumption. As they approach graduation, students also take on increasingly adult roles and responsibilities, such as an internship or job, marriage, or parenthood.

College Alcohol-Related Problems

The consequences of excessive drinking by students are more significant, more destructive, and more costly than many students or parents realize. As many as 10 to 30 percent of college students experience some negative consequences of drinking. Those at highest risk are men, fraternity or sorority members, and college athletes, who are more likely than other students to drive under the influence, engage in unplanned or unprotected sex, or participate in illegal activities while drunk.[22]

In the National College Health Assessment, 36 percent of students who drank did something they later regretted; 30 percent forgot who they were with or what they did. Men were more likely than women to injure themselves, have unprotected sex, get involved in a fight, or physically injure another person. Women were more likely to have someone use force or threat of force to have sex with them.[23] (See Table 12.2.) Students who drink heavily also are much more likely to abuse prescription drugs (see Chapter 11).[24]

Consequences of Drinking
Among the other problems linked to drinking are:

- **Atypical behavior.** Under the influence of alcohol, students behave in ways they normally wouldn't. Many become more outgoing and sociable. Others become more emotional and cry, tell secrets, or

TABLE 12.2 Most Common Consequences Students Experience After Drinking

Did something they later regretted	36%
Forgot where they were or what they did	30%
Physically injured themselves	18%
Had unprotected sex	14%
Involved in a fight	6%
Physically injured another person	4%
Had someone use or threaten force to have sex with them	1%

Source: American College Health Association. "American College Health Association National College Health Assessment Spring 2006 Reference Group Data Report (Abridged)." *Journal of American College Health,* Vol. 55, No. 4, January–February 2007, pp. 195–206.

become verbally aggressive. Male heavy drinkers are more prone to behave in ways that are considered "antisocial," or contrary to the standards of our society, such as forcing or trying to force unwanted sexual contact, driving drunk, exposing themselves, or having sex with a stranger.[25]

- **Academic problems.** The more that students drink, the more likely they are to fall behind in schoolwork, miss classes, have lower GPAs, and face suspensions.[26] In general, students with an A average have three to four drinks per week, while students with D or F averages drink almost 10 drinks a week. About 30 percent of students who drink and 68 percent of binge drinkers say they have missed a class because of alcohol use.[27]

- **Risky sexual behavior.** About one in five college students reports engaging in unplanned sexual activity, including having sex with someone they just met, while drunk. In one study, 15 percent reported having unprotected sex as a result of drinking.[28]

- **Sexual assault.** Alcohol plays a role in 9 of 10 rapes on campus. In one survey, 1.4 percent of students were forced or threatened by force to have sex. Some 97,000 students are victims of alcohol-related sexual assaults or date rapes every year.[29]

- **Unintentional injury.** More than 30 percent of college drinkers have been hurt or injured as a result of drinking. They also are more likely to cause injury to others, to have a car accident, to suffer burns, and to suffer a fall serious enough to require medical attention. Alcohol-related injuries result in more than 1,700 deaths every year.[30]

- **Consequences beyond college.** The majority of student drinkers do not develop alcohol abuse disorders. However, heavy drinkers are at greater risk for alcohol dependence. Alcohol-related convictions, including carrying a false I.D. or driving under the influence of alcohol, remain on an individual's criminal record and could affect a student's graduate school and professional opportunities.

- **Illness and death.** Many students suffer short-term health consequences of drinking, such as headaches and hangovers. Heavy alcohol use in college students is associated with immunological problems and digestive and upper respiratory disorders. Even moderate drinking can contribute to infertility in women. Longer term consequences of heavy drinking include liver disease, stroke, heart disease, and certain types of cancer.[31] About 300,000 of today's college students will eventually die from alcohol-related causes, including drunk-driving accidents, cirrhosis of the liver, various cancers, and heart disease.

"Secondhand" Drinking Problems

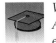 Heavy alcohol use can endanger both drinkers and others. Secondhand problems caused by other's alcohol use include loss of sleep, interruption of studies, assaults, vandalism, and unwanted sexual advances. Students living on campuses with high rates of binge drinking are two or more times as likely to experience these secondhand effects as those living on campuses with low rates. In one study, nearly three-quarters of campus rapes happened when the victims were so intoxicated that they were unable to consent or refuse.

Changing the Culture of Campus Drinking

Wasting the Best and the Brightest: Substance Abuse at America's Colleges—the most extensive examination ever of alcohol, drug, and tobacco use by college students—concluded that excessive student drinking is not a rite of passage but a culture of abuse that has been tolerated for too long by college administrators, parents, and students. Alarmed by the high toll that alcohol takes on young lives and campus communities, more schools are instituting programs to end dangerous drinking. Many strategies, such as scheduling Friday morning classes to discourage Thursday night drinking, have led to lower drinking rates.

The National Institute on Alcohol Abuse and Alcoholism has studied interventions that effectively deal with college drinking problems. Programs that address alcohol-related attitudes and behaviors, use survey data to counter students' misconceptions about their fellow students' drinking practices, and increase students' motivation to change their drinking habits have proved effective.[32]

The social norm approach, which communicates actual facts about drinking behavior to dispel myths, is simple, cost-efficient, and effective. Its positive message is that most students on virtually every campus believe in and practice safety, responsibility, and moderation, rather than excess drinking.

Motivational enhancement, a nonjudgmental, supportive approach to personal change, also has proved beneficial. In brief interventions, specially trained counselors help build students' self-efficacy (discussed in Chapter 2), in this case, their belief in their ability to change their drinking behavior.

Since first-year students are at particular risk for alcohol-related problems, some schools focus on incoming freshmen with interventions that include self-surveys, group discussions about normal drinking behavior, and practical strategies for high-risk situations. An online web course called College Alc, is an effective tool for reducing heavy drinking, drunkenness, and negative alcohol-related consequences in freshmen who were regular drinkers before college.[33]

In one study of high-risk college student drinkers, two daily twenty-minute sessions of meditation (described in Chapter 3 and the lab on antistress strategies, "Rx: Relax" in *IPC*) **IPC** or muscle relaxation significantly reduced alcohol use and drinking problems.[34] Instruction in protective behavioral strategies, such as those described earlier in this chapter, also can reduce alcohol use and alcohol-related problems.[35] Some schools have tried sending text messages designed to boost self-efficacy.[36] Others provide feedback on blood-alcohol concentrations when students return to their dorms at night,[37] and some use posters and T-shirts with messages such as "Seize the Keys" to encourage students not to let friends drive after drinking.[38]

Other university alcohol policies include campus alcohol bans, no alcohol at university-sponsored events, prohibition of beer kegs, limits on the maximum number of drinks served per student, and dry sorority and fraternity initiation activities. Studies suggest that students who attend schools that ban alcohol are less likely to engage in heavy binge drinking, more likely to abstain from using alcohol, and less likely to experience the secondhand effects of drinking.

There has been an increase in on-campus chapters of national support groups such as AA, Al-Anon, Adult Children of Alcoholics, and a peer-education program called BACCHUS: Boost Alcohol Consciousness Concerning the Health of University Students.

Has your school taken steps to change the drinking culture on your campus? Do you think the approaches are working?

motivational enhancement   A nonjudgmental but directive method for supporting motivation to change.

Your Life Change Coach

Taking Charge of Alcohol Use

Drinking, like other behaviors, is a choice. You—and no one else but you—have the right to decide not to drink, and you owe no one an explanation if you say no to alcohol. As with other risk-taking behaviors, never let anyone intimidate you into doing anything that violates your values. (See "Your Alcohol Audit" in *IPC*.) **IPC**

Protecting Yourself from Unsafe Drinking

Smart choices can help you avoid many of the negative consequences of drinking. Various "self-protective" behaviors, such as designating a driver, eating before or during drinking, and keeping track of the number of drinks consumed, have proved effective in reducing alcohol-related problems. Women employ these strategies more often when partying or socializing than men; black students use them more often than white students. The students who used these strategies most often had the fewest problem behaviors.

How do you compare with the students surveyed by the National College Health Assessment?

Behavior	Students Who Always or Usually Use the Strategy
Eat before and/or during drinking	79%
Use a designated driver	75%
Keep track of how many drinks you're having	65%
Avoid drinking games	42%
Decide in advance how many drinks to have	36%
Alternate alcoholic and nonalcoholic beverages	30%
Pace yourself to no more than one drink an hour	29%
Have a friend let you know when you've had enough	27%
Choose not to drink	25%

Staying in Control of Your Drinking

If you do drink, take responsibility for how much and how often you drink. Here are some guidelines that can help:

- **Keep a diary.** Writing down how much you drink each day can make you more aware of exactly how much you drink.

Understanding Alcohol

Pure alcohol is a colorless liquid obtained through the fermentation of a liquid containing sugar. **Ethyl alcohol,** or *ethanol*, is the type of alcohol in alcoholic beverages. Another type—methyl, or wood, alcohol—is a poison that should never be drunk. Any liquid containing .5 to 80 percent ethyl alcohol by volume is an alcoholic beverage. However, different drinks contain different amounts of alcohol.

 Do you know what a "drink" is? Most students don't. In one experiment undergraduates defined a "drink" as one serving, regardless of how big it was or how much alcohol it contained.[39] In fact, one standard drink can be any of the following:

- **One bottle or can** (12 ounces) of beer, which is 5 percent alcohol.
- **One glass** (4 or 5 ounces) of table wine, such as burgundy, which is 12 percent alcohol.
- **One small glass** (2 ½ ounces) of fortified wine, which is 20 percent alcohol.
- **One shot** (1 ounce) of distilled spirits (such as whiskey, vodka, or rum), which is 50 percent alcohol.

All of these drinks contain close to the same amount of alcohol—that is, if the number of ounces in each drink is multiplied by the percentage of alcohol, each drink contains the equivalent of approximately ½ ounce of 100 percent ethyl alcohol.

- **Pace yourself.** Try having a "spacer," a nonalcoholic drink every second or third drink.
- **Stay busy.** You will drink less if you play pool or dance rather than just sitting and drinking.
- **Try low-alcohol alternatives,** such as light beers and low- or no-alcohol wines.
- **Have alcohol-free days.** Don't drink at all at least two days a week.
- **Start with a soft drink.** You will drink much faster if you are thirsty, so have a nonalcoholic drink to quench your thirst before you start drinking alcohol.
- **Use standard drinks.** Monitor how much alcohol you drink. By converting what you drink into standard drinks, it is easier to keep track. (see page 350.)
- **Drink slowly.** Take sips and not gulps. Put your glass down between sips.
- **Avoid salty snacks.** Salty food like chips or nuts make you thirsty so you drink more.
- **Have one drink at a time.** Don't let people top up your drinks. It makes it harder to keep track of how much alcohol you're consuming.
- **Be assertive.** Don't be pressured into drinking more than you want or intend to. Say "Thanks, but no thanks."
- **Pay attention.** Watch as your drink is poured. Don't let your drink out of your sight.
- **Never leave a party with someone you don't know.** This is especially true if you've been drinking and are feeling somewhat intoxicated.
- **Abstain for 48 hours** if you do have an episode of heavy drinking to let your body recover.
- **When you throw a party, be a responsible host.** Collect car keys from your guests. Serve high-protein food like pepperoni pizza, shrimp, or spareribs. Serve nonalcoholic beverages. Do not force drinks on your guests or rush to refill their glasses when empty. Stop serving alcohol about two hours before the party is over.

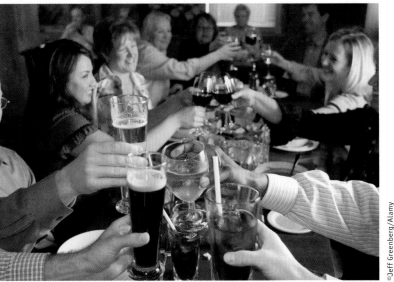

You can share in the fun and toast a happy occasion with non-alcoholic or alcoholic beverages.

But the words *bottle* and *glass* can be deceiving. Drinking a 16-ounce bottle of malt liquor, which is 6.4 percent alcohol, is not the same as drinking a 12-ounce glass of light beer (3.2 percent alcohol): The malt liquor contains 1 ounce of alcohol and is the equivalent of two drinks. Two bottles of high-alcohol wines (such as Cisco), packaged to resemble much less powerful wine coolers, can lead to alcohol poisoning, especially in those who weigh less than 150 pounds.

With distilled spirits (such as bourbon, scotch, vodka, gin, and rum), alcohol content is expressed in terms of **proof,** a number that is twice the percentage of alcohol: 100-proof bourbon is 50 percent alcohol; 80-proof gin is 40 percent alcohol. Many mixed drinks are equivalent to one and a half or two standard drinks; for instance, see the margarita in Figure 12.3.

Blood-Alcohol Concentration

The amount of alcohol in your blood at any given time is your **blood-alcohol concentration (BAC).** It is expressed in terms of the percentage of alcohol in the blood and is often measured from breath or urine samples.

Law enforcement officers use BAC to determine whether a driver is legally drunk. All the states have followed the recommendation of the federal Department of

---

ethyl alcohol   The intoxicating agent in alcoholic beverages; also called ethanol.

proof   The alcoholic strength of a distilled spirit, expressed as twice the percentage of alcohol present.

blood-alcohol concentration (BAC)   The amount of alcohol in the blood, expressed as a percentage.

Margarita:

1¹/2 oz. tequila (80 proof) = 1.5 oz. × 40 percent alcohol = 0.6 oz. alcohol

³/4 oz. triple sec (60 proof) = 0.75 oz. × 30 percent alcohol = 0.23 oz. alcohol

Splash of sour mix   0.83 oz. alcohol = 1¹/2 drinks

Dash of lime juice

Salt for the rim

Malt liquor:

16 oz. × 6.4 percent alcohol = 1 oz. alcohol = 2 drinks

MALT LIQUOR

Figure 12.3   How many standard drinks are you drinking?

Transportation to set .08 percent—the BAC that a 150-pound man would have after consuming about three mixed drinks within an hour—as the threshold at which a person can be cited for drunk driving (Figure 12.4).

 Using a formula for blood-alcohol concentration developed by highway transportation officials, researchers calculate that when college students drink, their typical BAC is .079, dangerously close to the legal limit.[40]

A BAC of .05 percent indicates approximately 5 parts alcohol to 10,000 parts other blood components. Most people reach this level after consuming one or two drinks and experience all the positive sensations of drinking—relaxation, euphoria, and well-being—without feeling intoxicated. If they continue to drink past the .05 percent BAC level, they start feeling worse rather than better, gradually losing control of speech, balance, and emotions. At a BAC of .2 percent, they may pass out. At a BAC of .3 percent, they could lapse into a coma; at .4 percent, they could die.

Many factors affect an individual's BAC and response to alcohol, including the following:

- **How much and how quickly you drink.** The more alcohol you put into your body, the higher your BAC. If you chug drink after drink, your liver, which metabolizes about ¹/₂ ounce of alcohol an hour, won't be able to keep up—and your BAC will soar.

- **What you're drinking.** The stronger the drink, the faster and harder the alcohol hits. Straight shots of liquor and cocktails such as martinis will get alcohol into your bloodstream faster than beer or table wine. Beer and wine not only contain lower concentrations of alcohol, but they also contain nonalcoholic substances that slow the rate of **absorption** (passage of the alcohol into your body tissues). If the drink contains water, juice, or milk, the rate of absorption will be slowed. However, carbon dioxide—whether in champagne, ginger ale, or a cola—whisks alcohol into your bloodstream. Also, the alcohol in warm drinks—such as a hot rum toddy or warmed sake—moves into your bloodstream more quickly than the alcohol in chilled wine or scotch on the rocks.

- **Your size.** If you're a large person (whether due to fat or to muscle), you'll get drunk more slowly than someone smaller who's drinking the same amount of alcohol at the same rate. Heavier individuals have a larger water volume, which dilutes the alcohol they drink.

- **Your gender.** Women have lower quantities of a stomach enzyme that neutralizes alcohol, so one drink for a woman has the impact that two drinks have for a man. Hormone levels also affect the impact of alcohol. Women are more sensitive to alcohol just before menstruation, and birth control pills and other forms of estrogen can intensify alcohol's impact.

- **Your age.** The same amount of alcohol produces higher BACs in older drinkers, who have lower volumes of body water to dilute the alcohol than younger drinkers do.

- **Your race.** Many members of certain ethnic groups, including Asians and Native Americans, are unable to break down alcohol as quickly as Caucasians. This can result in higher BACs, as well as uncomfortable reactions, such as flushing and nausea, when they drink.

- **Other drugs.** Some common medications—including aspirin, acetaminophen (Tylenol), and ulcer medications—can cause blood-alcohol levels to increase more rapidly. Individuals taking these drugs can be over the legal limit for blood-alcohol concentration after as little as a single drink.

- **Family history of alcoholism.** Some children of alcoholics don't develop any of the usual behavioral symptoms that indicate someone is drinking too much. It's not known whether this behavior is

Men	Approximate blood alcohol percentage								
	Body weight in pounds								
Drinks	100	120	140	160	180	200	220	240	
0	.00	.00	.00	.00	.00	.00	.00	.00	Only safe driving limit
1	.04	.03	.03	.02	.02	.02	.02	.02	Impairment begins
2	.08	.06	.05	.05	.04	.04	.03	.03	Driving skills significantly affected
3	.11	.09	.08	.07	.06	.06	.05	.05	
4	.15	.12	.11	.09	.08	.08	.07	.06	Possible criminal penalties
5	.19	.16	.13	.12	.11	.09	.09	.08	
6	.23	.19	.16	.14	.13	.11	.10	.09	
7	.26	.22	.19	.16	.15	.13	.12	.11	
8	.30	.25	.21	.19	.17	.15	.14	.13	Legally intoxicated
9	.34	.28	.24	.21	.19	.17	.15	.14	Criminal penalties
10	.38	.31	.27	.23	.21	.19	.17	.16	

Subtract 0.01 percent for each 40 minutes of drinking.
One drink is 1.25 oz. of 80 proof liquor, 12 oz. of beer, or 5 oz. of table wine.

Women	Approximate blood alcohol percentage									
	Body weight in pounds									
Drinks	90	100	120	140	160	180	200	220	240	
0	.00	.00	.00	.00	.00	.00	.00	.00	.00	Only safe driving limit
1	.05	.05	.04	.03	.03	.03	.02	.02	.02	Impairment begins
2	.10	.09	.08	.07	.06	.05	.05	.04	.04	Driving skills significantly affected
3	.15	.14	.11	.10	.09	.08	.07	.06	.06	
4	.20	.18	.15	.13	.11	.10	.09	.08	.08	Possible criminal penalties
5	.25	.23	.19	.16	.14	.13	.11	.10	.09	
6	.30	.27	.23	.19	.17	.15	.14	.12	.11	
7	.35	.32	.27	.23	.20	.18	.16	.14	.13	Legally intoxicated
8	.40	.36	.30	.26	.23	.20	.18	.17	.15	Criminal penalties
9	.45	.41	.34	.29	.26	.23	.20	.19	.17	
10	.51	.45	.38	.32	.28	.25	.23	.21	.19	

Subtract 0.01 percent for each 40 minutes of drinking.
One drink is 1.25 oz. of 80 proof liquor, 12 oz. of beer, or 5 oz. of table wine.

Figure 12.4   Alcohol Impairment Chart
Source: Adapted from data supplied by the Pennsylvania Liquor Control Board.

genetically caused or is a result of growing up with an alcoholic.

- **Eating.** Food slows the absorption of alcohol by diluting it, by covering some of the membranes through which alcohol would be absorbed, and by prolonging the time the stomach takes to empty.

- **Expectations.** In various experiments, volunteers who believed they were given alcoholic beverages but were actually given nonalcoholic drinks acted as if they were guzzling the real thing and became more talkative, relaxed, and sexually stimulated.

- **Physical tolerance.** If you drink regularly, your brain becomes accustomed to a certain level of alcohol. You may be able to look and behave in a seemingly normal fashion, even though you drink as much as would normally intoxicate someone your size. However, your driving ability and judgment will still be impaired.

absorption   The passage of substances into or across membranes or tissues.

Once you develop tolerance, you may drink more to get the desired effects from alcohol. In some people, this can lead to abuse and alcoholism. On the other hand, after years of drinking, some people become exquisitely sensitive to alcohol. Such reverse tolerance means that they can become intoxicated after drinking only a small amount of alcohol.

Intoxication

If you drink too much, the immediate consequence is that you get drunk—or, more precisely, intoxicated. Alcohol *intoxication,* which can range from mild inebriation to loss of consciousness, is characterized by at least one of the following signs: slurred speech, poor coordination, unsteady gait, abnormal eye movements, impaired attention or memory, stupor, or coma.

Medical risks of intoxication include falls, hypothermia in cold climates, and increased risk of infections because of suppressed immune function. Time and a protective environment are the recommended treatments for alcohol intoxication. For more details, see Your Strategies for Prevention: "What to Do When Someone Is Intoxicated."

Alcohol Poisoning

 Because federal law requires colleges to publish all student deaths, the stories of young lives ended by alcohol poisoning have gained national attention. Yet many students remain unaware that alcohol, in large enough doses, can and does kill.

Alcohol depresses nerves that control involuntary actions, such as breathing and the gag reflex (which prevents choking). A fatal dose of alcohol will eventually suppress these functions. Because alcohol irritates the stomach, people who drink an excessive amount often vomit. If intoxication has led to a loss of consciousness, a drinker is in danger of choking on vomit, which can cause death by asphyxiation. Blood-alcohol concentration can rise even after a drinker has passed out because alcohol in the stomach and intestine continues to enter the bloodstream and circulate throughout the body.

The signs of alcohol poisoning include:

- Mental confusion, stupor, coma, or person cannot be roused.
- Vomiting.
- Seizures.
- Slow breathing (fewer than eight breaths per minute).
- Irregular breathing (10 seconds or more between breaths).
- Hypothermia (low body temperature), bluish skin color, paleness.

Alcohol poisoning is a medical emergency requiring immediate treatment. Black coffee, a cold shower, or letting a person "sleep it off" does not help. Without medical treatment, breathing slows, becomes irregular, or stops. The heart beats irregularly. Body temperature falls, which can cause cardiac arrest. Blood sugar plummets, which can lead to seizures. Vomiting creates severe dehydration, which can cause seizures, permanent brain damage, or death. Even if the victim lives, an alcohol overdose can result in irreversible brain damage.

Rapid binge drinking is especially dangerous because the victim can ingest a fatal dose before becoming unconscious. If you suspect alcohol poisoning, call 911 for help. Don't try to guess the level of drunkenness. Tell emergency medical technicians the symptoms and, if you know, how much alcohol the victim drank. Prompt action may save a life. Here's what to do:

- If the person is breathing less than twelve times per minute or stops breathing for periods of ten seconds or more, **call 911.**
- If the person is asleep and you are unable to wake him or her up, **call 911.**
- Look at the person's skin. If it is cold, clammy, pale, bluish in color, **call 911.**
- Stay with a person who is vomiting. Try to keep him or her sitting up. If the person must lie down, keep him on his side with head turned to the side. Watch for choking; if the person begins to choke, **call 911.**

YOUR STRATEGIES FOR PREVENTION *What to Do When Someone Is Intoxicated*

- Continually monitor the intoxicated person.
- If the person is "out," check breathing, waking the person often to be sure he or she is not unconscious.

- Do not force the person to walk or move around.
- Do not allow the person to drive a car or ride a bicycle.

- Do not give the person food, liquid (including coffee), medicines, or drugs to sober the person up.
- Do not give the person a cold shower; the shock of the cold could cause unconsciousness.

Drinking and Driving

Drunk driving is the most frequently committed crime in the United States. Alcohol impairs driving-related skills regardless of the age of the driver or the time of day it is consumed. However, younger drinkers and drivers are at greatest risk. Underage drinkers are more likely to drive after drinking, to ride with intoxicated drivers, and to be injured after drinking—at least in part because they believe that people can drive safely and legally after drinking.

The number of alcohol-related fatalities on American highways has dropped in recent years, but more than 42,000 people still die on the nation's highways each year. Safety groups attribute the decline in alcohol-related deaths to enforcement tools like sobriety checkpoints and to the states' adoption of a uniform drunken-driving standard of a BAC of .08 percent.

 However, among college students ages 18 to 24, deaths from alcohol-related accidents and other unintentional injuries have increased to more than 1,700 a year. In one survey, 29 percent of college students drove after drinking some alcohol; 10 percent after five or more drinks; 23 percent rode in a car with a driver who was high or drunk. The rates of drinking and driving are higher at larger schools and schools in the southern and north-central regions.

In the last two decades, families of the victims of drunk drivers have organized to change the way the nation treats its drunk drivers. Because of the efforts of MADD (Mothers Against Drunk Driving), SADD (Students Against Destructive Decisions), and other lobbying groups, cities, counties, and states are cracking down on drivers who drink. Since courts have held establishments that serve alcohol liable for the consequences of allowing drunk customers to drive, many bars and restaurants have joined the campaign against drunk driving. Many communities also provide free rides home on holidays and weekends for people who've had too much to drink. Designated drivers who refrain from drinking also can help save lives. (See Your Strategies for Prevention: "How to Prevent Drunk-Driving Disasters.")

The Impact of Alcohol on the Body

Unlike food or drugs in tablet form, alcohol is directly and quickly absorbed into the bloodstream through the stomach walls and upper intestine. The alcohol in a typi-

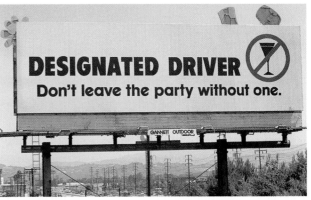

Public awareness campaigns like this one for designated drivers can help prevent the high incidence of fatalities caused by drunk drivers.

cal drink reaches the bloodstream in 15 minutes and rises to its peak concentration in about an hour. The bloodstream carries the alcohol to the liver, heart, and brain (Figure 12.5).

Most of the alcohol you drink can leave your body only after metabolism by the liver, which converts about 95 percent of the alcohol to carbon dioxide and water. The other 5 percent is excreted unchanged, mainly through urination, respiration, and perspiration.

Alcohol is a diuretic, a drug that speeds up the elimination of fluid from the body, so drink water when you drink alcohol to maintain your fluid balance. And alcohol lowers body temperature, so you should never drink to get or stay warm.

Digestive System

Alcohol reaches the stomach first, where it is partially broken down. The remaining alcohol is absorbed easily through the stomach tissue into the bloodstream. In the stomach, alcohol triggers the secretion of acids, which irritate the stomach lining. Excessive drinking at one sitting may result in nausea; chronic drinking may result in peptic ulcers (breaks in the stomach lining) and bleeding from the stomach lining.

The alcohol in the bloodstream eventually reaches the liver. The liver, which bears the major responsibility of fat metabolism in the body, converts this excess alcohol to fat. After a few weeks of four or five drinks a day, liver cells start to accumulate fat. Alcohol also stimulates liver cells to attract white blood cells, which normally travel throughout

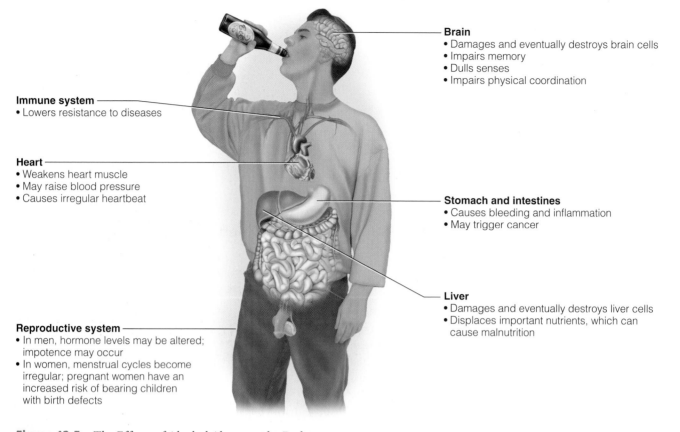

Immune system
• Lowers resistance to diseases

Heart
• Weakens heart muscle
• May raise blood pressure
• Causes irregular heartbeat

Reproductive system
• In men, hormone levels may be altered; impotence may occur
• In women, menstrual cycles become irregular; pregnant women have an increased risk of bearing children with birth defects

Brain
• Damages and eventually destroys brain cells
• Impairs memory
• Dulls senses
• Impairs physical coordination

Stomach and intestines
• Causes bleeding and inflammation
• May trigger cancer

Liver
• Damages and eventually destroys liver cells
• Displaces important nutrients, which can cause malnutrition

Figure 12.5 The Effects of Alcohol Abuse on the Body
Alcohol has a major effect on the brain, damaging brain cells, impairing judgment and perceptions, and often leading to accidents and altercations. Alcohol also damages the digestive system, especially the liver.

the bloodstream engulfing harmful substances and wastes. If white blood cells begin to invade body tissue, such as the liver, they can cause irreversible damage. More than 2 million Americans have alcohol-related liver diseases, such as alcoholic hepatitis and cirrhosis of the liver.

Weight and Waists

At 7 calories per gram, alcohol has nearly as many calories as fat (9 calories per gram) and significantly more than carbohydrates or protein (which have 4 calories per gram). Since a standard drink contains 12–15 grams of alcohol, the alcohol in a single drink adds about 100 calories to your daily intake. A glass of wine contains as many calories as some candy bars; you would have to walk a mile to burn them off. In addition to being a calorie-dense food, alcohol stimulates the appetite so you're likely to eat more.

"Beer bellies" earn their name. In a study of men and women over age 20 in Copenhagen, those who drank the most beer or spirits had wider waists on a ten-year follow-up. Wine did not have a similar impact.

Cardiorespiratory System

Alcohol gets mixed reviews regarding its effects on the cardiorespiratory system.

New research sponsored by the American Heart Association reveals that college students who drink excessively may double their levels of C-reactive protein (CRP), a biological marker for inflammation associated with a higher change of cardiorespiratory problems. Although the long-term impact is unknown, researchers caution that high CRP levels could predict future risk of heart disease.[41] However, several studies have shown, people who drink moderate amounts of alcohol have lower mortality rates after a heart attack, as well as a lower risk of heart attack compared to abstainers and heavy drinkers.

How do moderate amounts of alcohol enhance heart health? Researchers believe that it boosts beneficial high-density lipoproteins (HDL), lowers the risk of blood clots, and also may have an anti-inflammatory effect.

Some cardiologists contend that the benefits of moderate drinking may be overstated, especially because of alcohol's contribution to the epidemic of obesity around the world. Heavier drinking triggers the release of harmful oxygen molecules called free radicals, which can increase the risk of heart disease, stroke, and cirrhosis of the liver. Alcohol use can weaken the heart muscle directly, causing a disorder called cardiomyopathy. The combined use of alcohol and other drugs, including tobacco and cocaine, greatly increases the likelihood of damage to the heart.

Cancer

Long-term heavy drinking increases the risk of certain forms of cancer, especially cancer of the esophagus, mouth, throat, and larynx.

According to several large studies, women who have three drinks per day are 18 percent more likely to develop breast cancer than women who don't drink at all. The risk occurs with all forms of alcohol—beer, wine, and spirits—and increases the more women drink. In the Nurses' Health Study, breast cancer rates rose slightly even in women who took as little as half a drink per day. A single daily drink increases a woman's breast cancer risk slightly—perhaps 3 or 4 percent. Every additional daily drink increases the risk by 7 percent.

Brain and Behavior

At first when you drink, you feel up. In low dosages, alcohol affects the regions of the brain that inhibit or control behavior, so you feel looser and act in ways you might not otherwise. However, you also experience losses of concentration, memory, judgment, and fine motor control; and you have mood swings and emotional outbursts.

Moderate amounts of alcohol can have disturbing effects on perception and judgment, including the following:

- **Impaired perceptions.** You're less able to adjust your eyes to bright lights because glare bothers you more. Although you can still hear sounds, you can't distinguish between them or judge their direction well.
- **Dulled smell and taste.** Alcohol itself may cause some vitamin deficiencies, and the poor eating habits of heavy drinkers result in further nutrition problems.
- **Diminished sensation.** On a freezing winter night, you may walk outside without a coat and not feel the cold.
- **Altered sense of space.** You may not realize, for instance, that you have been in one place for several hours.
- **Impaired motor skills.** Writing, typing, driving, and other abilities involving your muscles are impaired. This is why law enforcement officers

sometimes ask suspected drunk drivers to touch their nose with a finger or to walk a straight line. Drinking large amounts of alcohol impairs reaction time, speed, accuracy, and consistency, as well as judgment.
- **Impaired sexual performance.** While drinking may increase your interest in sex, it may also impair sexual response, especially a man's ability to achieve or maintain an erection. As Shakespeare wrote, "It provokes the desire, but it takes away the performance."

Moderate and heavy drinkers show signs of impaired intelligence, slowed-down reflexes, and difficulty remembering. Because alcohol is a central nervous system depressant, it slows down the activity of the neurons in the brain, gradually dulling the responses of the brain and nervous system. One or two drinks act as a tranquilizer or relaxant. Additional drinks result in a progressive reduction in central nervous system activity, leading to sleep, general anesthesia, coma, and even death.

Heavy alcohol use may pose special dangers to the brains of drinkers at both ends of the age spectrum. Adolescents who drink regularly show impairments in their neurological and cognitive functioning. Elderly people who drink heavily appear to have more brain shrinkage, or atrophy, than those who drink lightly or not at all. In general, moderate drinkers have healthier brains and a lower risk of dementia than those who don't drink and those who drink to excess.

Interaction with Other Drugs

Alcohol can interact with other drugs—prescription and nonprescription, legal and illegal. Of the 100 most frequently prescribed drugs, more than half contain at least one ingredient that interacts adversely with alcohol. Because alcohol and other psychoactive drugs may work on the same areas of the brain, their combination can produce an effect much greater than that expected of either drug by itself. The consequences of this synergistic interaction can be fatal. Alcohol is particularly dangerous when combined with other depressants and anti-anxiety medications. (See the Savvy Consumer feature in this chapter.)

Immune System

Chronic alcohol use can inhibit the production of both white blood cells, which fight off infections, and red blood cells, which carry oxygen to all the organs and tissues of the body. Alcohol may increase the risk of infection with human immunodeficiency virus (HIV), by altering the judgment of users so that they more readily

▼ *Savvy*Consumer Alcohol and Drug Interactions

Drug	Possible Effects of Interaction
Allergies, colds, flu medicines (Allegra, Benadryl, Carlitin, Dimetapp, Sudafed, Tylenol Cold & Flu)	Drowsiness, dizziness, increased risk for overdose.
Analgesics (painkillers)	
Narcotic (Codeine, Demerol, Percodan, Vicodin)	Increase in central nervous system depression, possibly leading to respiratory failure and death.
Nonnarcotic (aspirin, acetaminophen, ibuprofen)	Irritation of stomach resulting in bleeding and increased susceptibility to liver damage.
Antabuse (disulfiram; an aid to quit drinking)	Nausea, vomiting, headache, high blood pressure, and erratic heartbeat.
Antianxiety drugs (Valium, Librium, Ativan, Xanax)	Increase in central nervous system depression; decreased alertness and impaired judgment.
Antidepressants (Prozac, Zoloft, Celexa, Lexapro, Paxil, Wellbutrin, Luvox, and others)	Increase in central nervous system depression; certain antidepressants in combination with red wine could cause a sudden increase in blood pressure.
Antihistamines (Actifed, Dimetap, and other cold medications)	Increase in drowsiness; driving more dangerous.
Antibiotics	Nausea, vomiting, headache; some medications rendered less effective.
Central nervous system stimulants (caffeine, Dexedrine, Ritalin)	Stimulant effects of these drugs may reverse depressant effect of alcohol but do not decrease its intoxicating effects.
Sedatives (Dalmane, Nembutal, Quaalude)	Increase in central nervous system depression, possibly leading to coma, respiratory failure, and death.

engage in activities such as unsafe sex that put them in danger. If you drink when you have a cold or the flu, alcohol interferes with the body's ability to recover. It also increases the chance of bacterial pneumonia in flu sufferers.

Increased Risk of Dying

Alcohol kills. Alcohol is responsible for 100,000 deaths each year and is the third-leading cause of death after tobacco and improper diet and lack of exercise. The leading alcohol-related cause of death is injury. Alcohol plays a role in almost half of all traffic fatalities, half of all homicides, and a quarter of all suicides. The second leading cause of alcohol-related deaths is cirrhosis of the liver, a chronic disease that causes extensive scarring and irreversible damage. In addition, as many as half of patients admitted to hospitals and 15 percent of those making office visits seek or need medical care because of the direct or indirect effects of alcohol.

Young drinkers—teens and those in their early twenties—are at highest risk of dying from injuries, mostly car accidents. Older drinkers over age 50 face the greatest danger of premature death from cirrhosis of the liver, hepatitis, and other alcohol-linked illnesses.

Most studies of the relationship between alcohol consumption and death from all causes show that moderate drinkers—those who consume approximately seven drinks per week—have a lower risk of death than abstainers, while heavy drinkers have a higher risk than either group. In one 10-year study, never-drinkers showed no elevated risk of dying, while consistent heavier drinkers were at higher risk of dying of any cause than other men.

Alcohol, Gender, and Race

Experts in alcohol treatment are increasingly recognizing racial and ethnic differences in risk factors for drinking problems, patterns of drinking, and most effective types of treatment.

Gender

According to conventional gender stereotypes, drinking is a symbol of manliness. In the past, far more men than women drank. In the United States today, both genders are likely to consume alcohol. However, there are well-documented differences in how often and how much men and women drink. In general, men drink more frequently, consume a larger quantity of alcohol per drinking occasion, and report more problems related to drinking. More than half of women drink: Of these, 45 percent are light drinkers; 3 percent, moderate drinkers; 2 percent, heavy drinkers; and 21 percent, binge drinkers.

The bodies of men and women respond to alcohol in different ways. Because they have a far smaller quantity of a protective enzyme in the stomach to break down alcohol before it's absorbed into the bloodstream, women absorb

TABLE 12.3 How Alcohol Discriminates

	Women	Men
Ability to Dilute Alcohol	Average total body water: 52%	Average total body water: 61%
Ability to Metabolize Alcohol	Women have a smaller quantity of dehydrogenase, an enzyme that breaks down alcohol.	Men have a larger quantity of dehydrogenase, which allows them to break down the alcohol they take in more quickly.
Hormonal Factors, Part 1	Premenstrual hormonal changes cause intoxication to set in faster during the days right before a woman gets her period.	Their susceptibility to getting drunk does not fluctuate dramatically at certain times of the month.
Hormonal Factors, Part 2	Alcohol increases estrogen levels. Birth control pills or other medicine with estrogen increase intoxication.	Alcohol also increases estrogen levels in men. Chronic alcoholism has been associated with loss of body hair and muscle mass, development of swollen breasts and shrunken testicles, and impotence.

Source: www.factsontap.org/factsontap/risky/discrimination.htm.

about 30 percent more alcohol into their bloodstream than men—see Table 12.3. The alcohol travels through the blood to the brain, so women become intoxicated much more quickly. And because there's more alcohol in the bloodstream to break down, the liver may also be adversely affected. In alcoholic women, the stomach seems to completely stop digesting alcohol, which may explain why female alcoholics are more likely to suffer liver damage than men.

An estimated 15 percent of women drink alcohol while pregnant, most having one drink or less per day. Even light consumption of alcohol can lead to **fetal alcohol effects (FAE):** low birthweight, irritability as newborns, and permanent mental impairment.

The babies of women who consume three or more ounces of alcohol (the equivalent of six or seven cocktails) are at risk of more severe problems. One of every 750 newborns has a cluster of physical and mental defects called **fetal alcohol syndrome (FAS):** small head, abnormal facial features, jitters, poor muscle tone, sleep disorders, sluggish motor development, failure to thrive, short stature, delayed speech, mental retardation, and hyperactivity.

About a third of the symptoms of alcohol abuse are gender-specific, but men exhibit more obvious ones, such as violent behavior. Because women develop more subtle problems such as feelings of guilt about alcohol consumption, they are less likely to be diagnosed as early as men.[42]

Both men and women experience blackouts after heavy drinking, but women black out after consuming half as much alcohol as men. Women also may be more susceptible to alcohol-induced memory problems when given comparable amounts of alcohol. In addition, they are at greater risk of engaging in risky behavior, including unprotected sex, than men.

Alcohol interferes with male sexual function and fertility through direct effects on testosterone and the testicles.

In half of alcoholic men, increased levels of female hormones lead to breast enlargement and a feminine pubic hair pattern. Damage to the nerves in the penis by heavy drinking can lead to impotence. In women who drink heavily, a drop in female hormone production may cause menstrual irregularity and infertility.

As women age, their risk of osteoporosis, a condition characterized by calcium loss and bone thinning, increases. Alcohol can block the absorption of many nutrients, including calcium, and heavy drinking may worsen the deterioration of bone tissue.

Race

African American Community

Overall, African Americans consume less alcohol per person than whites, yet twice as many blacks die of cirrhosis of the liver each year. In some cities, the rate of cirrhosis is ten times higher among African American than white men. Alcohol also contributes to high rates of hypertension, esophageal cancer, and homicide among African American men.

Hispanic Community

The various Hispanic cultures tend to discourage any drinking by women but encourage heavy drinking by men as part of machismo, or feelings of manhood. Hispanic men have higher rates of alcohol use and abuse

fetal alcohol effects (FAE) Milder forms of FAS, including low birthweight, irritability as newborns, and permanent mental impairment as a result of the mother's alcohol consumption during pregnancy.

fetal alcohol syndrome (FAS) A cluster of physical and mental defects in the newborn, including low birthweight, smaller-than-normal head circumference, intrauterine growth retardation, and permanent mental impairment caused by the mother's alcohol consumption during pregnancy.

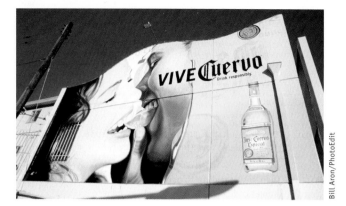

Bill Aron/PhotoEdit

Liquor advertisers use billboards like this to promote their products to Hispanic Americans.

than the general population and suffer a high rate of cirrhosis. Moreover, American-born Hispanic men drink more than those born in other countries.

Few Hispanics with severe alcohol problems enter treatment, partly because of a lack of information, language barriers, and poor community-based services.[43] Hispanic families generally try to resolve problems themselves, and their cultural values discourage the sharing of intimate personal stories, which characterizes Alcoholics Anonymous and other support groups. Churches often provide the most effective forms of help.

Native American Community

European settlers introduced alcohol to Native Americans. Because of the societal and physical problems resulting from excessive drinking, at the request of tribal leaders, the U.S. Congress in 1832 prohibited the use of alcohol by Native Americans. Many reservations still ban alcohol use, so Native Americans who want to drink may have to travel long distances to obtain alcohol, which may contribute to the high death rate from hypothermia and pedestrian and motor-vehicle accidents among Native Americans. (Injuries are the leading cause of death among this group.)

Certainly, not all Native Americans drink, and not all who drink do so to excess. However, they have three times the general population's rate of alcohol-related injury and illness. Cirrhosis of the liver is the fourth-leading cause of death among this cultural group. While many Native American women don't drink, those who do have high rates of alcohol-related problems, which affect both them and their children. Their rate of cirrhosis of the liver is 36 times that of white women. In some tribes, 10.5 out of every 1,000 newborns have fetal alcohol syndrome, compared with 1 to 3 out of 1,000 in the general population.

Asian American Community

Asian Americans tend to drink very little or not at all, in part because of an inborn physiological reaction to alcohol that causes facial flushing, rapid heart rate, lowered blood pressure, nausea, vomiting, and other symptoms. A very high percentage of women of all Asian American nationalities abstain completely. Some sociologists have expressed concern, however, that as Asian Americans become more assimilated into American culture, they'll drink more—and possibly suffer very adverse effects from alcohol.

Alcohol Problems

By the simplest definition, problem drinking is the use of alcohol in any way that creates difficulties, potential difficulties, or health risks for an individual. Like alcoholics, problem drinkers are individuals whose lives are in some way impaired by their drinking. The only difference is one of degree. Alcohol becomes a problem, and a person becomes an alcoholic, when the drinker can't "take it or leave it." He or she spends more and more time anticipating the next drink, planning when and where to get it, buying and hiding alcohol, and covering up secret drinking. As many as one in six adults in the United States may have a problem with drinking. To determine if you have a problem, see Your Strategies for Prevention: "How to Recognize the Warning Signs of Alcoholism."

Alcohol abuse involves continued use of alcohol despite awareness of social, occupational, psychological, or physical problems related to drinking, or drinking in dangerous ways or situations (before driving, for instance). A diagnosis of alcohol abuse is based on one or more of the following occurring at any time during a 12-month period:

- **A failure to fulfill major role obligations** at work, school, or home (such as missing work or school).

- **The use of alcohol in situations in which it is physically hazardous** (such as before driving).

- **Alcohol-related legal problems** (such as drunk-driving arrests).

- **Continued alcohol use despite persistent or recurring social or interpersonal problems** caused or exacerbated by alcohol (such as fighting while drunk).

Alcohol dependence is a separate disorder in which individuals develop a strong craving for alcohol because it produces pleasurable feelings or relieves stress or anxiety. Over time they experience physiological changes that lead to *tolerance* of its effects; this means that they must consume larger and larger amounts to achieve intoxication. If they abruptly stop drinking, they suffer *withdrawal,* a state of acute physical and psychological discomfort. A diagnosis of alcohol dependence is based on three or more of the following symptoms occurring during any 12-month period:

- **Tolerance,** as defined by either a need for markedly increased amounts of alcohol to achieve intoxication or desired effect, or a markedly diminished effect with continued drinking of the same amount of alcohol as in the past.
- **Withdrawal,** including at least two of the following symptoms: sweating, rapid pulse, or other signs of autonomic hyperactivity; increased hand tremor; insomnia; nausea or vomiting; temporary hallucinations or illusions; physical agitation or restlessness; anxiety; or grand mal seizures.
- **Drinking to avoid** or relieve the symptoms of withdrawal.
- **Consuming larger amounts of alcohol,** or drinking over a longer period than was intended.
- **Persistent desire** or unsuccessful efforts to cut down or control drinking.
- **A great deal of time spent** in activities necessary to obtain alcohol, drink it, or recover from its effects.
- **Important social, occupational, or recreational activities given up** or reduced because of alcohol use.
- **Continued alcohol use** despite knowledge that alcohol is likely to cause or exacerbate a persistent or recurring physical or psychological problem.

 According to a survey of more than 14,000 undergraduates at four-year colleges, 6 percent of college students met criteria for a diagnosis of alcohol dependence or alcoholism, 31 percent for alcohol abuse. More than two of every five students reported at least one symptom of these conditions and were at increased risk of developing a true alcohol disorder. Few reported seeking treatment since coming to college.

Alcoholism, as defined by the National Council on Alcoholism and Drug Dependence and the American Society of Addiction, is a primary, chronic disease in which genetic, psychosocial, and environmental factors influence its development and manifestations. The disease is often progressive and fatal. Its characteristics include an inability to control drinking, a preoccupation with alcohol, continued use of alcohol despite adverse consequences, and distorted thinking, most notably denial. Like other diseases, alcoholism is not simply a matter of insufficient willpower but a complex problem that causes many symptoms, can have serious consequences, yet can improve with treatment.

A lack of obvious signs of alcoholism can be deceiving. A person who doesn't drink in the morning but feels that

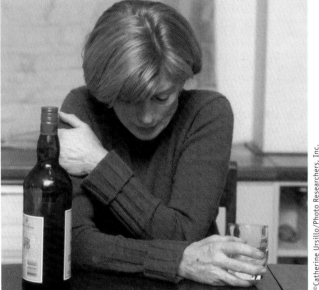

©Catherine Ursillo/Photo Researchers, Inc.

Daytime drinking and drinking alone can be signs of a serious problem, even though the drinker may otherwise appear to be in control.

alcohol abuse   Continued use of alcohol despite awareness of social, occupational, psychological, or physical problems related to its use, or use of alcohol in dangerous ways or situations, such as before driving.

alcohol dependence   Development of a strong craving for alcohol due to the pleasurable feelings or relief of stress or anxiety produced by drinking.

alcoholism   A chronic, progressive, potentially fatal disease characterized by impaired control of drinking, a preoccupation with alcohol, continued use of alcohol despite adverse consequences, and distorted thinking, most notably denial.

he or she must always have a drink at a certain time of the day may have lost control over his or her drinking. A person who never drinks alone but always drinks socially with others may be camouflaging loss of control. A person who is holding a job or taking care of the family may still spend every waking hour thinking about that first drink at the end of the day (preoccupation).

Causes of Alcohol Dependence and Abuse

Although the exact cause of alcohol dependence and abuse is not known, certain factors—including biochemical imbalances in the brain, heredity, cultural acceptability, and stress—all seem to play a role. They include the following:

- **Genetics.** Scientists have not yet identified conclusively a specific gene that puts people at risk for alcoholism. However, epidemiological studies have shown evidence of heredity's role. Studies of twins suggest that heredity accounts for two-thirds of the risk of becoming alcoholic in both men and women.

- **Stress and traumatic experiences.** Many people start drinking heavily as a way of coping with psychological problems.

- **Parental alcoholism.** According to researchers, alcoholism is four to five times more common among the children of alcoholics, who may be influenced by the behavior they see in their parents.

- **Drug abuse.** Alcoholism is also associated with the abuse of other psychoactive drugs, including marijuana, cocaine, heroin, amphetamines, and various antianxiety medications.

Medical Complications of Alcohol Abuse and Dependence

As previously discussed, excessive alcohol use adversely affects virtually every organ system in the body, including the brain, the digestive tract, the heart, muscles, blood, and hormones (look back at Figure 12.5, page 354). In addition, because alcohol interacts with many drugs, it can increase the risk of potentially lethal overdoses and harmful interactions. A summary of the major risks and complications follows:

- **Liver disease.** Chronic heavy drinking can lead to alcoholic hepatitis (inflammation and destruction of liver cells) and in the 15 percent of people who continue drinking beyond this stage, cirrhosis (irreversible scarring and destruction of liver cells).

The liver eventually may fail completely, resulting in coma and death.

- **Cardiorespiratory disease.** Heavy drinking can weaken the heart muscle (causing cardiac myopathy), elevate blood pressure, and increase the risk of stroke.

- **Cancer.** Heavy alcohol use may contribute to cancer of the liver, stomach, and colon, as well as malignant melanoma, a deadly form of skin cancer.

- **Brain damage.** Long-term heavy drinkers may suffer memory loss and be unable to think abstractly, recall names of common objects, and follow simple instructions. Chronic brain damage resulting from alcohol consumption is second only to Alzheimer's disease as a cause of cognitive deterioration in adults.

- **Vitamin deficiencies.** Alcoholism is associated with vitamin deficiencies, especially of thiamin (B_1). Lack of thiamin may result in Wernicke-Korsakoff syndrome, which is characterized by disorientation, memory failure, hallucinations, and jerky eye movements, and can be disabling enough to require life-long custodial care.

- **Digestive problems.** Alcohol triggers the secretion of acids in the stomach that irritate the mucous lining and cause gastritis. Chronic drinking may result in peptic ulcers (breaks in the stomach lining) and bleeding from the stomach lining.

- **Accidents and injuries.** Alcohol may contribute to almost half of the deaths caused by car accidents,

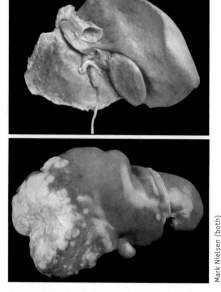

A normal liver (top) compared to one with cirrhosis.

Mark Nielsen (both)

burns, falls, and choking. Nearly half of those convicted and jailed for criminal acts committed these crimes while under the influence of alcohol.

- **Higher mortality.** As discussed earlier, the mortality rate for alcoholics is two to three times higher than that for nonalcoholics of the same age. Injury is the leading alcohol-related cause of death, chiefly in auto accidents involving a drunk driver. Alcohol is a factor in about 30 percent of all suicides.

Alcoholism Treatments

An estimated 8 million adults in the United States have alcohol dependence. Only a minority ever undergo treatment for alcohol-related problems. Until recent years, the only options for professional alcohol treatment were, as one expert puts it, "intensive, extensive, and expensive," such as residential programs at hospitals or specialized treatment centers. Today individuals whose drinking could be hazardous to their health may choose from a variety of approaches, including medication, behavioral therapy, or both. Treatment that works well for one person may not work for another. As research into the outcomes of alcohol treatments has grown, more attempts have been made to match individuals to approaches tailored to their needs and more likely to help them overcome their alcohol problems.[44]

Men and women who have seriously remained sober for more than a decade credit a variety of approaches, including Alcoholics Anonymous (AA), individual psychotherapy, and other groups, such as Women for Sobriety. There is no one sure path to sobriety—a wide variety of treatments may offer help and hope to those with alcohol-related problems.

Detoxification

The first phase of treatment for alcohol dependence focuses on **detoxification,** the gradual withdrawal of alcohol from the body. For 90 to 95 percent of alcoholics, withdrawal symptoms are mild to moderate. They include sweating; rapid pulse; elevated blood pressure; hand tremor; insomnia; nausea or vomiting; malaise or weakness; anxiety; depressed mood or irritability; headache; and temporary hallucinations or illusions. Withdrawal can be life-threatening when accompanied by medical problems, such as grand mal seizures, pneumonia, liver failure, or gastrointestinal bleeding. The standard treatment is a safer sedative, such as Valium or Ativan, with a gradual reduction in the dose.

Alcohol withdrawal delirium, commonly known as **delirium tremens,** or **DTs,** is most common in chronic

heavy drinkers who also suffer from a physical illness, fatigue, depression, or malnutrition. Delirium tremens are characterized by agitated behavior, delusions, rapid heart rate, sweating, vivid hallucinations, trembling hands, and fever. The symptoms usually appear over several days after heavy drinking stops. Individuals frequently report terrifying visual hallucinations, such as seeing insects all over their bodies. With treatment, most cases subside after several days, although delirium tremens has been known to last as long as four or five weeks. In some cases, complications such as infections or heart arrhythmias prove fatal.

Medical Treatments

Antianxiety and antidepressive drugs are sometimes used in early treatment for alcoholism, especially for those with underlying mental disorders. Three drugs—naltrexone, acamprosate, and topiramate—are approved to reduce the persistent craving for alcohol. Vitamin supplements, especially thiamin and folic acid, can help overcome some of the nutritional deficiencies linked with alcoholism.

The drug disulfiram (Antabuse), given to deter drinking, causes individuals to become nauseated and acutely ill when they consume alcohol. Antabuse interrupts the removal of acetaldehye by the liver, so this toxic substance accumulates and causes nausea or vomiting. If individuals taking Antabuse drink at all or consume foods with alcoholic content, they become extremely ill. They must avoid foods cooked or marinated in wine and cough syrup preparations containing alcohol. Some individuals have reactions to the alcohol in after-shave lotion. A large amount of alcohol can make them dangerously ill; fatalities have occurred. Side effects are usually mild and include drowsiness, bad breath, skin rash, and temporary impotence. Because Antabuse does not reduce cravings for alcohol, psychotherapy and support groups remain a necessary part of treatment.

Inpatient or Residential Treatment

In the past, 28-day treatment programs in a medical or psychiatric hospital or a residential facility were the cornerstone of early recovery treatment. According to outcome studies, inpatient treatment was effective, with as many as 70 percent of "graduates" remaining abstinent or stable, nonproblem drinkers for five years after.

detoxification The supervised removal of a poisonous or harmful substance (such as a drug) from the body; a therapy for alcoholics in which they are denied alcohol in a controlled environment.

delirium tremens (DTs) The delusions, hallucinations, and agitated behavior following withdrawal from long-term chronic alcohol abuse.

However, because of cost pressures from the insurance industry, the length of stay has been reduced, and there's been increasing emphasis on outpatient care.

Outpatient Treatment

Outpatient treatment may involve group therapy, individual supportive therapy, marital or family therapy, regular attendance at Alcoholics Anonymous (AA) or another support group, brief interventions, and relapse prevention. According to outcome studies, intensive outpatient treatment at a day hospital (with individuals returning home every evening) are as effective as inpatient care. Outpatient therapy continues for at least a year, but many individuals continue to participate in outpatient programs for the rest of their lives.

Brief Interventions

These methods include individual counseling, group therapy, and training in specific skills—such as assertiveness—all packed into a six- to eight-week period. Offered at a growing number of centers, brief interventions may be most helpful for problem drinkers who are not physically dependent on alcohol. They have proved effective in reducing alcohol consumption up to one year compared with no intervention or standard care. However, at ten years, there is no difference in alcohol consumption among those who had a brief intervention and those who did not. This indicates the need for follow-up advice and counseling.

Moderation Training

Highly controversial, this approach uses cognitive-behavioral techniques, such as keeping a diary to chart drinking patterns and learning "consumption management" techniques, such as never having more than one drink an hour.

Treatment programs in other countries, such as Great Britain and Canada, have long offered moderation training for problem drinkers who consume too much alcohol. However, most experts agree that the best—and perhaps only—hope for recovery for chronic alcoholics who are physically dependent on alcohol is complete abstinence.

12-Step Self-Help Programs

The best-known and most commonly used self-help program for alcohol problems is Alcoholics Anonymous (AA), which was founded more than 60 years ago and which has grown into an international organization that includes 2 million members and 185,000 groups worldwide. Acknowledging the power of alcohol, AA offers support from others struggling with the same illness, from a sponsor available at any time of the day or night, and from fellowship meetings that are held every day of the year. Because anonymity is a key part of AA, it has been diffi-cult for researchers to study its success, but it is generally believed to be a highly effective means of overcoming alcoholism and maintaining abstinence. Its 12 steps, which emphasize honesty, sobriety, and acknowledgment of a "higher power," have become the model for self-help groups for other addictive behaviors, including drug abuse (discussed in Chapter 11) and compulsive eating.

The average age of entry into AA is 30; about 60 percent of the members are men. Members encompass a wide range of ages, occupations, nationalities, and socioeconomic classes. People generally attend 12-step meetings every day when they first begin recovery; most programs recommend 90 meetings in 90 days. Many people taper off to one or two meetings a week as their recovery progresses. No one knows exactly how 12-step programs help people break out of addictions. Some individuals stop their drinking, or other destructive behavior, simply on the basis of the information they get at meetings. Others bond to the group and use it as a social support and refuge while they explore and release their inner feelings—a process similar to what happens in psychotherapy.

Many individuals recovering from substance abuse—as many as 1 in 10 Americans, by some estimates—will attend a 12-step meeting in their lifetime. For many with alcohol-related problems, AA is the first and only treatment they receive. Does AA work? Some studies have found that fewer than 1 in 30 people remain in AA after one year, although this may be because many are coerced to make their initial visits. However, continued AA attendance is modestly associated with abstinence and improved social functioning.

Spirituality is a key and controversial component of AA, with 11 of its 12 steps explicitly referring to the importance of God or a higher power for recovery. Yet both spiritually oriented and atheistic individuals benefit equally from AA programs. In a 10-year study, individuals involved with AA reported significantly larger gains in religious practices, such as prayer, compared with those without such exposure. Individuals who maintain consistent AA membership reported the greatest increases in "God consciousness" and religious practices.[45]

Harm Reduction Therapy

This controversial approach aims to help substance abusers reduce the negative impact of alcohol or drugs on their lives. Its fundamental principles include:

- While absolute abstinence may be preferable for many or most substance abusers, very few achieve it. Even these few will take time to reach this point and may relapse periodically.

- The field of medicine accepts and practices other types of treatments that preserve health and well-being even when people fail to comply with all recommended behaviors.

YOUR STRATEGIES FOR CHANGE *If Someone Close to You Drinks Too Much . . .*

- Try to remain calm, unemotional, and factually honest in speaking about the drinker's behavior. Include the drinker in family life.
- Discuss the situation with someone you trust: a member of the clergy, social worker, friend, or someone who has experienced alcoholism directly.

- Never cover up or make excuses for the drinker, or shield him or her from the consequences of drinking. Assuming the drinker's responsibilities undermines his or her dignity and sense of importance.
- Refuse to ride with the drinker if he or she is driving while intoxicated.

- Encourage new interests and participate in leisure-time activities that the drinker enjoys.
- Try to accept setbacks and relapses calmly.

- Therapists cannot make judgments for clients, even though they should present accurate information and may even express their own beliefs.
- There are many shades of improvement in every kind of therapy. If a certain level of improvement is all a person is capable of reaching, that person should be encouraged.

Alternatives to AA

Secular Organizations for Sobriety (SOS) was founded in 1986 as an alternative for people who couldn't accept the spirituality of AA. Like AA, SOS holds confidential meetings, celebrates sobriety anniversaries, and views recovery as a one-day-at-a-time process.

Rational Recovery, which also emphasizes anonymity and total abstinence, focuses on the self rather than spirituality. Members use reason instead of prayer and learn to control the impulse to drink by learning how to control the emotions that lead them to drink.

One of the most effective programs for women is Women for Sobriety, founded in 1975 by sociologist Jean Kirkpatrick, Ph.D. Its meetings focus on building self-esteem, self-confidence, and responsibility. "AA was started by men, and its message is very disempowering for women," said Kirkpatrick. "We view members as competent women who are struggling with issues that all women must face. Women don't need to recall the painful process of becoming alcoholics. They need to put the past behind them and move on, upward and onward."[46]

Recovery

Recovery from alcoholism is a lifelong process of personal growth and healing. The first two years are the most difficult, and relapses are extremely common. By some estimates, more than 90 percent of those recovering from substance use will use alcohol or drugs in any one 12-month period after treatment. However, approximately 70 percent of those who get formal treatment stop drinking for prolonged periods. Even without treatment, 30 percent of alcoholics are able to stop drinking for long periods. Those most likely to remain sober after treatment have the most to lose by continuing to drink: they tend to be employed, married, and upper-middle class. Recovering alcoholics who help other alcoholics stay sober are better able to maintain their own sobriety.[47]

Most recovering alcoholics experience urges to drink, especially during early recovery when they are likely to feel considerable stress. These urges are a natural consequence of years of drinking and diminish with time. Mood swings are common during recovery, and individuals typically describe themselves as alternately feeling relieved or elated and then discouraged or tearful. Such disconcerting ups and downs also decrease over time. Patience—learning to take "one day at a time"—is crucial.

Increasingly, treatment programs focus on **relapse prevention,** which includes the development of coping strategies and learning techniques that make it easier to live with alcohol cravings and rehearsal of various ways of saying "no" to offers of a drink. According to outcomes research, social skills training—a combination of stress management therapy, assertiveness and communication skills training, behavioral self-control training, and behavioral marital therapy—has proved effective in decreasing the duration and severity of relapses after one year in a group of alcoholics. A new approach to relapse behavior, "Mindfulness-Based-Relapse Prevention" teaches clients meditation techniques as a way of coping with cravings and high-risk relapse situations.[48]

Alcoholism's Impact on Relationships

Alcoholism shatters families and creates unhealthy patterns of communicating and relating. Separation and divorce rates are high among alcoholics. For tips on how to help a friend or family member, see Your Strategies for Change: "If Someone Close to You Drinks Too Much . . ."

relapse prevention An alcohol recovery treatment method that focuses on social skills training to develop ways of preventing or minimizing a relapse.

Growing Up with an Alcoholic Parent

An estimated 28 million children in the United States (or one of every four) are living in a household with an alcoholic adult. Parental alcoholism increases the likelihood of childhood ADHD, conduct disorder, and anxiety disorders. The experience often leads youngsters to play certain roles: The adjuster or "lost child" does whatever the parent says. The responsible child, or "family hero," typically takes over many household tasks and responsibilities. The acting-out child, or "scapegoat," shows his or her anger early in life by causing problems at home or in school and taking on the role of troublemaker. The "mascot" disrupts tense situations by focusing attention on himself or herself, often by clowning. Regardless of which roles they assume, the children of alcoholics are prone to learning disabilities, eating disorders, and addictive behavior.

Numerous studies have linked parental drinking to child abuse and neglect. Children of women who are problem drinkers have twice the risk of serious injury as children of mothers who don't drink. Children with two parents who are problem drinkers are at even higher risk. As teenagers, children of alcoholics are more likely to report early sexual intercourse and face a greater risk of adolescent pregnancy.

Adult Children of Alcoholics

Growing up with an alcoholic parent can have a long-lasting effect. Adult children of alcoholics are at risk for many problems. Some try to fill the emptiness inside with alcohol, drugs, or addictive habits. Others find themselves caught up in destructive relationships that repeat the patterns of their childhood. They are likely to have difficulty solving problems, identifying and expressing their feelings, trusting others, and being intimate. In addition to their own increased risk of addictive behavior, they are likely to marry individuals with some form of addiction and keep on playing out the roles of their childhood. They may feel inadequate, not know how to set limits or recognize normal behavior, be perfectionistic, and want to control all aspects of their lives. However, not all adult children are alike or necessarily suffer from psychological problems or face an increased risk of substance abuse themselves.

Because the impact of alcoholism can be so enduring, support groups—such as Adult Children of Alcoholics, Children of Alcoholics, and Adult Children of Dysfunctional Families—have spread throughout the country in the last decade. These organizations provide adult children of alcoholics a mutually supportive group setting to discuss their childhood experiences with alcoholic parents and the emotional consequences they carry into adult life. Through such groups or other forms of therapy, individuals may learn to move beyond anger and blame, see the part they themselves play in their current state of unhappiness, and create a future that is healthier and happier than their past.

Learn It : Live It

Responsible Drinking

Problems with drinking aren't just the serious ones such as drunk driving and alcoholism. They can start with minor problems, such as missing classes and term paper deadlines. Or they can start with the belief that a party is no fun unless there is a bottle or a six-pack.

As you decide about the role alcohol should play in your life, you might want to follow these guidelines, proposed by BACCHUS, a volunteer college student organization that promotes responsible alcohol-related behavior:

- Set a limit on how many drinks you're going to have ahead of time—and stick to it.
- When you're mixing a drink, measure the alcohol.
- Alternate nonalcoholic and alcoholic drinks.

- Drink slowly; don't guzzle.
- Eat before and while drinking.
- Develop alternatives to drinking so you don't turn to alcohol whenever you're depressed or upset. Exercise is a wonderful release for tension; meditation or relaxation techniques can also help you cope.
- Avoid performing tasks that require skilled reactions during or after drinking.
- Don't encourage or reinforce others' irresponsible behavior.

Above all, keep in mind that drinking should not be the primary focus of any activity. Responsible drinking is a matter of you controlling your drinking rather than the drinking controlling you.

SELFSURVEY : *Do You Have a Drinking Problem?*

This self-assessment, the Michigan Alcoholism Screening Test (MAST), is widely used to identify potential problems. This test screens for the major psychological, sociological, and physiological consequences of alcoholism.

Answer Yes or No to the following questions, and add up the points shown in the right column for your answers.

	Yes	No	Points
1. Do you enjoy a drink now and then?			(0 for either)
2. Do you think that you're a normal drinker? (By normal, we mean that you drink less than or as much as most other people.)			(2 for no)
3. Have you ever awakened the morning after some drinking the night before and found that you couldn't remember part of the evening?			(2 for yes)
4. Does your wife, husband, a parent, or other near relative ever worry or complain about your drinking?			(1 for yes)
5. Can you stop drinking without a struggle after one or two drinks?			(2 for no)
6. Do you ever feel guilty about your drinking?			(1 for yes)
7. Do friends or relatives think that you're a normal drinker?			(2 for no)
8. Do you ever try to limit your drinking to certain times of the day or to certain places?			(0 for either)
9. Have you ever attended a meeting of Alcoholics Anonymous?			(2 for yes)
10. Have you ever gotten into physical fights when drinking?			(1 for yes)
11. Has your drinking ever created problems for you and your wife, husband, a parent, or other relative?			(2 for yes)
12. Have your wife, husband, or other family members ever gone to anyone for help about your drinking?			(2 for yes)
13. Have you ever lost friends because of your drinking?			(2 for yes)
14. Have you ever gotten into trouble at work or school because of your drinking?			(2 for yes)

15. Have you ever lost a job because of your drinking? _____ _____ (2 for yes)

16. Have you ever neglected your obligations, your family, or your work for two or more days in a row because of drinking? _____ _____ (2 for yes)

17. Do you drink before noon fairly often? _____ _____ (1 for yes)

18. Have you ever been told you have liver trouble? Cirrhosis? _____ _____ (2 for yes)

19. After heavy drinking, have you ever had delirium tremens (DTs) or severe shaking, or heard voices or seen things that weren't actually there? _____ _____ (2 for yes*)

20. Have you ever gone to anyone for help about your drinking? _____ _____ (5 for yes)

21. Have you ever been in a hospital because of your drinking? _____ _____ (5 for yes)

22. Have you ever been a patient in a psychiatric hospital or on a psychiatric ward of a general hospital where drinking was part of the problem that resulted in hospitalization? _____ _____ (2 for yes)

23. Have you ever been seen at a psychiatric or mental health clinic or gone to any doctor, social worker, or clergyman for help with any emotional problem where drinking was part of the problem? _____ _____ (2 for yes)

24. Have you ever been arrested for drunk driving, driving while intoxicated, or driving under the influence of alcoholic beverages? _____ _____ (2 for yes)

25. Have you ever been arrested, or taken into custody, even for a few hours, because of drunken behavior _____ _____ (2 for yes)

    (If Yes, how many times? _____ **)

*Five points for delirium tremens
**Two points for each arrest

Scoring

In general, five or more points places you in an alcoholic category; four points suggests alcoholism; while three or fewer points indicates that you're *not* an alcoholic.

Your Health Action Plan for Avoiding Destructive Decisions

Students Against Destructive Decisions (originally founded as Students Against Driving Drunk) developed the following statement and contract for college students to discuss and sign. Use it as your health action plan for making responsible decisions about alcohol, drugs, and other behaviors that could put your health at risk:

Despite increased public and legislative awareness, the abuse of legal and illegal alcohol and other drugs is rampant in our society. The consequences of alcohol abuse and drug addiction are devastating and pose a major threat to young people in our society. No age group is more vulnerable to the tragic consequences of this abuse and addiction than are college students and other young adults.

College students across the nation have begun to band together to fight the substance abuse problems affecting their campuses. Innovative SADD programs have highlighted the power of college students to effectively deal with critical problems. The SADD College Contract for Life is designed to facilitate communication between college friends about potentially destructive decisions related to alcohol, drug use, HIV/AIDS, sexuality, date rape, impaired driving, and many more challenges. The Contract provides a practical tool for opening discussion, raising awareness, and demonstrating the desire to help friends find any assistance they need.[49]

Source: www.sadd.org/contract.htm#collegecfl

CENGAGENOW™ If you want to write your own goals for more nutritious choices, go to the Wellness Journal at HealthNow: **academic.cengage.com/login.**

COLLEGE CONTRACT FOR LIFE

Between Friends
STUDENTS AGAINST DESTRUCTIVE DECISIONS

As students at _____,
we recognize that we will be faced with many difficult decisions.
Throughout our college experience we may encounter issues such as
alcohol and other drug use, HIV/AIDS, risky sexual behaviors, date rape,
impaired driving, abusive relationships, and many more challenges.

By signing below, we have entered into a contract in which we agree
that we will always attempt to choose the best option that considers
our own well-being, health, and safety. In addition, we will help
friends whom we see making destructive decisions find any assistance
they need.

When I find myself in a situation that makes me uncomfortable or
that I feel unequipped to handle, I will discuss it with someone I trust.

_____

SIGNATURE OF 1ST PARTY   DATE

_____

SIGNATURE OF 2ND PARTY   DATE

Students Against Destructive Decisions

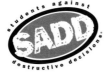

SADD, Inc. | **255 Main Street** | **Marlborough, MA 01752**
877-SADD-INC TOLL-FREE | **508-481-3568** | **508-481-5759** FAX
www.sadd.org

Review Questions

1. Which of the following statements about drinking on college campuses is true?
   a. The federal government has a goal to reduce the binge-drinking rate among college students to 20 percent.
   b. The number of women who binge-drink has decreased.
   c. Because of peer pressure, students in fraternities and sororities tend to drink less than students in dormitories.
   d. Students who attend two-year institutions tend to binge-drink when alcohol is available.

2. Responsible drinking includes which of the following behaviors?
   a. Avoid eating while drinking because eating speeds up absorption of alcohol.
   b. Limit alcohol intake to no more than four drinks in an hour.
   c. Take aspirin while drinking to lower your risk of a heart attack.
   d. Socialize with individuals who limit their alcohol intake.

3. Which of these is a standard drink?
   a. a margarita
   b. a 12-oz regular beer
   c. a double martini
   d. a 16-oz can of malt liquor

4. An individual's response to alcohol depends on all of the following *except*
   a. the rate at which the drink is absorbed into the body's tissues.
   b. the blood alcohol concentration.
   c. socioeconomic status.
   d. gender and race.

5. Which of the following statements about the effects of alcohol on the body systems is true?
   a. In most individuals, alcohol sharpens the responses of the brain and nervous system, enhancing sensation and perception.
   b. Moderate drinking may have a positive effect on the cardiorespiratory system.
   c. French researchers have found that drinking red wine with meals may have a positive effect on the digestive system.

   d. The leading alcohol-related cause of death is liver damage.

6. Racial and ethnic patterns related to alcohol use include which of the following?
   a. Asian American women tend to have higher rates of alcoholism than Asian American men.
   b. Socioeconomic conditions increase the likelihood of alcohol problems in African Americans and Native Americans.
   c. White Americans tend to have higher rates of cirrhosis of the liver than African Americans or Native Americans.
   d. The Hispanic culture discourages men from drinking because heavy drinking indicates a lack of machismo.

7. Alcoholism
   a. is considered a chronic disease with genetic, psychosocial, and environment components.
   b. is characterized by a persistent lack of willpower.
   c. may be classified as either Type A, which affects people who are high-strung, or Type B, which affects people who are more mild mannered.
   d. is easily controlled by avoiding exposure to social situations where drinking is common.

8. Which of the following statements about alcohol abuse and dependence is *false*?
   a. Alcohol dependence involves a persistent craving for and an increased tolerance to alcohol.
   b. An individual may have a genetic predisposition for developing alcoholism.
   c. Alcoholics often abuse other psychoactive drugs.
   d. Alcohol abuse and alcohol dependence are different names for the same problem.

9. Health risks of alcoholism include all of the following *except*
   a. hypertension.   c. peptic ulcers.
   b. lung cancer.   d. hepatitis.

10. Which of the following statements about alcoholism treatment is true?
   a. Inpatient treatment has been shown to be more effective than outpatient treatment.
   b. Alcoholism can be cured by detoxifying or ridding the body of all traces of alcohol.
   c. Antabuse is a medication given to alcoholics with underlying mental disorders.
   d. A combination of medical, behavioral, and self-help approaches may be necessary to treat alcohol abuse and dependence.

Answers to these questions can be found on page 583.

Critical Thinking

1. Driving home from his high school graduation party, 18-year-old Rick has had too much to drink. As he crosses the dividing line on the two-lane road, the driver of an oncoming car—a young mother with two young children in the backseat—swerves to avoid an accident. She hits a concrete wall and dies instantly, but her children survive. Rick has no record of drunk driving. Should he go to prison? Is he guilty of manslaughter? How would you feel if you were the victim's husband? If you were Rick's friend?

2. Some groups concerned about alcohol abuse advocate greater restrictions on availability, such as prohibiting the sale of alcoholic beverages in supermarkets, convenience stores, and gas stations. They would like to see a ban on advertisements, especially those aimed at young people. Opponents argue that laws have never been effective in controlling alcohol abuse. Do you think our society is too permissive in the way we allow alcohol to be promoted or sold? Would you support anti-alcohol laws? Why or why not?

3. Have you ever been around people who have been intoxicated when you have been sober? What did you think of their behavior? Were they fun to be around? Was the experience not particularly enjoyable, boring, or difficult in some way? Have you ever been intoxicated? How do you behave when you are drunk? Do you find the experience enjoyable? What do the people around you think of your actions when you are drunk?

4. What effects has alcohol use had in your life? Try making a list of the positive and negative effects your own alcohol use has had. Be specific. If you continue to drink at your current rate, what positive and negative effects do you think it will have on your future? What effects has other people's drinking had on your life? List family members and friends who drink regularly and how their drinking has affected you.

Media Menu

CENGAGENOW™ Go to the HealthNow website at **academic.cengage .com/ login** that will:

- Help you evaluate your knowledge of the material.
- Allow you to take an exam-prep quiz.
- Provide a Personalized Learning Plan targeting resources that address areas you should study.
- Coach you through identifying target goals for behavioral change and creating and monitoring your personal change plan throughout the semester.

INTERNET CONNECTIONS

Facts on Tap: Alcohol and Your College Experience
www.factsontap.org
This excellent site is geared to college students. Sections include Alcohol & Student Life, Alcohol & Sex, Alcohol & Your Body.

College Drinking: Changing the Culture
www.collegedrinkingprevention.gov
This website, sponsored by the National Institute of Alcohol Abuse and Alcoholism, focuses on the college alcohol culture with information for students, parents, college health administrators, and more. The site also features information about alcohol prevention, college alcohol policies, research topics, and factual information about the consequences of alcohol abuse and alcoholism.

Al-Anon Family Group Headquarters
www.al-anon.alateen.org
This site provides information and referrals to local Al-Anon and Alateen groups. It also includes a self-quiz to determine if you are affected by someone who has an alcohol problem.

National Association for Children of Alcoholics
www.nacoa.org
This association provides information about and for children of alcoholics. Their website contains numerous links to relevant support groups.

Key Terms

The terms listed are used and defined on the page indicated. Definitions are also found in the Glossary at the end of this book.

absorption	351	
alcohol abuse	359	
alcohol dependence	359	
alcoholism	359	
binge drinking	341	
blood-alcohol concentration (BAC)	349	
delirium tremens (DTs)	361	
detoxification	361	
ethyl alcohol	349	
fetal alcohol effects (FAE)	357	
fetal alcohol syndrome (FAS)		357
motivational enhancement		347
proof	349	
relapse prevention	363	

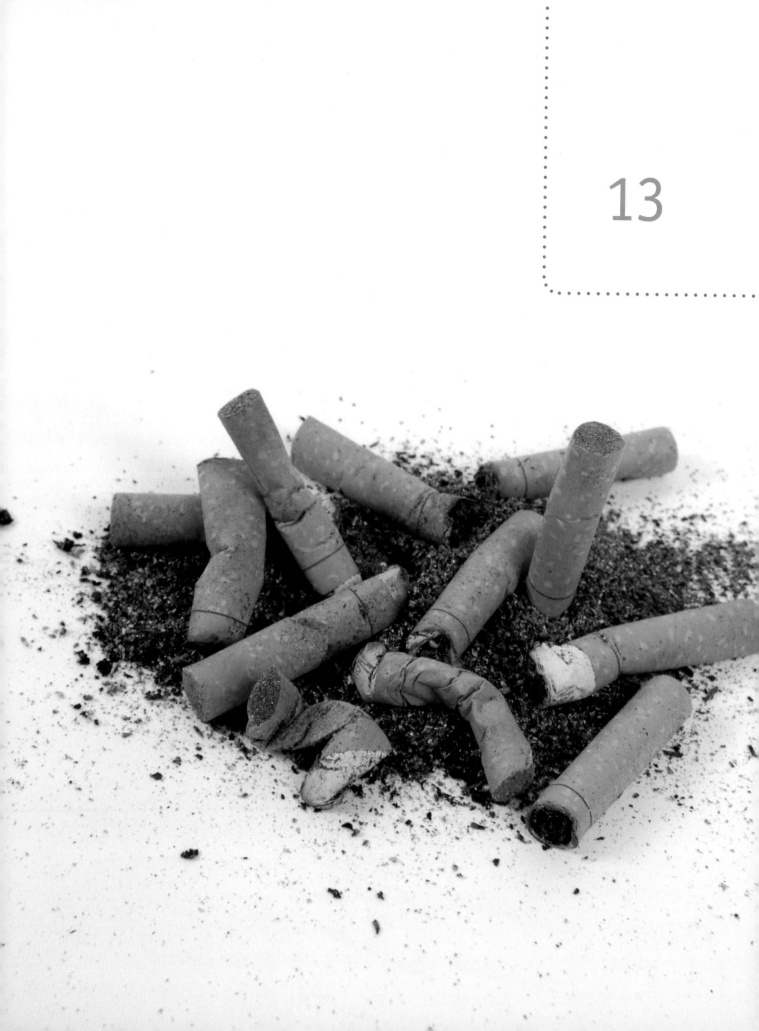

13

Tobacco Use, Misuse, and Abuse

ANDREA didn't really want her first cigarette. Her tent mate at camp had snatched one from a counselor's pack, and the two of them had climbed to a remote rock to share it. Andrea hated everything about her first drag: the taste, the smell, the horrible burning in her throat and lungs. But she loved feeling more grown-up and sophisticated than other seventh graders. By the time she reached high school, Andrea would sneak off to smoke with friends at least once a week. By graduation, she was smoking daily.

As a college freshman, Andrea discovered that she was part of an unpopular minority. Even though her dorm didn't ban smoking, her roommate declared their room a smoke-free zone. Her college didn't allow smoking in any classrooms or public areas. And many of her new friends reacted as if smoking was a sign of impaired intelligence. Andrea has decided to quit, but she's discovered that nicotine dependence is very difficult to overcome. "I just wish I'd never started smoking in the first place," she says.

According to the Centers for Disease Control and Prevention (CDC), 21 percent of American adults smoke.[1] The more and the longer they smoke, the greater their risks of heart disease, respiratory problems, several types of cancer, and a shortened lifespan.

Despite widespread awareness of the dangers of tobacco, smoking continues to kill more people than AIDS, alcohol, drug abuse, car crashes, murders, suicides, and fires combined. The worldwide death toll is 5 million people a year.

This chapter discusses smoking in America and on campus, the effects of tobacco on the body, tobacco dependence, quitting smoking, smokeless tobacco, and environmental tobacco smoke. The information it provides may help you to breathe easier today—and may help ensure cleaner air for others to breathe tomorrow.

After studying the material in this chapter, you should be able to:

- **Describe** today's tobacco smokers and the common reasons why they smoke.

- **Describe** some of the tobacco-control policies on college campuses.

- **List** the health effects of smoking tobacco or using smokeless tobacco.

- **Discuss** the health problems that can be prevented by quitting smoking.

- **Identify** the different types of tobacco products.

- **Discuss** several recommended ways to quit smoking.

- **Describe** the health effects of environmental, or secondhand, tobacco smoke.

- **Assess** the health risks you may have experienced as a result of your own or others' use of tobacco.

CENGAGENOW Log on to HealthNow at **academic.cengage.com/login** to find your Behavior Change Planner and to explore self-assessments, interactive tutorials, and practice quizzes.

Smoking in America

Americans are snuffing out cigarettes. The prevalence of smoking in the United States has declined more than 40 percent in recent decades. According to federal surveys, 21 percent of Americans smoke. Of these, about 8 in 10 smoke every day. More men (23 percent) than women (19 percent) are current smokers. Native Americans have the highest smoking rates, while Asians and Hispanics have the lowest. Individuals with undergraduate and graduate degrees are least likely to smoke.[2]

The drop in smoking in the overall population still falls short of the national health objective of reducing cigarette smoking among adults to 12 percent by 2010. However, some groups have met this goal. They include women with undergraduate or graduate degrees, men with graduate degrees, Hispanic and Asian women, and people over age 65. Smoking among high school sophomores and seniors has fallen to an all-time low.[3]

Another big drop has occurred in young adults between ages 18 and 24. This was the only age group in which smoking increased from 1993 to 2002, when 28.5 percent of college-age Americans reported smoking. According to the National College Health Assessment, 65 percent of students have never smoked.[4]

Tobacco Use on Campus

About one in every four to five students currently smoke. (See Reality Check.) Still, college students smoke much less than their same-age peers who aren't in school. However, many students who had never tried smoking may experiment with cigarettes in college. Eight in ten college smokers started smoking before age 18. They report smoking on twice as many days and smoke nearly four times as many cigarettes as those who began smoking at an older age.[5]

White students have the highest smoking rates, followed by Hispanic, Asian, and African American students. (See Figure 13.1.) Although black students are least likely to smoke, more are doing so than in the past. Smoking rates remain consistently lower at predominantly black colleges and universities, however.[6] About equal percentages of college men and women smoke. However, women are somewhat more likely than men to report smoking daily.[7]

Many college students say they smoke as a way of managing depression or stress. (See Figure 13.2.) Studies consistently link smoking with depression and low life satisfaction. Smokers are significantly more likely to have higher levels of perceived stress than nonsmokers. In one study, students who had been diagnosed or treated for depression were seven times as likely as other students to use tobacco.

Male students who smoke are more likely to say that smoking makes them feel more masculine and less anxious. More than half of female smokers feel that smoking helps them control their weight, although only 3 percent say it is their primary reason for smoking. Overweight female students are more likely to smoke to lose weight and to see weight gain as a barrier to quitting.

Students can and do change their smoking behavior. In one study, over the course of four years of college, about half of students who smoked every few days, every few

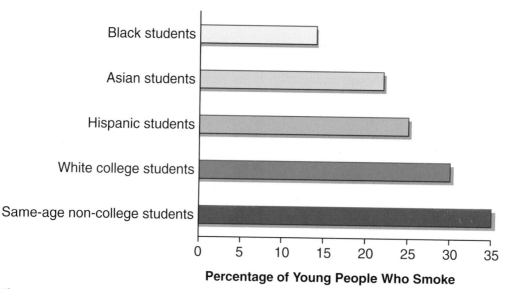

Figure 13.1 Who Smokes More?

Source: *Wasting the Best and the Brightest: Substance Abuse at America's Colleges and Universities.* New York: National Center on Addiction and Substance Abuse at Columbia University, March 2007.

weeks, or every few months quit, as did 13 percent of daily smokers. More than a quarter of daily smokers cut back. On the other hand, 12 percent of nonsmokers took up the habit, and most daily smokers continued to smoke through the end of college.[8]

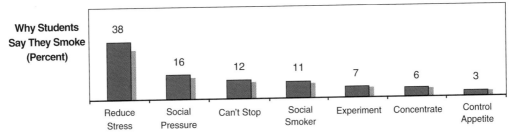

REALITYCHECK

- *How many college students smoke?* _____
- *How many smoked every day in the last month?* _____
- *How many smoked half a pack or more a day in the last month?* _____

Answers on next page.

Why Students Say They Smoke (Percent)

38 — Reduce Stress
16 — Social Pressure
12 — Can't Stop
11 — Social Smoker
7 — Experiment
6 — Concentrate
3 — Control Appetite

Figure 13.2 Why Students Smoke

Source: *Wasting the Best and the Brightest: Substance Abuse at America's Colleges and Universities.* New York: National Center on Addiction and Substance Abuse at Columbia University, March 2007.

Social Smoking

Some college students who smoke say they are "social smokers" who average less than one cigarette a day and smoke mainly in the company of others. On the positive side, social smokers smoke less often and less intensely than other smokers and are less dependent on tobacco. However, they are still jeopardizing their health. The more they smoke, the greater the health risks they face. Even smokers who don't inhale or nonsmokers who breathe in secondhand smoke are at increased risk for negative health effects.

In research studies, smoking less than a pack a week of cigarettes has proved to damage the lining of blood vessels and to increase the risk of heart disease as well as of cancer. In women taking birth control pills, even a few cigarettes a week can increase the likelihood of heart disease, blood clots, stroke, liver cancer, and gallbladder disease. Pregnant women who smoke only occasionally still run a higher risk of giving birth to unhealthy babies. Another risk is addiction. Social smokers are less motivated to quit and make fewer attempts to do so. Many end up smoking more cigarettes for many more years than they intended.

College Tobacco-Control Policies

Other than religious institutions, colleges and universities have traditionally had few smoking restrictions. This has changed. Several national health organizations, including the American College Health Association and National Center on Addiction and Substance Abuse, have recommended that colleges ban smoking in and around all campus buildings,

including student housing, and prohibit the sale, advertisement, and promotion of tobacco products on campus. Although some schools, particularly large public universities, have made progress in adopting such policies, most still fall short of the national recommendations.[9]

Although many colleges now provide smoke-free housing, others have not done so because of concern about increased costs, such as the need for outdoor ciga-

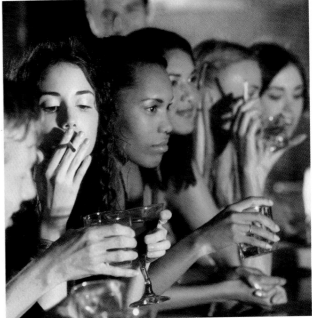

Social smoking has negative short- and long-term health effects and can lead to dependence.

©Jim Arbogast/Photodisc/Getty Images

REALITYCHECK

PART II: *Just the Facts*

- **24** *percent of college students smoke.*
- **12** *percent of students smoked every day in the last month.*
- **7** *percent smoked half a pack or more every day in the last month.*

Source: *Wasting the Best and the Brightest: Substance Abuse at America's Colleges and Universities.* New York: National Center on Addiction and Substance Abuse at Columbia University, March 2007.

rette receptacles. However, universities that have banned smoking from designated residence halls report decreased damage to the buildings, increased retention of students, and improved enforcement of marijuana policies. In general, schools in the West have done the most to implement tobacco policies. Those in the South, particularly in the major tobacco-growing states, have done the least.

Why People Start Smoking

Most people are aware that an enormous health risk is associated with smoking, but many don't know exactly what that risk is or how it might affect them.

The two main factors linked with the onset of a smoking habit are age and education. The majority of white men with less than a high school education are current or former daily cigarette smokers. White women with a similar educational background are also very likely to smoke or to have smoked every day. Hispanic men and women without a high school education are less likely to be or become daily smokers. These factors are associated with reasons for smoking.

Limited Education

People who have graduated from college are much less likely to smoke than high school graduates; those with fewer than 12 years of education are more likely to smoke. An individual with 8 years or less of education is 11 times more likely to smoke than someone with postgraduate training.

Adolescent Experimentation and Rebellion

For teenagers, smoking may be a coping mechanism for dealing with boredom and frustration; a marker of the transition into high school or college; a bid for adult status; a way of gaining admission to a peer group; or a way to have fun, reduce stress, or boost energy. The teenagers most likely to begin smoking are those least likely to seek help when their emotional needs are not met. They might smoke as a means of gaining social acceptance or to self-

medicate when they feel helpless, lonely, or depressed. Depressed teens are more susceptible to cigarette ads than their counterparts. For example, they are more likely to have a favorite cigarette ad or own clothing with cigarette logos.

Stress

In studies that have analyzed the impact of life stressors, depression, emotional support, marital status, and income, researchers have concluded that an individual with a high stress level is approximately 15 times more likely to be a smoker than a person with low stress. About half of smokers identify workplace stress as a key factor in their smoking behavior.

Parental Role Models

Children who start smoking are 50 percent more likely than youngsters who don't smoke to have at least one smoker in their family. A mother who smokes seems a particularly strong influence on making smoking seem acceptable. The majority of youngsters who smoke say that their parents also smoke and are aware of their own tobacco use.

Adolescents are more likely to smoke, express an intention to smoke, or smoke longer if their parents smoke.

Addiction

Nicotine addiction is as strong or stronger than addiction to drugs such as cocaine and heroin. The first symptoms of nicotine addiction can begin within a few days of starting to smoke and after just a few cigarettes, particularly in teenagers. Smoking a single cigarette before age 11 increases the odds of becoming dependent on nicotine. (See Self Survey: "Are You Addicted to Nicotine?")

Mental Disorders

The percentage of smokers jumps to more than 90 percent among those with alcoholism and other addictions, 85 percent among schizophrenia patients, and 80 percent among depressed patients. The relationship between depression and smoking is complex. Smokers are more likely to be depressed, while adults who are depressed are 40 to 50 percent more likely to smoke than adults who are not depressed. Research has identified biological connections between smoking and depression, suggesting a biological similarity between substance use and depressive disorders.

Genetics

Researchers speculate that genes may account for about 50 percent of smoking behavior, with environment playing an equally important role. Studies have shown that identical twins, who have the same genes, are more likely to have matching smoking profiles than fraternal twins. If one identical twin is a heavy smoker, the other is also likely to be; if one smokes only occasionally, so does the other.

 According to NIDA research, genetic factors play a more significant role for initiation of smoking in women than men, but they play a less significant role in smoking persistence for women.

Weight Control

Concern about weight is a significant risk factor for smoking among young women. Daily smokers are two to four times more likely to fast, use diet pills, and purge to control their weight than nonsmokers. Although black girls smoke at substantially lower rates than white girls, the common factor in predicting daily smoking among all girls, regardless of race, is concern with weight.

Aggressive Marketing

Cigarette companies spend more than $13 billion dollars each year on advertisements and promotional campaigns, with manufacturers targeting ads especially at women, teens, minorities, and the poor. Most controversial are cigarette advertisements in magazines and media aimed at teenagers and even younger children.[10]

Why People Keep Smoking

Whatever the reasons for lighting up that first cigarette, very different factors keep cigarettes burning pack after pack, year after year. In national polls, 7 in 10 smokers say that they want to quit but can't. The reason isn't a lack of willpower. Medical scientists have recognized tobacco dependence as an addictive disorder that may be more powerful than heroin dependence and that may affect more than 90 percent of all smokers.

Pleasure

According to the American Cancer Society, 9 in 10 regular smokers find smoking pleasurable. Nicotine—the addictive ingredient in tobacco—is the reason. Researchers have shown that nicotine reinforces and strengthens the desire to smoke by acting on brain chemicals that influence feelings of well-being. This drug also can improve memory, help in performing certain tasks, reduce anxiety, dampen hunger, and increase pain tolerance.

Mental Disorders

Individuals with mental disorders are twice as likely to smoke as others, and people with mental illness may account for nearly one-half of the tobacco market in the United States. Heavy smoking also is linked with an almost elevenfold risk of anxiety disorders in early adulthood.

Smokers with a history of depression are about half as likely to quit as others. Even after a recovery from major depression, smokers often continue to report some symp-

toms of depression. Smokers who are depressed tend to smoke more cigarettes than other smokers, are less successful in their efforts to stop smoking, and are more prone to depression after quitting. The longer people smoke, the more likely they are to develop symptoms of depression and anxiety.

Fear of Weight Gain

Smokers burn up an extra 100 calories a day—the equivalent of walking a mile—probably because nicotine increases metabolic rate. Once they start smoking, many individuals say they cannot quit because they fear they'll gain weight. The CDC estimates that women who stop smoking gain an average of 8 pounds, while men put on an average of 6 pounds. One in eight women and one in ten men who stop smoking put on 29 pounds or more. The reasons for this weight gain include nicotine's effects on metabolism as well as emotional and behavioral factors, such as the habit of frequently putting something into one's mouth. Yet as a health risk, smoking a pack and a half to two packs a day is a greater danger than carrying 60 pounds of extra weight.

Weight gain for smokers who quit is not inevitable. Aerobic exercise helps increase metabolic rate, and limiting alcohol and foods high in sugar and fat can help smokers control their weight as they give up cigarettes.

Dependence

Nicotine has a much more powerful hold on smokers than alcohol does on drinkers. Whereas about 10 percent of alcohol users lose control of their intake of alcohol and become alcoholics, as many as 80 percent of all heavy smokers have tried to cut down on or quit smoking but cannot overcome their dependence.

 About 8 percent of full-time college students meet the diagnostic criteria for past-30-day nicotine dependence, much lower than the rate of the general population (15 percent).[11]

Nicotine causes dependence by at least three means:

- It provides a strong sensation of pleasure.
- It leads to fairly severe discomfort during withdrawal.
- It stimulates cravings long after obvious withdrawal symptoms have passed.

Few drugs act as quickly on the brain as nicotine does. It travels through the bloodstream to the brain in seven seconds—half the time it takes for heroin injected into a blood vessel to reach the brain. And a pack-a-day smoker gets 200 hits of nicotine a day—73,000 a year.

After a few years of smoking, the most powerful incentive for continuing to smoke is to avoid the discomfort of withdrawal. Generally, 10 cigarettes a day will prevent withdrawal effects. For many who smoke heavily, signs of

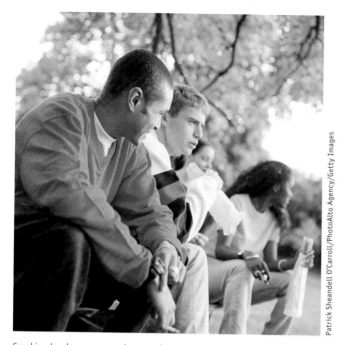

Smoking has become more inconvenient, expensive, and socially unacceptable, but many smokers continue to light up.

Patrick Sheandell O'Carroll/PhotoAlto Agency/Getty Images

withdrawal, including changes in mood and performance, occur within two hours after smoking their last cigarette. Smokeless tobacco users also get constant doses of nicotine. However, absorption of nicotine by the lungs is more likely to lead to dependence than absorption through the linings of the nose and mouth. As with other drugs of abuse, continued nicotine intake results in tolerance (the need for more of a drug to maintain the same effect), which is why only 2 percent of all smokers smoke just a few cigarettes a day, or smoke only occasionally.

Use of Other Substances

Many smokers also drink or use drugs. According to the Addiction Research Foundation in Canada, tobacco smokers say cigarettes are harder to abandon than other drugs, even when they find them less pleasurable than their preferred drug of abuse. Individuals who drink excessively also find their cigarette habit a hard one to break.

Smoking, Gender, and Race

On average, girls who begin smoking during adolescence continue smoking for 20 years, four years longer than boys. Women are at greater risk for developing smoking-related illnesses compared with men who smoke the same amount. Lung cancer now claims more women's lives than breast cancer. In men, cigarette smoking increases the risk of aggressive prostate cancer.

Smoking is a risk factor for developing rheumatoid arthritis for men, but not for women. Women who smoke are more likely to develop osteoporosis, a bone-weakening disease.

According to the U.S. Surgeon General, women account for 39 percent of smoking-related deaths each year, a proportion that has doubled since 1965. Each year, American women lose an estimated 2.1 million years of life due to premature deaths attributable to smoking. If she smokes, a woman's annual risk of dying more than doubles after age 45 compared with a woman who has never smoked.

High nicotine intake may affect male hormones, including testosterone. Smoking also can reduce blood flow to the penis, impairing a man's sexual performance and increasing the likelihood of erectile dysfunction.

Smoking directly affects women's reproductive organs and processes. Women who smoke are less fertile and experience menopause one or two years earlier than women who don't smoke. Smoking also greatly increases the possible risks associated with taking oral contraceptives.

Women who smoke during pregnancy increase their risk of miscarriage and pregnancy complications, including bleeding, premature delivery, and birth defects such as cleft lip or palate. Smoking during the third trimester affects the baby's physical and intellectual development. In one study, the more cigarettes a mother smoked, the lower her son's birth weight and IQ as he matured.

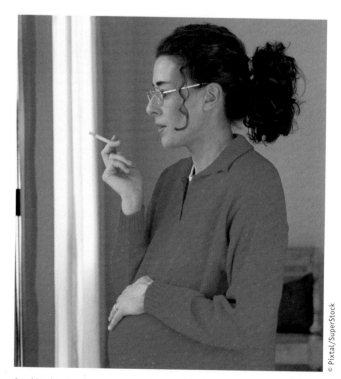

Smoking late in pregnancy can endanger the physical and intellectual development of the unborn child.

© Pixtal/SuperStock

Cigarette smoking is a major cause of disease and death in all population groups. However, tobacco use varies within and among racial and ethnic minority groups. Among adults, Native Americans and Alaska Natives have the highest rates of tobacco use. African American and Southeast Asian men also have a high smoking rate. Asian American and Hispanic women have the lowest rates of smoking. Tobacco use is significantly higher among white college students than among Hispanic, African American, and Asian American students.

Tobacco is the substance most abused by Hispanic youth, whose smoking rates have soared in the last ten years. In general, smoking rates among Hispanic adults increase as they adopt the values, beliefs, and norms of American culture. Recent declines in the prevalence of smoking have been greater among Hispanic men with at least a high school education than among those with less education.

Tobacco's Immediate Effects

Tobacco, an herb that can be smoked or chewed, directly affects the brain. While its primary active ingredient is nicotine, tobacco smoke contains almost 400 other compounds and chemicals, including gases, liquids, particles, tar, carbon monoxide, cadmium, pyridine, nitrogen dioxide, ammonia, benzene, phenol, acrolein, hydrogen cyanide, formaldehyde, and hydrogen sulfide.

How Nicotine Works

A colorless, oily compound, **nicotine** is poisonous in concentrated amounts. If you inhale while smoking, 90 percent of the nicotine in the smoke is absorbed into your body. Even if you draw smoke only into your mouth and not into your lungs, you still absorb 25 to 30 percent of the nicotine. The FDA has concluded that nicotine is a dangerous, addictive drug that should be regulated. Yet in recent years tobacco companies have increased the levels of addictive nicotine by an average of 1.6 percent per year.[12]

Faster than an injection, smoking speeds nicotine to the brain in seconds (Figure 13.3). Nicotine affects the brain in much the same way as cocaine, opiates, and amphetamines, triggering the release of dopamine, a neurotransmitter associated with pleasure and addiction, as well as other messenger chemicals. Because nicotine acts on some of the same brain regions stimulated by interactions with loved ones, smokers come to regard cigarettes as a friend that they turn to when they're stressed, sad, or mad.

Nicotine may enhance smokers' performance on some tasks but leaves other mental skills unchanged. Nicotine also acts as a sedative. How often you smoke and how you

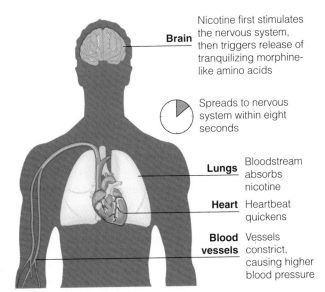

Figure 13.3   The Immediate Effects of Nicotine on the Body
The primary active ingredient in tobacco is nicotine, a fast-acting and potent drug.

Source: American Cancer Society, National Cancer Institute.

smoke determine nicotine's effect on you. If you're a regular smoker, nicotine will generally stimulate you at first, then tranquilize you. Shallow puffs tend to increase alertness because low doses of nicotine facilitate the release of the neurotransmitter *acetylcholine*, which makes the smoker feel alert. Deep drags, on the other hand, relax the smoker because high doses of nicotine block the flow of acetylcholine.

Nicotine stimulates the adrenal glands to produce adrenaline, a hormone that increases blood pressure, speeds up the heart rate by 15 to 20 beats a minute, and constricts blood vessels (especially in the skin). Nicotine also inhibits the formation of urine, dampens hunger, irritates the membranes in the mouth and throat, and dulls the taste buds so foods don't taste as good as they would otherwise.

Nicotine withdrawal usually begins within hours. Symptoms include craving, irritability, anxiety, restlessness, and increased appetite.

Tar and Carbon Monoxide

As it burns, tobacco produces **tar,** a thick, sticky dark fluid made up of several hundred different chemicals—many of them poisonous, some of them *carcinogenic* (enhancing the growth of cancerous cells). As you inhale

---

nicotine   The addictive substance in tobacco; one of the most toxic of all poisons.

tar   A thick, sticky dark fluid produced by the burning of tobacco, made up of several hundred different chemicals, many of them poisonous, some of them carcinogenic.

tobacco smoke, tar and other particles settle in the forks of the branchlike bronchial tubes in your lungs, where precancerous changes are apt to occur. In addition, tar and smoke damage the mucus and the cilia in the bronchial tubes, which normally remove irritating foreign materials from your lungs.

Smoke from cigarettes, cigars, and pipes also contains **carbon monoxide,** the deadly gas that comes out of the exhaust pipes of cars, in levels 400 times those considered safe in industry. Carbon monoxide interferes with the ability of the hemoglobin in the blood to carry oxygen, impairs normal functioning of the nervous system, and is at least partly responsible for the increased risk of heart attacks and strokes in smokers.

Health Effects of Cigarette Smoking

Figure 13.4 shows a summary of the physiological effects of tobacco and the other chemicals in tobacco smoke. If you're a smoker who inhales deeply and started smoking before the age of 15, you're trading a minute of future life for every minute you now spend smoking. On average, smokers die nearly seven years earlier than nonsmokers. Smoking not only eventually kills, it also ages you: Smokers get more wrinkles than nonsmokers.

But the effects of smoking are far more than skin-deep. A cigarette smoker is 10 times more likely to develop lung cancer than a nonsmoker and 20 times more likely to have a heart attack. Daily smokers also are more likely to have suicidal thoughts or attempt suicide, although the reasons are not clear (see Chapter 4).

Health Effects on Students

Although little research has focused specifically on college students, young people who smoke are less physically fit and suffer diminished lung function and growth. Young smokers frequently report symptoms such as wheezing, shortness of breath, coughing, and increased phlegm. They also are more susceptible to respiratory diseases. Young smokers are three times more likely to have consulted a doctor or mental health professional because of an emotional or psychological problem and almost twice as likely to develop symptoms of depression. Frequent smoking also has been linked to panic attacks and panic disorder in young people.[13]

Long-term health consequences of smoking in young adulthood include dental problems, lung disorders (including asthma, chronic bronchitis, and emphysema), heart disease, and cancer. Young women who smoke may develop menstrual problems, including irregular periods

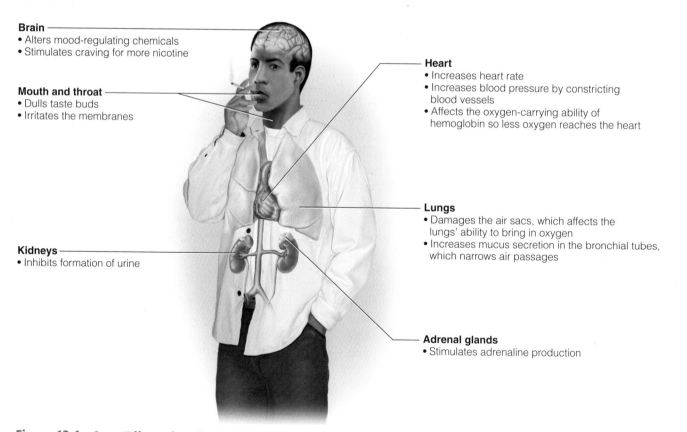

Brain
• Alters mood-regulating chemicals
• Stimulates craving for more nicotine

Mouth and throat
• Dulls taste buds
• Irritates the membranes

Kidneys
• Inhibits formation of urine

Heart
• Increases heart rate
• Increases blood pressure by constricting blood vessels
• Affects the oxygen-carrying ability of hemoglobin so less oxygen reaches the heart

Lungs
• Damages the air sacs, which affects the lungs' ability to bring in oxygen
• Increases mucus secretion in the bronchial tubes, which narrows air passages

Adrenal glands
• Stimulates adrenaline production

Figure 13.4 Some Effects of Smoking on the Body
Smoking harms the respiratory system and the cardiorespiratory system. The leading cause of death for smokers is heart attack.

and painful cramps. If they use oral contraceptives, they are at increased risk of heart disease or stroke.

Heart Disease and Stroke

The toxic chemicals in tobacco signal the heart to beat faster and harder. Blood vessels constrict, forcing blood to travel through a narrower space. Blood pressure increases—temporarily at first. Over time, smokers develop chronic high blood pressure. Smoking increases harmful cholesterol (LDL) and lowers beneficial cholesterol (HDL). It also leads to the buildup of plaque, or fatty deposits within the arteries; hardening of the arteries; and greater risk of blood clots.

Although a great deal of publicity has been given to the link between cigarettes and lung cancer, heart attack is actually the leading cause of death for smokers. Smoking doubles the risk of heart disease and increases the risk of sudden death two to four times. The effect of smoking on risk of heart attack is greater in younger smokers.

Smokers who suffer heart attacks have only a 50 percent chance of recovering. Smokers have a 70 percent higher death rate from heart disease than nonsmokers, and those who smoke heavily have a 200 percent higher death rate.

The federal Office of the Surgeon General blames cigarettes for one of every ten deaths attributable to heart disease. Smoking is more dangerous than the two most notorious risk factors for heart disease: high blood pressure and high cholesterol. If smoking is combined with one of these, the chances of heart attack are four times greater. Women who smoke and use oral contraceptives have a ten times higher risk of suffering heart attacks than women who do neither.

In addition to contributing to heart attacks, cigarette smoking increases the risk of stroke two to three times in men and women, even after other risk factors are taken into account.

Even people who have smoked for decades can reduce their risk of heart attack if they quit smoking. However, studies indicate some irreversible damage to blood vessels. Progression of atherosclerosis (hardening of the arteries) among former smokers continues at a faster pace than among those who never smoked.

Cancer

Smoking is linked to at least ten different cancers and accounts for 30 percent of all deaths from cancer. It is the cause of more than 80 percent of all cases of lung cancer. The more people smoke, the longer they smoke, and the earlier they start smoking, the more likely they are to develop lung cancer.

Smoking causes about 130,000 lung cancer deaths each year. Smokers of two or more packs a day have lung cancer mortality rates 15 to 25 times greater than nonsmokers.

If smokers stop smoking before cancer has started, their lung tissue tends to repair itself, even if there were already precancerous changes.

Chemicals in cigarette smoke and other environmental pollutants switch on a particular gene in the lung cells of some individuals. This gene produces an enzyme that helps manufacture powerful carcinogens, which set the stage for cancer. The gene seems more likely to be activated in some people than others, and people with this gene are at much higher risk of developing lung cancer. However, smokers without the gene still remain at risk, because other chemicals and genes also may be involved in the development of lung cancer.

Smokers who are depressed are more likely to get cancer than nondepressed smokers. Although researchers don't know exactly how smoking and depression may work together to increase the risk of cancer, one possibility is that stress and depression cause biological changes that lower immunity, such as a decline in natural killer cells that fight off tumors.

Respiratory Diseases

Smoking quickly impairs the respiratory system, including the cough reflex, a vital protective response. Even some teenage smokers show signs of respiratory difficulty—breathlessness, chronic cough, excess phlegm production—when compared with nonsmokers of the same age. Cigarette smokers are up to 18 times more likely than nonsmokers to die of noncancerous diseases of the lungs.

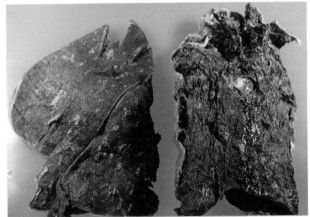

© Arthur Glauberman/Photo Researchers, Inc.

Healthy nonsmoker's lung (left) and smoker's lung (right). Healthy lungs are pink, with a smooth but porous texture. A smoker's lungs show obvious signs of impairment. Bronchial tubes are inflamed, air passages are constricted, and tar coats the bronchial tubes.

carbon monoxide A colorless, odorless gas produced by the burning of gasoline or tobacco; displaces oxygen in the hemoglobin molecules of red blood cells.

Cigarette smoking is the major cause of chronic obstructive pulmonary disease (COPD), which includes emphysema and chronic bronchitis. COPD is characterized by progressive limitation of the flow of air into and out of the lungs. In emphysema, the limitation of air flow is the result of disease changes in the lung tissue, affecting the bronchioles (the smallest air passages) and the walls of the alveoli (the tiny air sacs of the lung). Eventually, many of the air sacs are destroyed, and the lungs become much less able to bring in oxygen and remove carbon dioxide. As a result, the heart has to work harder to deliver oxygen to all organs of the body.

In chronic bronchitis, the bronchial tubes in the lungs become inflamed, thickening the walls of the bronchi, and the production of mucus increases. The result is a narrowing of the air passages. Smoking is more dangerous than any form of air pollution, at least for most Americans, but exposure to both air pollution and cigarettes is particularly harmful.

Other Smoking-Related Problems

Smokers are more likely than nonsmokers to develop gum disease, and they lose significantly more teeth. Even those who quit have worse gum problems than people who never smoked at all. Smoking may also contribute to the loss of teeth and teeth supporting bone, even in individuals with good oral hygiene.

Cigarette smoking is associated with stomach and duodenal ulcers; mouth, throat, and other types of cancer; and cirrhosis of the liver. Smoking may worsen the symptoms or complications of allergies, diabetes, hypertension, peptic ulcers, and disorders of the lungs or blood vessels. Some men who smoke 10 cigarettes or more a day may experience erectile dysfunction. Cigarette smokers also tend to miss work one-third more often than nonsmokers, primarily because of respiratory illnesses. In addition, each year cigarette-ignited fires claim thousands of lives.

Smoking is an independent risk factor for high-frequency hearing loss and also adds to the danger of hearing loss for those exposed to noise (Chapter 19). Cigarette smoking also may increase the likelihood of anxiety, panic attacks, and social phobias.

Other Forms of Tobacco

Two percent of Americans smoke cigars; 2 percent use smokeless tobacco.[14] Ingesting tobacco may be less deadly than smoking cigarettes, but it is dangerous. Smoking cigars, clove cigarettes, and pipes and chewing or sucking on smokeless tobacco all put the user at risk of cancer of the lip, tongue, mouth, and throat, as well as other diseases and ailments. Despite claims of lower risk, "safer" cigarettes still jeopardize smokers' health. (See "Savvy Consumer: Are Safer Cigarettes Really Safe?")

Cigars

 Cigar use has declined in the last few years. However, after cigarettes, cigars are the tobacco product most widely used by college students.

Savvy Consumer Are "Safer" Cigarettes Really Safe?

Tobacco companies are producing low-tar and "lower-risk" cigarettes that they claim reduce secondhand smoke or have fewer carcinogens and less nicotine. For example, Eclipse cigarettes heat rather than burn tobacco inside a cigarette-like tube to reduce the release of carbon monoxide, a big contributor to heart disease. Users of another product, Accord, insert special cigarettes into a small electronic device about the size of a pager that ignites the cigarette when the smoker puffs and sucks up secondhand smoke. Other brands claim to use genetic engineering or a chemical process to remove major carcinogens.

Are these products truly safer? The answer is no. For example, low-tar, "lite" cigarettes impair blood flow just as severely as regular cigarettes.[16] So-called safer cigarettes may actually lead to increased addiction. In one experiment, smokers puffed on their own brand and then on a so-called safer cigarette brand called Advance. While Advance cigarettes supposedly contain less of a type of cancer-causing substance called nitrosamines, they delivered 25 percent more nicotine, the addictive substance in cigarettes, into the blood than the smokers' own brands.

Accord cigarettes deliver less nicotine and boost smokers' heart rates and carbon monoxide levels less than traditional cigarettes. However, they aren't as satisfying to smokers, who may smoke more of them to reduce withdrawal symptoms such as anxiety, restlessness, and irritability.

Eclipse cigarettes suppress withdrawal symptoms about as well as conventional cigarettes. However, they deliver about 30 percent more carbon monoxide than regular cigarettes.

The bottom line: "Safer" cigarettes may reduce some toxins that are associated with smoking-related diseases, but they may increase levels of other dangerous substances and boost the likelihood of addiction. Don't think that you're protecting your health by switching to a "safe" cigarette. There is no such thing. The only proven way to avoid smoking-related risks of disease and death is to stop smoking.

About 16 percent of college men (and 4 percent of women) smoke cigars. White and African American students are more likely to smoke cigars than Hispanic or Asian American students.[15]

Cigar smoking is as dangerous as cigarette smoking even though cigar smokers do not inhale. Cigars can cause cancer of the lung and the digestive tract. The risk of death related to cigars approaches that of cigarettes, depending on the number of cigars smoked and the amount of cigar smoke inhaled. Cigar smoking can lead to nicotine addiction, even if the smoke is not inhaled. The nicotine in the smoke from a single cigar can vary from an amount roughly equivalent to that in a single cigarette to that in a pack or more of cigarettes.

Clove Cigarettes

Sweeteners have long been mixed with tobacco, and clove, a spice, is the latest ingredient to be added to the recipe for cigarettes. Clove cigarettes typically contain two-thirds tobacco and one-third clove. Consumers of these cigarettes are primarily teenagers and young adults.

Many users believe that clove cigarettes are safer because they contain less tobacco, but this isn't necessarily the case. The CDC reports that people who smoke clove cigarettes may be at risk of serious lung injury.

Clove cigarettes deliver twice as much nicotine, tar, and carbon monoxide as moderate-tar American brands. Eugenol, the active ingredient in cloves (which dentists have used as an anesthetic for years), deadens sensation in the throat, allowing smokers to inhale more deeply and hold smoke in their lungs for a longer time. Chemical relatives of eugenol can produce the kind of damage to cells that may lead to cancer.

Bidis

Skinny, sweet-flavored cigarettes called **bidis** (pronounced "beedees") have become a smoking fad among teens and young adults. For centuries, bidis were popular in India, where they are known as the poor man's cigarette and sell for less than five cents a pack. They look strikingly like clove cigarettes or marijuana joints and are available in flavors like grape, strawberry, and mandarin orange. Bidis are legal for adults and even minors in some states and are sold on the Internet as well as in stores.

Although bidis contain less tobacco than regular cigarettes, their unprocessed tobacco is more potent. Smoke from bidis has about three times as much nicotine and carbon monoxide and five times as much tar as smoke from regular filtered cigarettes. Because bidis are wrapped in nonporous brownish leaves, they don't burn as easily as cigarettes, and smokers have to inhale harder and more

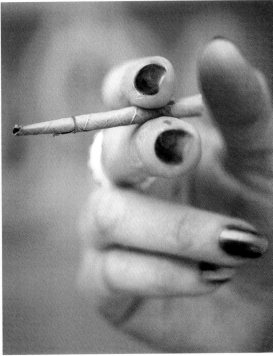

The smoke produced by bidis—skinny, flavored cigarettes—can contain higher concentrations of toxic chemicals than the smoke from regular cigarettes.

often to keep them lit. In one study, smoking a single bidi required 28 puffs, compared to 9 puffs for cigarettes.

Pipes

Many cigarette smokers switch to pipes to reduce their risk of health problems. But former cigarette smokers may continue to inhale, even though pipe smoke is more irritating to the respiratory system than cigarette smoke. People who have smoked only pipes and who do not inhale are much less likely to develop lung and heart disease than cigarette smokers. However, they are as likely as cigarette smokers to develop—and die of—cancer of the mouth, larynx, throat, and esophagus.

Smokeless Tobacco

An estimated 3 percent of adults in the United States use smokeless tobacco products (sometimes called "spit").[17]

 About 9 percent of college men (and .4 percent of women) are smokeless tobacco users.[18] These substances include snuff, finely ground tobacco that can be sniffed or placed inside the cheek and sucked, and chewing tobacco, tobacco leaves mixed with flavoring

bidis Skinny, sweet-flavored cigarettes.

Your Life Change Coach

Quitting

Smoking is a remarkably difficult habit to kick. However, half of all Americans who ever smoked have quit. Half of current smokers try to quit each year, but only 7 percent succeed on their first attempt.[19] (See the "Butt Out" lab in *IPC*.) **IPC**

 About half of whites who have smoked were able to kick the habit, compared with 45 percent of Asian Americans, 43 percent of Hispanics, and 37 percent of African Americans. Men and women with college and graduate degrees were much more likely to quit successfully than high school dropouts.

 Compared with men, women seem to have a higher behavioral dependence on cigarettes. For them, wearing a nicotine patch or chewing nicotine gum does not substitute for the "hand-to-mouth" behaviors associated with smoking, such as lighting a cigarette, inhaling, and handling the cigarette. Some investigators have found that women are more likely to quit successfully when they receive a combination of nicotine replacement and the use of a device like a nicotine inhaler to substitute for smoking behaviors.

One campus-based program that employed peer facilitators to help smokers quit and avoid relapse reported a success rate of 88 percent. Being "in the group" was the single most powerful contributor to quitting, and participants said their sense of connectedness helped them quit and stay smoke-free.

Nicotine withdrawal symptoms can behave like characters in a bad horror flick: Just when you think you've killed them, they're back with a vengeance. In recent studies, some people who tried to quit smoking reported a small improvement in withdrawal symptoms over two weeks, but then their symptoms leveled off and persisted. Others found that their symptoms intensified rather than lessened over time. For reasons scientists cannot yet explain, former smokers who start smoking again put their lungs at even greater jeopardy than smokers who never quit.

Once a former smoker takes a single puff, the odds of a relapse are 80 to 85 percent. Smokers are most likely to quit in the third, fourth, or fifth attempt. But thanks to new products and programs, it may be easier now than ever before to become an ex-smoker (Figure 13.5).

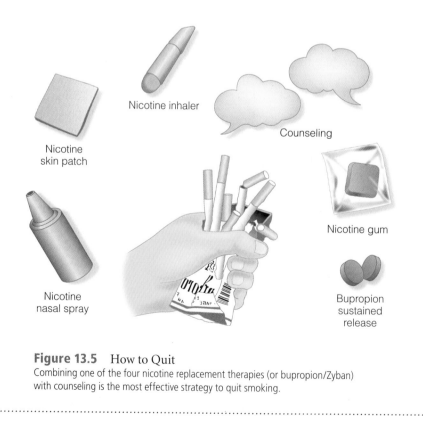

Figure 13.5 How to Quit
Combining one of the four nicotine replacement therapies (or bupropion/Zyban) with counseling is the most effective strategy to quit smoking.

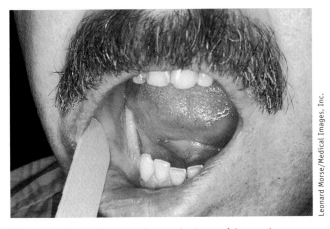

Chewing smokeless tobacco can damage the tissues of the mouth and lead to cancer of the lip, pharynx, larynx, esophagus, kidney, pancreas, and bladder.

Leonard Morse/Medical Images, Inc.

agents such as molasses. With both, nicotine is absorbed through the mucous membranes of the nose or mouth.

Smokeless tobacco causes a user's heart rate, blood pressure, and epinephrine (adrenaline) levels to jump. In addition, it can cause cancer and noncancerous oral conditions and lead to nicotine addiction and dependence. Smokeless tobacco users are more likely than nonusers to become cigarette smokers.

Powerful carcinogens in smokeless tobacco include nitrosamines, polycyclic aromatic hydrocarbons, and radiation-emitting polonium. Its use can lead to the development of white patches on the mucous membranes of the mouth, particularly on the site where the tobacco is placed. Most lesions of the mouth lining that result from the use of smokeless tobacco dissipate six weeks after the use of the tobacco products is stopped. However, when first found, about 5 percent of these lesions are cancerous or exhibit changes that progress to cancer within 10 years if not properly treated. Cancers of the lip, pharynx, larynx, and esophagus have all been linked to smokeless tobacco.

Nicotine replacement with gum or patches (see Your Life Change Coach: "Quitting") decreases cravings for smokeless tobacco and helps with short-term abstinence. However, it does not improve long-term abstinence. Behavioral approaches are more effective for long-term quitting.

Ways to Quit

Quitting on Your Own

More than 90 percent of former smokers quit on their own—by throwing away all their cigarettes, by gradually cutting down, or by first switching to a less potent brand. One characteristic of successful quitters is that they see themselves as active participants in health maintenance and take personal responsibility for their own health.

Often they experiment with a variety of strategies, such as learning relaxation techniques. In women, exercise has proved especially effective for quitting and avoiding weight gain. Making a home a smoke-free zone also increases a smoker's likelihood of successfully quitting.

Stop-Smoking Groups

Joining a support group doubles your chances of quitting for good. The American Cancer Society's FreshStart program runs about 1,500 stop-smoking clinics, each with about 8 to 18 members meeting for eight two-hour sessions over four weeks. Instructors explain the risks of smoking, encourage individuals to think about why they smoke, and suggest ways of unlearning their smoking habit. A quitting day is set for the third or fourth session.

The American Lung Association's Freedom from Smoking program consists of eight one- to two-hour sessions over seven weeks. The approach is similar to the American Cancer Society's, but smokers keep diaries and team up with buddies. Ex-smokers serve as advisers on quitting day. Both groups estimate that 27 or 28 percent of their participants successfully stop smoking.

Stop-smoking classes are also available through science departments and student health services on many college campuses, as well as through community public health departments. The Seventh-Day Adventists sponsor a four-week Breathe Free Plan, in which smokers commit themselves to clean living (no smoking, alcohol, tea, or coffee, along with a balanced diet and regular exercise).

Many businesses sponsor smoking-cessation programs for employees, which generally follow the approaches of professional groups. Motivation may be even higher in these programs than in programs outside the workplace because some companies offer attractive incentives to participants, such as lower rates on their health insurance.

Some smoking-cessation programs rely primarily on **aversion therapy,** which provides a negative experience every time a smoker has a cigarette. This may involve taking drugs that make tobacco smoke taste unpleasant, undergoing electric shocks, having smoke blown at you, or rapid smoking (the inhaling of smoke every six seconds until you're dizzy or nauseated).

Nicotine Anonymous, a nonprofit organization based on the 12 steps to recovery developed by Alcoholics Anonymous (see Chapter 12), acknowledges the power of nico-

aversion therapy A treatment that attempts to help a person overcome a dependence or bad habit by making the person feel disgusted or repulsed by that habit.

tine and provides support to help smokers, chewers, and dippers live free of nicotine. New members are encouraged to abstain from using nicotine "one day at a time" and to attend meetings regularly. In addition to local meetings, NicA offers online support and networking, which puts people in touch with others in their region who share their desire to quit using nicotine.

Telephone-counseling "quit lines," which advise smokers on how to restructure their lives and deal with urges, are helpful because people can get counseling without leaving their homes. The quality of online smoking cessation websites is not consistent, and information is often hard to find, incomplete, or not based on research.[20]

Nicotine Replacement Therapy (NRT)

This approach uses a variety of products that supply low doses of nicotine in a way that allows smokers to taper off gradually over a period of months. Nicotine replacement therapies include nonprescription products (nicotine gum and nicotine patches) and prescription products (nicotine nasal spray and nicotine inhaler). The nasal spray, dispensed from a pump bottle, delivers nicotine to the nasal membranes and reaches the bloodstream faster than any other nicotine replacement therapy product. The inhaler delivers nicotine into the mouth and enters the bloodstream much more slowly than the nicotine in cigarettes.[21]

Smokers who use NRT are 1.5 to 2 times more likely to quit.[22] Because nicotine is a powerful, addictive substance, using nicotine replacements for a prolonged period is not advised. Pregnant women and individuals with heart disease shouldn't use them.

The most effective approaches combine medication—nicotine patches or Zyban, for instance—with psychological intervention. Each doubles a person's chance of quitting successfully.

 Nicotine replacement therapy has proved more beneficial for men than women—particularly with higher doses of nicotine. Men who receive more nicotine achieve a higher quit rate than men getting lower doses.

For women, the nicotine "dose" does not have an impact on successful quitting. They are no more likely to stop smoking with high doses than with lower ones, indicating that they may be less dependent on nicotine than men.

Nicotine Gum

Nicotine gum (now available in generics as well) contains a nicotine resin that's gradually released as the gum is chewed. Absorbed through the mucous membrane of the mouth, the nicotine doesn't produce the same rush as a deeply inhaled drag on a cigarette. However, the gum maintains enough nicotine in the blood to diminish withdrawal symptoms.

Although this gum is lightly spiced to mask nicotine's bitterness, many users say that it takes several days to become accustomed to its unusual taste. Its side effects include mild indigestion, sore jaws, nausea, heartburn, and stomachache. Also, because nicotine gum is heavier than regular chewing gum, it may loosen fillings or cause problems with dentures. Drinking coffee or other beverages may block absorption of the nicotine in the gum; individuals trying to quit smoking shouldn't ingest any substance immediately before or while chewing nicotine gum.

Most people use nicotine gum as a temporary crutch and gradually taper off until they can stop chewing it relatively painlessly. However, 5 to 10 percent of users transfer their dependence from cigarettes to the gum. When they stop using nicotine gum, they experience withdrawal symptoms, although the symptoms tend to be milder than those prompted by quitting cigarettes. Intensive counseling to teach smokers coping methods can greatly increase success rates.

Nicotine Patches

Nicotine transdermal delivery system products, or patches, provide nicotine, their only active ingredient, via a patch attached to the skin by an adhesive. Like nicotine gum, the nicotine patch minimizes withdrawal symptoms, such as intense craving for cigarettes. Nicotine patches help nearly 20 percent of smokers quit entirely after six weeks, compared with 7 percent on a placebo patch. Some insurance programs pay for patch therapy. Nicotine patches, which cost between $3.25 and $4 each, are replaced daily during therapy programs that run between 6 and 16 weeks. There is no evidence that continuing their use for more than 8 weeks provides added benefit.

Some patches deliver nicotine around the clock and others for just 16 hours (during waking hours). Those most likely to benefit from nicotine patch therapy are people who smoke more than a pack a day, are highly motivated to quit, and participate in counseling programs. While using the patch, 37 to 77 percent of people are able to abstain from smoking. When combined with counseling, the patch can be about twice as effective as a placebo, enabling 26 percent of smokers to abstain for six months.

Patch wearers who smoke or use more than one patch at a time can experience a nicotine overdose; some users have even suffered heart attacks. Occasional side effects include redness, itching, or swelling at the site of the patch application; insomnia; dry mouth; and nervousness.

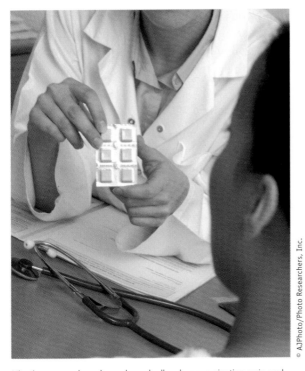

Nicotine gum, when chewed, gradually releases a nicotine resin and helps some smokers break their habit.

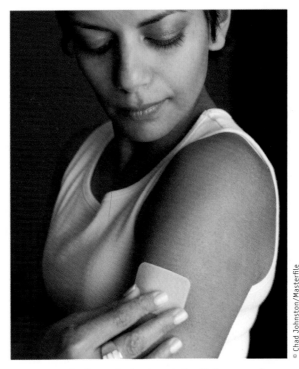

A nicotine patch releases nicotine through the skin in measured amounts, which are gradually decreased over time.

Nicotine Inhaler

Available only by prescription, the Nicotine Inhaler consists of a mouthpiece and a cartridge containing a nicotine-impregnated plug. The smoker inhales through the mouthpiece, using either shallow or deep puffs. The inhaled air becomes saturated with nicotine, which is absorbed mainly through the tissues of the mouth. The inhaler releases less nicotine per puff than a cigarette and does not contain a cigarette's harmful tars, carbon monoxide, and smoke. Treatment is recommended for three months with a gradual reduction over the next six to twelve weeks. Total treatment should not exceed six months.[23]

Bupropion (Zyban)

Another alternative to the patch is *bupropion*, a drug initially developed to treat depression, that is marketed in a slow-release form for nicotine addiction as Zyban. In studies that have combined Zyban with nicotine replacement and counseling, 40 to 60 percent of those treated have remained smoke-free for at least a year after completing the program. This success rate is much higher than the 10 to 26 percent reported among smokers who try to quit by using nicotine replacement alone. The combination of Zyban and nicotine replacement also prevented the initial weight gain that often accompanies quitting. Other medications used to treat nicotine addiction are clonidine, mecamylamine, and buspirone.

Other Ways to Quit

Hypnosis may help some people quit smoking. Hypnotherapists use their techniques to create an atmosphere of strict attention and give smokers in a mild trance positive suggestions for breaking their cigarette habit.

Acupuncture, in which a circular needle or staple is inserted in the flap in front of the opening to the ear, has also had some success. When smokers feel withdrawal symptoms, they gently move the needle or staple, which may increase the production of calming chemicals in the brain.

Since 1976, a November day has been set aside in the United States for the annual Great American Smoke-Out, an idea promoted by the American Cancer Society to encourage smokers to give up cigarettes for 24 hours. As many as 36 percent of American smokers have given up cigarettes on Smoke-Out Day; about 5 to 6 percent have quit permanently; 15 percent reduced smoking for extended periods. In addition, the World Health Organization has established World No-Tobacco Days in May to call on nations to urge tobacco users to abstain for at least one day and perhaps quit for good.

Quitting and the Risks Associated with Smoking

Not smoking another cigarette is a gift to your body and your life. It is not a guarantee that there will be no consequences of the cigarettes you've already smoked.

Within a year of quitting, an ex-smoker's risk of heart disease drops to half that of active smokers. After 15 years, it approaches that of people who've never smoked. This is great news because the risk of dying prematurely from heart disease is far greater than that of dying from cancer.

The risk of lung cancer from smoking fades more slowly, perhaps because of permanent DNA damage to lung cells. Even 10 to 15 years after quitting, an ex-smoker is several times more likely to die of lung cancer than someone who has never smoked. Former smokers are also more vulnerable to the effects of secondhand smoke in the workplace, even if they haven't lit up for the last ten years.[24]

Does the lung cancer risk ever go away? That may depend partly on how old you are when you quit. Women who quit before age 30 are no more likely to die from lung cancer than those who never smoked. However, a study of American veterans started in the 1950s showed that, even 40 years later, former smokers had a 50 percent greater chance of dying from lung cancer than lifetime nonsmokers.

While quitting sooner is better than later, later is better than never. Even smokers who quit in their sixties significantly reduce their lung cancer risk—and add several years to their life expectancy.

Environmental Tobacco Smoke

Maybe you don't smoke—never have, never will. That doesn't mean you don't have to worry about the dangers of smoking, especially if you live or work with people who smoke. **Environmental tobacco smoke,** or secondhand cigarette smoke, the most hazardous form of indoor air pollution, ranks behind cigarette smoking and alcohol as the third-leading preventable cause of death.

On average, a smoker inhales what is known as **mainstream smoke** eight or nine times with each cigarette, for a total of about 24 seconds. However, the cigarette burns for about 12 minutes, and everyone in the room (including the smoker) breathes in what is known as **sidestream smoke.**

According to the American Lung Association, incomplete combustion from the lower temperatures of a smoldering cigarette makes sidestream smoke dirtier and chemically different from mainstream smoke. It has twice as much tar and nicotine, five times as much carbon monoxide, and 50 times as much ammonia. And because the particles in sidestream smoke are small, this mixture of irritating gases and carcinogenic tar reaches deeper into the lungs. If you're a nonsmoker sitting next to someone smoking seven cigarettes an hour, even in a ventilated room, you'll take in almost twice the maximum amount of carbon monoxide set for air pollution in industry—and it will take hours for the carbon monoxide to leave your body.

The Risks of Secondhand Smoke

Even a little secondhand smoke is dangerous. According to the CDC, nonsmokers exposed to environmental tobacco smoke increase their heart disease risk by 25 to 30 percent and their lung cancer risk by 20 to 30 percent.[25] As a cancer-causing agent, secondhand smoke may be twice as dangerous as radon gas and more than a hundred times more hazardous than outdoor pollutants regulated by federal law. Secondhand smoke also increases the sick leave rates among employees.

Numerous epidemiological and autopsy studies have linked environmental tobacco smoke with lung cancer and other disorders. The nonsmoking spouses of smokers, for instance, are 30 percent more likely to die of heart disease than other nonsmokers.

Prenatal exposure to tobacco can have significant effects that may extend from infancy into adulthood. A mother's smoking during pregnancy affects a child's growth, cognitive development, and behavior both before and after birth. Birthweight decreases in direct proportion to the number of cigarettes smoked. The babies of teenage mothers who smoke have lower birthweight, length, head circumference, and chest circumference. As they grow, children of smokers tend to be shorter and weigh less than children of nonsmokers.

A mother's smoking during pregnancy may have cognitive and behavioral effects on the child as well. These include abnormal neurological responses, such as more tremors and startles. Among older children, researchers have found deficits in language and reading abilities

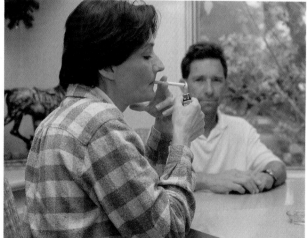

Secondhand smoke is the most common and hazardous form of indoor air pollution.

POINT COUNTERPOINT *Are Smokers Victims of Discrimination?*

POINT

State and federal civil rights laws prevent discrimination based on age, race, color, gender, marital status, national origin, weight, height, and religion. No-smoking bans in public and private places violate the rights of smokers and encourage discriminatory treatment of the victims of nicotine dependence.

COUNTERPOINT

As science has conclusively shown, tobacco is hazardous to non-smokers as well as smokers. No one has the right to jeopardize the health of others. Nicotine dependence may be very difficult to break, but individuals who chose to start smoking must face all the consequences, including restrictions on where they can light up.

YOUR VIEW

Should smokers be singled out for exclusion from certain places? Are they a threat to public health? Do you smoke or not? If you do, how do you feel about smoking restrictions? If not, how do you feel when someone lights up next to you? Do you ever ask smokers to move or put out their cigarettes? Do you feel you have a right to do so?

---

and poorer visual perception. Youngsters whose mothers smoked during pregnancy also tend to have problems with hyperactivity, inattention, and impulsivity. Some of these behavior problems persist through the teenage years and even into adulthood. At ages 16 to 18, children exposed to prenatal smoking have higher rates of conduct disorder, substance use, and depression than others.

Even if their mothers don't smoke, children exposed to secondhand smoke before birth also are likely to weigh less and to perform more poorly on tests of speech, language skills, intelligence, and visual-spatial abilities and to develop behavior problems. These youngsters perform at a level between that of children of active smokers and children of nonsmokers.

Exposure to smoke after birth increases the risk of sudden infant death syndrome (SIDS) and is associated with lower IQ scores and deficits in cognitive development.

Children who breathe environmental tobacco smoke suffer from more asthma, wheezing, and bronchitis than children in smoke-free homes. They also face increased risk of lung cancer, heart disease, and stroke. African American children may be more susceptible to the toxins in secondhand smoke.[26]

 The negative effects of early exposure to environmental tobacco smoke persist even after youngsters leave home. In recent research at Ohio State University, college students who grew up in a smokers' household had higher resting heart rates and blood pressure at rest and during psychological stress than those who grew up in smoke-free homes. Teen exposure to cigarette smoke increases the risk of metabolic syndrome (discussed in Chapter 14).[27]

The Politics of Tobacco

More than three decades after U.S. government health authorities began to warn of the dangers of cigarette smoking, tobacco remains a politically hot topic. However, a majority of people support tobacco control strategies, including creation of smoke-free environments, an increase in cigarette excise taxes, more funds to prevent people from smoking and to help smokers quit, and restriction of youth access to tobacco. (See Point/Counterpoint.)

The Tobacco Industry Payout

After many years of difficult negotiations, the tobacco industry and attorneys general from nearly 40 states reached a historic settlement. Major tobacco companies have agreed to pay more than $200 billion to settle smoking-related lawsuits filed by 46 states, to finance antismoking campaigns, to restrict marketing, to permit federal regulation of tobacco, and to pay fines if tobacco use by minors does not decline.

The funds from the U.S. state tobacco settlement, won in 1998, were supposed to support antismoking programs, but the majority of that funding is not being spent on anything related to smoking. Most of the money has gone to make up for budget shortfalls.

Increasing the price of cigarettes by 10 percent reduces the number of smokers by about 2 percent. Many states have raised taxes on cigarettes; some now charge more than a dollar a pack. Although personal health warnings are not particularly effective, new in-your-face warning labels are grabbing smokers' attention; for example, extra-large Canadian cigarette labels show rotting lungs and decaying teeth. The stronger, more graphic warning labels on cigarettes sold in Canada have proved more effective with young adults than the print-only warnings the United States uses.[28]

---

environmental tobacco smoke Secondhand cigarette smoke; the third-leading preventable cause of death.

mainstream smoke The smoke inhaled directly by smoking a cigarette.

sidestream smoke The smoke emitted by a burning cigarette and breathed by everyone in a closed room, including the smoker; contains more tar and nicotine than mainstream smoke.

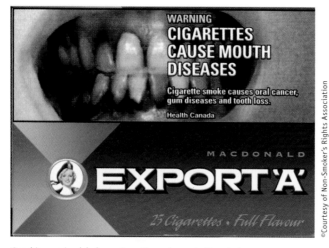

Graphic warning labels on cigarette packages in Canada have proven effective in discouraging smoking.

The Fight for Clean Air

Nonsmokers, realizing that their health is being jeopardized by environmental tobacco smoke, have increasingly turned to legislative and administrative measures to clear the air and protect their rights (Figure 13.6). (See also Your Strategies for Prevention: "How to Clear the Air.") Most states now have some restrictions on smoking in bars, restaurants, and workplaces. Nationally, the airlines have banned smoking on domestic flights. Many institutions, including medical centers and some universities, no longer allow smoking on their premises. States that have launched comprehensive antismoking programs, including higher cigarette taxes and a media campaign, have lowered smoking prevalence[29] and secondhand smoke levels.[30]

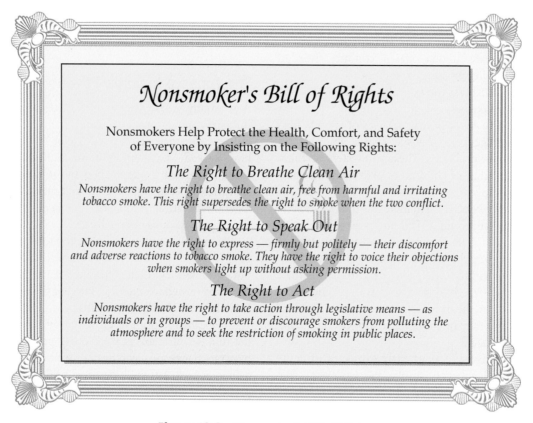

Nonsmoker's Bill of Rights

Nonsmokers Help Protect the Health, Comfort, and Safety of Everyone by Insisting on the Following Rights:

The Right to Breathe Clean Air

Nonsmokers have the right to breathe clean air, free from harmful and irritating tobacco smoke. This right supersedes the right to smoke when the two conflict.

The Right to Speak Out

Nonsmokers have the right to express — firmly but politely — their discomfort and adverse reactions to tobacco smoke. They have the right to voice their objections when smokers light up without asking permission.

The Right to Act

Nonsmokers have the right to take action through legislative means — as individuals or in groups — to prevent or discourage smokers from polluting the atmosphere and to seek the restriction of smoking in public places.

Figure 13.6 Nonsmoker's Bill of Rights

YOUR STRATEGIES FOR PREVENTION *How to Clear the Air*

- Let people know your feelings in advance by putting up "No Smoking" signs in your office, home, or car. If you're in a car and someone pulls out a cigarette, ask politely if the smoker can hold off until you reach your destination or stop for a break.

- If you're about to participate in a long meeting or class, find out if there are smoking restrictions. If there are, ask that they be enforced. If not, ask for a voluntary moratorium on smoking.

- At restaurants, always ask for a table in the nonsmoking section or, if there is none, one in a well-ventilated part of the restaurant.

- If someone's smoke is bothering you, speak up. Be polite, not pushy. Say something like, "Excuse me, but smoke bothers me."

Learn It : Live It

Becoming Smoke-Free

If you smoke—even just a few cigarettes a few times a week—you are at risk of nicotine addiction. Here is how to get back into control:

- **Use delaying tactics.** Have your first cigarette of the day 15 minutes later than usual, then 15 minutes later than that the next day, and so on.
- **Distract yourself.** When you feel a craving for a cigarette, talk to someone, drink a glass of water, or get up and move around.
- **Establish nonsmoking hours.** Instead of lighting up at the end of a meal, for instance, get up immediately, brush your teeth, wash your hands, or take a walk.
- **Never smoke two packs of the same brand in a row.** Buy cigarettes only by the pack, not by the carton.
- **Make it harder to get to your cigarettes.** Lock them in a drawer, wrap them in paper, or leave them in your coat or car.

- **Change the way you smoke.** Smoke with the hand you don't usually use. Smoke only half of each cigarette.
- **Stop completely for just one day at a time.** Promise yourself 24 hours of freedom from cigarettes; when the day's over, make the same commitment for one more day. At the end of any 24-hour period, you can go back to smoking and not feel guilty.
- **Spend more time in places where you can't smoke.** Take up bike-riding or swimming. Shower often. Go to movies or other places where smoking isn't allowed.
- **Go cold turkey.** If you're a heavily addicted smoker, try a decisive and complete break. Smokers who quit completely are less likely to light up again than those who gradually decrease their daily cigarette consumption, switch to low-tar and low-nicotine brands, or use special filters and holders.
- If these tactics don't work, talk to your doctor about nicotine replacement options or prescription medications.

SELFSURVEY : *Are You Addicted to Nicotine?*

Answer the following questions as honestly as you can by placing a check mark in the appropriate column.

	Yes	No
1. Do you smoke every day?	_____	_____
2. Do you smoke because of shyness and to build up self-confidence?	_____	_____
3. Do you smoke to escape from boredom and worries or while under pressure?	_____	_____
4. Have you ever burned a hole in your clothes, carpet, furniture, or car with a cigarette?	_____	_____
5. Have you ever had to go to the store late at night or at another inconvenient time because you were out of cigarettes?	_____	_____
6. Do you feel defensive or angry when people tell you that your smoke is bothering them?	_____	_____
7. Has a doctor or dentist ever suggested that you stop smoking?	_____	_____
8. Have you ever promised someone that you would stop smoking, then broken your promise?	_____	_____
9. Have you ever felt physical or emotional discomfort when trying to quit?	_____	_____
10. Have you ever successfully stopped smoking for a period of time, only to start again?	_____	_____
11. Do you buy extra supplies of tobacco to make sure you won't run out?	_____	_____
12. Do you find it difficult to imagine life without smoking?	_____	_____

	Yes	No
13. Do you choose only those activities and entertainments during which you can smoke?	_____	_____
14. Do you prefer, seek out, or feel more comfortable in the company of smokers?	_____	_____
15. Do you inwardly despise or feel ashamed of yourself because of your smoking?	_____	_____
16. Do you ever find yourself lighting up without having consciously decided to?	_____	_____
17. Has your smoking ever caused trouble at home or in a relationship?	_____	_____
18. Do you ever tell yourself that you can stop smoking whenever you want to?	_____	_____
19. Have you ever felt that your life would be better if you didn't smoke?	_____	_____
20. Do you continue to smoke even though you are aware of the health hazards posed by smoking?	_____	_____

If you answered Yes to one or two of these questions, there's a chance that you are addicted or are becoming addicted to nicotine. If you answered Yes to three or more of these questions, you are probably already addicted to nicotine.

Source: Nicotine Anonymous World Services, San Francisco.

Your Health Action Plan for Kicking the Habit

Here's a six-point program to help you or someone you love quit smoking. (Caution: Don't undertake the quit-smoking program until you have a two- to four-week period of relatively unstressful work and study schedules or social commitments.)

1. *Identify your smoking habits.* Keep a daily diary (a piece of paper wrapped around your cigarette pack with a rubber band will do) and record the time you smoke, the activity associated with smoking (after breakfast, in the car), and your urge for a cigarette (desperate, pleasant, or automatic). For the first week or two, don't bother trying to cut down; just use the diary to learn the conditions under which you smoke.

2. *Get support.* It can be tough to go it alone. Phone your local chapter of the American Cancer Society or Nicotine Anonymous or otherwise get the names of some ex-smokers who can give you support.

3. *Begin by tapering off.* For a period of one to four weeks, aim at cutting down to, say, 12 or 15 cigarettes a day; or change to a lower-nicotine brand and concentrate on not increasing the number of cigarettes you smoke. As indicated by your diary, begin by cutting out those cigarettes you smoke automatically. In addition, restrict the times you allow yourself to smoke. Throughout this period, stay in touch, once a day or every few days, with your ex-smoker friend(s) to discuss your problems.

4. *Set a quit date.* At some point during the tapering-off period, announce to everyone—friends, family, and ex-smokers—when you're going to quit. Do it with flair. Announce it to coincide with a significant date, such as your birthday or anniversary.

5. *Stop.* A week before Q-day, smoke only five cigarettes a day. Begin late in the day, say after 4:00 P.M. Smoke the first two cigarettes in close succession. Then, in the evening, smoke the last three, also in close succession, about 15 minutes apart. Focus on the negative aspects of cigarettes, such as the rawness in your throat and lungs. After seven days, quit and give yourself a big reward on that day, such as a movie or a fantastic meal or new clothes.

6. *Follow up.* Stay in touch with your ex-smoker friend(s) during the following two weeks, particularly if anything stressful or tense occurs that might trigger a return to smoking. Think of the person you're becoming—the very person cigarette ads would have you believe smoking makes you. Now that you're quitting smoking, you're becoming healthier, sexier, more sophisticated, more mature, and better looking—and you've earned it!

Sources: American Cancer Society, National Cancer Institute.

CENGAGENOW™ If you want to write your own goals for tobacco use, go to the Wellness Journal at HealthNow: **academic.cengage.com/login.**

Making This Chapter Work for YOU

Review Questions

1. Which of the following statements about smoking is *false?*
   a. Smoking behavior may have a genetic component.
   b. People who graduate college are less likely to smoke than those who complete only high school.
   c. Most regular smokers enjoy smoking.
   d. Nicotine addiction doesn't take hold until six months after a person starts smoking.

2. Tobacco use on college campuses
   a. is higher among black students.
   b. continues to increase despite no-smoking policies by all schools.
   c. less than that of same-age peers who aren't in school.
   d. is most often in the form of smokeless tobacco.

3. Which of the following statements about smoking and race is true?
   a. Hispanic men are less likely to smoke than Hispanic women.
   b. Native Americans smoke less than African Americans and Asian Americans.
   c. Smoking is culturally unacceptable among Southeast Asian American men.
   d. Caucasian college students smoke more than African American and Asian American students.

4. Women smokers
   a. are more likely to die from breast cancer than lung cancer.
   b. are less fertile than nonsmokers.
   c. are less likely to develop osteoporosis.
   d. bear children with fewer birth defects.

5. Which of the following statements about tobacco and its components is true?
   a. Nicotine affects the central nervous system in eight seconds.
   b. Tobacco stimulates the kidneys to form urine.
   c. Carbon monoxide contained in tobacco smoke is an addictive substance.
   d. The tar in burning tobacco impairs oxygen transport in the body.

6. Cigarette smokers
   a. are more likely to die of lung cancer than heart disease.
   b. usually develop lung problems after years of tobacco use.
   c. have two to three times the risk of suffering a stroke than nonsmokers.
   d. may completely reverse the damage to their blood vessels if they quit smoking.

7. Which of the following statements is *false?*
   a. Using chewing tobacco can lead to lesions on the mucous membranes of the mouth.
   b. Bidis come in several flavors.
   c. The active ingredient in cloves lowers sensation in the throat, so clove-cigarette smokers inhale more deeply.
   d. Smoking cigars is safe if you don't inhale.

8. Quitting smoking
   a. usually results in minor withdrawal symptoms.
   b. will do little to reverse the damage to the lungs and other parts of the body.
   c. can be aided by using nicotine replacement products.
   d. is best done by cutting down on the number of cigarettes you smoke over a period of months.

9. Ways to help yourself quit include all of the following *except*
   a. join a support group.
   b. make your home a smoke-free zone.
   c. try acupuncture.
   d. switch to bidis.

10. Secondhand tobacco smoke is
    a. the smoke inhaled by a smoker.
    b. more hazardous than outdoor pollution as a cancer-causing agent.
    c. less hazardous than mainstream smoke.
    d. less likely to cause serious health problems in children than in adults.

Answers to these questions can be found on page 583.

Critical Thinking

1. Has smoking become unpopular among your friends or family? What social activities continue to be associated with smoking? Can you think of any situation in which smoking might be frowned upon?

2. How would you motivate someone you care about to stop smoking? What reasons would you give for them to stop? Describe your strategy.

3. According to the chapter, environmental tobacco smoke is even more dangerous than mainstream smoke. If you're a nonsmoker, how would you react to someone who's smoking in the same room you occupy? Define the rights of smokers and nonsmokers.

Media Menu

CENGAGENOW™ Go to the HealthNow website at **academic**
.cengage.com/login that will:

- Help you evaluate your knowledge of the material.
- Allow you to take an exam-prep quiz.
- Provide a Personalized Learning Plan targeting resources that address areas you should study.
- Coach you through identifying target goals for behavioral change and creating and monitoring your personal change plan throughout the semester.

INTERNET CONNECTIONS

Smoking & Tobacco Use, CDC

www.cdc.gov/tobacco

This comprehensive feature on the Centers for Disease Control and Prevention (CDC) website provides educational information, research, a report from the U.S. Surgeon General, tips on how to quit, and much more.

Joe Chemo—an antismoking site

http://joechemo.org

Based on the character Joe Chemo, an antismoking parody of Joe Camel, this site is highly interactive and allows visitors to test their "Tobacco IQ," get a personalized "Smoke-o-Scope," and send free Joe Chemo e-cards. There is also extensive information for teachers, antismoking activists, health-care providers, journalists, and smokers who wish to quit.

Tobacco Facts

www.tobaccofacts.org

This excellent site provides access to many facts and resources regarding tobacco use.

Tobacco Control Resource Center and Tobacco Products Liability Project (TPLP)

www.tobacco.neu.edu

This site provides current information on tobacco-related litigation and legislation.

Key Terms

The terms listed are used and defined on the page indicated. Definitions are also found in the Glossary at the end of this book.

aversion therapy 383
bidis 381
carbon monoxide 379
environmental tobacco smoke 387
mainstream smoke 387
nicotine 377
sidestream smoke 387
tar 377

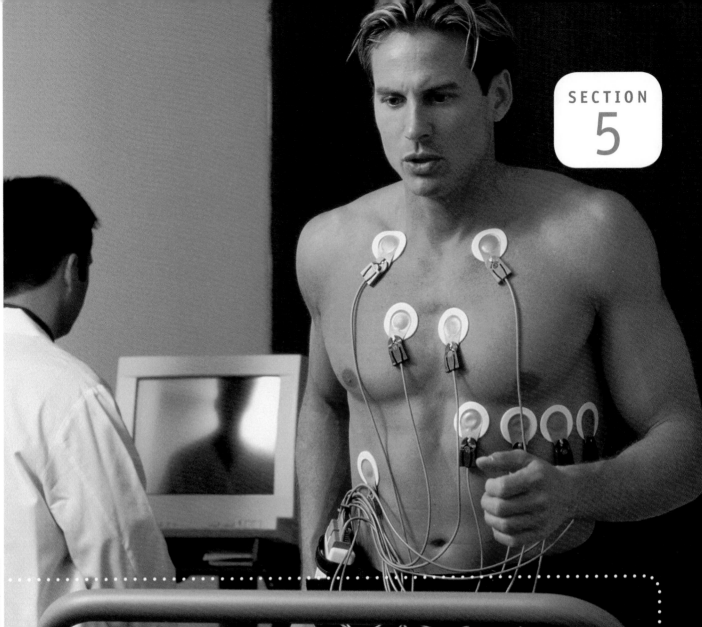

Protecting Your Health

E **VERY** day you make choices that affect both the quantity and the quality of your life. The right choices aren't always easy to make or to sustain. The chapters in this section can help by providing information you can use in making and implementing healthful decisions. By understanding the risks to your health, you can take steps to eliminate or overcome them—and not simply live life, but celebrate it every day.

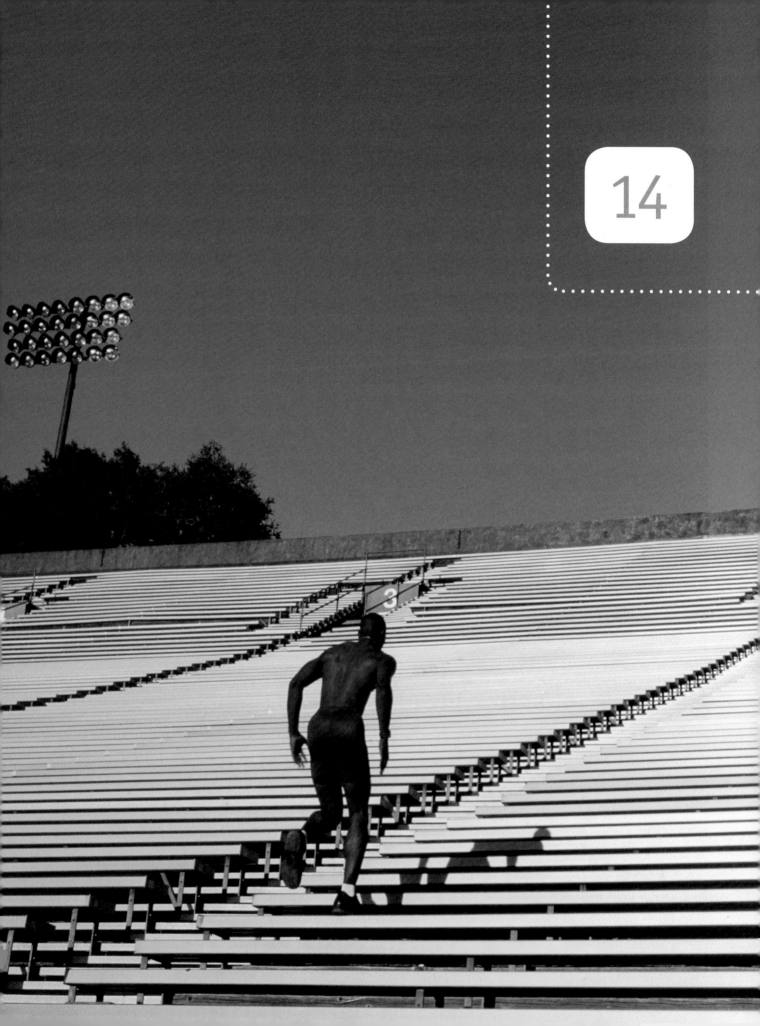

14

Preventing Major Diseases

JAMAL never forgot the terror he felt when his Dad had his first heart attack. Only ten, he couldn't understand why this towering giant of a man had fallen to the ground, his face twisted in pain, his fist pressed against his chest. His father seemed different when he came home from the hospital, as if something had gone out of him. But his face would still light up with an impish grin, especially when he'd sneak a cigarette and wink at Jamal so he wouldn't tell his mother. The second heart attack came four years later. This time Jamal's Dad didn't come home.

Jamal promised his mother that he'd take better care of his heart. He wouldn't smoke; he'd watch his blood pressure and weight; he'd keep tabs on his diet; he'd exercise regularly. Jamal didn't forget these promises as time passed. But like many college students, he felt invincible. He was shocked when a sports physical revealed that his blood pressure was high and his levels of the most dangerous type of cholesterol were elevated. But he also felt lucky: "I got my wake-up call," he explains. "And I'm not going to ignore it."

As Jamal realizes, it's never too soon, or too late, to start protecting your health and your future. Whether or not you will get a serious disease at some time in your life may seem to be a matter of odds. Genetic tendencies, environmental factors, and luck affect your chances of having to face many health threats. However, often you can prevent or delay major illnesses, such as heart disease, for years, even decades.

The time to start protecting your health is now. People mistakenly think of heart disease, cancer, and other disorders as illnesses of middle and old age. But the events leading up to these diseases often begin in childhood, progress in adolescence, and become a health threat to men in their thirties and forties and to women in their forties and fifties. This chapter provides the information about the risk factors, silent dangers, and medical advances that can improve your chances of a healthier, longer life.

After studying the material in this chapter, you should be able to:

- **Define** cardiometabolic health, and **list** actions for lowering cardiometabolic risk.

- **Explain** the disease process of diabetes mellitus, and **describe** the early symptoms and treatment for this disease.

- **Define** hypertension, and **discuss** why it is dangerous and ways to prevent it.

- **Describe** the types of cholesterol that compose your lipoprotein profile and the effects of each on cardiometabolic health.

- **Explain** how the heart functions, and **define** a myocardial infarction.

- **Define** stroke and transient ischemic attacks.

- **Discuss** the most common types of cancer, and **describe** the treatments for each.

- **List** your cardiometabolic and cancer risk factors.

© bread & butter/Photographer's Choice/Getty Images

The Power of Prevention

Deaths from the two major killers of Americans—cancer and heart disease—have dropped sharply in recent decades. According to an analysis of the decline in heart-related mortality, preventive steps to reduce the risk of disease were responsible for 44 percent of the decrease.[1] Despite the gains that have been made, more people are still dying of illnesses than should be, many at young ages. Two in three deaths could be delayed and one in three hospitalizations could be avoided by basic preventive steps, such as weight management, not smoking, and regular screenings.

Many chronic problems begin early in life. An estimated one in four college students already has at least one risk factor, such as excess weight or physical inactivity, that increases the risk of conditions affecting the heart and metabolism. The habits you develop now—regular exercise, sensible eating, responsible drinking—can keep you healthy for decades to come.

Your Cardiometabolic Health

In recent years medical scientists have focused on the complex connections between various risk factors, symptoms, and diseases. Physical inactivity, for instance, increases the risk of obesity, which in turn leads to greater risk of many diseases. This new awareness has led to a focus on **cardiometabolic** health. "Cardio" refers to the heart and blood vessels of the cardiovascular system; "metabolic," to the biochemical processes involved in the body's functioning.

Cardiometabolic Risk Factors

Specific risk factors determine your cardiometabolic health. Once you understand your risk, you can start making changes to lower your odds of developing metabolic syndrome, diabetes, and heart disease. Although you may have no signs of these illnesses, you may have at least one cardiometabolic risk factor. This alone increases the likelihood of having others. The more cardiometabolic risk factors you have, the greater risk you face of developing a serious health problem. However, you can reduce most cardiometabolic risk factors by making healthy changes in your lifestyle.

Risk Factors You Can Control

The choices you make and the habits you follow can have a significant impact on whether or not you remain healthy. Avoid the following potential risks for the sake of your cardiometabolic health.

Overweight/Obesity

Excess weight has emerged as an increasingly common and dangerous cardiometabolic risk factor in both men and women. BMI and measurement of waist circumference, discussed in Chapter 5, are good indicators of increased risk.

Waist Circumference

As discussed in Chapter 5, apple-shaped people who carry most of their excess weight around their waists are at greater risk of cardiometabolic conditions than are pear-shaped individuals who carry most of their excess weight below their waist.[2] The more visceral fat that you have, the more resistant your body's cells become to the effects of your own insulin. A measurement of more than 40 inches in men and more than 35 inches in women indicates increased health risks. A "pot belly" raises risk even when a person's weight is normal.[3]

Physical Inactivity

As discussed in Chapter 5, about one-quarter of U.S. adults are sedentary and another third are not active enough to reach a healthy level of fitness. The risk for cardiometabolic conditions is higher for people who are inactive compared with those who engage in regular physical activity.

 Fitness may be more important than overweight or obesity per se for women's cardiometabolic risk. A minimum of 30 minutes a day of moderate activity at least five days a week, can lift a woman from the "low-fitness category" and lessen her cardiometabolic risk.

 The greater the exercise "dose," the more benefits it yields. In studies that compared individuals of different fitness levels, the least fit were at much greater risk of dying. In men, more rigorous exercise, such as jogging, produces greater protection against heart disease and boosts longevity.

Tobacco Use

Smoking may be the single most significant risk factor for cardiometabolic conditions. Each year smoking causes more than 250,000 deaths from cardiovascular disease—far more than it causes from cancer and lung disease. Smokers who have heart attacks are more likely to die from them than are nonsmokers. Smoking is the major risk factor for *peripheral arterial disease,* in which the vessels that carry blood to the leg and arm muscles become hardened and clogged.

Both active and passive smoking accelerate the process by which arteries become clogged and increase the risk of heart attacks and strokes. Overall, nonsmokers exposed to environmental tobacco smoke are at a 25 percent higher relative risk of developing coronary heart disease than nonsmokers not exposed to environmental tobacco smoke.

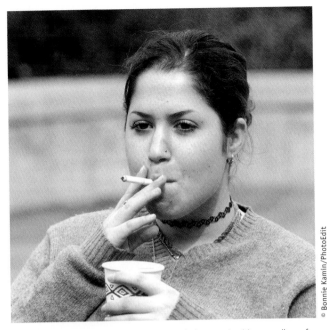

Quitting smoking is the best thing you can do for your health, regardless of how long or how much you've smoked.

High Blood Glucose

As discussed in greater detail on page 401, your stomach and digestive system break down the food you eat into glucose, a type of sugar. The hormone insulin acts like a key, letting glucose into cells and providing energy. "Insulin resistant" cells no longer respond well to insulin, and then glucose, unable to enter the cells, builds up in the bloodstream. Frequent thirst, blurry vision, weakness, unexplained weight loss, or unusual hunger can be signs of high blood glucose. A simple blood test will tell you if your glucose levels are too high. Here is what the readings mean:

Healthy blood glucose	Under 100
Prediabetes	100–125
Diabetes	More than 125

High Blood Pressure (Hypertension)

Blood pressure is a result of the contractions of the heart muscle, which pumps blood through your body, and the resistance of the walls of the vessels through which the blood flows. Each time your heart beats, your blood pressure goes up and down within a certain range. It's highest when the heart contracts; this is called **systolic blood pressure.** It's lowest between contractions; this is called **diastolic blood pressure.** A blood pressure reading consists of the systolic measurement "over" the diastolic measurement, recorded in millimeters of mercury (mm Hg).

High blood pressure, or **hypertension,** occurs when the artery walls become constricted so that the force exerted as the blood flows through them is greater than it should be. Physicians see blood pressure as a continuum:

The higher the reading, the greater the risk of stroke and heart disease.

As a result of the increased work in pumping blood, the heart muscle of a person with hypertension can become stronger and also stiffer. This stiffness increases resistance to filling up with blood between beats, which can cause shortness of breath with exertion. Hypertension can also act on the kidney arteries, which can lead to kidney failure in some cases. In addition, hypertension accelerates the development of plaque buildup within the arteries. Especially when combined with obesity, smoking, high cholesterol levels, or diabetes, hypertension increases the risks of cardiovascular problems several times. However, you can control high blood pressure through diet, exercise, and if necessary, medication. (See page 406.)

Lipoprotein Levels

Cholesterol is a fatty substance found in certain foods and also manufactured by the body. The measurement of cholesterol in the blood is one of the most reliable indicators of the formation of plaque, the sludgelike substance that builds up on the inner walls of arteries. You can lower blood cholesterol levels by cutting back on high-fat foods and exercising more, thereby reducing the risk of a heart attack.

Lipoproteins are compounds in the blood that are made up of proteins and fat. The different types are classified by their size or density. The heaviest are *high-density lipoproteins,* or HDLs, which have the highest proportion of protein. These "good guys," as some cardiologists refer to them, pick up excess cholesterol in the blood and carry it back to the liver for removal from the body. An HDL level of 40 mg/dL or lower substantially increases the risk of heart disease. (Cholesterol levels are measured in milligrams of cholesterol per deciliter of blood—mg/dL.) The average HDL for men is about 45 mg/dL; for women, it is about 55 mg/dL.

Low-density lipoproteins, or (LDLs), and very low-density lipoproteins (VLDLs) carry more cholesterol than HDLs and deposit it on the walls of arteries—they're the "bad guys." The higher your LDL cholesterol, the greater

cardiometabolic Referring to the heart and to the biochemical processes involved in the body's functioning.

systolic blood pressure Highest blood pressure when the heart contracts.

diastolic blood pressure Lowest blood pressure between contractions of the heart.

hypertension High blood pressure occurring when the blood exerts excessive pressure against the arterial walls.

cholesterol An organic substance found in animal fats; linked to cardiovascular disease, particularly atherosclerosis.

lipoprotein A compound in blood that is made up of proteins and fat; a high-density lipoprotein (HDL) picks up excess cholesterol in the blood; a low-density lipoprotein (LDL) carries more cholesterol and deposits it on the walls of arteries.

your risk for heart disease. If you are at high risk of heart disease, any level of LDL higher than 100 mg/dL may increase your danger. (See "What You Need to Know About Your Lipoprotein Profile" later in this chapter.)

Triglycerides are fats that flow through the blood after meals and have been linked to increased risk of coronary artery disease, especially in women. Triglyceride levels tend to be highest in those whose diets are high in calories, sugar, alcohol, and refined starches. High levels of these fats may increase the risk of obesity, and cutting back on these foods can reduce high triglyceride levels.

Figure 14.1 summarizes the factors to ask your doctor about at your next checkup.

Risk Factors You Can't Control

Family History

Certain cardiometabolic risk factors, such as abnormally high blood levels of lipids, can be passed down from generation to generation. Although you can't rewrite your family history, individuals with an inherited vulnerability can lower the danger by changing the risk factors within their control. Your cardiometabolic health depends to a great extent on your behavior, including the decisions you make about the foods you eat or the decision not to smoke.

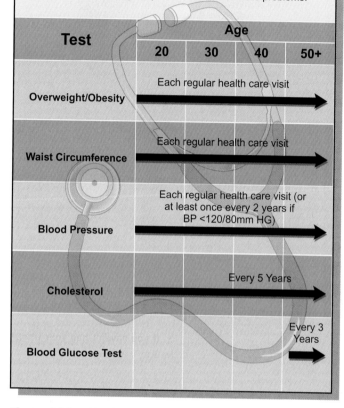

Checkup Chart

Use these guidelines to help you know when to ask your doctor about screenings to prevent cardiometabolic problems.

Test	Age			
	20	**30**	**40**	**50+**
Overweight/Obesity	Each regular health care visit →			
Waist Circumference	Each regular health care visit →			
Blood Pressure	Each regular health care visit (or at least once every 2 years if BP <120/80mm HG) →			
Cholesterol			Every 5 Years →	
Blood Glucose Test				Every 3 Years →

Figure 14.1 Checkup Chart
Source: Adapted from CheckUpAmerica.org.

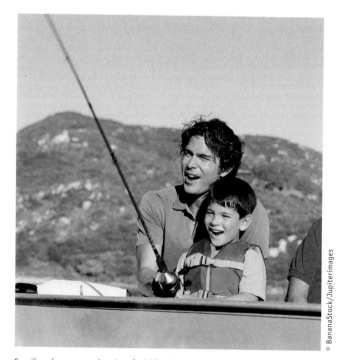

Families share more than just facial features and happy memories. Certain cardiometabolic risk factors can be passed down from one generation to another.

triglyceride A blood fat that flows through the blood after meals and is linked to increased risk of coronary artery disease.

Race and Ethnicity

Cardiometabolic risk factors occur at higher rates among ethnic minority populations such as African Americans, Hispanic Americans, and Native Americans. For reasons that aren't entirely clear, people of some races are more likely to develop diabetes. Blacks and Hispanics have double the rate for whites. The incidence is even higher among American Indians. Among the Pima Indians of Arizona, half of all adults have type 2 diabetes, one of the highest rates of diabetes in the world. Nearly four in every ten black adults have cardiovascular disease. Among Hispanic Americans, nearly three in ten have cardiovascular disease.

African Americans are twice as likely to develop high blood pressure as whites. African Americans also suffer strokes at an earlier age and of greater severity. Poverty may be an unrecognized risk factor for members of this minority group, who are less likely to receive medical treatments or undergo corrective surgery. Family history, lifestyle, diet, and stress may also play a role, starting early

Lowering Your Cardiometabolic Risks

Yes, advances in treatment can help if you eventually develop a cardiometabolic condition. But changes in lifestyle can do even more: To make healthy changes, select some of the behavioral modifications that follow.

Changes You Can Make Today

- Eat a good breakfast: whole-grain cereal, juice, yogurt, and so forth.
- Take a walk after lunch.
- Skip dessert at dinner.
- Eat one more serving of vegetables.
- Eat one more piece of fruit.
- Drink one more glass of water.
- Take the stairs for one or two flights rather than riding the elevator in your dorm or classroom building.
- Get seven to eight hours of sleep tonight.
- Don't smoke.

Changes You Can Make This Week

- **Block out time for exercise on your calendar.** Try for at least 30 minutes of physical activity most days.
- **If you haven't had your lipoproteins checked** within the last year, schedule a test.
- **If you don't know your blood pressure,** find out what it is. If you know it, compare your reading with those in Table 14.1 (page 405) to determine if it is too high.
- **Make a list of stress-reducing activities,** such as meditation or listening to music. Select two or three to do this week.
- **Get in touch with an old friend,** and enjoy catching up on each other's lives.

Changes You Can Make This Term

- **Learn your family history.** Inheriting a predisposition to high blood pressure, diabetes, or heart disease means that you need extra preventive care.
- **Be patient.** Don't get discouraged if change seems harder and slower than you thought it would be.
- **If you slip up and smoke again or blow your diet, don't give up.** Analyze what triggered your relapse. Was it the smell of smoke at the party Saturday night? Did you try to console yourself for a poor grade with a carton of chocolate ice cream? Think of how you might handle similar situations differently in the future, such as staying away from smokers at parties or taking a walk to lift your mood rather than turning to food.
- **Develop and use a support system of friends and family members.** Identify individuals you can talk to, work out with, or call.

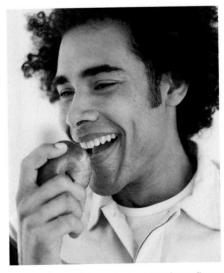

You can do something today to prevent heart disease in your future: Eat some fruit.

© Stockdisc/Jupiter Images

in life. However, researchers have found no single explanation for why African American youngsters, like their parents, tend to have higher blood pressure than white children.

 Black women are twice as likely as white women to suffer heart attacks and to die from heart disease. Common cardiometabolic risk factors—high blood pressure, diabetes, and high cholesterol—account for this increased jeopardy. In addition, black women are less likely to receive common medications, such as cholesterol-lowering drugs, to lower their risk.

Age

Cardiometabolic risk factors increase as people get older, especially past the age of 45. This may be because many individuals tend to exercise less, lose muscle mass, and gain weight as they age. However, cardiometabolic conditions are also increasing dramatically among younger people.

Metabolic Syndrome

Metabolic syndrome, once called Syndrome X or insulin-resistant syndrome, is not a disease but a cluster of disorders of the body's metabolism—including high blood pressure, high insulin levels, abdominal obesity, and abnormal cholesterol levels—that make a person more likely to develop diabetes, heart disease, or stroke. Each of these conditions is by itself a risk factor for other diseases. In combination, they dramatically boost the chances of potentially life-threatening illnesses.[4]

 This dangerous syndrome has become so widespread that health officials describe it as an epidemic that affects one in four Americans, especially Hispanic men and women.

 College-age men and women who maintain their weight as they get older are much less likely to develop metabolic syndrome. About one in four undergraduates already has one risk factor for metabolic syndrome. Young adults with metabolic syndrome are more likely than others their age to have thicker neck arteries, an indicator of atherosclerosis, the buildup of fatty plaques in arteries. As discussed in Chapter 6, drinking more than one soft drink (diet or regular) a day increases the risk of metabolic syndrome.[5] Losing 7 to 10 percent of your initial body weight may

reverse the symptoms of the metabolic syndrome.[6] For more ideas on how to undo these symptoms, see Your Strategies for Prevention: "How to Overcome Metabolic Syndrome."

Three or more of the following characteristics indicate metabolic syndrome:[7]

- **A larger-than-normal waist measurement—** 40 inches or more in men and 35 inches or more in women (for Asians and individuals with a genetic predisposition to diabetes, 37 to 39 inches in men and 31 to 35 inches in women).
- **A higher-than-normal triglyceride level—** 150 mg/dL or more.
- **A lower-than-normal high-density lipoprotein (HDL) level—**less than 40 mg/dL in men or 50 mg/dL in women.
- **A higher-than-normal blood pressure—** 130 mmHg systole over 85 mm Hg diastole (130/85), or higher.
- **A higher-than-normal fasting blood sugar—** 110 mg/dL or higher.

People with three factors of metabolic syndrome are nearly twice as likely to have a heart attack or stroke and more than three times more likely to develop heart disease than those with none.

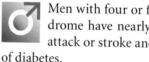 Men with four or five characteristics of the syndrome have nearly four times the risk of heart attack or stroke and more than 24 times the risk of diabetes.

Diabetes Mellitus

About 100 million people around the world, including about 21 million in the United States, have **diabetes mellitus,** a disease in which the body doesn't produce or respond properly to insulin, a hormone essential for daily life. In those with diabetes, the pancreas, which produces insulin (the hormone that regulates carbohydrate and fat metabolism) doesn't function as it should. When the pancreas either stops producing insulin or doesn't produce sufficient insulin to meet the body's needs, almost every body system can be damaged.

The prevalence of diabetes has nearly doubled in the last three decades, and health experts describe it as a global epidemic. About 6.3 percent of Americans have diabetes; a third are not aware that they have it because certain types develop insidiously with no visible symptoms.

Diabetes shortens life expectancy by an average of 8 years—7.8 years for men, 8.4 years for women.[8] The risk of premature death among people with diabetes is about twice that of people without the disease. According to

metabolic syndrome A cluster of disorders of the body's metabolism that make diabetes, heart disease, or stroke more likely.

diabetes mellitus A disease in which the inadequate production of insulin leads to failure of the body tissues to break down carbohydrates at a normal rate.

the American Diabetes Association, the total economic cost of diabetes is more than $132 billion a year. Diabetes accounts for $1 of every $10 spent on health care in the United States. An estimated 48 million Americans may develop diabetes by 2050.[9]

Understanding Diabetes

Glucose is the primary form of sugar that the body cells use for energy. When a person without diabetes eats a meal, the level of glucose in the blood rises, triggering the production and release of insulin by special cell clusters in the pancreas. Insulin enhances the movement of glucose into various body cells, bringing down the level of glucose in the blood. In those who have diabetes, however, insulin secretion is either nonexistent or deficient. Without sufficient insulin, the glucose in the blood is unable to enter most body cells, so the cells' energy needs aren't met. The levels of glucose in the blood rise higher and higher after each meal. This unused glucose eventually passes through the kidneys, which are unable to process the excessive glucose, and out of the body in urine (Figure 14.2).

Deprived of the fuel it needs, the body begins to break down stored fat as a source of energy. This process produces weak acids, called ketones. A buildup of ketones leads to ketoacidosis, an upheaval in the body's chemical balance that brings on nausea, vomiting, abdominal pain, lethargy, and drowsiness. Severe ketoacidosis can lead to coma and eventual death.

Before the development of insulin injections, diabetes was a fatal illness. Today diabetics can have normal lifespans. However, diabetes still can lead to devastating complications. Uncontrolled glucose levels slowly damage blood vessels throughout the body; thus, individuals who become diabetic early in life may face devastating complications even before they reach middle age.[10] Diabetes is the number one cause of blindness, nontraumatic amputations, and kidney failure, and diabetes increases by two or three times the risk of heart attack or stroke.

Diabetic women who become pregnant face higher risks of miscarriage and babies with serious birth defects; however, precise control of blood sugar levels before conception and in early pregnancy can lower the likelihood of these problems.

Types of Diabetes

Diabetes includes several conditions in which the body has difficulty controlling levels of glucose in the bloodstream. After an overnight fast, most people have blood

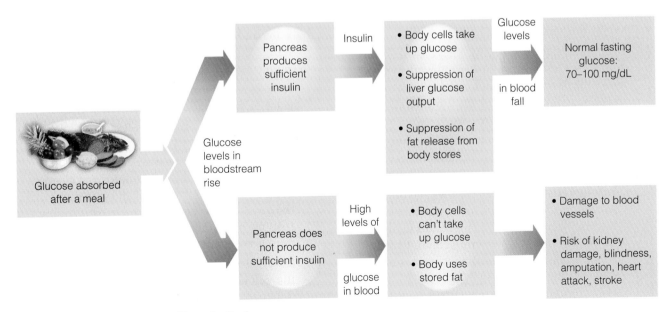

Figure 14.2 How Diabetes Affects the Body
Diabetes affects almost every organ system of the body in complex and often subtle ways.

glucose levels between 70 and 100 milligrams of glucose per deciliter of blood (mg/dL). This is considered normal. Abnormal readings can indicate the following:

- **Prediabetes.** In this condition, blood glucose levels are higher than normal but are not high enough for a diagnosis of diabetes. If your fasting blood glucose is consistently 126 mg/dL or higher, you have diabetes. However, if your fasting blood glucose level is between 101 and 125 mg/dL, you have prediabetes, which also is called hyperglycemia or glucose intolerance.

  An estimated 56 million Americans have prediabetes and are at increased risk for developing type 2 diabetes and for heart disease and stroke. Recent research has shown that some long-term damage to the body, especially the heart and circulatory system, already may be occurring during prediabetes. If people with prediabetes take action to manage their blood glucose, they can delay or prevent type 2 diabetes from developing. Diets rich in cereal fiber, magnesium, calcium, and Vitamin D may help.[11] Lifestyle changes also have shown promise.[12] (See Your Strategies for Prevention: "How to Lower Your Risk of Prediabetes and Type 2 Diabetes.")

- **Type 1 diabetes.** In this form of diabetes (once called juvenile-onset or insulin-dependent diabetes), the body's immune system attacks the insulin-producing beta cells in the pancreas and destroys them. The pancreas then produces little or no insulin and therefore blood glucose cannot enter the cells to be used for energy. Type 1 diabetes develops most often in young people but can appear in adults. Individuals with type 1 diabetes require insulin therapy because their own bodies no longer supply this vital hormone.

- **Type 2 diabetes.** In type 2 diabetes (once called adult-onset or non-insulin-dependent diabetes), either the pancreas does not make enough insulin or the body is unable to use insulin correctly. Its two characteristic problems are:

  - **Insufficient insulin** produced by the pancreas. Over time the body produces less and less insulin and eventually none at all.

  - **Insulin resistance.** When muscles and body tissue become resistant to insulin, glucose accumulates in the bloodstream. This results in high blood glucose levels (hyperglycemia). Exactly why the cells become insulin resistant is uncertain, although excess weight, inactivity, and fatty tissue seem to be important factors.

  Type 2 diabetes, which accounts for 90 percent of cases of diabetes, develops most often in middle-aged and older adults, but increasingly is appearing in young people, including adolescents and children. Diet, weight loss, exercise, and medications are the first line of treatment for type 2 diabetes, but insulin also may be required.

- **Gestational diabetes.** Women who get diabetes while they are pregnant are more likely to have a family history of diabetes, especially on their mothers' side; they are at greater risk of developing diabetes later in life.

Although type 1 and type 2 diabetes have different causes, two factors are important in both: an inherited predisposition to the disease and something in the environment that triggers diabetes. Genes alone are not enough. In most cases of type 1 diabetes, people need to inherit risk factors from both parents and to experience some environmental trigger, which might involve prenatal nutrition, a virus, or an unknown agent.

In type 2 diabetes, family history is one of the strongest risk factors for getting the disease, but only in Westernized countries. African Americans, Mexican Americans, and Native Americans have the highest rates, but people who live in less developed nations tend not to get type 2 diabetes, no matter how high their genetic risk.

Diabetes Signs and Symptoms

About a third of individuals with type 2 diabetes do not realize they have the illness. If you have risk factors for the disease, watch for the following warning signs:

- **Increased thirst and frequent urination.** Excess glucose circulating in your body draws water from your tissues, making you feel dehydrated. Drinking water and other beverages to quench thirst leads to more frequent urination.

- **Flu-like symptoms.** Type 2 diabetes can sometimes feel like a viral illness, with such symptoms as extreme fatigue and weakness. When glucose, your body's main fuel, doesn't reach cells, you may feel tired and weak.

- **Weight loss or weight gain.** Because your body is trying to compensate for lost fluids and glucose, you may eat more than usual and gain weight, or the opposite may occur. Although eating more than normal, you may lose weight because your muscle tissues don't get enough glucose to generate growth and energy.

- **Blurred vision.** High levels of blood glucose pull fluid from body tissues, including the lenses of the eyes, which affects ability to focus. Vision should improve with treatment of diabetes.

YOUR STRATEGIES FOR PREVENTION *How to Lower Your Risk of Prediabetes and Type 2 Diabetes*

The Diabetes Prevention Program (DPP), a landmark study sponsored by the National Institutes of Health, found that people at increased risk for type 2 diabetes can prevent or delay the onset of the disease by taking the following steps:

- Exercise 30 minutes on at least five days of the week.

- If you're overweight or obese, lose weight. Aim for 5 to 7 percent of your initial weight.
- Eat a diet rich in complex carbohydrates (bread and other starches) and high-fiber foods, and low in sodium and fat.

- Eat fruits and vegetables that are rich in antioxidants, substances that prevent oxygen damage to cells.
- If your doctor advises, take medications, such as metformin (Glucophage), to help lower your blood sugar.

- **Slow-healing sores or frequent infections.** Diabetes affects the body's ability to heal and fight infection. Bladder and vaginal infections can be a particular problem for women.
- **Nerve damage (neuropathy).** Excess blood glucose can damage the small blood vessels to your nerves, leading to symptoms such as tingling and loss of sensation in hands and feet.
- **Red, swollen, tender gums.** Diabetes increases the risk of infection in your gums and in the bones that hold your teeth in place.

Detecting Diabetes

To identify individuals with this disease as early as possible, the American Diabetes Association now recommends screening every three years for all men and women beginning at age 45. The American College of Endocrinology recommends screening at age 30 for individuals at risk, including those who are overweight, sedentary, have a family history of diabetes, or have high blood pressure or heart disease.

Tests that can detect diabetes include:

- **Random blood sugar test.** Because you don't necessarily fast for this test, your blood glucose may be high because you've just eaten. Even so, it shouldn't be higher than 200 mg/dL.
- **Fasting blood glucose test.** In general, glucose is lowest after an overnight fast. That's why the preferred way to test your blood sugar is after you've fasted overnight or for at least eight hours.
- **Glucose challenge test.** Often used to screen pregnant women for gestational diabetes, this test measures glucose before drinking eight ounces of an extremely sweet liquid after fasting for six hours, then every hour for a three-hour period. If your blood sugar rises more than expected and doesn't return to normal by the third hour, you likely have diabetes.

Diabetes Management

Unlike many other medical conditions, patients must take charge of their diabetes and monitor their blood glucose regularly to prevent or delay the serious complications of the disease. Diabetes educators teach patients a new set of ABCs: Manage your **A**1c (blood glucose or sugar), **B**lood pressure, and **C**holesterol:

- **A is for the A1c test.** This test measures the amount of glucose attached to hemoglobin molecules, the iron-rich molecules in red blood cells that deliver oxygen to the body. The higher your blood glucose levels, the more hemoglobin molecules you will have with glucose attached—and the greater the risk of damage to eyes, kidneys, and feet. In general, the life cycle of a red blood cell is 75 to 90 days, which is why the A1c test shows average blood glucose levels for the past two to three months. The American Diabetes Association recommends a goal for A1c of less than 7 percent. The American College of Endocrinology recommends a goal of 6.5 percent. (Normal A1c levels are below 6.) Individuals with diabetes should have their A1c levels checked at least twice a year.
- **B is for blood pressure.** As discussed on page 405, the goal for most people is 115/75. High blood pressure can cause heart attack, stroke, and kidney disease.
- **C is for cholesterol.** The LDL goal for most people is less than 160 mg/dL (see Table 14.2 on page 408). Bad cholesterol, or LDL, can build up and clog your blood vessels.

Treatment

The goal for diabetics is to keep blood sugar levels as stable as possible to prevent complications, such as kidney damage. Home glucose monitoring including new continuous glucose monitors, allow diabetics to check their blood sugar levels as many times a day as necessary and to adjust their diet or insulin doses as appropriate.

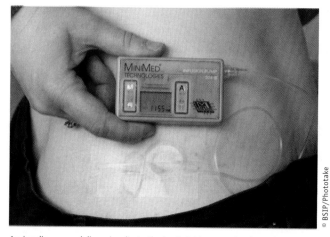

© BSIP/Phototake

An insulin pump delivers insulin to the body 24 hours a day through a thin plastic tube inserted just under the skin, usually on the abdomen.

Types of insulin differ in how long it takes to start working after injection (onset), when it works hardest (peak), and how long it lasts in the body (duration). Individuals with diabetes may use different types in various combinations, depending on time of day and timing of meals. New insulin inhalers offer an alternative to injections for those with type 2 diabetes.

Those with type 1 diabetes require daily doses of insulin via injections, an insulin infusion pump, or oral medication. Those with type 2 diabetes often can control their disease through a well-balanced diet, exercise, and weight management. However, insulin therapy may be needed to keep blood glucose levels near normal or normal, thereby reducing the risk of damage to the eyes, nerves, and kidneys. New medications help control weight and lower blood pressure and cholesterol.

Medical advances hold out bright hopes for diabetics. Laser surgery, for instance, is saving eyesight. Bypass operations are helping restore blood flow to the heart and feet. Dialysis machines and kidney and pancreas transplants save many lives. Researchers are exploring various approaches to prevention, including antibody therapies that delay the onset of type 1 diabetes.[13] Transplanting insulin-producing cells from healthy pancreases has helped a small number of patients, but many problems with this treatment remain.

Hypertension

Blood pressure refers to the force of blood against the walls of arteries. When blood pressure remains elevated over time—a condition called hypertension—it forces

prehypertension A condition of slightly elevated blood pressure, which is likely to worsen in time.

the heart to pump harder than is healthy. Because the heart must force blood into arteries that are offering increased resistance to blood flow, the left side of the heart becomes enlarged. If untreated, high blood pressure can cause a variety of cardiovascular complications, including heart attack and stroke—two of the three leading causes of death among U.S. adults—as well as kidney failure and blindness (Figure 14.3).

In a young person even mild hypertension can cause organs such as the heart, brain, and kidneys to start to deteriorate. By age 50 or 60, the damage may be irreversible.

Who Is at Risk?

The World Health Organization estimates that hypertension causes one in every eight deaths globally, making it the third leading killer in the world. In the United States, high blood pressure is responsible for about a third of cardiovascular problems like heart attack or stroke and a quarter of all premature deaths.

 About a third of adults age 18 and older in the United States—some 65 million men and women—have high blood pressure. Blood pressure has increased among children and adolescents as well as adults, with the highest rates among black and Mexican American children. The primary culprit is the increase in obesity in the young. No one knows why African Americans are more vulnerable, although some speculate that overweight or dietary factors may contribute.

Different races also suffer different consequences of high blood pressure. An African American with the same elevated blood pressure reading as a Caucasian faces a greater risk of stroke, heart disease, and kidney problems.

 Family history also plays a role. "If you study healthy college students with normal blood pressures, those who have one parent with hypertension will have blood pressure that's a little higher than average," notes Rose Marie Robertson, M.D., of the American Heart Association. "If two parents have high blood pressure, their levels will be a little higher, and they're destined to go higher still. If your parents have high blood pressure, have yours checked regularly."[14]

Men and women are equally likely to develop hypertension, but in women blood pressure tends to rise around the time of menopause. Half of all women over age 45 have hypertension.

For individuals who smoke, are overweight, don't exercise, or have high cholesterol levels, hypertension multiplies the risk of heart disease and stroke. Overweight people with high blood pressure have twice the risk of dying of a heart attack or stroke as those with normal blood pressure. At ultrahigh risk are people with diabetes or kidney disease.

What Is a Healthy Blood Pressure?

Current guidelines (Table 14.1) categorize a reading of 120/80 as **prehypertension,** a condition that is likely to worsen in time. A healthy reading is 115/75 mm Hg. Once blood pressure rises above this threshold, the risk of cardiovascular disease may increase.

In healthy adults, blood pressure screening should begin at age 21, with repeat evaluations at least every two

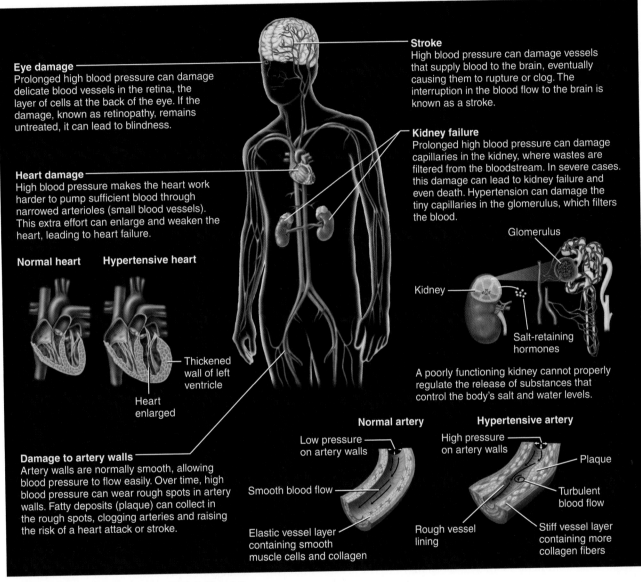

Stroke
High blood pressure can damage vessels that supply blood to the brain, eventually causing them to rupture or clog. The interruption in the blood flow to the brain is known as a stroke.

Eye damage
Prolonged high blood pressure can damage delicate blood vessels in the retina, the layer of cells at the back of the eye. If the damage, known as retinopathy, remains untreated, it can lead to blindness.

Kidney failure
Prolonged high blood pressure can damage capillaries in the kidney, where wastes are filtered from the bloodstream. In severe cases. this damage can lead to kidney failure and even death. Hypertension can damage the tiny capillaries in the glomerulus, which filters the blood.

Heart damage
High blood pressure makes the heart work harder to pump sufficient blood through narrowed arterioles (small blood vessels). This extra effort can enlarge and weaken the heart, leading to heart failure.

Glomerulus

Kidney

Salt-retaining hormones

Normal heart   **Hypertensive heart**

A poorly functioning kidney cannot properly regulate the release of substances that control the body's salt and water levels.

Thickened wall of left ventricle

Heart enlarged

Normal artery   **Hypertensive artery**

Low pressure on artery walls

High pressure on artery walls

Plaque

Smooth blood flow

Turbulent blood flow

Damage to artery walls
Artery walls are normally smooth, allowing blood pressure to flow easily. Over time, high blood pressure can wear rough spots in artery walls. Fatty deposits (plaque) can collect in the rough spots, clogging arteries and raising the risk of a heart attack or stroke.

Elastic vessel layer containing smooth muscle cells and collagen

Rough vessel lining

Stiff vessel layer containing more collagen fibers

Figure 14.3   Consequences of High Blood Pressure
If left untreated, elevated blood pressure can damage blood vessels in several areas of the body and lead to serious health problems.

TABLE 14.1   What Your Blood Pressure Means

Top Number (systolic)		Bottom Number (diastolic)	Your Group	What to Do
Below 120	and	Below 80	Normal blood pressure	Maintain a healthy lifestyle
120–139	or	80–89	Prehypertension	Adopt a healthy lifestyle
140–159	or	90–99	Stage 1 hypertension	Adopt a healthy lifestyle; take medication
160 or more	or	100 or more	Stage 2 hypertension	Adopt a healthy lifestyle; take more than one medication

Numbers are expressed in millimeters of mercury (mm Hg).

years, or more often depending on your current health, medical history, and risk factors for cardiovascular disease. According to the National College Health Assessment survey, about nine in ten students have done so. (See Reality Check.)

To get an accurate blood pressure reading, you should visit the doctor's office at least twice and have your blood pressure taken two or more times while you're seated. The average of those measurements determines how your blood pressure is classified.

The current guidelines classify hypertension into two categories:

- **Stage 1.** This consists of a systolic pressure ranging from 140 to 159 or a diastolic pressure ranging from 90 to 99.
- **Stage 2.** The most severe form of hypertension occurs with a systolic pressure of 160 or higher or a diastolic reading of 100 or higher.

Only one of the numbers—the top or bottom—needs to be high to meet these criteria. In people over age 50, systolic pressure is more important than diastolic. If it rises to 140 mm Hg or higher, doctors advise treatment regardless of the diastolic pressure.

Lowering High Blood Pressure

Lifestyle changes are a first-line weapon in the fight against high blood pressure. Rather than making a single change, a combination of behavioral changes, including losing weight, eating heart-healthy foods, reducing sodium, and exercising more, yields the best results.

High intake of folate, a B vitamin, can significantly reduce the risk of hypertension. In a study of women under age 35, those who consumed the most folate had one-third the risk of developing high blood pressure as those consuming very little. Among the approaches that have not proved effective are dietary supplements, such as calcium, magnesium, potassium, and fish oil.

The National Heart, Lung and Blood Institute has developed what is known as the DASH diet. Following DASH, which stands for Dietary Approaches to Stop Hypertension, has proved as effective as drug therapy in lowering blood pressure. An additional benefit: The DASH diet also lowers harmful blood fats, including cholesterol and low-density lipoprotein, and the amino acid homocysteine (one of the new suspects in heart disease risk).

Too much sodium and too little potassium boost blood pressure in people who are sensitive to salt. The American Medical Association is calling for food makers and restaurants to cut the sodium content of food by 50 percent by 2016. For a healthful diet, aim for less than 1.5 grams of sodium a day, and at least 4.7 grams of potassium. The lower the amount of sodium in the diet, the lower the blood pressure for both those with and those without hypertension and for both genders and all racial and ethnic groups. However, reducing dietary sodium has an even greater effect on blood pressure in blacks than whites, and in women than men.

Making healthy lifestyle modifications (see Your Strategies for Change: "How to Lower Your Blood Pressure") can help reduce Stage 1 hypertension, but most people also require a medication. Drugs for lowering blood pressure come in a range of regimens (once a day to several times a day) with a range of effects on other conditions, interactions with other drugs, and potential side effects. Current guidelines state that the first choice should be an inexpensive diuretic (water pill). Some experts argue that an ACE inhibitor or a calcium-channel blocker is a better place to start. Most people need more than one medication to get their blood pressure under control.

Those with Stage 2 hypertension typically need at least two types of high blood pressure medications (antihypertensives) to reduce blood pressure to a safer level. The goal for most people with hypertension is to reduce blood pressure to below 140/90 mm Hg.

Only about one-third of people with hypertension have it effectively controlled—below 140/90 mm Hg. Reducing systolic blood pressure 12 mm Hg for 10 years

---

YOUR STRATEGIES FOR CHANGE *How to Lower Your Blood Pressure*

- **Get moving.** Regular exercise can lower blood pressure by 10 points, prevent the onset of high blood pressure, or let you reduce your dosage of blood pressure medications.

- **Eat your way** to better blood pressure. Choose more fruits, vegetables, low-fat dairy products, whole grains, poultry, fish, and nuts. Cut down on red meat, sweets, sugar-containing beverages, and saturated fat and cholesterol.

- **Lose ten.** Shedding 10 percent of your current weight—or even 10 pounds—can make a big difference.

- **Don't smoke.** A single cigarette can cause a 20-point spike in systolic blood pressure. Don't light up. See Chapter 13 for tips on quitting.

- **Hold the salt.** If you're salt sensitive, you may be spiking your blood pressure as you spice your food.

- **Stick with your medications.** If your doctor has prescribed medication to lower your blood pressure, take it conscientiously. Your future health may depend on it.

can prevent 1 death in every 11 people treated for hypertension. In those with existing cardiovascular disease or organ damage, such as kidney disease, that reduction has an even bigger benefit, preventing one death in every nine people treated.

Your Lipoprotein Profile

Medical science has changed the way it views and targets the blood fats that endanger the healthy heart. In the past, the focus was primarily on total cholesterol in the blood. The higher this number was, the greater the risk of heart disease. The NHLBI's National Cholesterol Education Program has recommended more comprehensive testing, called a *lipoprotein profile,* for all individuals age 20 or older (see Savvy Consumer: "What You Need to Know About Your Lipoprotein Profile").

This blood test, which should be performed after a 9- to 12-hour fast and repeated at least once every five years, provides readings of:

- **Total cholesterol.**
- **LDL (bad) cholesterol,** the main culprit in the buildup of plaque within the arteries.
- **HDL (good or *Healthy*) cholesterol,** which helps prevent cholesterol buildup.
- **Triglycerides,** the blood fats released into the bloodstream after a meal.

What Is a Healthy Cholesterol Reading?

Total cholesterol is the sum of all the cholesterol in your blood. Less than 200 mg/dL total cholesterol is ideal, and 200–239 mg/dL is borderline-high. Total cholesterol above 240 mg/dL is high and doubles your risk of heart disease. However, total cholesterol is not the only crucial number you should know. Because LDL increases your risk for heart disease, you always should find out your LDL level. Even if your total cholesterol is higher than 200, you may not be at high risk for a heart attack. Some people—such as women before menopause and young, active men who have no other risk factors—may have high HDL cholesterol and desirable LDL levels. Ask your doctor to interpret your results so you both know your numbers and understand what they mean.

The updated guidelines of the National Cholesterol Education Program (NCEP) set lower target goals for LDL cholesterol, particularly for those at greatest risk of a heart attack or death from cardiovascular disease (Table 14.2).

Savvy Consumer | ## What You Need to Know About Your Lipoprotein Profile

- Go to your primary health-care provider to get a lipoprotein profile. Although cholesterol tests at shopping malls or health fairs can help identify people at risk, the analyzers are often not certified technicians, and the readings may be inaccurate. In addition, without a health expert to counsel them, some people may be unnecessarily frightened by a high reading—or falsely reassured by a low one.

- Ask about accuracy. Even at first-rate laboratories, cholesterol readings are often inaccurate. Find out if the lab is using the National Institutes of Health standards, and ask about the lab's margin for error (which should be less than 5 percent).

- Fast beforehand. Cholesterol tests are most accurate after a 9- to 14-hour fast. Schedule the test before breakfast if you can. Women may not want to get tested at the end of their menstrual cycles, when minor elevations in cholesterol levels occur because of lower estrogen levels.

- Cholesterol levels can also rise 5 to 10 percent during periods of stress. Reschedule the test if you come down with an intestinal flu because the viral infection could interfere with the absorption of food and thus with cholesterol levels. Let your doctor know if you're taking any drugs. Common medications, including birth control pills and hypertension drugs, can affect cholesterol levels.

- Sit down before allowing blood to be drawn or your finger to be pricked; fluids pool differently in the body when you're standing than when you're sitting. Don't let a technician squeeze blood from your finger, which forces fluid from cells, diluting the blood sample and possibly leading to a falsely low reading.

- Get real numbers. Don't settle for "normal" or "high," because laboratories can inaccurately label results. Find out exactly what your reading is: your LDL, HDL, and triglyceride levels.

TABLE 14.2   Targets for Lowering LDL

Risk Category	LDL Goal
Low Risk (1 or 0 risk factors for heart disease)	Less than 160 mg/dL
Moderate Risk (2 or more risk factors that create a 10 percent or lower risk of a heart attack in the next 10 years)	Less than 130 mg/dL
Moderately High Risk (2 or more risk factors that create a 10 to 20 percent chance of a heart attack in next 10 years)	Less than 130 mg/dL
High Risk (heart disease or diabetes, diseased blood vessels, 2 or more risk factors)	Less than 100 mg/dL
Very High Risk (heart disease and multiple, severe, or poorly controlled risk factors, especially smoking, or a history of heart attack or angina)	Less than 70 mg/dL

Source: Based on the National Cholesterol Education Program Adult Treatment Panel III Guidelines, www.circulationaha.org.

HDL, good cholesterol, also is important, particularly in women. Federal guidelines define an HDL reading of less than 40 mg/dL as a major risk factor for developing heart disease. HDL levels of 60 mg/dL or more are protective and lower the risk of heart disease.

Triglycerides, the free-floating molecules that transport fats in the bloodstream, ideally should be below 150 mg/dL. Individuals with readings of 150 to 199 mg/dL, considered borderline, as well as those with higher readings, may benefit from weight control, physical activity, and if necessary, medication.

Lowering Cholesterol

According to federal guidelines, about one in five Americans may require treatment to lower their cholesterol level. However, nearly half of people who need cholesterol treatment, which can reduce the risk of heart disease by 30 percent over five years, don't get it.[15] The National Cholesterol Education Program (NCEP) estimates that some 36 million Americans should be watching their diet and exercising more. Another 65 million should be taking cholesterol-lowering drugs. Depending on your lipoprotein profile and an assessment of other risk factors, your physician may recommend that you take steps to lower your LDL cholesterol.

Lifestyle Changes

Some individuals with elevated cholesterol can improve their lipoprotein profile with lifestyle changes:

- **Dietary changes.** In the past, dietary changes produced relatively modest improvements compared to the effects of medications, which can cut cholesterol by as much as 35 percent. However, a diet consisting of cholesterol-lowering foods, including nuts, soy, oats, and plant sterols (in margarine and green leafy vegetables), reduced LDL cholesterol by about 30 percent. An added benefit: a reduction in C-reactive protein, discussed later in this chapter. Researchers are recommending this diet as an effective first treatment for individuals with high cholesterol levels, particularly when coupled with exercise and weight loss.

- **Weight management.** For individuals who are overweight, losing weight can help lower LDL. This is especially true for those with high triglyceride levels and/or low HDL levels and those who have a large waist measurement (more than 40 inches for a man and more than 35 inches for a woman).

- **Physical activity.** Regular activity can help lower LDL, lower blood pressure, reduce triglycerides, and particularly important, raise HDL. Again, these benefits are especially important for those with high triglyceride levels or large waist measurements.

Lifestyle changes can lower harmful LDL levels by 5 to 10 percent. However, a greater reduction of 30 to 40 percent requires either intensive lifestyle changes, including an extremely low-fat diet, or the addition of cholesterol-lowering medication. (See "Unclogging the Arteries" on page 414.)

Medications

The last decade has seen a revolution in treatment for high cholesterol, thanks to a new class of drugs called statins—better known by brand names such as Lipitor, Mevacor, Pravachol, and Zocor. These medications can

atrium (plural **atria**)   Either of the two upper chambers of the heart, which receive blood from the veins.

ventricle   Either of the two lower chambers of the heart, which pump blood out of the heart and into the arteries.

cut the risk of dying of a heart attack by as much as 40 percent. Initially tested in men, statins have proved equally beneficial for women, including those whose cholesterol levels rise after menopause.

Statins work in the liver to block production of cholesterol. When the liver can't make cholesterol, it draws LDL cholesterol from the blood to use as raw material. This means that less LDL is available to trigger or promote the artery-clogging process known as atherosclerosis. Statins also appear to stabilize cholesterol-filled deposits in artery walls and to cool down inflammation. Long-term therapy with statins reduces the risk for death, heart attack, and stroke among people with heart disease, even when LDL levels are not elevated. The lower the LDL, the lower the risk.

Cardiovascular (Heart) Disease

In the United States, death rates from cardiovascular disease have dropped by 60 percent since 1950, one of the major U.S. health achievements of the twentieth century.

The medical advances described in this chapter have contributed to this decline, but much of the credit goes to lifestyle changes, such as quitting smoking and making dietary changes that lower blood pressure and cholesterol levels.

Yet we still have a long way to go to keep the hearts of all Americans healthy. Nearly 2,600 Americans die of heart disease every day—that's one every 34 seconds. More than 64 million Americans have heart disease.[16] Each year an estimated one million Americans suffer a heart attack; nearly half of them die.

How the Heart Works

The heart is a hollow, muscular organ with four chambers that serve as two pumps (see Figure 14.4). It is about the size of a clenched fist. Each pump consists of a pair of chambers formed of muscles. The upper two—each called an **atrium**—receive blood, which then flows through valves into the lower two chambers, the **ventricles,** which contract to pump blood out into

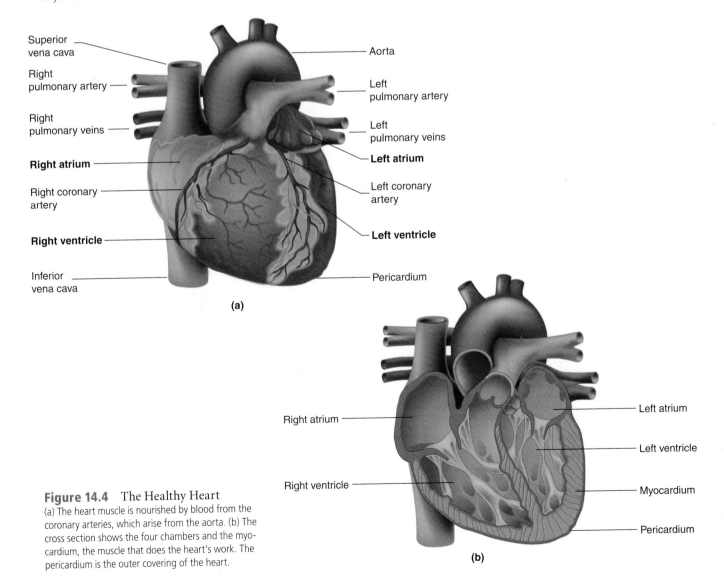

Figure 14.4   The Healthy Heart

(a) The heart muscle is nourished by blood from the coronary arteries, which arise from the aorta. (b) The cross section shows the four chambers and the myocardium, the muscle that does the heart's work. The pericardium is the outer covering of the heart.

the arteries through a second set of valves. A thick wall divides the right side of the heart from the left side; even though the two sides are separated, they contract at almost the same time. Contraction of the ventricles is called **systole;** the period of relaxation between contractions is called **diastole.** The heart valves, located at the entrance and exit of the ventricular chambers, have flaps that open and close to allow blood to flow through the chambers of the heart.

The *myocardium* (heart muscle) consists of branching fibers that enable the heart to contract, or beat, between 60 and 80 times per minute, or about 100,000 times a day. With each beat, the heart pumps about 2 ounces of blood. This may not sound like much, but it adds up to nearly 5 quarts of blood pumped by the heart in one minute, or about 75 gallons per hour.

The heart is surrounded by the *pericardium,* which consists of two layers of a tough membrane. The space between the two contains a lubricating fluid that allows the heart muscle to move freely. The *endocardium* is a smooth membrane lining the inside of the heart and its valves.

Blood circulates through the body by means of the pumping action of the heart, as shown in Figure 14.5. The right ventricle (on your own right side) pumps blood, via the *pulmonary arteries,* to the lungs, where it picks up oxygen (a gas essential to the body's cells) and gives off carbon dioxide (a waste product of metabolism). The blood returns from the lungs via the *pulmonary veins* to the left side of the heart, which pumps it, via the **aorta,** to the arteries in the rest of the body.

The arteries divide into smaller and smaller branches and finally into **capillaries,** the smallest blood vessels of all (only slightly larger in diameter than a single red blood cell). The blood within the capillaries supplies oxygen and nutrients to the cells of the tissues and takes up various waste products. Blood returns to the heart via the veins: The blood from the upper body (except the lungs) drains into the heart through the superior vena cava, while blood from the lower body returns via the *inferior vena cava.*

The workings of this remarkable pump affect your entire body. If the flow of blood to or through the heart or to the rest of the body is reduced, or if a disturbance occurs in the small bundle of highly specialized cells in the heart that generate electrical impulses to control heartbeats, the result may at first be too subtle to notice. However, without diagnosis and treatment, these changes could develop into a life-threatening problem.

Perhaps the biggest breakthrough in the field of cardiology has been not a test or a treatment but a realization: Heart disease is not inevitable. We can keep our hearts healthy for as long as we live, but the process of doing so must start early and continue throughout life.

Heart Risks on Campus

Many people, including college students and other young adults, are unaware of habits and conditions that put their hearts at risk. Many undergraduates view heart disease as mainly a problem for white men and underestimate the risks for women and ethnic groups. Students rate their own knowledge of heart disease as lower than that of sexually transmitted infections and psychological disorders. Yet heart disease is the third-leading cause of death among adults aged 25 to 44. Diabetes, family history, and other risk factors increase their likelihood of heart disease.

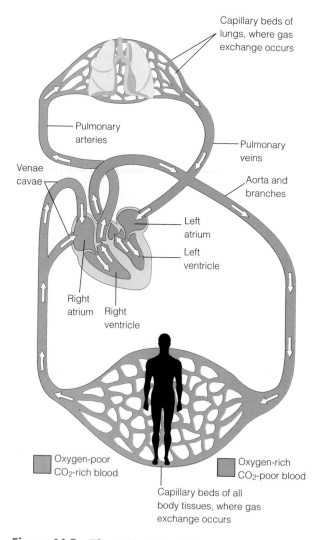

Figure 14.5 The Path of Blood Flow

Blood is pumped from the right ventricle into the pulmonary arteries, which lead to the lungs, where gas exchange (oxygen for carbon dioxide) occurs. Oxygenated blood returning from the lungs drains into the left atrium and is then pumped into the left ventricle, which sends the blood into the aorta and its branches. The oxygenated blood flows through the arteries, which extend to all parts of the body. Again, gas exchange occurs in the body tissues; this time oxygen is "dropped off" and carbon dioxide "picked up."

A single semester at college can put a student's heart at risk. Laboratory tests on 31 freshmen ages 18 to 22 at the beginning and end of their first term revealed a negative impact on total cholesterol, LDL cholesterol, and fasting glucose levels.[17]

Young athletes face special risks. Each year seemingly healthy teens or young adults die suddenly on playing fields and courts. The culprit in one of every three cases of sudden cardiac death in young athletes is a silent condition called hypertrophic cardiomyopathy (HCM), an excessive thickness of the heart muscle. Because of HCM, the heart is more prone to dangerous heart irregularities.

Hearts and Minds: Psychological Risk Factors

How you respond to everyday sources of stress can affect your heart as well as your overall health. While you may not be able to control the sources of stress, you can change how you habitually respond to it.

Researchers classify psychological risk factors for heart disease into three categories: chronic, episodic, and acute. Chronic factors, such as job strain or lack of social support, play an important role in the buildup of artery-clogging plaque and may increase blood pressure.[18] Even feeling that life has treated you unfairly boosts a person's chance of having a heart attack.[19]

Episodic factors, such as depression, can last from several weeks to two years and may lead to the creation of "unstable" plaque, which is more likely to break off and block a blood vessel within the heart. Short-term or acute psychological risk factors, such as an angry outburst, can directly trigger a heart attack in people with underlying heart disease.

These factors may act alone or combine and exert different effects at different ages and stages of life. They may influence behaviors such as smoking, diet, alcohol consumption, and physical activity, as well as directly cause changes in physiology.

Depression

Depression and heart disease often occur together. People with heart disease are more likely to be depressed, and some seemingly healthy people with depression are at 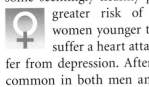 greater risk of heart problems. Depressed women younger than age 60 are more likely to suffer a heart attack than those who do not suffer from depression. After a heart attack, depression is common in both men and women, but physicians are less likely to recognize and treat depression in women.

Patients who suffer heart attacks and develop clinical depression have higher rates of complications and an increased risk of dying from another heart attack or other heart problems. People who are physically healthy with no risk factors for heart disease but who are prone to anger, hostility, and mild depression have higher levels of C-reactive protein, a substance linked to increased risk of heart disease.

Anger and Hostility

Anger and hostility have both short- and long-term consequences for the heart, particularly for men. In general the angriest men are three times more likely to develop heart disease than the most placid ones. Hostility more than doubles the risk of recurrent heart attacks in men (but not women). Research has linked hostility to increased cardiac risk factors, to decreased survival in men with coronary artery disease below the age of 61, to an increased risk of heart attack in men with metabolic syndrome, and to an increased risk of abnormal heart rhythms. Adults whose spouses rate them high in "antagonism"—a tendency to be argumentative, competitive, or cold—are more likely to have calcium buildup in their heart arteries.[20]

Angry young men may be putting their future heart health in jeopardy. In a study that tracked more than 1,000 physicians for 36 years and took into account other physical and psychological risk factors, the angriest young men were six times more likely to suffer heart attacks by 55 and three times more likely to develop any form of cardiovascular disease.[21] (See the lab on "Taming a Toxic Temper" in *IPC*.) **IPC**

How does hostility harm the heart? Anger triggers a surge in stress hormones that can provoke abnormal and potentially lethal heart rhythms and activates platelets, the

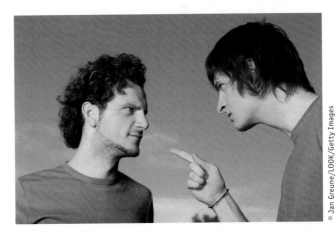

Hostility in men of any age can increase their risk of heart attacks and heart disease later in life.

systole The contraction phase of the cardiac cycle.

diastole The period between contractions in the cardiac cycle, during which the heart relaxes and dilates as it fills with blood.

aorta The main artery of the body, arising from the left ventricle of the heart.

capillary A minute blood vessel that connects an artery to a vein.

tiny blood cells that trigger blood clotting. High levels of anger can also trigger a spasm in a coronary artery, which results in the additional narrowing of a partially blocked blood vessel.

In women, anger and hostility do not always lead to heart troubles. However, women who outwardly express anger may be at increased risk if they also have other risk factors for heart disease, such as diabetes or unhealthy levels of lipoproteins.

Personality Types

In addition to stress, anger, and depression, other psychological traits can increase the risk of heart disease. Based on more than a decade of research, Dutch scientists have identified a "Type D" (for distressed) personality type. Type D people tend to be anxious, self-conscious, irritable, insecure, negative, and go to great lengths not to say or do anything that others might not like. In the Dutch study, almost four times as many Type D individuals as others in cardiac rehabilitation programs died within an eight-year period.

In the past, other personality types have been linked to disease, for example, hard-charging, hostile Type As to heart disease and conflict-avoiding, emotion-suppressing Type Cs to cancer. However, these traits have not proved to be significant risk factors for these illnesses.

Other Risk Factors

Inflammation and C-Reactive Protein

Inflammation—the process by which the body responds to fever, injury, or infection—plays an essential role in healing and recovering from infection. However, chronic low-grade inflammation may contribute to atherosclerosis and set the stage for heart attacks, strokes, and other forms of cardiovascular disease. The most common triggers of inflammation are smoking, lack of exercise, high-fat and high-calorie meals, and highly processed foods.

C-reactive protein (CRP), produced in the liver, rises whenever the body responds to inflammation. As scientists recognized the role of inflammation in heart disease, they developed the high-sensitivity CRP test (hsCRP), which detects coronary artery inflammation by measuring small changes in CRP. Several investigations have shown that CRP can predict heart disease before any other risk factors become evident, particularly in women. Individuals with the highest CRP levels are two to seven times more likely to develop heart disease than those with the lowest levels (see Table 14.3). High concentrations of CRP also may predict greater risk of sudden death. The test seems most useful in combination with a lipoprotein profile and assessments of other blood components.

Various strategies can reduce CRP levels. These include lifestyle changes (healthful diet, exercise, weight control, and not smoking) and medications (aspirin and, as needed, drugs to lower cholesterol and blood pressure). For more details, see Your Strategies for Change: "How to Lower Your C-Reactive Protein Level."

Homocysteine

High levels of *homocysteine*—an amino acid in the blood—have been linked to a greater risk of heart disease and stroke. Homocysteine may have an effect on atherosclerosis by damaging the inner lining of arteries and promoting blood clots. Several clinical trials are under way to test whether lowering homocysteine will reduce the risk of heart disease.

Illegal Drugs

Illegal drugs pose many dangers—one of the most serious is their potentially deadly impact on the cardiovascular system. Ecstasy, amphetamines, and cocaine can cause a sudden rise in blood pressure, heart rate, and contractions of the left ventricle (the pumping chamber) of the heart, which can increase the risk of a heart attack.

TABLE 14.3 C-Reactive Protein (CRP) Levels and Cardiovascular Risk

CRP (milligrams per liter)	Level of Cardiovascular Risk
Less than 0.5 mg/L	Lowest
Less than 1 mg/L	Low
1–3 mg/L	Moderate
Greater than 3 mg/L	High (risk doubles)

YOUR STRATEGIES FOR CHANGE *How to Lower Your C-Reactive Protein Level*

- Don't smoke.
- Eat a diet rich in fruit and vegetables.
- Increase your daily servings of whole grains and bran-containing foods.
- Switch from saturated fats and/or trans fats to olive oil, which has potent anti-inflammatory properties.
- Avoid highly refined carbohydrates (white bread, white rice, French fries, sugar-laden soda, etc.), which increase levels of inflammatory messengers called cytokines. Instead, eat whole grains, which dampen cytokine production.
- Munch on walnuts, peanuts, almonds, and other nuts and seeds that ease inflammation.
- Spice up your food with herbs and spices such as turmeric, ginger, garlic, basil, pepper, and many others with anti-inflammatory properties.

The hallucinogens lysergic acid diethylamide (LSD) and psilocybin (psychoactive mushrooms) also have the potential for triggering irregular heartbeats and heart attacks, although less serious cardiac complications, such as a temporary rise in blood pressure, are more common. Morphine and heroin, which account for almost half of drug-related deaths, can lower blood pressure and affect the heart rate. Inhalants can produce fatal heartbeat irregularities. Marijuana, the most widely used illegal drug among young adults, can affect blood pressure and heart rate, but it is not known whether it can trigger a heart attack.

Bacterial Infection

Certain bacteria may indeed put the heart at risk. *Streptococcus sanguis,* the bacterium found in dental plaque, has been implicated in the buildup of atherosclerotic plaque. Individuals with periodontal disease are at increased risk of heart disease and stroke. Regular brushing, flossing, and dental visits can reduce this danger.

Another common bacterium, *Chlamydia pneumoniae,* long linked to respiratory infections, also may threaten the heart. Individuals with high levels of antibodies to this bacteria are more likely to suffer a heart-related problem. Researchers have reported that antibiotics, taken to treat common infections, may protect against first-time heart attacks. A national clinical trial to determine whether antibiotics can reduce the risk of heart attack and stroke is under way.

The Heart of a Woman

Many people still think of heart disease as a "guy problem." Men do have a higher incidence of cardiovascular problems than women before age 45. Although women develop heart problems later in life, by about age 65, their risk is about the same as men's. Heart disease, which now kills one in four women in the United States, is the largest single cause of death of women worldwide.[22] American women are four to six times more likely to die of heart disease than of breast cancer.

New guidelines from the American Heart Association identify all women with at least one major cardiometabolic risk factor as being at risk for heart disease. Nine in ten women may meet this standard.[23] Many women don't get a proper diagnosis because they have a form of heart disease that doesn't show up on the usual diagnostic tests. In women with *vascular dysfunction,* the blood vessels—both the large coronary arteries and the small microvessels—supplying the heart do not expand properly to accommodate increased blood flow. Standard diagnostic procedures, including stress tests and coronary angiograms, do not reveal this condition. However, newer tests, including ultrasound of the blood vessels, can reveal heart problems that angiograms fail to pick up.

Because research has long focused on men, it also is not clear if women benefit equally from standard therapies. Aspirin, for instance, lowers the risk of heart attack in men of all ages, but not in women under age 65 (although it does reduce their stroke risk).[24] In women over 65, however, aspirin reduces both strokes and heart attacks.

Women are less likely to survive heart attacks than men, perhaps because they don't seek or receive treatment as soon as men. That's why women need to know the early signs and symptoms of female heart disease:

- Tiredness, even after getting adequate sleep.
- Trouble breathing.
- Trouble sleeping.
- Feeling sick to the stomach.
- Feeling scared or nervous.
- New or worse headaches.
- An ache in the chest.
- Feeling "heavy" or "tight" in the chest.
- A burning feeling in the chest.
- Pain in the back, between the shoulders.
- Pain or tightness in the chest that spreads to the jaw, neck, shoulders, ear, or the inside of the arms.
- Pain in the belly, above the belly button.

Researchers long believed that postmenopausal hormone therapy (HT) protected women from heart disease. However, more recent large-scale studies have shown little, if any, benefit. In fact, in older women HT increases the risk of cardiovascular problems and blood clots. However, women in their 50s who take estrogen therapy have lower levels of dangerous calcium deposits in their arteries, suggesting that supplemental estrogen for younger women with menopausal symptoms may benefit their hearts.[25]

In light of these inconclusive and contradictory results, the AHA guidelines recommend against use of hormone therapy simply to prevent heart disease. They also recommend not using antioxidant supplements or folic acid, which have proven ineffective.[26]

Aspirin and the Heart

Daily low-dose aspirin has been recommended as a preventive step for men at high risk of cardiovascular disease because it reduces the stickiness of platelets (cells that cause blood clotting). This lowers the risk of blood clots, which can block a blood vessel and trigger a heart attack or stroke. Several research studies have demonstrated an association between aspirin use and reductions in heart attacks in men.[27] However, while aspirin lowers the likelihood of heart attack, it may slightly increase stroke risk. As mentioned in the previous section, aspirin has not proved equally beneficial for women.

Who should consider aspirin therapy? Patients and their doctors should always make the decision, but in general those who might benefit include:

- Men over age 40 with several risk factors for having a heart attack.
- Men in their 50s, even if they don't have any risk factors.
- Women age 65 or older.
- Men and women with diabetes and at least one other risk factor.
- Anyone who has cardiovascular disease.

Aspirin can produce side effects, including gastrointestinal bleeding, allergic reactions, and peptic ulcers. However, the very low doses recommended for heart disease prevention generally do not cause serious problems. Aspirin is not advised for people taking anticlotting medication, who have stomach ulcers, or who have kidney or liver disease. Some individuals are aspirin-resistant and do not benefit from its protective effects.

Crises of the Heart

Coronary Artery Disease

The general term for any impairment of blood flow through the blood vessels, often referred to as "hardening of the arteries," is **arteriosclerosis.** The most common form is **atherosclerosis,** a disease of the lining of the arteries in which **plaque**—deposits of fat, fibrin (a clotting material), cholesterol, other cell parts, and calcium—narrows the artery channels. Twenty-first century research has revealed that inflammation also plays a crucial role.

Atherosclerosis

This process begins when LDL cholesterol penetrates the wall of an artery. Ideally, HDL cholesterol carries the cholesterol out of the artery wall to the liver for disposal. However, if LDL accumulates, the artery responds by releasing chemical messengers called cytokines, which trigger active inflammation in the artery wall. T-lymphocytes and macrophages, specialized white blood cells that are part of the body's defensive immune system, move from the bloodstream into the artery and engulf the LDL. As they ingest the LDL, the macrophages enlarge and become foam cells, which rupture, releasing cholesterol into the artery wall, where the cycle of damage begins again. In response, the smooth muscle cells in the artery wall create a fibrous cap over the inflamed area (Figure 14.6).

These hard-capped plaques are dangerous: They narrow arteries, reduce the flow of blood, and produce angina (chest pain). However, the usual culprits in heart attacks are smaller, softer plaques that can rupture. As the body responds with clotting factors, platelets, and blood cells, a blood clot, or thrombus, forms on the disrupted plaque's surface. The clot ultimately blocks the artery and kills heart muscle cells. Similar clots can block blood flow to the brain and lead to other complications, including kidney failure and circulation problems in the legs and feet.

Unclogging the Arteries

Reversing the buildup of plaque inside the arteries is possible with cholesterol-lowering drugs and a low-fat diet. A strict program of dietary and lifestyle change without any medication, developed by Dean Ornish, M.D., of the

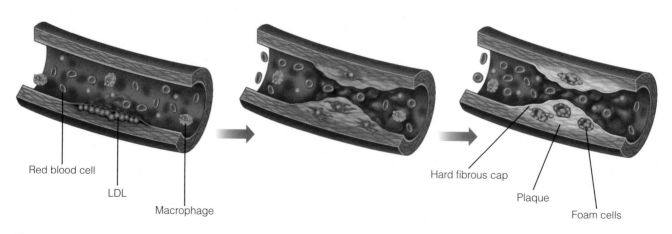

Red blood cell

LDL

Macrophage

Hard fibrous cap

Plaque

Foam cells

Figure 14.6 How Atherosclerosis Happens
LDL cholesterol penetrates an artery wall, and the accumulation of LDL cholesterol triggers an inflammation. Macrophages engulf the LDL and become foam cells. The artery wall creates a fibrous cap over this plaque, and the artery is narrowed. If the plaque ruptures, blood clots can block blood flow to the heart or to the brain.

University of California, San Francisco, also has proved effective in reversing coronary artery disease. The following are the key elements of this approach:

- **A very low-fat, vegetarian diet,** including nonfat dairy products and egg whites, keeping fat intake to below 8 percent of total calories consumed. Ornish's recommended diet allows no meat, poultry, fish, butter, cheese, ice cream, or any form of oil.
- **Moderate exercise,** consisting of an hour of aerobic activity three times a week. Walking is recommended because more rigorous exercise might be dangerous for heart patients, who may develop increased risk of blood clots, irregular heartbeats, or coronary artery spasms during exertion.
- **Stress counseling.** Ornish's patients learn how the body's stress response can cause a rapid heartbeat and narrowing of the arteries, and how stress reduction can reduce cholesterol levels.
- **An hour a day of yoga, meditation, breathing, and progressive relaxation.** Some patients use visualization, for instance, imagining their arteries being cleared by a tunneling machine.

Angina Pectoris

A temporary drop in the supply of oxygen to the heart tissue causes feelings of pain or discomfort in the chest known as **angina pectoris.** Some people suffer angina only when the demands on their hearts increase, such as during exercise or when under stress. Many people have angina for years and yet never suffer a heart attack; in some, the angina even disappears. However, angina should be considered a warning of danger if it becomes more severe or more frequent, occurs with less activity or exertion, begins to waken a person from a sound sleep at night, persists for more than ten to fifteen minutes, or causes unusual perspiration.

Heart Attack (Myocardial Infarction)

Each year, about 1.5 million Americans suffer a heart attack. About 500,000 die. Half of the deaths occur within an hour of the start of symptoms and before the person reaches the hospital. The medical name for a heart attack, or coronary, is **myocardial infarction (MI).** The *myocardium* is the cardiac muscle layer of the wall of the heart. It receives its blood supply, and thus its oxygen and other nutrients, from the coronary arteries. If an artery is blocked by a clot or plaque, or by a spasm, the myocardial cells do not get sufficient oxygen, and the portion of the myocardium deprived of its blood supply begins to die.

Although such an attack may seem sudden, usually it has been building up for years, particularly if the person has ignored risk factors and early warning signs. According to research, 80 to 90 percent of those who develop heart disease and 95 percent of those who suffer a fatal heart attack have at least one major risk factor.

Is It a Heart Attack?

If they experience the following symptoms, individuals should seek immediate medical care and take an aspirin (325 milligrams) to keep the blood clot in a coronary artery from getting any bigger:

- A tight ache, heavy, squeezing pain, or discomfort in the center of the chest, which may last for 30 minutes or more and is not relieved by rest.
- Chest pain that radiates to the shoulder, arm, neck, back, or jaw.
- Anxiety.
- Sweating or cold, clammy skin.
- Nausea and vomiting.
- Shortness of breath.
- Dizziness, fainting, or loss of consciousness.

As noted on page 413, women often experience heart attacks differently than men. In the month before an attack, many report unusual fatigue and disturbed sleep. Far fewer women than men experience chest pain. More common symptoms are shortness of breath, weakness and fatigue, a clammy sweat, dizziness, and nausea.

If you're with someone who's exhibiting the classic signs of heart attack, and if they last for two minutes or more, act at once. Expect the person to deny the possibility of anything as serious as a heart attack, but insist on taking prompt action.

Time is of the essence when a heart attack occurs. If you develop symptoms or if you're with someone who does, call 911 immediately. The sooner emergency personnel get to a heart attack victim and administer cardiac life support, the greater the odds of survival. Yet according to the American Heart Association, most patients wait three hours after the initial symptoms begin before seeking help. By that time, half of the affected heart muscle may already be lost.

---

arteriosclerosis Any of a number of chronic diseases characterized by degeneration of the arteries and hardening and thickening of arterial walls.

atheriosclerosis A form of arteriosclerosis in which fatty substances (plaque) are deposited on the inner walls of arteries.

plaque The sludgelike substance that builds up on the inner walls of arteries.

angina pectoris A severe, suffocating chest pain caused by a brief lack of oxygen to the heart.

myocardial infarction (MI) A condition characterized by the dying of tissue areas in the myocardium, caused by interruption of the blood supply to those areas; the medical name for a heart attack.

Cardiac Arrest

Cardiac arrest occurs when the heart stops beating. If circulation isn't restored within four or five minutes, the brain shuts down completely, and the person dies. **Cardiopulmonary resuscitation (CPR),** a combination of mouth-to-mouth breathing and chest compressions, can keep individuals with cardiac arrest alive until they can be treated in a hospital.

Only about one in twenty people who have a cardiac arrest outside a hospital survive, even if they receive CPR. The reason may be that even trained health professionals do not perform CPR correctly. CPR is most effective when started within minutes of a cardiac arrest by trained medical personnel who arrive within 8 to 12 minutes. Chest compression, not mouth-to-mouth resuscitation, seems to be the key to helping someone recover from a cardiac arrest.

Automated external defibrillators (AEDs), portable computerized devices, can actually restart a heart with a lethal rhythm (ventricular fibrillation) or that is not beating at all. The machines, widely available on airplanes and in public places like stadiums and terminals, also can be purchased by individuals. Written and voice instructions allow lay people as well as trained professionals to use them in case of emergency. A combination of CPR and defibrillation boosts the survival rate much higher than from CPR alone.

Saving Hearts

State-of-the-art treatments for heart attacks include clot-dissolving drugs, early administration of medications to thin the blood, intravenous nitroglycerin, and in some cases, a beta-blocker (which blocks many of the effects of adrenaline in the body, particularly its stimulating impact on the heart).

Percutaneous transluminal coronary angioplasty (PTCA), also called balloon angioplasty, is the most often performed heart operation. Less costly and less risky than bypass surgery, PTCA opens blood vessels in the heart that are narrowed but not completely blocked. PTCA involves a precise, time-consuming technique called *cardiac catheterization*—the threading of a narrow tube or catheter through an artery to the heart. An X-ray taken with a special dye injected into the arteries reveals the location and extent of a blockage. By inflating a tiny balloon at the tip of the catheter, physicians can break up the clog and widen the narrowed artery. When they deflate the balloon, circulation is restored. Stents can help prevent balloon-opened arteries from clogging again.

A *coronary bypass* is a procedure in which an artery from the patient's leg or chest wall is grafted onto a coronary artery to detour blood around the blocked area. Each year hundreds of thousands of coronary bypasses are performed in the United States; about 1 to 5 percent of these patients die as a result of surgical complications. Surgery or angioplasty to improve blood flow in patients with moderate to severe levels of blood flow restriction to the heart reduces the risk of cardiac death more than drugs alone.

Stroke

When the blood supply to a portion of the brain is blocked, a cerebrovascular accident, or **stroke,** occurs. More than a quarter of those who have strokes are under age 65. About two-thirds of the 750,000 strokes that occur every year in the United States strike women. However, before age 85, men experience more strokes. Nonetheless, women of every age fare worse than men in the prevention, diagnosis, treatment, and outcome of stroke.[28] An estimated 20 percent of stroke victims die within three months; 50 to 60 percent are disabled. About half of those who have a stroke are partially paralyzed on one side of their body; between a quarter and a half are partially or completely dependent on others for daily living; a third become depressed; a fifth cannot walk. Quick treatment with a clot-busting drug at a hospital can reduce the chance of disability after a stroke, but few people recognize the signs of a stroke (see Your Strategies for Prevention: "How to Recognize a Stroke") and seek medical care within three hours of the first symptoms.[29]

Strokes rank third, after heart disease and cancer, as a cause of death in this country. Worldwide, stroke is second only to heart disease as a cause of death. After decades of steady decline, the number of strokes per year has begun to rise. The main reasons seem to be that more people in the United States are living longer, advanced medical care is allowing more people to survive heart disease, and doctors are better able to diagnose and detect strokes. Yet 80 percent of strokes are preventable, and key risk factors can be modified through either lifestyle changes or drugs. The most important steps are treating hypertension, not smoking, managing diabetes, lowering cholesterol, and taking aspirin, which reduces stroke risk in women, but not men.

Causes of Stroke

There are two types of stroke: *ischemic stroke,* which is the result of a blockage that disrupts blood flow to the brain, and *hemorrhagic stroke,* which occurs when blood vessels rupture. One of the most common causes of ischemic stroke is the blockage of a brain artery by a thrombus, or blood clot—a *cerebral thrombosis.* Clots generally form around deposits sticking out from the arterial wall. Sometimes a wandering blood clot (embolus), carried in the bloodstream, becomes wedged in one of the cerebral arteries. This is called a *cerebral embolism*, and it can completely plug up a cerebral artery.

In hemorrhagic stroke, a diseased artery in the brain floods the surrounding tissue with blood. The cells nourished by the artery are deprived of blood and can't function, and the blood from the artery forms a clot that may interfere with brain function. This is most likely to occur if the patient suffers from a combination of hypertension and atherosclerosis. Hemorrhage (bleeding) may also be caused by a head injury or by the bursting of an aneurysm, a blood-filled pouch that balloons out from a weak spot in the wall of an artery.

Brain tissue, like heart muscle, begins to die if deprived of oxygen, which may then cause difficulty speaking and walking, and loss of memory. These effects may be slight or severe, temporary or permanent, depending on how widespread the damage and whether other areas of the brain can take over the function of the damaged area. About 30 percent of stroke survivors develop dementia, a disorder that robs a person of memory and other intellectual abilities.

Risk Factors

Risk factors for stroke, like those for heart disease, include some that can't be changed (such as gender, race, and age) and some that can be controlled:

- **Gender.** Men have a greater risk of stroke than women. However, women are at increased risk at times of marked hormonal changes, particularly pregnancy and childbirth. Past studies have shown an association between oral contraceptive use and stroke, particularly in women over age 35 who smoke. The newer low-dose oral contraceptives have not shown an increased stroke risk among women ages 18 to 44.

- **Race.** The incidence of strokes is two to three times greater in blacks than whites in the same communities. Hispanics also are more likely to develop hemorrhagic strokes than whites.

- **Age.** A person's risk of stroke more than doubles every decade after age 55.

- **Hypertension.** Detection and treatment of high blood pressure are the best means of stroke prevention.

- **High red blood cell count.** A moderate to marked increase in the number of a person's red blood cells increases the risk of stroke.

- **Heart disease.** Heart problems can interfere with the flow of blood to the brain; clots that form in the heart can travel to the brain, where they may clog an artery.

- **Blood fats.** Although the standard advice from cardiologists is to lower harmful LDL levels, what may be more important to lower stroke risk is an increase in the levels of protective HDL.

- **Diabetes mellitus.** Diabetics have a higher incidence of stroke than nondiabetics.

- **Estrogen therapy.** In the Women's Health Initiative—a series of clinical trials of hormone therapy for postmenopausal women—estrogen-only therapy significantly increased the risk of stroke.

- **A diet high in fat and sodium.** Individuals consuming the largest amounts of fatty foods and sodium are at much greater risk then those eating low-fat, low-salt diets.

Transient Ischemic Attacks (TIAs)

Sometimes a person will suffer **transient ischemic attacks (TIAs)**, "little strokes" that cause minimal damage but serve as warning signs of a potentially more severe stroke. One of three people who suffer TIAs will have a stroke during the following five years if they don't get treatment. The two major types of TIAs are:

cardiopulmonary resuscitation (CPR) A method of artificial stimulation of the heart and lungs; a combination of mouth-to-mouth breathing and chest compression.

stroke A cerebrovascular event in which the blood supply to a portion of the brain is blocked.

transient ischemic attack (TIA) A cerebrovascular event in which the blood supply to a portion of the brain is blocked temporarily; repeated attacks are predictors of more severe strokes.

- **Transient monocular blindness.** Blurring, a black-out or whiteout of vision, a sense of a shade coming down, or another visual disturbance in one eye.
- **Transient hemispheral attack.** Diminished blood flow to one side of the brain, causing numbness or weakness of one arm, leg, or side of the face, or problems speaking or thinking.

Many TIAs are caused by a narrowing of blood vessels in the neck (carotid arteries) because of a buildup of plaque. Specialists can diagnose this problem by feeling and listening to the arteries, by ultrasound, by measuring the pressure or circulation rate from the carotid arteries to the eyes, or by arterial angiography (injection of a dye into the arteries as X-rays are taken), a procedure that can be either dangerous, even deadly, or lifesaving.

Surgery to widen the carotid arteries may be recommended for individuals under age 60 with significant narrowing (50 to 80 percent or more). For other patients, aspirin and other drugs that make platelets less sticky and interfere with clotting may be effective.

Treatments for Strokes

Daily low-dose aspirin cuts in half the risk of strokes caused by abnormal heartbeats, which strike 75,000 Americans each year. Extremely rapid beating of the heart's upper chambers causes blood clots to form; they may enter the bloodstream and travel to the brain, where they can get stuck and choke off the blood supply. In the past, the only way to prevent such strokes was regular use of a medication called warfarin, which inhibits blood clotting and therefore increases the risk of severe bleeding. However, aspirin proved as effective as warfarin—without that dangerous side effect.

It now seems possible to save brain cells during a brief period immediately after a thrombotic stroke occurs. Thrombolytic drugs such as tissue-type plasminogen activator (tPA) can restore brain blood flow after a thrombotic stroke; other medications called heparinoids can reduce the blood's tendency to clot. For thrombolytic drugs to be effective, they must be administered within three hours after the stroke; heparinoids must be given within 24 hours. However, the average person does not seek help for 22 hours or longer.

 Men are more likely than women to benefit from clot-busting drugs.[30]

Cancer

Cancer has overtaken heart disease as the number-one killer of Americans under age 85. Yet many of the more than half a million deaths caused by cancer each year could be prevented. A third of cancers are related to smoking; another third, to obesity, poor diet, and lack of exercise.

Understanding Cancer

The uncontrolled growth and spread of abnormal cells causes cancer. Normal cells follow the code of instructions embedded in DNA (the body's genetic material); cancer cells do not. Think of the DNA within the nucleus of a cell as a computer program that controls the cell's functioning, including its ability to grow and reproduce itself. If this program or its operation is altered, the cell goes out of control. The nucleus no longer regulates growth. The abnormal cell divides to create other abnormal cells, which again divide, eventually forming *neoplasms* (new formations), or tumors.

How Cancer Spreads

Tumors can be either *benign* (slightly abnormal, not considered life-threatening) or *malignant* (cancerous). The only way to determine whether a tumor is benign is by microscopic examination of its cells. Cancer cells have larger nuclei than the cells in benign tumors; they vary more in shape and size; and they divide more often.

At one time cancer was thought to be a single disease that attacked different parts of the body. Now scientists believe that cancer comes in countless forms, each with a genetically determined molecular "fingerprint" that indicates how deadly it is. With this understanding, doctors can identify how aggressively a tumor should be treated.

Without treatment, cancer cells continue to grow, crowding out and replacing healthy cells. This process is called **infiltration,** or invasion. Cancer cells may also **metastasize,** or spread to other parts of the body via the bloodstream or lymphatic system (Figure 14.7). For many cancers, as many as 60 percent of patients may have metastases (which may be too small to be felt or seen without a microscope) at the time of diagnosis. Early detection and treatment result in the highest rate of cure—see Your Strategies for Prevention: "Seven Warning Signs of Cancer."

YOUR STRATEGIES FOR PREVENTION *Seven Warning Signs of Cancer*

If you note any of the following seven warning signs, immediately schedule an appointment with your doctor:

- Change in bowel or bladder habits.
- A sore that doesn't heal.
- Unusual bleeding or discharge.
- Thickening or lump in the breast, testis, or elsewhere.
- Indigestion or difficulty swallowing.
- Obvious change in a wart or mole.
- Nagging cough or hoarseness.

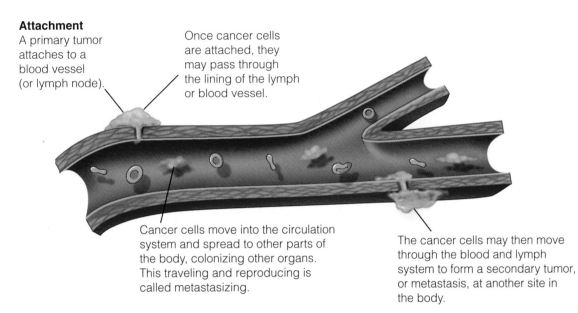

Attachment
A primary tumor attaches to a blood vessel (or lymph node).

Once cancer cells are attached, they may pass through the lining of the lymph or blood vessel.

Cancer cells move into the circulation system and spread to other parts of the body, colonizing other organs. This traveling and reproducing is called metastasizing.

The cancer cells may then move through the blood and lymph system to form a secondary tumor, or metastasis, at another site in the body.

Figure 14.7 Metastasis, or Spread of Cancer
Cancer cells can travel through the blood vessels to spread to other organs or through the lymphatic system to form secondary tumors.

Risk Factors for Cancer

Annual cancer deaths in the United States are falling. According to the American Cancer Society, 1.4 million individuals are diagnosed with cancer each year; about 559,000 die of it. The five-year survival rate for all cancer is 66 percent, up from 50 percent three decades ago.[31]

Since the occurrence of cancer increases over time, most cases affect adults who are middle-aged or older. In the United States, men have a one in two lifetime risk of developing cancer; for women, the risk is one in three (Figure 14.8).

The term **relative risk** compares the risk of developing cancer in people with a certain exposure or trait to the risk in those who do not have this exposure or trait. Smokers, for instance, have a ten-times-greater relative risk of developing lung cancer than nonsmokers. Most relative risks are smaller. For example, women who have a first-degree (mother, sister, or daughter) family history of breast cancer have about a twofold increased risk of developing breast cancer compared with women who do not have a family history of the disease. This means that they are about twice as likely to develop breast cancer.

Heredity

An estimated 13 to 14 million Americans may be at risk of a hereditary cancer. In hereditary cancers, such as retinoblastoma (an eye cancer that strikes young children) or certain colon cancers, a specific cancer-causing gene is passed down from generation to generation. The odds of any child with one affected parent inheriting this gene and developing the cancer are fifty/fifty.

Other people are born with genes that make them susceptible to having certain cells grow and divide uncontrol-

lably, which may contribute to cancer development. The most well-known are mutations of the BRCA gene, linked with increased risk of breast, colon, and ovarian cancer.

Genetic tests can identify some individuals who are born with an increased susceptibility to cancer. By spotting a mutated gene in an individual, doctors can sometimes detect cancer years earlier through increased cancer screening. The most likely sites for inherited cancers to

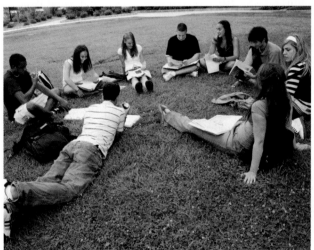

By age 39, 1 in 64 men and 1 in 51 women will develop cancer. As you look ahead to your future, consider your risk factors and lifestyle: What do you think are your odds of getting cancer?

infiltration A gradual penetration or invasion.

metastasize To spread to other parts of the body via the bloodstream or lymphatic system.

relative risk The risk of developing cancer in persons with a certain exposure or trait compared to the risk in persons who do not have the same exposure or trait.

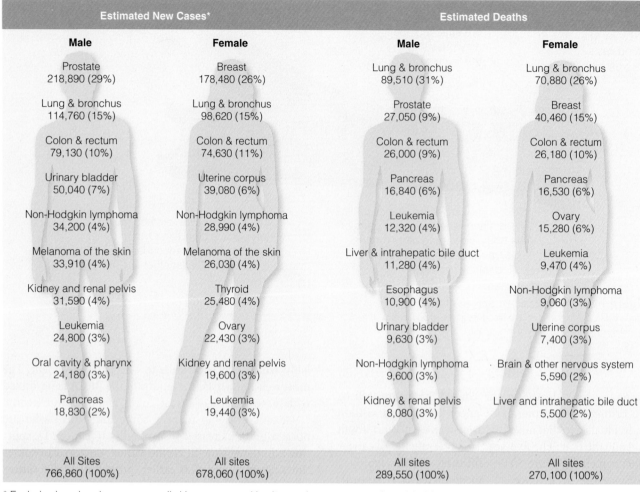

Estimated New Cases*		Estimated Deaths	
Male	**Female**	**Male**	**Female**
Prostate 218,890 (29%)	Breast 178,480 (26%)	Lung & bronchus 89,510 (31%)	Lung & bronchus 70,880 (26%)
Lung & bronchus 114,760 (15%)	Lung & bronchus 98,620 (15%)	Prostate 27,050 (9%)	Breast 40,460 (15%)
Colon & rectum 79,130 (10%)	Colon & rectum 74,630 (11%)	Colon & rectum 26,000 (9%)	Colon & rectum 26,180 (10%)
Urinary bladder 50,040 (7%)	Uterine corpus 39,080 (6%)	Pancreas 16,840 (6%)	Pancreas 16,530 (6%)
Non-Hodgkin lymphoma 34,200 (4%)	Non-Hodgkin lymphoma 28,990 (4%)	Leukemia 12,320 (4%)	Ovary 15,280 (6%)
Melanoma of the skin 33,910 (4%)	Melanoma of the skin 26,030 (4%)	Liver & intrahepatic bile duct 11,280 (4%)	Leukemia 9,470 (4%)
Kidney and renal pelvis 31,590 (4%)	Thyroid 25,480 (4%)	Esophagus 10,900 (4%)	Non-Hodgkin lymphoma 9,060 (3%)
Leukemia 24,800 (3%)	Ovary 22,430 (3%)	Urinary bladder 9,630 (3%)	Uterine corpus 7,400 (3%)
Oral cavity & pharynx 24,180 (3%)	Kidney and renal pelvis 19,600 (3%)	Non-Hodgkin lymphoma 9,600 (3%)	Brain & other nervous system 5,590 (2%)
Pancreas 18,830 (2%)	Leukemia 19,440 (3%)	Kidney & renal pelvis 8,080 (3%)	Liver and intrahepatic bile duct 5,500 (2%)
All Sites 766,860 (100%)	All sites 678,060 (100%)	All sites 289,550 (100%)	All sites 270,100 (100%)

* Excludes basal and squamous cell skin cancers and in situ carcinoma except urinary bladder.

Figure 14.8 Sex Differences in Cancer Rates and Deaths

Source: © 2007, American Cancer Society, Inc., Surveillance Research.

develop are the breast, brain, blood, muscles, bones, and adrenal glands. (See Point/Counterpoint: "Would You Want to Know?")

The telltale signs of inherited cancers include:

- **Early development.** Genetic forms of certain diseases strike earlier than noninherited cancers. For example, the average age of women diagnosed with breast cancer is 62. But if breast cancer is inherited, the average age at diagnosis is 44, an 18-year difference.

- **Family history.** Anyone with a close relative (mother, father, sibling, child) with cancer has about three times the usual chance of getting the same type of cancer.

- **Multiple targets.** The same type of hereditary cancer often strikes more than once—in both breasts or both kidneys, for instance, or in two separate parts of the same organ.

- **Unusual gender pattern.** Genes may be responsible for cancers that generally don't strike a certain gender—for example, breast cancer in a man.

- **Cancer family syndrome.** Some families, with unusually large numbers of relatives affected by cancer, seem clearly cancer-prone. For instance, in Lynch syndrome (a form of colon cancer), more than 20 percent of the family members in at least two generations develop cancer of both the colon and the endometrium.

Racial and Ethnic Groups

 More cases of cancer occur in African Americans than in any other racial or ethnic group.[32] Blacks are 30 percent more likely to die of cancer than whites. African American women have the highest incidence of colorectal and lung cancers of any ethnic group, while black men have the highest rates of prostate, colorectal, and lung cancer. African Americans

POINT COUNTERPOINT *Would You Want to Know?*

POINT
Medical science can already detect the genes that put some individuals at risk of serious, potentially fatal diseases. Women who find out that they carry particular genes may, for instance, decide to undergo surgery to remove their breasts or ovaries before cancer develops. As more tests become available, people should take advantage of the opportunity to peer into their medical futures.

COUNTERPOINT
The presence of certain genes does not predict with 100 percent certainty that an individual will develop the disease. And there

are no preventive measures or cures for some illnesses, such as Huntington's disease (a severe degenerative neurological disorder). Thus, the results of genetic testing could lead to unnecessary procedures or have a devastating psychological impact.

YOUR VIEW
Do any major illnesses run in your family? Would you like to know your odds of developing them? What if prevention required something as drastic as removal of an organ? What if nothing could be done to prevent the disease? Would you still want to know?

---

also have higher rates of incidence and deaths from other cancers, including those of the mouth, throat, esophagus, stomach, pancreas, and larynx.

Cancer rates also vary in other racial and ethnic groups. Hispanics have a six times lower risk of developing melanoma than Caucasians, yet tend to have a worse prognosis than Caucasians when they do develop this skin cancer. The incidence of female breast cancer is highest among white women and lowest among Native American women. Cervical cancer is most common in Hispanic women.

Asian Americans, both those born in the United States and immigrants, generally have lower cancer rates than other ethnic groups. Vietnamese men have much higher rates of liver cancer than whites, while Korean men and women are much more likely to develop stomach cancer. Compared with other Asian Americans, Chinese and Vietnamese women have higher rates of lung cancer. Asian Americans who have lived in the United States the longest are likely to develop the cancers that are most common here, such as breast and colon cancer, although at lower rates than whites.[33]

Obesity

Long recognized as threats to cardiovascular health, overweight and obesity may play a role in an estimated 90,000 cancer deaths each year. According to American Cancer Society researchers who examined the relationship between body mass index (BMI) and risk of dying from cancer, 14 percent of cancer deaths in men and 20 percent of cancer deaths in women may stem from excess weight.

The higher an individual's BMI, the greater the likelihood of dying of cancer. An unhealthy body weight increases the risk of many types of cancer, including breast (in postmenopausal women), colon and rectum, kidney, cervix, ovary, uterus, esophagus, gallbladder, stomach (in men), liver, pancreas, prostate, non-Hodgkin's lymphoma, and multiple myeloma.

The degree to which extra pounds affect cancer risk varies by site. Obesity elevates the risk of esophageal can-

cer fivefold; increases the risk of breast or uterine cancer by two to four times; and boosts the risk for colon cancer by 35 percent to twofold.

Infectious Agents

Worldwide, an estimated 17 percent of cancers can be attributed to infection. In economically developing countries, infections cause or contribute to 26 percent of cancers. In developed countries, they play a role in 7 percent of new cases of cancer.

Among the cancers that have been linked with infectious agents are human papilloma virus (HPV) with cervical cancer and *Helicobacter pylori* with stomach cancer. Viruses have been implicated in certain leukemias (cancers of the blood system) and lymphomas (cancers of the lymphatic system), cancers of the nose and pharynx, liver cancer, and cervical cancer. (See Chapter 16 for details on the human papilloma virus.) Human immune deficiency virus (HIV) can lead to certain lymphomas and leukemias and to a type of cancer called Kaposi's sarcoma.

Generally, the presence of a bacterium or a virus per se is not enough to cause cancer. A predisposing environment and other cofactors—most still unknown—are needed for cancer development and growth.

Common Types of Cancer

Cancer refers to a group of more than a hundred diseases characterized by abnormal cell growth. Although all cancers have similar characteristics, each is distinct. Some cancers are relatively simple to cure, whereas others are more threatening and mysterious. The earlier any cancer is found, the easier it is to treat and the better the patient's chances of survival.

Cancers are classified according to the type of cell and the organ in which they originate, such as the following:

- **Carcinoma,** the most common kind, which starts in the epithelium, the layers of cells that cover the body's surface or line internal organs and glands.

- **Sarcoma,** which forms in the supporting, or connective, tissues of the body: bones, muscles, blood vessels.
- **Leukemia,** which begins in the blood-forming tissues: bone marrow, lymph nodes, and the spleen.
- **Lymphoma,** which arises in the cells of the lymph system, the network that filters out impurities.

Skin Cancer

One of every five Americans can expect to develop skin cancer in their lifetimes. Once scientists thought exposure to the B range of ultraviolet light (UVB), the wavelength of light responsible for sunburn, posed the greatest danger. However, longer-wavelength UVA, which penetrates deeper into the skin, also plays a major role in skin cancers. An estimated 80 percent of total lifetime sun exposure occurs during childhood, so sun protection is especially important in youngsters. Tanning salons and sunlamps also increase the risk of skin cancer because they produce ultraviolet radiation. A half-hour dose of radiation from a sunlamp can be equivalent to the amount you'd get from an entire day in the sun.

 Young adults spend the most time in the sun and also frequent tanning salons. Even when they perceive the seriousness of skin cancer, college students—particularly women—describe suntanned skin as attractive, healthy, and athletic-looking and view the benefits of getting a suntan as outweighing the risks of skin cancer or premature aging. Some students actually become addicted to tanning.[34] (See Your Strategies for Change: "Are You Addicted to Tanning?") However, a CDC report concluded that indoor tanning is "simply not safe" and causes sunburn, infection, eye damage, and increased risk of skin cancer.[35]

The most common skin cancers are *basal cell* (involving the base of the epidermis, the top level of the skin) and *squamous cell* (involving cells in the epidermis). Their incidence is increasing among men and women under the age of 40. Long-term exposure to the sun is the biggest risk factor for these cancers.

Every year more than 5 million Americans develop skin lesions known as actinic keratoses (AKs), rough red or brown scaly patches that develop in the upper layer of the skin, usually on the face, lower lip, bald scalp, neck, and back of the hands and forearms. Forty percent of squamous cell carcinomas, the second leading cause of skin cancer deaths, begin as AKs. Treatments include surgical removal, cryosurgery (freezing the skin), electrodesiccation (heat generated by an electric current), topical chemotherapy, and removal with lasers, chemical peels, or dermabrasion.

Smoking and exposure to certain hydrocarbons in asphalt, coal tar, and pitch may increase the risk of squamous cell skin cancer. Other risk factors include occupational exposure to carcinogens and inherited skin disorders, such as xeroderma pigmentosum and familial atypical multiple-mole melanoma.

Malignant *melanoma,* the deadliest type of skin cancer, causes 1 to 2 percent of all cancer deaths. During the 1930s, the lifetime risk of melanoma was about 1 in 1,500. Today it is 1 in 75. This increase in risk is due mostly to overexposure to UV radiation. The use of a tanning bed ten times or more a year doubles the risk for individuals over age 30.

Both the amount and the intensity of lifetime sun exposure play key roles in determining risk for melanoma. People living in areas where the sun's ultraviolet rays reach Earth with extra intensity, such as tropical or high-altitude regions, are at increased risk. Although melanoma occurs more often among people over 40, it is increasing in younger people, particularly those who had severe sunburns in childhood. The rate of increase in melanoma also has risen more in men (4.6 percent a year) than in women (3.2 percent). Men are more likely than women to be diagnosed with melanoma after age 40.

Individuals with any of the following characteristics are at increased risk:

- **Fair skin,** light eyes, or fair hair.
- **A tendency to develop freckles** and to burn instead of tan.

YOUR STRATEGIES FOR CHANGE *Are You Addicted to Tanning?*

You know that exposure to ultraviolet rays increases your risk of developing skin cancer, but maybe you still can't stay out of the sun or a tanning booth. Why? Researchers theorize that repetitive tanning behavior may be the result of a kind of addiction.[36]

Texas beachgoers, asked questions about their tanning habits, gave replies similar to those who gamble or drink compulsively.

About a quarter of those interviewed were classified as "ultraviolet light (UVL) dependent" because of their answers to the CAGE screening test, which asks the following questions:

- **C**ut: Ever felt you ought to cut down on your behavior?
- **A**nnoyed: Have people annoyed you by criticizing your behavior?

- **G**uilt: Ever felt bad or guilty about your behavior?
- **E**ye Opener: Ever engaged in your behavior to steady your nerves in the morning?

Answering yes to two of the CAGE questions is a strong indication for an addictive behavior; answering yes to three confirms it.

- **A history of childhood sunburn** or intermittent, intense sun exposure.
- **A personal or family history** of melanoma.
- **A large number of nevi,** or moles (200 or more, or 50 or more if under age 20), or dysplastic (atypical) moles.

For tips on overcoming these risks, see Your Strategies for Prevention: "How to Save Your Skin."

Detection   The most common predictor for melanoma is a change in an existing mole or development of a new and changing pigmented mole. The most important early indicators are change in color, an increase in diameter, and changes in the borders of a mole (Figure 14.9). An increase in height signals a corresponding growth in depth under the skin. Itching in a new or long-standing mole also should not be ignored.

Treatment   If caught early, melanoma is highly curable, usually with surgery alone. Once it has spread, chemotherapy with a single drug or a combination can temporarily shrink tumors in some people. However, the five-year survival rate for metastatic melanoma is only 14 percent.

Breast Cancer

Every 3 minutes, a woman in the United States learns that she has breast cancer. Every 12 minutes, a woman dies of breast cancer. Many women misjudge their own likelihood of developing breast cancer, either overestimating or underestimating their susceptibility. In a national poll, 1 in every 10 surveyed considered herself at no risk at all. This is never the case. Every woman is at risk for breast cancer simply because she's female.

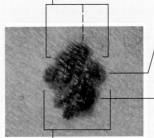

Asymmetry: One half doesn't match the other half

Border irregularity: The edges are ragged, notched, or blurred

Color: Rather than uniform pigmentation, there are shades of tan, brown, and black, with possible dashes of red, white, and blue.

Diameter: The mole is larger than 6 mm (about the size of a pencil eraser). (The melanoma shown here is magnified about 20 times its actual size.)

Courtesy of the Skin Cancer Foundation

Figure 14.9   ABCD: The Warning Signs of Melanoma
An estimated 95 percent of cases of melanoma arise from an existing mole. A normal mole is usually round or oval, less than 6 millimeters (about ¼ inch) in diameter, and evenly colored (black, brown, or tan). Seek prompt evaluation of any moles that change in ways shown in the photo.

Source: American Academy of Dermatology. All rights reserved.

However, not all women's risks are equal. The National Cancer Institute (NCI) has developed a computerized Breast Cancer Risk Assessment Tool, based on data from more than 280,000 women, that allows a woman to sit down with her doctor and discuss her own odds of developing breast cancer within the next five years and over her entire lifetime.

The most common risk factors include the following:

- **Age.** As shown in Figure 14.10, at 25, a woman's chance of developing breast cancer is 1 in 19,608; by age 45, it has increased to 1 in 93; by 65, it is 1 in 17. The mean age at which women are diagnosed is 63.

- **Family history.** The overwhelming majority of breast cancers—90 to 95 percent—are not due to strong genetic factors. However, having a first-degree relative—mother, sister, or daughter—with breast cancer does increase risk, and if the relative developed breast cancer before menopause, the cancer is more likely to be hereditary.

- **Long menstrual history.** Women who had their first period before age 12 are at greater risk than women who began menstruating later. The reason is that the more menstrual cycles a woman has, the longer her exposure to estrogen, a hormone known to increase breast cancer danger. For similar reasons, childless women, who menstruate continuously for several decades, are also at greater risk. Neither miscarriage nor induced abortion increases the risk of breast cancer.[37]

- **Age at birth of first child.** An early pregnancy—in a woman's teens or twenties—changes the actual maturation of breast cells and decreases risk. But if a woman has her first child in her forties, precancerous cells may actually flourish with the high hormone levels of the pregnancy.

- **Breast biopsies.** Even if laboratory analysis finds no precancerous abnormalities, women who require such tests are more likely to develop breast cancer. Fibrocystic breast disease, a term often used for "lumpy" breasts, is not a risk factor.

- 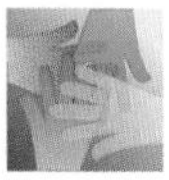 **Race.** Breast cancer rates are lower in Hispanic and Asian American populations than in whites and in African American women. Caucasian women over 40 have the highest incidence rate for breast cancer in this country, but African American women at every age have a greater likelihood of dying from breast cancer.

- **Occupation.** Based on two decades of following more than a million women, Swedish researchers have developed a list of jobs linked with a high risk of breast cancer. These include pharmacists, certain types of teachers, schoolmasters, systems analysts and programmers, telephone operators, telegraph and radio operators, metal platers and coaters, and beauticians.

- **Alcohol.** Women's risk of breast cancer increases with the amount of alcohol they drink. Those who take two or more drinks per day are 40 percent

By age 25	1 in 19,608
By age 30	1 in 2,525
By age 35	1 in 622
By age 40	1 in 217
By age 45	1 in 93
By age 50	1 in 50
By age 55	1 in 33
By age 60	1 in 24
By age 65	1 in 17
By age 70	1 in 14
By age 75	1 in 11
By age 80	1 in 10
By age 85	1 in 9
Ever	1 in 8

Figure 14.10 A Woman's Risk of Developing Breast Cancer

Source: Surveillance Program, National Cancer Institute.

more likely to develop breast cancer than women who don't drink at all. For a nondrinking woman, the lifetime risk of breast cancer by age 80 is 1 in 11. For heavy drinkers it's about 1 in 7, regardless of race, education, family history, use of hormone therapy, or other risk factors.

- **Hormone therapy (HT).** Several studies confirm an increased risk with a combination of estrogen and progestin, particularly in women who use combination HT for five years or longer. Women taking combination HT are more likely to have abnormal mammograms requiring further testing and to be diagnosed at a more advanced stage of breast cancer. Women taking only estrogen for shorter periods did not have an elevated rate of breast cancer, but their risk increased significantly after 15 years of use. In African American women, estrogen use has been linked to higher breast cancer risk, particularly in leaner women.

- **Obesity.** Excess weight, particularly after menopause, increases the risk of getting breast cancer. Overweight women, both pre- and postmenopausal, with breast cancer are more likely to die of their disease.

- **Sedentary lifestyle.** According to the World Health Organization, regular physical activity may cut the risk of developing breast cancer by 20 to 40 percent, regardless of a woman's menopausal status or the type or intensity of the activity. The reason may be that exercise lowers levels of circulating ovarian hormones.

Detection Doctors have long advised women to perform monthly breast self-exams (BSE) after their periods (Figure 14.11). In its newest guidelines, the American Cancer Society now describes BSE as "an option" for

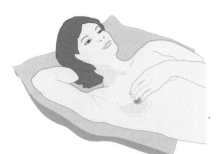

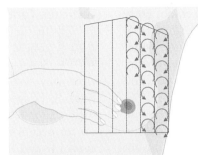

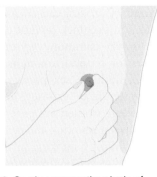

1. Lie flat on your back. Place a pillow or towel under one shoulder, and raise that arm over your head. With the opposite hand, you'll feel with the pads, not the fingertips, of the three middle fingers, for lumps or any change in the texture of the breast or skin.

2. The area you'll examine is from your collarbone to your bra line and from your breastbone to the center of your armpit. Imagine the area divided into vertical strips. Using small circular motions (the size of a dime), move your fingers up and down the strips. Apply light, medium, and deep pressure to examine each spot. Repeat this same process for your other breast.

3. Gently squeeze the nipple of each breast between your thumb and index finger. Any discharge, clear or bloody, should be reported to your doctor immediately.

Figure 14.11   Breast Self-Exam
The best time to examine your breasts is after your menstrual period every month.

women starting in their twenties and urges all women to report any breast changes promptly. It recommends a breast exam by a trained practitioner every three years for women in their twenties and thirties and every year for women 40 and over and a yearly mammogram for all women, starting at age 40.

The best tool for early detection is the diagnostic X-ray exam called **mammography.** Women whose breast cancer is detected by screening mammography have a significantly better prognosis than those whose cancer is found another way—even if the cancer has already spread to their lymph nodes. A likely reason is that mammography can detect tumors that are both slower growing and less biologically lethal than others.

Magnetic Resonance Imaging may be more accurate than mammography for detecting early forms of breast cancer before they progress to more aggressive forms.[38] The American Cancer Society now recommends MRI screening for women with a strong family history of breast or ovarian cancer and those who have been treated for Hodgkin's disease.[39] Women who've had cancer in one breast or those with extremely dense breasts may also benefit.[40]

Treatment   Breast cancer can be treated with surgery, radiation, and drugs (chemotherapy and hormonal therapy). Doctors may use one of these options or a combination, depending on the type and location of the cancer and whether the disease has spread.

Most women undergo some type of surgery. **Lumpectomy,** or breast-conserving surgery, removes only the cancerous tissue and a surrounding margin of normal tissue. A modified radical **mastectomy** includes the entire breast and some of the underarm lymph nodes. Removing underarm lymph nodes is important to determine if the cancer has spread, but a technique called sentinel node biopsy allows physicians to pinpoint the first lymph node into which a tumor drains (the sentinel node) and remove only the nodes most likely to contain cancer cells.

Radiation therapy is treatment with high-energy rays or particles to destroy cancer. In almost all cases, lumpectomy is followed by six to seven weeks of radiation. Chemotherapy is used to reach cancer cells that may have spread beyond the breast—in many cases even if no cancer is detected in the lymph nodes after surgery.

The use of drugs such as tamoxifen and aromatase inhibitors, in addition to standard chemotherapy, can significantly lower the risk of recurrence.

Cervical Cancer

An estimated 11,150 cases of invasive cervical cancer are diagnosed in the United States every year. The highest incidence rate occurs among Vietnamese women; Alaskan Native, Korean, and Hispanic women also have higher rates than the national average. The mortality rate for African American women is more than twice that of whites, largely because of a high number of deaths among older black women.

The primary risk factor for cervical cancer is infection with certain types of the human papilloma virus (HPV), discussed in Chapter 16. HPV occurs in more than

mammography   A diagnostic X-ray exam used to detect breast cancer.

lumpectomy   The surgical removal of a breast tumor and its surrounding tissue.

mastectomy   The surgical removal of an entire breast.

99.7 percent of cervical cancer cases. However, not every HPV infection becomes cervical cancer, and while HPV infection is very common, cervical cancer is not. Other risk factors for cervical cancer include early age of first intercourse, multiple sex partners, genital herpes, and smoking or significant exposure to passive smoke.

 College women are generally aware of the link between smoking and cervical cancer, but those who report smoking in the past month do not see themselves as personally at greater risk. They also are no more likely to have had a Pap test.[41]

The CDC has recommended vaccination of all girls by age 13 with Gardasil, the first vaccine developed to prevent cervical cancer. It targets four HPV types that together cause 70 percent of cervical cancers and 90 percent of genital warts. It does not protect against all HPV types that cause cervical cancer. Gardasil is most effective when given before first sexual contact and exposure to HPV. In girls and women who have never been infected with HPV, the vaccine can prevent almost all cases of disease caused by the four targeted types of HPV, including cancers of the genitals, cervix, and anus.[42]

The standard screening test for cervical cancer is the Pap smear. New, more precise forms of Pap testing and new screening tests for HPV may help detect cases of cervical cancer at earlier stages. The American Cancer Society now recommends that cervical cancer screening begin approximately three years after the onset of vaginal intercourse but no later than 21 years of age.[43] Warning signs for cervical cancer include irregular bleeding or unusual vaginal discharge. Precancerous cervical cells can be destroyed by laser surgery or freezing during a visit to a doctor's office.

The National Cancer Institute (NCI) recommends a combination of chemotherapy and radiation rather than the standard use of radiation alone for invasive tumors. For women whose cervical cancer is detected early, cryotherapy (use of extreme cold), electrocoagulation (intense heat), or surgery are standard treatments.

Ovarian Cancer

Ovarian cancer is the leading cause of death from gynecological cancers. Risk factors include a family history of ovarian cancer; personal history of breast cancer; obesity; infertility (because the abnormality that interferes with conception may also play a role in cancer development); and low levels of transferase, an enzyme involved in the metabolism of dairy foods. Often women develop no obvious symptoms until the advanced stages, although they may experience painless swelling of the abdomen, irregular bleeding, lower abdominal pain, digestive and urinary abnormalities, fatigue, backache, bloating, and weight gain. Ovarian cancer may be diagnosed by pelvic examination, ultrasound, MRI, computed tomography, or PET (positron emission tomography) scan.

Testicular Cancer

In the last 20 years the incidence of testicular cancer has risen 51 percent in the United States—from 3.61 to 5.44 per 100,000. It is not clear why testicular cancer is on the rise, although researchers speculate that changing environmental or socioeconomic risk factors could have a role. Testicular cancer occurs mostly among young men between the ages of 18 and 35, who are not normally at risk of cancer. At highest risk are men with an undescended testicle (a condition that is almost always corrected in childhood to prevent this danger). To detect possibly cancerous growths, men should perform monthly testicular self-exams, as shown in Figure 14.12.

Often the first sign of this cancer is a slight enlargement of one testicle. There also may be a change in the way it feels when touched. Sometimes men with testicular cancer report a dull ache in the lower abdomen or groin, along with a sense of heaviness or sluggishness. Lumps on the testicles also may indicate cancer.

A man who notices any abnormality should consult a physician. If a lump is indeed present, a surgical biopsy is necessary to find out if it is cancerous. If the biopsy is positive, a series of tests generally is needed to determine whether the disease has spread.

Treatment for testicular cancer generally involves surgical removal of the diseased testis, sometimes along with radiation therapy, chemotherapy, and the removal of nearby lymph nodes. The remaining testicle is capable of maintaining a man's sexual potency and fertility. Only in rare cases is removal of both testicles necessary. Testosterone injections following such surgery can maintain

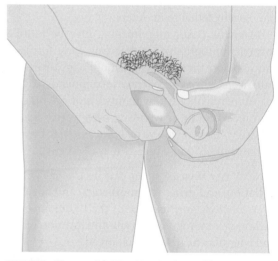

Figure 14.12 Testicular Self-Exam
The best time to examine your testicles is after a hot bath or shower, when the scrotum is most relaxed. Place your index and middle fingers under each testicle and the thumb on top, and roll the testicle between the thumb and fingers. If you feel a small, hard, usually painless lump or swelling, or anything unusual, consult a urologist.

potency. The chance for a cure is very high if testicular cancer is spotted early.

Colon and Rectal Cancer

 Colon and rectal, or colorectal, cancer is the third most common cancer and accounts for 10 percent of cancer deaths. Most cases occur after age 50. Both age and gender influence the risk of colon cancer. Older individuals and men are more likely to develop polyps (nonmalignant growths that may turn cancerous at some point) and tumors in the colon than young people and women.

Risk factors include age (over 50), personal or family history of colon and rectal cancer, polyps in the colon or rectum, ulcerative colitis, smoking, alcohol consumption, prolonged high consumption of red and processed meat, high-fat or low-fiber diet, and inadequate intake of fruits and vegetables. In the landmark Women's Health Initiative trials, a low-fat diet did not reduce the risk of colon and rectal cancer in postmenopausal women. Federal health officials recommend against the routine use of aspirin and nonsteroidal anti-inflammatory drugs to prevent colon cancer.[44]

New guidelines recommend screening for colon cancer beginning at age 50, earlier for those at higher risk based on personal, family, or medical history. The initial screening is crucial because it detects the largest, most dangerous polyps, which can then be removed.

Early signs of colorectal cancer are bleeding from the rectum, blood in the stool, or a change in bowel habits. Treatment may involve surgery, radiation therapy, and/or chemotherapy.

Prostate Cancer

 After skin cancer, prostate cancer is the most common form of cancer in American men. The risk of prostate cancer is 1 in 6; the risk of death due to metastatic prostate cancer is 1 in 30. More than a quarter of men diagnosed with cancer have prostate cancer. The disease strikes African American men more often than white; Asian and American Indian men are affected less often.

The risk of prostate cancer increases with age, family history, exposure to the heavy metal cadmium, high number of sexual partners, and history of frequent sexually transmitted infections. An inherited predisposition may account for 5 to 10 percent of cases. A purported link between vasectomy and prostate cancer has been disproved. Statin drugs, commonly prescribed to lower cholesterol, also may lower the risk of prostate cancer.[45]

The development of a simple annual screening test that measures levels of a protein called prostate-specific antigen (PSA) in the blood has revolutionized the diagnosis of prostate cancer. PSA testing is recommended for men at high risk (African Americans and men with close relatives

with prostate cancer) starting at age 45 and for all men at age 50. It remains controversial, however. Some claim that PSA testing saves lives; others, that it leads to unnecessary and potentially harmful treatments.

Treatment may include hormones, chemotherapy, and radiation. About 60,000 men undergo radical prostate surgery in the United States every year. The five-year survival rate has increased from 67 percent to 99 percent over the past 20 years.

Young people often feel immune to such serious diseases as cancer. But cancer can strike anyone. Regardless of your age, being in tune with your body is one of your best defenses against cancer. (See Reality Check.)

Other Major Illnesses

Other noninfectious diseases have a debilitating effect on many people. But most of the diseases discussed in this section can be controlled, if not cured.

Epilepsy and Seizure Disorders

About 10 percent of all Americans will have at least one seizure at some time. Between 0.5 and 1 percent of all Americans have recurrent seizures. Derived from the Greek word for seizure, **epilepsy** is the term used to refer to a variety of neurological disorders characterized by sudden attacks (seizures) of violent muscle contractions and unconsciousness. Epilepsy is rarely fatal; the primary danger to life is to suffer an attack while driving or swimming.

Seizures can be major, referred to as *grand mal;* minor, referred to as *petit mal;* or psychomotor. In a grand-mal seizure, the person loses consciousness, falls to the ground, and experiences convulsive body movements. Petit-mal seizures are brief, characterized by a loss of consciousness

epilepsy A variety of neurological disorders characterized by sudden attacks (seizures) of violent muscle contractions and unconsciousness.

for 10 to 30 seconds, by eye or muscle flutterings, and occasionally by a loss of muscle tone. About 90 percent of all epileptics have grand-mal seizures; 40 percent suffer both petit-mal and grand-mal seizures. The frequency of attacks defines the severity of the epilepsy. Diagnosis is based on a history of recurring attacks and a study of the brain's electrical activity, called an electroencephalogram (EEG).

About half of all cases of epilepsy have no known cause and are therefore classified as *idiopathic.* All others stem from conditions that affect the brain, such as trauma, tumors, congenital malformations, or inflammation of the membranes covering the brain. *Idiopathic* epilepsy usually begins between the ages of 2 and 14. Seizures before age 2 are usually related to developmental defects, birth injuries, or a metabolic disease affecting the brain. (Fever-induced convulsions are not related to epilepsy.) Seizures after age 14 are generally symptoms of brain disease or injury.

Seizure disorders don't reflect or affect intellectual or psychological soundness; people who suffer from them have normal intelligence. Therapy with anticonvulsant drugs can control seizures in most people, and once seizures are under control, epileptics can live full, normal lives by continuing to take their medications.

If you're with a person who suffers a grand-mal seizure, make sure he or she isn't injured during the attack. Don't try to restrain the person or interfere with his or her movements, and don't try to force anything into the person's mouth.

Asthma

Asthma is a disease characterized by constriction of the breathing passages. As with allergy, asthma rates have skyrocketed in the last two decades. Approximately 20 million Americans have asthma. Asthma-related problems account for more than half a million hospital stays each year and 14 deaths each day in the United States, according to the Asthma and Allergy Foundation of America.

 Asthma is more common among inner-city residents and blacks. The disease disproportionately affects African Americans. A black man in New York City is 11 times more likely to die from asthma than other men in the city.

While asthma is not always linked to allergy, the two are related. Among people with asthma, 90 percent of the children, 70 percent of young adults, and 50 percent of older adults also have allergies. According to epidemiologic research, 23 percent of youngsters diagnosed with allergies by age 1 develop asthma by age 6. Of those diagnosed after age 1, 13 percent eventually become asthmatic. Symptoms include wheezing, coughing, shortness of breath, and chest tightness. If the symptoms are untreated or undertreated, they can worsen and damage the lungs.

 The number of people with asthma continues to increase into adulthood. However, as shown by a study that followed college students for 23 years, most report that their symptoms improve or disappear.

The two main approaches to asthma treatment are control of the underlying inflammation by means of anti-inflammatory drugs, such as corticosteroids, cromolyn sodium, and nedocromil, and short-term relief of symptoms with bronchodilators, such as albuterol, which expand the breathing passages. In its most recent official

---

YOUR STRATEGIES FOR CHANGE *What to Do in Case of an Asthma Attack*

If you have asthma, here are some steps you should take:

- **Get away from the asthma trigger** (cigarette smoke, cat, pollen, etc.).
- **Assess the severity of the attack.** The most precise way to do so is with a peak flow meter. If your peak flow is less than half your best value, the attack is severe.

- **Use a quick reliever.** The fastest way to relieve an asthma attack is to use a quick-acting bronchodilator such as albuterol.
- **Suppress inflammation.** Quick-relief bronchodilators treat only the constricted muscles surrounding the bronchial tubes. Treating the overproduction of mucus requires an anti-inflammatory

medication, typically a corticosteroid, such as prednisone.

- **Know when to call for help.** Severe asthma attacks can be dangerous. If you don't feel improvement, get help immediately from your doctor or an urgent care or emergency health care center, or call 911.

guidelines, the National Heart, Lung and Blood Institute encouraged more frequent use of inhaled steroids and less reliance on bronchodilators, which have little effect on the underlying inflammation.

Although medications can help relieve asthma symptoms in the short term, prolonged use of the most popular drugs, the short-acting beta-agonists, actually can produce the opposite effect by closing air passages. Many people with severe asthma use more medication as their symptoms worsen—but the drugs actually exacerbate their condition. The reason, researchers theorize, may be that continuous use of asthma medications changes how the airway contracts in ways that intensify the constriction and make breathing more difficult.

Ulcers

Open sores, often more than an inch wide, that develop in the lining of the stomach or the duodenum (the first part of the small intestine) are called **ulcers.** They are caused by excessive acidic digestive juices. The major symptom is a burning pain felt throughout the upper abdomen. The pain may come and go, lasting up to three hours. It may begin either right after eating or several hours later.

One in five men and one in ten women get ulcers of the stomach or duodenum, but the number of ulcers is declining. Risk factors include heavy use of cigarettes, alcohol, or caffeine; the ingestion of large amounts of painkillers that contain aspirin or ibuprofen; and advanced age. Bleeding is not common but may be dangerous, even life-threatening. An untreated stomach ulcer can lead to serious weight loss and anemia.

Researchers have identified a bacterium, *Helicobacter pylori*, that may infect the digestive system and set the stage for ulcers. According to various studies, most ulcer patients carry this organism. One theory is that infection leads to an inflammation of the stomach lining called gastritis, which increases vulnerability to other stressors, such as smoking, alcohol, or anxiety. Treatment with antibiotics leads to improvement in most patients.

Conventional therapy for ulcers includes self-help measures, such as avoiding aspirin; eating small, frequent meals; taking antacids; and not smoking or drinking alcohol or caffeine. Drugs such as cimetidine, ranitidine, and sucralfate can reduce the amount of acid produced by the stomach and relieve ulcer symptoms.

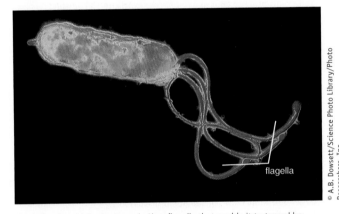

flagella

© A.B. Dowsett/Science Photo Library/Photo Researchers, Inc.

The bacterium *Helicobacter pylori* has flagella that enable it to tunnel beneath the protective layer coating the stomach lining.

Learn It : Live It

Preventing Serious Illness

You may not be able to control every risk factor in your life or environment, but you can protect yourself from the obvious ones.

- **Don't smoke.** There's no bigger favor you can do for your heart or lungs.
- **Cut down on saturated fats and cholesterol.** This can help prevent high blood cholesterol levels, obesity, and heart disease.
- **Watch your weight.** Even relatively modest gains can have a big effect on your risk of heart disease. Overweight and obesity are associated with increased risks for cancers at several sites: breast (among postmenopausal women), colon, endometrium, esophagus (adenocarcinoma), and kidney.

- **Get moving.** Regular exercise can help lower your blood pressure, lower LDLs, and reduce triglycerides.
- **Lower your stress levels.** If too much stress is a problem in your life, try the relaxation techniques described in Chapter 3.
- **Get your blood pressure checked regularly.** Knowing your numbers can alert you to a potential problem long before you develop any symptoms.
- **Avoid excessive exposure to ultraviolet light.** if you spend a lot of time outside, protect your skin by using sunscreen and wearing long-sleeve shirts and a hat. Also, wear sunglasses to protect your eyes.

asthma A disease or allergic response characterized by bronchial spasms and difficult breathing.

ulcer A lesion in, or an erosion of, the mucous membrane of an organ.

Don't purposely put yourself at risk by binge-sunbathing or by using sunlamps.

- **Control your alcohol intake.** The risk of cancers of the mouth, pharynx, larynx, esophagus, liver, and breast increases substantially with intake of more than two drinks per day for men or one drink for women.

- **Be alert to changes in your body.** You know your body's rhythms and appearance better than anyone else, and only you will know if certain things aren't right. Changes in bowel habits, skin changes, unusual lumps or discharges—anything out of the ordinary—may be clues that require further medical investigation.

SELFSURVEY : *Are You at Risk of Cancer?*

Answer the following questions:

1. Do you protect your skin from overexposure to the sun? _____
2. Do you abstain from smoking or using tobacco in any form? _____
3. If you're over 40 or if family members have had colon cancer, do you get routine digital rectal exams? _____
4. Do you eat a balanced diet that includes the recommended Daily Value for vitamins A, B, and C? _____
5. If you're a woman, do you have regular Pap tests and pelvic exams? _____
6. If you're a man over 40, do you get regular prostate exams? _____
7. If you have burn scars or a history of chronic skin infections, do you get regular checkups? _____
8. Do you avoid smoked, salted, pickled, and high-nitrite foods? _____
9. If your job exposes you to asbestos, radiation, cadmium, or other environmental hazards, do you get regular checkups? _____
10. Do you limit your consumption of alcohol? _____
11. Do you avoid using tanning salons or home sunlamps? _____
12. If you're a woman, do you examine your breasts every month for lumps? _____
13. Do you eat plenty of vegetables and other sources of fiber? _____
14. If you're a man, do you perform regular testicular self-exams? _____
15. Do you wear protective sunglasses in sunlight? _____
16. Do you follow a low-fat diet? _____
17. Do you know the cancer warning signs? _____

Scoring

If you answered no to any of the questions, your risk for developing various kinds of cancer may be increased.

Your Health Action Plan for Early Detection of Cancer

Site	Recommendation
Breast	• Yearly mammograms are recommended starting at age 40. The age at which screening should be stopped should be individualized by considering the potential risks and benefits of screening in the context of overall health status and longevity.
	• Clinical breast exam should be part of a periodic health exam, about every 3 years for women in their twenties and thirties, and every year for women 40 and older.
	• Women should know how their breasts normally feel and report any breast change promptly to their health care providers. Breast self-exam is an option for women starting in their twenties.
	• Women at increased risk (e.g., family history, genetic tendency, past breast cancer) should talk with their doctors about the benefits and limitations of starting mammography screening earlier, having additional tests (i.e., breast ultrasound and MRI), or having more frequent exams.

Site	Recommendation
Colon and Rectum	Beginning at age 50, men and women should begin screening with one of the examination schedules that follow: • A fecal occult blood test (FOBT) or fecal immunochemical test (FIT) every year • A flexible sigmoidoscopy (FSIG) every 5 years • Annual FOBT or FIT and flexible sigmoidoscopy every 5 years* • A double-contrast barium enema every 5 years • A colonoscopy every 10 years
Prostate	The PSA test and the digital rectal examination should be offered annually, beginning at age 50, to men who have a life expectancy of at least 10 years. Men at high risk (African American men and men with a strong family history of one or more first-degree relatives diagnosed with prostate cancer at an early age) should begin testing at age 45. For both men at average risk and high risk, information should be provided about what is known and what is uncertain about the benefits and limitations of early detection and treatment of prostate cancer so that they can make an informed decision about testing.
Uterus	**Cervix:** Screening should begin approximately 3 years after a woman begins having vaginal intercourse, but no later than 21 years of age. Screening should be done every year with regular Pap tests or every 2 years using liquid-based tests. At or after age 30, women who have had three normal test results in a row may get screened every 2 to 3 years. Alternatively, cervical cancer screening with human papilloma virus (HPV) DNA testing and conventional or liquid-based cytology could be performed every 3 years. However, doctors may suggest that a woman get screened more often if she has certain risk factors, such as HIV infection or a weak immune system. Women 70 years and older who have had three or more consecutive normal Pap tests in the last 10 years may choose to stop cervical cancer screening. Screening after total hysterectomy (with removal of the cervix) is not necessary unless the surgery was done as a treatment for cervical cancer. **Endometrium:** The American Cancer Society recommends that at the time of menopause all women should be informed about the risks and symptoms of endometrial cancer, and strongly encouraged to report any unexpected bleeding or spotting to their physicians. Annual screening for endometrial cancer with endometrial biopsy beginning at age 35 should be offered to women with or at risk for hereditary nonpolyposis colon cancer (HNPCC).
Cancer-Related Checkup	For individuals undergoing periodic health examinations, a cancer-related checkup should include health counseling, and, depending on a person's age and gender, might include examinations for cancers of the thyroid, oral cavity, skin, lymph nodes, testes, and ovaries, as well as for some nonmalignant diseases.

*Combined testing is preferred over either annual FOBT or FIT, or FSIG every 5 years, alone. People who are at moderate or high risk for colorectal cancer should talk with a doctor about a different testing schedule.

Source: American Cancer Society, Cancer Facts and Figures 2007. © 2007 American Cancer Society, Inc. *www.cancer.org.*

CENGAGENOW If you want to write your own goals for lowering your risk for major diseases, go to the Wellness Journal at HealthNow: **academic.cengage.com/login**

Making This Chapter Work
for YOU

Review Questions

1. You can control all of these cardiometabolic risk factors *except*
   a. lipoprotein levels.
   b. high blood glucose.
   c. family history.
   d. overweight.

2. Which of the following statements about diabetes mellitus is *false?*
   a. Individuals with type 2 diabetes can often control the disease without taking insulin.
   b. The incidence of diabetes has decreased in the last decade, especially among African Americans, Native Americans, and Latinos.

   c. Individuals with diabetes must measure the levels of glucose in their blood to ensure that it does not rise to unsafe levels.
   d. Untreated or uncontrolled diabetes can lead to coma and eventual death.

3. Hypertension
   a. is diagnosed when blood pressure is consistently lower than 130/85 mm Hg.
   b. may be treated with dietary changes, which include eating low-fat foods and avoiding sodium.
   c. can cause fatty deposits to collect on the artery walls.
   d. usually does not respond to medication, especially in severe cases.

4. In your lipoprotein profile, having a high level of this blood element is a good thing.
   a. HDL cholesterol
   b. LDL cholesterol
   c. C-reactive protein
   d. triglyceride

5. The heart
   a. has four chambers, which are responsible for pumping blood into the veins for circulation through the body.
   b. pumps blood first to the lungs where it picks up oxygen and discards carbon dioxide.
   c. beats about 10,000 times and pumps about 75 gallons of blood per day.
   d. has specialized cells that generate electrical signals to control the amount of blood that circulates through the body.

6. A heart attack
   a. occurs when the myocardium receives an excessive amount of blood from the coronary arteries.
   b. is typically suffered by individuals who have irregular episodes of atherosclerosis.
   c. can be treated successfully up to four hours after the event.
   d. occurs when the myocardial cells are deprived of oxygen-carrying blood, causing them to die.

7. You can protect yourself from certain types of cancer by
   a. not smoking.
   b. avoiding people who have had cancer.
   c. wearing sunscreen with an SPF of less than 15.
   d. using condoms during sexual intercourse.

8. Which of the following statements about skin cancer is true?
   a. Individuals with a large number of moles are at decreased risk for melanoma.
   b. The most serious type of skin cancer is squamous cell carcinoma.
   c. The safest way to get a tan and avoid skin cancer is to use tanning salons and sunlamps instead of sunbathing in direct sunlight.
   d. Individuals with a history of childhood sunburn are at increased risk for melanoma.

9. A woman's risk of developing breast cancer increases if
   a. she is Caucasian over the age of 40.
   b. she had her first child when in her teens or twenties.
   c. her husband's mother had breast cancer.
   d. she began menstruating when she was 15 or 16.

10. Prostate cancer
    a. occurs mostly among men between the ages of 18 and 35.
    b. is usually more aggressive in white men.
    c. has a low survival rate.
    d. can be detected through a screening test that measures the levels of prostate-specific antigen in the blood.

Answers to these questions can be found on page 583.

Critical Thinking

1. Have you had your blood pressure checked lately? If your reading was high, what steps are you now taking to help reduce your blood pressure?

2. Have you had a lipoprotein profile lately? Do you think it's necessary for you to obtain one? If your reading was/is borderline or high, what lifestyle changes can you make to help control your cholesterol level?

3. Do you have family members who have had cancer? Were these individuals at risk for cancer because of specific environmental factors, such as long-term exposure to tobacco smoke? If no particular cause was identified, what other factors could have triggered their diseases? Are you concerned that you might have inherited a genetic predisposition to any particular type of cancer because of your family history?

4. A friend of yours, Karen, discovered a small lump in her breast during a routine self-examination. When she mentions it, you ask if she has seen a doctor. She tells you that she hasn't had time to schedule an appointment; besides, she says, she's not sure it's really the kind of lump one has to worry about. It's clear to you that Karen is in denial and procrastinating about seeing a doctor. What advice would you give her?

Media Menu

CENGAGENOW™ Go to the HealthNow website at **academic.cengage .com/login** that will:

- Help you evaluate your knowledge of the material.
- Allow you to take an exam-prep quiz.
- Provide a Personalized Learning Plan targeting resources that address areas you should study.
- Coach you through identifying target goals for behavioral change and creating and monitoring your personal change plan throughout the semester.

Internet Connections

American Diabetes Association

www.diabetes.org

Here you will find the latest information on both type 1 and type 2 diabetes mellitus, including suggestions regarding diet and exercise. The online bookstore features meal planning guides, cookbooks, and self-care guides. Type in your zip code to find community resources.

American Heart Association

www.americanheart.org

This comprehensive site features a searchable database of all major cardiovascular diseases, plus information on healthy lifestyles, current research, CPR, cardiac warning signs, risk awareness, low-cholesterol diets, and family health. The interactive Heart Profilers® provides personalized information about treatment options for common cardiovascular conditions such as hypertension, heart failure, and cholesterol.

The Heart: An Online Exploration

www.fi.edu/biosci/heart.html

This interesting site, developed by the Franklin Institute of Science, provides an interactive multimedia tour of the heart, as well as statistics, resources, links, and information on how to monitor your heart's health by becoming aware of your vital signs.

Cancer Prevention and Control

www.cdc.gov/cancer/

This site, sponsored by the Centers for Disease Control and Prevention (CDC), features current information on cancer of the breast, cervix, prostate, skin, and colon. The site also provides monthly spotlights on specific cancers, as well as links to the National Comprehensive Cancer Control Program and the National Program of Cancer Registries.

Key Terms

The terms listed are used and defined on the page indicated. Definitions are also found in the Glossary at the end of this book.

angina pectoris	415
aorta	411
arteriosclerosis	415
asthma	429
atherosclerosis	415
atrium	408
capillary	411
cardiometabolic	397
cardiopulmonary resuscitation (CPR)	417
cholesterol	397
diabetes mellitus	400
diastole	411
diastolic blood pressure	397
epilepsy	427
hypertension	397
infiltration	419
lipoprotein	397
lumpectomy	425
mammography	425
mastectomy	425
metabolic syndrome	400
metastasize	419
myocardial infarction (MI)	415
plaque	415
prehypertension	404
relative risk	419
stroke	417
systole	411
systolic blood pressure	397
transient ischemic attack (TIA)	417
triglyceride	398
ulcer	429
ventricle	408

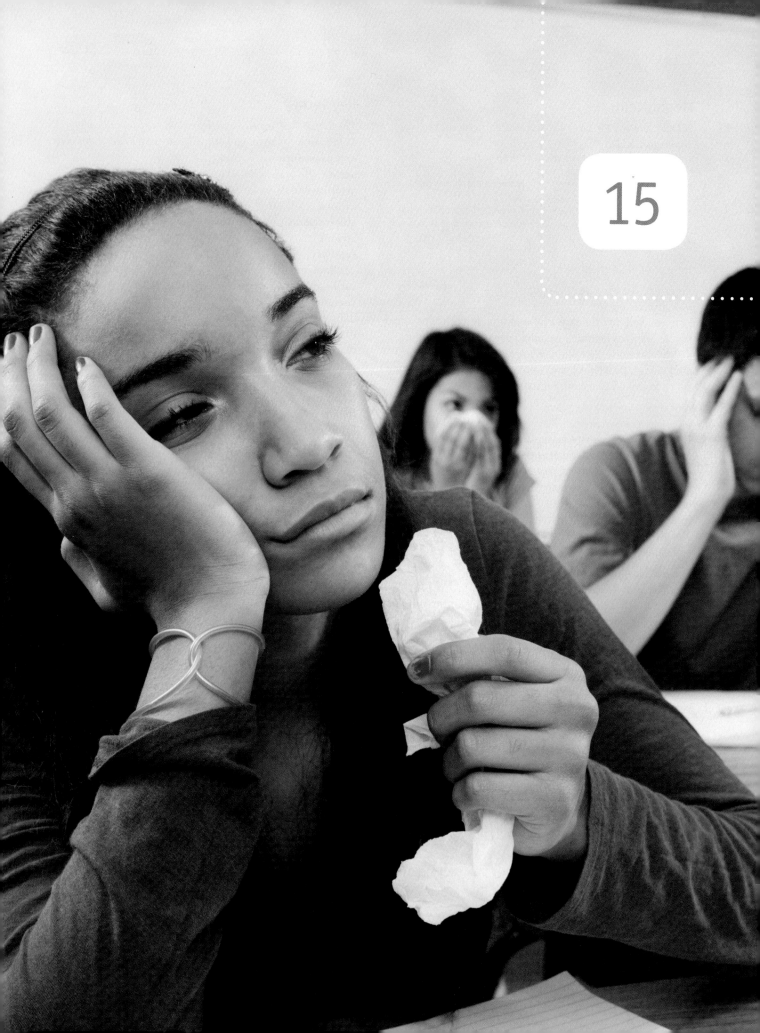

15

Avoiding Infectious Diseases

ZACH shrugged off the headache and sore throat he woke up with and rushed to class. During the lecture he started shivering. When he got up to leave, his legs felt shaky, and it hurt to walk. His entire body seemed stiff. Back in his dorm, Zach collapsed onto his bed. He felt feverish. His head throbbed. He started vomiting. Dark blotches broke out on his forehead, arms, and legs.

That evening his resident advisor drove Zach to the emergency room. The pain in his legs was excruciating, but his blood pressure was so low that the doctors couldn't give him pain medication. A spinal tap revealed that Zach had bacterial meningitis, a potentially deadly infection that causes swelling in the brain and spinal cord. Intensive treatment saved Zach's life, although he suffered hearing loss and severe nerve damage that required months of rehabilitation. Zach considers himself lucky. Bacterial meningitis can strike so unexpectedly and worsen so quickly that it can kill a healthy young person within days.

Throughout history, infectious diseases have claimed more lives than any military conflict or natural disaster. Although modern medicine has won many victories against the agents of infection, we remain vulnerable to a host of infectious illnesses. Drug-resistant strains of tuberculosis and *Staphylococcus* bacteria challenge current therapies. New infectious diseases, such as avian (bird) flu are emerging and traveling around the world. Agents of infection also can be used as weapons of war and terrorism.

This chapter is a lesson in self-defense against all forms of infection. The information it provides can help you boost your defenses, recognize and avoid enemies, shield yourself from infections, and realize when to seek help.

After studying the material in this chapter, you should be able to:

- **Explain** how the different agents of infection spread disease.

- **Describe** how your body protects itself from infectious disease.

- **List** ways to protect yourself from catching a cold or the flu and ways to feel better if you do catch one.

- **Name** and **describe** some common infectious diseases.

- **Explain** the dangers of overuse or misuse of antibiotics.

- **Name** the infectious diseases for which you are most at risk, and **list** your strategies for avoiding them.

CENGAGENOW™ Log on to HealthNow at **academic.cengage.com/login** to find your Behavior Change Planner and to explore self-assessments, interactive tutorials, and practice quizzes.

Understanding Infection

We live in a sea of microbes. Most of them don't threaten our health or survival; some, such as the bacteria that inhabit our intestines, are actually beneficial. Yet in the course of history, disease-causing microorganisms have claimed millions of lives. The twentieth century brought the conquest of infectious killers such as cholera and scarlet fever. Although modern science has won many victories against the agents of infection, infectious illnesses remain a serious health threat.

Infection is a complex process, triggered by various **pathogens** (disease-causing organisms) and countered by the body's own defenders. Physicians explain infection in terms of a **host** (either a person or a population) that contacts one or more agents in an environment. A **vector**—a biological or physical vehicle that carries the agent to the host—provides the means of transmission.

Agents of Infection

The types of microbes that can cause infection are viruses, bacteria, fungi, protozoa, and helminths (parasitic worms).

Viruses

The tiniest pathogens—**viruses**—are also the toughest; they consist of a bit of nucleic acid (DNA or RNA, but never both) within a protein coat. Unable to reproduce on its own, a virus takes over a body cell's reproductive machinery and instructs it to produce new viral particles, which are then released to enter other cells. The common cold, the flu, herpes, hepatitis, and AIDS are viral diseases.

The most common viruses are these types:

- **Rhinoviruses and adenoviruses,** which get into the mucous membranes and cause upper-respiratory tract infections and colds.

- **Coronaviruses,** named for their corona, or halo-like appearance, are second only to rhinoviruses in causing the common cold and other respiratory infections. A coronavirus is the cause of severe acute respiratory syndrome (SARS).

- **Influenza viruses,** which can change their outer protein coats so dramatically that individuals resistant to one strain cannot fight off a new one.

- **Herpes viruses,** which take up permanent residence in the cells and periodically flare up.

- **Papilloma viruses,** which cause few symptoms in women and almost none in men but may be responsible, at least in part, for a rise in the incidence of cervical cancer among younger women.

- **Hepatitis viruses,** which cause several forms of liver infection, ranging from mild to life-threatening.

- **Slow viruses,** which give no early indication of their presence but can produce fatal illnesses within a few years.

- **Retroviruses,** which are named for their backward (retro) sequence of genetic replication compared to other viruses. One retrovirus, human immunodeficiency virus (HIV), causes acquired immune deficiency syndrome (AIDS).

- **Filoviruses,** which resemble threads and are extremely lethal.

The problem in fighting viruses is that it's difficult to find drugs that harm the virus and not the cell it has commandeered. **Antibiotics** (drugs that inhibit or kill bacteria) have no effect on viruses. **Antiviral drugs** don't completely eradicate a viral infection, although they can decrease its severity and duration. Because viruses multiply very quickly, antiviral drugs are most effective when taken before an infection develops or in its early stages.

Bacteria

Simple one-celled organisms, **bacteria** are the most plentiful microorganisms as well as the most pathogenic. Most kinds of bacteria don't cause disease; some, like certain strains of *Escherichia coli* that aid in digestion, play important roles within our bodies. Even friendly bacteria, however, can get out of hand and cause acne, urinary tract infections, vaginal infections, and other problems.

Bacteria harm the body by releasing either enzymes that digest body cells or toxins that produce the specific effects of such diseases as diphtheria or toxic shock syndrome. In self-defense, the body produces specific proteins (called *antibodies*) that attack and inactivate the invaders. Tuberculosis, tetanus, gonorrhea, scarlet fever, and diphtheria are examples of bacterial diseases.

Because bacteria are sufficiently different from the cells that make up our bodies, antibiotics can kill them without harming our cells. Antibiotics work only against specific types of bacteria. If your doctor thinks you have a bacterial infection, tests of your blood, pus, sputum, urine, or stool can identify the particular bacterial strain.

Fungi

Single-celled or multicelled organisms, **fungi** consist of threadlike fibers and reproductive spores. Fungi lack chlorophyll and must obtain their food from organic material, which may include human tissue. Fungi release enzymes that digest cells and are most likely to attack hair-covered areas of the body, including the scalp,

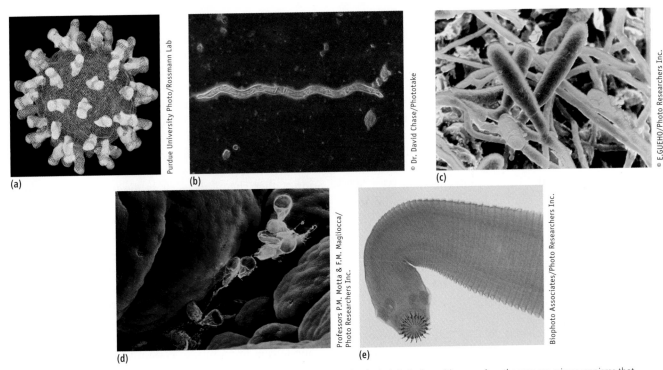

Examples of the major categories of organisms that cause disease in humans. Except for the helminths (parasitic worms), pathogens are microorganisms that can be seen only with the aid of a microscope. (a) Viruses: common cold, (b) Bacteria: syphilis, (c) Fungi: athlete's foot fungus, (d) Protozoa: Giardia lamblia, (e) Helminths: tapeworm.

beard, groin, and external ear canals. They also cause athlete's foot. Treatment consists of antifungal drugs.

Protozoa

These single-celled, microscopic animals release enzymes and toxins that destroy cells or interfere with their function. Diseases caused by **protozoa** are not a major health problem in this country, primarily because of public health measures. Around the world, however, some 2.24 billion people (more than 40 percent of the world's population) are at risk for acquiring malaria—a protozoan-caused disease. Up to 3 million die from this disease annually. Many more come down with amoebic dysentery. Treatment for protozoa-caused diseases consists of general medical care to relieve the symptoms, replacement of lost blood or fluids, and drugs that kill the specific protozoan.

The most common disease caused by protozoa in the United States is *giardiasis,* an intestinal infection caused by microorganisms in human and animal feces. It has become a threat at day-care centers, as well as among campers and hikers who drink contaminated water. Symptoms include nausea, lack of appetite, gas, diarrhea, fatigue, abdominal cramps, and bloating. Many people recover in a month or two without treatment. However, in some cases the microbe causes recurring attacks over many years. Giardiasis can be life-threatening in small children and the elderly, who are especially prone to severe dehydration from diarrhea. Treatment usually consists of antibiotics.

Helminths (Parasitic Worms)

Small parasitic worms that attack specific tissues or organs and compete with the host for nutrients are called **helminths.** One major worldwide health problem is *schistosomiasis,* a disease caused by a parasitic worm, the fluke, that burrows through the skin and enters the circulatory system. Infection with another helminth, the tapeworm, may be contracted from eating undercooked beef, pork, or fish containing larval forms of the tapeworm. Helminthic diseases are treated with appropriate medications.

How Infections Spread

The major *vectors,* or means of transmission, for infectious disease are animals and insects, people, food, and water.

pathogen A microorganism that produces disease.

host A person or population that contracts one or more pathogenic agents in an environment.

vector A biological or physical vehicle that carries the agent of infection to the host.

virus A submicroscopic infectious agent; the most primitive form of life.

antibodies Substances produced by microorganisms, or synthetic agents, that are toxic to bacteria.

antiviral drug A substance that decreases the severity and duration of a viral infection if taken prior to or soon after onset of the infection.

bacteria (singular, **bacterium**) One-celled microscopic organisms; the most plentiful pathogens.

fungi (singular, **fungus**) Organisms that reproduce by means of spores.

protozoa Microscopic animals made up of one cell or a group of similar cells.

helminth A parasitic roundworm or flatworm.

Animals and Insects

Disease can be transmitted by house pets, livestock, birds, and wild animals. Insects also spread a variety of diseases. The housefly may spread dysentery, diarrhea, typhoid fever, or trachoma (an eye disease rare in the United States but common in other parts of the world). Other insects, including mosquitoes, ticks, mites, fleas, and lice, can transmit such diseases as malaria, yellow fever, encephalitis, dengue fever (a growing threat in Mexico), and Lyme disease.

New threats in the United States include West Nile virus (WNV), which can be spread to humans by mosquitoes that bite infected birds, and monkeypox virus, carried by various animals, including prairie dogs. Concern has grown about avian influenza, or bird flu, which has spread to wild and domestic birds around the world. (These illnesses are discussed later in this chapter.)

People

The people you're closest to can transmit pathogens through the air, through touch, or through sexual contact. To avoid infection, stay out of range of anyone who's coughing, sniffling, or sneezing, and don't share food or dishes. Carefully wash your dishes, utensils, and hands, and abstain from sex or make self-protective decisions about sexual partners. (See Chapter 16 on Sexually Transmitted Infections.)

Food

Every year foodborne illnesses strike millions of Americans, sometimes with fatal consequences. Bacteria account for two-thirds of foodborne infections, and thousands of suspected cases of infection with *Escherichia coli* bacteria in undercooked or inadequately washed food have been reported. (See Chapter 6 for more on *E. coli* outbreaks.)

Every year as many as 4 million Americans have a bout with *Salmonella* bacteria, which have been found in about a third of all poultry sold in the United States. These infections can be serious enough to require hospitalization and can lead to arthritis, neurological problems, and even death. Consumers can greatly reduce the number of salmonella infections by proper handling, cooking, and refrigeration of poultry (see Chapter 6).

Water

Waterborne diseases, such as typhoid fever and cholera, are still widespread in less developed areas of the world. They have been rare in the United States, although outbreaks caused by inadequate water purification have occurred.

The Process of Infection

If someone infected with the flu sits next to you on a bus and coughs or sneezes, tiny viral particles may travel into your nose and mouth. Immediately, the virus finds or creates an opening in the wall of a cell, and the process of infection begins. During the **incubation period,** the time between invasion and the first symptom, you're unaware of the pathogen multiplying inside you. In some diseases, incubation may go on for months, even years; for most, it lasts several days or weeks.

The early stage of the battle between your body and the invaders is called the *prodromal period.* As infected cells die, they release chemicals that help block the invasion. Other chemicals, such as *histamines,* cause blood vessels to dilate, thus allowing more blood to reach the battleground. During all of this, you feel mild, generalized symptoms, such as headache, irritability, and discomfort. You're also highly contagious. At the height of the battle—the typical illness period—you cough, sneeze, sniffle, ache, feel feverish, and lose your appetite.

Recovery begins when the body's forces gain the advantage. With time, the body destroys the last of the invaders and heals itself. However, the body is not able to develop long-lasting immunity to certain viruses, such as colds, flu, or HIV.

How Your Body Protects Itself

Various parts of your body safeguard you against infectious diseases by providing **immunity,** or protection, from these health threats. Your skin, when unbroken, keeps out most potential invaders. Your tears, sweat, skin oils, saliva, and mucus contain chemicals that can kill bacteria. Cilia, the tiny hairs lining your respiratory passages, move mucus, which traps inhaled bacteria, viruses, dust, and foreign matter, to the back of the throat, where it is swallowed; the digestive system then destroys the invaders.

When these protective mechanisms can't keep you infection-free, your body's immune system, which is on constant alert for foreign substances that might threaten the body, swings into action. The immune system includes structures of the lymphatic system—the spleen, thymus gland, lymph nodes, and lymph vessels—that help filter impurities from the body (Figure 15.1). The **lymph nodes,** or glands, are small tissue masses in which some protective cells are stored. If pathogens invade your body, many of them are carried to the lymph nodes to be destroyed. This is why your lymph nodes often feel swollen when you have a cold or the flu.

More than a dozen different types of white blood cells (lymphocytes) are concentrated in the organs of the lymphatic system or patrol the entire body by way of the blood and lymph vessels. Some of these white blood cells are generalists and some are specialists. The generalists include *macrophages,* which are large scavenger cells with insatiable appetites for foreign cells, diseased and

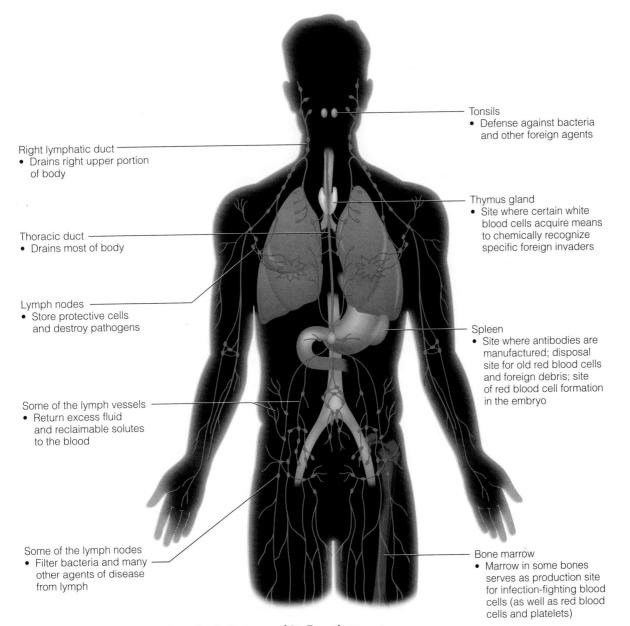

Tonsils
• Defense against bacteria and other foreign agents

Right lymphatic duct
• Drains right upper portion of body

Thymus gland
• Site where certain white blood cells acquire means to chemically recognize specific foreign invaders

Thoracic duct
• Drains most of body

Lymph nodes
• Store protective cells and destroy pathogens

Spleen
• Site where antibodies are manufactured; disposal site for old red blood cells and foreign debris; site of red blood cell formation in the embryo

Some of the lymph vessels
• Return excess fluid and reclaimable solutes to the blood

Some of the lymph nodes
• Filter bacteria and many other agents of disease from lymph

Bone marrow
• Marrow in some bones serves as production site for infection-fighting blood cells (as well as red blood cells and platelets)

Figure 15.1   The Human Lymphatic System and Its Functions
The lymphatic system helps filter impurities from the body.

run-down red blood cells, and other biological debris (Figure 15.2). The specialists are the *B cells* and *T cells,* which respond to specific invaders.

An *antigen* is any substance the white blood cells recognize as foreign. B cells create antibodies, which are proteins that bind to antigens and mark them for destruction by other white blood cells. Antigens are specific to the pathogen, and the antibody to a particular antigen binds only to that antigen (Figure 15.2). Once the human body produces antibodies against a specific antigen—the mumps virus, for instance—you're protected against that antigen for life. If you're again exposed to mumps, the antibodies previously produced prevent another episode of the disease.

But you don't have to suffer through an illness to acquire immunity. Inoculation with a vaccine containing synthetic or weakened antigens can give you the same protection. The type of long-lasting immunity in which the body makes its own antibodies to a pathogen is called *active immunity.* Immunity produced by the injection of **gamma globulin,** the antibody-containing part of the

incubation period   The time between a pathogen's entrance into the body and the first symptom.
immunity   Protection from infectious diseases.

lymph nodes   Small tissue masses in which some immune cells are stored.
gamma globulin   The antibody-containing portion of the blood fluid (plasma).

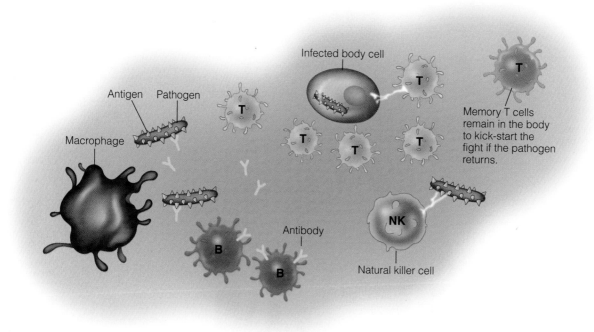

Figure 15.2 The Immune Response
Some T cells can kill infected body cells. B cells churn out antibodies to tag pathogens for destruction by macrophages and other white blood cells.

blood from another person or animal that has developed antibodies to a disease, is called *passive immunity.*

Immune Response

Attacked by pathogens, the body musters its forces and fights. Sometimes the invasion is handled like a minor border skirmish; other times a full-scale battle is waged throughout the body. Together, the immune cells work like an internal police force. When an antigen enters the body, the T cells aided by macrophages engage in combat with the invader. Certain T cells (cytotoxic T cells) can destroy infected body cells or tumor cells by "touch-killing." Meanwhile, the B cells churn out antibodies, which rush to the scene and join in the fray. Also busy at surveillance are natural killer cells that, like the elite forces of a SWAT team, seek out and destroy viruses and cancer cells (Figure 15.2).

If the microbes establish a foothold, the blood supply to the area increases, bringing oxygen and nutrients to the fighting cells. Tissue fluids, as well as antibacterial and antitoxic proteins, accumulate. You may develop redness, swelling, local warmth, and pain—the signs of **inflammation.** As more tissue is destroyed, a cavity, or **abscess,** forms and fills with fluid, battling cells, and dead white blood cells (pus). If the invaders aren't killed or inactivated, the pathogens are able to spread into the bloodstream and cause what is known as **systemic disease.**

Some people have an **immune deficiency**—either inborn or acquired. A very few children are born without an effective immune system; their lives can be endangered by any infection. Although still experimental, therapy to implant a missing or healthy gene may offer new hope for a normal life.

Immunity and Stress

Whenever we confront a crisis, large or small, our bodies produce powerful hormones that provide extra energy. However, this stress response dampens immunity, reducing the number of some key immune cells and the responsiveness of others.

Stress affects the body's immune system in different ways, depending on two factors: the controllability or uncontrollability of the stressor and the mental effort required to cope with the stress. An uncontrollable stressor that lasts longer than 15 minutes may interfere with cytokine interleukin-6, which plays an essential role in activating the immune defenses. Uncontrollable stressors also produce high levels of the hormone cortisol, which suppresses immune system functioning. The mental efforts required to cope with high-level stressors produce only brief immune changes that appear to have little consequence for health. However, stress has been shown to slow pro-inflammatory cytokine production, which is essential for healing.

Immunity and Gender

When the flu hits a household, the last one left standing is likely to be Mom. The female immune system responds more vigorously to common infections, offering extra protection against viruses, bacteria, and parasites.

The genders also differ in their vulnerability to allergies and autoimmune disorders. Although both men and women frequently develop allergies, allergic women are twice as likely to experience potentially fatal anaphylactic shock. A woman's robust immune system also is more likely to overreact and turn on her own organs and tissues. On average, three of four people with autoimmune disorders, such as multiple sclerosis, Hashimoto's thyroiditis, and scleroderma, are women.

Why are there such large gender differences in susceptibility? Scientists believe that the sex hormones have a great impact on immunity. Through a woman's childbearing years, estrogen, which protects heart, bone, brain, and blood vessels, also bolsters the immune system's response to certain infectious agents. Women produce greater numbers of antibodies when exposed to an antigen.

In contrast, testosterone may suppress this response—possibly to prevent attacks on sperm cells, which might otherwise be mistaken as alien invaders. When the testes are removed from mice and guinea pigs, their immune systems become more active.

Pregnancy dampens a woman's immune response, probably to ensure that her natural protectors don't attack the fetus as a foreign invader. This impact is so great that pregnant women with transplanted kidneys may require lower doses of drugs to prevent organ rejection. Pregnant women with multiple sclerosis and rheumatoid arthritis typically experience decreased symptoms during the nine months of gestation, then return to their prepregnancy state after giving birth. Oral contraceptives also can diminish symptoms of multiple sclerosis and rheumatoid arthritis. Neither pregnancy nor birth control pills has such an impact on lupus.

Immune Disorders

Sometimes our immune system overreacts to certain substances, mistakes the body's own tissues for enemies, or doesn't react adequately. The result is immune disorders such as allergies and autoimmune disorders.

Allergies

An **allergy** represents a hypersensitivity to a substance in our environment or diet. More than half of Americans between ages 6 and 59 are sensitive to one or more allergens. Allergies consistently rate as one of the top health problems among college students.[1]

According to the National Institute of Allergy and Infectious Diseases, more than 50 million Americans suffer from allergies. In one study, almost half of college students reported a problem with allergies in the previous year.[2] Allergies are the sixth leading cause of chronic disease and cost the U.S. healthcare system approximately $18 billion annually.[3]

Allergy sufferers run annual tabs of up to $2 billion in doctor visits, diagnostic tests, prescriptions, and decreased productivity. Every year allergies account for more than 10 million workdays missed; every day they keep 10,000 children out of school.

Thanks to treatment breakthroughs, allergy sufferers no longer have to choose between feeling better or feeling alert. Treatment options include nonsedating oral medications, nasal sprays, and **immunotherapy,** which consists of a series of injections of small but increasing doses of an allergen.

Autoimmune Disorders

Sometimes the body's defenses go awry, and the immune system declares war on the cells, tissues, or organs it normally protects. **Autoimmune disorders** rank among the top ten killers and disablers of American adults, particularly women. They strike about three times as many women as men, possibly because of the effects of female hormones on the immune system. Women are most vulnerable in the prime of life, during their reproductive years. (See Table 15.1).

For many people with autoimmune disorders, the biggest challenge is finding out what's wrong. Early symptoms, such as low-grade fever or achiness, often wax and wane and are dismissed or misdiagnosed by doctors. New blood tests for lupus and multiple sclerosis are promising faster, more accurate diagnoses, but for many autoimmune disorders, there are no conclusive laboratory tests.

Patients should keep a detailed record of when symptoms start, recur, flare, or subside, and seek a specialist—a rheumatologist, dermatologist, immunologist, or gastroenterologist, depending on symptoms—who has expertise in autoimmune disorders. New treatments are revolutionizing treatments for many autoimmune disorders, including rheumatoid arthritis.

---

inflammation A localized response by the body to tissue injury, characterized by swelling and the dilation of the blood vessels.

abscess A localized accumulation of pus and disintegrating tissue.

systemic disease A pathologic condition that spreads throughout the body.

immune deficiency Partial or complete inability of the immune system to respond to pathogens.

allergy A hypersensitivity to a particular substance in one's environment or diet.

immunotherapy A series of injections of small but increasing doses of an allergen, used to treat allergies.

autoimmune disorder Resulting from the attack on body tissue by an immune system that fails to recognize the tissue as self.

TABLE 15.1 Autoimmune Disorders

Disorder	Characteristics	Prevalence in Women vs. Men	Common Symptoms
Systemic lupus erythematosus (lupus)	A chronic autoimmune disorder that can affect any tissue or organ system including the joints, kidneys, heart, lungs, brain, blood, or skin.	9:1	Achy joints; frequent fever of 100°F or higher; anemia; fatigue; arthritis; skin rash; butterfly-shaped rash across cheek and nose; hair loss.
Graves' disease	A thyroid condition characterized by an overactive thyroid gland, which produces too much thyroid hormone.	7:1	Nervousness and irritability; weight loss; fast/irregular heart rate; heat intolerance/increased perspiration; increased appetite; sleep disturbances (such as insomnia); muscle weakness; trembling hands; irregular menstrual periods; exophthalmos (bulging eyes); appearance of a goiter (a swelling in the neck caused by enlargement of the thyroid gland).
Scleroderma	Proliferation of immune cells that produce scar tissue in the skin, some internal organs, and small blood vessels.	3:1	Reynaud's phenomenon, a condition characterized by decreased blood flow, usually to the fingers, and often brought on by cold temperatures; swelling and puffiness of the fingers or hands, followed by skin thickening a few months later; skin ulcers on the fingers; joint stiffness in the hands; sore throat; diarrhea.
Rheumatoid arthritis	Develops when the immune system attacks the synovium (the membranes that surround joints) causing inflammation, which gradually destroys cartilage, making movement of the joints painful and difficult. May also affect muscles, lungs, and liver	2.5:1	Inflamed, swollen, and tender joints that may eventually become deformed; weakness or loss of function of joints; morning stiffness, fatigue, or general sense of malaise. Often affects joints in a symmetrical pattern: If one knee or hand is affected, usually the other one also is impaired.
Multiple sclerosis	Occurs when the immune system attacks the myelin sheath—the fatty insulation surrounding nerve cells in the brain and spinal cord. The myelin sheath enables high-speed transmission of messages between these centers and the rest of the body; gradually, as scar tissue develops in different areas of myelin, nerve messages are disrupted, affecting the body in a variety of ways.	2:1	Fatigue; short-term memory problems; temporary weakness, tingling, or paralysis in one or more limbs; loss of coordination or unsteady gait; balance problems; swallowing; any or all symptoms may appear and then subside, then appear again, weeks, months, or years later.

Sources: American Autoimmune Related Diseases Association, Inc.; American Diabetes Association; American Thyroid Association; Lupus Foundation of America; National Graves' Disease Foundation; National Institute of Diabetes and Digestive and Kidney Diseases; National Institute of Arthritis and Musculoskeletal and Skin Diseases; National Multiple Sclerosis Society.

Immunizations for Adults

One of the great success stories of modern medicine has been the development of vaccines that provide protection against many infectious diseases. Immunization has reduced cases of measles, mumps, tetanus, whooping cough, and other life-threatening illnesses by more than 95 percent.

Although many people think that vaccines are only for children, they remain an important part of protection throughout life. Table 15.2 lists the vaccines recommended for college students and Figure 15.3 shows the recommended adult immunization schedule. One increased risk for adults is pertussis, or whooping cough, which has been steadily increasing. Because immunity typically wanes five to ten years after vaccination, adolescents and young adults are at risk. With the development of safer new vaccines, the CDC is recommending a "Tdap" (tetanus, diph-

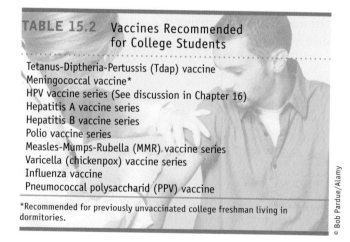

TABLE 15.2 Vaccines Recommended for College Students

Tetanus-Diptheria-Pertussis (Tdap) vaccine
Meningococcal vaccine*
HPV vaccine series (See discussion in Chapter 16)
Hepatitis A vaccine series
Hepatitis B vaccine series
Polio vaccine series
Measles-Mumps-Rubella (MMR) vaccine series
Varicella (chickenpox) vaccine series
Influenza vaccine
Pneumococcal polysaccharid (PPV) vaccine

*Recommended for previously unvaccinated college freshman living in dormitories.

© Bob Pardue/Alamy

theria, and pertussis) booster vaccination every ten years for everyone aged 19 to 64.[4] Immunity against measles also may wane; check with your doctor about a booster.[5]

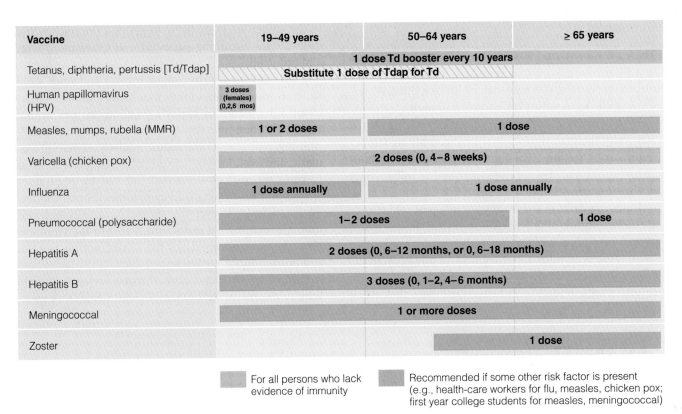

Vaccine	19–49 years	50–64 years	≥ 65 years
Tetanus, diphtheria, pertussis [Td/Tdap]	1 dose Td booster every 10 years		
	Substitute 1 dose of Tdap for Td		
Human papillomavirus (HPV)	3 doses (females) (0,2,6 mos)		
Measles, mumps, rubella (MMR)	1 or 2 doses	1 dose	
Varicella (chicken pox)	2 doses (0, 4–8 weeks)		
Influenza	1 dose annually	1 dose annually	
Pneumococcal (polysaccharide)	1–2 doses		1 dose
Hepatitis A	2 doses (0, 6–12 months, or 0, 6–18 months)		
Hepatitis B	3 doses (0, 1–2, 4–6 months)		
Meningococcal	1 or more doses		
Zoster		1 dose	

For all persons who lack evidence of immunity

Recommended if some other risk factor is present (e.g., health-care workers for flu, measles, chicken pox; first year college students for measles, meningococcal)

Figure 15.3   Recommended Adult Immunization

Source: Centers for Disease Control and Prevention. Prevention of varicella: recommendations of the Advisory Committee on Immunization Practices (ACIP). MMWR 2007; 56(No. RR-4). www.cdc.gov/mmwr/preview/mmwrhtml/mm5641a7.htm

Infectious Diseases

Although infections can be unavoidable at times, the more you know about their causes, the more you can do to protect yourself.

Who Is at Highest Risk of Infectious Diseases?

Like human bullies, the viruses responsible for the most common infectious illnesses tend to pick on those least capable of fighting back. Among the most vulnerable are the following groups:

- **Children and their families.** Youngsters get up to a dozen colds annually; adults average two a year. When a flu epidemic hits a community, about 40 percent of school-age boys and girls get sick, compared with only 5 to 10 percent of adults. But parents get up to six times as many colds as other adults.

- **The elderly.** Statistically, fewer older men and women are likely to catch a cold or flu, yet when they do, they face greater danger than the rest of the population. People over 65 who get the flu have a one in ten chance of being hospitalized for pneu-

monia or other respiratory problems, and a one in fifty chance of dying from the disease.

- **The chronically ill.** Lifelong diseases, such as diabetes, kidney disease, or sickle-cell anemia, decrease an individual's ability to fend off infections. Individuals taking medications that suppress the immune system, such as steroids, are more vulnerable to infections, as are those with medical conditions that impair immunity, such as infection with HIV.

- **Smokers and those with respiratory problems.** Smokers are a high-risk group for respiratory infections and serious complications, such as pneumonia. Chronic breathing disorders, such as asthma and emphysema, also greatly increase the risk of respiratory infections.

- **Those who live or work in close contact with someone sick.** Health-care workers who treat high-risk patients, nursing home residents, and others living in close quarters—such as students in dormitories—face greater odds of catching others' colds and flus.

- **Residents or workers in poorly ventilated buildings.** Building technology has helped spread certain airborne illnesses, such as tuberculosis, via recirculated air. Indoor air quality can be closely linked with disease transmission in winter, when people spend a great deal of time in tightly sealed rooms.

Common Cold

There are more than 200 distinct cold viruses. Although in a single season you may develop a temporary immunity to one or two, you may then be hit by a third. Americans come down with 1 billion colds annually.

Every year, about 25 million cold sufferers in the United States visit their family doctors with uncomplicated upper respiratory infections. The common cold results in about 20 million days of absence from work and 22 million days of absence from school.

Colds can strike in any season, but different cold viruses are more common at different times of years. Rhinoviruses cause most spring, summer, and early fall colds and tend to cause more symptoms above the neck (stuffy nose, headache, runny eyes). Adenoviruses, para-influenza viruses, coronaviruses, influenza viruses, and others that strike in the winter are more likely to get into the trachea and bronchi (the breathing passages) and cause more fever and bronchitis.

Cold viruses spread by coughs, sneezes, and touch. Cold sufferers who sneeze and then touch a doorknob or countertop leave a trail of highly contagious viruses behind them. The best preventive tactics are frequent hand-washing, replacing toothbrushes regularly, exercising regularly, and avoiding stress overload. High levels of stress increase the risk of becoming infected by respiratory viruses and developing cold symptoms. People who feel unable to deal with everyday stresses have an exaggerated immune reaction that may intensify cold or flu symptoms once they've contracted a virus. Those with a positive emotional outlook are less vulnerable.

Although colds and sore throats—a frequent cold symptom—are caused by viruses, many people seek treat-

---

Your Life Change Coach

Cold Comfort

Your own immune system can do something modern science cannot: cure a cold. All it needs is time, rest, and plenty of fluids. Usually, cold symptoms last for one to two weeks, although chest colds (bronchitis) may last two or three weeks.

To Avoid Getting a Cold

- Wash your hands often. (See Your Strategies for Prevention: "Smart Hand-Washing.") You can pick up cold germs easily, even when shaking someone's hand or touching doorknobs or handrails.
- Avoid people with colds when possible.
- Sneeze or cough into a tissue and then throw the tissue away.
- Clean surfaces you touch with a germ-killing disinfectant.
- Don't touch your nose, eyes, or mouth. Germs can enter your body easily by these paths.

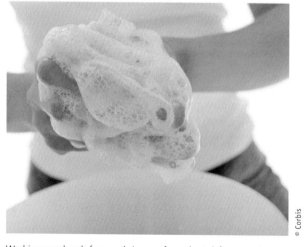

© Corbis

Washing your hands frequently is one of your best defenses against cold and flu viruses.

To Avoid Getting the Flu

A flu shot can greatly lower your chance of getting the flu. The best time to get the shot is from the middle of October to the middle of November, because most people get the flu in the winter. Although the shot can't cause the flu, you may feel sore or weak or have a fever for a few days.

Know The Difference Between a Cold and the Flu

A cold and the flu are alike in many ways. However, the flu can sometimes lead to more serious problems, such as pneumonia.

A stuffy nose, sore throat, and sneezing are usually signs of a cold. Tiredness, fever, headache, and major aches and pains probably mean you have the flu. Coughing can be a sign of either a cold or the flu, but a bad cough usually points to the flu.

ment with antibiotics, which are effective only against bacteria. Unless you're coughing up green or foul yellow mucus (signs of a secondary bacterial infection), antibiotics won't help. They have no effect against viruses and may make your body more resistant to such medications when you develop a bacterial infection in the future. An estimated 5 to 17 percent of sore throats in adults are caused by bacteria (*Group A streptococci*).

Excess prescribing for antibiotics accounts for more than half of all prescriptions and costs more than $700 million a year. In addition to their costs, antibiotics may increase risks to users and their contacts. An increasing number of studies show that antibiotics foster the growth of one or more strains of antibiotic-resistant bacteria for at least two to six months inside the person taking the pills—who can pass on this drug-resistant bug to family, roommates, and others.

According to a recent review of 30 published studies, taking vitamin C every day does not ward off the common cold or shorten its length or severity. However, some people might indeed benefit—those exposed to short bouts of extreme physical exercise or cold temperatures. Tests of high-dose vitamin C after the onset of cold symptoms showed no consistent effect on either the length of a cold or the severity of its symptoms.[6]

The latest findings on *Echinacea* are more positive. According to a new review of previous studies, the herbal supplement can cut the chances of catching a cold by more than half and shorten the duration of a cold by an average of 1.4 days. The combination of vitamin C and *Echinacea* may be even more effective. In the studies, the herbal supplement reduced the risk of catching a cold by 58 percent, while the combination of *Echinacea* and vitamin C reduced cold incidence by 86 percent.[7]

Help Yourself Feel Better While You Are Sick

- **Drink plenty of fluids,** particularly warm ones. Warmth is important because the aptly named "cold" viruses replicate at lower temperatures. Hot soups and drinks (particularly those with a touch of something pungent, like lemon or ginger) raise body temperature and help clear the nose. Tea may enhance the immune system.
- **Get plenty of rest.** Taking it easy reduces demands on the body, which helps speed recovery.
- **Do not take antibiotics.** They are ineffective against colds and flu.
- **Do not take aspirin or acetaminophen** (Tylenol), which may suppress the antibodies the body produces to fight cold viruses and increase symptoms such as stuffiness. Children, teenagers, and young adults should never take aspirin for a cold or flu because of the danger of Reye's syndrome, a potentially deadly disorder that can cause convulsions, coma, swelling of the brain, and kidney damage. A better alternative for achiness is ibuprofen (brand names include Motrin, Advil, and Nuprin), which doesn't seem to affect immune response.
- **Choose the right medicines for your symptoms.**

If you want to:	Choose medicine with:
Unclog a stuffy nose	Nasal decongestant
Quiet a cough	Cough suppressant
Loosen mucus so that you can cough it up	Expectorant
Stop runny nose and sneezing	Antihistamine
Ease fever, headaches, minor aches and pains	Pain reliever (Analgesic)

- **Know when to call your doctor.**
  You usually do not have to call a doctor right away if you have signs of a cold or flu. But be sure to call in these situations:
  - Your symptoms get worse.
  - Your symptoms last a long time.
  - After feeling a little better, you show signs of a more serious problem. Some of these signs are a sick-to-your-stomach feeling, vomiting, high fever, shaking, chills, chest pain, or coughing with thick, yellow-green mucus.

Influenza

Although similar to a cold, **influenza**—or the flu—causes more severe symptoms that last longer. Every year 10 to 20 percent of Americans develop influenza, more than 200,000 are hospitalized, and 36,000 die.

Flu viruses, transmitted by coughs, sneezes, laughs, and even normal conversation, are extraordinarily contagious, particularly in the first three days of the disease. The usual incubation period is two days, but symptoms can hit hard and fast. Two varieties of viruses—influenza A and influenza B—cause most flus. In recent years, the deadliest flu epidemics have been caused by various forms of influenza A viruses.

The CDC has set priorities for individuals who should get a flu shot because they are at higher risk for flu complications, such as heart disease, diabetes, and asthma. They are:

- **Individuals aged 65 years and older,** with and without chronic health conditions.
- **Residents of long-term care facilities.**
- **Individuals aged 2 to 64 years** with chronic health conditions.
- **Children aged 6 to 23 months.**
- **Pregnant women.**
- **Health-care personnel** who provide direct patient care.
- **Household contacts and caregivers** of children under six months.

In older individuals, flu shots may offer significant protection against strokes and heart disease. The only individuals who should steer clear are those allergic to eggs, since the inactivated flu viruses are grown in chick embryos.

Vaccination with the live, nasal-spray flu vaccine (FluMist®) is an option for healthy people aged 5 to 49 years who are not pregnant. The aerosol vaccine significantly reduces flu severity, days lost from work, health-care visits, and the use of over-the-counter medication. The spray represents a particular advantage for children since more than 30 percent of youngsters get the flu, but most don't receive a flu shot.

For those who don't get vaccinated, antiviral drugs, which must be taken within 36 to 48 hours of the first flu symptom, have provided the next best line of defense. Two of the oldest of these medications, amantadine and rimantadine, which work only against the type A flu virus, are no longer effective, possibly because the flu virus has mutated and become resistant.[8] Two newer agents, Tamiflu (oseltamivir) and Relenza (zanamivir), which fight both type A and type B influenza, still work. Tamiflu is approved by the FDA to prevent as well as treat the flu, particularly when there is a serious outbreak in a community. The other three drugs can also be used preventively, but Relenza, which is inhaled rather than swallowed, can cause wheezing.

Colds and Flus on Campus

College and university students are at increased risk for colds and influenza-like illnesses (see Reality Check). In one study that followed

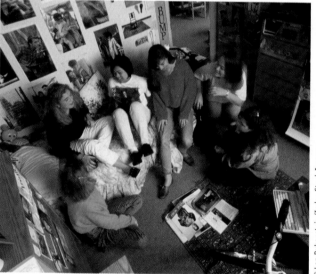

© Len Rubenstein/Index Stock Imagery

Students living in dormitories are more likely to catch the flu. The more roommates you have, the higher the risk.

YOUR STRATEGIES FOR PREVENTION *Smart Hand-Washing*

- Use hot water and lather up, covering the backs of your hands as well as your fingers and palms. Scrub for at least 15 seconds—about the time it takes to sing one chorus of "Happy Birthday to You."
- Don't think antibacterial soaps provide added protection. The research to date

suggests that they do not, and they may worsen the problem of antibiotic resistance.

- Don't switch to alcohol-based hand sanitizers. While they are handy when you can't get to a sink, they must come into contact with all surfaces of your hands in

order to be effective. Even then, they cleanse no better than plain soap and water.

- Dry your hands thoroughly. Wet hands are more likely to spread germs than dry ones.

more than 3,000 students from fall to spring, nine in ten had at least one cold or flu-like illness. These infections were responsible for 6,023 days in bed, 4,263 days of missed class, 3,175 days of missed work, and 45,219 days of illness.

Flu shots are now advised for almost everyone, but the majority of college health centers report vaccinating fewer than 20 percent of their students. Those living in dormitories are at higher risk of influenza than those in nondormitory settings. The specific aspects of dormitory life that increase the risk of flu symptoms include the number of roommates and the presence/absence of carpeting. Students living in "triples," with three beds to a room; those sleeping in the same room with a roommate in a double; and those with uncarpeted floors have higher rates of flu symptoms, such as fever, sore throat, and fatigue.

Meningitis

Meningitis, or invasive meningococcal disease, attacks the membranes around the brain and spinal cord and can result in hearing loss, kidney failure, and permanent brain damage. One of the most common types is caused by the bacterium *Neisseria meningitidis.* Viral meningitis is typically less severe.

Most common in the first year of life, the incidence of bacterial meningitis rises in young people between ages 15 and 24. Adolescents and young adults account for nearly 30 percent of all cases of meningitis in the United States. If not treated early, meningitis can lead to death or permanent disabilities. One in five of those who survive suffers from long-term side effects, such as brain damage, hearing loss, seizures, or limb amputation. Fatality rates are five times higher among 15- to 24-year-olds.[9]

 Each year 100 to 125 cases of meningitis occur on college campuses. An estimated 5 to 15 students die as a result. One in five survivors suffers long-term side effects. Individuals living in crowded living situations, such as dormitories, sleep-away camps, and barracks are at increased risk.

Meningitis spreads through the exchange of respiratory droplets, which can come from sharing a drink, cigarette, or silverware; kissing; coughing; or sneezing. Even inhaling secondhand smoke can infect you with the disease.

Preventing Meningitis

Vaccination protects against four of the five most common types of meningococcal bacteria. These four strains cause more than 80 percent of cases in adolescents and young adults. As with other immunizations, minor reactions may occur. These include pain and swelling at the injection site, headache, fatigue, or a vague sense of discomfort.

REALITYCHECK
- *How many college students report being vaccinated against meningitis?* _____
- *How many college students report getting a flu shot in the last year?* _____
- *How many college students report that a cold, flu, or sore throat affected their academic performance in the last year?* _____

Answers on nex page.

The CDC and other major health organizations, such as the American College Health Association, recommend routine vaccination with a new type of meningococcal vaccine, which provides longer-lasting protection than the previous type.[10] However, vaccinations are not advisable as the following lists indicate.[11]

Who should be vaccinated:

- All children when they turn 11 or 12 or when they enter high school, if they have not been previously vaccinated.
- College freshmen living in dorms.
- Military recruits.
- People who may have been exposed to meningitis during an outbreak.

Who should not get vaccinated or should wait:

- Anyone who has had a severe, life-threatening reaction or allergy to any vaccine component.
- Anyone who is moderately or severely ill at the time of the scheduled immunization.
- Anyone who had ever had Guillain-Barre syndrome (a neurological disorder).
- Pregnant women.

Recognizing Meningitis

The early symptoms of meningitis may be mild and resemble symptoms of flu or other less severe infections. Bacterial meningitis symptoms may develop within hours; viral meningitis symptoms may develop quickly or over several days. Fever, headache, and neck stiffness are the hallmark symptoms of meningitis. Not all symptoms may appear, but they can progress very quickly,

influenza   Any type of fairly common, highly contagious viral diseases.

meningitis   An extremely serious, potentially fatal illness that attacks the membranes around the brain and spinal cord; caused by the bacterium *Neisseria meningitis.*

killing an otherwise healthy person in 48 hours or less, so it is critical to seek medical attention quickly.

The most common symptoms of meningitis are:

- Sudden high fever.
- Severe, persistent headache.
- Neck stiffness and pain that makes it difficult to touch the chin to the chest.
- Nausea and vomiting, sometimes along with diarrhea.
- Confusion and disorientation (acting "goofy").
- Drowsiness or sluggishness.
- Eye pain or sensitivity to bright light.
- Pain or weakness in the muscles or joints.

Other possible signs and symptoms include:

- Abnormal skin color.
- Stomach cramps.
- Ice-cold hands and feet.
- Dizziness.
- Reddish or brownish skin rash or purple spots.
- Numbness and tingling.
- Seizures.

When to Seek Medical Care

If two or more of the symptoms of meningitis appear at the same time or if the symptoms are very severe or appear suddenly, seek medical care right away. If a red rash appears along with fever, see if the rash disappears when a glass is pressed against it. If it does not, this could be a sign of blood infection, which is a medical emergency. Call 911 without delay. Other symptoms that might require emergency treatment include loss of consciousness, seizures, muscle weakness, or sudden severe dementia.

A new rapid test can determine the presence of viral meningitis in just 2.5 hours. Because it can help quickly distinguish between viral and bacterial meningitis, the test could help reduce the unnecessary use of antibiotics.[12] About one in ten people who get meningitis dies from it. Of those who survive, another 11 to 19 percent lose fingers, arms, or legs, become deaf, have problems with their nervous systems, or suffer seizures, strokes, or brain damage.[13] Thus it is critical to seek medical care for this infection.

Hepatitis

An estimated 500,000 Americans contract hepatitis each year. At least five different viruses, referred to as **hepatitis** A, B, C, Delta, and E, can cause this inflammation of the liver. Newly identified viruses also may be responsible for some cases of what is called "non-A, non-B" hepatitis. Thanks largely to effective vaccines, rates of hepatitis A and hepatitis B infections have declined to their lowest rates in decades. Although there is no vaccine for hepatitis C, its incidence also has declined significantly.[14]

All forms of hepatitis target the liver, the body's largest internal organ. Symptoms include headaches, fever, fatigue, stiff or aching joints, nausea, vomiting, and diarrhea. The liver becomes enlarged and tender to the touch; sometimes the yellowish tinge of jaundice develops. Treatment consists of rest, a high-protein diet, and the avoidance of alcohol and drugs that may stress the liver. Alpha interferon, a protein that boosts immunity and prevents viruses from replicating, may be used for some forms.

Most people begin to feel better after two or three weeks of rest, although fatigue and other symptoms can linger. As many as 10 percent of those infected with hepatitis B and up to two-thirds of those with hepatitis C become carriers of the virus for several years or even life. Some have persistent inflammation of the liver, which may cause mild or severe symptoms and increase the risk of liver cancer.

Hepatitis A

Hepatitis A, a less serious form, is generally transmitted by poor sanitation, primarily fecal contamination of food or water, and is less common in industrialized nations than in developing countries. As many as 30 percent of individuals in the United States show evidence of past infection with the virus. Among those at highest risk in the United States are children and staff at day-care centers, residents of institutions for the mentally handicapped, sanitation workers, and workers who handle primates such as monkeys. Gamma globulin can provide short-term immunity; vaccines against hepatitis A have been approved by the FDA. The CDC recommends routine immunization against hepatitis A in states with high rates, as well as for travelers to countries

POINT COUNTERPOINT *Athletes at Risk*

POINT

Dangerous microbes such as hepatitis B have been found in the sweat of unexpectedly high numbers of athletes and high-intensity exercisers. Because of this potential threat, particularly in contact sports such as wrestling and football, schools should require screening of intramural and intercollegiate athletes and vaccination against HBV.

COUNTERPOINT

We live in a sea of microbes and should not over-react to the theoretical risks they pose. Athletes should be informed of the potential dangers of infection and of practical methods, such as the use of anti-microbial wipes, to reduce the risk of transmission. However, the decision to undergo screening and vaccination should be an individual one.

YOUR VIEW

Should colleges and universities, along with professional sports organizations, take every step possible to safeguard the health of their athletes? Or is there a point when required screening becomes an invasion of personal privacy and rights? What would you choose to do if you played a contact sport? What do you think your teammates should be required to do to ensure your safety?

---

where hepatitis A is common, men who have sex with men, and persons who use illegal drugs.

Hepatitis B

Hepatitis B, a potentially fatal disease transmitted through the blood and other bodily fluids, infects an estimated 400,000 people around the world each year. Once spread mainly by contaminated tattoo needles, needles shared by drug users, or transfusions of contaminated blood, hepatitis B is now transmitted mostly through sexual contact. It can cause chronic liver infection, cirrhosis, and liver cancer. Medications for hepatitis B often must be taken long-term, or the disease comes back even stronger.[15]

Hepatitis B is a particular threat to young people; 75 percent of new cases are diagnosed in those between ages 15 to 39. They usually contract hepatitis B through high-risk behaviors such as multiple sex partners and use of injected drugs. Athletes in contact sports, such as wrestling and football, may transmit the hepatitis B virus in sweat. With the discovery that HBV is more common in athletes than had been suspected, health experts are calling for mandatory HBV testing and vaccination against hepatitis B for all athletes.[16] (See Point/Counterpoint.)

Individuals who have tattoos or body piercing may also be at risk if procedures are not done under regulated conditions. At highest risk are male homosexuals, heterosexuals with multiple sex partners, health-care workers with frequent contact with blood, injection drug users, and infants born to infected mothers. Vaccination can prevent hepatitis B and is recommended for all newborns.

Hepatitis C

Hepatitis C virus (HCV) is four times as widespread as HIV, infecting about 2 percent of Americans. A simple blood test can show if you are infected with HCV. However, few of the estimated 3 to 4 million carriers in the United States realize they are infected. Of those infected with HCV, 80 percent have no symptoms.

The risk factors for HCV infection are blood transfusion or organ transplant before 1992, exposure to infected blood, illegal drug use, tattoos, or body piercing. If you choose to have a body piercing, avoid piercing guns, and make certain that the piercing equipment has been sterilized (see Savvy Consumer: "Before You Get a Tattoo or Piercing"). Hepatitis C virus is not spread by casual

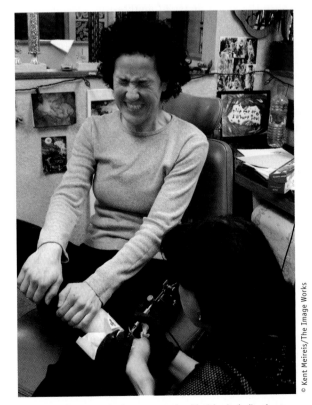

© Kent Meireis/The Image Works

Getting a tattoo or a piercing can pose health risks, including bacterial infection and hepatitis.

hepatitis An inflammation and/or infection of the liver caused by a virus, often accompanied by jaundice.

Before You Get a Tattoo or Piercing

"Body art"—tattoos and piercings—may seem harmless, but health officials warn of hidden risks, including hepatitis B and C infection and transmission of HIV. In a survey of undergraduates at a university in New York, 51 percent reported body piercings, and 23 percent had gotten tattoos. Almost one in five of those with piercings reported medical complications. Bacterial infection was the most common, followed by bleeding and injury or tearing at the site.

With no state or federal regulations of "body artists," unsafe tattooing and piercing practices can put consumers in danger. In one survey of "skin-penetration operators," only half said that they followed governmental guidelines for infection control. Many were not knowledgeable about standard infection-control principles and practices.

Epidemiologists have identified tattooing as a strong, independent risk factor for testing positive for hepatitis C virus (HCV) but not with development of acute hepatitis. In other words, individuals with tattoos may acquire HCV but may not develop symptoms themselves. This does not mean that they will never become symptomatic or that they cannot transmit HCV to others.

Even so-called temporary tattooing with henna is not without risk. Dermatologists have reported an increasing number of skin reactions. The culprit is an ingredient in many henna preparations called paraphenylenediamine (PPD). Allergic reactions to henna itself can occur, but are much rarer. Piercings of the tongue, lips, or cheeks present different dangers, including recessed gums; loose, chipped, or fractured teeth; pain; infection; inflammation; nerve damage; and tooth loss.

You may think you're safe if you go to a licensed tattoo or piercing salon. However, there are no formal schools, no certification requirements, and no diplomas for these practitioners. In many states it is possible to get a license without the benefit of any kind of training. Your best assurance of quality is making sure that basic safety principles are followed:

- **Ask to see certification that the autoclave, a high-temperature pressure cooker used for medical instruments, has been sterilized.** Ask to see the autoclave itself. Is it clean? More importantly, are the shop personnel happy to show it to you, or do they seem to have something to hide? Autoclaves need to be regularly tested to ensure that they are working properly. Ask to see the results of their latest spore test. Check the date. The results should be no more than two months old.

- **Make sure the artist is wearing standard medical latex gloves.** Check the fit. If the gloves are too big or too small, the artist runs the risk of either poking a hole in the gloves or tearing them. All it takes is a pinhole to run the risk of cross-contamination.

- **Find out if the artist is vaccinated for hepatitis B.** As this infection has spread, vaccination has become essential for a tattoo artist's own safety as well as that of clients. If artists claim to be vaccinated, never just take their word for it. Can they show you proof, such as a doctor's record, that they were vaccinated? If they tell you they don't remember if they've been vaccinated, they're probably lying. Most people vividly remember the vaccinations.

- **Make sure the artist uses only new sterile needles.** The needles should not be removed from the autoclave bag, the sort of pouch you see in dentists' offices, until you are ready for your tattoo. Ask to see the sterile confirmation logo on the bag itself. Usually the name of the company that made the bag will be visible on the front of the bag only when the equipment has been properly autoclaved. To determine if the needles are new and not just sterilized after previous use, check the color. They should be bright silver, not stained with ink or brownish looking.

- **Make sure the artist doesn't "double-dip."** The ink should be new, used on only one client—you.

- **Ask how the artist disposes of used needles.** They should be placed in a sharps container—a plastic container, usually red, with a biohazard symbol on the outside—and removed in a timely manner.

- **Always ask to see photos of the artist's finished work.** Examine the designs up close to check precision and skill. If you have the time, watch the artist work on another client before you go ahead with your tattoo.

- **If you require prophylactic antibiotics for dental cleanings or other procedures, do not get a tattoo.** Consumers with rheumatic heart disease and other conditions that increase their risk of infections have died as a result of bacterial infection contracted from a tattoo.

contact, such as hugging, kissing, or sharing food utensils. There is controversy over whether HCV also can be transmitted sexually.

About three-quarters of those infected with HCV develop chronic or long-term hepatitis. About one-quarter develop progressive, irreversible liver damage, with scar tissue (cirrhosis) gradually replacing healthy liver tissue. If the liver no longer functions adequately, a patient may require liver transplantation. Hepatitis C infection also increases the risk of non-Hodgkin's lymphoma by up to 30 percent.[17]

The most common treatment for hepatitis C is a combination of interferon, which stops the virus from making copies of itself; and ribavirin, an antiviral medication. The treatment lasts for 6 to 12 months, and can be extremely difficult to endure.

Mononucleosis

You can get **mononucleosis** through kissing—or any other form of close contact. "Mono" is a viral disease that targets people 15 to 24 years old. Its symptoms include a sore throat, headache, fever, nausea, and prolonged weakness. The spleen is swollen and the lymph nodes are enlarged. You may also develop jaundice or a skin rash similar to rubella (German measles).

The major symptoms usually disappear within two to three weeks, but weakness, fatigue, and often depression may linger for at least two more weeks. The greatest danger is from physical activity that might rupture the spleen, resulting in internal bleeding. The liver may also become inflamed. A blood test can determine whether you have mono. However, there's no specific treatment other than rest.

Chronic Fatigue Syndrome (CFS)

More than a million Americans have the array of symptoms known as **chronic fatigue syndrome (CFS).** CF Syndrome is a complex disorder characterized by profound fatigue that does not improve with bed rest and that may get worse with physical or mental activity. Other symptoms include weakness, muscle pain, impaired memory or concentration, insomnia, and postexertion fatigue that lasts for more than 24 hours. Symptoms can persist for years. CFS affects four times as many women as men.

Diagnosis of CFS remains difficult, although numerous studies have found significant immune abnormalities, such as high levels of certain immune cells (B lymphocytes and cytokines) that act as if they were constantly battling a viral infection. There is no known cure, but a combination of therapies can help relieve symptoms.

Tuberculosis

A bacterial infection of the lungs that was once the nation's leading killer, **tuberculosis (TB)** still claims the lives of more people than any acute infectious disease other than pneumonia (Figure 15.4). About 30 percent of the world's population is infected with the TB organism, although not all develop active disease. In the United States, immigration from countries where TB is common, poverty, homelessness, alcoholism and drug abuse, the HIV/AIDS epidemic, and the emergence of resistant strains of TB account for most new cases of TB. Approximately 15 million Americans have the disease.

Although TB is most prevalent among high-risk groups, the overall danger increases as more people develop active disease because TB is highly contagious. TB outbreaks have occurred throughout the country in hospitals, nursing homes, prisons, and office buildings, where inadequate ventilation increases the risk of infection.

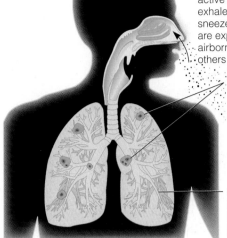

When someone with active tuberculosis exhales, coughs, or sneezes, TB bacteria are expelled in tiny airborne droplets that others may inhale.

The TB bacteria lodge mainly in the lungs, where they slowly multiply, creating patches, then cavities.

Other parts of the lung are affected, including the bronchi and the lining of the lung.

If untreated, TB can eventually spread to and damage the brain, bone, eyes, liver and kidneys, spine, and skin.

Figure 15.4   How Tuberculosis Spreads
If untreated, TB can eventually spread to and damage the brain, bone, eyes, liver, kidneys, spine, and skin.

Symptoms vary, depending on the organs that are infected. They include fever and sweating (particularly at night), unexplained weight loss, loss of appetite, fatigue, persistent cough that may produce bloody sputum, and difficulty breathing or chest pain when breathing.

Most TB patients recover completely after six months of taking a combination of three different medicines. Drug-resistant forms of the tuberculosis microorganism strike mostly patients who start drug treatment but don't follow through with it. Because they don't take enough of the medication to kill all the TB bacteria in their system, those that survive become resistant. Even with full treatment, the risk of dying from drug-resistant tuberculosis is 50 percent. HIV infection greatly increases susceptibility to infection with TB and the risk of dying if infected with treatment-resistant forms.

If you think you may have been exposed to TB or if you develop suspicious symptoms (loss of appetite and weight, low-grade fever, fatigue, chills, night sweats, coughing), see your doctor for a TB test. This consists of an injection just under the skin. The area of the arm where the

mononucleosis   An infectious viral disease characterized by an excess of white blood cells in the blood, fever, bodily discomfort, a sore throat, and kidney and liver complications.

chronic fatigue syndrome (CFS)   A cluster of symptoms whose cause is not yet known; a primary symptom is debilitating fatigue.

tuberculosis (TB)   A highly infectious bacterial disease that primarily affects the lungs and is often fatal.

test was administered should be checked by a health-care professional to determine the presence of the TB bacteria; further tests confirm the diagnosis. If the skin test is positive, indicating that TB is present, you'll be monitored with yearly chest X-rays. You may also require treatment, which usually requires three to four antibiotics taken daily for at least 6 to 9 months.

Group A and Group B Strep Infection

Sore throats are common winter complaints, but those caused by group A streptococcus bacteria—*strep throats*—are more than a trivial threat. If not treated promptly with antibiotics, strep bacteria can travel to the kidneys, the liver, or the heart, where they can cause rheumatic fever—an inflammation of the heart that can cause weakness, shortness of breath, joint pain, and an abnormal heartbeat. In recent years clusters of rheumatic fever have sprung up in several major cities. Pediatricians are urging parents to consult their doctors if a youngster complains of a sore throat or if strep is widespread in the community. Rapid new diagnostic tests can identify strep within minutes. If the test is positive, treatment with penicillin or a similar antibiotic is indicated. Brief treatment (five days) with Omnicef, a newer antibiotic, has proved as effective as ten days of oral penicillin.

Toxic streptococcal shock syndrome, or toxic strep, is an invasive form of the disease in which strep gains access to the blood and causes a drop in blood pressure, a very high fever, and the production of exotoxins (substances that can attack various organs, such as the kidneys, heart, or in rare cases, flesh). Toxic strep is rather rare and usually doesn't occur with strep throats. Prompt treatment is critical.

Group B streptococcus (GBS), the leading cause of life-threatening perinatal infections in the United States, is primarily a threat to newborns. Because some 15 to 40 percent of pregnant women carry GBS but have no symptoms, the American Academy of Pediatrics has called for universal screening of expectant mothers. Each year 12,000 newborns are infected, most of them during childbirth; more than 1,600 die; and another 1,600 suffer permanent brain damage from meningitis. Women at high risk of infecting their newborns with GBS are those who have premature labor, early rupture of their amniotic membranes, fever, and a high group B strep count before or during pregnancy, or who have previously borne an infant infected with GBS. Also at risk are diabetics, low-income women, and those under age 20.

Toxic Shock Syndrome

As discussed in Chapter 9, toxic shock syndrome (TSS) is a potentially deadly disease associated with the use of tampons, particularly high-absorbency types. It is caused by *Staphylococcus aureus* and group A *Streptococcus pyo-genes* bacteria that release toxins (poisonous waste products) into the bloodstream. Symptoms include a high fever; a rash that leads to peeling of the skin on the fingers, toes, palms, and soles; dizziness; dangerously low blood pressure; and abnormalities in several organ systems (the digestive tract and the kidneys) and in the muscles and blood.

In addition to women who use high-absorbency tampons, or leave their tampons in too long, those who have given birth within the preceding six to eight weeks are at greater risk. Children (including newborns), men, and postmenopausal women also have developed TSS, which usually has been traced to bacteria in skin abscesses, boils, cuts, or postsurgical wounds.

Without prompt treatment, TSS can cause severe and permanent damage, including muscle weakness, partial paralysis, amnesia, disorientation, an inability to concentrate, and impaired lung and kidney function. Sometimes toxic shock weakens the blood vessels, increasing the risk of heart problems. Victims can enter the life-threatening crisis called shock, in which blood flow throughout the body is inadequate to sustain life. Treatment usually consists of immediate hospitalization, intravenous administration of fluids, medications to raise blood pressure, and powerful antibiotics; intravenous administration of immunoglobins that attack the toxins produced by these bacteria may also be beneficial.

The "Superbug" Threat: MRSA

For decades most strains of the bacterium *Staphylococcus aureus* responded to treatment with penicillin. When the bacterium became resistant to penicillin, physicians switched to a newer antibiotic, methicillin. Within a year the first case of methicillin-resistant *S. aureus* (MRSA) was detected. This "superbug," which fights off traditional antibiotics, has become a major health threat.[18]

One in three healthy people carry *S. aureus* bacteria on their skin. Of these as many as one in 100 may be carrying MRSA. In medical terms, these individuals are "colonized" but not infected. For infection to occur, MRSA must enter the body through an accidental injury such as a scrape or burn or via a deliberate break in the skin such as a surgical incision.

The rate of MRSA infections is highest in hospitals and health-care facilities, but MRSA also can develop among sports teams, child care attendees, and prison inmates.[19] Rates of MRSA infection among hospital patients are quite high. According to a recent study, as many as 1.2 million hospital patients in the United States may be infected every year.[20] Nearly 119,000 hospital patients may die as a result.[21]

MRSA spreads by touch. In health-care settings, it can spread from patient to patient through contact with doctors and nurses with unwashed hands or contaminated

YOUR STRATEGIES FOR PREVENTION *How to Avoid MRSA*

- Wash hands thoroughly and frequently.
- Ask health-care professionals if they've washed their hands before examining or treating you.
- Keep cuts and scrapes clean. Cover them with a band-aid.

- Avoid touching other people's cuts, incisions, or dressings.
- Don't share personal items such as towels or razors.
- If you go to a gym, wipe the equipment before working out. Use a clean towel to

prevent your skin from coming into direct contact with the machines. Shower after each workout.

gloves or contact with unsterile medical equipment. Health advocates are calling for increased screening of patients for MRSA, isolating and treating MRSA carriers, more conscientious hand washing, and more diligent use of gowns, gloves, and masks to prevent transmission of MRSA.

Outside of hospitals, community-associated MRSA (CA-MRSA) is a growing threat that can occur in people without any established risks. This form of MRSA can be spread by sexual contact and contact sports.[22]

Who Is at Highest Risk?

People at high risk of becoming infected with MRSA are those in close contact with carriers, as hospital patients are. MRSA poses the greatest danger to individuals who have/are:

- A weakened immune system.
- A pre-existing infection.
- Open wounds, cuts, or burns.
- Other types of wounds, such as skin breaks from an intravenous drug line.

- Undergone surgery.
- Athletes in contact sports.
- Elderly
- Premature or newborn babies.
- Taken antibiotics recently or for a long period.[23]

For ways to protect yourself, see Your Strategies for Prevention: "How to Avoid MRSA."

The Dangers of MRSA Infections

MRSA bacteria can infiltrate a range of tissues and body systems causing problems such as wound infections, deep abscesses, lung infections, and blood poisoning, which can be fatal. Because of its antibiotic resistance, MRSA is difficult, but not impossible to treat. Most strains of the bacteria are responding to newer antibiotics.

Insect- and Animal-Borne Infections

Common insects and animals, including ticks and mosquitoes, can transmit dangerous infections. Lyme disease is the most widespread in the United States. Other threats include West Nile virus, monkeypox virus, and avian influenza, or bird flu. For ways to protect yourself, see Your Strategies for Prevention: "How to Avoid Insect-Borne Diseases."

Lyme Disease

Lyme disease, a bacterial infection, is spread by ticks carrying a particular bacterium—the spirochete *Borrelia burgdorferi*. An infected person may have various symptoms, including joint inflammation, heart arrhythmias, blinding headaches, and memory lapses. The disease can also cause miscarriages and birth defects. Lyme disease is by far the most commonly reported vector-borne infectious disease in the United States.

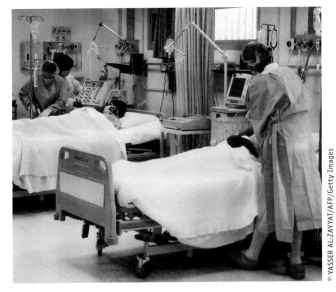

© YASSER AL-ZAYYAT/AFP/Getty Images

Hospitals can be dangerous places. MRSA spreads from patient to patient when hand-washing is inadequate or when gloves or equipment are contaminated.

Lyme disease   A disease caused by a bacterium carried by a tick; it may cause heart arrhythmias, neurological problems, and arthritis symptoms.

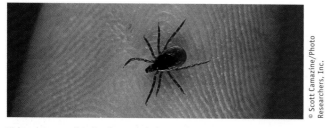

Ticks are responsible for the spread of Lyme disease. If you spot a tick, remove it as soon as possible with tweezers or small forceps. Put it in a plastic bag or sealed bottle and save it. If you develop a rash or other symptoms, take it with you to the doctor.

You are not likely to get Lyme disease if a tick is attached to your skin for less than 24 to 48 hours. About 70 to 80 percent of infected individuals will develop a red rash at the site of the tick bite. Over a period of days to weeks, the rash grows larger. The center may fade, creating a ring or "bulls-eye" appearance. The rash may rarely burn or itch. Once diagnosed, Lyme disease is treated with antibiotics. Nonsteroidal anti-inflammatory drugs, such as aspirin or ibuprofen, can relieve fever and pain.

The FDA has licensed a vaccine to prevent Lyme disease in individuals 15 to 70 years old. LYMErix, like most vaccines, stimulates the immune system to produce antibodies, in this case against the bacterium that causes Lyme disease. But the vaccine, administered in three doses over a one-year period, is not 100 percent effective and should not be considered a substitute for protective clothing and tick repellent.

The primary culprit in most cases of Lyme disease is the deer tick, although other ticks, including the western black-legged tick, the dog tick, and the Lone Star tick, also may transmit the bacterium that causes Lyme disease.

About 60 percent of untreated individuals develop arthritis, and their joints become swollen and painful. If Lyme disease spreads to the nervous system, it can cause neurological symptoms, including memory loss, inability to concentrate, muscle weakness with tingling and numbness in the arms and legs, and Bell palsy, a facial droop caused by muscle paralysis.[24]

West Nile Virus

West Nile virus (WNV) is transmitted by a mosquito that feeds on an infected bird and then bites a human. The first cases in the United States occurred in 1999. Experts now see WNV as a seasonal epidemic that flares up in the summer and continues into the fall. WNV also can be spread through blood transfusions, organ transplants, breast-feeding, and from mother to fetus during pregnancy.

WNV interferes with normal central nervous system functioning and causes inflammation of brain tissue. The risk of catching WNV is low. Relatively few mosquitoes carry WNV, and fewer than 1 percent of people who are bitten by mosquitoes experience any symptoms. Repellents that contain DEET, picaridin, and oil of lemon eucalyptus can protect against these mosquitoes.

There is no specific treatment for WNV infection. People with more severe cases usually require hospitalization and supportive treatment, including intravenous fluids and help with breathing. An antiviral drug, interferon, which might lessen the symptoms and duration of the illness in infected patients, is undergoing testing.

Monkeypox Virus

This rare viral disease occurs mainly in Africa, where it was first identified in monkeys. Researchers have since recovered monkeypox from other animals, including rats, mice, and rabbits, as well as humans.

The signs and symptoms of monkeypox are similar to those of smallpox but milder. People can catch monkeypox from an infected animal's bite, blood, or body fluids. It can spread from person to person during long periods of face-to-face contact or by touching the body fluids of a sick person or bedding or clothing contaminated with the virus. There is no specific treatment.

Avian Influenza

Avian influenza, or bird flu, is caused by viruses that occur naturally among wild birds. Most strains of bird flu virus cannot infect humans, but a few can, usually

---

YOUR STRATEGIES FOR PREVENTION *How to Avoid Insect-Borne Diseases*

- Apply insect repellent containing DEET (N,N-diethyl-meta-toluamide), which provides the longest-lasting protection against bites, when you're outdoors.

- When possible, wear long-sleeved clothes and long pants treated with repellents containing permethrin or DEET since insects may bite through thin clothing. Do not apply repellents containing permethrin directly to exposed

skin. If you spray your clothing, there is no need to spray repellent containing DEET on the skin under your clothing.

- Consider staying indoors at dawn, dusk, and in the early evening, which are peak mosquito-biting times.

- After spending time outdoors, examine yourself for ticks or bites every day. Check less obvious places, such as the scalp and behind the ears.

- If you do spot a tick, remove it right away. Using tweezers or forceps, grasp the tick firmly as close to its head and as near to your skin as possible. Gently pull backward, without squeezing the tick's body, until its hold is released. Wash your hands thoroughly. Treat the wound with rubbing alcohol.

with great difficulty. Influenza viruses jumped from birds to humans three times in the twentieth century. In each case a mutation in the genes of the virus allowed it to infect humans. Then a further change allowed the virus to pass easily from one human to another, rapidly spreading around the world in a deadly pandemic.

A virus called H5N1, previously found only in birds, spread to domestic poultry and infected people who had worked closely with sick birds in Hong Kong in 1997. The H5N1 virus has spread to wild migratory birds, which have carried it to other countries and continents.

The H5N1 virus has infected millions of wild and domestic birds and animals such as pigs and cats. The humans who have developed this strain of bird flu handled sick birds in the process of plucking or butchering them or were exposed to the birds' feces. The United States has banned the importation of all birds and bird products from countries known to have bird flu outbreaks.

So far the H5N1 virus has not mutated into a form that can easily infect humans or that humans can transmit to another person. Experts disagree as to whether H5N1 will ever mutate in such a way as to cause a pandemic. Some worry because the virus has already evolved to infect cats, pigs, and humans. Others note that the virus is unlikely to spread easily from one person to another because it clusters in the deepest branches of the respiratory tract and cannot be spread easily by coughs and sneezes.

Bird flu can be very severe, and even healthy young adults who contracted it have died. However, others have developed only mild symptoms; some exposed to the virus developed no symptoms at all. The initial symptoms are similar to those of ordinary influenza, but people with bird flu are likely to have high fevers, more severe coughing, and muscle and joint pain; feel out of breath even when resting; become confused; and feel too weak to get out of bed.

The FDA has approved the first vaccine that could be used in the event of an avian flu outbreak in the United States.[25] It also has outlined a preparedness plan to find potential food or feed contamination, identify FDA-regulated substances (including dietary supplements) at risk of contamination, and take other steps to lower the risk to the public.[26]

The Threat of a Pandemic

Pandemic flu is a virulent human flu that causes a global outbreak, or pandemic, of serious illness. Influenza pandemics tend to occur when disease-causing organisms that typically affect only animals adapt and infect humans, then further adapt so they can pass easily from human to human. The flu pandemic of 1918–1919 claimed half a million lives.

Concern about the spread of avian flu has spawned fears of a deadly new pandemic. The virus can be (but is rarely) transmitted from birds to humans, but there have not been any cases of human-to-human transmission.[27] Although experts disagree about the probability of an avian flu pandemic, a worldwide influenza epidemic may occur.[28]

Here are some ways you can protect yourself:

- **Stay informed.** Check reliable sources of information, such as the federal website **www.pandemicflu.gov**.
- **Get an annual flu shot.** It won't protect you from a pandemic flu virus, but it can prevent simultaneous infections.
- **See your doctor** within two days of developing flu symptoms.
- **Wash your hands frequently,** particularly after being in crowded public places.
- **Stay healthy.** Eating right, working out, and getting enough sleep keep your immune system strong.
- **Think carefully about travel in flu season.** Viruses are easily transmitted in confined spaces such as airplanes, trains, and buses. If possible, don't travel to places with outbreaks of deadly viruses.

Emerging Infectious Diseases

The twenty-first century has ushered in new agents of infection and new apprehension about the potential use of infectious diseases as instruments of terror and mass destruction.

SARS

Severe acute respiratory syndrome (SARS) became a new global health threat in 2003, with major outbreaks in several Asian countries, including China and Hong Kong, and in Toronto.

Another outbreak occurred in China in 2004. SARS-associated coronavirus (SARS-CoV) spreads by close face-to-face contact, most often by droplets expelled into the air when an infected person coughs or sneezes. The virus is believed capable of living outside the body for at least 24 hours. A few persons may be especially infectious and are more likely to spread the SARS virus to others in the same airplane, household, school, workplace, or hospital. Doctors do not know how long a person remains contagious.

The average incubation period for SARS is six to ten days. Symptoms include high fever, coughing, headache, chills, muscle aches, and shortness of breath. Most of those infected develop pneumonia. There are no specific treatments for SARS. Patients receive supportive care, such as fluids to prevent dehydration and ventilators to aid breathing. Scientists are developing possible vaccines and antiviral agents.

Bioterror Threats

Americans have learned firsthand that certain infectious agents can be used as weapons of terrorism and war. Bioterror agents, such as anthrax and, potentially, smallpox, botulism and tularemia, have been added to the ranks of emerging infectious diseases.

Anthrax Anthrax, which is found naturally in wild and farm animals, can also be produced in a laboratory. The disease is spread through exposure to anthrax spores, not through exposure to an infected person.

Smallpox Smallpox is a serious, contagious, and sometimes fatal infectious disease. Smallpox was eradicated decades ago after a successful worldwide vaccination program. The last case of smallpox in the United States was in 1949. The last naturally occurring case in the world was in Somalia in 1977. There is no treatment, and up to 30 percent of those infected with smallpox die.

Because of fear that terrorists might use smallpox as a biological weapon, the U.S. government has stockpiled enough vaccine to inoculate everyone in the event of an emergency. Most individuals vaccinated before 1972, when mandated smallpox immunization ended in the United States, retain some immunity for many years, some for up to 75 years. However, half of all Americans have never received the smallpox vaccine, and many scientists believe protection wanes over time for those who did. Those vaccinated in the past can safely be revaccinated for optimum protection. An Institute of Medicine committee has recommended against vaccinating the entire population at this time.

Botulism Botulism is a muscle-paralyzing disease caused by a toxin made by the bacterium *Clostridium botulinum*. Botulinum toxin is among the most lethal substances known, and it can kill within 24 hours. Botulism causes muscle weakness and eventual paralysis that starts at the top of the body and works its way down. The disease kills by paralyzing muscles used to breathe. The CDC and some state health departments keep an antidote to botulinum toxin in storage. Treatment includes taking the antidote and possibly using a ventilator for breathing until the toxin works its way out of the system.

Tularemia Tularemia is an illness that normally infects wild animals, such as rabbits and squirrels. Humans can acquire the illness by coming in contact with the blood or body fluids of infected animals, from the bite of a fly or tick that carries blood from an infected animal, or from contaminated food or water. As a biological weapon, tularemia-causing bacteria could be dispersed through the air to be inhaled. Signs and symptoms vary but include fever, headache, chills, weakness, enlarged and tender lymph nodes, and an ulcerated sore if bitten by an infected fly or tick. Intravenous (IV) antibiotics can be used to treat tularemia. Even without treatment, it's fatal in less than 2 percent of cases. Tularemia is not passed from person to person.

Reproductive and Urinary Tract Infections

Reproductive and urinary tract infections are very common. Many are not spread exclusively by sexual contact, so they are not classified as sexually transmitted diseases.

Vaginal Infections

Vaginal complaints account for approximately 10 million medical office visits a year. The most common are trichomoniasis, candidiasis, and bacterial vaginosis (Table 15-3).

Protozoa (*Trichomonas vaginalis*) that live in the vagina can multiply rapidly, causing itching, burning, and discharge—all symptoms of **trichomoniasis.** Male carriers usually have no symptoms, although some may develop urethritis or an inflammation of the prostate and seminal vesicles. Anyone with this infection should be screened for syphilis, gonorrhea, chlamydia, and HIV. Sexual partners must be treated with oral medication (metronidazole, trade name Flagyl), even if they have no symptoms, to prevent reinfection.

TABLE 15.3 Common Reproductive Tract Infections

Infection	Transmission	Symptoms	Treatment
Bacterial vaginosis	Most common causative agent, *Gardnerella vaginalis* bacterium, sometimes transmitted through coitus	Women: Fishy- or musty-smelling, thin discharge, like flour paste in consistency and usually gray Men: Mostly asymptomatic	Metronidazole (Flagyl) by mouth or intravaginal applications of topical metronidazole gel or clindamycin cream
Candidiasis (yeast infection)	*Candida albicans* fungus may accelerate growth when the chemical balance of the vagina is disturbed; also transmitted through sexual interaction	Women: White, "cheesy" discharge; irritation of vaginal and vulval tissues	Vaginal suppositories or topical cream, such as clotrimazole (GyneLotrimin) and miconazole (Monistat), or oral fluconazole
Trichomoniasis	Protozoan parasite *Trichomonas vaginalis,* usually passed through genital sexual contact	Women: White or yellow vaginal discharge with an unpleasant odor; sore and irritated vulva Men: No symptoms	Metronidazole (Flagyl) for both women and men

Populations of a yeast called *Candida albicans*—normal inhabitants of the mouth, digestive tract, and vagina—are usually held in check. Under certain conditions, however (such as poor nutrition, stress, or antibiotic use), the microbes multiply, causing burning, itching, and a whitish discharge, and producing what is commonly known as a yeast infection. Common sites for **candidiasis,** which is also called *moniliasis,* are the vagina, vulva, penis, and mouth.

 The women most likely to test positive for candidiasis have never been pregnant, use condoms for birth control, have sexual intercourse more than four times a month, and have taken antibiotics in the previous 15 to 30 days. Vaginal medications, such as GyneLotrimin and Monistat, are nonprescription drugs that provide effective treatment. Women should keep the genital area dry and wear cotton underwear.

Male sexual partners may be advised to wear condoms during outbreaks of candidiasis.

Bacterial vaginosis is characterized by alterations in the microorganisms that live in the vagina, including depletion of certain bacteria and overgrowth of others. It typically causes a white or gray vaginal discharge with a distinctive fishy odor similar to that of trichomoniasis. Its underlying cause is unknown, although it occurs most frequently in women with multiple sex partners. Long-term dangers include pelvic inflammatory disease (PID, discussed in Chapter 16) and pregnancy complications. Metronidazole, either in the form of a pill or a vaginal gel, is the primary treatment. According to CDC guidelines, treatment for male sex partners appears to be of little benefit, but some health practitioners recommend treatment for both partners in cases of recurrent infections. Antibiotic therapy may help prevent an infected woman from acquiring an STI.[29]

Urinary Tract Infections

A urinary tract infection (UTI) can be present in any of the three parts of the urinary tract: the urethra, the bladder, or the kidneys. An infection involving the urethra is known as **urethritis.** If the bladder is also infected, it's called **cystitis.** If it reaches the kidneys, it's called *pyelonephritis.*

 An estimated 40 percent of women report having had a UTI at some point in their lives. Three times as many women as men develop UTIs, probably for anatomical reasons. A woman's urethra is only 1.5 inches long; a man's is 6 inches. Therefore, bacteria, the major cause of UTIs, have a shorter distance to travel to infect a woman's bladder and kidneys. About one-fourth to one-third of all women between ages 20 and 40 develop UTIs, and 80 percent of those who experience one infection develop recurrences.

Conditions that can set the stage for UTIs include irritation and swelling of the urethra or bladder as a result of pregnancy, bike riding, irritants (such as bubble bath, douches, or a diaphragm), urinary stones, enlargement of the prostate gland in men, vaginitis, and stress. Early diagnosis is critical because infection can spread to the kidneys and, if unchecked, result in kidney failure. Symptoms include frequent burning, painful urination, chills, fever, fatigue, and blood in the urine.

Recurrent UTIs, a frequent problem among young women, have been linked with a genetic predisposition, sexual intercourse, and the use of diaphragms.

trichomoniasis An infection of the protozoan *Trichomonas vaginalis;* females experience vaginal burning, itching, and discharge, but male carriers may be asymptomatic.

candidiasis An infection of the yeast *Candida albicans,* commonly occurring in the vagina, vulva, penis, and mouth and causing burning, itching, and a whitish discharge.

bacterial vaginosis A vaginal infection caused by overgrowth and depletion of various microorganisms living in the vagina, resulting in a malodorous white or gray vaginal discharge.

urethritis Infection of the urethra.

cystitis Inflammation of the urinary bladder.

Learn It ⋮ **Live It**

The Best Defense

Microorganisms such as bacteria and viruses greatly outnumber humans on the planet. Yet despite their vast numbers, relatively few invade, multiply, and cause illness in people. Many microorganisms, such as those living in your intestine, actually play a role in keeping you healthy. The goal isn't to wipe out all microbes but to recognize those with a potential to harm us and take steps to defend ourselves.

The three steps to infection protection are:

- **Immunizations.** Keep track of the vaccinations you've received and the dates you received them. Check with your doctor about any booster shots you may require. Get a tetanus booster every five years (an easy way not to forget: get one every time you celebrate a birthday ending in a 5 or 0, such as 25 and 30). Get your flu shot or spray. As discussed in the following chapter, if you're a woman and have not been vaccinated against human papilloma virus (HPV), talk to your doctor about the potential benefits for you.

- **Good health habits.** Take this chapter's Self-Survey to check your infection protection IQ. Identify the areas where you may need to boost your defenses, and follow the guidelines in Your Health Action Plan.

- **Prompt treatment.** The early symptoms of many infectious diseases are similar. Yes, it may just be a bad cold or the flu, but you can't rule out the possibility of a more deadly threat, such as bacterial meningitis. Don't ignore severe or persistent symptoms.

SELFSURVEY ⋮ *What's Your Infection IQ?*

Check the items that apply to you.

_____ I wash my hands with soap and water after I use the restroom.

_____ I wash my hands with soap and water before I eat.

_____ Before and after using exercise equipment, I wipe the handles.

_____ I wash my hands with soap and water after working out with weights or exercise equipment at a gym.

_____ I avoid contact with people who are coughing and sneezing.

_____ I wash my hands with soap and water more often during the cold and flu season.

_____ All of my vaccinations are current.

_____ I eat at least 3 balanced meals a day.

_____ I get 6 to 8 hours of sleep at night.

_____ I use relaxation techniques to lower my stress level.

_____ I do not smoke.

_____ I do not drink or keep alcohol consumption to a minimum.

_____ I do not use drugs of any kind, including steroids.

_____ I throw leftovers out after 3 days.

_____ I wash fruits and vegetables before eating.

_____ I check expiration dates on food items.

_____ I apply insect spray (containing DEET) when I am outdoors.

_____ I wear long-sleeved clothing and long pants when hiking.

_____ I check myself for ticks after a hike.

Scoring

Add up your checkmarks, and look for patterns in your protective behaviors. Are you conscientious about exercise and sleep, but careless about washing your hands or wiping down gym equipment? Do you protect yourself against food infections (discussed in Chapter 6) but not against sexually transmitted infections (discussed in Chapter 16)? Identify the aspects of infection protection that need the most work, and start practicing the defensive behaviors that will lower your risk.

Your Health Action Plan for Better Infection Protection

Some day medical science may develop vaccines or other means of providing total protection against infectious diseases. Until then your best defense is to take commonsense steps to promote well-being and reduce the risks of infection. Here are some basic principles of self-defense:

- **Eat a balanced diet** to be sure you get essential vitamins and minerals. Severe deficiencies in vitamins B_6, B_{12}, and folic acid impair immunity. Keep up your iron and zinc intake. Iron influences the number and vigor of certain immune cells, whereas zinc is crucial for cell repair. Too little vitamin C also may increase susceptibility to infectious diseases.
- **Avoid fatty foods.** A low-fat diet can increase the activity of immune cells that hunt down and knock out cells infected with viruses.
- **Get enough sleep.** Without adequate rest, your immune system cannot maintain and renew itself. (See the lab "Sleep Power" in *IPC*.) **IPC**
- **Exercise regularly.** Aerobic exercise stimulates the production of an immune-system booster called interleukin-2.
- **Don't smoke.** Smoking decreases the levels of some immune cells and increases susceptibility to respiratory infections.

- **Control your alcohol intake.** Heavy drinking interferes with normal immune responses and lowers the number of defender cells.
- **Wash your hands frequently** with hot water and soap. In a public restroom, use a paper towel to turn off the faucet after you wash your hands, and avoid touching the doorknob. Wash objects used by someone with a cold.
- **Don't share food, drinks, silverware, glasses,** and other objects that may carry infectious microbes.
- **Spend as little time as possible in crowds** during cold and flu season, especially closed places, such as elevators and airplanes. When out, keep your distance from sneezers and coughers.
- **Don't touch your eyes, mouth, and nose,** especially after being with someone who has cold symptoms.
- **Use tissues** rather than cloth handkerchiefs, which may harbor viruses for hours or days.
- **Avoid irritating air pollutants** whenever possible.

CENGAGENOW If you want to write your own goals for preventing infectious diseases, go to the Wellness Journal at HealthNow: **academic.cengage.com/login.**

Making This Chapter Work for YOU

Review Questions

1. Which of the following statements about disease-causing microbes is *false?*
   a. Helminths cause malaria, one of the major worldwide diseases.
   b. AIDS is caused by a virus.
   c. In the United States, the most common protozoan disease is giardiasis.
   d. Salmonella is a foodborne illness caused by bacteria.

2. Which of the following statements about the immune system is *false?*
   a. The immune system has two types of white blood cells: B cells, which produce antibodies that fight bacteria and viruses, and T cells, which protect against other invaders.
   b. Immune system structures include the spleen, tonsils, thymus gland, and lymph nodes located throughout the body.
   c. Inoculation with a vaccine confers active immunity.
   d. The effect of stress on the human immune system depends on whether you can control the stressor and on the mental effort required to cope.

3. College students should have all of the following immunizations *except*
   a. hepatitis A.
   b. pertussis.
   c. measles.
   d. tetanus.

4. Which of the following statements about the common cold and influenza is true?
   a. Influenza is just a more severe form of the common cold.
   b. Aspirin should be avoided by children and young adults who have a cold or influenza.
   c. The flu vaccine is also effective against most of the viruses that cause the common cold.
   d. Antibiotics are appropriate treatments for colds but not for influenza.

5. The meningitis vaccination
   a. is recommended for all college freshmen.
   b. protects against four of the five most common types of meningococcal bacteria.
   c. also protects against gonorrhea.
   d. may cause minor reactions such as fever or hives.

6. Hepatitis B
   a. is spread mainly through contaminated needles.
   b. infects mostly middle-aged people.
   c. does not have a preventive vaccine.
   d. can be spread in the sweat of athletes.

7. Which statement about methicillin-resistant *Staphylococcus aureus* (MRSA) is *false*?
   a. MRSA can be spread by doctors in a hospital.
   b. MRSA can be spread by athletes playing contact sports.
   c. MRSA is carried on the skin of as many as 1 in 100 people.
   d. MRSA can cause lung infections.

8. Which of the following statements is true?
   a. The Lyme disease vaccine stimulates the immune system to produce antibodies against the bacterium *Borrelia burgdorferi*.
   b. West Nile virus is transmitted to humans by birds.

   c. West Nile virus is the most commonly reported vector-borne infectious disease in the United States.
   d. Avian flu has been transmitted from human to human.

9. Which of the following statements about specific infectious diseases is *false*?
   a. Symptoms of SARS include high fever, coughing, headache, and chills.
   b. Anthrax can be found in wild and farm animals.
   c. Hepatitis A is usually transmitted through contaminated needles, transfusions, and sexual contact.
   d. College freshmen are at higher risk for contracting meningitis than the general population of young people between the ages of 18 and 23.

10. Which statement about reproductive and urinary tract infections is *false*?
    a. Yeast infections can be treated with nonprescription drugs.
    b. Symptoms of UTIs include burning urination, chills, fever, and blood in the urine.
    c. Three times as many women as men develop UTIs.
    d. Bacterial vaginosis usually causes a vaginal discharge with a rotten-egg odor.

Answers to these questions can be found on page 583.

Critical Thinking

1. Prior to reading this chapter, describe what you did to avoid contracting infectious disease. Now that you have read the chapter, will you be making any changes in your practices? Briefly explain the convenience, advantages, and disadvantages of each practice that you have and/or will be using to prevent infection.

2. At the pharmacy, the shelves are full of medications for cold and flu. How do you sort through them? Do you get recommendations from family and friends? Do you study the labels? Do you keep track of what works for you?

3. Did you get vaccinated for meningitis? Why or why not? Where did you get your information on the disease and the vaccine, and how did you make your decision?

Media Menu

CENGAGENOW™ Go to the HealthNow website at **academic.cengage .com/login** that will:

- Help you evaluate your knowledge of the material.
- Allow you to take an exam-prep quiz.
- Provide a Personalized Learning Plan targeting resources that address areas you should study.
- Coach you through identifying target goals for behavioral change and creating and monitoring your personal change plan throughout the semester.

INTERNET CONNECTIONS

Immunization Action Coalition

www.immunize.org

This site features comprehensive vaccination information for children, adolescents, and adults.

National Institute of Allergy and Infectious Diseases

www3.niaid.nih.gov

This institute is part of the National Institutes for Health. Its website provides information about current research and includes fact sheets about all manner of topics related to allergies and infectious diseases.

National Center for Infectious Diseases

www.cdc.gov/ncidod

This comprehensive site, sponsored by the Centers for Disease Control and Prevention (CDC), features an infectious disease index, news on emerging infectious diseases, and a section for travelers.

Key Terms

The terms listed are used and defined on the page indicated. Definitions are also found in the Glossary at the end of this book.

abscess	441
allergy	441
antibiotics	437
antiviral drug	437
autoimmune disorder	441
bacteria	437
bacterial vaginosis	457
candidiasis	457
chronic fatigue syndrome (CFS)	451
cystitis	457
fungi	437
gamma globulin	439
helminth	437
hepatitis	449
host	437
immune deficiency	441
immunity	439
immunotherapy	441
incubation period	439
inflammation	441
influenza	447
Lyme disease	453
lymph nodes	439
meningitis	447
mononucleosis	451
pathogen	437
protozoa	437
systemic disease	441
trichomoniasis	457
tuberculosis (TB)	451
urethritis	457
vector	437
virus	437

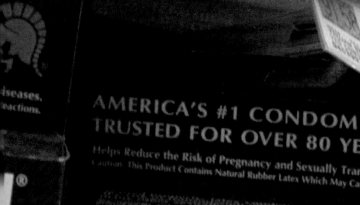
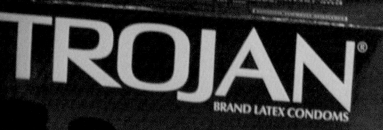

Lowering Your Risk of Sexually Transmitted Infections

"THERE'S something I have to tell you." Anise knew, just by the sound of her boyfriend's voice, that the "something" wasn't good news. "My herpes is back."

Stunned, Anise tried to absorb all the information packed into this short sentence: She'd had no idea that the man she'd been sleeping with for several months had a sexually transmitted infection (STI). How did he get it? What else hadn't he told her about his past? What did he mean that it was "back"? Could she have caught it? And, finally, she asked the all-too-human question: How could this have happened to me?

By their very nature, infectious diseases take people by surprise. Some of today's most common and dangerous infectious illnesses spread primarily through sexual contact, and their incidence has skyrocketed. The federal government estimates that 65 million Americans have a sexually transmitted infection (STI). These diseases cannot be prevented in the laboratory. Only you, by your behavior, can prevent and control them.

All human beings are sexual from birth to death. Whether you are male or female, single or married, straight, gay, lesbian, bisexual, or transgender, sexuality is a normal, natural part of your life. You are just as responsible for your sexual health as for any other aspect of your well-being. To safeguard your sexual health, you need to be aware of and protect yourself from sexually transmitted infections and diseases.

After studying the material in this chapter, you should be able to:

- **Recite** the ABCs of safer sex, and **explain** some specific steps for safeguarding sexual health.
- **Describe** the methods of STI transmission.
- **Name** the sexually transmitted infections, and **describe** the symptoms and treatment for each.
- **Define** HIV infection, **list** five facts about sexual transmission of HIV, and **name** strategies for reducing the risk of HIV infection.
- **Review** your sexual history, **assess** the risks you have taken in the past, and **describe** your strategies for the future.

CENGAGENOW™ Log on to HealthNow at **academic.cengage.com/login** to find your Behavior Change Planner and to explore self-assessments, interactive tutorials, and practice quizzes.

Sexually Transmitted Infections and Diseases

In medical terms **sexually transmitted infection (STI)** refers to the presence of an infectious agent that can be passed from one sexual partner to another. If the infection causes symptoms, it becomes a **sexually transmitted disease (STD)**. Many health organizations prefer to use the term STI because sexual infections can be—and often are—transmitted by people who do not have symptoms.

STIs occur in all animals (and even plants) that reproduce sexually. By some estimates, as many as 75 percent of sexually active women and men will develop an STI of some kind. Some people view sexual infections in moral terms. By attaching stigma and shame to STIs, these individuals may not seek treatment and thereby jeopardize their sexual health. However, embarrassment should never justify putting your health at risk.

Remember, STIs can:

- Last a lifetime.
- Put stress on relationships.
- Cause serious medical complications.
- Impair fertility.
- Cause birth defects.
- Lead to major illness and death.

Although each STI is distinct, they are all transmitted mainly through:

- Direct sexual contact with someone's symptoms (like genital ulcers) or sexual contact with someone's infected semen, vaginal fluids, blood, and other body fluids.
- Sharing contaminated needles through injectable drug use.
- Maternal transfer (mother to fetus during pregnancy or childbirth).

All STI pathogens like dark, warm, moist body surfaces, particularly the mucous membranes that line the reproductive organs; they hate light, cold, and dryness. Figure 16.1 shows how STIs in body fluids spread from person to person and how a barrier can help prevent their entry.

Table 16.1 lists the common STIs, their transmission, symptoms, and treatment. It is possible to catch or have more than one STI at a time. Curing one doesn't necessarily cure another, and treatments don't prevent another bout with the same STI.

Many STIs, including early HIV infection and gonorrhea in women, may not cause any symptoms. As a result, infected individuals may continue their usual sexual activity without realizing that they're jeopardizing anothers' well-being.

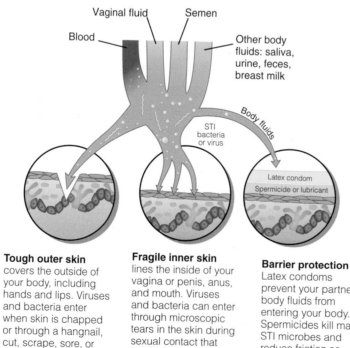

Figure 16.1 How STIs Spread
Most STIs are spread by viruses or bacteria carried in certain body fluids.

TABLE 16.1   Common Sexually Transmitted Infections (STIs): Mode of Transmission, Symptoms, and Treatment

STI	Transmission	Signs and Symptoms	Treatment
Human papilloma virus (HPV) (genital warts) (p. 469)	Spread primarily through vaginal, anal, or oral sex	Cauliflowerlike growths in genital and rectal areas	Removal of lesions by laser surgery or chemicals
Herpes simplex (p. 471)	Genital herpes virus (HSV-2) transmitted by vaginal, anal, or oral sex. Oral herpes virus (HSV-1) transmitted primarily by kissing	Small, painful red bumps (papules) to the genital region (genital herpes) or mouth (oral herpes). The papules become painful blisters that eventually rupture to form wet, open sores.	No known cure. Treatment may reduce symptoms; acyclovir, famcyclovir, or valacyclovir promote healing and suppress recurrent outbreaks
Chlamydia (p. 472)	*Chlamydia trachomatis* bacterium transmitted primarily through sexual contact (can also be spread by fingers from one body site to another)	Men: Watery discharge; pain when urinating Women: Usually asymptomatic; sometimes a similar discharge to men's; leading cause of pelvic inflammatory disease (PID)	Antibiotics: doxycycline, azithromycin, ofloxacin, levofloxacin
Gonorrhea ("clap") (p. 474)	*Neisseria gonorrhoeae* bacterium ("gonococcus") spread through genital, oral-genital, or genital-anal contact	Men: Pus discharge from urethra; burning during urination Women: Usually asymptomatic; can lead to PID and sterility in both men and women	Antibiotics: cephalosporins
Nongonococcal urethritis (NGU) (p. 475)	Bacteria, most commonly transmitted through sexual intercourse	Men: Discharge from the penis and irritation during urination Women: Mild discharge of pus from the vagina but often no symptoms	A single dose of azithromycin or doxycycline for seven days
Syphilis (p. 475)	*Treponema pallidum* bacterium ("spirochete") transmitted from open lesions during genital, oral-genital, or genital-anal contact	Primary: Chancre Secondary: Rash Latent: Asymptomatic Late: Irreversible damage to central nervous system, cardiovascular system	Penicillin or other antibiotic
Chancroid (p. 476)	*Haemophilus ducrevi* bacterium transmitted by sexual interaction	Men: Painful irregular chancre on penis Women: Chancre on labia	Tetracycline
Pubic lice ("crabs") (p. 476)	*Phthirus pubis* spread easily through body contact or through shared clothing or bedding	Persistent itching; visible lice often located in public hair or other body hairs	1% permethrin cream for body areas; 1% lindane shampoo for hair
HIV/AIDS (p. 476)	HIV transmitted in blood and semen, primarily through sexual contact or needle sharing among injection drug users	Asymptomatic at first; opportunistic infections	Combination of three or more antiretroviral drugs (termed highly active antiretroviral therapies, or HAART) plus other specific treatment for opportunistic infections and tumors

STIs in Society

More Americans are infected with STIs now than at any other time in history. According to the Institute of Medicine, the odds of acquiring an STI during a lifetime are one in four. STIs are among the top ten most frequently reported diseases in the United States. The major cause of preventable sterility in America, STIs have tripled the rate of ectopic (tubal) pregnancies, which can be fatal if not detected early. STI complications, including miscarriage, premature delivery, and uterine infections after delivery, annually affect more than 100,000 women.

Infection with an STI greatly increases the risk of HIV transmission (discussed later in this chapter). The incidence of STIs is highest in 16- to 24-year-olds—particularly older teenagers—and homosexual men. Others affected by STIs include unborn and newborn children who can "catch" potentially life-threatening infections in the womb or during birth.

Around the world, some 50 million cases of curable STIs occur each year (not including HIV and herpes). Almost 700,000 people are infected every day with one of the over 20 STIs tracked by world health officials. STIs are much more widespread in developing nations because of lack of adequate health standards, prevention practices, and access to treatment.

sexually transmitted infection (STI) The presence in the human body of an infectious agent that can be passed from one sexual partner to another.

sexually transmitted disease (STD) A disease that is caused by a sexually transmitted infection that produces symptoms.

STIs on Campus

Young people of college age account for about half of new cases of sexually transmitted infections. The college years are a prime time for contracting STIs. According to the American College Health Association, chlamydia and HPV have reached epidemic levels at many schools—although many of those infected aren't even aware of it.

In the National College Health Assessment, infection with human papilloma virus (HPV) was the most commonly reported STI on campus; 2.3 percent of stu-

dents said they had HPV in the past school year. Genital herpes, reported by 0.9 percent, ranked second, while 0.8 percent of students had chlamydia and 0.3 percent had pelvic inflammatory disease.[1] All of these infections are discussed in this chapter.

Contracting STIs may increase the risk of being infected with HIV. Because college students have more opportunities to have different sexual partners and may use drugs and alcohol more often before sex, they are at greater risk. Half of new HIV infections occur in people under age 25.

Colleges and universities vary in the STI services, including screening, diagnosis, and treatment, that they

---

Your Life Change Coach

The ABCs of Safer Sex

Making smart, healthy choices about sex is the key to preventing sexual illnesses. (See the lab on "The Seduction of Safer Sex" in *IPC*.) **IPC** As you will discover in this chapter, there are many specific steps to take to safeguard your sexual health. However, the three key fundamentals are as simple as A, B, C.

A is for Abstain

Abstinence from vaginal and anal intercourse and oral sex is free, available to everyone, extremely effective at preventing both pregnancy and sexually transmitted infections, and has no medical or hormonal side effects. If you decide to abstain only from vaginal or anal penetration, remember that other sexual activity such as oral sex can also expose you to STIs. If you have oral sex, make it safer by using effective barrier methods such as condoms or latex dental dams. (A dental dam is a square piece of latex that can be stretched across the vulva or anus to prevent the transmission of STI.) In the absence of barrier methods, men should avoid ejaculating in their partners' mouths. Also,

- Be aware of sores and discharge or unpleasant odors from your partner's genitals. These are signs to avoid oral sex.
- Don't floss or brush teeth before oral sex. It might tear the lining of the mouth, increasing exposure to viruses.

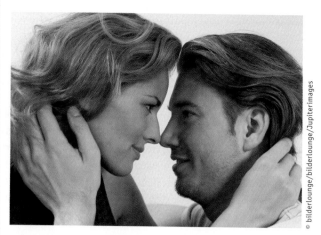

Abstain, *Be* faithful, or use *Condoms.* Following the ABC's of safer sex doesn't mean you can't have an intimate, loving relationship.

- Avoid aggressive and deep thrusting in oral sex, which can damage throat tissues and increase susceptibility for throat-based gonorrhea, herpes, and abrasions.
- Remember that oral sex can transmit various STIs, including HPV, herpes, gonorrhea, syphilis, and HIV.

B is for Be Faithful

For men and women who are sexually active, a mutually faithful sexual relationship with just one healthy partner is the safest option. Women and men in a committed relationship don't need to worry about getting sexually transmitted infections if:

- Neither partner ever had sex with anyone else.
- Neither partner ever shared needles.
- Neither partner currently has or ever had an STI.

© bilderlounge/bilderlounge/Jupiterimages

offer. In a national survey, about half of colleges and universities made condoms available to students—some free in an open display, some free on request, and some for a fee or in vending machines. Larger schools, those with health centers, and those with on-campus housing are more likely to provide STI education and services.

STIs and Gender

Both men and women can develop STIs, but their risks are not the same. Here is some gender-specific information.

If You Are a Woman

• Keep in mind that your risk of getting an infection is greater than a man's. STIs can be transmitted through breaks in the mucous membranes, and women have more mucosal area exposed and experience more trauma to these tissues during sexual activity than men.[2]

• Don't think you don't have to worry just because you have no symptoms. Symptoms of STIs also tend to be more "silent" in women, so they often go undetected and untreated, leading to potentially

If these criteria fail to apply, two partners should be sure that neither has an STI before giving up on safer-sex practices. Some infections, like HIV, may take years to develop symptoms. The only way to know is by testing.

Of course, a committed relationship remains safe only as long as both partners remain committed. Most women who get HIV from having sex think they are their sex partners' only lover and never suspect that their partners' other lovers are men.

C is for Condoms

Condoms are the only contraceptive that helps prevent both pregnancy and STIs when used properly and consistently. Male condoms reduce the risk of transmission of an STI by 50 to 80 percent. They are more effective against STIs transmitted by bodily fluids (chlamydia, gonorrhea, HIV, etc.) than those transmitted by skin-to-skin contact (HPV, syphilis, herpes, chancroid). Inexpensive and widely available in pharmacies, supermarkets, and convenience stores, condoms don't require a doctor visit or a prescription.

Most physicians recommend prelubricated, American-made latex or polyurethane condoms. Check the package for FDA approval. Also check the expiration (Exp) or manufacture (MFG) date on the box or individual package to see until when it is safe to use the condom. Make sure the package and the condom appear in good condition. If the package does not state that the condoms are meant to prevent disease, they may not provide adequate protection even if they are the most expensive ones on the shelf.

Condoms can deteriorate if not stored properly since they are affected by both heat and light. Don't use a condom that has been stored in your back pocket, your wallet, or the glove compartment of your car. Keep fresh condoms handy at all times. If a condom feels sticky or very dry don't use it; the packaging has probably been damaged.

Although it can be awkward to bring up the subject of condoms, don't let your embarrassment put your health at risk. Discuss using a condom before having sex; don't wait until you're on the brink of a sexual encounter.

See Chapter 10 for instructions on how to put on a condom. Here are some additional guidelines:

• **Use a new condom** each and every time you engage in any form of intercourse.
• **Do not use spermicide containing nonoxynol-9.** According to recent research, nonoxynol-9 without condoms is ineffective against HIV transmission. Even with condoms, it does not protect women from the bacteria that cause gonorrhea and chlamydia.
• **If a condom fails** during vaginal or anal intercourse, remove it carefully. If you continue sexual activity, replace it with a new condom.

serious complications. For instance, pelvic inflammatory disease has no symptoms but puts you at risk of infertility and ectopic pregnancy.

- At your checkup talk to your doctor about whether you should be tested for sexually transmitted infections. You need to ask for these tests, or else they won't be done.

If You Are a Man

- After potential exposure to an STI, give yourself a little extra protection by urinating and washing your genitals with an antibacterial soap.
- At your checkup talk to your doctor about whether you should be tested for sexually transmitted infec-

tions. You need to ask for these tests, or else they won't be done.

STI Risk Factors and Risk Continuums

Various factors put young people at risk of STIs, including:

- **Feelings of invulnerability,** which lead to risk-taking behavior. Even when they are well informed of the risks, adolescents and young adults may remain unconvinced that anything bad can or will happen to them.
- **Multiple partners.** Figure 16.2 illustrates how STI risks increase as relationships become less familiar and exclusives.

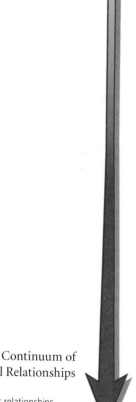

RELATIONSHIPS

Celibacy/Abstinence

Monogamy
lifetime
less than lifetime
(with negative STI/HIV tests)

less than lifetime
(with no tests)

A few well-known partners

Multiple well-known partners

A few anonymous partners

Multiple anonymous partners

BEHAVIORS

Noninsertive

Kissing/Making out
Petting/Fondling
Masturbation
Sex toy use
Outercourse

Insertive and protected
(condoms, other barriers)
Cunnilingus
Fellatio
Vaginal intercourse (i)
Vaginal intercourse (r)
Anal intercourse (i)
Anal intercourse (r)

Insertive and
not protected
(withdrawal)

Fellatio
Cunnilingus
Anilingus
Vaginal intercourse (i)
Vaginal intercourse (r)
Anal intercourse (i)
Anal intercourse (r)

Insertive, not protected,
including ejaculation
Fellatio
Vaginal intercourse (r)
Anal intercourse (r)

i = insertive partner
r = receptive partner

Low risk

High risk

Figure 16.2 Continuum of Risk for Sexual Relationships and Behaviors
STI risks increase as relationships become less familiar and exclusive and as sexual activities bexome unprotected and receptive.

In surveys of students, a significant number report having had four or more sexual partners during their lifetime.

- **Failure to use condoms.** Among those who reported having had sexual intercourse in the previous three months, fewer than half of the students reported condom use. (See Reality Check.) Figure 16.3 shows the risk continuum for protected and nonprotected sexual behaviors. STI risks increase as sexual activities become unprotected and receptive.

 Students who'd had four or more sexual partners were significantly less likely to use condoms than those who'd had fewer partners.

- **Substance abuse.** Individuals who drink or use drugs are more likely to engage in sexually risky behaviors, including sex with partners whose health status and history they do not know, and unprotected intercourse.

Rate your own sexual health risk by taking this chapter's Self Survey.

 By age 50 at least 80 percent of women will have acquired HPV. Young women who engage in sexual intercourse at an early age are more likely than those with later sexual debuts to become infected with HPV. Their risk also increases if they have multiple sexual partners or a history of a sexually transmitted infection, use drugs, or have partners with multiple sexual partners.

College-age women are among those at greatest risk of acquiring HPV infection. In various studies conducted in college health centers, 10 to 46 percent of female students (mean age 20 to 22) had

Human Papilloma Virus

Human papilloma virus (HPV) is the most common sexually transmitted infection in the United States.[3] Most people who become infected with HPV do not have any symptoms, and the infection clears on its own. However, HPV infection can cause cervical cancer in women and genital warts and other types of cancers in both sexes.

Of the 100 or more different strains, or types, of HPV, approximately 40 are sexually transmitted. Some "high-risk" HPV strains may lead to cancer of the cervix, vulva, vagina, anus, or penis. If transmitted via oral sex, they increase the risk of mouth and throat cancers. In a recent study, individuals with HPV infections were 32 times more likely to develop such cancers. The risk increases along with the number of oral sex partners.[4]

The "low-risk" types of HPV may cause Pap test abnormalities or genital warts. Genital warts are single or multiple growths or bumps, sometimes shaped like cauliflower, that appear in the genital area.

Incidence

Approximately 20 million people in the United States are currently infected with HPV, and 6.2 million Americans get a new HPV infection each year. Worldwide there are more than 440 million individuals with HPV infection.[5] At least 50 percent of sexually active men and women acquire HPV at some point in their lives. According to recent data, 25 percent of 14- to 19-year-olds and 45 percent of 20- to 24-year-olds are infected with HPV.[6]

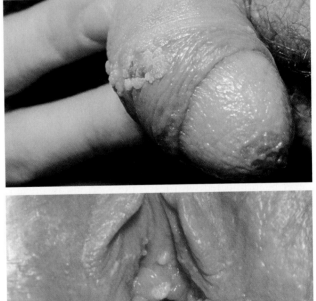

Human papilloma virus, which causes genital warts, is the most common viral STI.

© Marazzi/Photo Researchers, Inc.

© Bart's Medical Library/Phototake

human papilloma virus (HPV) A pathogen that causes genital warts and increases the risk of cervical cancer.

a cervical HPV infection—and increased risk of precancerous cell changes.

Yet college students' awareness of HPV and their potential risk is very low. In one study, both sexes did not see themselves as susceptible to HPV. Male students were more likely than female students to think that only women could acquire HPV.[7] In another report, even women with adequate to high levels of knowledge about HPV did not take steps such as using condoms or having regular Pap tests to protect themselves.[8]

The HPV Vaccine

Gardasil, the first vaccine developed to prevent cervical cancer, targets four HPV types that together cause 70 percent of cervical cancers and 90 percent of genital warts.[9] It does not protect against all HPV types that cause cervical cancer. Gardasil is most effective when given before first sexual contact and exposure to HPV.[10] In girls and women who have never been infected with HPV, the vaccine can prevent almost all cases of disease caused by the four targeted types of HPV, including cancers of the genitals, cervix, and anus.[11] In women with prior infection—with the HPV strains targeted by the vaccine, other strains, or both—Gardasil's efficacy falls from almost 100 percent to as low as 17 percent.[12]

The CDC has recommended HPV vaccination for all girls before they turn 13, and some states are considering mandatory immunization. However, there is continuing controversy over the timing and need for universal vaccination.[13] (See Savvy Consumer: "Who Should Get the HPV Vaccine?")

Women who get the HPV vaccine must still take safersex precautions because they are not protected against all forms of HPV or other STIs. They also still need regular Pap smear testing to detect early changes that may lead to cervical cancer.

Symptoms

Most people with HPV infection do not know they are infected. The virus lives in the skin or mucous membranes and usually causes no symptoms. Some people get visible genital warts or have precancerous changes in the cervix, vulva, anus, or penis. After contact with an infected individual, genital warts may appear within three weeks to eighteen months, with an average period of about three months.

HPV infection may invade the urethra and cause urinary obstruction and bleeding. It greatly increases a woman's risk of developing a precancerous condition called cervical *intraepithelial neoplasia*, which can lead to cervical cancer. Adolescent girls infected with HPV appear to be particularly vulnerable to developing cervical cancer. It is not known if HPV itself causes cancer or acts in conjunction with cofactors (such as other infections, smoking, or suppressed immunity). A woman's risk of cervical cancer is strongly related to the number of her partner's current and lifetime female partners.[14] Women are five to eleven times as likely to get cervical cancer if their steady sex partner has had 20 or more previous partners.

Most HPV infections are asymptomatic in men, who may unwittingly increase their partners' risk. Men who test positive for HPV typically report significantly more sex partners than those who do not. HPV may also cause genital warts in men and increase the risk of cancer of the penis. People with visible genital warts also may have asymptomatic or subclinical HPV infections that are extremely difficult to treat.

Diagnosis and Treatment

After sexual contact with an infected person, warts may appear within weeks or months. Genital warts are diagnosed by visual inspection.

Most women are diagnosed with HPV after an abnormal Pap test. Further testing can detect HPV DNA in women. The results of HPV DNA testing can help healthcare providers decide if treatment is necessary to prevent or treat cervical cancer. (See Chapter 14 for a discussion of cervical cancer.)

No form of therapy has been shown to completely eradicate HPV, nor has any single treatment been uniformly effective in removing warts or preventing their recurrence. CDC guidelines suggest treatments that focus on the removal of visible warts—laser therapy, cryotherapy (freezing), and topical applications of podofilox, podophyllin, or trichloroacetic acid—and then eradication of the virus. At least 20 to 30 percent of treated individuals experience recurrence.

Savvy Consumer — Who Should Get the HPV Vaccine?

The HPV vaccine, Gardasil, which consists of three shots given over a six-month period, has been extensively tested in thousands of young women worldwide and is considered safe. However, the longest study so far has lasted only five years, so long-term effects are not known.[15] Gardasil confers immunity for at least five years, but no one yet knows whether a booster shot or shots will be necessary. The vaccine is still being tested in boys, men, and women over age 26.

The CDC has recommended vaccination for the following groups:

- All girls ages 11 to 12 years of age, although doctors may give it to girls as young as nine.
- Girls and women ages 13 to 26 who did not receive it when they were younger.[16]

Some states are considering legislation to make HPV vaccination mandatory for all girls because the vaccine is most effective when given before a girl becomes sexually active. Some religious groups oppose mandatory immunization because they feel that vaccinating girls against an STI gives them the wrong message about sexual responsibility. Consumer advocates worry about the unknown long-term effects. Others feel that the decision should be made privately by parents in consultation with their pediatricians.

Gardasil costs about $120 per shot, or $360 for the three-shot series. Most insurance companies cover recommended vaccines, but since this one is new, consumers need to check with their insurance provider to be certain. The most common side effects are pain at the injection site and fever. There have been cases of tingling, numbness, and loss of sensation in young girls receiving the vaccine.

Who should *not* get the HPV vaccine?

- Women older than 26 (the vaccine is still being tested in women in this age group).
- Pregnant women.
- Girls or women who have ever had a life-threatening allergic reaction to any component of HPV vaccine.
- Girls or women who are moderately to severely ill at the time of vaccination.

Herpes Simplex

Herpes (from the Greek word that means *to creep*) collectively describes some of the most common viral infections in humans. Characteristically, **herpes simplex** causes blisters on the skin or mucous membranes.

Herpes simplex exists in several varieties. *Herpes simplex virus 1 (HSV-1)* can be transmitted by kissing and generally causes cold sores and fever blisters around the mouth. *Herpes simplex virus 2 (HSV-2)* is sexually transmitted and may cause blisters on the penis, inside the vagina, on the cervix, in the pubic area, on the buttocks, on the thighs, or in the mouth and throat (transmitted via oral sex).

HSV transmission occurs through close contact with mucous membranes or abraded skin. Condoms help prevent infection but aren't foolproof. When herpes sores are present, the infected person is highly contagious and should avoid bringing the lesions into contact with someone else's body through touching, sexual interaction, or kissing.

Individuals without any obvious symptoms shed the virus subclinically, whether or not they have lesions. Most people with herpes contract it from partners who were not aware of any symptoms or of their own contagiousness. Standard methods of diagnosing genital herpes in women, which rely primarily on physical examination and viral cultures, may miss as many as two-thirds of all cases. Blood tests are more effective in detecting unrecognized infections with HSV-2.

The herpes virus is present in genital secretions even when patients do not notice any signs of the disease, and people infected with genital herpes can spread it even between flare-ups when they have no symptoms. There is growing evidence that genital herpes promotes the spread of HIV.

A newborn can be infected with genital herpes while passing through the birth canal, and the frequency of mother-to-infant transmission seems to be increasing. Most infected infants develop typical skin sores, which can be cultured to confirm a herpes diagnosis. Some physicians recommend treatment with acyclovir. Because of the risk of severe damage and possible death, caesarean delivery may be advised for a woman with active herpes lesions.

herpes simplex A condition caused by one of the herpes viruses and characterized by lesions of the skin or mucous membranes; herpes simplex virus 2 is sexually transmitted and causes genital blisters or sores.

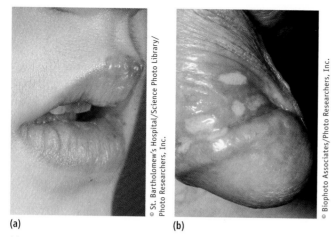

(a) Herpes simplex virus (HSV-1) as a mouth sore; (b) Herpes simplex virus (HSV-2) as a genital sore.

Incidence

Genital herpes has skyrocketed during the last three decades, yet only a minority of infections with HSV-2 are recognized by those infected. About 40 percent of new cases of genital herpes occur in young people aged 15 to 24. An estimated 4.2 million young adults in this age range—11 percent of the population—have been infected.

Symptoms

Most people with genital herpes have no symptoms or very mild symptoms that go unnoticed or are not recognized as a sign of infection. The most common is a cluster of blistery sores, usually on the vagina, vulva, cervix, penis, buttocks, or anus. They may last several weeks and go away. They may return in weeks, months, or years.

Other symptoms include: blisters, burning feelings if urine flows over sores, inability to urinate if severe swelling of sores blocks the urethra, itching and pain in the infected area. Severe first episodes of herpes may also cause swollen, tender lymph glands in the groin, throat, and under the arms, fever, chills, headache, and achy flu-like feelings.

The virus that causes herpes never entirely goes away; it retreats to nerves near the lower spinal cord, where it remains for the life of the host. Herpes sores can return without warning weeks, months, or even years after their first occurrence, often during menstruation or times of stress, or with sudden changes in body temperature. Of those who experience HSV recurrence, 10 to 35 percent do so frequently—that is, about six or more times a year. In most people, attacks diminish in frequency and severity over time. Herpes, like other STIs, can trigger feelings of shame, guilt, and depression.

Treatment

The three antiviral medications approved for the treatment of genital herpes are:

- *Acyclovir.* The oldest antiviral medication for herpes, acyclovir is sold as a generic drug and under the brand name Zovirax®. Available as an ointment and pill, acyclovir has been shown to be safe in persons who have used it continuously (every day) for as long as 10 years.
- *Valacyclovir.* Sold as Valtrex®, this medication delivers acyclovir more efficiently so that the body absorbs more of the drug and medication can be taken fewer times during the day.
- *Famciclovir.* Sold as Famvir®, this drug utilizes penciclovir as its active ingredient to stop HSV. Like valacyclovir, it is well absorbed, persists for a longer time in the body, and can be taken less frequently than acyclovir.

These antiviral medications are prescribed for initial and recurrent episodes of herpes. In episodic therapy, a person begins taking medication at the first sign of recurrence and continues for several days to hasten the healing or prevent a full outbreak from occurring. In suppressive therapy, people with genital herpes take antiviral medication daily to prevent symptoms. For individuals who have frequent recurrences (six or more per year), suppressive therapy can reduce the number of outbreaks by at least 75 percent. Suppressive therapy may also reduce asymptomatic shedding of HSV.

Various treatments—compresses made with cold water, skim milk, or warm salt water; ice packs; or a mild anesthetic cream—can relieve discomfort. Herpes sufferers should avoid heat, hot baths, or nylon underwear. Some physicians have used laser therapy to vaporize the lesions. Clinical trials of an experimental vaccine to protect people from herpes infections are underway.

Chlamydia

The most widespread sexually transmitted bacterium in the United States is *Chlamydia trachomatis*, which causes an estimated 3 million cases of **chlamydia** each year. The use of condoms with spermicide can reduce, but not eliminate, the risk of chlamydial infection.

Incidence

One in 25 young Americans is infected with chlamydia. Chlamydia is six times more prevalent in young black adults than in young white adults, with almost 14 percent of young black women and more than 11 percent of black men testing positve. Chlamydial infections are more common in younger than in older women, and they also occur more often in both men and women with gonorrhea.

Those at greatest risk of chlamydial infection are individuals 25 years old or younger who engage in sex with more than one new partner within a two-month period and women who use birth control pills or other nonbarrier contraceptive methods. The U.S. Preventive Services Task Force recommend regular screening for chlamydia for all sexually active women under age 25 and for older women with multiple sexual partners, a history of STIs, or inconsistent use of condoms.

Symptoms

As many as 75 percent of women and 50 percent of men with chlamydia have no symptoms or symptoms so mild that they don't seek medical attention. Without treatment, up to 40 percent of cases of chlamydia can lead to pelvic inflammatory disease, a serious infection of the woman's fallopian tubes that also can damage the ovaries and uterus. Also, women infected with chlamydia may have three to five times the risk of getting infected with HIV if exposed. Babies exposed to chlamydia in the birth canal during delivery can be born with pneumonia or with an eye infection called conjunctivitis, both of which can be dangerous unless treated early with antibiotics. Symptomless women who are screened and treated for chlamydial infection are almost 60 percent less likely than unscreened women to develop pelvic inflammatory disease. Chlamydia may also be linked to cervical cancer.

 When women have symptoms of chlamydia they may experience

- Abdominal pain.
- Abnormal vaginal discharge.
- Bleeding between menstrual periods.
- Cervical or rectal inflammation.
- Low-grade fever.
- Yellowish discharge from the cervix that may have a foul odor.
- Vaginal bleeding after intercourse.
- Painful intercourse.
- Painful urination.
- The urge to urinate more than usual.

 When men have symptoms of chlamydia, they may experience

- Pain or burning while urinating.
- Pus or watery or milky discharge from the penis.
- Swollen or tender testicles.
- Rectal inflammation.

Men often don't take these symptoms seriously because the symptoms may appear only early in the day and can be very mild.

Chlamydia, which can spread from a man's urethra to his testicles, can also cause a condition called epididymitis, which can cause sterility. Symptoms include fever, swelling, and extreme pain in the scrotum. Six percent of men with epididymitis develop reactive arthritis, which causes swelling and pain in the joints and can progress and become disabling.

In women and men, chlamydia may cause the rectum to itch and bleed. It can also result in a discharge and diarrhea. If it infects the eyes, it may cause redness, itching, and a discharge. If it infects the throat, it may cause soreness.

Treatment

Various antibiotics kill *chlamydia*. Some are taken in a single dose; others over several days. Both partners must be treated to avoid reinfections.

The CDC, in its most recent guidelines, recommends that all women with chlamydia be rescreened three to four months after treatment is completed. The reason is that re-infection, which often happens because a patient's sex partners were not treated, increases the risk of pelvic inflammatory disease and other complications. Immediately treating the partners of people infected with gonorrhea or chlamydia can reduce rates of recurrence of these infections.

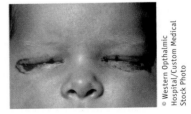

© Western Opthalmic Hospital/Custom Medical Stock Photo

A baby exposed to chlamydial infection in the birth canal during delivery may develop an eye infection. Symptoms include a bloody discharge and swollen eyelids.

chlamydia   A sexually transmitted infection caused by the bacterium *Chlamydia trachomatis*, often asymptomatic in women, but sometimes characterized by urinary pain; if undetected and untreated, may result in pelvic inflammatory disease (PID).

Pelvic Inflammatory Disease (PID)

 Infection of a woman's fallopian tubes or uterus, called **pelvic inflammatory disease (PID),** is not actually an STI, but rather a complication of STIs. About one in every seven women of reproductive age has PID; half of all adult women may have had it. Each year, about 1 million new cases are reported.

Ten to 20 percent of initial episodes of PID lead to scarring and obstruction of the fallopian tubes severe enough to cause infertility. Other long-term complications are ectopic pregnancy and chronic pelvic pain. The risk of these complications rises with subsequent PID episodes, bacterial vaginosis (discussed in Chapter 15), and use of an IUD. Smoking also may increase the likelihood of PID. Two bacteria—*Gonococcus* (the culprit in gonorrhea) and *Chlamydia*—are responsible for one-half to one-third of all cases of PID. Other organisms are responsible for the remaining cases.

Most cases of PID occur among women under age 25 who are sexually active. *Gonococcus*-caused cases tend to affect poor women; those caused by *Chlamydia* range across all income levels. One-half to one-third of all cases are transmitted sexually, and others have been traced to some IUDs that are no longer on the market. Several studies have shown that women with PID are more likely to have used douches than those without the disease. Consistent condom use may decrease PID risk.

PID is a silent disease that in half of all cases produces no noticeable symptoms as it progresses and causes scarring of the fallopian tubes. Experts are encouraging women with mild symptoms, such as abdominal pain or tenderness, to seek medical evaluation and are encouraging physicians to test these patients for infections. Urine testing is a cost-effective method of detecting gonorrhea and chlamydia in young women and can prevent development of PID. For women with symptoms, magnetic resonance imaging (MRI) is highly accurate in establishing a diagnosis of PID and detecting other diseases that may be responsible for the symptoms. Treatment may require hospitalization and intensive antibiotics therapy. PID causes an estimated 15 to 30 percent of all cases of infertility every year and about half of all cases of ectopic pregnancy.

Gonorrhea

Gonorrhea (sometimes called "the clap" in street language) is one of the most common STIs in the United States. After steady declines from the 1970s to the late 1990s, gonorrhea infections have increased, with about 60 percent of new cases occurring in young adults. The incidence is highest among teenagers and young adults.

Sexual contact, including oral sex, is the primary means of transmission.

 Most men who have gonorrhea know it. Thick, yellow-white pus oozes from the penis and urination causes a burning sensation. These symptoms usually develop two to nine days after the sexual contact that infected them. Men have a good reason to seek help: It hurts too much not to.

In men, untreated gonorrhea can spread to the prostate gland, testicles, bladder, and kidneys. Among the serious complications are urinary obstruction and sterility caused by blockage of the vas deferens (the excretory duct of the testis).

Women also may experience discharge and burning on urination. However, as many as eight out of ten infected women have no symptoms.

Gonococcus, the bacterium that causes gonorrhea, can live in the vagina, cervix, and fallopian tubes for months, even years, and continue to infect the woman's sexual partners. Approximately 5 percent of sexually active American women have positive gonorrhea cultures but are unaware that they are silent carriers.

If left untreated in men or women, gonorrhea spreads through the urinary-genital tract. In women, the inflammation travels from the vagina and cervix, through the uterus, to the fallopian tubes and ovaries. The pain and fever are similar to those caused by stomach upset, so a woman may dismiss the symptoms. Eventually these symptoms diminish, even though the disease spreads to the entire pelvis. Pus may ooze from the fallopian tubes or ovaries into the peritoneum (the lining of the abdominal cavity), sometimes causing serious inflammation. However, this, too, can subside in a few weeks.

Gonorrhea, the leading cause of sterility in women, can cause PID. In pregnant women, gonorrhea becomes a threat to the newborn. It can infect the infant's external genitals and can cause a serious form of conjunctivitis. As a preventive step, newborns may have penicillin dropped into their eyes at birth.

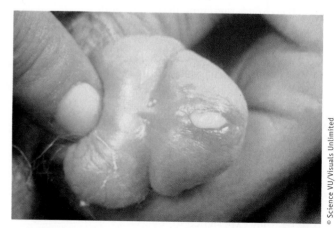

A cloudy discharge is symptomatic of gonorrhea.

In both sexes, gonorrhea can develop into a serious, even fatal, bloodborne infection that can cause arthritis in the joints, attack the heart muscle and lining, cause meningitis, and attack the skin and other organs.

Although a blood test has been developed for detecting gonorrhea, the tried-and-true method of diagnosis is still a microscopic analysis of cultures from the male's urethra, the female's cervix, and the throat and anus of both sexes.

Because gonorrhea often occurs along with chlamydia, practitioners often prescribe an agent effective against both, such as ofloxacin. Fluoroquinolones are no longer advised for use in its treatment. The cephalosporin antibiotics are now the recommended treatment.[17] Antibiotics taken for other reasons may not affect or cure gonorrhea, because of their dosage or type. And you can't develop immunity to gonorrhea; within days of recovering from one case, you can catch another.

Nongonococcal Urethritis (NGU)

The term **nongonococcal urethritis (NGU)** refers to any inflammation of the urethra that is not caused by gonorrhea. NGU is the most common STI in men, accounting for 4 to 6 million visits to a physician every year. Three microorganisms—*Chlamydia trachomatis, Ureaplasma urealyticum,* and *Mycoplasma genitalium*—are the primary causes; the usual means of transmission is sexual intercourse. Other infectious agents, such as fungi or bacteria, allergic reactions to vaginal secretions, or irritation by soaps or contraceptive foams or gels also may lead to NGU.

In the United States, NGU is more common in men than gonococcal urethritis. The symptoms in men are similar to those of gonorrhea, including discharge from the penis (usually less than with gonorrhea) and mild burning during urination. Women frequently develop no symptoms or very mild itching, burning during urination, or discharge. Symptoms usually disappear after two or three weeks, but the infection may persist and cause cervicitis or PID in women and, in men, may spread to the prostate, epididymis, or both. Treatment usually consists of doxycycline or azithromycin and should be given to both sexual partners.

Syphilis

A corkscrew-shaped, spiral bacterium called *Treponema pallidum* causes **syphilis.** This frail microbe dies in seconds if dried or chilled but grows quickly in the warm, moist tissues of the body, particularly in the mucous membranes of the genital tract. Entering the body through any tiny break in the skin, the germ burrows its way into the bloodstream. Sexual contact, including oral sex or intercourse, is a primary means of transmission. Genital ulcers caused by syphilis may increase the risk of HIV infection, while individuals with HIV may be more likely to develop syphilis.

Public education programs, expanded screening and surveillance, increased tracing of contacts, and condom promotion have helped control the spread of syphilis in some areas. Syphilis rates have fallen to the lowest ever reported in the United States, but reported cases are on the rise in New York City and other areas.

Syphilis has clearly identifiable stages:

- **Primary syphilis.** The first sign of syphilis is a lesion, or *chancre* (pronounced "shanker"), an open lump or crater the size of a dime or smaller, teeming with bacteria. The incubation period before its appearance ranges from 10 to 90 days; three to four weeks is average. The chancre appears exactly where the bacteria entered the body: in the mouth, throat, vagina, rectum, or penis. Any contact with the chancre is likely to result in infection.

- **Secondary syphilis.** Anywhere from one to twelve months after the chancre's appearance, secondary-stage symptoms may appear. Some people have no symptoms. Others develop a skin rash or a small, flat rash in moist regions on the skin; whitish patches on the mucous membranes of the mouth or throat; temporary baldness; low-grade fever; headache; swollen glands; or large, moist sores around the mouth and genitals. These sores are loaded with bacteria; contact with them, through kissing or intercourse, may transmit the infection. Symptoms may last for several days or several months. Even without treatment, symptoms eventually disappear as the syphilis microbes go into hiding.

- **Latent syphilis.** Although there are no signs or symptoms, no sores or rashes at this stage, the bacteria are invading various organs inside the body, including the heart and brain. For two to four years, there may be recurring infectious and highly

pelvic inflammatory disease (PID) An inflammation of the internal female genital tract, characterized by abdominal pain, fever, and tenderness of the cervix.

gonorrhea A sexually transmitted infection caused by the bacterium *Neisseria gonorrhoeae;* symptoms include discharge from the penis; women are generally asymptomatic.

nongonococcal urethritis (NGU) Inflammation of the urethra caused by organisms other than the *Gonococcus* bacterium.

syphilis A sexually transmitted infection caused by the bacterium *Treponema pallidum* and characterized by early sores, a latent period, and a final period of life-threatening symptoms, including brain damage and heart failure.

contagious lesions of the skin or mucous membranes. However, syphilis loses its infectiousness as it progresses: After the first two years, a person rarely transmits syphilis through intercourse.

After four years, even congenital syphilis is rarely transmitted. Until this stage of the disease, however, a pregnant woman can pass syphilis to her unborn child. If the fetus is infected in its fourth month or earlier, it may be disfigured or even die. If infected late in pregnancy, the child may show no signs of infection for months or years after birth, but may then become disabled with the symptoms of tertiary syphilis.

- **Tertiary syphilis.** Ten to 20 years after the beginning of the latent stage, the most serious symptoms of syphilis emerge, generally in the organs in which the bacteria settled during latency. Syphilis that has progressed to this stage has become increasingly rare. Victims of tertiary syphilis may die of a ruptured aorta or of other heart damage, or may have progressive brain or spinal cord damage, eventually leading to blindness, insanity, or paralysis. About a third of those who are not treated during the first three stages of syphilis enter the tertiary stage later in life.

Health experts are urging screening for syphilis for everyone who seeks treatment for an STI, especially adolescents; for everyone using illegal drugs; and for the partners of these two groups. They also recommend that anyone diagnosed with syphilis be screened for other STIs and be counseled about voluntary testing for HIV.

Penicillin is the drug of choice for treating primary, secondary, and latent syphilis. The earlier treatment begins, the more effective it is. Those allergic to penicillin may be treated with doxycycline, ceftriaxone, or erythromycin. An added danger of not getting treatment for syphilis is an increased risk of HIV transmission.

Chancroid

A **chancroid** is a soft, painful sore or localized infection caused by the bacterium *Haemophilus ducrevi* and usually acquired through sexual contact. Half of the cases heal by themselves. In other cases, the infection may spread to the lymph glands near the chancroid, where large amounts of pus can accumulate and destroy much of the local tissue. The incidence of this STI, widely prevalent in Africa and tropical and semitropical regions, is rapidly increasing in the United States, with outbreaks in several states, including Louisiana, Texas, and New York. Chancroids, which may increase susceptibility to HIV infection, are believed to be a major factor in the heterosexual spread of HIV. This infection is treated with antibiotics (ceftriaxone, azithromycin, or erythromycin) and can be prevented by keeping the genitals clean and washing them with soap and water in case of possible exposure.

Pubic Lice and Scabies

These infections are sometimes, but not always, transmitted sexually. *Pubic lice* (or "crabs") are usually found in the pubic hair, although they can migrate to any hairy areas of the body. Lice lay eggs called nits that attach to the base of the hair shaft. Irritation from the lice may produce intense itching. Scratching to relieve the itching can produce sores. *Scabies* is caused by a mite that burrows under the skin, where they lay eggs that hatch and undergo many changes in the course of their life cycle, producing great discomfort, including intense itching.

Lice and scabies are treated with applications of permethrin cream and lindane shampoo to all the areas of the body where there are concentrations of body hair (genitals, armpits, scalp). You must repeat treatment in seven days to kill any newly developed adults. You must also wash or dry-clean clothing and bedding.

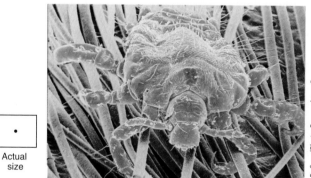

Actual size

A pubic louse, or "crab."

© E. Gray/Photo Researchers, Inc.

HIV and AIDS

Thirty years ago, no one knew about **human immunodeficiency virus (HIV).** No one had ever heard of **acquired immune deficiency syndrome (AIDS).** Once seen as an epidemic affecting primarily gay men and injection drug users, AIDS has taken on a very different form. Today, heterosexuals in developing countries have the highest rates of infection and mortality. And HIV infection continues to spread, doubling at an estimated rate of every ten years.

Incidence

About 39.4 million people worldwide are infected with HIV; 15,000 more individuals are infected every day. AIDS now claims about 3 million lives—more than half children—around the world a year. According to the CDC, 1,039,000 to 1,185,000 people are living with HIV or AIDS in the United States, with about 43,000 new infections every year.

Gay men account for 65 percent of AIDS diagnoses among men. Homosexual and bisexual men, particularly those who are young or nonwhite and living in metropolitan areas, are at particularly high risk. The percentage of individuals who acquired HIV through heterosexual contact has increased to 31 percent. Many heterosexuals are not aware of their partners' HIV status and may not see themselves as being at risk of HIV infection. According to the CDC, about a third of the HIV-infected individuals in the United States have not been diagnosed.

 African Americans and Hispanics account for a disproportionate share of new AIDS diagnoses. Almost half of all those living with HIV/AIDS in the United States are African American (Figure 16.4). The AIDS case rate per 100,000 people is 9.5 times that of whites. African Americans are less likely to survive after a diagnosis of AIDS than other ethnic or racial groups. HIV/AIDS is the third-leading cause of death among African Americans between ages 25 and 34 and the sixth leading cause of death for whites and Hispanics in this age group.[18]

HIV/AIDS is seen as a threat to men, but 26 percent of new HIV infections in the United States occur among women (see Figure 16.4). About a quarter of Americans living with HIV/AIDS are women. Nonwhite women, particularly African Americans, have been hardest hit. While African American women make up just 13 percent of the female population of the United States, they account for 67 percent of newly diagnosed female cases. HIV/AIDS is most prevalent among women in their childbearing years.[19]

Reducing the Risk of HIV Transmission

HIV/AIDS can be so frightening that some people have exaggerated its dangers, whereas others understate them. The fact is that although no one is immune to HIV, you can reduce the risk if you abstain from sexual activity or remain in a monogamous relationship with an uninfected partner, and do not inject drugs.

If you're not in a long-term monogamous relationship with a partner you're sure is safe, and you're not willing to abstain from sex, there are things you can do to lower your risk of HIV infection. Remember that the risk of HIV transmission depends on sexual behavior, not sexual orientation. Among young men, the prevalence and frequency of sexual risk behaviors are similar regardless of sexual orientation, ethnicity, or age. Homosexual, heterosexual, and bisexual individuals all need to know about the kinds of sexual activity that increase their risk.

Sexual Transmission

Here's what you should know about sexual transmission of HIV:

- Casual contact does *not* spread HIV infection. You cannot get HIV infection from drinking from a water fountain, contact with a toilet seat, or touching an infected person.

- Compared to other viruses, HIV is extremely difficult to get.

- HIV can live in blood, semen, vaginal fluids, and breast milk.

Sex of adults and adolescents with HIV/AIDS diagnosed

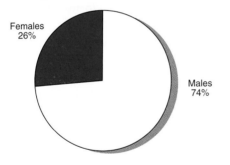

Females 26%

Males 74%

Race/ethnicity of persons (including children) with HIV/AIDS

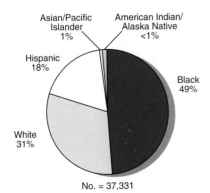

Asian/Pacific Islander 1%

American Indian/ Alaska Native <1%

Hispanic 18%

Black 49%

White 31%

No. = 37,331

Figure 16.3   HIV/AIDS by Gender and Race

Source: Kaiser Family Foundation.

chancroid   A soft, painful sore or localized infection usually acquired through sexual contact.

human immunodeficiency virus (HIV)   A type of virus that causes a spectrum of health problems, ranging from a symptomless infection to changes in the immune system, to the development of life-threatening diseases because of impaired immunity.

acquired immune deficiency syndrome (AIDS)   The final stages of HIV infection, characterized by a variety of severe illnesses and decreased levels of certain immune cells.

- Many chemicals, including household bleach, alcohol, and hydrogen peroxide, can inactivate HIV.

- In studies of family members sharing dishes, food, clothing, and frequent hugs with people with HIV infection or AIDS, those who have contracted the virus have shared razor blades, toothbrushes, or had other means of blood contact.

- You cannot tell visually whether a potential sexual partner has HIV. A blood test is needed to detect the antibodies that the body produces to fight HIV, thus indicating infection. As noted in Chapter 9, circumcision greatly reduces the risk for HIV infection.[20]

- HIV can be spread in semen and vaginal fluids during a single instance of anal, vaginal, or oral sexual contact between heterosexuals, bisexuals, or homosexuals. The risk increases with the number of sexual encounters with an infected partner.

- Teenage girls may be particularly vulnerable to HIV infection because the immature cervix is easily infected.

- Anal intercourse is an extremely high-risk behavior because HIV can enter the bloodstream through tiny breaks in the lining of the rectum. HIV transmission is much more likely to occur during unprotected anal intercourse than vaginal intercourse.

- Other behaviors that increase the risk of HIV infection include having multiple sexual partners, engaging in sex without condoms or virus-killing spermicides, sexual contact with persons known to be at high risk (for example, prostitutes or injection drug users), and sharing injection equipment for drugs.

- Individuals are at greater risk if they have an active sexual infection. Sexually transmitted infections, such as herpes, gonorrhea, and syphilis, facilitate transmission of HIV during vaginal or rectal intercourse.

- No cases of HIV transmission by deep (French) kissing have been reported, but it could happen. Studies have found blood in the saliva of healthy people after kissing; other lab studies have found HIV in saliva. Social (dry) kissing is safe.

- Oral sex can lead to HIV transmission. The virus in any semen that enters the mouth could make its way into the bloodstream through tiny nicks or sores in the mouth. A man's risk in performing oral sex on a woman is smaller because an infected woman's genital fluids have much lower concentrations of HIV than does semen.

- HIV infection is not widespread among lesbians, although there have been documented cases of possible female-to-female HIV transmission. However, in each instance, one partner had had sex with a bisexual man or male injection drug user or had injected drugs herself.

Federal health officials fear that a new generation may not be using adequate safer sex precautions, because they have grown complacent about the dangers of HIV/AIDS. Efforts to prevent sexual transmission of HIV have taken a new focus: counseling those who already have HIV in an attempt to get them to stop spreading it. Those who knowingly transmit HIV may face legal prosecution. (See Point/Counterpoint.)

Nonsexual Transmission

Efforts to prevent nonsexual forms of HIV transmission have been very effective. Screening the blood supply has reduced the rate of transfusion-associated HIV transmission by 99.9 percent. Treatment with antiretroviral drugs during pregnancy and birth has reduced transmission by about 90 percent in optimal conditions. Among drug users in some settings, programs that combine addiction treatment and needle exchange reduced the incidence of HIV infection by 30 percent.

HIV Infection

HIV infection refers to a spectrum of health problems that results from immunologic abnormalities caused by the virus when it enters the bloodstream. In theory, the

---

POINT COUNTERPOINT *Is Spreading an STI a Crime?*

POINT

Individuals diagnosed with an STI that could cause serious, even life-threatening illness, such as HIV, should abstain from sex or inform any potential sex partner of their condition. If they fail to do so, they should face legal prosecution for endangering the health of another person. The penalties in cases involving HIV should be severe.

COUNTERPOINT

Failing to inform a potential sexual partner of an STI is morally wrong. However, many circumstances, such as drinking, can interfere with clear communication. As long as two people mutually consent to sex, failure to disclose should not be viewed as a crime.

YOUR VIEW

Do you think individuals who jeopardize their partner's health by not informing them of an STI deserve punishment? Or is it the responsibility of every person engaging in sexual activity to ask about a potential partner's history and insist on safer-sex practices? How would you feel if you found out after the fact that a partner has an STI and that you may be infected?

body may be able to resist infection by HIV. In reality, in almost all cases, HIV destroys the cell-mediated immune system, particularly the CD4+ T-lymphocytes (also called *T4 helper cells*). The result is greatly increased susceptibility to various cancers and opportunistic infections (infections that take hold because of the reduced effectiveness of the immune system).

HIV triggers a state of all-out war within the immune system. Almost immediately following infection with HIV, the immune system responds aggressively by manufacturing enormous numbers of CD4+ cells. It eventually is overwhelmed, however, as the viral particles continue to replicate, or multiply. The intense war between HIV and the immune system indicates that the virus itself, not a breakdown in the immune system, is responsible for disease progression.

Shortly after becoming infected with HIV, individuals may experience a few days of flu-like symptoms, which most ignore or attribute to other viruses. Some people develop a more severe mononucleosis-type syndrome. After this stage, individuals may not develop any signs or symptoms of disease for a period ranging from weeks to more than 12 years.

HIV symptoms, which tend to increase in severity and number the longer the virus is in the body, may include any of the following:

- Swollen lymph nodes.
- Fever, chills, and night sweats.
- Diarrhea.
- Weight loss.
- Coughing and shortness of breath.
- Persistent tiredness.
- Skin sores.
- Blurred vision and headaches.
- Development of other infections, such as certain kinds of pneumonia.

HIV infection is associated with a variety of HIV-related diseases, including different cancers and dangerous infections including tuberculosis. HIV-infected individuals may develop persistent generalized lymphadenopathy, enlargement of the lymph nodes at two or more different sites in the body. This condition typically persists for more than three months without any other illness to explain its occurrence. Diminished mental function may appear before other symptoms. Tests conducted on infected but apparently healthy men have revealed impaired coordination, problems in thinking, or abnormal brain scans.

For ways to protect yourself, see Your Strategies for Prevention: "How to Reduce Your Risk for HIV Infection."

HIV Testing

The CDC recommends screening for all patients ages 13 to 64. This means that anyone receiving routine medical care and testing can be screened for HIV without giving specific informed consent. The goal is to identify the estimated 250,000 Americans who have undiagnosed HIV.[21]

All HIV tests measure antibodies, cells produced by the body to fight HIV infection. A negative test indicates no exposure to HIV. It can take three to six months for the body to produce the telltale antibodies, however, so

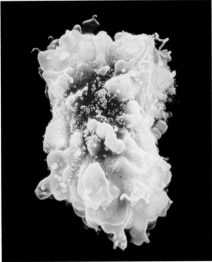

Electron micrograph of a white blood cell being attacked by HIV *(light blue particles)*, the virus that causes AIDS.

Lennart Nilsson © Boehringer Ingelheim International GmbH

a negative result may not be accurate, depending on the timing of the test.

HIV testing can be either confidential or anonymous. In confidential testing, a person's name is recorded along with the test results, which are made available to medical personnel and in 32 states, the state health department. In anonymous testing, no name is associated with the test results. Anonymous testing is available in 39 states.

The only home HIV test approved by the FDA, Home Access, is available in drug stores or online for $40 to $50. An individual draws a blood sample by pricking a finger and sends it to a laboratory along with a personal identification number. Results are given over the phone by a trained counselor, usually within several days.

Newly developed blood tests can determine how recently a person was infected with HIV and distinguish between long-standing infections and those contracted within the previous four to six months.

Diagnosing AIDS

A diagnosis of AIDS applies to anyone with HIV whose immune system is severely impaired, as indicated by a CD4+ count of less than 200 cells per cubic millimeter of blood, compared to normal CD4+ cell counts in healthy people not infected with HIV of 800 to 1,200 per cubic millimeter of blood. In addition, AIDS is diagnosed in persons with HIV infection who experience recurrent pneumonia, invasive cervical cancer, or pulmonary tuberculosis.

People with AIDS also may experience persistent fever, diarrhea that persists for more than one month, or involuntary weight loss of more than 10 percent of normal body weight. Neurological disease—including dementia (confusion and impaired thinking) and other problems with thinking, speaking, movement, or sensation—may occur. Secondary infectious diseases that may develop in people with AIDS include *Pneumocystis carinii* pneumonia, tuberculosis, or oral candidiasis (thrush). Secondary cancers associated with HIV infection include Kaposi's sarcoma and cancer of the cervix.

Treating HIV/AIDS

New forms of therapy have been remarkably effective in boosting levels of protective T cells and reducing *viral load*—the amount of HIV in the bloodstream. People with high viral loads are more likely to progress rapidly to AIDS than people with low levels of the virus.

The current "gold-standard" approach to combating HIV is known as HAART (highly active antiretroviral therapies), which dramatically reduces viral load even though it does not eradicate the virus. This complex regimen uses one of 250 different combinations of three or more antiretroviral drugs. Since the development of HAART, the number of deaths among persons with AIDS in the United States has declined by 70 percent, and the number of those living with AIDS has risen.

Because HAART can drastically lower viral load, there is some evidence that it also may reduce the risk of infectiousness of HIV-positive individuals. Fearing that this could lead to unsafe sex, researchers did a meta-analysis of HAART recipients and found no increased sexual risk behavior. Even when HIV levels are undetectable, they note, this does not mean the infected person is "cured," nor does it eliminate the possibility of transmitting HIV.

In the last few years, several new drugs have become available, and many of these antiretroviral agents can be taken just once or twice a day. New antiretroviral agents and new types of drugs are currently in clinical trials. Work is also continuing toward an HIV vaccine. As more effective therapies have emerged, there has been a major shift in attitude: Physicians are more optimistic about long-term treatments, and hope is replacing despair as more individuals are living productive lives with HIV.

Breakthrough drugs are indeed allowing HIV-infected people to live longer. However, new dangers have emerged. Up to 15 percent of new HIV cases in the country may stem from drug-resistant strains of the virus. "Superinfection" with more than one strain of HIV seems more common than previously thought. As a result, HIV-infected people who initially were doing well without drugs may become ill after contracting a second strain of the AIDS virus.

Learn It : **Live It**

Protecting Your Sexual Health

As with other aspects of your well-being, your sexual health depends on your choices and behaviors. Here are some basic guidelines:

- **Talk first.** Get to know your partner. Before having sex, establish a committed relationship that allows trust and open communication. You should be able to discuss past sexual histories and any previous STIs or IV drug use. You should not feel coerced or forced into having sex.

- **Stay sober.** Alcohol and drugs impair your judgment, make it harder to communicate clearly, and can lead to forgetting or failing to use condoms properly.

- **Be honest.** If you have an STI, like HPV or herpes, advise any prospective sexual partner. Allow him or her to decide what to do. If you mutually agree on engaging in sexual activity, use latex condoms and other protective measures.

- **Don't feel you have to have sex** for fear of hurting someone's feelings or fear of being the "only one" who isn't doing it. If you don't want to have sex, be honest, discuss the reasons behind your decision with your partner, and stay true to you.

- **Respect** everyone's right to make his or her own personal decision—including yours. There is no perfect point in a relationship where sex has to happen. If your partner tells you that he or she is not ready to have sex, respect this decision, discuss the reasons behind it, and be supportive.

- **Be prepared for a sex emergency.** Consider carrying two condoms with you just in case one breaks or tears. Both men and women are equally responsible for preventing STIs, and both should carry condoms.

- **Abstinence doesn't mean less affection.** Practicing abstinence—the most effective way to protect against STIs—doesn't mean you can't have an intimate relationship with someone. It just means you don't have vaginal or anal intercourse or oral sex.

- **Make your sexual health a priority.** Whether you are having sex or not, both men and women need regular check-ups to make sure they are sexually healthy.

SELFSURVEY : *Assessing Your STI Risk*

This Self Survey looks at your risk of acquiring or transmitting any sexually transmitted infection (STI).

STI Quiz

1. **True** or **False:** A person can have an STI and not know it.

2. **True** or **False:** It is normal for women to have some vaginal discharge.

3. **True** or **False:** Once you have had an STI and have been cured, you can't get it again.

4. **True** or **False:** HIV is mainly present in semen, blood, vaginal secretions, and breast milk.

5. **True** or **False:** Chlamydia and gonorrhea can cause pelvic inflammatory disease.

6. **True** or **False:** A pregnant woman who has an STI can pass the disease on to her baby.

7. **True** or **False:** Most STIs go away without treatment, if people wait long enough.

8. **True** or **False:** STIs that aren't cured early can cause sterility.

9. **True** or **False:** Birth control pills offer excellent protection from STIs.

10. **True** or **False:** Condoms can help prevent the spread of STIs.

11. **True** or **False:** If you know your partner, you can't get an STI.

12. **True** or **False:** Chlamydia is the most common bacterial STI.

13. **True** or **False:** A sexually active woman should get an annual pap test from her doctor.

Answers

1. **True** Some of the most common symptoms of an STI infection include: Abnormal discharge, painful urination, burning, itching or tingling in the genital area, but it is important to remember that many women and men who have an STI often do not experience any symptoms at all. Chlamydia, for example, often has no symptoms.

2. **True** Normal vaginal discharge has several purposes: cleaning and moistening the vagina and helping to prevent and fight infections. Although it's normal for the color, texture, and amount of vaginal fluids to vary throughout a woman's menstrual cycle, some changes in discharge may indicate a problem.

   If you think you may have a problem, you should see a doctor as soon as possible. First, though, it helps to learn some of the differences between what is normal and abnormal vaginal discharge for you.

3. **False** Having an STI and being cured from it does not mean that your body now has a built in immunity to the bacteria that causes the infection. You must protect yourself from becoming infected again by using a condom. Remember, it is your body!

4. **True** Although small traces of HIV can be found in tears, saliva, urine and perspiration, extensive studies have shown that there is not enough of the virus or the virus is not strong enough to be transmitted. Only blood, semen, vaginal secretions, and breast milk have been proven to transmit the HIV virus and hepatitis B. HIV cannot be passed on by casual contact.

5. **True** Many different organisms can cause PID, but most cases are associated with gonorrhea and genital chlamydial infections, two very common STIs. Scientists have found that bacteria normally present in small numbers in the vagina and cervix also may play a role.

6. **True** STIs can be passed from a pregnant woman to the baby before, during, or after the baby's birth. Some STIs (like syphilis) cross the placenta and infect the baby while it is in the uterus (womb). Other STIs (like gonorrhea, chlamydia, hepatitis B, and genital herpes) can be transmitted from the mother to the baby during delivery as the baby passes through the birth canal. HIV can cross the placenta during pregnancy, infect the baby during the birth process, and unlike most other STIs, can infect the baby through breastfeeding.

7. **False** Even if symptoms appear to go away, the infected person will still have the infection and is able to pass the infection on to others until he/she gets treatment. STIs that aren't cured early can cause sterility.

8. **True** If the fallopian tubes are blocked at one or both ends, the egg can't travel through the tubes into the uterus. Blocked tubes may result from pelvic inflammatory disease, which is often caused by untreated STIs.

9. **False** The birth control pill does not protect against sexually transmitted infections. For those having sex, condoms must always be used along with birth control pills to protect against STIs. Abstinence (the decision to not have sex) is the only method that always prevents pregnancy and sexually transmitted infections.

10. **True** Most condoms are made of latex. Those made of lambskin may offer less protection against some sexually transmitted infections, including HIV, so use of latex condoms is recommended. For people who may have an allergic skin reaction to latex, both male and female condoms made of polyurethane are available.

When properly used, latex and plastic condoms are effective against most STIs. Condoms do not protect against infections spread from sores on the skin not covered by a condom (such as the base of the penis or scrotum).

11. **False** As stated in question number 1, a person can have an STI and not know it. If they can't tell, how can you?

12. **True** The U.S. Centers for Disease Control and Prevention estimates that more than 4 million new cases of chlamydia occur each year. The highest rates of chlamydial infection are in 15- to 19-year-old adolescents regardless of demographics or location.

13. **True** The Pap test is a way to find cell changes on the cervix. Abnormal cells may lead to cancer, so having a Pap test can find and treat them early, before they have time to progress to cancer.

    Although Pap tests do not test for STIs, some STIs such as HPV (human papillomavirus infection) can cause abnormal Pap test results. Certain types of HPV are linked to cancer in both women and men.

Copyright 2002 by SmarterSex.org.

Your Health Action Plan for Coping with STIs

What to Do If You Have an STI

- If you suspect that you have an STI, don't feel too embarrassed to get help through a physician's office or a clinic. Treatment relieves discomfort, prevents complications, and halts the spread of the disease.

- Following diagnosis, take oral medication (which may be given instead of or in addition to shots) exactly as prescribed.

- Try to figure out from whom you got the STI. Be sure to inform that person, who may not be aware of the problem.

- If you have an STI, never deceive a prospective partner about it. Tell the truth—simply and clearly. Be sure your partner understands exactly what you have and what the risks are.

Telling a Partner You Have an STI

Even though the conversation can be awkward and embarrassing, you need to talk honestly about any STI that you may have been exposed to or contracted. What you don't say can be hazardous to your partner's health. Here are some guidelines:

- **Talk before you become intimate.** A good way to start is simply by saying, *"There is something we need to talk over first."*

- **Be honest.** Don't downplay any potential risks.

- **Don't blame.** Even if you suspect that your partner was the source of your infection, focus on the need for medical attention.

- **Be sensitive to your partner's feelings.** Anger and resentment are common reactions when someone feels at risk. Try to listen without becoming defensive.

- **Seek medical attention.** Do not engage in sexual intimacies until you obtain a doctor's assurance that you are no longer contagious.

Source: Bacchus and Gamma Peer Education Network, www.smartersex.org.

CENGAGENOW™ If you want to write your own goals for preventing STIs, go to the Wellness Journal at HealthNow: **academic.cengage.com/login**.

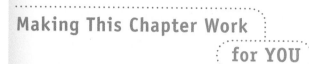

Making This Chapter Work for YOU

Review Questions

1. Sexually transmitted infections
   a. are the major cause of preventable sterility in the United States.
   b. are declining in incidence on college campuses.
   c. have declined in incidence in developing nations due to improving health standards.
   d. do not increase the risk of being infected with HIV.

2. Viral agents cause all of the following STIs *except*
   a. herpes.
   b. genital warts.
   c. HIV.
   d. chlamydia.

3. Jake is sexually active but doesn't want to use a condom. His other choices to protect himself against STIs include all of these *except*
   a. abstinence.
   b. a sexual relationship with a longtime friend.
   c. a sexual relationship with one STI-free partner.
   d. masturbation only.

4. Which of these activities cannot transmit an STI?
   a. having oral sex
   b. hugging
   c. sharing a needle with a fellow athlete using steroids
   d. sharing a razor

5. Which statement about HPV infection is *false*?
   a. HPV cannot be transmitted through oral sex.
   b. HPV increases a woman's risk of developing cervical cancer.
   c. HPV causes genital warts.
   d. HPV increases a man's risk of cancer of the penis.

6. The herpes simplex virus HSV-2
   a. cannot be transmitted through oral sex.
   b. cannot be transmitted if a condom is used.
   c. can be transmitted even when the infected person shows no symptoms.
   d. can be permanently killed with antiviral medications.

7. Chlamydial infections
   a. are caused by a virus.
   b. can cause eye infections in men.
   c. usually display no symptoms in women.
   d. are more common in older women.

8. Which statement is true?
   a. Gonorrhea is mostly symptomless in men.
   b. Secondary syphilis usually occurs 10 to 20 years after the latent stage.
   c. Pubic lice can be killed with regular shampoo.
   d. African Americans account for a disproportionate share of new AIDS diagnoses.

9. Which of the following statements about HIV transmission is true?
   a. Individuals are not at risk for HIV if they are being treated for chlamydia or gonorrhea.
   b. HIV can be transmitted between lesbians.
   c. Heterosexual men who do not practice safe sex are at less risk for contracting HIV than homosexual men who do practice safe sex.
   d. HIV cannot be spread in a single instance of sexual intercourse.

10. A person with AIDS
    a. has a low viral load and a high number of T4 helper cells.
    b. can no longer pass HIV to a sexual partner.
    c. may suffer from secondary infectious diseases and cancers.
    d. will not respond to treatment.

Answers to these questions can be found on page 583.

Critical Thinking

1. Your friend Shayla recently broke up after a five-year relationship with her first boyfriend. How would you counsel Shayla on re-entering the dating scene and becoming intimate with a new partner?

2. When reading this chapter, did the photos gross you out? Do you think they will have an impact on your sexual behavior? Would you advocate more media coverage of these symptoms and consequences of STIs? How do the photos in this chapter differ from the smoking warning at the end of Chapter 13 or "meth-mouth" in Chapter 11?

3. Have you ever dated someone with an STI? If so, when did you find out about it? How did you feel? Did it affect your sex life? In what way?

4. Any time a person has a blood test, an HIV screening can be performed without asking permission. Do you see this as a violation of privacy or as a good public health practice? Explain.

Media Menu

CENGAGENOW™ Go to the HealthNow website at **academic.cengage .com/login** that will:
- Help you evaluate your knowledge of the material.
- Allow you to take an exam-prep quiz.
- Provide a Personalized Learning Plan targeting resources that address areas you should study.
- Coach you through identifying target goals for behavioral change and creating and monitoring your personal change plan throughout the semester.

INTERNET CONNECTIONS

Centers for Disease Control and Prevention
www.cdc.gov/std
www.cdc.gov/hiv

These sites at the CDC feature current information, fact sheets, treatment guides, surveillance, and statistics on sexually transmitted infections and HIV/AIDS.

National Institute of Allergy and Infectious Diseases
www3.niaid.nih.gov/research/topics/STI/
This site, is part of the National Institutes of Health, features research on STIs, including basic and clinical research and activities related to vaccine development.

HIV InSite: Gateway to AIDS Knowledge
http://hivinsite.ucsf.edu
This site, sponsored by the University of California San Francisco School of Medicine, provides statistics, education, prevention, and new developments related to HIV/AIDS.

Key Terms

The terms listed are used and defined on the page indicated. Definitions are also found in the Glossary at the end of this book.

acquired immune deficiency syndrome (AIDS) 477
chanchroid 477
chlamydia 473
gonorrhea 475
herpes simplex 471
human immunodeficiency virus (HIV) 477
human papilloma virus (HPV) 469
nongonococcal urethritis (NGU) 475
pelvic inflammatory disease (PID) 475
sexually transmitted disease (STD) 465
sexually transmitted infection (STI) 465
syphilis 475

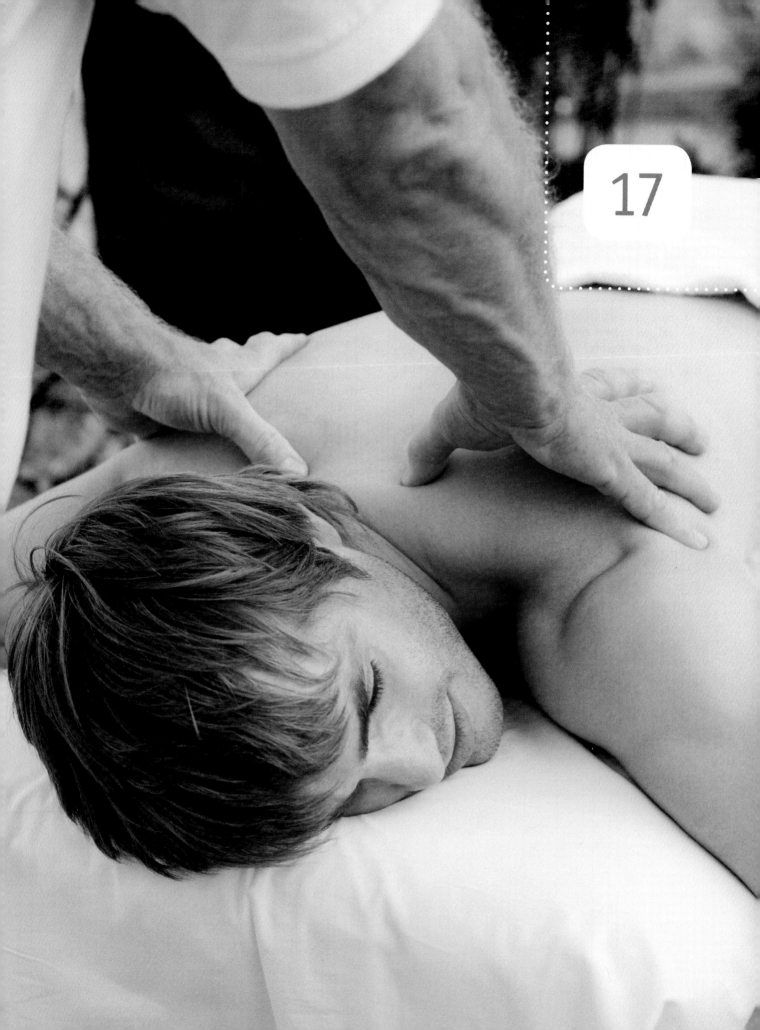

Getting Quality Traditional and Nontraditional Health Care

LONG after she immigrated to the United States from India, Tapu's grandmother refused to go to Western doctors. She preferred practitioners who used the herbs and techniques she had relied on in her homeland. Tapu's father, an American-trained physician, would argue with his mother-in-law about what he considered her old-fashioned views. As a doctor's son, Tapu grew up believing in the superiority of Western medicine.

In his sophomore year at college, Tapu found out that he needed oral surgery. To his surprise, the oral surgeon suggested an alternative method of controlling postoperative pain: acupuncture. "My dad's never going to approve," he said. "And he's the one who's still paying my medical bills." The doctor referred Tapu—and his father—to recent studies conducted by National Institute of Health researchers on acupuncture's efficacy in relieving postsurgical pain. After doing more research online, Tapu agreed to try acupuncture following his operation.

Like Tapu, millions of Americans are turning to complementary and alternative medicine (CAM), a term that includes a broad range of healing philosophies, approaches, and therapies not traditionally taught in medical schools or provided in hospitals. But consumers are learning that they have to be just as savvy—and skeptical—about these therapies and practitioners as they are with any other form of health care.

Because there are so many health-care choices, you face a greater responsibility for your personal well-being. Whether you are monitoring your blood pressure, taking medication, or deciding whether to try an alternative therapy, you need to gather information, ask questions, weigh advantages and disadvantages, and take charge of your health. The reason: No one cares more about your health than you do, and no one will do more to promote your well-being than you.

After studying the material in this chapter, you should be able to:

- **List** ways of becoming an informed health-care consumer.
- **Discuss** strategies for self-care.
- **Describe** common medical exam procedures and medical tests.
- **Identify** strategies for maintaining good oral health.
- **List** your rights as a medical consumer.
- **Describe** the different types of complementary and alternative therapies and explain what research has shown about their effectiveness.
- **Compare** and **contrast** the different types of health-care practitioners and health-care facilities.
- **Describe** how you can get the best information from your next medical exam.

CENGAGENOW™ Log on to HealthNow at **academic.cengage.com/login** to find your Behavior Change Planner and to explore self-assessments, interactive tutorials, and practice quizzes.

© Botanica/Jupiterimages

Quality Health Care

Quality matters in health care perhaps more than anywhere because your life may depend on it. Yet the quality of health care varies greatly in this country. Some physicians, some hospitals, some health-care plans do a better job of helping people stay healthy or get better if they become ill.

But quality begins with you. By learning how to maintain your health, evaluate medical information, and spot early signs of a problem, you're more likely to get the best possible care—and to keep down your medical bills. Self-care means head-to-toe maintenance, including good oral care, appropriate screening tests, knowing your medical rights, and understanding the health-care system.

Chances are that you've tried—or will try—alternative therapies. Many use a "whole-person" approach that addresses all the dimensions of health. You need to be just as savvy a consumer when considering a complementary or alternative treatment as you would with a more mainstream one. You also need to continue your best healthy practices throughout your life so you can function at your best for as long as possible. But your future begins with the healthy choices you make today and every day.

Your Life Change Coach

Making Quality Health-Care Decisions

Although you may not realize it, you make crucial decisions that affect your health every day. You choose what you eat, whether you exercise, if you smoke or drink, when to fasten your seat belt. You decide when to see health professionals, what to tell them, and whether to follow their advice. (See the lab on "Health Assurance" in *IPC*.) **IPC**

The responsibility for making smart choices about your health lies with you. Never before has so much information about health been available in so many forms and formats. However, not all of it is accurate, objective, or helpful. In order to base your decisions on a solid scientific basis, you have to develop and apply your critical-thinking skills.

The following sections can help.

Finding Good Advice Online

Three in four Internet users are "e-health" consumers who seek information or support, communicate with health-care providers, or buy medical products online. "They use the Internet as an adjunct to physicians, who remain their primary source of health advice," says Mark Bard, president of Manhattan Research, a health-care marketing firm.[1] As noted in this chapter's Reality Check, about 3 in 4 college students have used the Internet to get health information, but many are skeptical of what they find.

If you go to websites for medical information, here are some guidelines for evaluating them:

- **Check the creator.** Websites are produced by health agencies, health support groups, school health programs, health-product advertisers, health educators, and health-education organizations. Read site headers and footers carefully to distinguish biased commercial advertisements from unbiased sites created by scientists and health agencies.

- **If you are looking for the most recent research,** check the date the page was created and last updated as well as the links. Several nonworking links signal that the site isn't carefully maintained or updated.
- **Check the references.** As with other health-education materials, web documents should provide the reader with references. Unreferenced suggestions may be scientifically unsound and possibly unsafe.
- **Consider the author.** Is he or she recognized in the field of health education or otherwise qualified to publish a health-information web document? Does the author list his or her occupation, experience, and education?
- **Look for possible bias.** Websites may be attempting to provide health information to consumers, but they also may be attempting to sell a product. Many sites are merely disguised advertisements. (See Table 17.1 for some doctor-endorsed websites.)

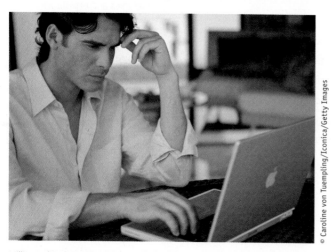

© Caroline von Tuempling/Iconica/Getty Images

Millions of Americans go online to learn about medical problems and treatments and to chat with others who have similar conditions.

Health Care and the College Student

 All of the more than 14 million men and women enrolled in institutions of higher learning need some health-care services, regardless of their age or general health. The Preventive Services Task Force of the U.S. Public Health Service recommends that all adolescents and young adults have periodic screenings for high blood pressure, obesity, and problem alcohol consumption and that they receive regular counseling concerning the use of drugs, tobacco, and alcohol; sexually transmitted infections; effective contraception; a healthy diet; exercise; oral health; and prevention of motor vehicle injuries and other accidents.

In addition to the medical services available at student health centers, colleges provide health information.

REALITYCHECK

- *How many college students turn to the Internet for health-related information?* _____
- *How many college students consider health-related information on the Internet reliable?* _____

Answers on next page.

Getting Medical Facts Straight

Cure! Breakthrough! Medical miracle! These words make headlines. Remember that although medical breakthroughs and cures do occur, most scientific progress is made one small step at a time. Rather than putting your faith in the most recent report or the hottest trend, try to gather as much background information and as many opinions as you can.

When reading a newspaper or magazine story or listening to a radio or television report about a medical advance, look for answers to the following questions:

- **Who are the scientists involved?** Are they recognized, legitimate health professionals? What are their credentials? Are they affiliated with respected medical or scientific institutions? Be wary of individuals whose degrees or affiliations are from institutions you've never heard of, and be sure that the person's educational background is in a discipline related to the area of research reported.
- **Where did the scientists report their findings?** The best research is published in peer-reviewed professional journals, such as the *New England Journal of Medicine*. Research developments also may be reported at meetings of professional societies.
- **Is the information based on personal observations?** Does the report include testimonials from cured patients or satisfied customers? If the answer to either question is yes, be wary.
- **Does the article, report, or advertisement include words like** *amazing, secret,* **or** *quick?* Does it claim to be something the public has never seen or been offered before? Such sensationalized language is often a tip-off to a dubious treatment.

TABLE 17.1 Doctor-Recommended Websites

National Library of Medicine: MedlinePlus http://medlineplus.gov

MedlinePlus contains links to information on hundreds of health conditions and issues. The site also includes a medical dictionary, an encyclopedia with pictures and diagrams, and links to physician directories.

FDA Center for Drug Evaluation and Research www.fda.gov

Click on Drugs@FDA for information on approved prescription drugs and some over-the-counter medications.

WebMD www.webmd.com

WebMD is full of information to help you manage your health. The site's quizzes and calculators are a fun way to test your medical knowledge. Get diet tips, information on drugs and herbs, and check out special sections on men's and women's health.

Mayo Clinic http://mayoclinic.com

The renowned Mayo Clinic offers a one-stop health resource website. Use the site's Health Decision Guides to make decisions about prevention and treatment. Learn more about complementary and alternative medicine, sports medicine, and senior health in the Healthy Living Centers.

Centers for Disease Control www.cdc.gov

Stay up to date on the latest public health news and get the CDC's recommendations on travelers' health, vaccines and immunizations, and protecting your health in case of a disaster.

Medscape www.medscape.com

Medscape delivers news and research specifically tailored to your medical interests. The site requires (free) registration.

REALITYCHECK

PART II: *Just the Facts*

- **72** *percent of college students turn to the Internet for health-related information.*
- **23** *percent of college students consider health-related information on the Internet reliable.*

Source: American College Health Association. "American College Health Association National College Health Assessment Spring 2006 Reference Group Data Report (Abridged)." *Journal of American College Health*, Vol. 55, No. 4, January–February 2007, pp. 195–206.

According to a CDC survey of approximately 4,600 undergraduates at 136 colleges and universities, about three-quarters of undergraduates have received some form of health information. About half of all students surveyed had been given some information on prevention of alcohol and drug use and HIV infection and AIDS.

 Black students were more likely than white students to say they'd been taught about AIDS and HIV in college classes. African American, Hispanic, or students of other racial and ethnic groups also were more likely than whites to report receiving information on any health topic. More traditional full-time students between ages 18 and 24 who had never been married and were not working full-time had received health information, compared to part-time, older, non-traditional students.

 Because undergraduates are remarkably diverse, they also vary in their health beliefs and practices, particularly when born outside the United States in countries with different medical traditions. A study that compared the health beliefs of undergraduates born in the United States, China, and India found unexpected similarities and differences. Regardless of their origins, students identified the same four factors as very important for keeping healthy: enough rest and sleep, physical exercise, proper weight, and eating proper foods.

Your Life Change Coach, *Continued*

- **Is someone trying to sell you something?** Manufacturers who cite studies to sell a product have been known to embellish the truth.
- **Does the information defy all common sense?** Be skeptical. If something sounds too good to be true, it probably is.

Making Sense of Medical Research

Medical research is the only way that anyone, physician or consumer, can assess the quality of diagnostic methods, medications, or surgical treatments. The principal rule of science is that nothing works until it's been proved.

Researchers rely on a variety of studies to determine whether a new approach to prevention, diagnosis, or treatment works. These include:

- **Epidemiological studies,** in which scientists assess the health status of a large, defined group of people, such as the population of a country or region. They may look at various health habits, such as alcohol consumption, to determine whether those who practice these habits have a higher likelihood of developing certain diseases.
- **Animal studies, or preclinical trials,** in which scientists administer a drug or try a procedure on various laboratory animals to assess its safety and determine its effects.
- **Clinical trials,** in which volunteers agree to act as test subjects—"human guinea pigs," as it were. Patients must give written permission in order to participate. Clinical trials generate data for the purpose of evaluating one or more diagnostic or therapeutic approaches in a population. Well-designed clinical trials, which must have strict eligibility criteria, a standardized intervention, follow-up, and measures of outcome, set the "gold standard" for new diagnostic tests or medical or surgical treatments.

In *controlled studies,* the group receiving an experimental drug or treatment is compared with a group receiving no treatment or standard therapy. In *single-blind studies,* the subjects don't know whether they're receiving the experimental drug or treatment, or an inactive substance. In *double-blind studies,* neither the subjects nor the researchers have this information. In *prospective studies,* patients are selected, assessed, participate in the trial, and are then followed for a preset period. In *retrospective studies,* investigators look back at their past experiences with a certain group of patients.

The results of even the most careful studies aren't considered conclusive in and of themselves. The FDA reviews every new drug, as well as the research methods used to test it, before it's allowed on the market. And a new therapy is widely accepted (or rejected) only after publication of study results in a *peer-reviewed* journal (one in which scientists

The students also agreed on the need for rest and sleep in recovering from an illness. Only 20 percent of American-born students—compared with 40 percent of those born in China and 48 percent of those born in India—said seeing a nurse or doctor promptly was very important for recovering from illness. More of the India-born students placed great importance on eating proper foods, taking vitamins, and religious faith for recovery. The largest proportion of each group placed their greatest faith in doctors and in their families to help them when sick.[2]

Self-Care

Most people do treat themselves. You probably prescribe aspirin for a headache, chicken soup or orange juice for a cold, or a weekend trip to unwind from stress. At the very least, you should know what your **vital signs** are and how they compare against normal readings (Table 17.2).

Once a thermometer was the only self-testing equipment found in most American homes. Now hundreds of home tests are available to help consumers monitor everything from fertility to blood pressure to cholesterol levels (Table 17-3). More convenient and less expensive than a visit to a clinic or doctor's office, the new tests are generally as accurate as those administered by a professional.

Self-care also can mean getting involved in the self-help movement, which has grown into a major national trend. An estimated 20 million people participate in self-help support groups. Millions of others join virtual support communities online.

meta-analysis Summarization and review of research in a particular area to evaluate the results of several large clinical trials in a uniform manner.

vital signs Measurements of physiological functioning; specifically, temperature, blood pressure, pulse rate, and respiration rate.

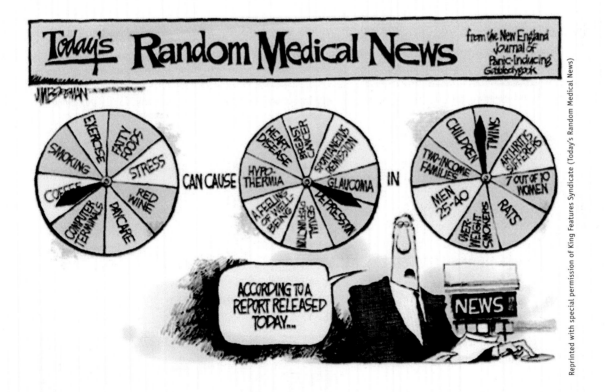

Reprinted with special permission of King Features Syndicate (Today's Random Medical News)

in the same field critique the research methods before accepting the paper) and after *replication* (the repetition of the same investigation by other researchers with similar results). In recent years, a technique called **meta-analysis,** which summarizes and reviews research in a particular area, has been used to evaluate the results of several large trials in a uniform manner.

One reason why study results must be confirmed is that, no matter what treatment patients receive, one-third to one-half of all patients improve temporarily. This well-documented but little-understood phenomenon is called the *placebo effect.* Scientific trials of a new treatment must show that the patients receiving the experimental medication or therapy improve *more* than those receiving a sugar pill or mock procedure (the placebo).

TABLE 17.2 Take Your Own Vital Signs

Vital Sign	Normal Values
Temperature	98.9° F in the morning or 99.9° F later in the day is upper limit of the normal oral temperature for people 40 years old or younger. • Women's temperatures are slightly higher than men's. • African-Americans' temperatures are slightly higher than white Americans. Measure your temperature with a mercury or digital thermometer.
Blood pressure	Below 120 (systolic) and below 80 (diastolic). You can measure your own blood pressure if you want to invest in blood pressure equipment. Check your local drugstore to purchase a blood pressure cuff or digital blood presure monitor.
Pulse	72 beats per minute. Take your pulse rate at your wrist or at the carotid artery in your neck.
Respiration rate	15-20 breaths per minute.

TABLE 17.3 Home Health Tests: A Consumer's Guide

Type of Test	What It Does
Pregnancy	Determines if a woman is pregnant by detecting the presence of human chorionic gonadotropin in urine. Considered 99 percent accurate.
Fertility	Measures levels of luteinizing hormone (LH), which rise 24 to 36 hours before a woman conceives. Can help women increase their odds of conceiving.
Blood pressure	Measures blood pressure by means of an automatically inflating armband or a cuff for the finger or wrist; helps people taking hypertension medication or suffering from high blood pressure monitor their condition.
Cholesterol	Checks cholesterol in blood from a finger prick; good for anyone concerned about cholesterol.
Colon cancer	Screening test to detect hidden blood in stool; recommended for anyone over 40 or concerned about colorectal disease.
Urinary tract infection	Diagnoses infection by screening for certain white blood cells in urine; advised for women who get frequent UTIs and whose doctors will prescribe antibiotics without a visit.
HIV infection	Detects antibodies to HIV in a blood sample sent anonymously to a lab. Controversial because no face-to-face counseling is available for those who test positive.

Oral Health

Oral health involves more than healthy teeth—it refers to the entire mouth, including all the structures that allow us to talk, bite, chew, taste, swallow, smile, scream, or scowl. Oral health is a critical part of overall health. Research has revealed links between chronic oral infection and heart and lung diseases, stroke, low birthweight, premature births, and diabetes.

Poor oral health can lead to a variety of health problems. People with gum disease are at higher risk for developing heart disease, stroke, uncontrolled diabetes, preterm births, and respiratory disease. One recent study found an increased risk of pancreatic cancer in individuals who had experienced tooth loss.[3]

Thanks to fluoridated water and toothpaste and improved dental care, Americans' oral health is better than in the past. However, without good self-care, you probably will lose some teeth to decay and gum disease. The best way to prevent such problems is through proper and regular brushing and flossing. For more tips, see Your Strategies for Prevention: "How to Take Care of Your Mouth."

Gum, or periodontal, **disease** is an inflammation that attacks the gum and bone that hold your teeth in place. The culprit is **plaque,** the sticky film of bacteria that forms on teeth. More than 300 species of bacteria live under the gum line, and about half a dozen have been linked to serious gum problems. The early stage of gum disease is called **gingivitis.** If untreated, it develops into a more serious form known as **periodontitis,** in which plaque moves down the tooth to the roots, which then become infected. In advanced periodontitis, the infection destroys the bone and fibers that hold teeth in place.

Symptoms of gum disease include bleeding during brushing or flossing, redness and puffiness of gums,

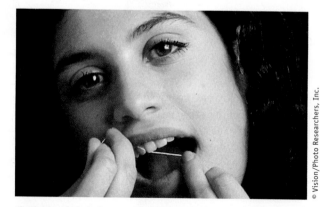

Flossing every day helps prevent gum disease and other health problems. Using a gentle sawing motion, work the floss down to your gum line. Move the floss up and down to scrape the sides of each tooth. Clean between all your teeth, using a fresh section of floss for each tooth.

© Vision/Photo Researchers, Inc.

YOUR STRATEGIES FOR PREVENTION *How to Take Care of Your Mouth*

- Brush your teeth every morning and every night. Oral bacteria reach their highest count during sleep because fluids in the mouth accumulate. Night-time cleaning reduces the bacterial population; morning cleaning lets you reduce the buildup.

- Use a toothpaste that has the American Dental Association (ADA) seal of acceptance and a toothbrush with soft, rounded bristles. Replace your toothbrush every three months.

- Hold the brush at a 45-degree angle from your gums. Pay particular attention to the space between your teeth and gums, especially on the inside, toward your tongue. Brush for two to five minutes. Don't brush too vigorously. If you scrub as hard as you can, you may damage your teeth and gums. Abrasion—a problem for more than half of American adults—erodes tooth surfaces, weakens teeth, and increases sensitivity to hot and cold foods. There is some evidence that powered toothbrushes are better at removing plaque and reducing the risk of gum disease than are ordinary manual toothbrushes.

- Because brushing can't reach plaque and food trapped between teeth, daily flossing is essential. Using waxed or unwaxed floss, start behind the upper and lower molars at one side of your mouth and work toward the other side.

- See your dentist twice a year for routine cleaning and examination. Your dentist should take a complete medical history from you and update it every six months, examine your mouth for signs of cancer, and thoroughly outline all treatment options.

- Make sure that everyone who works on the inside of your mouth wears a mask and rubber gloves to reduce the risk of disease transmission (that is, bacterial and viral infections, such as hepatitis, herpes, and HIV).

---

tenderness or pain, persistent bad breath or a bad taste in the mouth, receding gums, shifted or loosened teeth, and changes in the way your teeth fit together when you bite. New treatments, which offer an alternative to traditional gum surgery, include a single antibiotic injection or the implant of a small antibiotic chip in the periodontal pockets to promote healing.

Taking care of your mouth isn't important only for dental health: It may affect how long you live. Gingivitis and periodontitis trigger an inflammatory response that causes the arteries to swell, which leads to a constriction of blood flow that can increase the incidence of cardiovascular disease. Periodontal disease also leads to a higher white blood cell count, an indicator that the immune system is under increased stress. The good news: You can prevent these problems by flossing daily and brushing your teeth and your tongue (to get rid of bacteria that can cause gum disease and bad breath).

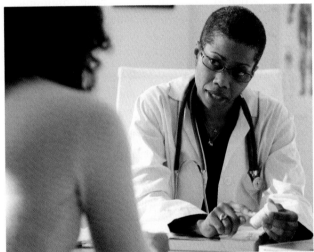

Take charge of your health by educating yourself and asking your doctor questions about your health and treatments.

Getting Quality Health Care

Once patients simply put their faith in physicians and assumed that they knew best and would make the correct medical decisions. Today health care has become far more complex and impersonal. Increasingly, doctors as well as consumer advocates insist that patients need to take responsibility for their own care. Rather than assuming that health-care providers will do whatever is necessary and appropriate, you must take the initiative to ensure that you get quality care.

The Doctor-Patient Partnership

Once the family doctor was indeed part of the family. The family doctor brought babies into the world, shepherded them through childhood, comforted and coun-seled them, stood by their bedside in their darkest hours. Patients entrusted the doctor with their cares, their confidences, their very lives. Dramatic breakthroughs in diagnosing and treating illness shifted the focus in medicine from the family physician to the specialist, from basic caring to high-tech medical care. Patients today are more likely to be cured of a vast array of illnesses than were patients a century ago. However, they often complain of insensitive, uncaring physicians who focus on their diseases rather than on them as individuals.

---

gum disease Inflammation of the gum and bones that hold teeth in place.

plaque The sticky film of bacteria that forms on teeth.

gingivitis Inflammation of the gums.

periodontitis Severe gum disease in which the tooth root becomes infected.

As more physicians have joined managed-care organizations (discussed later in this chapter), which emphasize efficiency, they sometimes feel pressure to see more patients a day, to spend less time with each, and to discourage expensive tests and treatments.

Because physicians have less time and less autonomy, patients today must do more. Your first step should be learning more about your body, any medical conditions or problems you develop, and your options for treatment. You can find a great deal of information via computer online services, patient advocacy and support organizations (see the Hales Health Almanac at the end of this book for listings), and libraries.

This information can help you know what questions to ask and how to evaluate what your doctor says. But you have to be willing to speak up. Busy doctors give patients less than a minute on average during a routine visit to say what's bothering them before they interrupt. This doesn't mean your doctor isn't interested, but it does mean that you have to develop good communication skills so you can tell physicians what they need to know to help you.

Choosing a Primary Care Physician

Why does a healthy young adult need a doctor? To stay healthy as long as possible. At some point in early adulthood, you should establish a relationship with a physician who will do basic screening tests (Table 17.4), record your family history, and help you prevent problems down the road. The primary care physicians who are playing increasingly important roles in American health care include family practitioners, general internists, and pediatricians.

Obstetrician-gynecologists serve as the primary providers of health care for more than half of all women. If you're a woman and your gynecologist is the only physician you see, make sure that he or she performs other tests, such as measuring your blood pressure, in addition to a pelvic and breast exam. If you develop other symptoms or health concerns, ask for an appropriate referral.

At college health centers, clinics, and some health-care organizations, consumers may be assigned to a primary physician or restricted to certain doctors. Even if your

---

TABLE 17.4 Screening Tests and Recommendations

Anemia

Beginning in adolescence, all nonpregnant women should be screened every five to ten years until menopause.

Clinical Breast Exam/Mammography

Women ages 20 to 39 should receive a clinical breast exam every three years. Women age 40 and older should receive an annual clinical breast exam and mammography.

Cervical Cancer Screening (Pap Smear)

Three years after first sexual intercourse or by age 21, whichever comes first, until age 30, women should receive an annual Pap smear. After age 30, the screening rate may decrease. See "Your Health Action Plan for Early Detection of Cancer" in Chapter 14.

Cholesterol and Lipids

Adults over age 20 should have a lipoprotein panel test every five years.

Colorectal Cancer Screening

Adults age 50 and older should receive an annual fecal occult blood test and colonoscopy every ten years.

Type 2 Diabetes

Beginning at age 45, adults should have a fasting blood glucose test every three years.

Hypertension Screening

Adults age 18 and older should have an annual blood pressure (BP) check. If the BP is less than 130/85, it should be checked every two years. If the blood pressure is between 130–139/85–89, it should be checked annually. After age 60, blood pressure should be checked annually.

Osteoporosis

Women age 65 and older should have a baseline bone mineral density test. To reduce the risk of fractures, women should increase dietary calcium and vitamin D, perform weight-bearing exercise, stop smoking, and moderate alcohol intake.

Prostate Cancer Screening

Men age 50 and older should discuss potential benefits and known harms of screening with PSA and digital rectal exam.

Skin Cancer Screening

Adults should receive an annual skin exam.

Visual Exam

Adults age 18 to 40 should have a complete visual examination every two to three years; ages 41 to 60, every 2 years; and ages 61 and older, every year.

YOUR STRATEGIES FOR CHANGE *How to Talk to Your Doctor*

- Prepare in advance. Write down your questions, organize them in a logical fashion, and select the top ten queries you want answered. Make a copy of all your questions to review and leave with your doctor.
- Ask about a "question hour." Many health-care practitioners set aside a specific time

of day for patients with call-in questions. Find out if your college health center offers this service. Does a nurse field all calls? Can you get specific advice?

- Go online. Many doctors' offices answer queries by email. Ask your doctor if you can email follow-up questions or progress reports on how you're feeling.

- Interrupt the interrupter. If you're having difficulty explaining what's wrong, say so. If your doctor tries to put words in your mouth, say, "Please just listen so I can tell you the whole story without getting sidetracked."

---

choices are limited, don't suspend your critical judgment. If your assigned physician does not listen to your concerns or is not providing adequate care, you can—and should—request another physician. Your rapport with your primary physician and the feelings of mutual trust and respect that develop between you can have as much of an impact on your well-being as your doctor's technical expertise. For ideas on how to establish rapport, see Your Strategies for Change: "How to Talk to Your Doctor."

One key to making the health-care system work for you lies in choosing a good physician. After seeing your primary care physician, ask yourself the following questions to evaluate the quality of care you are getting.

- Did your physician take a comprehensive history? Was the physical examination thorough?
- Did your physician explain what he or she was doing during the exam?
- Did he or she spend enough time with you?
- Did you feel free to ask questions? Did your physician give you straight answers? Did he or she reassure you when you were worried?
- Does your physician seem willing to admit that he or she doesn't know the answers to some questions?
- Does your physician hesitate to refer you to a specialist even when you have a complex problem that warrants such care?

Look back at your answers. If they make you feel uneasy, have a talk with your physician. Or find a physician or a health plan that provides better service.

Your Medical Exam

Although analysts have not found evidence that an annual screening physical is warranted for healthy adults, primary care physicians feel differently. In a recent survey about two-thirds agreed that an annual physical examination is necessary. The benefits, as doctors see them, include time to counsel patients about preventive health services, detection of underlying illnesses before symptoms develop, and improved patient-physician relationships.[4]

Your physician will want a past **medical history**, including major illnesses, surgery, and treatments. Report any allergies you have, particularly to drugs, and the medications you take, including aspirin, antacids, sleeping pills, oral contraceptives, and recreational drugs, even if illegal. Your physician may also want to know about topics you consider private, such as sexually transmitted infections. Remember that he or she needs all this information to provide you with comprehensive treatment. Note, too, that a physician must report certain information—for example, certain sexually transmitted diseases—to health authorities.

After the physician has asked you questions about your complaints, medical history, and lifestyle, he or she will probably perform the standard tests described next (Figure 17.1). During the examination, point out any pains, lumps, or skin growths you've noticed. If you feel pain when the physician palpates (feels) any part of your body, say so.

- **Head.** Using a flashlightlike instrument called an *ophthalmoscope*, the physician will look at the lens, retina, and blood vessels of your eyes. For patients over 40, he or she may test for a treatable eye disease called glaucoma (a disorder characterized by increased pressure within the eye), which can cause blindness if not detected early: A puff of air against the surface of each eye measures the pressure within the eye. The physician also will examine your ears, mouth, tongue, teeth, and gums.
- **Neck.** Feeling around your neck, the physician will check for enlarged lymph glands (a sign of infection), for lumps in the thyroid gland, and for warning signs of stroke in the neck arteries.

medical history   The health-related information collected during the interview of a client by a health-care professional.

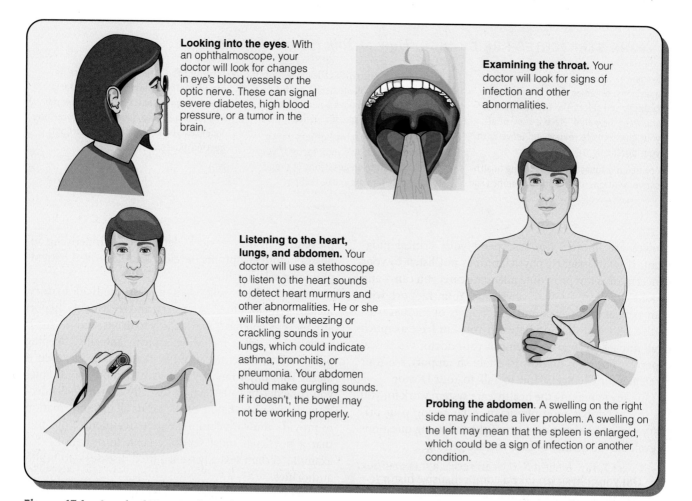

Looking into the eyes. With an ophthalmoscope, your doctor will look for changes in eye's blood vessels or the optic nerve. These can signal severe diabetes, high blood pressure, or a tumor in the brain.

Examining the throat. Your doctor will look for signs of infection and other abnormalities.

Listening to the heart, lungs, and abdomen. Your doctor will use a stethoscope to listen to the heart sounds to detect heart murmurs and other abnormalities. He or she will listen for wheezing or crackling sounds in your lungs, which could indicate asthma, bronchitis, or pneumonia. Your abdomen should make gurgling sounds. If it doesn't, the bowel may not be working properly.

Probing the abdomen. A swelling on the right side may indicate a liver problem. A swelling on the left may mean that the spleen is enlarged, which could be a sign of infection or another condition.

Figure 17.1   Standard Tests Performed During a Medical Checkup

- **Chest.** With a *stethoscope,* the physician will listen to the sounds made by your heart, to detect heart murmurs and irregular contractions, and by your lungs, to detect asthma or emphysema. By tapping on your chest and back with his or her fingers, the physician can tell the size and shape of your heart, which may reveal some forms of heart disease, and whether any fluid has collected in your lungs. The physician will also check for abnormal lumps in a woman's breasts.

- **Abdomen.** Here the physician uses his or her fingers to probe for tender spots and malformations of the liver and other organs, which may reveal signs of alcoholism, hepatitis, or hernias.

- **Rectum and genitals.** With a gloved hand, the physician can feel in the rectum for growths and hemorrhoids. A rectal examination can also reveal enlargement of the male's prostate gland. The physician will check male testicles and spermatic cords for abnormalities.

- **Pelvic examination.** During a pelvic examination, a woman lies on her back, with her heels in stirrups

at the end of the examining table and her legs spread out to the sides. The physician inspects the labia, clitoris, and vaginal opening. Using two gloved, lubricated fingers, the physician will check for abnormalities in the vagina, uterus, fallopian tubes, and ovaries. Many physicians will also perform a rectal or rectovaginal (one finger in the rectum and one in the vagina) examination. A nurse or other health-care worker should be present throughout the exam.

The *speculum* is a medical instrument that spreads the walls of the vagina so that the inside can be seen. The physician will gently scrape cells from the cervix for a **Pap smear,** a procedure that identifies abnormal cells that may indicate an infection or, more seriously, cervical cancer, a slow-growing cancer that's usually curable if detected early (see Chapter 14). All women should start having regular Pap smears once they begin having intercourse, or at age 18. While there has been debate about how often women should have Pap smears, many health-care providers recommend Pap smears every year for women who are sexually active or have other risk factors, such as infection with human papilloma virus (see Chapter 16).

- **Extremities.** The physician may check your knees and other joints for reflexes, which can indicate nerve disorders, and look for tremors in outstretched hands or in the face. The color, elasticity, and wetness or dryness of your skin can alert him or her to nutritional problems, or can indicate diabetes or skin cancer. Hair and nails can give indications of internal health, such as blood disorders. Swelling of the ankles can be an indication of heart, kidney, or liver disease.

- **Pulse and blood pressure.** Your physician may check your pulse in various places, looking for signs of poor circulation. The rhythm and speed of the heart may also signal diseases of the heart or thyroid gland. High blood pressure can be an early warning sign of possible heart attack, stroke, or kidney damage.

Medical Tests

Besides the diagnostic tests just listed, the physician may order some laboratory and other tests, including the following:

- **Chest X-ray.** A chest X-ray can reveal abnormalities of the heart and lungs; if you're a smoker, the physician may insist on one.

- **Electrocardiogram.** The *electrocardiogram,* performed while you're at rest, records the electrical activity of your heart. It can show irregularities in heart rhythm or muscle damage, as well as hardening of the arteries.

- **Urinalysis.** Your urine may be analyzed by a medical laboratory. If sugar (glucose) is found in your urine, your physician may order a separate blood test to check for diabetes. The presence of blood cells may indicate infection of the bladder or kidneys. Abnormal amounts of albumin (protein) in the urine may also suggest kidney disease.

- **Blood tests.** The physician or laboratory technician may draw blood to do a blood cell count. An excess of white blood cells may indicate an infection or, occasionally, leukemia. A deficiency of red blood cells may indicate anemia. Your blood also may be analyzed to measure the levels of its various components. High levels of glucose can indicate diabetes, and high levels of uric acid may mean gout or kidney stones. Your lipoprotein profile may indicate cardiac risk (see Chapter 14).

See the Hales Health Almanac at the back of this book for a comprehensive guide to medical tests.

Evidence-Based Medicine

One of the ways in which physicians are working to improve the quality of care is by basing diagnostic testing and treatments on solid evidence produced by rigorous research studies (usually randomized controlled trials). Evidence-based medicine is not an entirely new concept of medical care but a methodical approach that establishes a solid and conscientious scientific basis for decision making about health care. Evidence-based medicine pays particular attention to **outcomes,** that is, the impact that a specific medication or treatment has on a patient's condition, overall health, and quality of life.

Outcomes research is designed to answer questions such as: Is treatment better or worse than no treatment? Is one treatment better than another? If a treatment is effective, is a little just as good as a lot? Does quality of life change because of treatment? Are the benefits of treatment worth the cost or the risks to the patient?

Studies of outcomes look at how patients fared with or without a specific treatment, the costs involved, and the impact of undergoing or not undergoing treatment in terms of the patients' quality of life. Outcomes research can help determine which of several therapies or approaches provides the best results at the most reasonable costs.

When you are diagnosed with a health problem, ask your doctor if your treatment is based on the latest evidence and clinical guidelines. The National Guideline Clearinghouse provides a comprehensive database of evidence-based clinical practice guidelines for many common health problems, available at **www.guideline.gov**.

Preventing Medical Errors

More people die from medical errors than from motor vehicle accidents, breast cancer, or AIDS.[5] Medical errors occur when a planned part of medical care doesn't work properly or when the wrong plan was used in the first place. They can happen anywhere in the health-care system, from doctors' offices to pharmacies to hospitals to patients' homes. They may involve medications, diagnoses, tests, lab equipment, surgery, or infection. They are most likely to occur when doctors and patients have problems communicating.

Your best defense against medical errors is information. "Questions are the answer," is the theme of a prevention campaign by the Agency for Healthcare Research and Quality.[6] Your questions can keep you safe and ensure you get quality health care. See Your Strategies for Prevention: "Inform Yourself."

Pap smear   A test in which cells removed from the cervix are examined under a microscope for signs of cancer; also called a Pap test.

outcomes   The ultimate impacts of particular treatments or absence of treatment.

Asserting Your Medical Rights

As a consumer, you have basic rights that help ensure that you know about any potential dangers, receive competent diagnosis and treatment, and retain control and dignity in your interactions with health-care professionals. Many hospitals publish a patient's bill of rights, including your rights to know whether a procedure is experimental; to refuse to undergo a specific treatment; to designate someone else to make decisions about your care if and when you cannot; and to leave the hospital, even against your physician's advice.

You have the right to be treated with respect and dignity, including being called "Mr." or "Ms." or whatever you wish, rather than by your first name. Make clear your preferences. If you feel that health-care professionals are being condescending or inconsiderate, say so—in the same tone and manner that you would like others to use with you. If you're hospitalized, find out if there's a

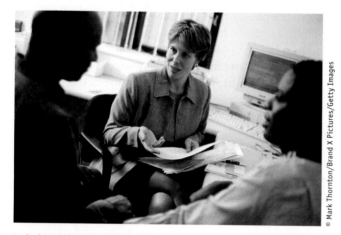

In the hospital, you can discuss the patient's rights and other individual concerns with a patient advocate.

patient advocate or representative at your hospital. These individuals can help you communicate with physicians, make any special arrangements, and get answers to questions or complaints.

Your Right to Information

By law, a patient must give consent for hospitalization, surgery, and other major treatments. **Informed consent** is a right, not a privilege. Use this right to its fullest. Ask questions. Seek other opinions. Make sure that your expectations are realistic and that you understand the potential risks, as well as the possible benefits, of a prospective treatment.

Your Right to Privacy and Access to Medical Records

Your medical records are your property. You have the right to see them whenever you choose and to limit who else can see them. Federal standards protecting the privacy of patients' medical information guarantee patients access to their medical records, give them more control over how personal health information is disclosed, and limit the ways that health plans, pharmacies, and hospitals can use personal medical information.

Key provisions include:

- **Access to medical records.** As a patient, you should be able to see and obtain copies of your medical records and request corrections if there are errors. Health-care providers must provide these within 30 days; they may charge for the cost of copying and mailing records.

- **Notice of privacy practices.** Your providers must inform you of how they use personal medical information. Doctors, nurses, and other providers may not disclose information for purposes not related to your health care.

- **Prohibition on marketing.** Pharmacies, health plans, and others must obtain specific authorization before disclosing patient information for marketing.

informed consent Permission (to undergo or receive a medical procedure or treatment) given voluntarily, with full knowledge and understanding of the procedure or treatment and its possible consequences.

quackery Medical fakery; unproven practices claiming to cure diseases or solve health problems.

- **Confidentiality.** Patients can request that doctors take reasonable steps to ensure confidential communications, such as calling a cell phone rather than home or office.

Your Right to Quality Health Care

The essence of a *malpractice* suit is the claim that the physician failed to meet the standard of quality care required of a reasonably skilled and careful medical doctor. Although physicians don't have to guarantee good results to their patients and aren't held liable for unavoidable errors, they are required to use the same care and judgment in treatment that other physicians in the same specialty would use under similar circumstances. To protect themselves financially, physicians, particularly those in surgical specialties who are most likely to be sued, pay tens of thousands of dollars a year in malpractice insurance premiums. Some of this cost is passed on to patients.

Most lawsuits are based on negligence and assert that a physician failed to render diagnosis and treatment with appropriate professional knowledge and skill. Other cases are brought for failure to provide information, obtain consent, or respect a patient's confidentiality. However, analysis of malpractice cases has shown that, in 70 to 80 percent, a doctor's attitude and inability to communicate effectively—by devaluing patients' views, delivering information poorly, failing to understand patients' perspectives, or displaying an air of superiority—also played a role.

The Public Citizen Health Research Group has compiled a national directory of "questionable physicians," which lists physicians disciplined by state medical boards or the federal government for offenses ranging from overprescribing drugs to sexual misconduct to negligent or substandard care. Some of these physicians committed minor misdeeds, such as failing to complete continuing medical education requirements. Consumer advocates urge patients to find out why a particular name appears on the list by calling the state licensing board. At the federal level, the agencies most involved in ensuring quality health care are the Food and Drug Administration (FDA), which approves the production and labeling of drugs, and the Federal Trade Commission (FTC), which oversees advertising and prohibits deceptive or false claims. (See the Savvy Consumer feature.)

✓Savvy Consumer   Protecting Yourself from Quackery and Health Hoaxes

Every year millions of Americans go searching for medical miracles that never happen. In all, they spend more than $10 billion on medical **quackery,** unproven health products and services. Those who lose only money are the lucky ones. Many also waste precious time, during which their conditions worsen. Some suffer needless pain, along with crushed expectations.

To keep from risking your life on false hope, follow these guidelines:

- Arm yourself with up-to-date information about your condition or disease from appropriate organizations, such as the American Cancer Society or the Arthritis Foundation, which keep track of unproven and ineffective methods of treatment.

- Ask for a written explanation of what a treatment does and why it works, evidence supporting all claims (not just testimonials), and published reports of the studies, including specifics on numbers treated, doses, and side effects. Be skeptical of self-styled "holistic practitioners," treatments supported by crusading groups, and endorsements from self-proclaimed experts or authorities.

- Don't part with your money quickly. Insurance companies won't reimburse for unproven therapies.

- Don't discontinue your current treatment without your physician's approval. Many physicians encourage supportive therapies—such as relaxation exercises, meditation, or visualization—as a supplement to standard treatments.

Promoters of fraudulent health products often use similar claims and practices to trick consumers into buying their products. Be suspicious when you see:

- Claims that a product is a "scientific breakthrough," "miraculous cure," "secret ingredient," or "ancient remedy."

- Claims that the product is an effective cure for a wide range of ailments. No product can cure multiple conditions or diseases.

- Claims that use impressive-sounding medical terms. They're often covering up a lack of good science.

- Undocumented case histories of people who've had amazing results. It's too easy to make them up. And even if true, they can't be generalized to the entire population. Anecdotes are not a substitute for valid science.

- Claims that the product is available from only one source and payment is required in advance.

- Claims of a "money-back" guarantee.

- Websites that fail to list the company's name, physical address, phone number, or other contact information.

To file a complaint with the Federal Trade Commission (FTC) or to get free information on consumer topics, call 1-877-FTC-HELP (1-877-382-4357), or use the complaint form at www.ftc.gov.

Source: Federal Trade Commission, www.ftc.gov/bcp/consumer.shtm.

Men and Women as Health-Care Consumers

 The genders differ significantly in the way they use health-care services in the United States. Women see more doctors than men, take more prescription drugs, are hospitalized more, and control the spending of three of every four health-care dollars. In a national telephone poll, 76 percent of American women—but only 60 percent of men—said they had had a health exam in the last 12 months.

Many experts believe that the need for birth control and reproductive health services gets women into the habit of making regular visits to health-care professionals, primarily gynecologists. There are no comparable specialists for men, who tend to visit urologists, specialists in male reproductive organs, only when they develop problems. Men also are conditioned to take a stoic, tough-it-out attitude to early symptoms of a disease.

Men feel they are not allowed to manifest illness unless it's overt, says family practitioner Martin Miner, M.D., who has conducted research on men and health care. One reason men die earlier than women is because of the length of time they wait to go for treatment.

The genders also differ in the symptoms and syndromes they develop. For instance, men are more prone to back problems, muscle sprains and strains, allergies, insomnia, and digestive problems. Men develop heart disease about a decade earlier in life than women. More men develop ulcers and hernias; women are more likely to get gallbladder disease and irritable bowel syndrome. An estimated 3 to 6 percent of men suffer from migraines, compared with 15 to 17 percent of women. Yet women and men spend similar proportions of their lifetimes—about 81 percent—free of disability. For men, whose lifespans are shorter, this translates into an average of 58.8 years; for women, 63.9 years.

The genders also differ in access to health services. Women are more likely than men to lack health insurance, and the lower a woman's income and education, the less her likelihood of getting important preventive services, such as an annual Pap smear or prenatal care.

Women and men are about equally likely to use complementary and alternative medicine—but different types. Men outnumber women in use of chiropractic services and acupuncture, while women are more likely to try herbal medicine, mind-body remedies, folk remedies, movement and exercise techniques, and prayer or spiritual practices. Both genders turn to alternative treatments for the same reason: a desire for greater control over their health.

Elective Treatments

As medical technology has developed new options, millions of Americans are trying elective procedures and products that are not medically necessary but that promise to enhance health or appearance. Some are new alternatives for correcting common problems, such as poor vision, while others offer the promise of looking younger or more attractive.

Vision Surgery

Millions of people in the United States have undergone laser surgery to correct their vision. In LASIK (laser-assisted in situ keratomileusis), the most common technique, a surgeon uses a razorlike instrument to lift a flap of the cornea—the clear stiff outer layer over the colored iris—and then reshapes the exposed area using a laser. The surgery alters the way the eye focuses light, correcting nearsightedness, farsightedness, and some astigmatism. Laser surgery cannot make an aging eye's lens

---

YOUR STRATEGIES FOR PREVENTION *When Is LASIK Not for You?*

You are probably NOT a good candidate for refractive surgery if:

- **You are not a risk taker.** Certain complications are unavoidable in a percentage of patients, and there are no long-term data available for current procedures.

- **Cost is an issue.** Most medical insurance will not pay for refractive surgery. Although the cost is coming down, it is still significant.

- **You required a change in your contact lens or glasses prescription in the past year.** This is called refractive instability.

Patients who are in their early twenties or younger, whose hormones are fluctuating due to disease such as diabetes, who are pregnant or breastfeeding, or who are taking medications that may cause fluctuations in vision are more likely to have refractive instability and should discuss the possible additional risks with their doctor.

- **You have a disease or are on medications that may affect wound healing.** Certain conditions, such as autoimmune diseases and diabetes, and some medications may prevent proper healing after a refractive procedure.

- **You actively participate in contact sports.** If you participate in boxing, wrestling, martial arts, or other activities in which blows to the face and eyes are a normal occurrence, LASIK is probably not right for you.

- **You are under 18.** Currently, no lasers are approved for LASIK on persons under the age of 18.

- **It will jeopardize your career.** Some jobs, including certain military assignments, prohibit refractive procedures.

Source: Food and Drug Administration, www.fda.gov/cdrh/LASIK/when.htm.

flexible again to improve close-up vision in middle-aged adults. Numbing eye drops make the treatment painless, although burning and scratchiness are normal for a couple of hours afterward. An estimated 10 to 30 percent of patients require additional surgery, or "enhancements," to sharpen their vision. Other complications include glare, sensitivity to bright lights, and poor night vision. (See Your Strategies for Prevention: "When Is LASIK Not for You?")

Prices have fallen, but ophthalmologists have warned consumers that some laser surgery centers have cut corners to cut prices, such as hiring inexperienced surgeons or using optometrists or technicians rather than MDs for pre- and postoperative checkups. A qualified eye surgeon should have a record of 100 or more LASIK procedures and at least 25 enhancements—but no more than 20 percent of his or her patients should require enhancements. Ideally, the surgeon should also be the one doing your pre- and postprocedure checks.

Cosmetic Surgery

Approximately 11 million cosmetic treatments are performed every year.[7] About a quarter of those undergoing plastic surgery are between the ages of 18 and 29. The number of teenagers opting for cosmetic procedures—primarily liposuction, nose reshaping, and breast augmentation—is increasing. Nonsurgical cosmetic procedures such as injections of synthetic collagen and botulinum toxin (Botox®) also have become more popular. Health insurance rarely covers cosmetic procedures, which can run in to the tens of thousands of dollars.

The most common cosmetic operation is liposuction, the removal of fatty tissue by means of a vacuum device. It can be performed on many areas of the body, from sagging jowls to midsection "love handles." The doctor first flushes the target area with a solution of lidocaine (a local anesthetic with a numbing effect), saline, and epinephrine (a drug that reduces bleeding by constricting blood vessels). Inserting a hollow wandlike cannula under the skin, the doctor breaks up fatty deposits and suctions them, along with other body fluids, with a vacuum device.

Risks and complications include infection, numbness, bleeding, discoloration, lumpiness, and, if too much tissue is removed without proper cautions, potentially fatal complications. The American Society of Plastic and Reconstructive Surgeons estimates the mortality rate is one in 5,000 liposuction patients. Several states are considering legislation to tighten restrictions on training and credentialing doctors who perform liposuction.

Breast augmentation is the second most common cosmetic procedure, and surgeons report a 300 percent increase in demand in the last six years. The Institute of Medicine, after reviewing all available evidence, has reported that there appears to be no link between breast implants and autoimmune disease, connective tissue disorders, or cancer. However, today's surgeons use implants filled with a saltwater solution. Patients still face possible complications, including rupture, scarring, infection, and leaking or hardening of their implants.

Getting Quality Nontraditional Health Care

The medical research community uses the term **complementary and alternative medicine (CAM)** to apply to all health-care approaches, practices, and treatments not widely taught in medical schools and not generally used in hospitals. CAM includes many healing philosophies, approaches, and therapies, including preventive techniques designed to delay or prevent serious health problems before they start and **holistic** methods that focus on the whole person and the physical, mental, emotional, and spiritual aspects of well-being. Some approaches are based on the same physiological principles as traditional Western methods; others, such as acupuncture, are based on different healing systems.

According to a recent nationwide government survey of more than 31,000 adults aged 18 and over, 50 percent have used CAM at some time and 46 percent have tried some form of complementary and alternative medicine in the last year. When CAM includes megavitamins and prayer specifically for health, the number reporting they ever used some form of CAM rises to 75 percent; 62 percent did so in the past year.[8]

CAM use varies among different groups. Those most likely to use CAM include women, people with higher education, those hospitalized within the past year, and former smokers (compared to current smokers or those who never smoked). African American adults are more likely than white or Asian American adults to use CAM practices, including megavitamin therapy and prayer. Middle-aged people report using CAM more often than either younger or older individuals. In one study, the average age of a CAM user was 45, and men and women were equally likely to try a nontraditional therapy.[9]

Some states have mandated health insurance coverage for CAM therapies, which also are becoming more common in Canada and Europe. Many medical schools now

complementary and alternative medicine (CAM) A term used to apply to all health-care approaches, practices, and treatments not widely taught in medical schools, not generally used in hospitals, and not usually reimbursed by medical insurance companies.

holistic An approach to medicine that takes into account body, mind, emotions, and spirit.

include training in CAM in their curricula. **Integrative medicine,** which combines selected elements of both conventional and alternative medicine in a comprehensive approach to diagnosis and treatment, has gained greater acceptance within the medical community.

To determine whether CAM is right for you, see Your Strategies for Prevention: "Before You Try CAM."

Types of CAM

The National Center for Complementary and Alternative Medicine (NCCAM) has classified CAM therapies into five categories (Figure 17.2).

- Alternative medical systems.
- Mind-body medicine.
- Biologically based therapies.
- Manipulative and body-based methods.
- Energy therapies.

Alternative Medical Systems

Systems of theory and practice other than traditional Western medicine are included in this group. They include acupuncture, Eastern medicine, t'ai chi, external and internal qi, Ayurvedic medicine, naturopathy, and unconventional Western systems, such as homeopathy and orthomolecular medicine.

Acupuncture is an ancient Chinese form of medicine, based on the philosophy that a cycle of energy circulating

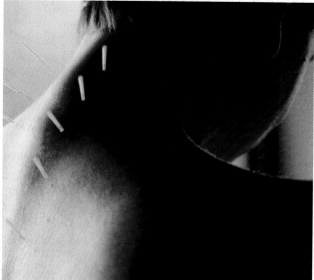

The ancient Chinese practice of acupuncture produces healing through the insertion and manipulation of needles at specific points, or meridians, throughout the body.

© Jon Feingersh/Corbis

through the body controls health. Pain and disease are the result of a disturbance in the energy flow, which can be corrected by inserting long, thin needles at specific points along longitudinal lines, or *meridians,* throughout the body. Each point controls a different corresponding part of the body. Once inserted, the needles are rotated gently back and forth or charged with a small electric current for a short time. Western scientists aren't sure exactly how acupuncture works, but some believe that the needles alter the functioning of the nervous system.

A National Institute of Health (NIH) consensus development panel that evaluated current research into acupuncture concluded that there is "clear evidence" that acupuncture can control nausea and vomiting in patients after surgery or while undergoing chemotherapy and can relieve postoperative dental pain. The panel said that acupuncture is "probably" also effective in the control of nausea in early pregnancy and that there were "reasonable" studies showing satisfactory treatment of addiction to illicit drugs and alcohol (but not to tobacco), stroke rehabilitation, headache, menstrual cramps, tennis elbow, general muscle pain, low back pain, carpal tunnel syndrome, and asthma. Ongoing studies are evaluating its efficacy for chronic headaches and migraines. Acupressure (applying pressure with the thumbs or fingertips to the same points on the body stimulated in acupuncture) seems more effective in reducing low-back pain and providing long-term relief than physical therapy.[10]

Considered alternative in this country, **Ayurveda** is a traditional form of medical treatment in India, where it has evolved over thousands of years. Its basic premise is that illness stems from incorrect mental attitudes, diet, and posture. Practitioners use a discipline of exercise,

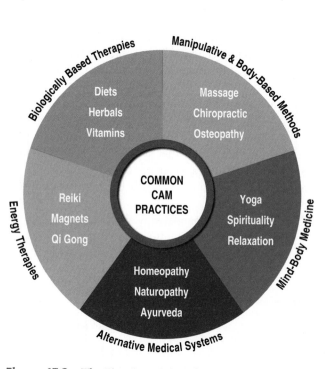

Figure 17.2 The Five Categories of CAM

Source: NCCAM, http://nccam.nih.gov.

YOUR STRATEGIES FOR PREVENTION *Before You Try CAM*

You should never decide on any treatment—traditional or CAM—without fully evaluating it. Here are some key questions to ask:

- **Is it safe?** Be particularly wary of un-regulated products.
- **Is it effective?** Check the website of the National Center for CAM: http://nccam.nih.gov.
- **Will it interact with other medicines or conventional treatments?** Many

widely used alternative remedies can interact with prescription medications in dangerous ways.

- **Is the practitioner qualified?** Find out if your state licenses practitioners who provide acupuncture, chiropractic services, naturopathy, herbal medicine, homeopathy, and other treatments.
- **What has been the experience of others?** Talk to people who have used CAM for a similar problem, both recently and in the past.

- **Can you talk openly and easily with the practitioner?** You should feel comfortable asking questions and confident in the answers you receive. And the practitioner's office should put you at ease.
- **What are the costs?** Many CAM services are not covered by HMOs or health insurers.

---

meditation, herbal medication, and proper nutrition to cope with such stress-induced conditions as hypertension, the desire to smoke, and obesity.

Homeopathy is based on three fundamental principles: like cures like; treatment must always be individualized; and less is more—the idea that increasing dilution (and lowering the dosage) can increase efficacy. By administering doses of animal, vegetable, or mineral substances to a large number of healthy people to see if they all develop the same symptoms, homeopaths determine which substances may be given, in small quantities, to alleviate the symptoms. Some of these substances are the same as those used in conventional medicine: nitroglycerin for certain heart conditions, for example, although the dose is minuscule.

Naturopathy emphasizes natural remedies, such as sun, water, heat, and air, as the best treatments for disease. Therapies might include dietary changes (such as more vegetables and no salt or stimulants), steam baths, and exercise. Some naturopathic physicians (who are not MDs) work closely with medical doctors in helping patients.

Mind-Body Medicine

Mind-body medicine uses techniques designed to enhance the mind's capacity to affect bodily function and symptoms. Some techniques that were considered alternative in the past have become mainstream (for example, patient support groups and cognitive-behavioral therapy). Other mind-body approaches are still considered CAM, including meditation, prayer (see Chapter 2), yoga, t'ai chi, visual imagery, mental healing, and therapies that use creative outlets such as art, music, or dance. About 30 percent of Americans report using relaxation techniques and imagery, biofeedback, and hypnosis; 50 percent use prayer.

The physical and emotional risks of using mind-body interventions are minimal. Although we need much more research on how these approaches work and when to apply

them most effectively, there is considerable evidence that mind-body interventions have positive effects on psychological functioning and quality of life and may be particularly helpful for patients coping with chronic illnesses.

Mind-body approaches definitely have won some acceptance in modern medical care. Techniques such as hypnosis have proved helpful in reducing discomfort and complications during and after various surgical procedures. With *biofeedback* (discussed in Chapter 3), people can learn to control usually involuntary functions, such as

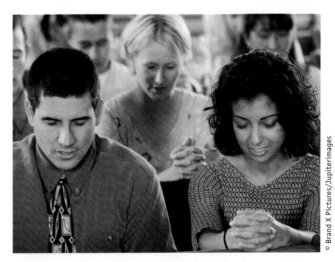

© Brand X Pictures/Jupiterimages

Prayer is the most commonly used of the CAM therapies.

---

integrative medicine An approach that combines traditional medicine with alternative/complementary therapies.

acupuncture A Chinese medical practice of puncturing the body with needles inserted at specific points to relieve pain or cure disease.

Ayurveda A traditional Indian medical treatment involving meditation, exercise, herbal medications, and nutrition.

homeopathy A system of medical practice that treats a disease by administering dosages of substances that would in healthy persons produce symptoms similar to those of the disease.

naturopathy An alternative system of treatment of disease that emphasizes the use of natural remedies such as sun, water, heat, and air. Therapies may include dietary changes, steam baths, and exercise.

circulation to the hands and feet, tension in the jaws, and heartbeat rates. Biofeedback has been used to treat dozens of ailments, including asthma, epilepsy, pain, and Raynaud's disease (a condition in which the fingers become painful and white when exposed to cold). Many health insurers now cover biofeedback treatments.

Creative *visualization,* (also discussed in Chapter 3) helps patients heal, including some diagnosed as terminally ill with cancer. Other patients use visualization to create a clear idea of what they want to achieve, whether the goal is weight loss or relaxation.

Biologically Based Therapies

Biologically based CAM therapies use substances such as herbs, foods, and vitamins. They include **herbal medicine** (botanical medicine or phytotherapy), the use of individual herbs or combinations; special diet therapies, such as macrobiotics, Ornish, McDougall, and high fiber; Mediterranean orthomolecular medicine (use of nutritional and food supplements for preventive or therapeutic purposes); and use of other products (such as shark cartilage) and procedures applied in an unconventional manner.

In the last ten years, sales of herbal supplements have skyrocketed by 100 percent, but most people don't consider evidence-based indications before trying them. According to recent research, two-thirds of people who use herbs do not do so in accordance with scientific guidelines.[11] Although more than 1,500 different preparations are on the U.S. market, just a few single-herb preparations account for about half the sales in the United States: echinacea, garlic, ginkgo biloba, ginseng, kava, St. John's wort, and valerian. Unlike medications, herbal products are exempt from the FDA's regulatory scrutiny. The ingredients and the potency of active ingredients can vary from batch to batch.

Rigorous research studies are producing the first scientific evidence on the safety and efficacy of herbal supplements. Their benefits generally have proved modest (Table 17.5). Echinacea may cut the risk and severity of a cold.[12] However, garlic has shown no effect on cholesterol.[13] Other agents, such as saw palmetto, produce slight benefits but far less than available medications.

Most of the herbs tested have proved generally safe, although side effects such as headache and nausea can occur. However, some herbs can cause serious, even fatal dangers. Echinacea may cause liver damage if taken in combination with anabolic steroids. Several widely used herbs, including ginger, garlic, and ginkgo biloba, are dangerous if taken prior to surgery.

The FDA has prohibited the sale of dietary supplements containing ephedra, which was linked with dozens of deaths and more than 1,000 adverse reactions. It has issued warnings on other potentially dangerous herbs, including chaparral, comfrey, yohimbe, lobelia, germander, willow bark, jin bu huan, and products containing magnolia or stephania.

Manipulative and Body-Based Methods

CAM therapies based on manipulation and/or movement of the body are divided into three subcategories:

- **Chiropractic medicine.**
- **Massage therapy and body work** (including osteopathic manipulation, Swedish massage, Alexander technique, reflexology, Pilates, acupressure, and rolfing).
- **Unconventional physical therapies** (including colonics, hydrotherapy, and light and color therapies).

Chiropractic is a treatment method based on the theory that many human diseases are caused by misalignment of the bones (subluxation). Chiropractors are licensed in all 50 states, but chiropractic is considered a mainstream

TABLE 17.5 Evidence-Based Evaluations of Herbal Supplements

Herb	Evidence
Saw Palmetto	Reduces an enlarged prostate, but the effect is small compared with prescription medication
Ginseng	Improves energy of cancer patients
Echinacea	Cuts risk of cold in half
Kava	May reduce anxiety, but can cause liver damage
Gingko biloba	No improvement in memory or thinking in the healthy elderly, but a small benefit for patients with dementia
Garlic	Not effective in lowering cholesterol
Black Cohosh	No more effective than placebo for hot flashes; long-term effects unknown

© David Young-Wolff/PhotoEdit, Inc.

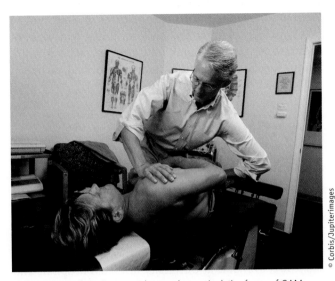

Chiropractic medicine is among the popular manipulative forms of CAM.

© Corbis/Jupiterimages

therapy by some and a form of CAM by others. Significant research in the last ten years has demonstrated its efficacy for acute lower-back pain. NIH is funding research on other potential benefits, including headaches, asthma, middle ear inflammation, menstrual cramps, and arthritis.

Chiropractors, who emphasize wellness and healing without drugs or surgery, may use X-rays and magnetic resonance imaging (MRI) as well as orthopedic, neurological, and manual examinations in making diagnoses. However, chiropractic treatment consists solely of the manipulation of misaligned bones that may be putting pressure on nerve tissue and affecting other parts of the body. Many HMOs offer chiropractic services, which are the most widely used alternative treatment among managed care patients.

Energy Therapies

Various approaches focus on energy fields believed to exist in and around the body. Some use external energy sources, such as electromagnetic fields. Magnets are marketed to relieve pain but there is little scientific evidence of their efficacy. Others, such as therapeutic touch, use a therapist's healing energy to repair imbalances in an individual's biofield.

The Health-Care System

As a college student, you can turn to the student health service if you get sick. There, a nurse, nurse practitioner, physician's assistant, or medical doctor may evaluate your symptoms and provide basic care. However, you may rely on a primary care physician in your hometown to perform regular checkups or manage a chronic condition like asthma. If you're injured

in an accident, you probably will be treated at the nearest emergency room. If you become seriously ill and require highly specialized care, you may have to go to a university-affiliated medical center to receive state-of-the-art treatment.

Students can often continue their health-care coverage under their parents' policy until the age of 23. However, if a parent belongs to an HMO with a local network of providers, the student may not be covered for anything outside the plan's service area except emergency care. A more open plan, like a preferred provider organization, may allow students to see doctors near school, but the costs may be high.

Most colleges offer some type of health insurance plan, with the student health center acting as the primary care provider. Many schools require enrollment if the student is not covered under any other plan. Check the plan carefully. Physicals, gynecological visits, and other preventive care may not be covered. College plans also may not cover preexisting conditions, such as asthma.

Heath-Care Practitioners

Fewer than 10 percent of health-care practitioners are physicians; other types of health professionals are assuming more important roles in delivering primary, or basic, health services. As a consumer, you should be aware of the range and special skills of the most common types of health-care providers.

Physicians

A medical doctor (M.D.) trained in American medical schools usually takes at least three years of premedical college courses (with an emphasis on biology, chemistry, and physics) and then completes four (but sometimes three or five) years of medical school. The first two years of medical school are devoted to the study of human anatomy, embryology, pharmacology, and similar basic subjects. During the last two years, students work directly with physicians in hospitals. Medical students who pass a series of national board examinations then enter a one-year internship in a hospital, followed by another two to five years of residency (depending on their specialty), which leads to certification in a particular field, or specialty.

About 500,000 of the nation's 700,000 physicians are specialists or subspecialists, who focus on a specific part of the body, organ system, type of disease, or type of treatment. Traditionally, they have had greater

herbal medicine An ancient form of medical treatment using substances derived from trees, flowers, ferns, seaweeds, and lichens to treat disease.

chiropractic A method of treating disease, primarily through manipulating the bones and joints to restore normal nerve function.

status and earned much larger incomes than primary care physicians—family practitioners, pediatricians, and internists—who provide preventive care, regular checkups, and routine treatments of uncomplicated medical conditions. However, changes in health policy (such as increases in Medicare payments to primary care physicians) and in the delivery of services have given a more prominent role to primary care physicians. They now often function as "gatekeepers" who decide whether a patient needs to see a medical specialist.

Nurses

A registered nurse (RN) graduates from a school of nursing approved by a state board and passes a state board examination. RNs may have a bachelor's or an associate degree and may specialize in certain areas, such as intensive care or nurse-midwifery. Nurse practitioners, RNs with advanced training and experience, may run community clinics or provide screening and preventive care at group medical practices. Some have independent practices.

Licensed practical nurses (LPNs), also called licensed vocational nurses, are licensed by the state. After graduating from state-approved schools of practical nursing, they must take a board exam. They work under the supervision of RNs or physicians. Certified nursing assistants (CNAs), nursing aides, and orderlies assist registered and practical nurses in providing services directly related to the comfort and well-being of hospitalized patients.

Specialized and Allied-Health Practitioners

More than 60 types of health practitioners work with physicians and nurses in providing medical services. Some, such as *occupational therapists,* have at least a bachelor's degree. Allied-health professionals may specialize in a variety of fields. *Clinical psychologists* have graduate degrees and provide a wide range of mental health services but don't prescribe medications—as do *psychiatrists. Optometrists,* trained in special schools of optometry, diagnose visual abnormalities and prescribe lenses or visual aids; however, they don't prescribe drugs, diagnose or treat eye diseases, or perform surgery—functions performed by *ophthalmologists. Podiatrists* are specially trained, licensed health-care professionals who specialize in problems of the feet.

Dentists

Most dental students earn a bachelor's degree and then complete two more years of training in the basic sciences and two years of clinical work before graduating with a degree of D.D.S. or D.M.D. (Doctor of Dental Surgery or Doctor of Medical Dentistry). To qualify for a license, graduates must pass both a written and a clinical examination. Dentists may work in general practice or choose a specialty, such as orthodontics (straightening teeth).

Chiropractors

Chiropractors hold the degree of Doctor of Chiropractic (D.C.), which signifies that they have had two years of college-level training, plus four years in a health-care school specializing in chiropractic, described earlier in this chapter.

Health-Care Facilities

As a prospective patient, you can choose from various options: a physician's office, a clinic, an emergency room, or a hospital. Most **primary care**—also referred to as ambulatory or outpatient care—is provided by a physician in an office, emergency room, or clinic. *Secondary care* usually is provided by specialists or subspecialists in either an outpatient or inpatient (hospital) setting. *Tertiary care,* available at university-affiliated hospitals and regional referral centers, includes special procedures such as kidney dialysis, open-heart surgery, and organ transplants.

College Health Centers

The American College Health Association estimates that 1,500 institutions of higher learning provide direct health services. Student health centers, initially developed by departments of physical education and hygiene, range in size from small dispensaries staffed by nurses to large-scale, multispecialty clinics that provide both inpatient and outpatient care and are fully accredited by the Joint Commission on Accreditation of Healthcare Organizations. Some serve only students; others provide services for faculty, staff, and family members.

On some campuses, health educators work with the student health centers to provide counseling on such topics as nutrition; tobacco, drug, and alcohol abuse; exercise and fitness; sexuality; and contraception. Some college health centers provide psychological counseling, as well as dental, pharmacy, and optometric services. Some campuses also provide sports-medicine services for student

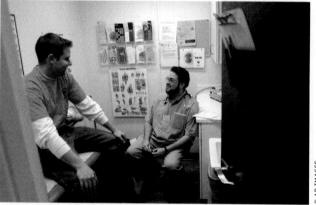

Student health centers on campus offer a variety of services.

athletes. Services are paid for by various combinations of prepaid health fees, general university funds, fee-for-service charges, and health-insurance reimbursements.

Outpatient Treatment Centers

Increasingly, procedures that once required hospitalization, such as simple surgery, are being performed at outpatient centers, which may be freestanding or affiliated with a medical center. Patients have any necessary tests performed beforehand, undergo surgery or receive treatment, and return home after a few hours to recuperate. Outpatient centers can handle many common surgical procedures, including cataract removal, tonsillectomy, breast biopsy, dilation and curettage (D and C), vasectomy, and face-lifts.

Without the high overhead costs of a hospital, outpatient surgery costs run only about 30 to 50 percent of standard hospital fees. Today, 70 percent of hospitals do outpatient, or "in-and-out," surgery. To cut health-care costs, insurance companies are encouraging, or in some cases requiring, their policyholders to choose outpatient surgery. However, operations requiring prolonged general anesthesia or extensive postoperative care still must be performed on an inpatient basis.

Freestanding emergency or urgent-care centers (those not part of a hospital) claim that they deliver high-quality medical treatment with maximum convenience in minimal time. Rather than going to crowded hospital emergency rooms when they slice a finger in the kitchen, patients can go to a freestanding emergency center and receive prompt attention.

Hospitals and Medical Centers

Different types of hospitals offer different types of care. The most common type of hospital is the *private*, or community, *hospital*, which may be run on a profit or a nonprofit basis, generally contains 50 to 400 beds and provides more personalized care than public hospitals do. The quality of care individual patients receive depends mostly on the physicians themselves. Public *hospitals* include city, county, public health service, military, and Veterans Administration hospitals. The quality of patient care depends on the overall quality of the institution.

Of the more than 6,500 hospitals nationwide, about 300 are major *academic medical centers* or teaching hospitals. Affiliated with medical schools, they generally provide the most up-to-date and experienced care, because staff physicians must stay current in order to teach their students. These centers, with the best equipment, researchers, and resources, offer high-technology care—at a price. The cost of treatment at all teaching hospitals averages approximately 20 percent higher than at nonteaching hospitals. At major teaching hospitals with large graduate training programs for physicians and other health providers, the

costs are as much as 45 percent higher than those at nonteaching hospitals.

The Joint Commission on the Accreditation of Healthcare Organizations (JCAH) reviews all hospitals every three years. Eighty percent of hospitals qualify for JCAH accreditation. If you have to enter a hospital and your health insurance or plan allows a choice, try to find out as much as you can about the alternatives available to you:

- Talk to your physician about a hospital and why he or she recommends it.

- As a cost-cutting strategy, many hospitals have cut back on the use of registered nurses. Check with the local nursing association about the ratio of patients to nurses, and the ratio of RNs to LPNs.

- Find out room rates and charges for ancillary services, including tests, lab work, X-rays, and medications. Check with your health plan to see whether you need preapproval for any of these costs and ask what you will be expected to pay.

- Ask how many times in the past year the hospital has performed the procedure recommended for you, and what the success and complication rates have been. Ask about the hospital's nosocomial (hospital-caused) infection rate and accident rate. You also have the right to information on the number and types of malpractice claims filed against a hospital.

- If possible, go on a tour of the hospital. Does the setting seem comfortable? Is the staff courteous? Does the hospital seem clean and efficiently run?

Emergency Services   Hospital emergency rooms should be used only in a true emergency. Most are overwhelmed, understaffed, and underfinanced—particularly in big cities. Patients usually see a different physician each time; he or she deals with the main complaints but doesn't have time for a full examination. Extensive tests and procedures are difficult to arrange in an emergency room, and patients who don't have truly urgent problems may have to wait for a long time. Emergency-room fees are higher than those for standard office visits and are not always covered by medical insurance.

Inpatient Care   Inpatient hospital care remains the most expensive form of health care. Health-insurance companies and health-care plans (described on pages 508–510) often demand a second opinion or make their own evaluation before approving coverage of an elective, or nonemergency, hospital admission. As another means

primary care   Ambulatory or outpatient care provided by a physician in an office, emergency room, or clinic.

of controlling costs, health insurers (including Medicare) may limit hospital stays or pay for hospital care on the basis of **diagnostic-related groups,** or **DRGs.** Under this system, hospitals are paid according to a patient's diagnosis—for example, a set number of dollars for every appendectomy. If the hospital can treat and discharge patients more quickly than the national average for that DRG, it makes money. On the other hand, if a patient develops unexpected complications or is slow to recover, the hospital loses money.

Because hospital stays are shorter than in the past, patients often leave "quicker and sicker"—after a shorter stay and not as far along in their recovery. Nevertheless, the benefits of shorter hospital stays, including reduced risk of infection and more rapid resumption of normal life activities, may outweigh the slightly increased risks associated with early discharge.

Home Health Care

With hospitals discharging patients sooner, **home health care**—the provision of equipment and services to patients in the home to restore or maintain comfort, function, and health—has become a major industry. Advances in technology have made it possible for treatments once administered only in hospitals—such as kidney dialysis, chemotherapy, and traction—to be performed at home at 10 to 40 percent of the cost. The physician's house call, once considered an anachronism, has also come back in fashion. According to various surveys, the majority of primary care physicians will see patients in their homes.

Hospital discharge planners usually arrange home health care for patients who've been hospitalized. Families can also contact health aides, nurses, and other needed professionals on their own. According to the Health Insurance Association of America, most private insurance policies offer some coverage for these home health-care costs.

Paying for Health Care

Many individuals with insurance are covered under an employer-based plan (options offered and partially funded by their employer). Individual health insurance coverage, though more costly, can be obtained through some companies. Uninsured persons depend on their own ability to pay, their qualifying for government insurance, or the care that physicians and institutions donate to those unable to pay.[14]

Your health plan affects many things, including:

- **Who** will care for you (doctors and other health-care providers), and how much choice you will have.
- **What** kind of care you will receive (for example, which preventive services are covered).

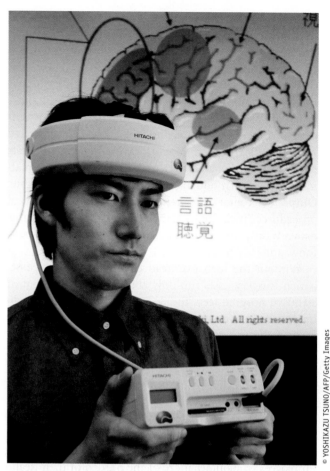

Innovations in medical technology are providing new options for the diagnosis and treatment of many disorders of the brain and body.

- **Where** you will receive your care (which hospitals, for example).
- **When** you will receive your care (will you receive it when you need it).
- **How** you will be cared for (the quality of care you receive).
- **How much** you will pay.

Indemnity Insurance

Indemnity insurance covers some health expenses (usually at a set percentage of the charge) and allows an individual to select a physician or a hospital without restrictions. Patients are responsible for paying the portion of the medical bill that is not covered by insurance. This type of coverage has become uncommon.

Managed Care

Managed care has become the predominant form of health care in the United States. Managed-care organizations, which take various forms, deliver care through a network of physicians, hospitals, and other health-care professionals who agree to provide their services at fixed or discounted rates. Nine in ten physicians in the United States have contracted with managed-care companies.

Consumers in a managed-care group must follow certain procedures in advance of seeking care (for example, getting prior approval for a test or treatment) and must abide by a limit on reimbursement for certain services. Some procedures may be deemed unnecessary and not be covered at all. Patients who choose to see a physician who is not a participating member of the medical-insurance coverage group may have to pay the entire fee themselves.

Managed-care plans have been criticized for pressuring providers to "undertreat" patients—for example, sending them home from the hospital too soon or denying them costly tests or treatments. Members have complained of long waits, the need to switch primary physicians if their doctor leaves the plan, difficulty getting approval for needed services, and a sense that providers pay more attention to the bottom line than to the health needs of their patients.

As dissatisfaction with managed care has grown, consumers have demanded more choice of physicians, direct access to specialists, and the ability to go "out of network." In response to patients' complaints, many states have approved "patient protection acts" or "comprehensive consumer bills of rights."

According to the National Committee for Quality Assurance, managed-care plans have shown improvement in the delivery of care, but health-care costs continue to rise. As a result, employers are cutting back coverage and asking employees to shoulder more of the burden of their health care in the belief that consumers will seek more efficient care when they are required to pay more out of pocket.

Health Maintenance Organizations (HMOs)

Health maintenance organizations, or **HMOs,** are managed-care plans that emphasize routine care and prevention by providing complete medical services in exchange for a predetermined monthly payment. In a *group-model* HMO, physicians provide care in offices at a clinic run by the HMO. In an *individual practice association (IPA),* or network HMO, independent physicians provide services in their own offices. HMOs generally pay a fixed amount per patient to a physician or hospital, regardless of the type and number of services actually provided. This is called *capitation.*

Members of HMOs pay a regular, preset fee that usually includes diagnostic tests, routine physical exams, and vaccinations as well as treatment of illnesses. HMOs usually do not require a deductible, and copayments for medications or services are small. The primary drawback of standard HMOs is that the consumer is limited to a particular health-care facility and staff.

Preferred Provider Organizations (PPOs)

In a **preferred provider organization (PPO),** a third party—a union, an insurance company, or a self-insured business—contracts with a group of physicians and hospitals to treat members at a discount. PPO members may choose any physician within the network, and usually pay a 10 percent copayment for care within the system and a higher percentage (20 to 30 percent) for care elsewhere. PPOs generally require prior approval for expensive tests or major procedures.

A *point-of-service (POS)* plan is a PPO that permits patients to use physicians outside the network. Consumers pay the difference between the preferred provider's discounted fee and the outside physician's fee. A *gatekeeper* plan requires members to choose a primary physician, as in an HMO, who must approve all referrals to specialists.

When deciding on an HMO or PPO, use these questions as a guide:

- How many doctors can I choose from?
- Is the network made up of private or group practice physicians?
- Which doctors are accepting new patients?
- Can I change my primary care physician?
- What is the procedure for referrals to specialists?
- How easy is it to get an appointment?
- How far in advance must routine visits be scheduled?
- What arrangements are there for handling emergency care?
- What health-care services are offered?
- Are there limits on medical tests, surgery, or other services?
- What if I want or need a special service that is not covered?
- Which hospitals are used?
- What happens if I'm out of town and need medical attention?
- What is the yearly total for monthly premiums?
- Are there any copayments? For which services and how much?

diagnostic-related group (DRG) A category of conditions requiring hospitalization for which the cost of care has been determined prior to a client's hospitalization.

home health care Provision of medical services and equipment to patients in the home to restore or maintain comfort, function, and health.

indemnity insurance A form of insurance that pays a major portion of medical expenses after a deductible amount is paid by the insured person.

managed care Health-care services and reimbursement predetermined by third-party insurers.

health maintenance organization (HMO) An organization that provides health services on a fixed-contract basis.

preferred provider organization (PPO) A group of physicians contracted to provide health care to members at a discounted price.

POINT COUNTERPOINT *Who Should Pay for the Uninsured?*

POINT

Almost one in five Americans—including many families and young adults—has no health insurance. Unable to pay for routine care, they are at risk of developing serious illnesses that will cost far more to treat than to prevent. It is in society's best interest to make health care available to all, regardless of ability to pay.

COUNTERPOINT

The costs of providing universal health coverage are too great. Taxpayers who obtain health coverage through jobs or who pay independently should not bear the additional burden of underwriting care for those who cannot afford it.

YOUR VIEW

Do you think the nation has a responsibility to ensure that all citizens get health-care insurance? Or should health insurance be a personal responsibility? Who pays for your health care? Who will pay after you graduate from college? What will you do if you can't afford health insurance?

Government-Financed Insurance Plans

The government, through programs like Medicare and Medicaid, funds 45 percent of total U.S. health spending. Under Medicare, the federal government pays 80 percent of most medical bills, after a deductible fee, for people over age 65. Medicare also offers options for coverage of prescription medications.

Medicaid, a federal and state insurance plan that protects people with very low or no incomes, is the chief source of coverage for the unemployed. However, many unemployed Americans don't qualify because their family incomes are above the poverty line. Publicly insured patients are more likely than those with private insurance to receive inadequate care and to experience adverse health outcomes.

The Uninsured

The United States is the only industrialized nation that does not have national health insurance. More Americans lack health insurance coverage than a decade ago—an estimated 47 million. Many more experience temporary lapses in coverage or are underinsured, meaning that they don't have adequate coverage and are less likely to receive preventive care or routine checkups. Uninsured individuals who experience a change in health caused by an injury or a new chronic condition have more difficulty obtaining recommended care and are more likely to suffer a greater decline in short-term health.[15]

Racial and ethnic minorities are much more likely to be uninsured than white Americans. More than a third of the Hispanic population and over a quarter of Native Americans are uninsured, compared to 12 percent of whites. The uninsured rates among African Americans and Asian Americans are also much higher than among whites. Nearly one-third of the uninsured are Hispanic, despite the fact that Hispanics make up just 13 percent of the population. This disparity results from several factors, including citizenship issues and language barriers.

Young adults, 18 to 24 years of age, are more likely than any other age group to be uninsured. Of Americans between the ages of 18 and 24 years, almost a third are without medical insurance. (See Point/Counterpoint.)

A committee of the Institute of Medicine (IOM), after years of exhaustive study, has urged federal leaders to provide health insurance for everyone living in the United States. The consequences of being uninsured, the IOM concluded, include "worse health and earlier death," including 18,000 deaths every year. It proposed that coverage be universal (for all residents, not just citizens), continuous, affordable, sustainable, and provided in such a way as to promote access to high-quality care.

Learn It : Live It

Taking Charge of Your Health

You can do more to safeguard and enhance your well-being than any health-care provider. Here are some recommendations to keep in mind:

- **Trust your instincts.** You know your body better than anyone else. If something is bothering you, it deserves medical attention. Don't let your health-care provider—or your health plan administrator—dismiss it without a thorough evaluation.

- **Do your homework.** Go to the library or online and find authoritative articles that describe what you're experiencing. The more you know about possible causes of your symptoms, the more likely you are to be taken seriously.

- **Find a good primary care physician who listens carefully and responds to your concerns.** Look for a family doctor or general internist who takes a careful history, performs a thorough exam, and listens and responds to your concerns.

- **See your doctor regularly.** If you're in your twenties or thirties, you may not need an annual exam, but it's important to get checkups at least every two or three years so you and your doctor can get to know each other and develop a trusting, mutually respectful relationship.

- **Get a second opinion.** If you are uncertain of whether to undergo treatment or which therapy is best, see another physician and listen carefully for any doubts or hesitation about what you're considering.

- **Seek support.** Patient support and advocacy groups can offer emotional support, information on many common problems, and referral to knowledgeable physicians.

- **If your doctor cannot or will not respond to your concerns, get another one.** Regardless of your health coverage, you have the right to replace a physician who is not meeting your health-care needs.

- **Speak up.** If you don't understand, ask. If you feel that you're not being taken seriously or being treated with respect, say so. Sometimes the only difference between being a patient or becoming a victim is making sure your needs and rights are not forgotten or overlooked.

- **Bring your own advocate.** If you become intimidated or anxious talking to physicians, ask a friend to accompany you, to ask questions on your behalf and to take notes.

SELFSURVEY : *Are You a Savvy Health-Care Consumer?*

1. You want a second opinion, but your doctor dismisses your request for other physicians' names as unnecessary. What do you do?

   a. Assume that he or she is right and you would merely be wasting time.

   b. Suspect that your physician has something to hide and immediately switch doctors.

   c. Contact your health plan and request a second opinion.

2. As soon as you enter your doctor's office, you get tongue-tied. When you try to find the words to describe what's wrong, your physician keeps interrupting. When giving advice, your doctor uses such technical language that you can't understand what it means. What do you do?

   a. Prepare better for your next appointment.

   b. Pretend that you understand what your doctor is talking about.

   c. Decide you'd be better off with someone who specializes in complementary/alternative therapies and seems less intimidating.

3. You feel like you're running on empty, tired all the time, worn to the bone. A friend suggests some herbal supplements that promise to boost energy and restore vitality. What do you do?

   a. Immediately start taking them.

   b. Say that you think herbs are for cooking.

   c. Find out as much as you can about the herbal compounds and ask your doctor if they're safe and effective.

4. Your hometown physician's office won't give you a copy of your medical records to take with you to college. What do you do?

   a. Hope you won't need them and head off without your records.

   b. Threaten to sue.

   c. Politely ask the office administrator to tell you the particular law or statute that bars you from your records.

5. Your doctor has been treating you for an infection for three weeks, and you don't seem to be getting any better. What do you do?

   a. Talk to your doctor, by phone or in person, and say, "This doesn't seem to be working. Is there anything else we can try?"

   b. Stop taking the antibiotic.

   c. Try an herbal remedy that your roommate recommends.

6. Your doctor suggests a cutting-edge treatment for your condition, but your health plan or HMO refuses to pay for it. What do you do?

   a. Try to get a loan to cover the costs.

   b. Settle for whatever treatment options are covered.

   c. Challenge your health plan.

7. You call for an appointment with your doctor and are told nothing is available for four months. What do you do?

   a. Take whatever time you can get whenever you can get it.

   b. Explain your condition to the nurse or receptionist, detailing any symptoms and pain you're experiencing.

   c. Give up and decide you don't need to see a doctor at all.

8. Even though you've been doing sit-ups faithfully, your waist still looks flabby. When you see an ad for waist-whittling liposuction, What do you do?

    a. Call for an appointment.

    b. Talk to a health-care professional about a total fitness program that may help you lose excess pounds.

    c. Carefully research the risks and costs of the procedure.

9. You have a condition that you do not want anyone to know about, including your health insurer and any potential employer. What do you do?

    a. Use a false name.

    b. Give your physician a written request for confidentiality about this condition.

    c. Seek help outside the health-care system.

10. Your doctor suggests a biopsy of a funny-looking mole that's sprouted on your nose. Rather than using a laboratory that specializes in skin analysis, your HMO requires that all samples be sent to a general lab, where results may not be as precise. What do you do?

    a. Ask your doctor to request that a specialty pathologist at the general lab perform the analysis.

    b. Hope that in your case, the general lab will do a good-enough job.

    c. Threaten to change HMOs.

Answers

1: c; 2: a; 3: c; 4: c; 5: a; 6: c; 7: b; 8: b and c; 9: b; 10: a

Your Health Action Plan for Protecting Yourself from Medical Mistakes and Misdeeds

Just as physicians practice "defensive" medicine to protect themselves from legal liability, today's patients should take preventive steps to defend themselves from potentially harmful health services.

The Whats, Whys, and Hows of Medical Testing

- Before undergoing any test, find out why you need it. Get a specific answer, not a "just in case" or "for your peace of mind." If you've had the test before could the earlier results be used? Would a follow-up exam be just as helpful?

- Get some practical information as well: Should you do specific things before the test (such as not eat for a specified period)? How long will the test take? What will the test feel like? Will you need help getting home afterward?

- Check out the risks. Any invasive test—one that penetrates the body with a needle, tube, or viewing instrument—involves some risk of infection, bleeding, or tissue damage. Tests involving radiation also present risks, and some people develop allergic reactions to the materials used in testing.

- Get information on the laboratory that will be evaluating the test. Ask how often false positives or false negatives occur. (False positives are abnormal results indicating that you have a particular condition when you really don't; false negatives indicate that you don't have a particular condition when you really do.) Find out about civil or criminal negligence suits filed against the laboratory on charges such as failing to diagnose cervical cancer because of incorrect reading of Pap smears.

- You'll also want to know what happens when the test indicates a problem: Will the test be repeated? Will a different test be performed? Will treatment begin immediately? Could any medications you're taking (including nonprescription drugs, like aspirin) affect the testing procedures or results?

- If you have a test don't assume that no news is good news. Check back to get the results.

CENGAGENOW™ If you want to write your own goals for getting quality medical care or using CAM, go to the Wellness Journal at HealthNow: **academic.cengage.com/login**.

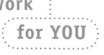

Making This Chapter Work for YOU

Review Questions

1. Which of the following statements about health information on the Internet is true?

    a. Chat rooms are the most reliable source of accurate medical information.

    b. Physicians who have websites must adhere to a strict set of standards set by the American Medical Association.

    c. Government-sponsored sites such as that of the Centers for Disease Control and Prevention are excellent sources of accurate health-care information.

    d. The Internet is a safe and cost-effective source of prescription drugs.

2. In a preclinical trial,

    a. researchers examine the cost-effectiveness of a specific treatment.

    b. animals are used to test new medical treatments.

    c. humans are used to test new medical treatments.

    d. the health status of a large group of people who exhibit certain health habits is reviewed.

3. Periodontal disease

    a. results from poor eating habits.

    b. can lead to cardiovascular problems.

c. in its early stage can be prevented by brushing alone.

d. is caused by a variety of bacteria and viruses.

4. During a medical exam, your doctor will
   a. check your cardiovascular system by listening to your heart and feeling your neck arteries.
   b. check your lungs by probing for tender spots and malformations.
   c. look into your eyes to see if you have vision problems that require glasses or contact lenses.
   d. evaluate your joints by tapping on the knees and elbows.

5. Informed consent means that
   a. the patient has informed the doctor of his or her symptoms and has consented to treatment.
   b. the physician has informed the patient about the treatment to be given and has consented to administer the treatment.
   c. the patient has informed the doctor of his or her symptoms, and the doctor has consented to administer treatment.
   d. the physician has informed the patient about the treatment to be given, and the patient has consented to the treatment.

6. Patients have all the rights below except which of the following? The right:
   a. to access their medical records.
   b. to medical care that meets accepted standards of quality.
   c. to donate a body part for compensation.
   d. to leave the hospital against their physician's advice.

7. People use complementary and alternative therapies
   a. to spend less money on health care.
   b. to take an active role in their own treatment.
   c. to show their disdain for the medical establishment.
   d. to take more prescription drugs.

8. Which statement is *false?*
   a. Acupuncture has been shown to control nausea in patients after surgery.
   b. Chiropractic has been shown to relieve acute lower-back pain.
   c. People can learn to control involuntary functions through biofeedback.
   d. Naturopathy is based on the premise that like cures like.

9. Which of the following statements about the health-care system is true?
   a. Primary care is usually provided by specialists in a hospital.
   b. Nurses can perform some surgical procedures once they are board certified.
   c. Most hospitals in the United States are teaching hospitals and affiliated with medical schools.

d. The length of hospital stays may be determined by a patient's diagnosis rather than the person's pace of recovery.

10. Managed care features all of the following except
    a. health maintenance organizations.
    b. a fee-for-service system of insurance.
    c. preferred provider organizations.
    d. limitations on reimbursement for certain health services.

Answers to these questions can be found on page 583.

Critical Thinking

1. Think about an experience you've had with a traditional medical practitioner. How did you feel during the physical examination? Did you trust the practitioner? Were you comfortable with the level of communication? Evaluate your experience and give your opinion of the value of the checkup.

2. Have you used any complementary or alternative approaches to health care? If so, were you satisfied with the results? How did your experience with the CAM therapist compare with your most recent experience with a traditional medical practitioner? Do you feel confident that you know the difference between alternative care and quackery?

3. If you're young and healthy, you'll have little problem getting health insurance. However, if you develop a chronic illness, sustain serious injuries in an accident, or simply get older, you may find insurance harder to get and more expensive to keep. What is your insurance coverage? Do you believe insurance companies have the right to turn down applicants with preexisting conditions, such as high blood pressure? Do they have the right to require screening for potentially serious health problems, such as HIV infection, or to cancel the policies of individuals who have run up high medical bills in the past?

4. Jocelyn has been experiencing a great deal of fatigue and frequent headaches for the past couple of months. She doesn't have health insurance and doesn't want to spend money on a doctor visit. So she did some research on the Internet about ways to relieve her symptoms and was considering taking a couple of herbal supplements that were touted as potential treatments. If she asked you for your advice, what would you tell her? Do you think that self-care is appropriate in this situation?

Media Menu

CENGAGENOW™ Go to the HealthNow website at **academic.cengage .com/login** that will:
- Help you evaluate your knowledge of the material.
- Allow you to take an exam-prep quiz.
- Provide a Personalized Learning Plan targeting resources that address areas you should study.

- Coach you through identifying target goals for behavioral change and creating and monitoring your personal change plan throughout the semester.

INTERNET CONNECTIONS

National Health Information Center

www.health.gov/nhic/

This excellent site, sponsored by the National Health Information Center (NHIC) of the U.S. Office of Disease Prevention and Health Promotion, is a health information referral service providing health professionals and consumers with a database of various health organizations. The site provides a searchable database, publications, and a list of toll-free numbers for health information.

National Center for Complementary and Alternative Medicine

http://nccam.nih.gov

This National Institutes of Health site features a variety of fact sheets on alternative therapies and dietary supplements, research, current news, and databases for the public as well as for practitioners.

MedicineNet

www.medicinenet.com

This comprehensive site is written for the consumer by board-certified physicians and contains medical news, a directory of procedures, a medical dictionary, a pharmacy, and first aid information. You can use the information at MedicineNet.com to prepare for a doctor visit, learn about a diagnosis, or understand a prescribed treatment or procedure.

U.S. Food and Drug Administration

www.fda.gov

In addition to providing information on regulation and legislation relating to food and drugs, the FDA website offers information on strategies for evaluating health products and services.

Key Terms

The terms listed are used and defined on the page indicated. Definitions are also found in the Glossary at the end of this book.

acupuncture	**503**
Ayurveda	**503**
chiropractic	**505**
complementary and alternative medicine (CAM)	**501**
diagnostic-related groups (DRGs)	**509**
gingivitis	**493**
gum disease	**493**
health maintenance organization (HMO)	**509**
herbal medicine	**505**
holistic	**501**
home health care	**509**
homeopathy	**503**
indemnity insurance	**509**
informed consent	**498**
integrative medicine	**503**
managed care	**509**
medical history	**495**
meta-analysis	**491**
naturopathy	**503**
outcomes	**497**
Pap smear	**497**
periodontitis	**493**
plaque	**493**
preferred provider organization (PPO)	**509**
primary care	**507**
quackery	**498**
vital signs	**491**

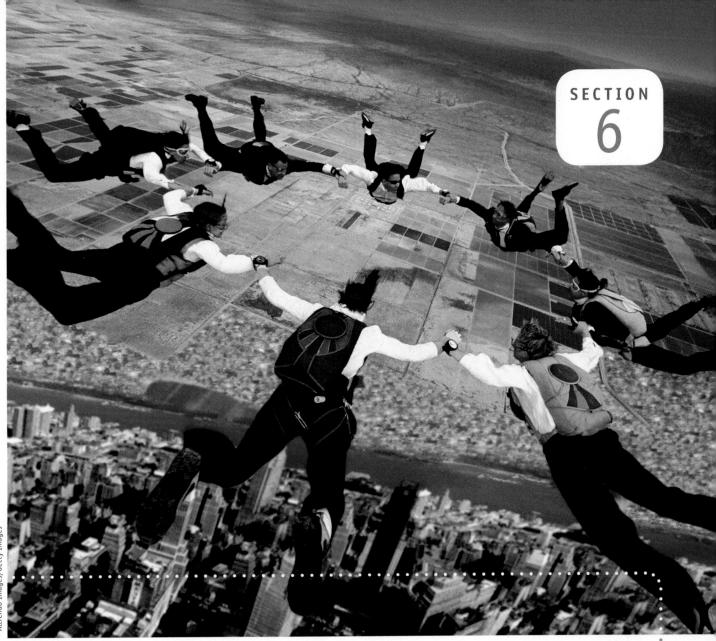

Health in Context

PERSONAL health involves more than a single individual. We are social beings, and we live our lives as part of a network of family, friends, acquaintances, colleagues, neighbors. Our actions affect others; others' behaviors have a significant impact on our well-being.

For college students, staying safe is an essential part of staying healthy. Injury claims more lives of young Americans than illness. Threats such as violence and terrorism are too serious and widespread to ignore.

All of us share something else: our planet. The problems of creating a healthy environment are many and complex. They too demand our attention and commitment.

Aging and dying are as much a part of the real world as life itself. The quest to find fulfillment in living and meaning in dying is one of the challenges of living.

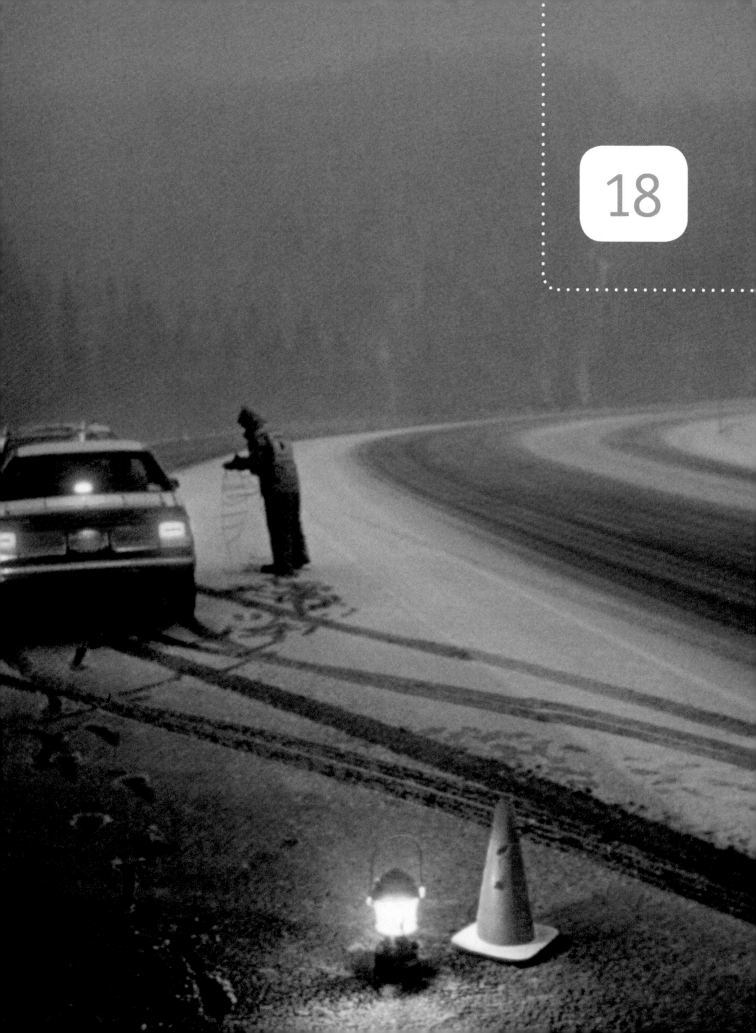

18

Protecting Yourself from Injury, Violence, and Victimization

THIS can't be happening to me!" This was the phrase that first ran through Parker's mind when the car swerved out of control. He kept repeating it to himself as he heard the sickening sound of metal hitting metal and felt a terrible crushing pain shoot up through his legs. Later at the hospital, when he woke up after surgery, it was his first thought. And all through the long months of rehabilitation, on the days when he thought life would never go back to normal, he'd try to tell himself that this too couldn't be happening to him.

Most young people think the same way. Accidents, injuries, assaults, crimes—all seem like things that happen only to other people, only in other places. But no one, regardless of how young, healthy, or strong, is immune from danger. The risks to college students include alcohol-associated injuries and illnesses, traffic accidents, and physical and sexual assaults.

Recognizing the threat of intentional and unintentional injury is the first step to ensuring your personal safety. You may think that the risk of something bad happening is simply a matter of chance, of being in the wrong place at the wrong time. That's not the case. Certain behaviors, such as using alcohol or drugs or not buckling your seat belt, greatly increase the risk of harm. Ultimately, you have more control over your safety than anyone or anything else in your life. (See "Your Guardian Angel" lab in *IPC*.) **IPC**

This chapter is a primer in self-protection that could help safeguard—perhaps even save—your life. Included are recommendations for common sense safety on the road, at home, and at work. This chapter also explores other serious threats to personal safety in our society: violence and sexual victimization.

After studying the material in this chapter, you should be able to:

- **List** and **explain** factors that increase the likelihood of an accident.

- **Name** four key factors in driving safely.

- **Describe** safety hazards at work and at home.

- **Define** sexual victimization, sexual harassment, stalking, and sexual coercion.

- **List** the different types of rape, and describe recommended actions for preventing rape.

- **Explain** the consequences of sexual violence.

- **Assess** your risk of sexual or social violence, and make a plan to lower that risk.

CENGAGENOW™ Log on to HealthNow at **academic.cengage.com/login** to find your Behavior Change Planner and to explore self-assessments, interactive tutorials, and practice quizzes.

© Bob Witkowski/Workbook Stock/Jupiter Images

Personal Safety

The major threat to the lives of college students isn't illness but injury. Almost 75 percent of deaths among Americans 15 to 24 years old are caused by "unintentional injuries" (a term public health officials prefer), suicides, and homicides. Accidents, especially motor vehicle crashes, kill more college-age men and women than all other causes combined; the greatest number of lives lost to accidents is among those 25 years of age.[1]

Unintentional Injury: Why Accidents Happen

Some of the many factors that influence an individual's risk of accident or injury are these:

- **Age.** Injury is the leading cause of death during the first four decades of life in the United States. Most victims of fatal accidents are males, often in their teens and twenties. Feeling full of life and energy, they may take dangerous risks because they think they're invulnerable.

- **Alcohol.** An estimated 40 percent of Americans are involved in an alcohol-related accident sometime during their lives. Alcohol plays a role in about a quarter of fatal motor vehicle accidents and half of fatal motorcycle crashes.

- **Stress.** When we're tense and anxious, we all pay less attention to what we're doing. One common result is an increase in accidents. If you find yourself having a series of small mishaps or near-misses, do something to lower your stress level, rather than wait for something more harmful to happen (see Chapter 3).

- **Situational Factors.** Some situations—such as driving on a curvy, wet road in a car with worn tires—are so inherently dangerous that they greatly increase the odds of an accident. But even when there's greater risk, you can lower the danger: For instance, you can make sure your tires and brakes are in good condition.

- **Thrill Seeking.** To some people, activities that others might find terrifying—such as skydiving or parachute jumping—are stimulating. These thrill seekers may have lower than normal levels of the brain chemicals that regulate excitement. Because the stress of potentially hazardous sports may increase the levels of these chemicals, they feel pleasantly aroused rather than scared.

Accidents can happen to anyone at any time, so it's important that you be prepared. See Your Strategies for Prevention: "What to Do in an Emergency."

Safe Driving

With more drivers and more vehicles on the roads than ever before, accidents kill 43,340 people a year.[2] Alcohol use is a factor in about 40 percent of these crashes; speeding, in about one-third. Rollovers caused by drivers who lose control of their vehicles kill about 25 people daily. Crashes involving teen drivers result in about 25 fatalities each day. Motor vehicle accidents injure almost three million people, more than any other form of unintentional injury.

College students aren't necessarily safer drivers than others their age. According to national data, full-time college students drink and drive more often than part-time students and other young adults, but they also are more likely to wear seat belts

---

YOUR STRATEGIES FOR PREVENTION *What to Do in an Emergency*

Life-threatening situations rarely happen more than once or twice in any person's life. When they do, you must think and act quickly to prevent disastrous consequences.

- **Stop, look, and listen.** Your immediate response to an emergency may be overwhelming fear and anxiety. Take several deep breaths. Start by assessing the circumstances. Look for any possible dangers to you or the victim, such as a live electrical wire or a fire. Listen for sounds, such as a cry for help or a siren. Don't attempt rescue techniques, such as cardiopulmonary resuscitation (CPR), unless you're trained.

- **Don't wait for symptoms to go away or get worse.** If you suspect that someone is having a heart attack or stroke, or has ingested something poisonous, *phone for help immediately.* A delay could jeopardize the person's life. Stay on the line long enough to give your name, address, and a brief description of the emergency.

- **Don't move a victim.** The person may have a broken neck or back, and attempting to move him or her could cause extensive damage or even death.

- **Don't drive.** Even if the hospital is just ten minutes away, you're better off waiting for a well-equipped ambulance with trained paramedics who can deliver

emergency care on the spot. People rushing to emergency rooms are more likely to get into accidents themselves.

- **Don't do too much.** Often well-intentioned good Samaritans make injuries worse by trying to tie tourniquets, wash cuts, or splint broken limbs. Also, don't give an injured person anything to eat or drink.

- **At home, keep a supply of basic first-aid items in a convenient place.** Beyond the emergency number 911, make sure that telephone numbers for your doctor and neighbors are handy.

while driving and riding in cars. How can you increase your odds of staying safe on the road? Some key factors are staying sober and alert, using your seat belt, making sure your vehicle has working air bags, and controlling road rage. The number-one culprit in car crashes is distraction—whether by chatting on the phone, fiddling with a radio, or eating.

Stay Sober and Alert

The number of fatalities caused by drunk driving, particularly among young people, has dropped. The National Highway Traffic Safety Administration (NHTSA) attributes this decline to increases in the drinking age, to educational programs aimed at reducing nighttime driving by teens, to the formation of Students Against Destructive Decisions (SADD; originally called Students Against Drunk Driving) and similar groups, and to changes in state laws that lowered the legal blood-alcohol concentration level for drivers under age 21 (some states have zero tolerance blood-alcohol level (BAC) for drivers under 21).

Falling asleep at the wheel is second only to alcohol as a cause of serious motor-vehicle accidents. About half of drivers in the United States drive while drowsy. Nearly 14 million have fallen asleep at the wheel in the past year, according to the National Sleep Foundation. Men and young adults between the ages of 18 and 29 are at the highest risk for driving while drowsy or falling asleep at the wheel.

Buckle Up

Seat belt use has reached an all-time high, with three in four Americans buckling up. States with seat belt laws have even higher rates of use: 80 percent. However, young people are less likely to use seat belts. Men between ages 19 and 29 are least likely to wear seat belts while driving or riding in a car. By official estimates, two-thirds of 15 to 20-year-olds killed in motor vehicle accidents were not wearing seat belts. Unbelted crash occupants are three times as likely to die in an emergency department while undergoing treatment.[3]

Seat belts save an estimated 9,500 lives in the United States each year. When lap-shoulder belts are used properly, they reduce the risk of fatal injury to front-seat passengers by 45 percent and the risk of moderate to critical injury by 50 percent. Because an unrestrained passenger can injure others during a crash, the risk of death is lowest when all occupants wear seat belts, according to federal analysts. Seat belt use by everyone in a car may prevent about one in six deaths that might otherwise occur in a crash.

Check for Air Bags

An air bag, either with or without a seat belt, has proved the most effective means of preventing adult death,

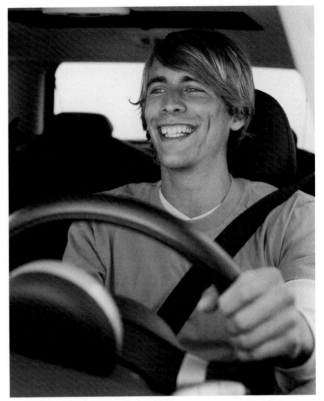

Buckling up is one of the simplest and most effective ways of protecting yourself from injury.

© Nick Clements/Digital Vision/Getty Images

somewhat more so for women than for men. However, they do not lower the risk of serious injury; seat belts do. Air bags used in conjunction with seat belts do not significantly reduce the risk of injury; without seat belts, they increase the risk of injury, particularly to the head and legs.

Because there is controversy over the potential hazard they pose to children, the American Academy of Pediatrics recommends that children be placed in the back seat, whether or not the car is equipped with a passenger air bag.

Rein in Road Rage

The emotional outbursts known as road rage are a factor in as many as two-thirds of all fatal car crashes and one-third of nonfatal accidents, according to the NHTSA. Psychologist Arnold Nerenberg of Whittier, California, a specialist in motorway mayhem, estimates 1.78 billion episodes of road rage occur each year, resulting in more than 28,000 deaths and 1 million injuries.[4]

Some strategies for reducing road rage include the following:

- **Lower the stress in your life.** Take a few moments to breathe deeply and relax your shoulders before putting the key in the ignition.

- **Consciously decide not to let other drivers get to you.** Decide that whatever happens, it's not going to make your blood pressure go up.

YOUR STRATEGIES FOR PREVENTION *How to Drive Safely*

- Don't drive while under the influence of alcohol or other drugs, including medications that may impair your reflexes, cause drowsiness, or affect your judgment. Never get into a car if you suspect the driver may be intoxicated or affected by a drug.

- Remain calm when dealing with drivers who are reckless or rude. Be alert and anticipate possible hazards. Don't let yourself be distracted by conversations, children's questions, arguments, food or drink, or scenic views.

- Don't get too comfortable. Alertness matters. Use the rearview mirror often. Don't let passengers or packages obstruct your view. Use turn signals when changing lanes or making a turn. If someone cuts you off, back off to a safe distance.

- Watch out for warning signs of fatigue, such as difficulty focusing, frequent blinking or heavy eyelids, trouble keeping one's head up; repeated yawning; trouble remembering the last few miles driven; and drifting from the lane or hitting the shoulder rumble strip.

- Drive more slowly if weather conditions are bad. Avoid driving at all during heavy rain, snow, or other conditions that affect visibility and road conditions. If you must drive in hazardous conditions, make sure that your car has the proper equipment, such as chains or snow tires, and that you know how to respond in case of a skid.

- Maintain your car properly, replacing windshield wipers, tires, and brakes when necessary. Keep flares and a fire extinguisher in your car for use in emergencies.

- **Slow down.** If you're going five or ten miles over the speed limit, you won't have the time you need to react to anything that happens.

- **Modify bad driving habits one at a time.** If you tend to tailgate slow drivers, spend a week driving at twice your usual following distance. If you're a habitual horn honker, silence yourself.

- **Be courteous—even if other drivers aren't.** Don't dawdle in the passing lane. Never tailgate or switch lanes without signaling. Don't use your horn or high beams unless absolutely necessary.

- **Never retaliate.** Whatever another driver does, keep your cool. Count to ten. Take a deep breath. If you yell or gesture at someone who's upset with you, the conflict may well escalate.

- **If you do something stupid, show that you're sorry.** On its website, the AAA Foundation for Traffic Safety solicited suggestions for automotive apologies. The most popular: slapping yourself on your forehead or the top of your head to indicate that you know you goofed. Such gestures can soothe a miffed motorist—and make the roads a slightly safer place for all of us.

For more tips on safe driving, see Your Strategies for Prevention, "How to Drive Safely."

Cell Phones and Safety

More than 231 million people use wireless communication devices such as cell phones—a drastic increase from the 4.3 million Americans who did so in 1990. According to a recent survey, most drivers—approximately seven in ten of those interviewed—talk on cell phones while driving, while about one in five sends and receives text messages.[5] In some states, it is now illegal to talk or text on a cell phone while driving.

Driver inattention is responsible for 25 to 30 percent of crashes. Drivers are most likely to be distracted by common activities, such as reaching for an item in the glove compartment or talking to passengers. However, motorists who use cell phones while driving are four times as likely to get into crashes serious enough to injure themselves. Even if the cell phone is a hands-free model, using it while driving is as dangerous as driving drunk.[6] The reason is that talking or texting while driving distracts the brain as well as the eyes—much more so than talking to another person in the vehicle. Conversation on any type of phone disrupts a driver's attention to the visual environment, leading to what researchers call "inattention blindness," the inability to recognize objects encountered in the driver's visual field. This form of cognitive impairment may distract drivers for up to two minutes after the phone conversation has ended.

On the other hand, cell phones are helpful in alerting authorities to road hazards, congestion, or problem drivers and in summoning help in case of a breakdown or other emergency.

Here are some tips for safer cell phone use:

- Find out if cell phone use while driving is legal in your state.

- Do not dial new calls until you're stopped.

- Keep calls short, less than 1 or 2 minutes.

- When you're on the phone, avoid difficult maneuvers, such as changing lanes, that require a lot of attention.

- Have a passenger send or receive calls.

- Invest in a hands-free model, especially if you use your phone regularly. While the cognitive distraction is the same, it helps to avoid the mechanical distraction.

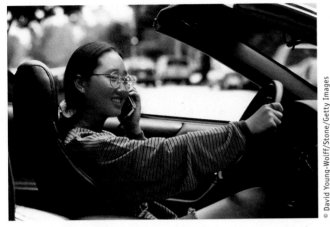

Any form of distraction, including talking on a cell phone, can put you and others at risk.

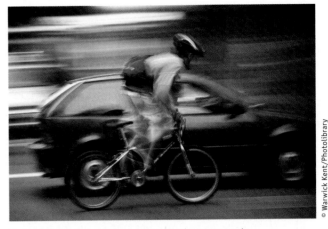

Wear a helmet whenever you get on a bicycle or motorcycle.

Safe Cycling

Mile for mile, motorcycling is far more risky than automobile driving. The most common motorcycle injury is head trauma, which can lead to physical disability, including paralysis and general weakness, as well as problems reading and thinking. It can also cause personality changes and psychiatric problems, such as depression, anxiety, uncontrollable mood swings, and anger. Complete recovery from head trauma can take four to six years, and the costs can be staggering. Head injury can also result in permanent disability, coma, and death. To prevent head trauma, motorcycle helmets are required in most states.

Approximately 80.6 million people ride bicycles. Each year, bicycle crashes kill about 750 to 1,500 of these individuals and send 450,000 to 587,000 to emergency rooms. Men are more likely to suffer cycling injuries. Head injury is the cause of 70 to 85 percent of bicycle crash deaths.

According to a national survey, 50 percent of all bicycle riders in the United States regularly wear bike helmets—43 percent every time they ride and 7 percent more than half the time. Wearing a helmet can reduce head injuries and deaths by an estimated 29 to 90 percent, depending on the type of helmet. (See Savvy Consumer: "How to Buy a Bicycle Helmet.")

Safety at Work

The workplace is second only to the home as the most frequent site of accidents. The industries with the highest fatality rates are mining; transportation, communication, and public utilities; construction; and agriculture, forestry, and fishing. Whatever your job, find out about potential hazards and learn the proper safety regulations. (Chapter 19 discusses some potential environmental hazards at work, including noise and toxic substances.)

According to a report by the National Research Council and Institute of Medicine, annually about one million workers suffer musculoskeletal disorders of the lower back and upper extremities as a result of their "particular jobs and working conditions—including heavy lifting, repeti-

▼Savvy_{Consumer} How to Buy a Bicycle Helmet

What should you look for when buying a helmet? Here are some basic guidelines:

- A government regulation requires all helmets produced after 1999 to meet the Consumer Product Safety Commission standard; look for a CPSC sticker inside the helmet. The ASTM (American Society for Testing and Materials) standard is comparable to CPSC. The Snell Memorial Foundation's B-90 standard is even better.
- Check the fit. The helmet should sit level on your head, touching all around, comfortably snug but not tight. The helmet should not move more than about an inch in any direction, regardless of how hard you tug at it.
- Pick a bright color for visibility. Avoid dark colors, thin straps, or a rigid visor that could snag in a fall.
- Look for a smooth plastic outer shell, not one with alternating strips of plastic and foam.
- Watch out for excessive vents, which put less protective foam in contact with your head in a crash.
- Mirrors should have a breakaway mount; the wire type mounted on eyeglasses can gouge an eye in a fall.

tive and forceful motions, and stressful working conditions." Many can be prevented.

Computers and Your Health

As computers have become part of daily life for everyone from preschoolers to seniors, health professionals have learned a great deal about potential health problems, including repetitive motion injuries and vision-related difficulties.

Repetitive Motion Injuries

Repetitive motion injuries (RMI) have surpassed back and neck injuries as the number one claim for workers compensation injuries. Repeated motions—such as the hand and arm movements made while using a computer keyboard—all day, every day, can result in muscle and tendon strain and inflammation. About 20 percent of people with pain, tingling, or numbness in the hands may have carpal tunnel syndrome, an overuse injury caused by repetitive motions in the hands and wrists. Symptoms include pain, swelling, and numbness and weakness in the hands or the arms. If these problems are identified early, permanent damage can generally be avoided by altering the work environment and allowing for more breaks during the day.

The slope and height of a computer keyboard can affect the likelihood of repetitive motion injuries. If you work at a computer, good posture and correct positioning of the computer screen and keyboard can help prevent repetitive motion injuries, eyestrain, and back strain (Figure 18.1). Here are some additional tips:

- Place the keyboard so that your elbows are bent at a 90° angle and you don't have to bend your wrists to type.
- Use a chair that provides ample back support. Keep your thighs parallel to the floor and your feet on the floor. If your feet don't reach the floor, use a footrest.
- If you experience neck strain, place a document holder next to your screen so that you can view the materials more easily.
- Every 15 minutes take a 30-second break, stretch your arms, and walk around the office. Take a 15-minute break at least once every two hours.

Vision Problems

Computer vision syndrome is a condition marked by tired and sore eyes, blurred vision, headaches, and neck, shoulder, and back pain. The American Optometric Association estimates that it afflicts nearly 90 percent of workers who use computers and also is common among children and students of all ages. The symptoms result

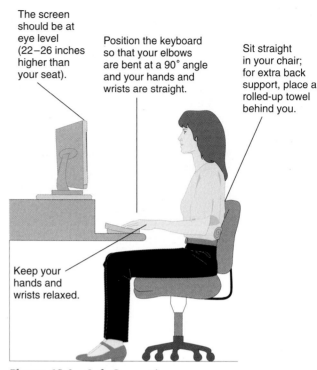

The screen should be at eye level (22–26 inches higher than your seat).

Position the keyboard so that your elbows are bent at a 90° angle and your hands and wrists are straight.

Sit straight in your chair; for extra back support, place a rolled-up towel behind you.

Keep your hands and wrists relaxed.

Figure 18.1 Safe Computing
By paying attention to your posture and your computer's position, you can help protect yourself from repetitive motion injury, back strain, and eyestrain.

from repeatedly stressing some aspect of the visual system, but they often disappear as soon as the person stops working at the computer.

The eye focuses on a computer image differently from the way it focuses on a printed one. The pixels that appear on a computer screen, unlike printed characters, are bright in the center and gradually fade away into the background color. This makes it difficult for the eye to sustain focus. Optometrists have developed a specific method, called a PRIO examination, that simulates how the eye responds to pixels on a computer screen. It can determine the need and proper prescription for computer-only eyeglasses.

Safety at Home

Every year home accidents cause nearly 25 million injuries. Poison poses the greatest threat, causing more than 17,000 deaths every year. Half a million children swallow poisonous materials each year; 90 percent are under age 5. Adults may also be poisoned by mistakenly taking someone else's prescription drugs or taking medicines in the dark and swallowing the wrong one. In most cities, you can call a poison control center for advice.

Falls of all kinds are the second leading cause of death from unintentional injury in the United States. High heels or worn footgear, poor lighting, slippery or uneven walkways, broken stairs and handrails, loose or worn rugs, and objects left where people walk all increase the likelihood of a slip.

You can prevent fires by making sure that the three ingredients of fire—fuel, a heat source, and oxygen—don't get a chance to mix. Almost anything can act as fuel for fire, including paper, wood, and flammable liquids such as oils, gasoline, and some paints. A heat source can be a spark from a lighted match, a pilot light, or an electrical wire. Oxygen is necessary for the chemical reaction between the fuel and heat source that causes combustion.

If a fire starts and it's small, you may be able to put it out with a portable fire extinguisher before it spreads. However, if the fire does get out of control, you might have only two to five minutes to get out of the house or building alive. A fire-escape plan can save time and lives. Sketch a plan of your house, apartment building, dormitory, or fraternity or sorority house. Identify two ways out of each room or apartment. Make sure everyone is familiar with these escape routes. Designate an area outside where all family members or dorm residents should meet after escaping from a fire.

In a national survey, 67 percent of colleges had at least one dorm without a sprinkler system. If a fire breaks out in your dorm room, get out as quickly as possible, but don't run. Before opening a room door, place your hand on it. If it's hot, don't open it. If the door feels cool, open it slightly to check for smoke; if there's none, leave by your planned escape route. If you're on an upper floor and your escape routes are blocked, open a window (top and bottom, if possible) and wait or signal from the window for help. Never try to use an elevator in a fire.

Which Gender Is at Greater Risk?

Just like illness, injury doesn't discriminate against either gender. Both men and women can find themselves in harm's way—but for different reasons. Here are some gender differences in vulnerability:

- Men are ten times more likely to die of an occupational injury than women.

- Males are most often the victims and the perpetrators of homicides in the United States. In about 68 percent of cases reported by the Bureau of Justice Statistics, both the offender and the victim were male.

- Overall, men are 3.6 times more likely than women to be murdered and 9 times more likely to commit murder. Both men and women are more likely to kill or attempt to kill male victims than female victims.

- Men are more likely than women to be assaulted as adults.

Living in a Dangerous World

The World Health Organization (WHO) defines violence as "the intentional use of physical force or power, threatened or actual, against oneself, another person, or a group or community, that either results in, or has a high likelihood of resulting in, injury, death, psychological harm, maldevelopment, or deprivation." A simpler way of putting it is that "violence is anything you wouldn't want someone to do to you."[7] Although anyone is capable of violent crime, being aware of certain behaviors in a person may keep you safer. See Your Strategies for Prevention: "How to Recognize Potentially Violent People."

After more than a decade of declining rates, violent crime in the United States seems to be increasing. Guns are the second-leading cause of injury-related death in the United States after car accidents. About 260 Americans are injured by firearms every day; one-third die from their wounds. Gun violence annually takes the lives of nearly 30,000 Americans. (See "Point-Counterpoint.")

Although men commit nine times more violent crimes than women, the rates are getting closer. Individuals with mental illness are somewhat more likely to become violent and to be the victims of violent crimes.

There are ethnic and racial differences in patterns of violence. African Americans are at greater risk of victimization by violent crime than whites or persons of other racial groupings. Hispanics are at greater risk of violent victimization than non-Hispanics. There is little difference between white women and nonwhite women in rape, physical assault, or stalking. Native American and Alaska Native women are significantly more likely than white women or African American women to report being raped. Mixed-race women also have a significantly higher incidence of rape than white women. Native American and Alaska Native men report significantly more physical assaults than Asian and Pacific Islander men.

Crime and Violence on Campus

According to the Bureau of Justice, college students are victims of almost half a million violent crimes a year, including assault, robbery, sexual assault, and rape. While this number may seem high, the overall violent crime rate has dropped from 88 to 41 victimizations per 1,000 students in the last decade.[8]

repetitive motion injury (RMI) Inflammation of or damage to a part of the body due to repetition of the same movements.

computer vision syndrome A condition caused by computer use marked by tired and sore eyes, blurred vision, headaches, and neck, shoulder, and back pain.

College students ages 18 to 24 are less likely to be victims of violent crime, including robbery and assault, than nonstudents of the same age. More than half (58 percent) of crimes against students are committed by strangers. More than nine in ten occur off campus, most often in an open area or street, on public transportation, in a place of business, or at a private home. In about two-thirds of the crimes, no weapon is involved. Most off-campus crimes occur at night, while on-campus crimes are more frequent in the day.[9]

Male college students are twice as likely to be victims of overall violence than female students. White undergraduates have higher rates of violent victimization than students of other races. Simple assault accounts for two-thirds of violent crimes against students; sexual assault or rape account for around 6 percent.[10]

About three in four campus crimes are never reported to the police. The main reasons students give for not reporting crimes are that they are too minor or private or they are not certain that it was a crime. Individuals also may be too ashamed or emotionally overwhelmed to contact authorities.

According to researchers, only 2 percent of victimized college women report crimes to the police. The most frequent reason for not reporting sexual and physical incidents is that they didn't seem serious enough. However, women who were sexually victimized also felt ashamed, feared that they would be held responsible, or didn't want anyone to know what happened. Nonwhite women were significantly more likely than white women to say that they did not report an incident to the police because they

thought they would be blamed or because they did not want the police involved.[11]

The Jeanne Clery Disclosure of Campus Security Policy and Campus Crime Statistics Act, originally known as the Student Right-to-Know and Campus Security Act, requires colleges to publish annual crime statistics for their campuses. However, the act excludes certain offenses, such as theft, threats, harassment, and vandalism, so the picture it presents may not be complete. The most recent crime statistics for the nation's colleges, universities, and career schools are posted on the Internet at **http://ope.ed.gov/security**. How safe is your school? Take the Self Survey: "How Safe Is Your School?" on page xxx.

Because of concerns about safety on campus, more schools are taking tougher stands on student behavior. Many have established codes of conduct barring the use of alcohol and drugs, fighting, and sexual harassment. Many also have instituted policies requiring suspension or expulsion for students who violate this code.

Hazing

Hazing refers to any activity that humiliates, degrades, or poses a risk of emotional or physical harm for the sake of joining a group or maintaining full status in that group. This behavior may occur in fraternities and sororities, athletic teams, or other campus organizations. Its forms include verbal ridicule and abuse, forced consumption of alcohol or ingestion of vile substances, sexual violation, sleep deprivation, paddling, beating, burning, or branding.

POINT COUNTERPOINT *Guns on Campus*

POINT

According to the American College Health Association, 8 percent of college students keep a weapon on campus. Many contend that guns have no place on campus, and schools often ban all firearms. Advocates of gun control view the presence of guns as increasing the danger to their owners and to others.

COUNTERPOINT

Although violent crime remains uncommon on campuses, some students argue that they need a gun for self-defense. Opponents of gun control contended that if students were allowed to carry weap-

ons on campus, they might be able to defend themselves in case of an armed attack.

YOUR VIEW

Gun control is one of the most controversial topics in our society. Do you think weapons should be banned from college campuses? Or do you believe that every American, on or off campus, should have the right to own a gun?

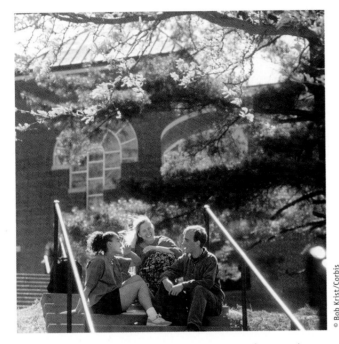

A peaceful scene like this doesn't mean that a campus is safe. Do you know the crime statistics for your college?

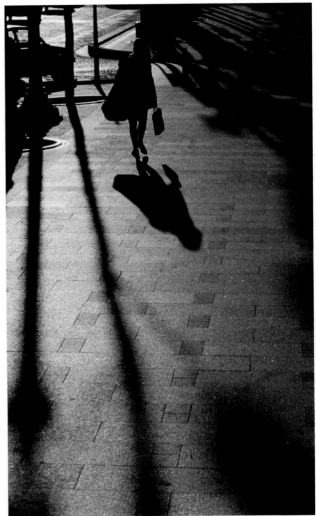

Does your campus have regular security patrols, surveillance cameras, or late-night escorts?

Hate or Bias Crimes

Recent years have seen the emergence of violent crimes motivated by hatred of a particular person's (or group of persons') race, ethnicity, religion, sexual orientation, or political values.

More than half of hate or bias crimes on campus are motivated by race. Twenty percent of students, faculty, and staff surveyed fear for their physical safety because of their sexual orientation or gender identity.[12] These crimes can take the form of graffiti; verbal slurs; bombings, threatening notes, emails, or phone calls; and physical attacks. They often generate fear and intimidation in large groups of students, undermining health, academic work, and the basic security of a campus.

Murders and Assaults

Mass shootings, such as the massacre at Virginia Tech University in 2007, are rare on college campuses. Murder and manslaughter also are uncommon. However, there are about 3,000 aggravated assaults—an attack with a weapon or one that causes serious injury—each year. Weapons were involved in about a third of violent college crimes. Firearms were used in 9 percent of all violent crimes and 8 percent of assaults.[13]

The American College Health Association, in its most recent "Campus Violence White Paper," has recommended various strategies to keep campuses safe, including:

* Enforcing codes of conduct.
* Tougher sanctions, including expulsion, for serious misconduct.
* Zero-tolerance policies for campus violence.
* Building a sense of community.
* Screening out students who pose a real threat.
* Warning students about criminal activity at orientation, through the campus newspaper, in residence halls, and through campus Internet communications devices.[14]

Consequences of Campus Violence

The toll of crime and violence at colleges and universities is high. Violence can cripple as well as claim lives. Moreover, the victims of violent crime often suffer lasting psychological and emotional effects. Some victims take a leave of absence or transfer to another school. Those who remain in school may have problems concentrating, studying, and attending classes, and may avoid academic and social activities. Some develop clinical symptoms that affect their mental and physical health (see Chapter 4).

Sexual Victimization and Violence

Sexual victimization refers to any situation in which a person is deprived of free choice and forced to comply with sexual acts. This is not only a woman's issue; in fact, men also are victimized. In recent years, researchers have come to view acts of sexual victimization along a continuum, ranging from street hassling, stalking, and obscene telephone calls to rape, battering, and incest.

Sexual Harassment

All forms of **sexual harassment** or unwanted sexual attention—from the display of pornographic photos to the use of sexual obscenities to a demand for sex by anyone in a position of power or authority—are illegal.

Nearly two-thirds of students experience sexual harassment at some point during college, including nearly one-third of first year students, according to a recent research report on campus sexual harassment. Nearly one-third of students say they have experienced physical harassment, such as being touched, grabbed, or pinched in a sexual way. Sexual comments and jokes are the most common form of harassment. More than half of female students and nearly half of male students say they have experienced this type of harassment. Lesbian, gay, bisexual, and transgender (LGBT) students are more likely than heterosexual students to be sexually harassed.[15]

Sexual harassment takes an especially heavy toll on female students, who often feel upset, self-conscious, embarrassed, or angry. Men are much less likely to admit to being very or somewhat upset. A third of harassed college women say they felt afraid; one-fifth say they were disappointed in their college experience as a result of sexual harassment.

More than a third of students who experience harassment tell no one; about half tell a friend. Only 7 percent of students say they reported sexual harassment to a faculty member or other college employee. More than half of students would like their college or university to offer a Web-based, confidential method for submitting complaints about sexual harassment. Nearly half would like their college or university to designate an office or person to contact about sexual harassment.

About half of college men and a third of women admit that they have sexually harassed someone on campus. Private college students are more likely than their public college peers to have ever done so. Students at large schools (population of 10,000 or more) are more likely than students at small schools with fewer than 5,000 students to say they have experienced sexual harassment. The most common rationale for harassment is "I thought it was funny." Harassment occurs in dorms or student housing

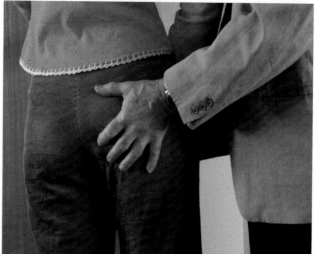

Sexual harassment can take many forms, ranging from suggestive comments to physical touching, and can occur in classrooms as well as workplaces.

as well as outside on campus grounds, in classrooms or lecture halls.[16]

If you encounter sexual harassment as a student, report it to the department chair or dean. If you don't receive an adequate response to your complaint, talk with the campus representatives who handle matters involving affirmative action or civil rights. Federal guidelines prevent any discrimination against you in terms of grades or the loss of a job or scholarship if you report harassment. Schools that do not take measures to remedy harassment could lose federal funds.

Stalking

The "willful, repeated, and malicious following, harassing, or threatening of another person," as stalking is defined, is common on college campuses—perhaps more so than in the general population. In studies, as many as 25 to 30 percent of female students and 11 to 17 percent of male students report having been stalked.

College students may be targeted for several reasons. Simply because they are young and still learning how to manage complex social relationships, some individuals may not recognize their behavior as stalking or even as disturbing. In addition, college students tend to live close to each other and to have flexible schedules and large amounts of unsupervised time.

Stalking is not a benign behavior and can result in emotional or psychological distress, physical harm, or sexual assault. By some estimates, 10 percent of stalking incidents result in forced or attempted sexual contact. The most common consequence is psychological, with victims reporting emotional or psychological distress.

Dating Violence

Actual or threatened physical or sexual violence or psychological and emotional abuse of a current or former dating partner is a form of violence. It can occur between heterosexual, homosexual, or bisexual partners.

 Over the course of five years (the national average for a college career), including summers and vacations, one of every four or five female students is raped. In a single academic year, 3 percent of coeds are raped—35 rapes for every 1,000 women. According to the Department of Justice, a campus with 6,000 coeds averages one rape a day every day for the entire school year. (See "Reality Check.")

In nine surveys of male university students, between 3 and 6 percent had been raped by other men; up to 25 percent had been sexually assaulted. Like female rape victims, male victims suffer long-term psychological problems, physical injuries, and are at risk of contracting a sexually transmitted infection.

Nonvolitional Sex and Sexual Coercion

Nonvolitional sex is sexual behavior that violates a person's right to choose when and with whom to have sex and what sexual behaviors to engage in. The more extreme forms of this behavior include sexual coercion or forced sex, rape, childhood sexual abuse, and violence against people with nonconventional sexual identities. Other forms, such as engaging in sex to keep one's partner or to pass as heterosexual, are so common that many think of them as normal.

Sexual coercion can take many forms, including exerting peer pressure, taking advantage of one's desire for popularity, threatening an end to a relationship, getting someone intoxicated, stimulating a partner against his or her wishes, or insinuating an obligation based on the time or money one has expended. Men may feel that they need to live up to the sexual stereotype of taking advantage of every opportunity for sex. Women are far more likely than men to encounter physical force.

 Eight in ten college students reported using verbal coercion and two in ten used physical coercion against a dating partner in one year.[17]

Rape

Rape refers to sexual intercourse with an unconsenting partner under actual or threatened force. Sexual intercourse between a male over the age of 16 and a female under the age of consent (which ranges from 12 to 21 in different states) is called *statutory rape*. In *acquaintance rape*, or *date rape*, the victim knows the rapist. In *stranger rape*, the rapist is an unknown assailant. Both acquain-

tance and stranger rapes are serious crimes that can have a devastating impact on their victims.

For many years, the victims of rape were blamed for doing something to bring on the attack. However, researchers have shown that women are raped because they encounter sexually aggressive men, not because they look or act a certain way. Although no woman is immune to attack, many rape victims are children or adolescents.

Women who successfully escape rape attempts do so by resisting verbally and physically, usually by yelling and fleeing. Women who use forceful verbal or physical resistance (screaming, hitting, kicking, biting, and running) are more likely to avoid rape than women who plead, cry, or offer no resistance.

Types of Rape

Although rape has long been viewed as an act of violence and domination, recent studies indicate that not all rapes fit into a single pattern. Within the broad category of rape are specific, but not mutually exclusive, subcategories of the crime, including anger rape, power rape, sadistic rape, gang rape, and sexual gratification rape.

Anger rape, usually on a total stranger, is motivated by hatred and a desire for revenge for the rejection the rapist feels he's suffered from women. Anger rapists often harbor long-standing hostility toward women, use far more physical violence than is needed for submission, and usually don't find the rape sexually gratifying.

Power rape is a generally premeditated attack motivated by a desire to dominate and control another person. Power rapists, unable to deal with stress and their sense of failure, may rape to regain a sense of power. They use only

sexual harassment Uninvited and unwanted sexual attention.

nonvolitional sex Sexual behavior that violates a person's right to choose when and with whom to have sex and what sexual behaviors to engage in.

sexual coercion Sexual activity forced upon a person by the exertion of psychological pressure by another person.

rape Sexual penetration of a female or a male by means of intimidation, force, or fraud.

REALITYCHECK

PART II: *Just the Facts*

- **20 to 25** *percent of college women are the victims of an attempted or completed rape.*

- **90** *percent of college women know the men who attacked them.*

- **5 to 15** *percent of college men say they've committed rape.*

- **43** *percent of college men say they have coerced women into having sex.*

Source: Carr, Joetta, et al. "Campus Violence White Paper." *Journal of American College Health*, Vol. 55, No. 5, March/April 2007, pp. 304–319.

as much force as needed to make their victims submit and may find the rape sexually gratifying, even though that's not their primary motive.

Sadistic rape is a premeditated assault that often involves bondage, torture, or sexual abuse. Sadistic rapists find power and anger sexually arousing and may subject victims to rituals of humiliation or torture. They're often preoccupied with violent pornography; their motives are more complex and difficult to understand than those of other types of rapists.

Gang rape involves three or more rapists. Men in close groups that drink and party together—such as fraternities or athletic teams—are more likely to participate in such assaults. The reasons may go beyond aggression and sexual gratification to the excitement and camaraderie the men feel while sharing the experience.

Sexual gratification rape is usually an impulsive attack by someone willing to use physical coercion for the sake of sex. These rapists generally use no more force than needed to get a partner to submit and may stop the attack if it becomes clear they'll have to use extreme violence to overcome resistance. Many acquaintance rapes fit into this category.

Acquaintance, or Date, Rape

The same factors that lead to other forms of sexual victimization can set the stage for date rape. Socialization into an aggressive role, acceptance of rape myths, and a view that force is justified in certain situations increase the likelihood of a man's committing date rape. Other factors can also play a role, including the following:

- **Personality and early sexual experiences.** Certain factors may predispose individuals to sexual aggression, including first sexual experience at a very young age, earlier and more frequent than usual childhood sexual experiences (both forced and voluntary), hostility toward women, irrespon-

sibility, lack of social consciousness, and a need for dominance over sexual partners.

- **Situational variables (what happens during the date).** Men who initiate a date, pay all expenses, and provide transportation are more likely to be sexually aggressive, perhaps because they feel they can call all the shots.

- **Rape-tolerant attitudes.** As several studies have confirmed, college men hold more rape-tolerant attitudes than do college women. For example, college men are significantly more likely than college women to agree with statements such as, "Some women ask to be raped and may enjoy it" and "If a woman says 'no' to having sex, she means 'maybe' or even 'yes.'"

  Some social groups, such as fraternities and athletic teams, may encourage the use of alcohol; reinforce stereotypes about masculinity; and emphasize violence, force, and competition. The group's shared values, including an acceptance of sexual coercion, may keep individuals from questioning their behavior.

- **Drinking.** Alcohol use is one of the strongest predictors of acquaintance rape. Men who've been drinking may not react to subtle signals, may misinterpret a woman's behavior as a come-on, and may feel more sexually aroused. At the same time, drinking may impair a woman's ability to effectively communicate her wishes and to cope with a man's aggressiveness.[18]

- **Date rape drugs.** Drugs such as Rohypnol (flunitrazepam) and GHB (gamma hydroxybutyrate) have been implicated in cases of acquaintance, or date,

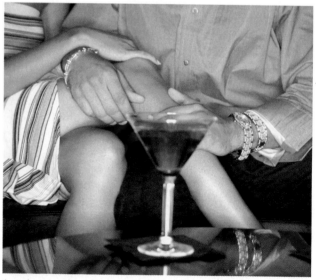

Acquaintance rape and alcohol use are very closely linked. Both men and women may find their judgment impaired or their communications unclear as a result of drinking.

© Masterfile

rape. Since both drugs are odorless and tasteless, victims have no way of knowing their drink has been tampered with. The subsequent loss of memory leaves victims with no explanation for where they've been or what's happened.

Rohypnol—which can cause impaired motor skills and judgment, lack of inhibitions, dizziness, confusion, lethargy, very low blood pressure, coma, and death—has been outlawed in the United States. Deaths also have been attributed to GHB overdoses.

- **Gender differences in interpreting sexual cues.** In research comparing college men and women, the men typically overestimated the woman's sexual availability and interest, seeing friendliness, revealing clothing, and attractiveness as deliberately seductive. In one study of date rape, the men reported feeling "led on," in part because their female partners seemed to be dressed more suggestively than usual.

Stranger Rape

Rape prevention consists primarily of making it as difficult as possible for a rapist to make you his victim:

- Don't advertise that you're a woman living alone. Use initials on your mailbox. Install and use secure locks on doors and windows, changing door locks after losing keys or moving into a new residence.

- Don't open your door to strangers. If a repairman or public official is at your door, ask him to identify himself and call his office to verify that he is a reputable person on legitimate business.

- Lock your car when it is parked, and drive with locked car doors. Should your car break down, attach a white cloth to the antenna and lock yourself in. If someone other than a uniformed officer stops to offer help, ask this person to call the police or a garage but do not open your locked car door.

- Avoid dark and deserted areas, and be aware of the surroundings where you're walking. Should a driver ask for directions when you're a pedestrian, avoid approaching his car. Instead, call out your reply from a safe distance.

- Have house or car keys in hand as you approach the door. Check the back seat before getting into your car.

- Carry a device for making a loud noise, like a whistle or, even better, a pint-sized compressed air horn available in many sporting goods and boat supply stores. Sound the noise alarm at the first sign of danger.

- Take a self-defense class to learn techniques of physical resistance that can injure the attacker or distract him long enough for you to escape.

Male Nonconsensual Sex and Rape

No one knows how common male rape is because men are less likely to report such assaults than women. Researchers estimate that the victims in about 10 percent of acquaintance rape cases are men. These hidden victims often keep silent because of embarrassment, shame, or humiliation, as well as their own feelings and fears about homosexuality and conforming to conventional sex roles.

Although many people think men who rape other men are always homosexuals, most male rapists consider themselves to be heterosexual. Young boys aren't the only victims. The average age of male rape victims is 24. Rape is a serious problem in prison, where men may experience brutal assaults by men who usually resume sexual relations with women once they're released.

Impact of Rape

Rape-related injuries include unexplained vaginal discharge, bleeding, infections, multiple bruises, and fractured ribs. Victims of sexual violence often develop chronic symptoms, such as headaches, backaches, high blood pressure, sleep disorders, pelvic pain, and sexual fertility problems. But sexual violence has both a physical and a psychological impact. The psychological scars of a sexual assault take a long time to heal. Therapists have linked sexual victimization with hopelessness, low self-esteem, high levels of self-criticism, and self-defeating relationships. An estimated 30 to 50 percent of women develop posttraumatic stress disorder (see Chapter 4) following a rape. Many do not seek counseling until a year or more after an attack, when their symptoms have become chronic or intensified.

Acquaintance rape may cause fewer physical injuries but greater psychological torment. Often too ashamed to tell anyone what happened, victims may suffer alone, without skilled therapists or sympathetic friends to reassure them. Women raped by acquaintances blame themselves more, see themselves less positively, question their judgment, have greater difficulty trusting others, and have higher levels of psychological distress. Nightmares, anxiety, and flashbacks are common. The women may avoid others, become less capable of protecting themselves, and continue to be haunted by sexual violence for years. A therapist can help these victims begin the slow process of healing.

What to Do in Case of Rape

Fewer than 5 percent of college rapes are reported.[19] Women who are raped should call a friend or a rape crisis center. A rape victim should not bathe or change her clothes before calling. Semen, hair, and material under her fingernails or on her apparel all may be useful in identifying the man who raped her.

A rape victim who chooses to go to a doctor or hospital should remember that she may not necessarily have to talk to police. However, a doctor can collect the necessary evidence, which will then be available if she later decides to report the rape to police. All rape victims should talk with a doctor or health-care worker about testing and treatment for sexually transmitted infections and postintercourse conception.

Even an unsuccessful rape attempt should be reported because the information a woman may provide about the attack—the assaulter's physical characteristics, voice, clothes, car, even an unusual smell—may prevent another woman from being raped.

Halting Sexual Violence

Sexual violence has its roots in social attitudes and beliefs that demean women and condone aggression. According to international research, much sexual violence takes place within families, marriage, and dating relationships. In many settings, rape is a culturally approved strategy to control and discipline women. In these places, laws and policies to improve women's status are critical to ending sexual coercion.

 Schools have developed more than 60 college sexual health prevention programs. Providing such experiences to incoming freshmen, according to researchers, has a positive impact on the behavior of most heterosexual women and men. However, both

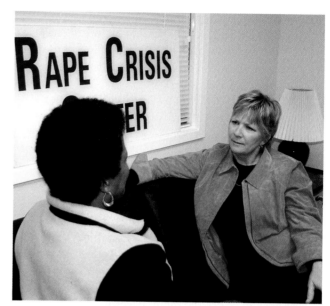

©Geri Engberg/The Image Works

Counseling from a trained professional can help ease the trauma suffered by a rape victim.

heterosexual students and homosexual students who have been sexually assaulted in the past remain vulnerable to more abuse.[20]

All men and women should recognize misleading rape myths and develop effective ways of communicating to avoid misinterpretation of sexual cues. Students should also know to whom they can turn to learn more about and seek help for sexual victimization: counselors, campus police, deans of student affairs, fraternity or sorority representatives, and campus ministers.

Your Life Change Coach

Preventing Date Rape

According to data from the U.S. Bureau of Justice, nine in ten reported rapes and sexual assaults in the United States involve a single offender with whom the victim had a prior relationship.

Both women and men report having been forced into sexual activity by someone they know. Many college students are in the age group most likely to face this threat: women aged 16 to 25 and men under 25. Women are most vulnerable and men are most likely to commit assaults during their senior year of high school and their first year of college.

Women who describe incidents of sexual coercion that meet the legal definition of rape often don't label it as such. They may have a preconceived notion that true rape consists of a blitzlike attack by a stranger. Or they may blame themselves for getting into a situation in which they couldn't escape. They may feel some genuine concern for others who would be devastated if they knew the truth (for example, if the rapist were the brother of a good friend or the son of a neighbor).

Here are strategies that can lower your risk of being involved in a date rape:

 For men:

- Remember that it's okay not to "score" on a date.
- Don't assume that a sexy dress or casual flirting is an invitation to sex.
- Be aware of your partner's actions. If she pulls away or tries to get up, understand that she's sending you a message—one you should acknowledge and respect.

While most campuses provide self-defense seminars for potential female victims of rape and general campus safety measures, some have tried innovative approaches, such as Men Against Violence, a peer-education program that confronts male students' conceptions of manhood and appropriate gender roles to reduce their likelihood of sexual or physical violence. Such all-male, peer-guided approaches that challenge myths about rape and rape victims also have proved effective with college fraternity men.

In addition, practical institutional steps—such as providing adequate lighting, escort services, and clear policies against both violence and drug and alcohol abuse—can help. Self-defense classes teach women how to avoid becoming victims either by escaping or protecting themselves. Follow-up studies of college women have found that self-defense training increased their sense of control over their life, confidence, security, independence, and physical prowess.

Campuses are also providing secondary prevention by getting help to victims of sexual violence as soon as possible through rape-crisis teams and emergency mental-health services, and tertiary prevention by working with victims to ameliorate the long-term effects of their experience through psychotherapy, educational services, and medical care.

Learn It : Live It

Helping the Victims of Violence

As their numbers have grown and their anguish has been recognized, the victims of violence have received greater attention. Hundreds of shelters for battered wives and their children have been set up across the country. They offer physical and psychological treatment and a haven where women can begin to rebuild their shattered self-esteem, as well as their daily lives. Rape counseling and crisis centers on college campuses and in the community provide various forms of assistance to victims of rape. In many cities, the telephone directory lists hot lines and resources. More than 400 victims' advocacy groups have been set up across the country to advise those hurt by crime. Support organizations help many survivors deal with the emotional aftermath of their experiences.

Sometimes well-intentioned friends and relatives add to the stress felt by the victims of violence. Here's how to offer comfort without implying criticism:

- **Don't try to deny that it happened.** Although it may be hard to talk about—or even listen to—what happened, the reality of the event must not be ignored. Denial makes victims doubt their own experience and question themselves at a time when they crave reassurance.

- **Don't pressure the victim to talk—or not to talk.** Some individuals need to go over every detail of what happened, again and again, until they work out their feelings of outrage and become ready to get on with their lives. Others find going into details too humiliating. Let the victim set the tone and limits for disclosure. Don't pry or prod.

- Restrict drinking, drug use, or other behaviors (such as hanging out with a group known to be sexually aggressive in certain situations) that could affect your judgment and ability to act responsibly.

- Think of the way you'd want your sister or a close female friend to be treated by her date. Behave in the same manner.

 For women:
  - If the man pays for all expenses, he may think he's justified in using force to get "what he paid for." If you cover some of the costs, he may be less aggressive.

- Back away from a man who pressures you into other activities you don't want to engage in on a date, such as chugging beer or drag racing with his friends.

- Avoid misleading messages and avoid behavior that may be interpreted as sexual teasing. Don't tell him to stop touching you, talk for a few minutes, and then resume petting.

- Despite your clearly stated intentions, if your date behaves in a sexually coercive manner, use a strategy of escalating forcefulness—direct refusal, vehement verbal refusal, and if necessary, physical force.

- Avoid using alcohol or other drugs when you definitely do not wish to be sexually intimate with your date.

- **Don't blame the victim.** Even when no one doubts that the victim is completely innocent, individuals may be plagued by regrets and self-accusation: Why didn't I lock the windows? Why did I park on that dark street? Any second-guessing or implied criticism adds to this burden of blame and shame.

- **Don't try to rush the victim to leave the past behind and get on with his or her life.** Recovery from any traumatic event takes time, and only the victim knows the appropriate pace. If, however, months pass without any lessening of symptoms or improvement in day-to-day functioning, family members and friends shouldn't hesitate to recommend that their loved one see a mental health professional.

SELFSURVEY : *How Safe Is Your School?*

Residence Hall Security

YES	NO	
—	—	Single-sex residence halls
—	—	Coed residence halls
—	—	Freshman residence halls
—	—	Substance-free residence halls
—	—	Senior residence halls
—	—	Alcohol prohibited
—	—	Drugs prohibited
—	—	Propped door alarms
—	—	Coed bathrooms
—	—	Card swipe—like hotels—for exterior and interior residence hall rooms
—	—	Patented keys
—	—	Standard keys
—	—	Automatic locked doors
—	—	Propped doors
—	—	Doors locked at night
—	—	Doors never locked
—	—	Doors always locked
—	—	Guards on duty 24 hours/day
—	—	Guards on duty at night
—	—	Apartments on campus
—	—	Fire sprinklers
—	—	Peep hole in room door
—	—	Dead bolt on room door
—	—	Safety chain on room door
—	—	Bath in room
—	—	Bathrooms down hallway
—	—	Single-sex bathrooms kept locked
—	—	Floors locked—all floors
—	—	Secure windows—all floors
—	—	Panic alarms in rooms

Visitors

YES	NO	
—	—	Phone/intercom at entrance
—	—	Leave ID with Guard
—	—	Guest passes with guard
—	—	Sign in guests with guard

Security Patrols in Residence Halls

YES	NO	
—	—	By police nightly
—	—	By security nightly
—	—	By students—RA or equivalent
—	—	By no one

Roommate Conflicts

YES	NO	
		Offending Roommate Quickly Transferred:
—	—	For using illegal drugs
—	—	For having sex while roommate present
—	—	For binge/underage drinking
—	—	For noisy parties
—	—	For hate speech
—	—	For physical abuse or violence
—	—	For vandalism

Health Services

YES	NO	
—	—	Rape crisis center
—	—	Alcohol–drug counselors
—	—	Student AA meetings on campus
—	—	Peer education programming
—	—	Safety education programming
—	—	Alcohol and other drug programming
—	—	Support groups—depression, eating disorders, etc.
—	—	Wellness center
—	—	Womens' center

Campus Security

YES	NO	
		Campus Security Force
—	—	Sworn police
—	—	Unsworn security
—	—	Security guards
—	—	Trained volunteer students
—	—	Arrest power
—	—	Patrolling day
—	—	Patrolling night
—	—	Carry firearms
—	—	Bicycle patrols
—	—	Surveillance cameras
—	—	Emergency phones in working condition
—	—	Escort services—24 hours
—	—	Shuttle services
—	—	Personal alarm devices

Parental Notification

YES	NO	
—	—	For suicide attempts
—	—	For depression
—	—	For alcohol poisoning
—	—	For DUI

_____ _____ For stalking
_____ _____ For acts of violence
_____ _____ For illegal drug use
_____ _____ For underage drinkers
_____ _____ For public drunkenness
_____ _____ For housing firearms
_____ _____ For sexual assault
_____ _____ For hate crimes or speech
_____ _____ For academic probation
_____ _____ For disciplinary probation
_____ _____ For residence hall violations
_____ _____ For off-campus citations

Campus Judicial System

YES NO

_____ _____ Releases results in hearings involving crimes of violence
_____ _____ Open campus judicial hearings
_____ _____ Reveals names of campus sex offenders

Get campus crime statistics from **www.ope.ed/gov/security** *or from your admissions office.*

Criminal Offenses

Murder _____
Forcible sex offenses _____
Nonforcible sex offenses _____
Robbery _____
Aggravated assault _____
Burglary _____
Arson _____
Motor vehicle theft _____
Hate crimes _____
Total criminal offenses _____
Per student crime ratio _____

Campus Arrests

Liquor law violations _____
Drug law violations _____
Weapons violations _____
TOTAL CAMPUS ARRESTS _____

Calculate campus crimes per thousand students and compare them with other schools. Also, attempt a balanced evaluation by combining your subjective impressions with any calculations.

Source: Security on Campus, Inc., www.securityoncampus.org.

Your Health Action Plan for Personal Safety on Campus

FUNDAMENTALS

- Freshmen should "respectfully decline" to have photo and personal information published for distribution to the campus community. Fraternities and upperclassmen have abused this type of publication to "target" naive freshmen.
- Study the campus and neighborhood with respect to routes between your residence and class/activities schedule. Know where emergency phones are located if you do not have a cell phone.
- Share your class/activities schedule with parents and a network of close friends, effectively creating a type of

"buddy" system. Give network telephone numbers to your parents, advisors, and friends.

- Always travel in groups. Use a shuttle service after dark. Never walk alone at night. Avoid shortcuts.
- Put the campus security number into your cell phone's fast-call numbers so you can access it with a single keystroke.
- Survey the campus, academic buildings, residence halls, and other facilities while classes are in session and after dark to see that buildings, walkways, quadrangles, and parking lots are adequately secured, lit, and patrolled. Are emergency phones, escorts, and shuttle services adequate?
- To gauge the social scene, drive down fraternity row on weekend nights and stroll through the student hangouts. Are people behaving responsibly, or does the situation seem reckless and potentially dangerous? Remember, alcohol and/or drug abuse is involved in about 90 percent of campus crime. Carefully evaluate off-campus student apartment complexes and fraternity houses if you plan to live off-campus.

RESIDENCE

- Doors and windows to your residence hall should be equipped with quality locking mechanisms. Room doors should be equipped with peep holes and deadbolts. Always lock them when you are absent. Do not loan out your key. Rekey locks when a key is lost or stolen.
- Card access systems are far superior to standard metal key and lock systems. Card access enables immediate lock changes when keys are lost, stolen, or when housing arrangements change. Most hotels and hospitals have changed to card access systems for safety reasons. Higher education institutions need to adopt similar safety features.
- Always lock your doors and first and second floor windows at night. Never compromise your safety for a roommate who asks you to leave the door unlocked.
- Dormitories should have a central entrance/exit lobby where nighttime access is monitored, as well as an outside telephone which visitors must use to gain access.
- Dormitory residents should insist that residential assistants and security patrols routinely check for propped doors—day and night.
- Do not leave your identification, wallets, checkbooks, jewelry, cameras, and other valuables in open view.
- Program your phone's speed dial memory with emergency numbers that include family and friends.
- Know your neighbors and don't be reluctant to report illegal activities and suspicious loitering.

OFF-CAMPUS RESIDENTS

Off-campus residents should contact their student legal aid representative to draft leases that stipulate minimum standards of security and responsibility. Students and parents should also consult any "Neighborhood Watch" association active in the community or the municipal police regarding local crime rates.

Source: Reprinted with permission by Security on Campus, Inc., www.securityoncampus.org. Security on Campus assists victims of campus crime.

CENGAGENOW If you want to write your own goals for staying safe, go to the Wellness Journal at HealthNow: **academic.cengage.com/login.**

Making This Chapter Work for YOU

Review Questions

1. When confronted with an emergency,
   a. move the victim to a safe place.
   b. move all electrical wires out of the way.
   c. wait to see whether someone else has taken matters in hand.
   d. assess the situation and call 911.

2. Which of the following factors affects an individual's risk of accident or injury?
   a. hunger level
   b. stress level
   c. amount of automobile insurance coverage
   d. knowledge of CPR

3. Which of the following is *not* a safe-driving tip?
   a. Avoid driving at night for the first year after getting a license.
   b. Make sure your car has snow tires or chains before driving in hazardous snowy conditions.
   c. If riding with an intoxicated driver, keep talking to him so that he doesn't fall asleep at the wheel.
   d. Don't let packages or people obstruct the rear or side windows.

4. Seat belt use
   a. is optional if your car has air bags.
   b. is higher in teenage men than women.
   c. reduces the risk of serious injury by about 50 percent.
   d. is declining in the United States.

5. Which of the following statements about home safety is true?
   a. Falls pose the greatest threat of injury in the home, followed by poison.
   b. The three ingredients of fire are fuel, a heat source, and oxygen.
   c. The risk of falls is lowest in the elderly.
   d. If you're on the top floor of the dorm when a fire breaks out, get to the elevator quickly.

6. You can avoid computer health hazards by
   a. positioning the monitor so that you are looking up at it.
   b. positioning the keyboard so that you don't have to bend your wrists to use it.
   c. sustaining focus on the screen with the PRIO method.
   d. taking a 15-minute break every 30 minutes.

7. Which statement about violence on college campuses is *false?*
   a. Campus hazing often involves activities that would be called torture if perpetrated elsewhere.
   b. Most crimes against students occur on campus.
   c. Many campuses have codes of conduct on alcohol, drugs, and fighting.
   d. Crime statistics for colleges and universities are posted on the Internet.

8. Sexual victimization
   a. includes sexual harassment, sexual coercion, and rape.
   b. is gender-specific, affecting women who are violated emotionally or physically by men.
   c. is rare in academic environments such as college campuses.
   d. most commonly takes the form of physical assault and stalking.

9. Which of the following statements about rape is true?
   a. When a person is sexually attacked by a stranger, it is referred to as *rape*. When a person is sexually attacked by an acquaintance, it is referred to as *sexual coercion.*
   b. Statutory rape is defined as sexual intercourse initiated by a woman under the age of consent.
   c. Men who rape other men usually consider themselves heterosexuals.
   d. Women who flirt and dress provocatively are typically more willing to participate in aggressive sex than women who dress conservatively and do not flirt.

10. Ways to protect or prevent rape include which of the following?
    a. Use alcohol and drugs only in familiar surroundings.
    b. Take a self-defense class.
    c. To avoid angering a sexually aggressive person, become passive and quiet.
    d. Do not discuss your sexual limits on a first or second date because just talking about sex will encourage your date to think you are interested in a sexual relationship.

Answers to these questions can be found on page 583.

Critical Thinking

1. Can you name two risk factors in your daily life that might increase the likelihood of accidental injury? What actions have you taken to keep yourself safe? Are there other risk factors you could minimize or eliminate? What might you do about them?

2. A friend of yours, Eric, frequently makes crude or derogatory comments about women. When you finally call him on this, his response is, "I didn't say anything wrong. I like women." What might you say to him?

3. At one college, women raped by acquaintances on dates scrawled the names of their assailants on the walls of women's restrooms on campus. Several young men whose names appeared on the list objected, protesting that they were innocent and were being unfairly accused. How do you feel about this method of fighting

back against date rape? Do you think it violates the rights of men? How do you feel about naming women who've been raped in news reports? Are there circumstances in which a woman's identity should be revealed? Would fewer women report a rape if not assured of privacy?

Media Menu

CENGAGENOW™ Go to the HealthNow website at **academic.cengage .com/login** that will:
- Help you evaluate your knowledge of the material.
- Allow you to take an exam-prep quiz.
- Provide a Personalized Learning Plan targeting resources that address areas you should study.
- Coach you through identifying target goals for behavioral change and creating and monitoring your personal change plan throughout the semester.

INTERNET CONNECTIONS

RAINN-Rape, Abuse & Incest National Network
www.rainn.org
This site provides great information from an organization fighting against rape, assault, and incest.

The Rape Crisis Center
www.rapecrisis.com
This private nonprofit organization provides support to victims of sexual violence and their families, including a 24/7 crisis hotline and several advocacy programs.

National Safety Council (NSC)
www.nsc.org
The mission of the NSC is to educate and influence society to adopt safety, health, and environmental policies, practices, and procedures that prevent human suffering and economic losses arising from preventable causes.

National Youth Violence Prevention Resource Center (NYVPRC)
www.safeyouth.org
This site is a gateway to resources for professionals, parents, youth, and individuals working to prevent and end violence committed by and against young people.

Key Terms

The terms listed are used and defined on the page indicated. Definitions are also found in the Glossary at the end of this book.

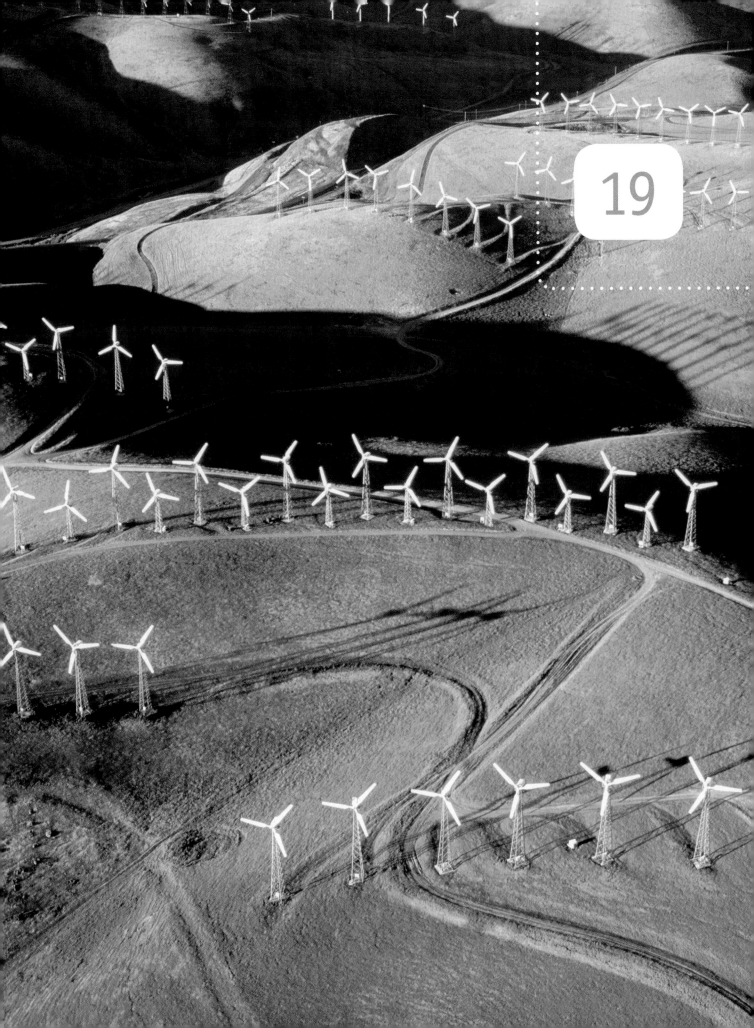

19

Working Toward a Healthy Environment

MANY college students study environmental threats such as global warming. Growing numbers are joining groups such as the Campus Climate Challenge to find solutions. "This is our problem, and it's up to us to solve it, starting right here on campus, right now," declare the leaders of the New Jersey student chapters. Rather than merely protesting or demanding action, these students pledge to find ways to reduce pollution and to work toward cutting their schools' contributions to global warming. Some have planted trees; some have set up recycling centers; other have launched energy-conservation makeovers for their campuses.

No one has more stake in the future of the planet than the next generation. Environmental concerns may seem so enormous that nothing any individual can do will have an effect. This is not the case. All of us, as citizens of the world, can help find solutions to the challenges confronting our planet. The first step is realizing that you have a personal responsibility for safeguarding the health of your environment and, thereby, your own well-being.

This chapter explores the complex interrelationships between your world and your well-being. It discusses major threats to the environment—including climate changes; atmospheric changes; air, water, and noise pollution; chemical risks; and radiation—and provides specific guidance on what you can do.

After studying the material in this chapter, you should be able to:

- **Name** some of the direct and indirect health risks associated with climate change.

- **List** the effects of ozone and particle pollution on lung health and functioning.

- **Identify** the major indoor pollutants.

- **Describe** the characteristics of the decibel scale.

- **List** the key sources and health risks of electromagnetic fields.

- **Write** a list of actions that you can take to protect the environment.

CENGAGENOW Log on to HealthNow at **academic.cengage.com/login** to find your Behavior Change Planner and to explore self-assessments, interactive tutorials, and practice quizzes.

The Environment and Your Health

Ours is a planet in peril. Glaciers are melting. Sea levels are rising. Forests are being destroyed. Droughts have become more frequent and more intense. Heat waves have killed tens of thousands of people. Hurricanes and floods have ravaged cities. Millions have died from the effects of air pollution and contaminated water.

The planet Earth—once taken for granted as a ball of rock and water that existed for our use for all time—is a single, fragile **ecosystem** (a community of organisms that share a physical and chemical environment). Our environment is a closed ecosystem, powered by the sun. The materials needed for the survival of this planet must be recycled over and over again. Increasingly, we're realizing just how important the health of this ecosystem is to our own well-being and survival.

For good or for ill, we cannot separate our individual health from that of the environment in which we live. The air we breathe, the water we drink, the chemicals we use all have an impact on the quality of our lives. At the same time, the lifestyle choices we make, the products we use, the efforts we undertake to clean up a beach or save wetlands affect the quality of our environment.

Climate Change

The International Panel on Climate Change of the United Nations, made up of leading scientists from around the world, has reported with absolute certainty that the world's climate is changing in significant ways and will continue to do so in the foreseeable future.[1] These experts predict an increase in extreme weather events (such as hurricanes and heat waves), greater weather variability, and rising water temperatures. The American Association for the Advancement of Science (AAAS) and other prestigious institutions around the world have issued warnings on the growing dangers of global climate change.

Global Warming

Earth's average temperature increased about 1 degree in the twentieth century to approximately 59 degrees, but the rate of warming in the last three decades has been three times the average rate since 1900. Seas have risen about six to eight feet globally over the last century and are rising at a higher rate.

Why is our planet getting warmer? Figure 19.1 shows the normal greenhouse effect: Certain gases in Earth's atmosphere trap energy from the sun and retain heat somewhat like the glass panels of a greenhouse. These "greenhouse" gases include carbon dioxide, methane, and nitrous oxide. Human activities, scientists now say with 90 percent certainty, have increased the greenhouse gases in our atmosphere.[2] We burn fossil fuels (oil, natural gas, coal) and wood products, which release carbon dioxide into the atmosphere. We produce coal, natural gas, and oil, which emit methane. Livestock and the decomposition of organic wastes also produce methane. Agricultural and industrial processes emit nitrous oxide. These emissions enhance the normal greenhouse effect, trapping more heat and raising the temperature of the atmosphere and Earth's surface.

After years of doubt and debate, most leading experts agree that the buildup of greenhouse gases is changing natural climate and weather patterns in new and potentially dangerous ways. Carbon dioxide levels are higher now than at any time in the past 800,000 years and, according to the AAAS, "is heading for levels not experienced for millions of years."[3]

The Health Risks

No individual is immune to the effects of climate change. The World Health Organization (WHO) estimates that climate change is already causing at least 150,000 excess deaths a year and that this number will climb to at least 300,000 annually by 2030.[4]

Climate change can imperil health directly—for example, as the result of floods or heat waves—and indirectly—by changing the patterns of infectious diseases, supplies of fresh water, and food availability. For example, as the planet continues to warm, infectious diseases—particularly mosquito-borne illnesses such as malaria, dengue fever, yellow fever, and encephalitis—may spread to more regions.[5] Already in the United States, mosquitoes and other insects that carry diseases such as West Nile virus, Rocky Mountain spotted fever, and Lyme disease are spreading to areas once considered too cold for these insects to survive.

Continued climate change could bring other health threats—such as increased air pollution, hunger, water shortages, and coastal flooding—to millions of people around the world. As scientists have issued more urgent alarms, citizen groups, corporations, and national and international agencies are devoting more resources to environmental health issues. The Kyoto Protocol, the first global environment standards, will expire in 2012, and the nations of the world have begun the process of negotiating new ones.

The Impact of Pollution

Any change in the air, water, or soil that could reduce its ability to support life is a form of *pollution*. Natural events, such as smoke from fires triggered by lightning,

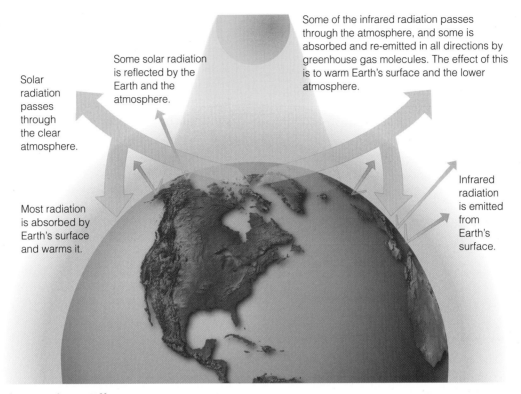

Figure 19.1   The Greenhouse Effect

The normal greenhouse effect warms Earth to a hospitable temperature. An increase in greenhouse gases intensifies the greenhouse effect, trapping more heat and raising Earth's temperature.

can cause pollution. The effects of pollution depend on the concentration (amount per unit of air, water, or soil) of the **pollutant,** how long it remains in the environment, and its chemical nature. An *acute effect* is a severe, immediate reaction, usually after a single, large exposure. For example, pesticide poisoning can cause nausea and dizziness, even death. A *chronic effect* may take years to develop or may be a recurrent or continuous reaction, usually after repeated exposure. The development of cancer after repeated exposure to a pollutant such as asbestos is an example of a chronic effect.

Environmental agents that trigger changes, or *mutations,* in the genetic material (the DNA) of living cells are called **mutagens.** The changes that result can lead to the development of cancer. A substance or agent that causes cancer is a **carcinogen:** All carcinogens are mutagens; most mutagens are carcinogens. Furthermore, when a mutagen affects an egg or a sperm cell, its effects can be passed on to future generations. Mutagens that can cross the placenta of a pregnant woman and cause a spontaneous abortion or birth defects in the fetus are called *teratogens.*

 Pollution is a hazard to all who breathe. Deaths caused by air pollution exceed those from motor vehicle injuries. Those with respiratory illnesses are at greatest risk during days when smog or allergen counts are high. However, as a recent study showed, even healthy college students suffer impairments in their heart and circulatory systems as a result of urban air pollution.[6] The effects of carbon monoxide are much worse in smokers, who already have higher levels of the gas in their blood.

As carbon dioxide levels in the air rise due to the greenhouse effect, air quality will worsen. Gases found in polluted air—such as ozone, sulfur dioxide, and nitrogen dioxide—contribute to heart disease and worsen the health of individuals who already have heart conditions. Poor air quality also contributes to breathing difficulties and may be responsible for the dramatic increase in asthma in recent decades. Elevated carbon dioxide levels can trigger asthma attacks and allergies by increasing ragweed pollen. Greater carbon dioxide in the air also stimulates the growth of poison ivy and other nuisance plants.

Toxic substances in polluted air can enter the human body in three ways: through the skin, through the digestive system, and through the lungs. The combined interaction of two or more hazards can produce an effect greater than

ecosystem   A community of organisms sharing a physical and chemical environment and interacting with each other.

pollutant   A substance or agent in the environment, usually the by-product of human industry or activity, that is injurious to human, animal, or plant life.

mutagen   An agent that causes alterations in the genetic material of living cells.

carcinogen   A substance or agent that causes cancer.

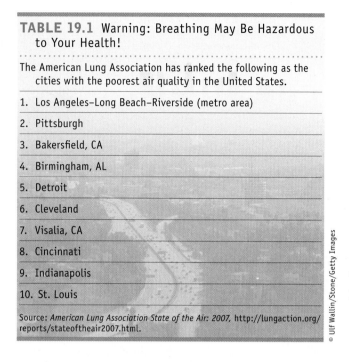

TABLE 19.1 Warning: Breathing May Be Hazardous to Your Health!

The American Lung Association has ranked the following as the cities with the poorest air quality in the United States.

1. Los Angeles–Long Beach–Riverside (metro area)
2. Pittsburgh
3. Bakersfield, CA
4. Birmingham, AL
5. Detroit
6. Cleveland
7. Visalia, CA
8. Cincinnati
9. Indianapolis
10. St. Louis

Source: *American Lung Association State of the Air: 2007,* http://lungaction.org/reports/stateoftheair2007.html.

© Ulf Wallin/Stone/Getty Images

that of either one alone. Pollutants can affect an organ or organ system directly or indirectly.

Among the health problems that have been linked with pollution are the following:

- Headaches and dizziness.
- Eye irritation and impaired vision.
- Nasal discharge.
- Cough, shortness of breath, and sore throat.
- Constricted airways.
- Constriction of blood vessels and increased risk of heart disease.
- Chest pains and aggravation of the symptoms of colds, pneumonia, bronchial asthma, emphysema, chronic bronchitis, lung cancer, and other respiratory problems.
- Birth defects and reproductive problems.
- Nausea, vomiting, and stomach cancer.
- Allergy and asthma from diesel fumes in polluted air.

The Air You Breathe

Remember the last time you stood at a busy intersection as a bus or truck spewed brownish fumes in your face? Maybe your eyes stung, or your throat burned. But breathing polluted air can do more than irritate: It can take months or even years off your life. As pollutants destroy the hairlike cilia that remove irritants from the lungs, individuals may suffer chronic bronchitis, characterized

by excessive mucus flow and continuous coughing. Emphysema may develop or worsen, as pollutants constrict the bronchial tubes and destroy the air sacs in the lungs, making breathing more difficult.

When air pollution levels are high, heart attacks, strokes, heart failure flare-ups, and lung troubles increase. Air contamination also has enduring effects on heart health and increases atherosclerosis and deaths due to heart disease. For the elderly and people with asthma or heart disease, polluted air can be life-threatening. Even healthy individuals can be affected, particularly if they exercise outdoors during high-pollution periods.

According to the American Lung Association, nearly half of the people in the United States live in counties with unhealthy levels of ozone or particle pollution. As shown in Table 19.1, the residents of the Los Angeles–Long Beach–Riverside metropolitan areas are breathing the worst air in the country.[7]

Ozone

Ozone, the primary ingredient of smog air pollution, can impair the body's immune system and cause long-term lung damage. (Ozone in the upper atmosphere protects us by repelling harmful ultraviolet radiation from the sun, but ozone in the lower atmosphere is a harmful component of air pollution.) Automobiles also produce carbon monoxide, a colorless and odorless gas that diminishes the ability of red blood cells to carry oxygen. The resulting oxygen deficiency can affect breathing, hearing, and vision in humans and stunt the growth of plants and trees.

Several large investigations have confirmed that ozone at levels currently found in the United States can shorten lives. Even on days when ozone levels are below the national standard, the risk of premature death is greater in areas with higher levels. The individuals most vulnerable to the effects of ozone are children, senior citizens, people who work or exercise outdoors, those with a respiratory disease such as asthma, and "responders" who are otherwise healthy but respond intensely to ozone.

 Ozone's other ill effects include shortness of breath, chest pain when inhaling deeply, wheezing, coughing, and increased susceptibility to respiratory infections. Studies of college freshmen who were lifelong residents of Los Angeles or the San Francisco Bay Area found that long exposure to elevated ozone levels had reduced their "lung function," that is, their lungs' ability to work efficiently.

Ozone pollution has decreased nationwide in recent years, but a third of Americans still live in areas with unhealthful levels. Among the cities with the highest ozone levels are Los Angeles, Houston, Dallas, New York, Washington DC, and Philadelphia.

Particle Pollution

Scientists refer to the mix of very tiny solid and liquid particles in the air as *particle pollution*. The particles themselves can range in size from microscopic to one-tenth the diameter of a strand of hair. Our natural defenses help us to cough or sneeze large particles out of our bodies, but they don't keep out smaller particles, which get trapped in the lungs. The smallest ones pass through the lungs into the bloodstream.

Particle pollution damages the body in ways similar to cigarette smoking. Even short-term exposure can be deadly because particle pollution increases the risk of heart attacks and strokes, especially among the elderly and those with heart conditions. It also diminishes lung function, causes inflammation of lung tissue in young, healthy adults, increases the number and severity of asthma attacks, and increases mortality in infants and young children.

Living near highways or spending time in heavy traffic, whether driving or taking public transportation, may be especially dangerous. Several studies have found an increased risk of premature death in those who live, work, drive, or ride in high-traffic areas. Air pollution may permanently impair the capacity of the lungs of 10- to 18-year-olds who live within about a third of a mile of a freeway, limiting their ability to breathe for the rest of their lives and increasing their risk of serious lung diseases.[8]

Particle pollution—considered the most dangerous because it can be an immediate as well as a long-term threat to life—has increased in the eastern part of the United States but decreased in the West. The cities that rank the worst in terms of particle pollution include Pittsburgh, Detroit, Chicago, Cleveland, Baltimore, Philadelphia, and New York.

The Water You Drink

Fears about the public water supply have led many Americans to turn off their taps. About two-thirds take steps to drink purer water, either by using filtration and distillation methods or by drinking bottled water. However, Consumer Union, a nonprofit advocacy group, maintains that the United States has the safest water supply in the world. The Environmental Protection Agency has set standards for some 80 contaminants. These include many toxic chemicals and heavy metals—including lead, mercury, cadmium, and chromium—that can cause kidney and nervous system damage and birth defects.

What's in *Your* Water?

Each year the CDC reports an average of 7,400 cases of illness related to the water people drink. The most common culprits include parasites, bacteria, viruses, chemicals, and lead. Health officials suggest having your water tested if you live near a hazardous waste dump or industrial park, if the pipes in your house are made of lead or joined together with lead solder, if your water comes from a well, or if you purchase water from a private company. Check to see if your state health department or local water supplier will provide free testing. If not, use a state-certified laboratory that tests water in accordance with EPA standards.

About two-thirds of Americans drink water containing fluoride, an additive to water and toothpaste that helps teeth resist decay. According to the American Dental Association, the incidence of tooth decay is lower among children and adolescents who drink fluoridated water.

Federal health officials have found no evidence that fluoride causes cancer in humans and have concluded that its benefits far outweigh any risks. However, excessive fluoride can increase bone loss and fractures in pre- and post-menopausal women. Health professionals advise consumers to use only small amounts of fluoridated toothpaste, rinse thoroughly after brushing, and use fluoride supplements only when the home water supply is known to be deficient.

Three-quarters of the population of the United States drinks water treated with chlorine to kill disease-causing bacteria. The Council on Environmental Quality has warned that people drinking chlorinated water have a 53 percent greater risk of getting colon and bladder cancer and a 13 to 93 percent greater risk of getting rectal cancer than those not drinking chlorinated water. There may even be a link between soft water and a higher rate of cardiovascular disease, perhaps because soft water in some areas tends to have more sodium in it.

Is Bottled Better?

Is bottled water better? That's what consumers have often assumed. Bottled water sales have tripled in the past ten years. Women and college-age Americans make up the majority of bottled-water drinkers. Yet in the past, the Food and Drug Administration (FDA) simply defined bottled water as "sealed in bottles or other containers and intended for human consumption." Bottled water wasn't required to be "pure" or even to be tested for toxic chemicals. One survey found chemical contaminants associated with cancer in 22 of 100 brands tested.

According to the Earth Policy Institute, producing plastic for the 8 billion gallons of bottled water consumed annually in the United States burns enough oil to power 100,000 cars for a year. Bottled water has not been proven healthier than tap water, and nutritionists contend that

ozone a form of oxygen that is a harmful component of air pollution.

POINT COUNTERPOINT *Environmental Action 101*

POINT

A growing number of colleges and universities are designing innovative buildings and creating programs to reduce energy usage and conserve national resources. Some, for instance, have bought alternative-fuel vehicles for campus transportation or installed solar panels to heat dormitories.

COUNTERPOINT

Institutions of higher education should focus on their mission of educating young people rather than committing resources to energy reduction. The government or corporations should take the lead in environmental innovation. Academics should primarily serve as consultants or advisors.

YOUR VIEW

Do you think students should support and participate in the search for innovative solutions to environmental problems? Should schools require students to limit their energy usage on campus?

"vitamin" waters provide no additional benefits. (See Chapter 6 for more on water and other beverages.) Dentists report an increase in cavities in children and teenagers who drink bottled water rather than fluoridated tap water.

Indoor Pollutants

Because people in industrialized nations spend more than 90 percent of their time in buildings, the quality of the air they breathe inside can have an even greater impact on their well-being than outdoor pollution.

Cigarette Smoke

The most hazardous form of indoor air pollution is cigarette smoke. Nearly half of all nonsmoking Americans are regularly exposed to secondhand smoke, which contains more than 50 cancer-causing chemicals. According to a major scientific report from the U.S. Surgeon General, secondhand smoke exposure can cause heart disease and lung cancer in nonsmoking adults and sudden infant death syndrome (SIDS), respiratory problems, ear infections, and asthma attacks in babies and children. Even brief exposure to secondhand smoke has immediate adverse effects on the cardiovas-

---

Your Life Change Coach

Going Green

More universities are developing programs to achieve **sustainability**, the use of as little as possible of resources that cannot be renewed. (See Point/Counterpoint.) Innovative programs include "green" dorms and campaigns to reduce energy waste.[9] Not all undergraduates share this concern, but higher numbers express commitment to environmental action than in the past. (See "Reality Check".)

By the choices you make and the actions you take, you can improve the state of the world. No one expects you to sacrifice every comfort or spend great amounts of money. However, for almost everyone, there's plenty of room for improvement. If enough people make small individual changes, they can have an enormous impact. (See "Our Space" lab in *IPC*.) **IPC**

One basic environmental action is **precycling**: buying products packaged in recycled materials. According to Earthworks, a consumer group, packaging makes up a third of what people in the United States throw away. When you precycle, you consider how you're going to dispose of a product and the packaging materials before purchasing it. For example, you might choose eggs in recyclable cardboard packages, rather than in Styrofoam cartons, and look for juice and milk in refillable bottles.

Recycling—collecting, reprocessing, marketing, and reusing materials once considered trash—serves several important functions, including:

- **Preserving natural resources.** Reprocessing used materials to make new products and packaging reduces the consumption of natural resources. Recycling steel saves iron ore, coal, and limestone. Recycling newsprint, office paper, and mixed paper saves trees.

- **Saving energy.** Recycling used aluminum cans, for instance, requires only about 5 percent of the energy needed to produce aluminum. Recycling just one can save enough electricity to light a 100-watt bulb for $3\frac{1}{2}$ hours.

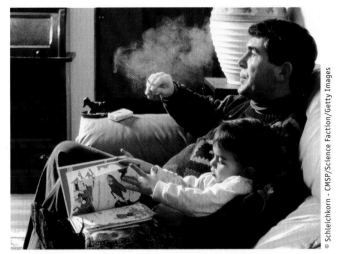

Nonsmokers exposed to secondhand smoke, including children, face increased risk of developing lung cancer and heart disease.

REALITYCHECK

- *What percentage of college freshmen say that "becoming involved in programs to clean up the environment" is essential or very important?*

- *Are women or men more committed to improving the environment?*

Answers on next page.

cular system and increases risk for heart disease and lung cancer.[10]

Formaldehyde

Some indoor pollutants come from the very materials that buildings are made of and from the appliances inside them. Formaldehyde is commonly used in building materials, carpet backing, furniture, foam insulation, plywood, and particle board, and it can cause nausea, dizziness, headaches, heart palpitations, stinging eyes, and burning lungs. Formaldehyde gas, which is colorless and odorless, has been shown to cause cancer in animals. Most manufacturers have voluntarily quit using it, but many homes already contain materials made with urea-formaldehyde, which can seep into the air. To avoid formaldehyde exposure, buy solid wood or nonwood products whenever possible, and ask about the formaldehyde content of building products, cabinets, and furniture before purchasing them.

- **Reducing greenhouse gas emissions.** Recycling cuts these gases by decreasing the amount of energy used to produce and transport new products.

- **Decreasing the need for landfill storage or incineration.** Both are more costly and can contribute to air pollution.

Different communities take different approaches to recycling. Many provide regular curbside pickup of recyclables, and others have drop-off centers. Buyback centers pay for recyclables. In some places, reverse vending machines accept returned beverage containers and provide deposit refunds.

Discarded computers, other electronic devices, and printer cartridges also should be recycled, by donating them to schools or charitable organizations. "Tech trash" buried in landfills is creating a new hazard because trace amounts of potentially hazardous agents, such as lead and mercury, can leak into the ground and water. Find out if your campus has a program to recycle electronic devices.

With *composting*—which some people describe as nature's way of recycling—the benefits can be seen as close as your backyard. Organic products, such as leftover food and vegetable peels, are mixed with straw or other dry material and kept damp. Bacteria eat the organic material and turn it into a rich soil. Some people keep a compost pile (which should be stirred every few days) in their backyard; others take their organic garbage (including mowed grass and dead leaves) to community gardens or municipal composting sites.

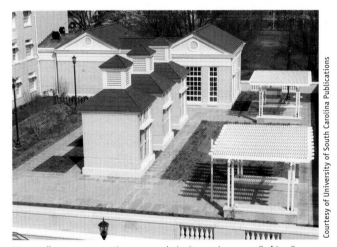

Many colleges are conserving energy, designing environmentally friendly buildings, restricting traffic, and limiting use of hazardous materials. Does your campus have a "green" program?

sustainability A method of using a resource so that the resource is not depleted or permanently damaged.

precycling The use of products that are packaged in recycled or recyclable material.

recycling The processing or reuse of manufactured materials to reduce consumption of raw materials.

Asbestos

Asbestos, a mineral widely used for building insulation, has been linked to lung and gastrointestinal cancer among asbestos workers and their families, although it may take 20 to 30 years for such cancers to develop. Fibers from asbestos home insulation or fireproofing that become airborne can cause progressive and deadly lung diseases, including thickening, plaques, and fibrosis (excess fibrous connective tissue) as well as various types of cancer.[11] The danger may be greatest for those who smoke and are also exposed to asbestos.

If you're concerned about asbestos in your home, don't waste money searching for asbestos in the air. The results of such tests are meaningless. To check a building material for asbestos, put three small pieces in a film canister and send it to a laboratory approved by the U.S. Environmental Protection Agency (EPA). If you find asbestos in your house, sealing the source (for example, an old linoleum floor) may be safer than removing it. Contact your state or city health department for advice. If asbestos must be removed, have it done by professionals.

Lead

A danger both inside and outside our homes is lead, which lurks in some 57 million American homes, most built before 1960, with walls, windows, doors, and banisters coated with more than 3 million metric tons of lead-based paint. The percentage of children aged one to five with elevated levels of lead in their blood has dropped to 2.2 percent, half of what it was in the early 1990s.

Fetuses and children under age 7 are particularly vulnerable to lead because their nervous systems are still developing and because their body mass is so small that they ingest and absorb more lead per pound than adults. Even 10 micrograms (millionths of a gram) of lead per deciliter of blood—the CDC standard for lead poisoning—can kill a child's brain cells and cause poor concentration, reduced short-term memory, slower reaction times, and learning disabilities.

Adults exposed to low levels of lead (which once were thought to be safe) may develop headaches, high blood pressure, irritability, tremors, and insomnia. Health effects increase with exposure to higher levels and include anemia, stomach pain, vomiting, diarrhea, and constipation. Long-term exposure can impair fertility and damage the kidneys. Workers exposed to lead may become sterile or suffer irreversible kidney disease, damage to their central nervous system, stillbirths, or miscarriages.

The CDC and the American Academy of Pediatrics recommend annual testing of blood levels of lead in all children from age 9 months to 6 years, regardless of where they live. High-risk youngsters—those who live or play in older housing (especially if a building is in poor condition or undergoing renovation), those who live with someone who uses lead for a job or hobby, and those who live near a lead smelter, a processing plant, or a heavily traveled road or highway—should be screened every two or three months until age 3 and every six months until age 6. High levels of ascorbic acid (vitamin C) have been associated with a lower rate of elevated blood lead levels.

Mercury

Exposure to mercury can damage the central nervous system, endocrine system, kidneys, and other organs and can result in brain damage and death. Mercury is particularly toxic to fetuses, infants, and young children, and it may damage development of the nervous system. Women exposed to mercury in pregnancy have sometimes given birth to children with serious birth defects.[12]

Some fish contain high levels of a form of mercury called methylmercury that can harm an unborn child's developing nervous system if eaten regularly. The FDA has advised that certain individuals—young children, women who are or might become pregnant, and nursing mothers—avoid eating shark, swordfish, king mackerel, and tilefish (all high in mercury); limit their consumption of fish and shellfish that are lower in mercury, such as shrimp, canned light tuna, salmon, pollock, and catfish, to 12 ounces (two average meals) a week; and keep consumption of canned albacore tuna (which is somewhat higher in mercury) to 6 ounces (one average meal) a week. They also should check local advisories about the safety of fish caught by family and friends in local lakes, rivers, and coastal areas. If no specific advice is available, the FDA advises eating a maximum of 6 ounces per week of local fish and no additional fish or shellfish.

Although free of lead, some popular latex paints may contain potentially hazardous mercury, which manufacturers routinely added until a 1990 ban, to prevent the growth of mold and mildew. The threat of mercury poisoning is greatest during painting and immediately after.

Even mercury in medical devices, such as sphygmomanometers that measure blood pressure, can be a hazard. Symptoms of mercury poisoning include a racing heartbeat, sweating, aching limbs, kidney problems, hand tremors, peeling skin, and emotional problems.

Mold

One of the oldest and most widespread substances on Earth, mold—a type of fungus that decomposes organic matter and provides plants with nutrients—has emerged as a major health concern. Common molds include *Aspergillus, Penicillium,* and *Stachybotrys,* a slimy, dark green mold that has been blamed for infant deaths and various illnesses, from Alzheimer's disease to cancer, in adults that breathe in its spores. Faulty ventilation systems and airtight buildings have been implicated as contributing to the increased mold problem.

Experts agree that mold may trigger or worsen a number of health problems, including dizziness, breathing problems, nausea, and asthma attacks. However, mold usually is harmful only to allergic or sensitive individuals.[13] In the last decade, high-profile lawsuits have resulted in multimillion dollar judgments, despite a lack of scientific evidence linking mold exposure and cancer or brain damage.

Mold problems can range from small patches to large infestations of entire rooms or even a whole building. The first step to reduce mold exposure is moisture control, which may require new methods of keeping rainwater and ground water away from the interior and maintaining the heating ventilation and air conditioning systems appropriately. Bleach or soap and water can clean up small infestations. Larger ones may require appropriate protective respiratory equipment or professionally trained, licensed, and experienced contractors.

Carbon Monoxide and Nitrogen Dioxide

Carbon monoxide (CO) gas—which is tasteless, odorless, colorless, and nonirritating—can be deadly. Produced by the incomplete combustion of fuel in space heaters, furnaces, water heaters, and engines, CO reduces the delivery of oxygen in the blood. Every year an estimated 10,000 Americans seek treatment for CO inhalation; at least 250 die because of this silent killer. Those most at risk are the chronically ill, the elderly, pregnant women, and infants. Typical symptoms of CO poisoning, which is most common in winter, are headache, nausea, vomiting, fatigue, and dizziness. More severe poisoning can damage the heart and cause respiratory distress, confusion, and coma. A blood test can measure CO levels; inhaling pure oxygen speeds removal of the gas from the body. Most people who don't lose consciousness as a result of CO poisoning recover completely.

Another dangerous gas, nitrogen dioxide, can reach very high levels if you use a natural gas or propane stove in a poorly ventilated kitchen. This gas may lead to respiratory illnesses. Pilot lights are a steady source of nitrogen dioxide; to reduce exposure, switch to spark ignition.

Radon

Radioactive radon—which diffuses from rock, brick, concrete building materials, and natural soil deposits under some homes—produces charged decay products that cling to dust particles. Once trapped inside a building, radon can reach levels that may increase the risk of lung cancer. The EPA estimates that the inhalation of indoor radon is responsible for approximately 14,000 lung cancer deaths per year. Radon levels tend to be highest in areas with granite and black shale topped with porous soil.

An estimated 10 million homes and over 30 million people are at risk from high levels of radon. If you live in a high-radon area, don't panic. Your hypothetical risk of dying from radon-caused lung cancer is about equal to the known risk of dying in a home fire or fall. Check with the geology department at the nearest university or with your state health department to find out if they've performed radon tests in your area. If there may be danger, you can buy a radon detector. In most homes, the readings turn out to be low. If not, your state health department can provide guidelines for bringing them down.

Your Hearing Health

Hearing loss is the third-most common chronic health problem, after high blood pressure and arthritis, among older Americans. Loud noises cause hearing loss in an estimated 10 million Americans every year. Only about one-fifth of the 28 million Americans suffering from hearing loss have sought professional help.[14]

How Loud Is That Noise?

Loudness, or the intensity of a sound, is measured in **decibels (dB).** A whisper is 20 decibels; a conversation in a living room is about 50 decibels. On this scale, 50 isn't two and a half times louder than 20, but 1,000 times louder: Each 10-dB rise in the scale represents a tenfold increase in the intensity of the sound. Very loud but short bursts of sounds (such as gunshots and fireworks) and quieter but longer-lasting sounds (such as power tools) can induce hearing loss.

decibel (dB) A unit for measuring the intensity of sounds.

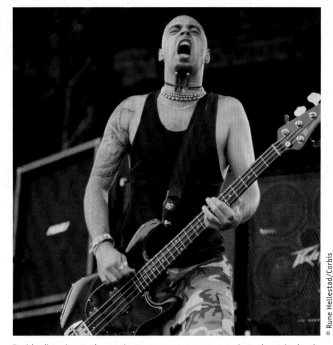

© Rune Hellestad/Corbis

Besides listening to the music at your next concert, tune in to the noise level and how your ears are feeling.

Decibels	Example	Zone
0	The softest sound a typical ear can hear	Safe
10 dB	Just audible	
20 dB	Watch ticking; leaves rustling	
30 dB	Soft whisper at 16 feet	
40 dB	Quiet office; suburban street (no traffic)	
50 dB	Interior of typical urban home; rushing stream	1,000 times louder than 20dB
60 dB	Normal conversation; busy office	
70 dB	Vacuum cleaner at 10 feet; hair dryer	
80 dB	Alarm clock at 2 feet; loud music; average daily traffic	1,000 times louder than 50dB
90 dB*	Motorcycle at 25 feet; jet 4 miles after takeoff	Risk of injury
100 dB*	Video arcade; loud factory; subway train	
110 dB*	Car horn at 3 feet; symphony orchestra; chain saw	1,000 times louder than 80dB
120 dB	Jackhammer at 3 feet; boom box; nearby thunderclap	Injury
130 dB	Rock concert; jet engine at 100 feet	
140 dB	Jet engine nearby; amplified car stereo; firearms	1,000 times louder than 110dB

Figure 19.2   Louder and Louder

The human ear perceives a 10-decibel increase as a doubling of loudness. Thus, the 100 decibels of a subway train sound much more than twice as loud as the 50 decibels of a rushing stream.

*Note: The maximum exposure allowed on the job by federal law, in hours per day: 90 decibels, 8 hours; 100 decibels, 2 hours; 110 decibels, 1/2 hour.

Sounds under 75 dB don't seem harmful. However, prolonged exposure to any sound over 85 dB (the equivalent of a power mower or food blender) or brief exposure to louder sounds can harm hearing. The noise level at rock concerts can reach 110 to 140 dB, about as loud as an air raid siren. Personal sound systems (boom boxes) can blast sounds of up to 115 dB. Cars with extremely loud music systems, known as boom cars, can produce an ear-splitting 145 dB—louder than a jet engine or thunderclap (Figure 19.2).

Common "sound offenders" are nightclubs (with sustained levels of well over 100 decibels), restaurants (with levels of 80 to 96 decibels), and street traffic (80 decibels or more). However, even low-level office noise can undermine well-being and increase health risks.

Effects of Noise

Noise-induced hearing loss is 100 percent preventable—and irreversible. Hearing aids are the only treatment, but they do not correct the problem; they just amplify sound to compensate for hearing loss.

The healthy human ear can hear sounds within a wide range of frequencies (measured in hertz), from the low-frequency rumble of thunder at 50 hertz to the high-frequency overtones of a piccolo at nearly 20,000 hertz. High-frequency noise damages the delicate hair cells that serve as sound receptors in the inner ear. Damage first begins as a diminished sensitivity to frequencies around 4,000 hertz, the highest notes of a piano.

Early symptoms of hearing loss include difficulty understanding speech and *tinnitus* (ringing in the ears). Brief, very loud sounds, such as an explosion or gunfire, can produce immediate, severe, and permanent hearing loss. Longer exposure to less intense but still hazardous sounds, such as those common at work or in public places, can gradually impair hearing, often without the individual's awareness.

Conductive hearing loss, often caused by ear infections, cuts down on perception of low-pitched sounds. Sensorineural loss involves damage or destruction of the

YOUR STRATEGIES FOR PREVENTION *How to Protect Your Ears*

- If you must live or work in a noisy area, wear hearing protectors to prevent exposure to blasts of very loud noise. Don't think cotton or facial tissue stuck in your ears can protect you; foam or soft plastic earplugs are more effective. Wear them when operating lawn mowers, weed trimmers, or power tools.
- Give your ears some quiet time. Rather than turning up the volume on your personal music player to blot out noise,

look for truly quiet environments, such as the library, where you can rest your ears and focus your mind.
- Soundproof your home by using draperies, carpets, and bulky furniture. Put rubber mats under washing machines, blenders, and other noisy appliances. Seal cracks around windows and doors.
- Beware of large doses of aspirin. Researchers have found that eight aspirin tablets a day can aggravate the damage

caused by loud noise; twelve a day can cause ringing in the ears (tinnitus).
- Don't drink in noisy environments. Alcohol intensifies the impact of noise and increases the risk of lifelong hearing damage.
- When you hear a sudden loud noise, press your fingers against your ears. Limit your exposure to loud noise. Several brief periods of noise seem less damaging than one long exposure.

sensory cells in the inner ear that convert sound waves to nerve signals.

Noise can harm more than our ears: High-volume sound has been linked to high blood pressure and other stress-related problems that can lead to heart disease, insomnia, anxiety, headaches, colitis, and ulcers. Noise frays the nerves; people tend to be more anxious, irritable, and angry when their ears are constantly barraged with sound. For suggestions for hearing health, see Your Strategies for Prevention: "How to Protect Your Ears."

Are Earbuds Hazardous to Hearing?

Although there is limited research, audiologists (who specialize in hearing problems) report seeing greater noise-induced hearing loss in young people. One probable culprit is extended use of earbuds, tiny earphones used with portable music players that deliver sound extremely close to the eardrum. Hearing loss can be temporary or permanent.

The dangers to your hearing depend on how loud the music is and how long you listen. Because personal music players have long-lasting rechargeable batteries, people—especially young ones—both listen for long periods and turn up the volume. As long as the sound level is within safety levels (see Figure 19.2), you can listen as long as

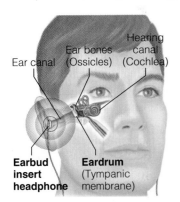

Ear canal | Ear bones (Ossicles) | Hearing canal (Cochlea)

Earbud insert headphone | **Eardrum** (Tympanic membrane)

you'd like. If you listen to music so loud that someone else can hear it two or three feet away, it's too loud.[15]

For safe listening, limit listening to a portable music player with earphones or earbuds at 60 percent of its potential volume to one hour a day. At the very least, take a

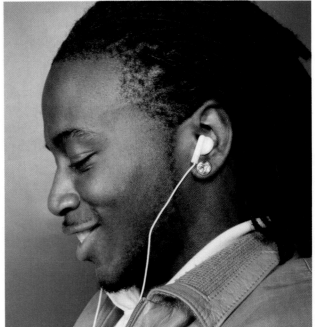

How loudly do you play your favorite music? How long do you use earbuds?

five-minute break after an hour of listening and keep the volume low.

Ask yourself the following questions to determine if you should have your hearing checked:

- Do you frequently have to ask people to repeat themselves?

- Do you have difficulty hearing when someone speaks in a whisper?

- Do people complain that you turn up the volume too much when watching television or listening to music?

- Do you have difficulty following conversation in a noisy environment?

- Do you avoid groups of people because of hearing difficulty?
- Have your friends or family suggested you might have hearing loss?

Chemical Risks

Various chemicals, including benzene, asbestos, and arsenic, have been shown to cause cancer in humans. Probable carcinogens include DDT and PCB. Risks can be greatly increased with simultaneous exposures to more than one carcinogen, for example, tobacco smoke and asbestos.[16]

According to the CDC, the levels of potentially harmful chemicals, including pesticides and lead, in Americans' blood have declined. Still, an estimated 50,000 to 70,000 U.S. workers die each year of chronic diseases related to past exposure to toxic substances, including lung cancer, bladder cancer, leukemia, lymphoma, chronic bronchitis, and disorders of the nervous system. **Endocrine disruptors,** chemicals that act as or interfere with human hormones, particularly estrogen, may pose a different threat. Scientists are investigating their impact on fertility, falling sperm counts, and cancers of the reproductive organs. Exposure to toxic chemicals causes about 3 percent of developmental defects.

Pesticides

High quantities of toxic chemical waste from unused or obsolete pesticides are posing a continuing and worsening threat to people and the environment in Eastern Europe, Africa, Asia, the Middle East, and Latin America. In the United States, the FDA estimates that 33 to 39 percent of our food supply contains residues of pesticides that may pose a long-term danger to our health. Scientists have detected traces of pesticides in groundwater in both urban and rural areas.

No relationship has been found between fertility, as measured by time to pregnancy (that is, the time taken for a couple to conceive once they decide they want to), and male exposure to pesticides. Exposure to pesticides may, however, pose a risk to pregnant women and their unborn children. Men whose jobs routinely expose them to pesticides may be at increased risk of prostate cancer. Parental exposure does not increase the likelihood of childhood brain cancer.

Chlorinated hydrocarbons include several high-risk substances—such as DDT, kepone, and chlordane—that have been restricted or banned because they may cause cancer, birth defects, neurological disorders, and damage to wildlife and the environment. They are extremely resistant to breakdown.

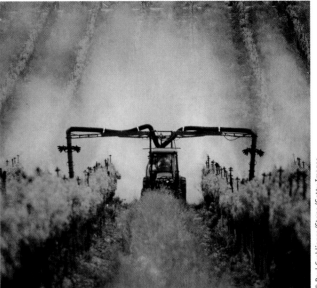

Pesticides protect crops from harmful insects, plants, and fungi but may endanger human health.

© Paul Greblianas/Stone/Getty Images

Organic phosphates, including chemicals such as malathion, break down more rapidly than the chlorinated hydrocarbons. Most are highly toxic, causing cramps, confusion, diarrhea, vomiting, headaches, and breathing difficulties. Higher levels in the blood can lead to convulsions, paralysis, coma, and death.

Farmworkers and those in the communities surrounding agricultural land are at greatest risk for pesticide exposure. However, even city dwellers aren't out of range. About half (52 percent) of the nation uses insect repellents, including some made with potent insecticides.

Chemical Weapons

Terrorist threats include the possibility of the use of chemical weapons. Possible bioterror agents include poison gases, herbicides, and other types of chemical substances that can kill, maim, or temporarily incapacitate. Chemical agents can be dispersed as liquids, vapors, gases, and aerosols that attack nerves, blood, skin, or lungs. In contrast to biological weapons, chemical weapons can kill rapidly, often within hours or minutes, and sometimes with just a small drop. Possible protection against chemical weapons includes gas masks, shelters, and sealed suits and vehicles. Treatment and antidotes can sometimes help after exposure. If contaminated, you need to flush your eyes and skin immediately for at least five to ten minutes while awaiting emergency help.

Some common chemical agents include ricin, which when inhaled causes weakness, fever, chest tightness, cough, and severe respiratory problems including potentially fatal fluid buildup in the lungs; sarin, a nerve gas that can cause death within minutes by paralyzing the muscles used for breathing; and VX, which kills within minutes by blocking the transmission of nerve impulses along the central nervous system, causing convulsions, respiratory paralysis, and death.

Multiple Chemical Sensitivity

The proliferation of chemicals in modern society has led to an entirely new disease, **multiple chemical sensitivity (MCS),** also called environmentally triggered illness, universal allergy, or chemical AIDS. MCS was first described almost a half century ago when a Chicago allergist treated a number of patients who reported becoming ill after being exposed to various petrochemicals. Since that time, many more cases of MCS have been reported, yet there is no agreed-upon definition of the condition, no medical test that can diagnose it, and no proven treatment.

According to medical theory, people become chemically sensitive in a two-step process: First, they experience a major exposure to a chemical, such as a pesticide, a solvent, or a combustion product. The sensitized person then begins to react to low-level chemical exposures from ordinary substances, such as perfumes and tobacco smoke. Symptoms include a runny nose, breathing difficulties, memory problems, chest pain, depression, dizziness, fatigue, headache, inability to concentrate, nausea, aches and pains in muscles and joints, and heart palpitations.[17]

Invisible Threats

Among the unseen threats to health are various forms of *radiation,* energy radiated in the form of waves or particles.

Electromagnetic Fields

Any electrically charged conductor generates two kinds of invisible fields: electric and magnetic. Together they're called **electromagnetic fields (EMFs).** For years, these fields, produced by household appliances, home wiring, lighting fixtures, electric blankets, and overhead power lines, were considered harmless. However, epidemiological studies have revealed a link between exposure to high-voltage lines and cancer (especially leukemia, a blood cancer) in electrical workers and children.

Laboratory studies on animals have shown that alternating current, which changes strength and direction 60 times a second (and electrifies most of North America), emits EMFs that may interfere with the normal functioning of human cell membranes, which have their own electromagnetic fields. The result may be mood disorders, changes in circadian rhythms (our inner sense of time), miscarriage, developmental problems, or cancer.

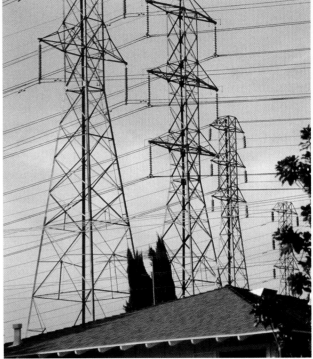

© Tony Freeman/PhotoEdit

Although laboratory studies on animals indicate that EMFs affect human cell membranes, research on humans has found only a weak connection between EMFs and disease.

Researchers have documented increases in breast cancer deaths in women who worked as electrical engineers, electricians, or in other high-exposure jobs, and a link between EMF exposure and increased risk of leukemia and possibly brain cancer.

After six years of congressionally mandated research, the National Institute of Environmental Health Sciences concluded that the evidence of a risk of cancer and other human disease from the electric and magnetic fields around power lines is "weak." This finding applies to the extremely low frequency electric and magnetic fields surrounding both the big power lines that distribute power and the smaller but closer electric lines in homes and

endocrine disruptors Synthetic chemicals that interfere with the ways that hormones work in humans and wildlife.

chlorinated hydrocarbons Highly toxic pesticides, such as DDT and chlordane, that are extremely resistant to breakdown; may cause cancer, birth defects, neurological disorders, and damage to wildlife and the environment.

organic phosphates Toxic pesticides that may cause cancer, birth defects, neurological disorders, and damage to wildlife and the environment.

multiple chemical sensitivity (MCS) A sensitivity to low-level chemical exposures from ordinary substances, such as perfumes and tobacco smoke, that results in physiological responses such as chest pain, depression, dizziness, fatigue, and nausea. Also known as environmentally triggered illness.

electromagnetic fields (EMFs) The invisible electric and magnetic fields generated by an electrically charged conductor.

appliances. However, the researchers also noted that EMF exposure "cannot be recognized as entirely safe."

Expectant mothers who often use electric blankets or heated water beds during winter have a higher miscarriage rate than nonusers. Babies conceived in the winter by electric blanket–users grow more slowly in the womb and tend to have a lower birthweight than others. Federal officials urge "prudent avoidance" of electric blankets for women who are pregnant or hoping to conceive.

Cell phones emit low levels of electromagnetic energy (see Savvy Consumer: "Are Cell Phones Safe to Use?").

Microwaves

Microwaves (extremely high frequency electromagnetic waves) increase the rate at which molecules vibrate; this vibration generates heat. There's no evidence that existing levels of microwave radiation encountered in the environment pose a health risk to people, and all home microwave ovens must meet safety standards for leakage.

A concern about the safety of microwave ovens stems from the chemicals in plastic wrapping and plastic containers used in microwave ovens. Chemicals may leak into food. In high concentrations, some of the chemicals (such as DEHA, which makes plastic more pliable) can cause cancer in mice. Consumers should be cautious about using clingy plastic wrap when reheating leftovers, and plastic-encased metal "heat susceptors" included in convenience foods such as popcorn and pizza. Although these materials seem safe when tested in conventional ovens at temperatures of 300° to 350° Fahrenheit, microwave ovens can boost temperatures to 500° Fahrenheit.

Ionizing Radiation

Radiation that possesses enough energy to separate electrons from their atoms, leaving charged ions, is called **ionizing radiation.** Its effects on health depend on many factors, including the amount, length of exposure, type, part of the body exposed, and the health and age of the individual.

We're surrounded by low-level ionizing radiation every day. Most comes from cosmic rays and radioactive minerals, which vary according to geography. (Denver has more than Atlanta, for instance, because of its altitude.) Man-made sources, including medical and dental X-rays, account for approximately 18 percent of the average person's lifetime exposure.

Radiation exposure in humans is measured in units called rads and rems. A *rad (radiation absorbed dose)* is a measure of the energy deposited by ionizing radiation when it's absorbed by an object. A *rem (roentgen equivalent man)* is a measure of the biological effect of ionizing radiation. Different types of radiation cause different amounts of damage. The rem measurement takes this into account. For X-rays, rads and rems are equivalent. A quantity of 1 rad or 1 rem is a substantial dose of radiation. Smaller doses are measured in *milliards* (thousandths of a rad) or *millirems* (thousandths of a rem). The average annual radiation exposure for a person in the United States is about one-tenth of a rem.

Virtually any part of the body can be affected by ionizing radiation, although bone marrow and the thyroid are especially vulnerable. Radon exposures in homes can increase the risk of lung cancer. Although high levels of radiation are most dangerous, even low-level radiation can be harmful to health. According to the National Research Council, the risk of getting cancer from small amounts of radiation is four times more than had been previously estimated, and there's much greater danger of mental retardation among babies exposed to radiation in the womb from eight to fifteen weeks after conception.

Diagnostic X-Rays

The EPA estimates that 30 to 50 percent of the 700 million X-rays taken every year in the United States are unnecessary. However, doctors sometimes prescribe X-rays or newer imaging techniques involving radiation, such as CT scans, to protect themselves from malpractice suits, and hospitals benefit financially from the heavy use of X-ray equipment.

Dental X-rays involve little radiation, but many people receive so many so often that they're second only to chest examinations in frequency. Dentists typically obtain radiographs of all the teeth at the beginning of a patient's care, and again every three to five years. However, you can cut down on total X-rays by bringing previous films with you or having your dentist forward copies when you switch dentists.

Always ask why an X-ray is being ordered. Don't give your consent unless there's a clear need. Keep a record of the date and location of every X-ray exam. Some of these X-rays may someday provide information that would make more X-rays unnecessary. Ask the radiologist to explain specifically how much radiation you'll be exposed to, and be sure to wear a protective leaded apron. There's no sense in refusing a needed medical X-ray just because you're afraid of the radiation exposure. Under certain circumstances, the benefits far outweigh the risks.

Irradiated Foods

The use of radiation on food, from either radioactive substances or devices that produce X-rays, is known as **irradiation.** It doesn't make the food radioactive—its primary benefit is to prolong the food's useful life. Like the heat in canning, irradiation can kill all the microorganisms that might grow in food; the sterilized food can

Savvy Consumer   Are Cell Phones Safe?

Since cellular phone service was introduced in the United States in 1984, mobile and handheld phones have become ubiquitous, and concern has grown about their possible health risks. The federal government sets upper exposure limits to electromagnetic energy from cell phones known as the specific absorption rate, or SAR. A phone emits the most radiation during a call, but it also emits small amounts periodically whenever it's turned on.

Can exposure to low levels of electromagnetic energy that the body absorbs from a cell phone be harmful? More than 70 research papers on the potentially harmful effects of cell phone use have raised concerns about cancer, neurological disorders, sleep problems, or headaches; others have shown no association or were inconclusive. The Food and Drug Administration (FDA) and Federal Communications Commission (FCC) have stated that "the available scientific evidence does not show that any health problems are associated with using wireless phones. There is no proof, however, that wireless phones are absolutely safe." Additional studies are underway.

Researchers have documented an increase in ear canal temperature with cell phone use, protein changes in human cells exposed to cell phone radiation, and an increased rate of benign brain tumors.[18] Some health experts have discouraged children from using cell phones largely because of concerns that their developing nervous systems may be especially vulnerable.

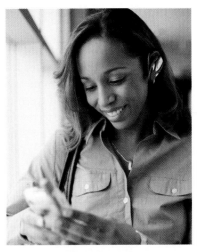

© Jim Craigmyle/CORBIS

A headset can keep the phone's antenna away from your head and body. Shields that claim to reduce exposure generally don't work as advertised, according to the FDA and FCC.

then be stored for years in sealed containers at room temperature without spoiling. In addition, low-dose irradiation can inhibit the sprouting of vegetables such as potatoes and onions, and delay the ripening of some fruits, such as bananas, mangoes, tomatoes, pears, and avocados—cost-saving benefits of great appeal to the food industry.

Irradiated foods are believed to be safe to eat, and the federal government has approved their distribution. Most research has focused on low-dose irradiation to delay ripening and destroy insects. Nutritional studies have shown no significant decreases in the quality of the foods, but high-dose treatments may cause vitamin losses similar to those that occur during canning. It's also possible that the ionizing effect of radiation creates new compounds in foods that may be mutagenic or carcinogenic. In meats, irradiation proved less effective than cooking in destroying bacteria.

microwaves   Extremely high frequency electromagnetic waves that increase the rate at which molecules vibrate, thereby generating heat.

ionizing radiation   A form of energy emitted from atoms as they undergo internal change.

irradiation   Exposure to or treatment by some form of radiation.

Learn It ┊ **Live It**

Taking Care of Mother Earth

Environmental problems can seem so complex that you may think there's little you can do about them. That's not the case. This world can be made better instead of worse. The job isn't easy, and all of us have to do our part. Just as many diseases of the previous century have been eradicated, so in time we may be able to remove or reduce many environmental threats. Your future—and our planet's future—may depend on it.

- **Plant a tree.** Even a single tree helps absorb carbon dioxide and produces cooling that can reduce the need for air conditioning.

- **Look for simply packaged items.** Whenever possible, choose items packed in recycled materials or something recyclable.

- **Bring your own bag.** Whenever possible, avoid using plastic or paper bags for items you could carry in a cloth or string carryall.

- **Hit the switch.** Turn off all electrical appliances (TVs, CD players, radios, lights, computers, printers) when you're not in the room or paying attention to them.

- **Avoid disposables.** Use a mug instead of a paper or Styrofoam cup, a sponge instead of a paper towel, a cloth napkin instead of a paper one.

- **Be water wise.** Turn off the tap while you shave or brush your teeth. Install water-efficient faucets, toilets, and shower heads. Wash clothes in cold water. Drink tap rather than bottled water.

- **Cancel junk mail.** It consumes 100 million trees a year. To get off mailing lists, write: Direct Mail Association, Mail Preference Service, P.O. Box 9008, Farmingdale, NY 11735-9008

- **Spare the seas.** If you live near the coast or are picnicking or hiking near the ocean, don't use plastic bags (which are often blown into the water) or plastic six-pack holders (which can get caught around the necks of sea birds).

- **Don't buy products made of endangered substances.** Examples include coral, ivory, tortoise shell, or wood from endangered forests (teak, mahogany, ebony, rosewood).

- **Speak out.** E-mail your senators and congressional representatives, who vote on pollution controls, budgets for the enforcement of safety regulations, and the preservation of forests and wildlife. Identify the particular bill or issue you're addressing. Be as specific, brief, and to the point as possible. Go to **www.senate.gov** and click on "Senators" to find the e-mail addresses. To find your congressional representative, go to **www.house.gov** and click on "Write Your Representative."

Are You Doing Your Part for the Planet?

You may think that there is little you can do, as an individual, to save Earth. But everyday acts can add up and make a difference in helping or harming the planet on which we live.

	Almost Never	Sometimes	Always
1. Do you walk, cycle, carpool, or use public transportation as much as possible to get around?	____	____	____
2. Do you recycle?	____	____	____
3. Do you reuse plastic and paper bags?	____	____	____
4. Do you try to conserve water by not running the tap as you shampoo or brush your teeth?	____	____	____
5. Do you use products made of recycled materials?	____	____	____
6. Do you drive a car that gets good fuel mileage and has up-to-date emission control equipment?	____	____	____
7. Do you turn off lights, televisions, and appliances when you're not using them?	____	____	____
8. Do you avoid buying products that are elaborately packaged?	____	____	____
9. Do you use glass jars and waxed paper rather than plastic wrap for storing food?	____	____	____
10. Do you take brief showers rather than baths?	____	____	____
11. Do you use cloth towels and napkins rather than paper products?	____	____	____
12. When listening to music, do you keep the volume low?	____	____	____
13. Do you try to avoid any potential carcinogens, such as asbestos, mercury, or benzene?	____	____	____
14. Are you careful to dispose of hazardous materials (such as automobile oil or antifreeze) at appropriate sites?	____	____	____
15. Do you follow environmental issues in your community and write your state or federal representatives to support "green" legislation?	____	____	____

Count the number of items you've checked in each column. If you've circled 10 or more in the "always" column, you're definitely helping to make a difference. If you've mainly circled "sometimes," you're moving in the right direction, but you need to be more consistent and more conscientious. If you've circled 10 or more in the "never" column, carefully read this chapter and "Your Health Action Plan for Protecting the Planet" to find out what you can do.

Your Health Action Plan for Protecting the Planet

Simple steps can help save energy, lower carbon dioxide (CO_2) emissions, and cut down on energy costs. Here are some recommendations from the Environmental Defense and World Wildlife Fund:

- Wash laundry in warm or cold water, not hot. *Average annual CO_2 reduction: up to 500 pounds for two loads of laundry a week.*

- Buy products sold in the simplest possible packaging. Carry a tote bag or recycle shopping bags. *Average annual CO_2 reduction: 1,000 pounds because garbage is reduced 25 percent.*

- Switch from standard light bulbs to energy-efficient fluorescent ones. *Average annual CO_2 reduction: about 500 pounds per bulb.*

- Set room thermostats lower in winter and higher in summer. *Average annual CO_2 reduction: about 500 pounds for each two-degree reduction.*

- Run dishwashers only when full, and choose the energy-saving mode rather than the regular setting. *Average annual CO_2 reduction: 200 pounds.*

- Bike, carpool, or take mass transit whenever possible. *Average annual CO_2 reduction: 20 pounds for each gallon of gasoline saved.*

- Drive a car that gets high gas mileage and produces low emissions. Keep your speed at or below the speed limit.

- Keep your tires inflated and your engine tuned. Recycle old batteries and tires. (Most stores that sell new ones will take back old ones.)

- Turn off your engine if you're going to be stopped for more than a minute.

- Collect all fluids that you drain from your car (motor oil, antifreeze) and recycle or properly dispose of them.

CENGAGENOW™ If you want to write your own goals for working toward a healthy environment, go to the Wellness Journal at HealthNow: **academic. cengage.com/login.**

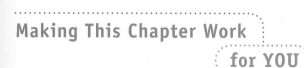

Making This Chapter Work for YOU

Review Questions

1. Threats to the environment include
   a. an open ecosystem.
   b. depletion of the oxygen layer.
   c. ecological processes.
   d. global warming.

2. Which of the following statements about climate change is true?
   a. Increasing carbon dioxide production will slow the progress of global warming.
   b. Most experts say that the buildup of greenhouse gases is changing natural climate and weather patterns.
   c. Climate change poses no health risks for humans in the next 20 years.
   d. Increasing tree cover and agricultural lands will contribute to global warming.

3. Mutagens
   a. are caused by birth defects.
   b. result in changes to the DNA of body cells.
   c. are agents that trigger changes in the DNA of body cells.
   d. are caused by repeated exposure to pollutants.

4. Which of the following statements about air pollution is *false?*
   a. More than 80 percent of the people in the United States live in counties with unhealthy levels of ozone or particle pollution.
   b. Ozone in the upper atmosphere protects us from harmful ultraviolet radiation from the sun, but in the lower atmosphere, it is a harmful air pollutant.
   c. Air pollution can cause the same types of respiratory health problems as smoking.
   d. Particle pollution diminishes lung function and increases the severity of asthma attacks.

5. One of the most important things you can do to help protect the environment is
   a. use as much water as possible to help lower the ocean water levels.
   b. recycle paper, bottles, cans, and unwanted food.
   c. avoid energy-depleting fluorescent bulbs.
   d. use plastic storage containers and plastic wrap to save trees from being cut down.

6. An example of the concept of sustainability is
   a. getting enough to eat at every meal.
   b. lowering the price of gas to 1990 levels.

   c. using wind power to generate electricity.
   d. maintaining our current levels of energy usage.

7. You can protect your hearing by
   a. avoiding prolonged exposure to sounds under 75 decibels.
   b. using foam earplugs when operating noisy tools or attending rock concerts.
   c. limiting noise exposure to short bursts of loud sounds such as fireworks.
   d. drinking alcohol in noisy environments to mute the sounds.

8. Drinking water safety
   a. may be compromised if your water comes from a well.
   b. is low in the United States because of chemical treatment.
   c. can be guaranteed by using bottled water, which is completely free of chemical contaminants.
   d. is measured by the cases of illness reported each year.

9. Pesticide risks to health include:
   a. reduced male fertility.
   b. higher incidence of childhood brain cancer if parents have been exposed.
   c. higher incidence of cancer and birth defects from chlorinated hydrocarbons such as DDT.
   d. higher incidence of diabetes.

10. Which statement about radiation is *false?*
    a. Evidence indicates a weak link between electromagnetic fields around power lines and cancer and other diseases.
    b. Radio frequency signals from cell phones cause brain cancer.
    c. Women who are pregnant should not use electric blankets.
    d. Chemicals in plastic wrap may leak into foods heated in microwave ovens.

Answers to these questions can be found on page 583.

Critical Thinking

1. How do you contribute to environmental pollution? How might you change your habits to protect the environment?

2. An excerpt from a recent newspaper article stated, "Children living in a public housing project near a local refinery suffer from a high rate of asthma and allergies, and an environmental group says the plant may be to blame." The refinery has met all the local air quality standards, employs hundreds in the community, and pays substantial city taxes, which support police, fire, and social services. If you were a city council member, how would you balance health and environmental concerns with the

need for industry in your community? What actions would you recommend in this particular situation?

3. In one Harris poll, 84 percent of Americans said that, given a choice between a high standard of living (but with hazardous air and water pollution and the depletion of natural resources) and a lower standard of living (but with clean air and drinking water), they would prefer clean air and drinking water and a lower standard of living. What about you? What exactly would you be willing to give up: air conditioning, convenience packaging and products, driving your own car rather than using public transportation? Do you think most people are willing to change their lifestyles to preserve the environment?

Media Menu

CENGAGENOW™ Go to the HealthNow website at **academic.cengage .com/login** that will:

- Help you evaluate your knowledge of the material.
- Allow you to take an exam-prep quiz.
- Provide a Personalized Learning Plan targeting resources that address areas you should study.
- Coach you through identifying target goals for behavioral change and creating and monitoring your personal change plan throughout the semester.

INTERNET CONNECTIONS

Envirolink

www.envirolink.org

Envirolink is a nonprofit organization that brings together individuals and groups concerned about the environment and provides access to a wealth of online environmental resources.

Student Environmental Action Coalition

www.seac.org

Since 1988, the Student Environmental Action Coalition has been empowering students and youth to fight for environmental and social justice in our schools and communities.

Campus Climate Challenge

www.campusclimatechallenge.org

The Challenge leverages the power of young people to organize on college campuses and high schools across Canada and the United States to win 100% Clean Energy policies at their schools.

The Stop Global Warming Virtual March

www.stopglobalwarming.org

This site is a nonpartisan effort to bring citizens together to declare that global warming is here now and that it is time to demand solutions.

National Center for Environmental Health (NCEH)

www.cdc.gov/nceh/

This site, sponsored by the U.S. Centers for Disease Control and Prevention, features a searchable database as well as fact sheets and brochures on a variety of environmental topics, from emergency preparedness and public health tracking to environmental hazards and lead poisoning prevention.

Key Terms

The terms listed are used and defined on the page indicated. Definitions are also found in the Glossary at the end of this book.

carcinogen   539
chlorinated hydrocarbons 549
decibel (dB)   545
ecosystem   539
electromagnetic fields (EMFs)   549
endocrine disruptors   549
ionizing radiation   549
irradiation   549
microwaves   549
multiple chemical sensitivity   549
mutagen   539
organic phosphates   549
ozone   541
pollutant   539
precycling   543
recycling   543
sustainability   543

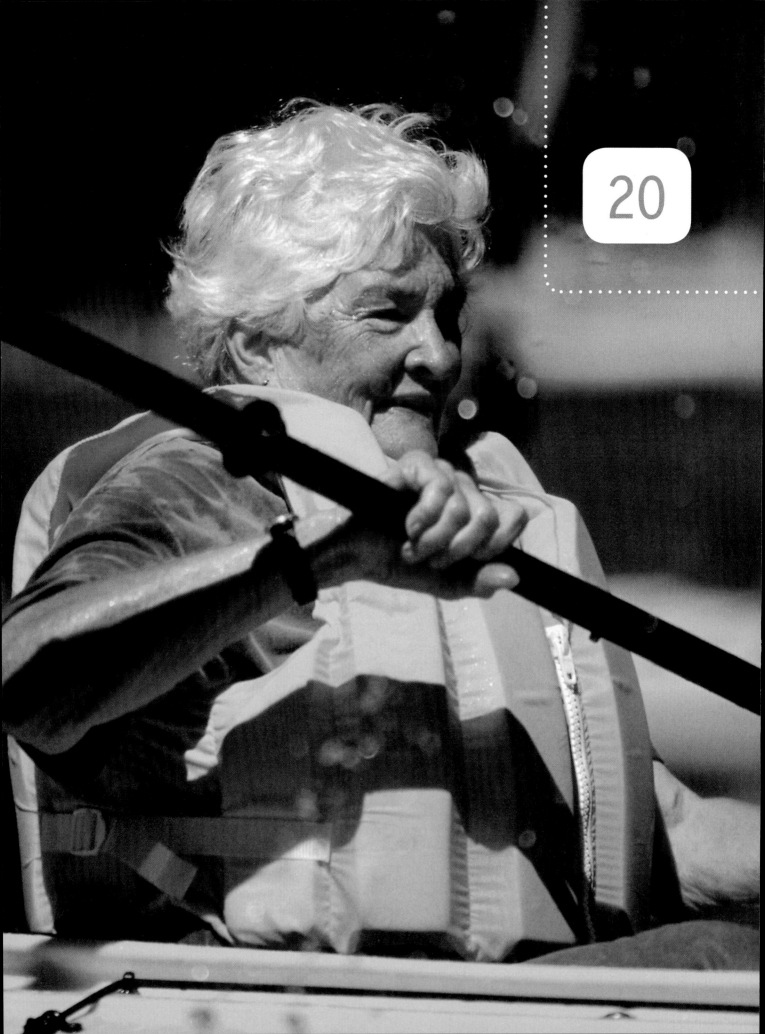

A Lifetime of Health

SHIRLEY didn't feel old until she enrolled in a college personal health course. Formal at first, the other students—young enough to be her children—started calling her "Mom." When the professor announced that the next week's topic would be aging, Shirley beamed, "I'll be the expert!"

More of us can expect to do the same. In the United States, the number of persons over age 65 is expected to increase to an estimated 71 million in 2030, more than the number of school-age children.

Although **aging**—the characteristic pattern of normal life changes that occurs as humans, plants, and animals grow older—remains inevitable, you can do a great deal to influence the impact that the passage of time has on you. Whether you're in your teens, twenties, thirties, or older, now is the time to start taking the steps that will add healthy, active, productive years to your life.

This chapter provides a preview of the changes age brings, the steps you can take to age healthfully, and the ways you can make the most of all the years of your life.

Invariably, though, no one gets out of this life alive. Death is the natural completion of things, as much a part of the real world as life itself. In time we all lose people we cherish: grandparents, aunts and uncles, parents, friends, neighbors, coworkers, siblings. With each loss, part of us may seem to die, yet each loss also reaffirms how precious life is. (See the lab called "Finity" in *IPC*.) **IPC**

This chapter explores the meaning of death, describes the process of dying, provides information on end-of-life issues, and offers advice on comforting the dying and helping their survivors.

After studying the material in this chapter, you should be able to:

- **List** the benefits that older Americans can gain from physical activity.

- **Name** three memory skills that diminish with age.

- **Discuss** the hormonal changes that occur in men and women at midlife.

- **Name** two challenges of aging and **discuss** their risk factors and possible ways of preventing them.

- **Explain** the purposes of advanced directives.

- **Define** death and **explain** the stages of emotional reaction experienced in facing death.

- **Name** a chapter topic that affects someone in your family, and **discuss** how your knowledge and attitude on the topic has changed.

CENGAGENOW™ Log on to HealthNow at **academic.cengage.com/login** to find your Behavior Change Planner and to explore self-assessments, interactive tutorials, and practice quizzes.

The Aging of America

About one in eight Americans—approximately 12 percent of the population—is over age 65. With millions of baby boomers reaching retirement age, one in every four Americans will be older than 65 by the year 2030. The number of centenarians has increased a whopping 88 percent since 1900.[1] (See Figure 20.1.)

 Older Americans are as diverse as other segments of our population. About one in five (19 percent) comes from a minority group. The largest percentage of these are African American (8 percent) or Hispanic (6 percent). Asians or Pacific Islanders make up about 3 percent of older Americans.[2]

Americans celebrating their 65th birthdays can expect to live an additional 18.4 years—19.8 years for women and 16.8 years for men. Older men are much more likely to be married than older women: 72 percent of men have spouses, compared with 42 percent of women. Over half of older Americans live with their husbands or wives. About 30 percent of Americans over age 65 live alone, as do half of women over age 75. About 1.57 million older people care for their grandchildren, either as primary caretakers or along with a parent.

About one in four older Americans—38 percent, compared with 67 percent of those between ages 18 and 64—describe their health as excellent or very good. Older African Americans, American Indians/Alaska Natives, and Hispanics are less likely to say they are in top health than are whites. Most older persons have at least one chronic condition; many have several health problems. Among the most frequent are hypertension, arthritis, heart disease, cancer, and diabetes.[3]

How Long Can You Expect to Live?

The answer depends on you. Statistically, you're likely to live longer than your parents or grandparents. Life

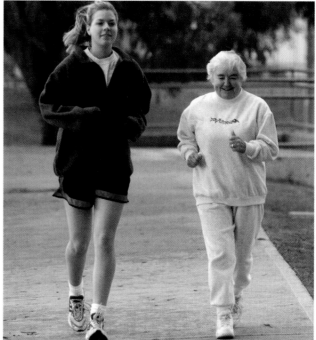

Why do you think this student would probably say "old" is about 60, while the woman on the right would likely say 70?

expectancy has been increasing steadily over the last century, reaching an all-time high in the United States of 77.6 years. According to the National Center for Health Statistics, life expectancy for American women now stands at 80.4 years; for men, it is a record high of 75.2 years.

Contrary to common belief, heredity doesn't determine how long you'll live or how well you'll age. Genes, as studies of identical twins have revealed, influence only about 30 percent of the rate and ways in which we age.

 When does a person become old? That answer may depend on your gender. In a survey of 441 undergraduates at a large southeastern university, men said that a person becomes "old" at age 58.

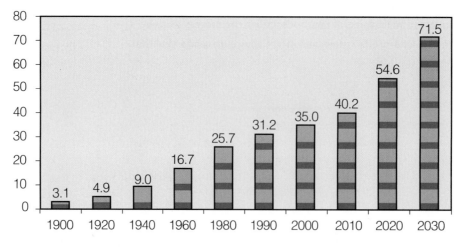

Figure 20.1 Number of Persons Age 65 and Over, 1900–2030 (in millions)

Source: *A Profile of Older Americans: 2006.* Washington, DC: Administration on Aging, 2007.

Women viewed a person becoming "old" at age 62. But "old," like beauty, may be in the eye of the beholder. In other studies individuals between the ages of 65 and 74 identified 70 as the age at which a person becomes "old."[4]

The Longevity Gender Gap

Women's lifespans average 5 to 10 percent longer than men's. No one knows exactly why. This longevity gender gap has been shrinking since 1990 and now stands at 5.2 years. Women in other developed nations—Australia, Canada, France, Greece, Italy, Japan, the Netherlands, Norway, Spain, Sweden, Switzerland—live up to two years longer than those in the United States and about seven years longer than men. In the former Soviet Union, life expectancy for females is 13 years longer than for males.

The gender gap in longevity also narrows over time. At birth a baby boy has a life expectancy about five years shorter than a girl's. By age 65, a man can expect to live an additional 16.8 years, just three years less than a woman. By age 85, the difference in projected life expectancies is down to 1.2 years.

The gender difference in mortality rates emerges from the moment of conception. Baby girls are less likely to die in the womb or after delivery than baby boys. Once past age 30, women consistently outnumber and outlive men. By age 85, there are three women for every man.

Why do men die sooner? The female edge may begin at conception with the extra X chromosome, which provides a backup for defects on the X gene and a double dose of the genetic factors that regulate the immune system. In addition, the female hormone estrogen bolsters immunity and protects heart, bone, brain, and blood vessels.

In some cancers, estrogen may somehow protect against distant metastases. In contrast, testosterone may dampen the immune response in males—possibly to prevent attacks on sperm cells that might otherwise be mistaken as alien invaders. When the testes are removed from mice and guinea pigs, their immune systems become more active. In men, lessened immunity may lower resistance to cancer as well as infectious disease. Half of all men—compared with a third of women—develop cancer. Smoking, which for a long time was much more prevalent among men, accounts for some of this difference. However, this is changing; 23 percent of American women smoke, and lung cancer rates in women have doubled since the early 1970s.

Testosterone also has been implicated in men's risk of heart disease and stroke. Originally designed to equip men with an instantaneous burst of power—essential for survival in Stone Age times—this potent male hormone may surge so intensely that it wreaks havoc throughout the cardiovascular system.

Males also die more often as a result of intentional and nonintentional injury. Overall, men are three times more likely than women to die in accidents, mainly in cars and on the job. Men also are four times more likely to die violently. Nine in ten murderers and eight in ten murder victims are men.

REALITYCHECK

Do you think the following statements are true or false?

• *Happiness usually peaks in young adulthood and declines throughout life.* _____

• *The happiest Americans are older than age 50.* _____

Answers on next page.

Successful Aging

Americans are living better as well as longer. Disability decreased steadily through the 1980s and 1990s, and the rate of improvement is accelerating. Nursing home use has fallen. Senior citizens are healthier and more independent. Among the factors contributing to a longer healthspan are improved medical care, diet, exercise, and public health advances.

 When surveyed, about half of Americans aged 65 to 69 say, "These are the best years of my life." Many people in their seventies and eighties agree. Sixty percent of older black and 57 percent of older Hispanic respondents say these are their best years. When asked about the keys to a meaningful and vital life, older adults rate having family and friends and taking care of their health as most important, followed by spiritual life. (See this chapter's Reality Check.)

Physical Activity: It's Never Too Late

The effects of ongoing activity are so profound that gerontologists sometimes refer to exercise as "the closest thing to an antiaging pill." Exercise slows many changes associated with advancing age, such as loss of lean muscle tissue, increase in body fat, and decreased work capacity. The bottom line: What you *don't* do may matter more than what you do do.

No one is ever too old to get in shape. The American College of Sports Medicine encourages seniors to engage in the full range of physical activities, including aerobic conditioning. With regular conditioning, 60-year-olds can regain the fitness they had at age 40 to 45. Adults over the age of 72 who exercise more and smoke less than their peers are most likely to enjoy long, healthy, and happy

aging The characteristic pattern of normal life changes that occur as living things grow older.

PART II: *Just the facts*

- **False.** *Happiness typically declines through adolescence and young adulthood, reaching its lowest point in a person's forties.*
- **True.** *Both women and men report greater happiness after age 50 and continue to do so until extreme old age.*

Sources: Based on the British Household Panel Survey, conducted by Andrew Oswald, Institute of Education, University of London. Several American studies have confirmed the same pattern of happiness increasing with age.

lives, according to a study that followed 1,000 seniors for nine years.

Exercise lowers the risk of heart disease and stroke in the elderly—and greatly improves general health. Male and female runners over age 50 have much lower rates of disability and much lower health-care expenses than less active seniors. Even less intense activities, such as gardening, dancing, and brisk walking, can delay chronic physical disability and cognitive decline.

According to the U.S. surgeon general, physical activity offers older Americans additional benefits, including the following:

- **Greater ability to live independently.**
- **Reduced risk of falling and fracturing bones.**
- **Lower risk of dying from coronary heart disease** and of developing high blood pressure, colon cancer, and diabetes.
- **Reduced blood pressure** in some people with hypertension.
- **Fewer symptoms of anxiety** and depression.
- **Improvements in mood** and feelings of well- being.

Despite these potential benefits, many seniors are not active. By age 75, about one in three men and one in two women engage in no physical activity. Yet even sedentary

---

Your Life Change Coach

Staying Healthy Longer

If you want to feel young when you're older, the time to start taking care of yourself is now—whether you're 25, 45, or 65. The healthier you become now, the longer you're likely to stay healthy in the future.

Since genes influence only about 30 percent of the aging process, "the rest is up to us," says Michael Roizen, M.D., coauthor of *You: The Owner's Manual,* who notes that it's possible to turn back the biological clock. "With relatively simple changes, someone whose chronological age is 69 can have a physiological age of 45. And the most amazing thing is that it's never too late to live younger—until one foot is six feet under."[5]

Keep Your Arteries Young

"You are as young—or as old—as your arteries," says Roizen. Problems like high blood pressure, high cholesterol, and buildup of atherosclerotic plaque increase the likelihood of stroke, heart disease, kidney problems, even memory impairment. If your arteries are healthy, you're much more likely to have a healthy heart and a healthy brain. People with "young" arteries tend to retain a higher level of cognitive functioning.

Premature aging of the arteries is largely self-inflicted; common culprits are a high-fat diet, lack of exercise, obesity, and a high-stress lifestyle. At any age, the unexercised body—though free of the symptoms of illness—will rust out long before it could ever wear out.

Avoid Illness

In studies of centenarians, most have had no serious chronic illnesses. Among the most important strategies: not smoking, avoiding weight gain in middle age, and recognizing and treating conditions like elevated cholesterol and high blood pressure.

Also important is keeping up with immunizations against diseases, such as influenza and pneumococcal pneumonia, that take a greater toll on the elderly. For women at risk of osteoporosis, new options, including "designer estrogens" like raloxifene, can preserve their bones' health. A healthy diet, chockful of fruits and vegetables, also can contribute to a healthy old age, in part because

individuals in their eighties and nineties can participate in an exercise program—and gain significant benefits.

Nutrition and Obesity

The most common nutritional disorder in older persons is obesity. Overweight men and women over age 65 face higher risk of diabetes, heart disease, stroke, and other health problems, including arthritis.

Many elderly people who live independently do not get adequate amounts of one or more essential nutrients. The reasons are many: limited income, difficulty getting to stores, chronic illness, medications that interfere with the metabolism of nutrients, problems chewing or digesting, poor appetite, inactivity, illness, depression. Nutritionists urge the elderly, like other Americans, to concentrate on eating healthful foods; many also recommend daily nutritional supplements, which may provide the added benefit of improving cognitive function in healthy people over 65.

The Aging Brain

Scientists used to think that the aging brain, once worn out, could never be fixed. Now they know that the brain can and does repair itself. When neurons (brain cells) die, the surrounding cells develop "fingers" to fill the gaps and establish new connections, or synapses, between surviving neurons. Although self-repair occurs more quickly in young brains, the process continues in older brains. Even victims of Alzheimer's disease, the most devastating form of senility, have enough healthy cells in the diseased brain to regrow synapses. Scientists hope to develop drugs that someday may help the brain repair itself.

Mental ability does not decline along with physical vigor. Researchers have been able to reverse the supposedly normal intellectual declines of 60- to 80-year-olds by tutoring them in problem solving. Reaction time, intellectual speed and efficiency, nonverbal intelligence, and maximum work rate for short periods may diminish by age 75. However, understanding, vocabulary,

they contain antioxidants that may ward off many age-related problems.

Maintain Your Zest for Living

Attitude matters. The healthiest seniors are "engaged" in life, resilient, optimistic, productive, and socially involved. While they are not immune to life's slings and arrows, successful agers bounce back after a setback and have a "can-do" attitude about the challenges they face. They also tend to be lifelong learners who may take up entirely new hobbies late in life—pursuits that stimulate production of more connections between neurons and may slow aging within the brain. Social interactions, such as entertaining friends and getting involved with religious activities, lead to greater life satisfaction as people get older.

Just as with muscles, the best advice to keep your brain healthy as you age is "use it or lose it." Some memory losses among healthy older people are normal—but reversible with training in simple methods, such as word associations, that improve recall.

Stay Strong

For years, experts assumed that older meant weaker. Landmark research with frail nursing home residents in their eighties and nineties showed this isn't so. After just eight to ten weeks of strength training, even the oldest seniors increased muscle and bone, sped up their metabolic rate, improved sleep and mobility, boosted their spirits, and gained in self-confidence. Other studies have found that exercise programs can increase lung capacity, double leg strength, and decrease the risk of disability and premature death.

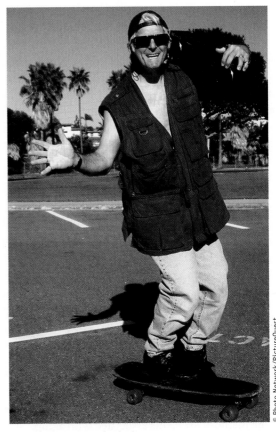

Age is partly a matter of attitude.

© Photo Network/PictureQuest

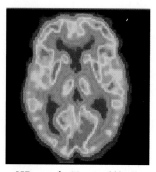
PET scan of a 20-year-old brain

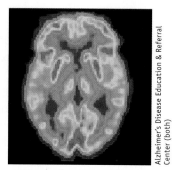
PET scan of a 80-year-old brain

Alzheimer's Disease Education & Referral Center (both)

In these PET scans, the red and yellow show greater neuron activity in the young adult. The brain of the older person shows less activity and more dark areas, indicating that the fluid-filled ventricles have grown larger.

ability to remember key information, and verbal intelligence remain about the same.

Aspirin, even at low doses, appears to prevent declines in key areas of the brain, according to brain-imaging studies.[6] However, long-term use of low-dose aspirin did not lead to improved thinking, memory, and other cognitive skills in women over age 65 participating in the landmark Women's Health Study.[7] In other research, nonsteroidal anti-inflammatory medications failed to prevent Alzheimer's disease in older men and women with a family history of the disorder.[8]

Memory

Between the ages of 30 and 90, the brain loses about 10 percent of its volume. Forgetfulness isn't an automatic result, however. Crossword puzzles, practicing the piano, and playing chess exercise the brain and can counteract natural changes in memory. Exercise also helps cognitive function.

Some memory skills, particularly the ability to retrieve names and quickly process information, inevitably diminish over time. What normal changes should you expect? Here is a preview:

- **Recalling information takes longer.** As individuals reach their mid- to late sixties, the brain slows down, but usually just by a matter of milliseconds. As long as they're not rushed, older adults eventually adapt and perform just as well as younger ones.

- **Multitasking becomes more difficult.** College students can study and listen to the stereo at the same time. Thirty-something moms can soothe the baby, field questions about homework, and prepare dinner all at once. But older individuals find it much more difficult to divide their attention or to remember details after having switched their attention to something else. Inability to ignore background information while focusing on a task may underlie the memory problems associated with aging.

- **"Accessing" names gets harder.** The ability to remember names, especially those you don't use

frequently, diminishes by as much as 50 percent between ages 25 and 65. Preventive strategies can help, such as repeating a person's name when introduced, writing down the name as soon as possible, and making obvious associations (the Golden Gate for a man named Bridges).

- **Learning new information is harder.** The quality of memory doesn't change, just the speed at which we receive, absorb, and react to information. That's why strategies like taking notes or outlining material become critical for older students, especially when learning new skills. However, adding to existing knowledge remains as easy as ever.

- **Wisdom matters.** In any memory test involving knowledge of the world, vocabulary, or judgment, older people outperform their younger counterparts.

Women at Midlife

In the next two decades some 40 million American women will end their reproductive years. "The primary misconception is that this is a terrible time when all women suffer horrible symptoms," says Sherry Sherman, M.D., project officer for the National Institute of Aging's Study of Women Across the Nation, which has followed 3,300 women through midlife since 1996. "When you look at healthy women in the community in terms of what actually affects their lives, their periods stop. That's it."[9]

Perimenopause

While the average age of **menopause**—defined as the complete cessation of menstrual periods for 12 consecutive months—is 51.5, a woman's reproductive system begins changing more than a decade earlier. "The change of life starts in our thirties with irregular menstrual cycles and then heats up in our forties with hot flashes and night sweats"[10] says psychiatrist Marsha Speller, M.D., author of *The Menopause Answer Book*.

For many women, **perimenopause**—the four-to-ten-year span before a woman's last period—is more baffling and bothersome than the years after. During this time the egg cells, or oocytes, in a woman's ovaries start to senesce or die off at a faster rate. Eventually, the number of egg cells drops to a tiny fraction of the estimated 2 million packed into her ovaries at birth. Trying to coax some of the remaining oocytes to ripen, the pituitary gland churns out extra follicle-stimulating hormone (FSH). This surge is the earliest harbinger of menopause, occurring six to ten years before a woman's final periods. Eventually, the other menstrual messenger, luteinizing hormone (LH), also increases, but at a slower rate.

These hormonal shifts can trigger an array of symptoms. The most common is night sweats (a *subdromal hot*

Savvy Consumer — Alternative Treatments for Menopause Symptoms

For Hot Flashes

- **Lifestyle changes.** These include dressing and eating to avoid being too warm, sleeping in a cool room, and reducing stress. Avoid spicy foods and caffeine. Try deep breathing and stress reduction techniques, including meditation and other relaxation methods.
- **Antidepressants,** such as Effexor, Paxil, and Prozac. These medications have been proved moderately effective in clinical trials.

For Vaginal Dryness

- **Vaginal lubricants** and moisturizers (available over the counter).
- **Products that release estrogen** locally (such as vaginal creams, a vaginal suppository, called Vagifem, and a plastic ring, called an Estring) are used for more severe dryness.

For Mood Swings

- **Lifestyle behaviors,** including getting enough sleep and being physically active.
- **Relaxation exercises.**
- **Antidepressant** or antianxiety drugs.

For Insomnia

- **Over-the-counter sleep aids.**
- **Milk products,** such as a glass of milk or cup of yogurt—choose low-fat or fat-free varieties—consumed at bedtime.
- **Physical activity** in the morning or early afternoon. Exercising later in the day may increase wakefulness.
- **Hot shower or bath** immediately before going to bed.

For Mental Problems

- **Mental exercises.**
- **Lifestyle behaviors,** especially getting enough sleep and being physically active.

---

flash, in medical terms), which can be just intense enough to disrupt sleep. The drop in estrogen levels also may cause hot flashes (bursts of perspiration that last from a few seconds to 15 minutes).

A woman's habits and health history also have an impact. Women with a lifelong history of depression are more likely to experience early perimenopause. The fluctuating hormones of perimenopause may increase depressive symptoms even in women who have never had previous depressions.[11] Smokers experience more symptoms at an earlier age than nonsmokers. Heavier women also have more severe symptoms.

Menopause

About 10 to 15 percent of women breeze through this transition with only trivial symptoms. Another 10 to 15 percent are virtually disabled. The majority fall somewhere in between these extremes. Women who undergo surgical or medical menopause (the result of removal of their ovaries or chemotherapy) often experience abrupt symptoms, including flushing, sweating, sleeplessness, early morning awakenings, involuntary urination, changes in libido, mood swings, perception of memory loss, and changes in cognitive function.

Race and ethnicity profoundly affect women's experience. African American women report more hot flashes and night sweats but have more positive attitudes toward menopause. Japanese and Chinese women experience more muscle stiffness and fewer hot flashes but view menopause more negatively. Hispanic women reach menopause a year or two earlier than Caucasian women; Asian women, a year or two later.

Dwindling levels of estrogen subtly affect many aspects of a woman's health, from her mouth (where dryness, unusual tastes, burning, and gum problems can develop) to her skin (which may become drier, itchier, and overly sensitive to touch). With less estrogen to block them, a woman's androgens, or male hormones, may have a greater impact, causing acne, hair loss, and according to some anecdotal reports, surges in sexual appetite. (Other women, however, report a drop in sexual desire.)

At the same time, a woman's clitoris, vulva, and vaginal lining begin to shrivel, sometimes resulting in pain or bleeding during intercourse. Since the thinner genital tissues are less effective in keeping out bacteria and other pathogens, urinary tract infections may become more common. Some women develop breast or ovarian cysts, which usually go away on their own. Eventually, a woman's ovaries don't respond at all to her pituitary hormones. After the last ovulatory cycle, progesterone is no longer secreted, and estrogen levels decrease rapidly. A woman's testosterone level also falls.

menopause The complete cessation of ovulation and menstruation for twelve consecutive months.

perimenopause The period from a woman's first irregular cycles to her last menstruation.

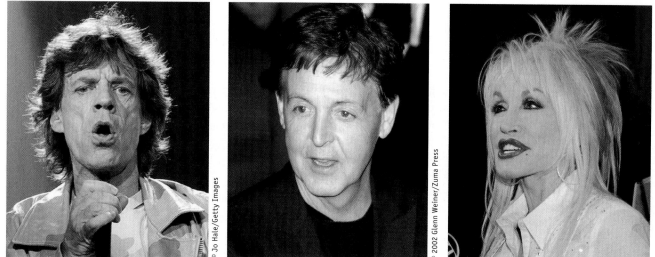

What life after 60 can look like.

In the United States, the average woman who reaches menopause has a life expectancy of about 30 more years. However, she faces risks of various diseases, including an increased risk of obesity, metabolic syndrome, heart disease, stroke, and breast cancer. Women can reduce these risks by exercise, good nutrition, and controlling weight both before and after menopause.

"Exercise is the best thing a woman can do for herself at midlife," says JoAnn Pinkerton, M.D., of the National Women's Health Resource Center. "It improves your heart function so you have less chance of heart disease. It improves your cognition so you think better. It decreases your risk of breast cancer. It helps your mood. It lessens the likelihood of depression. It increases energy and protects your bones."[12] Both walking and yoga have proven effective in easing the symptoms, boosting mood, and improving the quality of life of women during menopause.[13]

Hormone Therapy

 Hormone therapy (HT) was long believed to prevent heart disease and strokes and help women live longer. But medical thinking on HT, particularly a combination of estrogen and progestin, has changed completely in recent years. HT is no longer recommended for reasons other than short-term relief of symptoms such as hot flashes and night sweats.

The Women's Health Initiative (WHI)—a series of clinical trials begun in 1991 on postmenopausal women—halted its study of combination estrogen/progestin therapy in July 2002 and its study of estrogen-only therapy in 2004 because of safety concerns. Combination therapy slightly increased the risk of breast cancer, heart disease, blood clots, and stroke. Women taking only estrogen for shorter periods did not have an elevated rate of breast cancer, but their risk increased significantly after 15 years of use.[14]

The risk of heart disease may be lower if women begin treatment within ten years of menopause. Both estrogen therapy and estrogen-progestin therapy increase the risk of stroke in postmenopausal women. Neither has proven effective in preventing dementia or cognitive decline. Hormonal therapy does reduce the risk of postmenopausal osteoporosis, but its risks and benefits need to be weighed against those of other available treatments. Women who stop hormonal therapy have about a 50 percent chance that their menopausal symptoms will recur, regardless of their age or how long they used HT.[15] In controlled trials black cohosh, the most popular herbal treatment, either alone or with other herbs, proved no more effective than placebo in relieving hot flashes and other menopause symptoms.[16] For alternative treatments for menopause symptoms, see the Savvy Consumer feature.

Men at Midlife

Although men don't experience the dramatic hormonal upheaval that women do, they do experience a decline by as much as 30 to 40 percent in their primary sex hormone, testosterone, between the ages of 48 and 70. This change, sometimes called *andropause,* may cause a range of symptoms, including decreased muscle mass, greater body fat, loss of bone density, flagging energy, lowered fertility, and impaired virility. Some researchers are experimenting with testosterone supplements, which in tests with young men have been shown to increase lean body mass and decrease body fat—at least temporarily. However, other researchers warn that, particularly in older men, excess testosterone might raise the risk of prostate cancer and heart disease.

After age 40, the prostate gland, which surrounds the urethra at the base of the bladder, enlarges. This condition, called *benign prostatic hypertrophy,* occurs in every man. By age 50, half of all men have some enlargement of the gland; after 70, three-quarters do. As it expands, the prostate tends to pinch the urethra, decreasing urinary

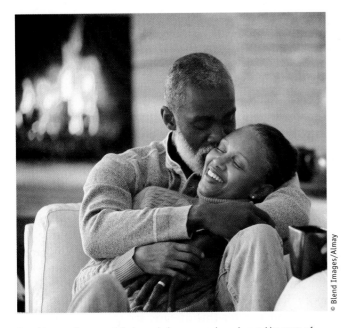

For older couples, sexual desire and pleasure can be enhanced by years of intimacy and affection.

flow and creating a sense of urinary urgency, particularly at night. Other warning signs of prostate problems include difficult urination, blood in the urine, painful ejaculation, or constant lower-back pain.

Medical treatments for benign prostate hypertrophy include drugs that improve urine flow and reduce obstruction of the bladder outlet as well as medications that partially shrink the enlarged prostate by lowering the level of the major male hormone inside the prostate. In some cases, surgical treatment is necessary.

Sexuality and Aging

Health and sexuality interact in various ways as we age. When they are healthy and have a willing partner, a substantial number of older men remain sexually active. The fittest men and women report more frequent sexual activity.

 Other research has found a relationship between sex and longevity. A Swedish study found that men, but not women, who had discontinued intercourse had higher death rates. A study of the entire male population of a small Welsh town found that the sexually active men had half the mortality of the inactive group. In a Duke University study, longevity in women correlated with enjoyment of sexual intercourse, rather than with its frequency.

Aging does cause some changes in sexual response: Women produce less vaginal lubrication. An older man needs more time to achieve an erection or orgasm and to attain another erection after ejaculating. Both men and women experience fewer contractions during orgasm. However, none of these changes reduce sexual pleasure or desire.

The Challenges of Age

No matter how well we eat, exercise, and take care of ourselves, some physical changes are inevitable as we age. Figure 20.2 shows some of these changes, but most of them are not debilitating, and people can remain active and vital into extreme old age. Aging brains and bodies do become vulnerable to diseases like Alzheimer's and osteoporosis. Other common life problems, such as depression, substance misuse, and safe driving, become more challenging as we age.

Alzheimer's Disease

About 15 percent of older Americans lose previous mental capabilities, a brain disorder called **dementia.** Sixty percent of these—a total of 5.1 million men and women over age 65—suffer from the type of dementia called **Alzheimer's disease,** a progressive deterioration of brain cells and mental capacity.

Age is the top risk factor for Alzheimer's.[17] Someone in America develops Alzheimer's every 72 seconds; by 2050 the rate will increase to every 33 seconds. The percentage of people with Alzheimer's doubles for every five-year age group beyond 65. By age 85, nearly half of men and women have Alzheimer's. A person with the disease typically lives eight years after the onset of symptoms, but some live as long as 20 years. Some 7.7 million older Americans will develop Alzheimer's disease by 2030. The greatest increase will be among people age 85 and older.

 Women are more likely to develop Alzheimer's than men, and women with Alzheimer's perform significantly worse than men in various visual, spatial, and memory tests. Initiating hormone therapy after age 60 increases the risk of Alzheimer's disease.

African Americans have higher rates of Alzheimer's disease than Africans living in Africa, according to the first study to find differences in the incidence of this illness in an industrial and a nonindustrial country.

The early signs of dementia—insomnia, irritability, increased sensitivity to alcohol and other drugs, and decreased energy and tolerance of frustration—are usually subtle and insidious. Diagnosis requires a comprehensive assessment of an individual's medical history, physical health, and mental status, often involving brain scans and a variety of other tests.

hormone therapy (HT) The use of supplemental hormones during and after menopause.

dementia Deterioration of mental capability.

Alzheimer's disease A progressive deterioration of intellectual powers due to physiological changes within the brain; symptoms include diminishing ability to concentrate and reason, disorientation, depression, apathy, and paranoia.

Even though medical science cannot restore a brain that is in the process of being destroyed by an organic brain disease like Alzheimer's, medications can control difficult behavioral symptoms and enhance or partially restore cognitive ability. Often physicians find other medical or psychiatric problems, such as depression, in these patients; recognizing and treating these conditions can have a dramatic impact.

The FDA has approved several prescription drugs for people with mild to moderate dementia, including Cognex, Aricept, Exelon, and Reminyl. All increase the level of the brain chemical acetylcholine. Researchers are studying other medications that might delay Alzheimer's or stop its progression.

Osteoporosis

Another age-related disease is *osteoporosis,* a condition in which losses in bone density become so severe that a bone will break after even slight trauma or injury (see photo). A chronic disease, osteoporosis is silent for years or decades before a fracture occurs.

Women, who have smaller skeletons, are more vulnerable than men; in extreme cases, their spines may become so fragile that just bending causes severe pain. But although commonly seen as an illness of women, osteoporosis occurs frequently in men. One in every two women and one in four men over 50 will have an osteoporosis-related fracture in their lifetimes (Figure 20.3).

Calcium and vitamin D supplements in healthy postmenopausal women provide a modest benefit in preserving bone mass and preventing hip fractures but do not prevent other types of fractures, according to the results of a major clinical trial, part of the Women's Health Initiative (WHI), which studied more than 36,000 women over age 50.[18] For tips on lowering your risk for this disease, see the Your Strategies for Prevention feature.

Hair and nails	Hair often turns gray and thins out. Men may go bald. Fingernails can thicken.
Brain	The brain shrinks, but it is not known if that affects mental functions.
The senses	The sensitivity of hearing, sight, taste, and smell can all decline with age.
Skin	Wrinkles occur as the skin thins and the underlying fat shrinks, and age spots often develop.
Glands and hormones	Levels of many hormones drop, or the body becomes less responsive to them.
Muscles	Strength usually peaks in the twenties, then declines.
Immune system	The body becomes less able to resist some pathogens.
Heart and blood vessels	Cardiovascular problems become more common. The heart grows less efficient; buildup within arteries decreases oxygen and nutrients to cells.
Breasts	Tissue degenerates after menopause, and breasts sag.
Lungs	Lung capacity drops; risk of bronchitis and pneumonia grows.
Kidneys and urinary tract	The kidneys become less efficient. The bladder can't hold as much, so urination is more frequent.
Digestive system	Digestion slows down as the secretion of digestive enzymes decreases.
Reproductive system	Women go through menopause, and testosterone levels drop for men.
Bones and joints	Wear and tear can lead to arthritic joints, and osteoporosis is common, especially in women.

Figure 20.2 The Effects of Aging on the Body

YOUR STRATEGIES FOR PREVENTION *How to Lower Your Risk of Osteoporosis*

Regardless of your age and gender, you can prevent future bone problems by taking some protective steps now. The most important guidelines are as follows:

- Get adequate calcium. Increased calcium intake, particularly during childhood and the growth spurt of adolescence, can produce a heavier, denser skeleton and reduce the risk of the complications of bone loss later in life. College-age women also can strengthen their bones and reduce their risk of osteoporosis by increasing their calcium intake and physical activity.

- If you do not get enough calcium in your diet, take daily supplements.

- Drink alcohol only moderately. More than two or three alcoholic beverages a day impairs intestinal calcium absorption.

- Don't smoke. Smokers tend to be thin and enter menopause earlier, thus extending the period of jeopardy from estrogen loss.

- Let the sunshine in (but don't forget your sunscreen). Vitamin D, a vitamin produced in the skin in reaction to sunlight, boosts calcium absorption.

- Exercise regularly. Both aerobic exercise and weight training can help preserve bone density.

Risk Factors

Osteoporosis doesn't begin in old age. The bone weakness that increases the risk of osteoporosis may actually begin before birth. Infants undernourished in the womb are small when born, remain smaller than their age peers at age 1, have low bone mass at 25, and have an increased risk of fractures in late adulthood. Other risk factors include:

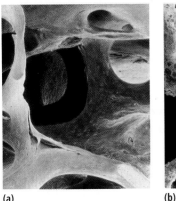
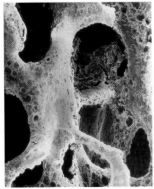

(a)   (b)

The Effect of Osteoporosis on Bone Density **(a)** Normal bone tissue. **(b)** After the onset of osteoporosis, bones lose density and become hollow and brittle.

Source: © Dr. P. Motta, Department of Anatomy, University "La Sapienza," Rome/ Science Photo Library/Photo Researchers, Inc.

- **Age.** Risk increases as you grow older.

- **Being female.** Women have less bone tissue than do men and tend to experience a rapid loss of bone in the first few years after menopause.

- **Body size.** Small, thin-boned women are at greatest risk.

- **Ethnicity.** White and Asian women are at highest risk.

- **Family history.** Having parents with a history of osteoporosis as well as fractures in adulthood can place you at increased risk.

- **Sex hormones.** Abnormal absence of menstrual periods (amenorrhea) or menopause can increase risk.

- **Anorexia.**

- **Lifetime diet low in calcium and vitamin D.**

Preparing for Medical Crises and the End of Life

Throughout this book, we have stressed the ways in which you can determine how well and how long you live. You can also make decisions about the end of your life.

Various racial and ethnic groups have different preferences for their end-of-life wishes. Many Arab Americans prefer not to go to nursing homes as they near the end of their lives, while many African Americans are comfortable with nursing homes and hospitals. Hispanic individuals express strong concerns about dying with dignity. Many white people don't want their families to take care of them, although they—like members of other racial and ethnic group—want their families nearby as they live out their last days.[19]

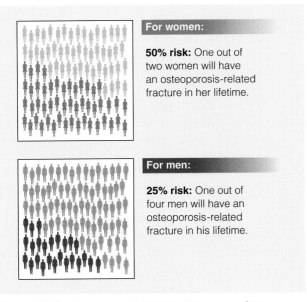

For women:

50% risk: One out of two women will have an osteoporosis-related fracture in her lifetime.

For men:

25% risk: One out of four men will have an osteoporosis-related fracture in his lifetime.

Figure 20.3 Osteoporosis Risk in Women and Men

Advance Directives

Every state and the District of Columbia has laws authorizing the use of **advance directives** to specify the kind of medical treatment individuals want in case of a medical crisis. These documents are important because, without clear indications of a person's preferences, hospitals and other institutions often make decisions on an individual's behalf, particularly if family members are not available or disagree.

The two most common advance directives are health-care proxies and living wills. Each state has different legal requirements for these forms. You can find state-specific forms at www.caringinfo.org. Once the forms are completed, make copies of your advance directives and give them to anyone who might have input in decisions on your behalf. Also give copies to your physician or health-care organization and ask that they be made part of your medical record.

Health-Care Proxy

A *health-care proxy* is an advance directive that gives someone else the power to make health decisions on your behalf. This advance directive is also called Medical Power of Attorney or Health-Care Power of Attorney (see the sample in Figure 20.4). People typically name a relative or close friend as their agent. Let family and friends know that you have completed a health-care proxy. Tell your primary physician, but you should not designate your doctor as your agent. Many states prohibit this. Even when allowed, it is not a good idea because your doctor's primary responsibility is to administer care.

Living Will

Individuals can use a **living will** (also called health-care directive or physician's directive) to indicate whether they want or don't want all possible medical treatments and technology used to prolong their lives. Living wills are most effective when they focus on priorities and goals, not so much on how to achieve them.

Most states recognize living wills as legally binding, and a growing number of health-care professionals and facilities offer patients help in drafting living wills. Figure 20.5 shows a physician's directive for Texas and notes where state laws may differ.

The Five Wishes

An innovative document called "Five Wishes" helps the aged, the seriously ill, their loved ones, and caregivers prepare for medical crises. Written with the help of the American Bar Association's Commission on the Legal Problems of the Elderly, the Five Wishes document has a health-care proxy, a health-care directive, and three other "wishes." Persons using this document can specify:

- Which person they want to make health-care decisions for them when they are no longer able to do so.
- Which kinds of medical treatments they do or don't want.
- How comfortable they want to be made.
- How they want people to treat them.
- What they want loved ones to know.

The Five Wishes document (at www.agingwithdignity. org) is legally valid in 38 states. Churches, synagogues, hospices, hospitals, physicians, social service agencies, and employers also are distributing the document to help people plan for their own care or that of aging parents.

DNR Order

You can also sign an advance directive specifying that you want to be allowed to die naturally—you do not want to be resuscitated in case your heart stops beating. **Do-not-resuscitate (DNR)** orders apply mainly to hospitalized, terminally ill patients and must be signed by a physician. However, in some states, it is possible to complete a *nonhospital DNR* form that specifies an individual's wish not to be resuscitated at home. Patients in the final stages of advanced cancer or AIDS may choose to use such forms to protect their rights in case paramedics are called to their home.

Holographic Wills

Perhaps you think that only wealthy or older people need to write wills. However, if you're married, have children, or own property, you should either hire a lawyer to draw up a will or at least write a **holographic will** yourself, specifying who should inherit your possessions. If you die *intestate* (without a will), the state will make these decisions for you. Even a modest estate can be tied up in court for a long period of time, depriving family members of money when they need it most.

A holographic will is a handwritten (not typed) statement that some states will recognize. You can:

- **Name a family member** or friend as the executor, the person who sees that your wishes are carried out.
- **List the things you own** and to whom you want them to go; include addresses and telephone numbers, if possible.

---

advance directives Documents that specify an individual's preferences regarding treatment in a medical crisis.

living will An advance directive providing instructions for the use of life-sustaining procedures in the event of terminal illness or injury.

do-not-resuscitate (DNR) An advance directive expressing an individual's preference that resuscitation efforts not be made during a medical crisis.

holographic will A will wholly in the handwriting of its author.

INSTRUCTIONS

TEXAS MEDICAL POWER OF ATTORNEY — PAGE 1

TEXAS MEDICAL POWER OF ATTORNEY

DESIGNATION OF HEALTH CARE AGENT.

PRINT YOUR NAME

I, _____, appoint:
(name)

PRINT THE NAME, ADDRESS AND HOME AND WORK TELEPHONE NUMBERS OF YOUR AGENT

_____
(name of agent)

_____
(address)

_____
(work telephone number)   *(home telephone number)*

as my agent to make any and all health care decisions for me, except to the extent I state otherwise in this document. This medical power of attorney takes effect if I become unable to make my own health care decisions and this fact is certified in writing by my physician.

STATE LIMITATIONS ON YOUR AGENT'S POWER (IF ANY)

LIMITATIONS ON THE DECISION MAKING AUTHORITY OF MY AGENT ARE AS FOLLOWS.

PRINT THE NAME, ADDRESS AND HOME AND WORK TELEPHONE NUMBERS OF YOUR FIRST AND SECOND ALTERNATE AGENTS

TEXAS MEDICAL POWER OF ATTORNEY — PAGE 2

DESIGNATION OF ALTERNATE AGENT.

(You are not required to designate an alternate agent but you may do so. An alternate agent may make the same health care decisions as the designated agent if the designated agent is unable or unwilling to act as your agent. If the agent designated is your spouse, the designation is automatically revoked by law if your marriage is dissolved.)

If the person designated as my agent is unable or unwilling to make health care decisions for me, I designate the following persons to serve as my agent to make health care decisions for me as authorized by this document, who serve in the following order:

FIRST ALTERNATE

A. First Alternate Agent

_____
(name of first alternate agent)

_____
(home address)

_____
(work telephone number)   *(home telephone number)*

SECOND ALTERNATE

B. Second Alternate Agent

_____
(name of second alternate agent)

_____
(home address)

_____
(work telephone number)   *(home telephone number)*

LOCATION OF ORIGINAL

The original of this document is kept at: _____

LOCATION OF COPIES

TEXAS MEDICAL POWER OF ATTORNEY — PAGE 3

The following individuals or institutions have signed copies:

Name: _____

Address: _____

Name: _____

Address: _____

DURATION.

I understand that this power of attorney exists indefinitely from the date I execute this document unless I establish a shorter time or revoke the power of attorney. If I am unable to make health care decisions for myself when this power of attorney expires, the authority I have granted my agent continues to exist until the time I become able to make health care decisions for myself.

EXPIRATION DATE (IF ANY)

(IF APPLICABLE) This power of attorney ends on the following date: _____

PRIOR DESIGNATIONS REVOKED.

I revoke any prior medical power of attorney.

ACKNOWLEDGMENT OF DISCLOSURE STATEMENT.

I have been provided with a disclosure statement explaining the effect of this document. I have read and understood that information contained in the disclosure statement.

(YOU MUST DATE AND SIGN THIS POWER OF ATTORNEY)

PRINT THE DATE

I sign my name to this medical power of attorney on _____
(date)

PRINT YOUR LOCATION

day of _____, at _____.
(month)   *(year)*   *(city and state)*

SIGN THE DOCUMENT

_____
(signature)

PRINT YOUR NAME

_____
(print name)

© 2000 PARTNERSHIP FOR CARING, INC.

...ESSING ...EDURE

...R TWO ...ESSES ...IGN AND ...YOUR ...UMENT ...LOW

...MUST ...PRINT ...NAMES ...ND ...ESSES

...ESS #1

...ESS #2

TEXAS MEDICAL POWER OF ATTORNEY — PAGE 4

STATEMENT OF FIRST WITNESS.

I am not the person appointed as agent by this document. I am not related to the principal by blood or marriage. I would not be entitled to any portion of the principal's estate on the principal's death. I am not the attending physician of the principal or an employee of the attending physician. I have no claim against any portion of the principal's estate on the principal's death. Furthermore, if I am an employee of a health care facility in which the principal is a patient, I am not involved in providing direct patient care to the principal and am not an officer, director, partner or business office employee of the health care facility or any parent organization of the health care facility.

Signature: _____

Print Name: _____ Date: _____

Address: _____

SIGNATURE OF SECOND WITNESS

Witness Signature: _____

Print Name: _____ Date: _____

Address: _____

© 2000 PARTNERSHIP FOR CARING, INC.

Courtesy of Partnership for Caring, Inc.   9/99
1620 Eye Street, NW, Suite 202, Washington, DC 20006 800-989-9455

Figure 20.4 Health-Care Proxy

A medical power of attorney is an advance directive. This example is from the state of Texas.

Source: Reprinted by permission of Partnership for Caring Inc., Washington, DC 20006. 800-889-9455.

Directives are effective until they're revoked. Still, it's considered a good idea to initial and date your directive every few years to show that it still expresses your wishes.

DIRECTIVE TO PHYSICIANS
For Persons 18 Years of Age and Over

I, _____, recognize that the best health care is based upon a partnership of trust and communication with my physician. My physician and I will make health care decisions together as long as I am of sound mind and able to make my wishes known. If there comes a time that I am unable to make medical decisions about myself because of illness or injury, I direct that the following treatment preferences be honored:

If, in the judgment of my physician, I am suffering with a terminal condition from which I am expected to die within six months, even with available life-sustaining treatment provided in accordance with prevailing standards of medical care:

_____ I request that all treatments other than those needed to keep me comfortable be discontinued or withheld and my physician allow me to die as gently as possible; OR

_____ I request that I be kept alive in this terminal condition using available life-sustaining treatment (THIS SELECTION DOES NOT APPLY TO HOSPICE CARE).

If, in the judgment of my physician, I am suffering with an irreversible condition so that I cannot care for myself or make decisions for myself and am expected to die without life-sustaining treatment provided in accordance with prevailing standards of care:

_____ I request that all treatments other than those needed to keep me comfortable be discontinued or withheld and my physician allow me to die as gently as possible; OR

_____ I request that I be kept alive in this irreversible condition using available life-sustaining treatment (THIS SELECTION DOES NOT APPLY TO HOSPICE CARE).

Additional requests: (After discussion with your physician, you may wish to consider listing particular treatments in this space that you do or do not want in specific circumstances, such as artificial nutrition and fluids, intravenous antibiotics, etc. Be sure to state whether you do or do not want the particular treatment).

After signing this DIRECTIVE, if my representative or I elect hospice care, I understand and agree that only those treatments needed to keep me comfortable would be provided and I would not be given available life-sustaining treatments.

If I do not have a Medical Power of Attorney and I am unable to make my wishes known, I designate the following person(s) to make treatment decisions with my physician compatible with my personal values.

Name _____

Address _____

Name _____

Address _____

(If a Medical Power of Attorney has been executed, then an agent already has been named and you should not list additional names in this document.)

If the above persons are not available, or if I have not designated a spokesperson, I understand that a spokesperson will be chosen for me following standards specified in the laws of Texas. If, in the judgment of my physician, my death is imminent within minutes to hours, even with the use of all available medical treatment provided within the prevailing standard of care, I acknowledge that all treatments may be withheld or removed except those needed to maintain my comfort.

I understand that under Texas law this Directive has no effect if I have been diagnosed as pregnant. This DIRECTIVE will remain in effect until I revoke it. No other person may do so. I understand that I may revoke this DIRECTIVE at any time.

I understand the full import of this DIRECTIVE and I am emotionally and mentally competent to make this DIRECTIVE.

Signed _____

City, County, and State of Residence _____

Date _____

Two competent witnesses must sign below, acknowledging your signature. The witness designated as "Witness 1" may not be a person designated to make a treatment decision for the patient and may not be related to the patient by blood or marriage. The witness may not be entitled to any part of the estate and may not have a claim against the estate of the patient. The witness may not be the attending physician or an employee of the attending physician. If this witness is an employee of the health care facility in which the patient is being cared for, this witness may not be involved in providing direct patient care to the patient. This witness may not be an officer, director, partner, or business office employee of the health care facility in which the patient is being cared for or of any parent organization of the health care facility.

Witness 1 _____

Witness 2 _____

TEXAS LAW DOES NOT REQUIRE THIS DIRECTIVE TO BE NOTARIZED.

In some states the directive is valid for pregnant women. Others exclude women during all or part of their pregnancy, although that has been challenged on the grounds that a woman's right to privacy doesn't end when she becomes pregnant.

You can revoke or amend your directive at any time simply by making a statement to a physician, nurse, or other health-care worker.

In most states, directives will have a space to specify treatment you do or don't want. Ask your physician what to include here. You can:

• Ask for or prohibit use of artificial feeding tubes, cardiopulmonary resuscitation, antibiotics, dialysis, and respirators.

• Ask for pain medication to keep you comfortable.

• State whether you would prefer to die in the hospital or at home.

• Designate a proxy—someone to make decisions about your treatment when you're unable.

• Donate organs or other body parts.

In some states your signature must be notarized. Elsewhere, the signature of the witnesses is adequate, although if you're in a hospital or nursing home, in some states you may need as an additional witness the chief of staff or medical director.

Figure 20.5 Preparing a Physician's Directive

Source: Texas Medical Association.

- **Select a guardian for your children** (if any), presumably someone whose ideas about raising children are similar to your own. Be sure that any named guardians are willing and able to accept this responsibility before writing them into your will.
- **Specify any funeral arrangements.**

Be sure to keep the will in a safe place, where your executor, family members, or closest beneficiary can find it quickly and easily; tell them where it is.

Ethical Dilemmas

Modern medicine can do more to delay or defy death than was once thought possible. However, the ability to sustain life in patients with no hope of recovery has created wrenching medical and moral dilemmas. Increasingly, lawyers, ethicists, and consumer advocates are arguing that health-care providers must recognize a fundamental right of patients: the right to die.

Health economists, noting that more than half of U.S. health-care dollars are spent in the last year of life, have questioned "heroic" measures to prolong the life of chronically ill elderly patients or those with fatal diseases. Policies on such aggressive measures vary from hospital to hospital and state to state; often medical staff are not aware of patients' wishes.

Some health-care facilities require that staff members try to resuscitate any patient whose heart stops unless a do-not-resuscitate (DNR) order has been written, usually with the family's permission.

Families may demand aggressive medical care near the end of life on the basis of religious grounds, such as a conviction that every moment of life is a gift from God worth preserving at any cost. However, doctors are not obliged to provide a treatment they consider medically inappropriate or inhumane simply because of the family's religious beliefs. Ideally, doctors and family members, perhaps with the aid of a chaplain, work together to reach a consensus on the appropriate limits to life-sustaining treatment.

Another major ethical concern is the fate of an estimated 5,000 to 10,000 unconscious Americans who are being kept alive by artificial means. Some are in a **coma,** a state of total unconsciousness. They may have no sense of where they are, no memory, and no experience of pain. Others are in a **persistent vegetative state,** in which they're awake and yet unaware. They open their eyes; their brain waves show the characteristic patterns of waking and sleep. They can usually breathe on their own after a few weeks on artificial respiration; they can cough; the pupils of their eyes respond to light; but they do not respond to pain. (See Point/Counterpoint: "The Right to Die.")

The Gift of Life

If you're at least 18 years old, you can fill out a donor card (Figure 20.6), agreeing to designate, in the event of your death, any organs or tissues needed for transplantation. Corneas may help a blind person see, for example. Kidneys, or even a heart, may be transplanted. The donation takes effect upon your death and is a generous way of giving others the possibilities for life that you have had yourself. The card should be filled out and signed; some must be signed

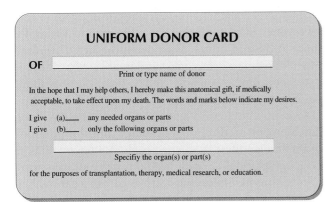

Figure 20.6   Example of a Uniform Donor Card

coma   A state of total unconsciousness.

persistent vegetative state   A state of being awake and capable of reacting to physical stimuli, such as light, while being unaware of pain or other environmental stimuli.

in the presence of two witnesses. Attach the donor card to the back of your driver's license or I.D. card. (Whole-body donations may require other arrangements.)

The reasons for becoming an organ donor or agreeing to donate a loved one's organs are complex. Older men and women generally have higher donation rates.[20] Families often base their decision on a loved one's explicit desire either to donate organs or not. Concerns about disfigurement and feelings of emotional exhaustion also play a role.[21]

Death and Dying

Some 2.4 million people die in the United States each year. Although most are older, death occurs in all age groups. The causes of death vary with both age and gender. Among those under age 35, intentional and nonintentional injury are the primary causes of death. Among older Americans, cancer and heart disease are the top killers. In fact, cancer, heart disease, and stroke continue to claim the most lives around the world.[22] (See Figure 20.7.) Men typically die at a younger age than women. College-age individuals are most likely to die as a result of accidents or assaults. (See Table 20.1.)

Defining Death

In our society, death isn't a part of everyday life, as it once was. Because machines can now keep alive people who, in the past, would have died, the definition of death has become more complex. Death has been broken down into the following categories:

- **Functional death.** The end of all vital functions, such as heartbeat and respiration.
- **Cellular death.** The gradual death of body cells after the heart stops beating. If placed in a tissue culture or, as is the case with various organs, transplanted to another body, some cells can remain alive indefinitely.

TABLE 20-1 Dying Young

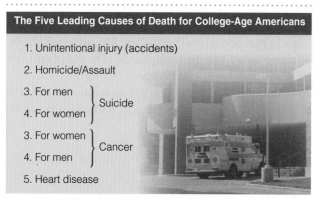

The Five Leading Causes of Death for College-Age Americans

1. Unintentional injury (accidents)
2. Homicide/Assault
3. For men ⎫
   ⎬ Suicide
4. For women ⎭
3. For women ⎫
   ⎬ Cancer
4. For men ⎭
5. Heart disease

Source: National Center for Injury Prevention and Control.

© 2006 Jupiter Images

- **Death.** The moment when the heart stops beating.
- **Brain death.** The end of all brain activity, indicated by an absence of electrical activity (confirmed by an electroencephalogram, or EEG) and a lack of reflexes. The notion of brain death is bound up with what we consider to be the actual person, or self. The destruction of a person's brain means that his or her personality no longer exists; the lower brain centers controlling respiration and circulation no longer function.
- **Spiritual death.** The moment when the soul, as defined by many religions, leaves the body.

When does a person actually die? The traditional legal definition of death is failure of the lungs or heart to function. However, because respiration and circulation can be maintained by artificial means, most states have declared that an individual is considered dead only when the brain, including the brain stem, completely stops functioning. Brain-death laws prohibit a medical staff from "pulling the plug" if there is any hope of sustaining life.

The Meaning of Death

Death is not a mystery to those who have died. The living are the ones who struggle to find meaning in it. As far back as 60,000 years ago, prehistoric people observed special ceremonies when burying their dead. Many early cultures believed that people continued to exist after death and had the same needs that they did in life; hence they buried their loved ones with food, dishes, weapons, and jewels. Some religions, such as Christianity, believe that the dead will rise again; to them, the burial of the body is symbolic, like the planting of a seed in the earth to await rebirth. Many Eastern religions share the belief that death marks the end only of physical existence and of the limited view of reality that human beings can grasp.

Death itself is a remote experience in most lives today, something that takes place off-stage in a hospital or nursing home. In earlier times, dying was a much more visible part of daily living. Families, friends, and other loved ones in a community would share in caring for those at the end of life. Most deaths occurred at home, often following a brief illness and unaffected by the limited medical care available. Today, the process of dying has become invisible.

Our attitudes toward dying also have changed with the development of medical technology and the extension of the human lifespan. Some people will do anything to delay aging or defeat death itself through medical science or other means. Others see death as part of a natural biological process and work toward the goal of dying well, with dignity and without undue suffering.

Denying Death

Most of us don't quite believe that we're going to die. A reasonable amount of denial helps us focus on the day-to-day realities of living. However, excessive denial can be life-threatening. Some drivers, for instance, refuse to buckle their seat belts because they refuse to acknowledge that a drunk driver might collide with them. Similarly, cigarette smokers deny that lung cancer will ever strike them, and people who eat high-fat meals deny that they'll ever suffer a heart attack.

One important factor in denial is the nature of the threat. It's easy to believe that death is at hand when someone's pointing a gun at you; it's much harder to think that cigarette smoking might cause your death 20 or 30 years down the road. The late Elisabeth Kübler-Ross, a psychiatrist who extensively studied the process of dying, described the downside of denying death in *Death: The Final Stage of Growth*:

> It is the denial of death that is partially responsible for people living empty, purposeless lives; for when you live as if you'll live forever, it becomes too easy to postpone the things you know that you must do. You live your life in preparation for tomorrow or in the remembrance of yesterday—and meanwhile, each today is lost. In contrast, when you fully understand that each day you awaken could be the last you have, you take the time that day to grow, to become more of who you really are, to reach out to other human beings.[23]

Emotional Responses to Dying

Kübler-Ross identified five typical stages of reaction that a person goes through when facing death (Figure 20.8).

1. **Denial ("No, not me").** At first knowledge that death is coming, a terminally ill patient rejects the news. The denial overcomes the initial shock and allows the person to begin to gather together his or her resources. Denial, at this point, is a healthy defense mechanism. It can become distressful, however, if it's reinforced by the relatives and friends of the dying patient.

2. **Anger ("Why me?").** In the second stage, the dying person begins to feel resentment and rage regarding imminent death. The anger may be directed at God or at the patient's family and caregivers, who can do little but try to endure any expressions of anger, provide comfort, and help the patient on to the next stage.

3. **Bargaining ("Yes, me, but . . .").** In this stage, a patient may try to bargain, usually with God, for a way to reverse or at least postpone dying. The patient may promise, in exchange for recovery, to do good works or to see family members more often. Alternatively, the patient may say, "Let me live long enough to see my grandchild born" or "to see the spring again."

4. **Depression ("Yes, it's me").** In the fourth stage, the patient gradually realizes the full consequences of

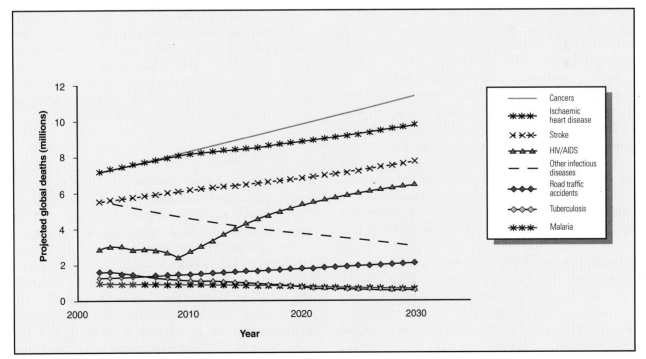

Figure 20.7   Global Causes of Death

According to the World Health Organization, cancer, heart disease, strokes, and HIV/AIDS will be the leading causes of death in the coming decades.

Source: *World Health Statistics 2007*. Geneva: World Health Organization, 2007.

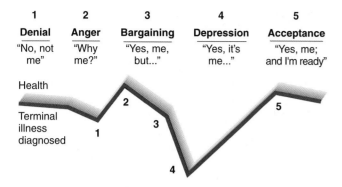

Figure 20.8 Kübler-Ross's Five Stages of Adjustment to Facing Death

his or her condition. This may begin as grieving for health that has been lost and then become anticipatory grieving for the loss that is to come of friends, loved ones, and life itself. This stage is perhaps the most difficult: The dying person should not be left alone during this period. Neither should loved ones try to cheer up the patient, who must be allowed to grieve.

5. **Acceptance ("Yes, me; and I'm ready").** In this last stage, the person has accepted the reality of death: The moment looms as neither frightening nor painful, neither sad nor happy—only inevitable. The person who waits for the end of life may ask to see fewer visitors, to separate from other people, or perhaps to turn to just one person for support.

Several stages may occur at the same time and some may happen out of sequence. Each stage may take days or only hours or minutes. Throughout, denial may come back to assert itself unexpectedly, and hope for a medical breakthrough or a miraculous recovery is forever present.

Some experts dispute Kübler-Ross's basic five-stage theory as too simplistic and argue that not all people go through such well-defined stages in the dying process. The way a person faces death is often a mirror of the way he or she has faced other major stresses in life: Those who have had the most trouble adjusting to other crises will have the most trouble adjusting to the news of their impending death.

An individual's will to live can postpone death for a while. In a study of elderly Chinese women, researchers found that their death rate decreased before and during a holiday during which the senior women in a household play a central role; it increased after the celebration. A similar temporary drop occurs among Jews at the time of Passover. However, different events may have different effects. The prospect of an upcoming birthday postpones death in women but hastens it in men. The will to live typically fluctuates in terminal patients, varying along with depression, anxiety, shortness of breath, and a sense of well-being.

The family of a dying person experiences a spectrum of often wrenching emotions. Family members, too, may deny the verdict of death, rage at the doctors and nurses who can't do more to save their loved one, bargain with God to give up their own health if necessary, sink into helplessness and depression, and finally accept the reality of their anticipated loss.

How We Die

Life can end in very different ways. Sudden death, by accident or murder, for instance, brings an abrupt end to life in individuals who may have been in optimal health. A terminal illness, such as an aggressive and fatal cancer, can lead to a steep drop in functioning prior to death. When organs such as the kidneys fail, a patient's well-being tends to plummet and then recover but in a downward pattern. The frailty of old age leads to a gradual decline to ever lower levels of functioning and eventual death.

Most people who have a fatal or **terminal illness** prefer to know the truth about their health and chances for recovery. Even when they're not officially informed by a doctor or relative, most fatally ill people know or strongly suspect that they're dying. Dying people usually make it clear whether they want to talk about death and to what extent. The most frequent concern is how much time is left. Usually physicians can give only a rough estimate, such as "several weeks or months."

Once death was a taboo topic even between doctors and patients. Filled with a zeal to heal, physicians viewed death as the enemy; it caused a sense of medical impotence and failure that often led them to pull away from dying patients. However, surveys of physicians show changes in the last decades. Today's doctors are much more open to communicating with dying patients and their families on issues concerning death. They, too, benefit from open, honest conversations with their patients.

A "Good" Death

As life expectancy has increased and high-technology interventions have multiplied, many health-care professionals as well as citizens and social organizations have begun to demand a better way of caring for those who are dying. The Center to Improve Care of the Dying, in Washington, DC, has set goals for reintegrating dying within living, thus enhancing the prospect for growth at the end of life. These experts talk of "dying well," "living while dying," and "physician-assisted living." They aim to change our way of thinking about dying so that we view the end of life as a time of love and reconciliation, and transcendence of suffering.

Physicians who care for the dying are being urged to do all that they can to eliminate pain. They are encouraged not to withhold opioid drugs, such as morphine, simply out of fear of addiction. More efforts are being made for patients to be taken care of at home, with appropriate support and well-informed guidance.

Various psychological factors can affect those at risk of dying. Elderly people who lack hope in the future are much more likely to die within the next few years. Researchers speculate that hopelessness may lead to biochemical and nervous system abnormalities or that hopeless individuals may not eat well, take medications as prescribed, or follow a doctor's recommendations.

Spirituality plays a major role. In various surveys, many patients say they want their doctors and nurses to address their spiritual concerns. In one survey, even 45 percent of nonreligious patients thought physicians should inquire politely about patients' spiritual needs. However, some worry that such queries may be inappropriate or detract from a doctor's primary mission.

There are few data on the impact of spiritual approaches on the dying. In a survey of relatives of deceased patients, 63 percent thought that their loved one's faith was of help at the time of death. In a study of nursing home residents, traditional religious beliefs and values affected acceptance, endurance, coping, and security in the face of impending death.

Caregiving

When someone becomes terminally ill, a woman—usually the patient's wife, daughter, or sister—is most likely to provide day-to-day care, often for periods longer than a year. Caregiving takes a different toll on men and women. In one study of adult daughters and husbands caring for terminally ill breast cancer patients, the daughters experienced more symptoms of anxiety and depression and greater family strain.

The impact of caregiving continues even after the death of an ill spouse. In one study, the health of older caregivers who had experienced strain prior to a spouse's death did not deteriorate. They showed no increase in depressive symptoms or use of antidepressant drugs and did not lose weight. Those who had not been caregivers were more likely to experience depression and weight loss.

Hospice: Caring When Curing Isn't Possible

A **hospice** is a homelike health-care facility or program that helps dying men and women who can afford such care to live their final days to the fullest, as free as possible from disabling pain and mental anguish. Hospice workers generally work in teams, usually consisting of a nurse, physician, social worker, chaplain, and trained volunteers. Other professionals, such as a physical therapist, may join the team when needed. These workers provide the comfort, support, and care dying patients need until they do die.

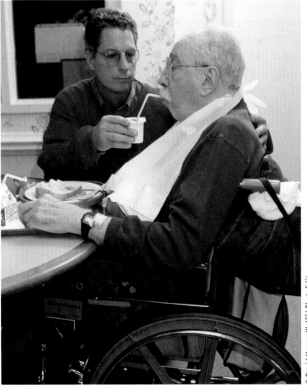

© David Young-Wolff/ PhotoEdit

Humanitarian caregiving for both critically ill patients and their loved ones can take some of the fear out of death.

Hospice programs offer a combination of medical and emotional care that involves not only the patient but also the family members or others concerned with caring for the patient. Most hospice patients have life expectancies of six months or less and are no longer receiving treatments aimed at curing their diseases. When someone is available to provide care, patients remain in their own homes. Hospice nurses regularly visit all home patients and are available around the clock.

For patients requiring care that the family cannot provide, round-the-clock care is available at the hospice facility. Unlike a traditional hospital, where the focus is on diagnosis, cure, and treatment, a hospice works to make what is left of life pain-free and comfortable. Visiting hours for relatives and friends are flexible, with no restrictions on visits by children and grandchildren. Hospice services are covered, in full or in part, by most major insurance companies.

Near-Death Experiences

Reports of near-death experiences have grown, thanks largely to advances in emergency medical care. Most are remarkably similar, whether they occur in children or

terminal illness An illness in which death is inevitable.

hospice A homelike health-care facility or program committed to supportive care for terminally ill people.

adults, whether they're the result of accidents or illnesses, even whether the individuals actually are near death or only think they are. Some individuals who have survived a close brush with death report **autoscopy** (watching, from several feet in the air, resuscitation attempts on their own bodies) or **transcendence** (the sense of passing into a foreign region or dimension). Some see light, often at the end of a tunnel. Their vision seems clearer; their hearing, sharper. Some recall scenes from their lives or feel the presence of loved ones who have died. Many report profound feelings of joy, calm, and peace. Fewer than 1 percent of those who've reported near-death experiences described them as frightening or distressing, although a larger number recall transitory feelings of fear or confusion.

Many near-death experiences occur in individuals who've been sedated or given other medications; however, many others do not. Several studies have shown that individuals who received medication or anesthesia were actually less likely to remember near-death experiences than those who hadn't had any drugs. Some scientists have speculated that lack of oxygen, changes in blood gases, altered brain functioning, or the release of neurotransmitters (messenger chemicals in the brain) may play a role in near-death experiences. However, there's little solid evidence that physiological events are responsible. There's also no proof that wishful thinking, cultural conditioning, posttraumatic stress, or other psychological mechanisms may be at work. For now, the most that scientists can say for sure about this medical mystery is that it needs further study.

Suicide

Suicide increases with age and is most common in persons aged 65 years and older. This age group accounts for 18 percent of all suicides in the United States. For every completed suicide, there are 10 to 40 unsuccessful attempts. (Chapter 4 presents a detailed discussion of the risk factors and warning signs of suicide.)

One of the main factors leading to suicide is illness, especially terminal illness. A great deal of debate centers on quality of life, yet there is no reliable or consistent way to measure this. Patients who are dying may feel some quality of life, even when others do not recognize it, or their evaluations of the quality of their lives may fluctuate. Dying patients who say their lives are not worth living may be suffering from depression; hopelessness is one of its characteristic symptoms.

"Rational" Suicide

An elderly widow suffering from advanced cancer takes a lethal overdose of sleeping pills. A young man with several AIDS-related illnesses shoots himself. A woman in her fifties, diagnosed as having Alzheimer's disease, asks a doctor to help her end her life. Are these suicides "rational" because these individuals used logical reasoning in deciding to end their lives?

The question is intensely controversial. Advocates of the right to "self-deliverance" argue that individuals in great pain or faced with the prospect of a debilitating, hopeless battle against an incurable disease can and should be able to decide to end their lives. As legislatures and the legal system tackle the thorny questions of an individual's right to die, mental health professionals worry that, even in those with fatal diseases, suicidal wishes often stem from undiagnosed depression.

Because depression may indeed warp the ability to make a rational decision about suicide, mental health professionals urge physicians and family members to make sure individuals with chronic or fatal illnesses are evaluated for depression and given medication, psychotherapy, or both. It is also important for everyone to allow enough time—an average of three to eight weeks—to see if treatment for depression will make a difference in their desire to keep living.

Physician-Assisted Suicide

According to U.S. surveys, there is greater support for physician-assisted suicide and euthanasia among patients and the general public than among physicians. More Caucasians support these practices than members of ethnic minority groups.

Oregon is the first state to legalize physician-assisted suicide for terminally ill patients. The Supreme Court has upheld the state's Death with Dignity Act, which bars suicide assistance for anyone whose judgment may be impaired by a mental disorder.

If patients have a right to die, should doctors help them end their lives? Physicians could stop any extraordinary efforts to sustain life (for example, by withholding oxygen or ending intravenous feedings); such actions are referred to as passive *euthanasia,* or *dyathanasia.* Euthanasia, the active form of so-called mercy killing, has generally been viewed as illegal and unethical. Euthanasia is tolerated and legally pardoned in the Netherlands but remains illegal in all European countries. The demand for physician-assisted death in the Netherlands has not risen; and patients and physicians have become more reluctant to ask for or offer this option over the past few years.[24]

Some medical groups, such as the American Medical Association, oppose as unethical any physician's involvement in euthanasia. Others argue that individuals have the right to end their own lives and that physicians who provide prescriptions for lethal doses of certain drugs are acting out of compassion and respect for patients' wishes.

The Practicalities of Death

At a time of great emotional pain, grieving family members must cope with medical, legal, and practical concerns, including obtaining a medical certificate of the cause of death, registering the death, and making funeral arrangements. They also may want to arrange for organ donations and, in some circumstances, an autopsy.

Funeral Arrangements

A body can be either buried or cremated. Burial requires the purchase of a cemetery plot, which many families do decades before death. A burial is typically the third most expensive purchase of a lifetime, behind the cost of a house and car. The average national costs range as high as $6,000, although they vary considerably. Memorial societies are voluntary groups that help people plan in advance for death. They obtain services at moderate cost, keep the arrangements simple and dignified, and—most important, perhaps—ease the emotional and financial burden on the rest of the family when death finally does come.

If the body is to be cremated, you must comply with some additional formalities, with which the funeral director can help you. After a *cremation* (incineration of the remains), you can either collect the ashes to keep, bury, or scatter yourself, or ask the crematorium to dispose of them.

The tradition of a funeral may help survivors come to terms with the death, enabling them to mourn their loss and to celebrate the dead person's life. Funerals are usually held two to four days after the death. Many have two parts: a religious ceremony at a church or funeral home, and a burial ceremony at the grave site.

Alternatively, the body may be disposed of immediately, through burial, cremation, or bequeathal to a medical school, and a memorial service held later. In a memorial service, the body is not present, which may change the focus of the service from the person's death to his or her life.

Autopsies

An autopsy is a detailed examination of a body after death, also called a postmortem exam. There are two types:

- **Medicolegal.** This type of autopsy is performed to establish the cause of death and to gather information about the death for use as evidence in any legal proceedings. It is done to detect any crimes and to help identify the proper person for prosecution, to investigate possible industrial hazards or contagious diseases that may endanger the public health, or to establish the cause of death for insurance purposes.

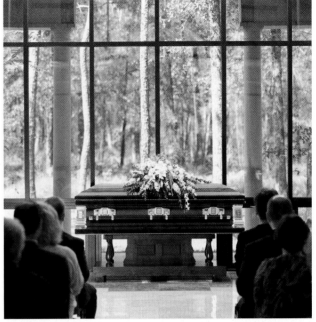

Funerals and memorial services help those in mourning to honor the deceased and to come to terms with their loss.

© Terry Vine/Stone/Getty Images

- **Medical/educational.** This type of autopsy is performed, usually in the hospital where the person died, to increase medical knowledge and to determine a more exact cause of death. It may be requested by the attending physician or the family, but it cannot be performed without the family's permission.

Autopsies can be extremely valuable in establishing an accurate cause of death, revealing a different diagnosis that might have led to a change in therapy and prolonged survival in about 10 percent of cases. Thirty years ago about 50 percent of patients who died in hospitals were autopsied. However, the autopsy rate in the United States has been steadily declining, and today about 10 to 20 percent of deaths in teaching hospitals are autopsied.

Grief

An estimated 8 million Americans lose a member of their immediate family each year. Each death leaves an average of five people bereaved. Such loss may be the single most upsetting and feared event in a person's life. It produces a wide range of reactions, including anxiety, guilt, anger, and financial concern. Many may see the

autoscopy The sensation of one's self being outside its body, often experienced by individuals in near-death medical crises.

transcendence The sense of passing into a foreign region or dimension, often experienced by a person near death.

YOUR STRATEGIES FOR CHANGE *How to Cope with Grief*

- **Accept your feelings**—sorrow, fear, emptiness, whatever—as normal. Don't try to deny emotions such as anger, guilt, despair, or relief.

- **Let others help you**—by bringing you food, taking care of daily necessities, providing companionship and comfort. (It will make them feel better, too.)

- **Face each day as it comes.** Let yourself live in the here-and-now until you're ready to face the future. Give yourself time—perhaps more than you ever imagined—for the pain to ebb, the scars to heal, and your life to move on.

- **Don't think there's a right or wrong way to grieve.** Mourning takes many forms,

and there's no set timetable for working through the various stages of grief.

- **Seek professional counseling** if you remain intensely distressed for more than six months or your grief does not ease over time. Therapy can help prevent potentially serious physical and psychological problems.

---

death of an old person as less tragic than the death of a child or young person. A sudden death is more of a shock than one following a long illness. A suicide can be particularly devastating, because family members may wonder whether they could have done anything to prevent it. The cause of death also can affect the reactions of friends and acquaintances. Some people express less sympathy and support when individuals are murdered or take their own lives.

According to the stage theory of grief, individuals respond to the loss of a loved one by progressing through several steps, just like people facing death. These consist of shock-numbness, yearning-searching, disorganization-despair, and reorganization. All these reactions can occur simultaneously, although most peak within six months. Acceptance continues to increase over time.[25] The most common and one of the most painful experiences is the death of a parent. When both parents die, even adult individuals may feel like orphaned children. They mourn not just for the father and mother who are gone, but also for their lost role of being someone's child.

The death of a child can be even more devastating. Eventually parents may be able to resolve their grief and accept the death as "God's will" or as "something that happens." Time erases their pain and they feel a desire to get on with their lives, consciously putting the loss behind them. Others deal with their grief by keeping busy or by substituting other problems or situations to take their minds off their loss. Yet many parents who lose a child continue to grieve for many years. Although the pain of their loss diminishes with time, they view it as part of themselves and describe an emptiness inside—even though most have rich, meaningful, and happy daily lives.

The loss of a mate can also have a profound impact, although men's and women's responses to the death—and their subsequent health risks—may depend on how their spouses died. Men whose wives die suddenly face a much greater risk of dying themselves than those whose wives die after a long illness. On the other hand, women whose husbands die after a long illness face greater risk of dying than other widows. The reason may be that men whose wives were chronically ill learned how to cope with the loss of their nurturers, while women who spend a long time caring for an

ill husband may be at greater risk because of the combined burdens of caregiving and loss of financial support.

 Bereavement is not a rare occurrence on college campuses, but it is largely an ignored problem. Counselors have called upon universities to help students who have lost a loved one through initiatives such as training nonbereaved students to provide peer support and raising consciousness about bereavement. For help in dealing with grief, see the Your Strategies for Change feature.

Grief's Effects on Health

Men and women who lose partners, parents, or children endure so much stress that they're at increased risk of serious physical and mental illness, and even of premature death. Studies of the health effects of grief have found the following:

- Grief produces changes in the respiratory, hormonal, and central nervous systems and may affect functions of the heart, blood, and immune systems.

- Grieving adults may experience mood swings between sadness and anger, guilt and anxiety.

- Grievers may feel physically sick, lose their appetite, sleep poorly, or fear that they're going crazy because they "see" the deceased person in different places.

- Friendships and remarriage offer the greatest protection against health problems.

- Some widows may have increased rates of depression, suicide, and death from cirrhosis of the liver. The greatest risk factors are poor previous mental and physical health and a lack of social support.

- Grieving parents, partners, and adult children are at increased risk of serious physical and mental illness, suicide, and premature death.

Sometimes grief progresses from an emotionally painful but normal experience to a more persistent problem, called *complicated grief*.[26] Individuals who experience very long-lasting or severe symptoms, including inability to accept a loved one's death, persistent thoughts about the death, and preoccupation with the lost loved one, can benefit from professional treatment.

Learn It : **Live It**

Living Long and Well

"Every man desires to live long," wrote Jonathan Swift, "but no man would be old." We all wish for long lives, yet we want to avoid the disease and disability that can tarnish our golden years. Here are the best ways to do so.

- **Exercise regularly.** By improving blood flow, staving off depression, warding off heart disease, and enhancing well-being, regular workouts help keep mind and body in top form.
- **Don't smoke.** Every cigarette you puff can snuff out seven minutes of your life, according to the Centers for Disease Control and Prevention.
- **Watch your weight and blood pressure.** Increases in these vital statistics can increase your risk of hypertension, cardiovascular disease, and other health problems.
- **Eat more fruits and vegetables.** These foods, rich in vitamins and protective antioxidants, can reduce your risk of cancer and damage from destructive free radicals.
- **Cut down on fat.** Fatty foods can clog the arteries and contribute to various cancers.
- **Limit drinking.** Alcohol can undermind physical health and sabotage mental acuity.
- **Cultivate stimulating interests.** Elderly individuals with complex and interesting lifestyles are most likely to retain sharp minds and memories beyond age 70.
- **Don't worry; be happy.** At any age, emotional turmoil can undermine well-being. Relaxation techniques, such as meditation, help by reducing stress.
- **Reach out.** Try to keep in contact with other people of all ages and experiences. Make the effort to invite them to your home or go out with them. On a regular basis, do something to help another person.
- **Make the most of your time.** Greet each day with a specific goal—to take a walk, write letters, visit a friend.

SELFSURVEY : *What Is Your Aging I.Q.?*

Answer True or False

T F **1.** Everyone becomes "senile" sooner or later, if he or she lives long enough.
T F **2.** American families have by and large abandoned their older members.
T F **3.** Depression is a serious problem for older people.
T F **4.** The numbers of older people are growing.
T F **5.** The vast majority of older people are self-sufficient.
T F **6.** Mental confusion is an inevitable, incurable consequence of old age.
T F **7.** Intelligence declines with age.
T F **8.** Sexual urges and activity normally cease around age 55–60.
T F **9.** If a person has been smoking for 30 or 40 years, it does no good to quit.
T F **10.** Older people should stop exercising and rest.
T F **11.** As you grow older, you need more vitamins and minerals to stay healthy.
T F **12.** Only children need to be concerned about calcium for strong bones and teeth.
T F **13.** Extremes of heat and cold can be particularly dangerous to old people.
T F **14.** Many older people are hurt in accidents that could have been prevented.
T F **15.** More men than women survive to old age.
T F **16.** Death from stroke and heart disease are declining.
T F **17.** Older people on the average take more medications than younger people.
T F **18.** Snake oil salesmen are as common today as they were on the frontier.
T F **19.** Personality changes with age, just like hair color and skin texture.
T F **20.** Sight declines with age.

Scoring

1. False. Even among those who live to be 80 or older, only 20–25 percent develop Alzheimer's disease or some other incurable form of brain disease. "Senility" is a meaningless term that should be discarded.
2. False. The American family is still the number-one caretaker of older Americans. Most older people live close to their children and see them often; many live with their spouses. In all, 8 out of 10 men and 6 out of 10 women live in family settings.
3. True. Depression, loss of self-esteem, loneliness, and anxiety can become more common as older people face retirement, the deaths of relatives and friends, and other such crises—often at the same time. Fortunately, depression is treatable.
4. True. By the year 2030, one in four people will be over 65 years of age.
5. True. Only a small percentage of the older population live in nursing homes. The rest live independently or with relatives or caregivers.
6. False. Mental confusion and serious forgetfulness in old age can be caused by Alzheimer's disease or other conditions that cause incurable damage to the brain, but some 100 other problems can cause the same symptoms. A minor head injury, a high fever, poor nutrition, adverse drug reactions, and depression can all be treated and the confusion will be cured.
7. False. Intelligence per se does not decline without reason. Most people maintain their intellect or improve as they grow older.
8. False. Most older people can lead an active, satisfying sex life.
9. False. Stopping smoking at any age not only reduces the risk of cancer and heart disease, it also leads to healthier lungs.
10. False. Many older people enjoy—and benefit from—exercises such as walking, swimming, and bicycle riding. Exercise at any age can help strengthen the heart and lungs, and lower blood pressure. See your physician before beginning a new exercise program.
11. False. Although certain requirements, such as that for "sunshine" vitamin D, may increase slightly with age, older people need the same amounts of most vitamins and minerals as younger people. Older people in particular should eat nutritious food and cut down on sweets, salty snack foods, high-calorie drinks, and alcohol.
12. False. Older people require fewer calories, but adequate intake of calcium for strong bones can become more important as you grow older. This is particularly true for women, whose risk of osteoporosis increases after menopause. Milk and cheese are rich in calcium as are cooked dried beans, collards, and broccoli. Some people need calcium supplements as well.
13. True. The body's thermostat tends to function less efficiently with age and the older person's body may be less able to adapt to heat or cold.
14. True. Falls are the most common cause of injuries among the elderly. Good safety habits, including proper lighting, nonskid carpets, and keeping living areas free of obstacles, can help prevent serious accidents.
15. False. Women tend to live 5 to ten percent longer than men.
16. True. Fewer men and women are dying of stroke or heart disease.
17. True. The elderly consume 25 percent of all medications and, as a result, have many more problems with adverse drug reactions.
18. True. Medical quackery is a $10 billion business in the United States. People of all ages are commonly duped into "quick cures" for aging, arthritis, and cancer.
19. False. Personality doesn't change with age. Therefore, all old people can't be described as rigid and cantankerous. You are what you are for as long as you live. But you can change what you do to help yourself to good health.
20. False. Although changes in vision become more common with age, any change in vision, regardless of age, is related to a specific disease. If you are having problems with your vision, see your doctor.

Source: National Institute on Aging, www.counselingnotes.com/seniors/age/age_iq.htm.

Your Health Action Plan
for Preparing for a Medical Crisis in an Aging Relative

"Medical crises are more common and more likely to lead to serious complications after age 60," says Kenneth Brummel-Smith, M.D., former president of the American Geriatrics Society. As your parents, grandparents, and other relatives get older, here is what you can do in advance:

- **Watch for warning signals.** If your relative begins stumbling or having near-misses on the highway, make sure he or she sees a doctor before a serious fall or accident occurs. There may be a cure or, if not a cure, a way to improve functioning.

- **Suggest a surrogate.** Even if a couple has been married for 40 years, neither has the legal right to make medical decisions for a spouse. The same is true for children and other relatives. The only way to get that right is to fill out a form, usually called an advance directive or medical power of attorney (discussed on page 568).

- **Talk to loved ones.** "Waiting for something bad to happen doesn't make it any easier to talk about," says Dr. Brummel-Smith, who suggests sitting down for a formal discussion at some point after a relative reaches age 65 "but definitely before age 75."

- **Focus on values.** "You don't have to discuss every possible drug or surgery or intervention," says Dr. Brummel-Smith. "What's important is that you understand the older person's values. What are fates worse than death? Independence may be more important than living a longer life." Many families use the "Five Wishes" form (available online at **www.agingwithdignity.org** and described on page 568) to discuss preferences for medical, personal, emotional, and spiritual care.

- **Involve the person's primary physician.** Often it's not a question of what doctors can do medically in a crisis, but of what they should do, which is the patient's decision.

Encourage loved ones to discuss "what ifs" with their doctors and make their desires clear. For instance, a primary physician should know which treatments patients want (such as resuscitation during surgery) as well as those they don't want (such as remaining on a ventilator if unable to breathe on their own).

- **Investigate alternative living options.** Aging parents should visit retirement communities or nursing homes while they're still healthy, not with the idea of moving into them, but of knowing what's available. They also should find out if their health plan provides services for seniors after a medical crisis.

- **Make sure you know where to find key documents.** An easily accessible folder with copies of the latest lab reports, consultations, and advance directives helps to avoid unnecessary tests and get faster treatment when a crisis does occur.

CENGAGENOW™ If you want to write your own goals for working toward a healthy environment, go to the Wellness Journal at HealthNow: **academic.cengage.com/login**.

Making This Chapter Work for YOU

Review Questions

1. Factors that contribute to staying healthy longer include all of the following *except*
   a. avoiding illness.
   b. moderate smoking.
   c. regular exercise.
   d. lifelong learning.

2. Physically fit people over age 60
   a. have lower risk of dying from chronic heart disease.
   b. can regain the fitness level of a 25-year-old.
   c. show no difference in levels of anxiety and depression.
   d. have higher health-care expenses.

3. Which statement about the aging brain is *false*?
   a. When brain cells die, surrounding cells can fill the gaps to maintain cognitive function.
   b. Remembering names and recalling information may take longer.
   c. "Use it or lose it."
   d. Mental ability and physical ability both decline with age.

4. Which statement about aging is *false*?
   a. The most common nutritional disorder in the elderly is obesity.
   b. In men, sexual activity and longevity are linked.
   c. Hormone therapy reduces the risk of heart disease in menopausal women.
   d. Seniors who take up new hobbies late in life may slow aging within the brain.

5. Which statement about age-related problems is correct?
   a. Osteoporosis affects only women.
   b. Alzheimer's disease is a form of dementia.
   c. Osteoporosis treatment includes surgery.
   d. Drug interactions do not occur in the elderly.

6. When should concern change to intervention?

   a. Uncle Charlie is 85 and continues to drive himself to the grocery store and to the Senior Center during the daytime.
   b. Nana takes pills at breakfast, lunch, and dinner but sometimes mixes them up.
   c. Mom's hot flashes have become a family joke.
   d. Your older brother can never remember where he put his car keys.

7. According to Elisabeth Kübler-Ross, an individual facing death goes through all of the following emotional stages except
   a. bargaining.
   b. acceptance.
   c. denial.
   d. repression.

8. The gender gap related to longevity
   a. is due to deficiencies in the Y chromosome.
   b. results from the presence of a mutant gene.
   c. may be due to the X chromosome and its hormonal influences on the immune system.
   d. is about 13 years in the United States.

9. An advance directive
   a. indicates who should have your property in the event you die.
   b. may authorize which individuals may not participate in your health care if you are unable to care for yourself.
   c. can specify your desires related to the use of medical treatments and technology to prolong your life.
   d. should specify which physician you designate to be your health-care proxy.

10. You can best help a friend who is bereaved by
   a. encouraging him to have a few drinks to forget his pain.
   b. simply spending time with her.
   c. avoiding talking about his loss because it is awkward.
   d. reminding her about all she still has in her life.

Answers to these questions can be found on page 583.

Critical Thinking

1. How are your parents or other mentors staying fit and alert as they age? Do you think you might use similar strategies?

2. Do you think that coming to terms with mortality allows an individual to live each day to its fullest, rather than putting off what he or she would like to do until tomorrow? How does this concept affect your own life? Explain. Do you believe in a next life? How does this affect your view of life and death?

3. Have your living parents and grandparents written advanced directives or a living will? Have you discussed with them their preferences regarding treatment in the event of a medical crisis? If you haven't had this discussion with your family, how can you begin the process of helping your parents or grandparents communicate their wishes?

4. As many as 10,000 people in this country are chronically unconscious, kept alive by artificial respirators and feeding tubes. If you were in an accident that left you in a vegetative state, would you want doctors to do everything possible to fight for your life? Would you want to spend months or even years totally unaware of your surroundings? Should health-care professionals have the right to declare that anyone is too old, too ill, or too frail to try to save? Should they have the right to insist that someone live on even if that person isn't experiencing much of a life?

Media Menu

CENGAGENOW™ Go to the HealthNow website at **academic.cengage .com/login** that will:
- Help you evaluate your knowledge of the material.
- Allow you to take an exam-prep quiz.
- Provide a Personalized Learning Plan targeting resources that address areas you should study.
- Coach you through identifying target goals for behavioral change and creating and monitoring your personal change plan throughout the semester.

INTERNET CONNECTIONS

National Institute on Aging

www.nia.nih.gov

This government site features a comprehensive array of resources on aging, including publications on a variety of geriatric health topics, current news events, and a resource directory for older people.

RealAge

www.realage.com

This site features diet and exercise assessment tools—such as a BMI calculator, exercise estimator, and RealAge assessment quizzes on a variety of health topics—to help you determine your risk of disease and what you can do to reduce this risk. The main feature is an interactive, online personal lifestyle assessment that also gives you options for "growing younger."

U.S. Administration on Aging

http://aoa.gov

This site, part of the Department of Health and Human Services, has information for seniors and their families on promoting healthy lifestyles and general aging topics.

The End of Life: Exploring Death in America

www.npr.org/programs/death/

This site, sponsored by National Public Radio, contains transcripts and resources from an *All Things Considered* series focusing on how Americans deal with death and dying. Features include personal stories, a place where you can tell your own story, and a comprehensive list of organizations that can help families who are coping with death, dying, and the diseases of old age.

Key Terms

The terms listed are used and defined on the page indicated. Definitions are also found in the Glossary at the end of this book.

advance directives   568
aging   559
Alzheimer's disease   565
autoscopy   577
coma   571
dementia   565
do-not-resuscitate (DNR) 568
holographic will 568
hormone therapy (HT)   565
hospice 575
living will   568
menopause   563
perimenopause   563
persistent vegetative state 571
terminal illness 575
transcendence   577

Making This Chapter Work for You

Answers to Review Questions

Chapter 1
1. d; **2.** c; **3.** b; **4.** c; **5.** a; **6.** b; **7.** c; **8.** d; **9.** c; **10.** c

Chapter 2
1. b; **2.** a; **3.** b; **4.** c; **5.** d; **6.** a; **7.** c; **8.** a; **9.** b; **10.** b

Chapter 3
1. b; **2.** d; **3.** a; **4.** a; **5.** c; **6.** b; **7.** a; **8.** c; **9.** d; **10.** b

Chapter 4
1. a; **2.** c; **3.** b; **4.** a; **5.** a; **6.** b; **7.** b; **8.** d; **9.** d; **10.** b

Chapter 5
1. c; **2.** b; **3.** c; **4.** b; **5.** c; **6.** b; **7.** b; **8.** b; **9.** a; **10.** d

Chapter 6
1. c; **2.** a; **3.** d; **4.** a; **5.** d; **6.** c; **7.** a; **8.** a; **9.** a; **10.** b

Chapter 7
1. c; **2.** b; **3.** c; **4.** c; **5.** d; **6.** a; **7.** c; **8.** c; **9.** a; **10.** c

Chapter 8
1. d; **2.** c; **3.** b; **4.** a; **5.** d; **6.** b; **7.** a; **8.** d; **9.** c; **10.** c

Chapter 9
1. b; **2.** d; **3.** c; **4.** d; **5.** d; **6.** b; **7.** d; **8.** c; **9.** a; **10.** a

Chapter 10
1. c; **2.** d; **3.** a; **4.** c; **5.** c; **6.** b; **7.** c; **8.** a; **9.** b; **10.** d

Chapter 11
1. a; **2.** c; **3.** d; **4.** b; **5.** c; **6.** c; **7.** d; **8.** a; **9.** b; **10.** d

Chapter 12
1. a; **2.** d; **3.** b; **4.** c; **5.** b; **6.** b; **7.** a; **8.** d; **9.** b; **10.** d

Chapter 13
1. d; **2.** c; **3.** d; **4.** b; **5.** a; **6.** c; **7.** d; **8.** c; **9.** d; **10.** b

Chapter 14
1. c; **2.** b; **3.** b; **4.** a; **5.** b; **6.** d; **7.** a; **8.** d; **9.** d; **10.** d

Chapter 15
1. a; **2.** c; **3.** a; **4.** b; **5.** b; **6.** d; **7.** c; **8.** a; **9.** c; **10.** d

Chapter 16
1. a; **2.** d; **3.** b; **4.** b; **5.** a; **6.** c; **7.** c; **8.** d; **9.** b; **10.** c

Chapter 17
1. c; **2.** b; **3.** b; **4.** a; **5.** d; **6.** c; **7.** b; **8.** d; **9.** d; **10.** b

Chapter 18
1. d; **2.** b; **3.** c; **4.** c; **5.** b; **6.** b; **7.** b; **8.** a; **9.** c; **10.** b

Chapter 19
1. d; **2.** b; **3.** c; **4.** a; **5.** b; **6.** c; **7.** b; **8.** a; **9.** c; **10.** b

Chapter 20
1. b; **2.** a; **3.** d; **4.** c; **5.** b; **6.** b; **7.** d; **8.** c; **9.** c; **10.** b

Hales Health Almanac

HEALTH INFORMATION ON THE INTERNET

YOUR HEALTH DIRECTORY

EMERGENCY!

A CONSUMER'S GUIDE TO MEDICAL TESTS

HEALTH INFORMATION ON THE INTERNET

Using the Internet

What are the very latest statistics on the incidence of the flu? Are any new drugs in the works for the treatment of diabetes? How can I get in touch with others who suffer from asthma? Is it possible to make a low-fat chocolate cake? You can answer these kinds of questions with the help of the Internet. A gold mine of information for the student of health, the Internet can help you with research for your schoolwork and also with personal questions and concerns about your own health.

What are the practical uses of the Internet for the student of health and the health care consumer?

- **Research.** The Internet is a repository for many health journals, government statistics, archives, and other sources of scholarly information. Subscribing to a mailing list or posting to a newsgroup in an area of interest can yield new sources of information that would be hard to get elsewhere.
- **Self-help and support.** Dozens of newsgroups and mailing lists offer support and advice for people dealing with all kinds of health-related issues, from Alzheimer's caregivers to people with eating disorders to athletes comparing training programs.
- **Goods and services.** Online shopping for health-related products is easy.
- **Graduate school and career information.** If you are interested in a career in a health-related field, most graduate schools have websites that list their programs, entrance requirements, faculty profiles, and other information of interest to prospective students. And you can consult online listings of jobs available in many areas of health care.

Searching the Web

One way to find websites of interest to you is to use a search engine. The large popular search engines are:

- **Google** *www.google.com*
- **Yahoo!** *www.yahoo.com*
- **AltaVista** *http://www.altavista.com*

To use a search engine, go to the home page for the site, type one or more keywords or phrases into the "search" box. The engine will then search all the sites in its index and return a list to you, with hyperlinks and sometimes short descriptions, of those that contain your keywords.

No single search engine contains all the contents of the Internet. After connecting to a search engine for the first time, it is a good idea to read the tool's description, search options, and rules and restrictions. Each engine offers a different "view" of the Web and you'll want to tailor your query to make the best use of that system.

The key to an effective search is picking the right keywords. Try to find distinctive words or combinations of words. If you use several keywords, check your search engine's searching tips—in most cases you can use the plus sign, the minus sign, quotation marks and the word OR to make your search more precise. For example, the word "OR" broadens the search results. You may try searching "pregnancy teen OR adolescent," to find sites that refer to teen or adolescent pregnancy.

Your search may turn up hundreds or even thousands of results—or only a few. If you have more results than you can handle, try making the keywords in your search more precise or go to your search engine's advanced search section. If you have too few results, try another search engine, using synonyms or variations on your keywords, or be less specific in your query.

News Groups/Discussion Forums

News groups and discussion forums are ways of discussing topics over the Internet with other people who share the same interests or concerns. They are a popular way to establish an online community, share information, and give and receive support. For example, a person suffering from a relatively rare disorder may not know anyone else with the same problems and concerns on campus or in town, but he or she can frequent a news group specifically for people with that disorder to learn about other peoples' experiences, the latest

treatments, and just to commiserate. Or a person who is trying to quit smoking can participate in a news group to share frustrations, tips, and successes. But, as always, be aware that not everything posted to a news group is necessarily true; you must be a critical thinker.

Many commercial online services offer members-only news groups to their subscribers, but many other news groups are available to anyone. To find a news group on a topic of interest to you, try going to http://groups.google.com.

News group addresses are grouped into several broad categories called hierarchies. Listed below are some of the standard hierarchies that relate to health.

- **alt** groups generally alternative in nature (i.e., alt.sex)
- **bionet** groups discussing biology and biological sciences (i.e., bionet.immunology)
- **misc** groups that don't fit into other categories (i.e., misc.fitness)
- **rec** groups discussing hobbies, sports, music, and art (i.e., rec.food)
- **sci** groups discussing subjects related to the science and scientific research (i.e., sci.epidemiology)
- **soc** groups discussing social issues including politics, social programs, etc. (i.e., soc.college)
- **talk** public debating forums on controversial issues (i.e., talk.abortion)

Before you make a posting to a news group, you may want to "lurk" for awhile, that is, read the discussion without contributing your own posting. Lurking will give you a sense of the kinds of postings that are appropriate for that news group and what the news group culture is like. Read the news group's "FAQ," or list of answers to frequently asked questions before joining the discussion.

Postings to many news groups are updated frequently, so if an item is of interest to you, you should print it or save it to your computer since it may be gone the next day. After lurking for awhile, you can join in the discussion by posting a message to the news group. You may also want to reply only to the originator of a certain message. You may want to join in on the discussion of an already-existing topic, or start your own "thread."

Be cautious when providing your e-mail address to a site or news group. Spam is junk e-mail, and spammers scoop up e-mail addresses in news groups and chat rooms.

Mailing Lists

You are probably already on a few mailing lists—they are used by retailers, organizations, politicians, educational institutions, and many other groups who e-mail large numbers of people. But mailing lists (or list serves) are also groups of people who "get together" via e-mail to discuss a specific topic. Mailing lists offer a way to participate in lively discussions, stay up on current research, or find out answers to burning questions. There are mailing lists on nearly every topic imaginable. Mailing lists are similar to news groups in that they are forums for discussion, but the messages are delivered to your e-mail account instead of to a public bulletin board. Here's how it works:

- First, find a mailing list dealing with a subject you are interested in discussing with others (i.e., attention deficit disorder).
- Then, you have to subscribe: send an e-mail to that mailing list's "subscribe" address with the word "subscribe" in the subject line and in the main body of the text.
- Usually, the mailing list will then subscribe you to the list and send you instructions on how to "post" to the group. "Posting" means that you send out a comment to the entire mailing list that you have subscribed to.

- Every time any member posts to the list serve, all the subscribers get that posting as an e-mail message.
- Once you have subscribed you will begin to receive e-mail messages from the mailing list. Be careful though: Some discussion groups have a large following and you may find your mailbox filling up faster than you can read the messages.
- Again, evaluate carefully any information you get from a mailing list to make sure it is accurate.

Thinking Critically About Health Information on the Internet

Unlike information in most books and journals, anyone can post information or advice on the Internet. Some of this information can be misleading or downright harmful, so it is important to use your best critical thinking skills to evaluate health information you find on the Internet. Ask yourself the following questions:

- **Who is the author or sponsor of the information?** The author of the site is usually listed at the top or bottom of a site's home page. Be very wary of any anonymous site. Sites that are maintained by established schools or universities, government agencies, professional organizations, or other established organizations like the American Cancer Society are probably trustworthy. Sites created by individuals or other groups may or may not contain valid information; see if you can verify their information in other places.

- **Is it current?** Many sites post the date of their last update. Look for sites where you can determine when the information was created or modified; many of the best sites are updated weekly or even daily.
- **What is the purpose of the site?** The hidden purpose of some health websites is to sell products or act as a vehicle for advertisements. Be wary of any site that tries to sell you things or get your money. Also beware of sites that seem to be trying to persuade you of things, promote "miracle cures" or anything that seems too good to be true. Some people also use news groups and other chat forums to sell or persuade. Be skeptical and use your common sense.
- **Who is the intended audience?** Some Internet information is intended for doctors and other health-care professionals; although the information may be accurate, it may be too difficult for a layperson to interpret. Other websites or Internet forums are targeted toward people with specific problems or disorders, students, or the general public.
- **Is the information verifiable?** To get a better perspective on information from the Internet, see if you can verify it with other sources. Before you follow any health advice you get from the Net, check it out with your physician.

Health Resources on the Internet

"Your Health Directory" (next pages) contains web addresses for many health-related organizations. And hundreds of health-related Internet addresses can be found at http://health.wadsworth.com.

In *An Invitation to Health*, I emphasize that you shoulder a great deal of responsibility for your health and the quality of your life. Given the complexity of our minds and bodies and the many social and environmental factors that affect us, this responsibility can be a very heavy burden. But your load can be made lighter if you know where to turn for health information, services, and support.

In this directory, you will find more than 100 health-related topics and about 250 resources, including addresses, phone numbers, and websites for government agencies, community organizations, professional associations, recovery groups, and Internet sources. Many of these organizations and groups have toll-free 800 or 888 phone numbers, and most have websites (one caution: as you may have experienced, website addresses—like street addresses and phone numbers—change on occasion). Much of the material available from these groups is free.

Also included in Your Health Directory are clearinghouses and information centers that are especially rich sources of health knowledge. Their main purpose is to collect, help manage, and disseminate information. Clearinghouses often perform other services as well, such as creating original publications and providing tailored responses to individual requests. These organizations also may provide referrals to other groups that can help you.

Many of the groups listed here have local offices or chapters. You can call, write, or visit the websites of these organizations to find out if there is a branch in your vicinity, or you can check your local telephone directory.

The purpose of this directory is to help you be in control of your health. If you know where to turn for answers to your questions and if you know what choices you have, you may find that you have more control over your life.

Resources by Topic

Abortion

National Abortion Federation
(provides information about abortion and referral for abortion services)
1600 L St. NW, Suite 40
Washington, DC 20036
(202) 667-5881
(800) 772-9100
E-mail: naf@prochoice.org
www.prochoice.org

Accident Prevention

Centers for Disease Control and Prevention
1600 Clifton Rd. N.E.
Atlanta, GA 30333
(800) CDC-INFO
(404) 639-3534
(800) 311-3435
E-mail: cdcinfo@cdc.gov
www.cdc.gov

National Safety Council
1121 Spring Lake Dr.
Itasca, IL 60143-3201
(630) 285-1121
(800) 621-7619
E-mail: info@nsc.org
www.nsc.org

Adoption

AASK (Adopt a Special Kid)
(provides assistance to families who adopt older and handicapped children)
700 Edgewater Drive, Suite 103, Building B
Oakland, CA 94621
E-mail: info@aask.org
www.aask.org

Aging

Administration on Aging
U.S. Department of Health and Human Services
One Massachusetts Ave.
Suites 4100 and 5100
Washington, DC 20201
(800) 677-1116 (Eldercare Locator—to find services for an older person in his or her locality)

(202) 619-0724 (AoA's National Aging Information Center)
Fax: (202) 357-3555
E-mail: aoainfo@aoa.hhs.gov
www.aoa.gov

American Association of Retired Persons
601 E St., N.W.
Washington, DC 20049
(888) OUR-AARP
www.aarp.org

Gray Panthers
1612 K Street, N.W., Suite 300
Washington, DC 20006
(800) 280-5362
(202) 737-6637
E-mail: info@graypanthers.org
www.graypanthers.org

AIDS (Acquired Immunodeficiency Syndrome)

National Center for HIV, STD, and TB Prevention (NCHSTP)

Centers for Disease Control and Prevention
1600 Clifton Rd. N.E.
Atlanta, GA 30333
(800) HIV-0440
E-mail: contactus@aidsinfo.nih.gov
www.cdc.gov/hiv/dhap.htm

University of California at San Francisco HIV Insite
UCSF Center for HIV Information
4150 Clement St., Bldg 16
VAMC IIIV-UCSF
San Francisco, CA 94121
Fax: (415) 379-5547
E-mail: info@chi.ucsf.edu
www.hivinsite.ucsf.edu

Gay Men's Health Crisis
The Tisch Building
119 West 24th St.
New York, NY 10011
(212) 367-1000
(212) 807-6655 (hotline)
(800) AIDS-NYC
www.gmhc.org

National AIDS Hotline
(800) CDC-INFO (800-232-4636)
E-mail: cdcinfo@cdc.gov

San Francisco AIDS Foundation
995 Market St. #200
San Francisco, CA 94103
(415) 487-3000
(800) 367-AIDS (hotline)
E-mail: feedback@sfaf.org
www.sfaf.org

Alcohol Abuse and Alcoholism

Al-Anon and Alateen
(support groups for friends and relatives
of alcoholics)
1600 Corporate Landing Pkwy.
Virginia Beach, VA 23454
(757) 563-1600
Fax: (757) 563-1655
E-mail: wso@al-anon.org
www.al-anon-alateen.org
See also white pages of telephone directory
for listing of local chapter

Alcohol Hotline
(800) ALCOHOL

Alcoholics Anonymous
Street Address:
475 Riverside Dr., 11th Floor
New York, NY 10115
Mailing Address:
Alcoholics Anonymous
Grand Central Station
P.O. Box 459
New York, NY 10163
(212) 870-3400
www.alcoholics-anonymous.org
See also white pages or telephone direc-
tory for listing of local chapter

**National Association of
Children of Alcoholics**
11426 Rockville Pike, Suite 301
Rockville, MD 20852
(888) 554-COAS (554-2627)
(301) 468-0985
E-mail: nacoa@nacoa.org
www.nacoa.org

**National Clearinghouse for
Alcohol and Drug Information**
P.O. Box 2345
Rockville, MD 20847-2345
(800) 729-6686
(240) 221-4019
www.health.org

**National Institute on Alcohol Abuse
and Alcoholism**
5635 Fishers Lane
MSC 9304
Bethesda, MD 20892-9304
(301) 443-3860
www.niaaa.nih.gov
See also Drug Abuse; Drinking & Driving
Groups

Allopathic Medicine

American Medical Association
515 N. State St.
Chicago, IL 60610
(800) 621-8335
www.ama-assn.org

Alternative Medicine

**National Center for Complementary
and Alternative Medicine (NCCAM)**
P.O. Box 7923
Gaithersburg , MD 20898
(888) 644-6226
International: (301) 519-3153
TTY: (866) 464-3615 (toll-free)
E-mail: info@nccam.nih.gov
www.nccam.nih.gov

Alzheimer's Disease

Alzheimer's Association National Office
125 N. Michigan Ave., Fl. 17
Chicago, IL 60601-7663
(800) 272-3900
312) 335-8700
Fax: (312) 335-1110
E-mail: info@alz.org
www.alz.org

Arthritis

Arthritis Foundation
P.O. Box 7669
Atlanta, GA 30357-0669
(800) 283-7800
(404) 872-7100
(404) 965-7888
www.arthritis.org

**National Institute of Arthritis and
Musculoskeletal and Skin Diseases**
National Institutes of Health
1 Ams Circle
Bethesda, MD 20892-3675
(301) 495-4484
(877) 22-NIAMS (226-4267)
E-mail: NIAMSInfo@mail.nih.gov
www.nih.gov/niams

Asthma

**Asthma and Allergy Foundation
of America**
1233 20th St., N.W., Suite 402
Washington, DC 20036
(800) 7-ASTHMA (727-8462)
(202) 466-7643
Fax: (202) 466-8940
E-mail: Info@aafa.org
www.aafa.org

Lung Line
National Jewish Medical Research Center
(information and referral service)
1400 Jackson St.
Denver, CO 80206
(800) 222-LUNG (5864)
(303) 388-4461
www.njc.org

Attention Deficit Disorder

**National Attention Deficit Disorder
Association (National ADDA)**
P.O. Box 543
Pottstown, PA 19464
(484) 945-2101
Fax: (610) 970-7520
www.add.org

**Children and Adults with Attention
Deficit Disorder (CHADD)**
8181 Professional Place, Suite 150
Landover, MD 20785
(800) 233-4050
(301) 306-7070
www.chadd.org

Automobile Safety

American Automobile Association (AAA)
1000 AAA Dr. #28
Heathrow, FL 32746-5080
(407) 444-4240
www.aaa.com
See also white or yellow pages of telephone
directory for listing of local chapter

Insurance Institute for Highway Safety
1005 North Glebe Rd., Suite 800
Arlington, VA 22201
(703) 247-1500
www.highwaysafety.org

**National Highway Traffic Safety
Administration**
1200 New Jersey Ave., SW
West Building
Washington, DC 20590
(888) 327-4236
(202) 366-0123
www.nhtsa.dot.gov

Auto Safety Hotline
(for consumer complaints about auto safety and child safety seats, and requests for information on recalls)
(800) 327-4236

Birth Control and Family Planning

Advocates for Youth
(develops programs and material to educate youth on sex and sexual responsibility)
2000 M Street N.W., Suite 750
Washington, DC 20036
(202) 419-3420
Fax: (202) 419-1448
E-mail: information@advocatesforyouth.org
www.advocatesforyouth.org

American College of Obstetricians and Gynecologists
(provides literature and contraceptive information)
409 12th Street, S.W.
P.O. Box 96920
Washington, DC 20090-6920
(202) 638-5577
www.acog.com

Engender Health
(provides information and referrals to individuals considering tubal ligation or vasectomy)
40 Ninth Ave.
New York, NY 10001
(212) 561-8000
E-mail: info@engenderhealth.org
www.engenderhealth.org

Planned Parenthood Federation of America (PPFA)
434 West 33rd St.
New York, NY 10001
(212) 541-7800
www.plannedparenthood.org
See also white or yellow pages of telephone directory for listing of local chapter

Birth Defects

Cystic Fibrosis Foundation (CFF)
6931 Arlington Rd.
Bethesda, MD 20814
(800) FIGHT-CF (344-4823)
(301) 951-4422
Fax: (301) 951-6378
E-mail: info@cff.org
www.cff.org

March of Dimes Birth Defects Foundation
1275 Mamaroneck Ave.
White Plains, NY 10605
(888) 663-4637
(914) 428-7100
www.modimes.org

Blindness

American Foundation for the Blind
11 Penn Plaza, Suite 300
New York, NY 10001
(800) AFB-LINE (232-5463)
(212) 502-7600
E-mail: afbinfo@afb.net
www.afb.org

National Federation of the Blind
1800 Johnson St.
Baltimore, MD 21230
(800) 638-7518
(410) 659-9314
www.nfb.org

National Library Service for the Blind and Physically Handicapped
Library of Congress
1291 Taylor St., N.W.
Washington, DC 20011
(888) NLS-READ
(202) 707-5100
E-mail: nls@loc.gov
www.loc.gov/nls

Blood Banks

American Red Cross
2025 E Street, N.W.
Washington, DC 20006
(202) 303-4498
To make a donation: (800) HELP-NOW
(800-435-7669)
www.redcross.org
See also white or yellow pages of telephone directory for listing of local chapter

Breast Cancer

Reach to Recovery
(support program for women who have undergone mastectomies as a result of breast cancer)
American Cancer Society
2200 Lake Blvd.
Atlanta, GA 30319
(800) 227-2345
(404) 816-7800
www.cancer.org

Cancer

American Cancer Society
American Cancer Society
3200 Lake Blvd.
Atlanta, GA 30319
(800) 227-2345
(404) 816-7800
www.cancer.org

Cancer Information Service
National Cancer Institute
Suite 3036A
6116 Executive Blvd.
Bethesda, MD 20892
(800) 4-CANCER (422-6237)
(301) 435-3848
www.cis.nci.nih.gov

Leukemia & Lymphoma Society
1311 Mamaroneck Ave.
White Plains, NY 10605
(914) 949-5213
Fax: (914) 949-6691
www.leukemia.org

National Coalition for Cancer Survivorship
1010 Wayne Ave., Suite 770
Silver Spring, MD 20910-5600
(301) 650-9127
(877) NCCS-YES (622-7937)
Fax: (301) 565-9670
E-mail: info@canceradvocacy.org
www.canceradvocacy.org

R. A. Bloch Cancer Foundation (Cancer Connection)
(support group that matches cancer patients with volunteers who are cured, in remission, or being treated for same type of cancer)
One H and R Block Way
Kansas City, MO 64105
(800) 433-0464
(816) 854-5050
www.blochcancer.org

Child Abuse

National Child Abuse Prevention
(provides services to children, adolescents, mentally retarded adults, and elderly)
606 Delsea Drive
Sewell, NJ 08080
(908) 369-8972
E-mail: patstan1@patmedia.net
www.ncap.org

National Child Abuse Hotline
(800) 422-4453

National Committee for the Prevention of Child Abuse
(provides literature on child abuse prevention programs)
200 S. Michigan Ave., 17th Floor
Chicago, IL 60604-2404
(312) 663-3520
E-mail: mailbox@preventchildabuse.org
www.preventchildabuse.org

Parents Anonymous
(self-help group for abusive parents)
75 W. Foothill Blvd., Suite 220
Claremont, CA 91711-3475
(909) 621-6184
Fax: (909) 625-6304
E-mail:Parentsanonymous@
parentsanonymous.org
www.parentsanonymous.org

Childbirth

American College of Nurse-Midwives
(R.N.s who provide services through the maternity cycle)
8403 Colesville Rd, Suite 1550
Silver Spring, MD 20910
www.midwife.org

American College of Obstetricians and Gynecologists
409 12th St., S.W.
P.O. Box 96920
Washington, DC 20090-6920
(202) 638-5577
www.acog.com

Lamaze International
2025 M St., Suite 800
Washington, DC 20036-3309
(800) 368-4404
(202) 367-1128
Fax: (202) 367-2128
E-mail: info@lamaze.org
www.lamaze.org

International Childbirth Education Association
P.O. Box 20048
Minneapolis, MN 55420
(952) 854-8660
Fax: (952) 854-8772
E-mail: info@icea.org
www.icea.org

Child Health and Development

National Center for Education in Maternal and Child Health
Georgetown University
Box 571272
Washington, DC 20007-2292
(202) 784-9770
Fax: (202) 784-9777
E-mail: mchlibrary@ncemch.org
www.ncemch.org

National Institute of Child Health & Human Development
Bldg. 31, Rm. 2A32, MSC 2425
31 Center Dr.
Bethesda, MD 20892-2425
(800) 370-2943
E-mail: NICHDInformationResource
Center@mail.nih.gov
www.nichd.nih.gov

Chiropractic

American Chiropractic Association
1701 Clarendon Blvd.
Arlington, VA 22209
(800) 986-4632
Fax: (703) 243-2593
E-mail: memberinfo@acatoday.org
www.amerchiro.org

Consumer Information

Federal Consumer Information Center
(catalog of publications developed by federal agencies for consumers)
Department WWW
Pueblo, CO 81009
(888) 878-3256
www.pueblo.gsa.gov

U.S. Consumer Product Safety Commission
U.S. Consumer Product Safety
Commission
4330 East West Hwy
Bethesda, MD 20814
(800) 638-2772
(301) 504-7923
Fax: (301) 504-0124 and (301) 504-0025
E-mail: info@cpsc.gov
www.cpsc.gov

Consumers Union of United States
(tests quality and safety of consumer products: publishes Consumer Reports magazine)
101 Truman Ave.

Yonkers, NY 10703
(914) 378-2000
www.consumerreports.org

Council of Better Business Bureaus
4200 Wilson Blvd., Suite 800
Arlington, VA 22203-1883
(703) 276-0100
Fax: (703) 525-8277
www.bbb.org
See also white or yellow pages of telephone directory for listing of local chapter

Food and Drug Administration (FDA)
Office of Consumer Affairs
Consumer Inquiries
5600 Fishers Lane
Rockville, MD 20857
(888) INFO-FDA (463-6332)
www.fda.gov

Crime Victims

Crisis Prevention Institute, Inc.
(offers programs on nonviolent physical crisis interventions)
3315-K North 124th St.
Brookfield, WI 53005
(800) 558-8976 (U.S. and Canada)
(262) 783-5787
E-mail: info@crisisprevention.com
www.crisisprevention.com

National Center for Victims of Crime
2000 M Street, N.W., Suite 480
Washington, DC 20010
(202) 467-8700
Fax: (202) 467-8701
www.ncvc.org

Death and Grieving

Share
(support group for parents who have lost a newborn)
c/o St. Joseph's Health Center
300 First Capitol Dr.
St. Charles, MO 63301-2893
(800) 821-6819
(636) 947-6164
E-mail: share@nationalshareoffice.com
www.nationalshareoffice.com

Dental Health

American Dental Association (ADA)
211 E. Chicago Ave.
Chicago, IL 60611
(312) 440-2500
www.ada.org

National Institute of Dental and Craniofacial Research
Public Information & Liaison Branch
45 Center Dr., MSC 6400
Bethesda, MD 20892-6400
(301) 496-4261
E-mail: nidcrinfo@mail.nih.gov
www.nidcr.nih.gov

Depressive Disorders

American Psychiatric Association
1000 Wilson Blvd., Suite 1825
Arlington, VA 22209-3901
(888) 357-7924
(202) 336-5500
E-mail: apa@psych.org
www.psych.org

American Psychological Association
750 First St., N.E.
Washington, DC 20002-4242
(800) 374-2721
(202) 336-5510
TDD/TTY: (202) 336-6123
www.apa.org

Depression & Bipolar Support Alliance
730 N. Franklin, Suite 501
Chicago, IL 60610-7204
(800) 826-3632
(312) 642-0049
Fax: (312) 642-7243
www.dbsalliance.org

DES (Diethylstibestrol)

DES Action, USA
(support group for persons exposed to DES)
158 S. Stanwood Rd
Columbus, OH 43209
(800) DES-9288
Fax: (510) 465-4815
E-mail: desaction@columbus.rr.com
www.desaction.org

Diabetes

American Diabetes Association
National Center
1701 North Beauregard St.
Alexandria, VA 22311
(800) DIABETES (342-2383)
(703) 549-1500
E-mail: AskADA@diabetes.org
www.diabetes.org

Juvenile Diabetes Research Foundation International (JDRFI)
120 Wall St.
New York, NY 10005-4001

(800) JDF-CURE (533-2873)
(212) 785-9500
Fax: (212) 785-9595
E-mail: info@jdrf.org
www.jdfcure.org

National Diabetes Information Clearinghouse
1 Information Way
Bethesda, MD 20892-3560
(800) 860-8747
(301) 654-3327
E-mail: ndic@info.niddk.nih.gov
www.diabetes.niddk.nih.gov/

Digestive Diseases

National Institute of Diabetes & Digestive & Kidney Diseases (NIDDK)
Office of Communication & Public Liaison
NIDDK, NIH, Building 31
Room 9A04 Center Dr., MSC 2560
Bethesda, MD 20892-2560
(301) 654-3810
www.niddk.nih.gov

Disabled Services

American Alliance for Health, Physical Education, Recreation & Dance (AAHPERD)
(provides information about recreation and fitness opportunities for the disabled)
1900 Association Drive
Reston, VA 20191-1598
(800) 213-7193
Fax: (703) 476-9527
www.aahperd.org

National Library Service for the Blind and Physically Handicapped
Library of Congress
1291 Taylor St., N.W.
Washington, DC 20011
(888) 657-7323
(202) 707-5100
TDD: (202) 707-0744
Fax: (202) 707-0712
E-mail: nls@loc.gov
www.loc.gov/nls

Special Olympics International (SOI)
1133 19th Street, N.W.
Washington, DC 20036
(202) 628-3630
Fax: (202) 824-0200
www.specialolympics.org

Domestic Violence

National Coalition Against Domestic Violence (NCADV)
1120 Lincoln Street
Suite 1603
Denver, CO 80203
(303) 839-1852
Fax: (303) 831-9251
E-mail: mainoffice@ncadv.org
www.ncadv.org

National Domestic Violence Hotline
(800) 799-SAFE (799-7233)

National Network to End Domestic Violence
660 Pennsylvania, SE, Suite 303
Washington, DC 20003
(202) 543-5566
www.nnedv.org

Down Syndrome

National Down Syndrome Society
666 Broadway, 8th Floor
New York, NY 10012-2317
(800) 221-4602
(212) 460-9330
E-mail: info@ndss.org
www.ndss.org

National Down Syndrome Congress
1370 Center Drive, Suite 102
Atlanta, GA 30338
(800) 232-6372
E-mail: NDSCcenter@aol.com
www.ndsccenter.org

Drinking and Driving Groups

Mothers Against Drunk Driving
511 E. John Carpenter Frwy., Suite 700
Irving, TX 75062
(800) GET-MADD (438-6233)
(214) 744-6233
www.madd.org
See also white or yellow pages of telephone directory for local chapter

Students Against Destructive Decisions (also Students Against Driving Drunk (SADD))
255 Main Street
Marlboro, MA 01752
(877) SADD-INC (723-3462)
(508) 481-3568
Fax: (508) 481-5759
E-mail: info@sadd.org
www.saddonline.com

Drug Abuse

Cocaine Anonymous World Services
P.O. Box 49200
Los Angeles, CA 90049-8000 or
3740 Overland Ave., Ste. C
Los Angeles, CA 90034
(800) 347-8998
(310) 559-5833
E-mail: Cawso@ca.org
www.ca.org

Narcotics Anonymous (NA)
(support group for recovering narcotics
addicts)
P.O. Box 9999
Van Nuys, CA 91409
(818) 773-9999
Fax: (818) 700-0700
www.na.org
See also white or yellow pages of telephone
directory for local chapter

National Cocaine Hotline
(800) COCAINE (262-2463)

National Institute on Drug Abuse
6001 Executive Blvd., Room 5213
Bethesda, MD 20892-9651
(301) 443-1124
Helpline: (800) 662-4357
E-mail: information@nida.nih.gov
www.nida.nih.gov

**Center for Substance Abuse Prevention
(CSAP)**
Substance Abuse and Mental Health
Administration
5600 Fishers Lane
Rockwall 2 Bldg.
Rockville, MD 20857
(301) 443-8956
www.prevention.samhsa.gov

Eating Disorders

**National Eating Disorders Association
(NEDA)**
(self-help groups that provide information and referrals to physicians and
therapists)
603 Stewart St., Suite 803
Seattle, WA 98101
(800) 931-2237
(206) 382-3587
E-mail: info@NationalEatingDisorders.org
www.nationaleatingdisorders.org

**Anorexia Nervosa and Related Eating
Disorders (ANRED)**
(provides information and referrals for
people with eating disorders)
P.O. Box 5102
Eugene, OR 97405
(541) 344-1144
www.anred.com

Environment

**U.S. Environmental Protection
Agency (EPA)**
Ariel Rios Bldg.
1200 Pennsylvania Ave., N.W.
Washington, DC 20460
(202) 272-0167
www.epa.gov

Greenpeace, USA
702 H St. N.W.
Washington, DC 20001
(800) 326-0959
(202) 462-1177
E-mail: info@wdc.greenpeace.org
www.greenpeace/usa.org

Natural Resources Defense Council
40 West 20th St.
New York, NY 10011
(212) 727-2700
Fax: (212) 727-1773
E-mail: nrdcinfo@nrdc.org
www.nrdc.org

Sierra Club
85 2nd St., 2nd Floor
San Francisco, CA 94105-3441
(415) 977-5500
(415) 977-5799
E-mail: Information@sierraclub.org
www.sierraclub.org

World Wildlife Fund
1250 24th St., N.W.
P.O. Box 97180
Washington, DC 20090-7180
(800) CALL-WWF (225-5993)
(202) 293-4800
Fax: (202) 293-2911
www.wwfus.org

Epilepsy

Epilepsy Foundation of America
4351 Garden City Drive
Landover, MD 20785-7223
(800) EFA-1000 (332-1000)
(301) 459-3700
www.efa.org

Gay and Lesbian Organizations and Services

Human Rights Campaign
1640 Rhode Island Avenue, N.W.
Washington, DC 20036-3278
(202) 628-4160
(800) 777-4723
Fax: (202) 347-5323
E-mail: hrc@hrc.org
www.hrc.org

**National Gay and Lesbian Task Force
(NGLTF)**
1325 Massachusetts Ave., N.W., Suite 600
Washington, DC, 20005
(202) 393-5177
Fax: (202) 393-2241
E-mail: Thetaskforce@thetaskforce.org
www.ngltf.org

**Parents, Families, and Friends of
Lesbians and Gays (PFLAG)**
1726 M St., N.W., Suite 400
Washington, DC 20036
(202) 467-8180
Fax: (202) 467-8194
E-mail: info@pflag.org
www.pflag.org

Genetics

American College of Medical Genetics
9650 Rockville Pike
Bethesda, MD 20814-3998
(301) 634-7127
Fax: (301) 571-0677
E-mail: acmg@faseb.org
www.acmg.net

The Human Genome Organization
HUGO Americas
Laboratory of Genetics
National Institute on Aging
NIH/NIA-IRP. GRC, Box 31
5600 Nathan Shock Dr.
Baltimore, MD 21224-6825
(410) 558-8337
Fax: (410) 558-8331
E-mail: schlessingerd@grc.nia.nih.gov

GeneTests—GeneClinics
(a database of information for patients
and families with genetic disorders, providing access to support groups)
University of Washington School of
Medicine
Seattle, WA
www.genetests.org

Hazardous Waste

Environmental Protection Agency (EPA)
Ariel Rios Bldg.
1200 Pennsylvania Ave., N.W.
Washington, DC 20460
(202) 260-2090
www.epa.gov

Hazardous Waste Hotline Information
(800) 424-9346

Health Care

Association for Applied and Therapeutic Humor (AATH)
(publishes a newsletter and sponsors seminars for people in the helping professions)
65 Enterprise
Aliso Viejo, CA 92656
(888) 747-AATH
Fax: (602) 995-1449
www.aath.org

American Medical Association
515 N. State St.
Chicago, IL 60610
(800) 621-8335
www.ama-assn.org

American Nurses Association
600 Maryland Ave., S.W.
Suite 100 West
Washington, DC 20024-2571
(800) 274-4ANA (274-4262)
(202) 651-7000
www.ana.org

Health Education

National Center for Chronic Disease Prevention and Health Promotion
Centers for Disease Control and Prevention
Mail Stop A34
1600 Clifton Rd., N.E.
Atlanta, GA 30333
(404) 639-3534
(800) 311-3435
E-mail: cdcinfo@cdc.gov
www.cdc.gov/nccdphp

Hearing Impairment

American Society for Deaf Children
(resource group for parents of hard of hearing and deaf children)
3820 Hartzdale
Camp Hill, PA 17011
(717) 334-7922
Fax: (717) 334-8808

(800) 942-ASDC (Parent Hotline)
www.deafchildren.org

Better Hearing Institute (BHI)
(provides educational and resource materials on deafness)
Better Hearing Institute
515 King St., Suite 420
Alexandria, VA 22314
(703) 684-3391
E-mail: mail@betterhearing.org
www.betterhearing.org

Heart Disease

American Heart Association (AHA)
7272 Greenville Ave.
Dallas, TX 75231
(800) 242-8721
(214) 373-6300
www.americanheart.org

National Heart, Lung, and Blood Institute
(provides information on cardiovascular risk factors and disease)
Bldg. 31, Room 5A52
31 Center Dr., MSC 2486
Bethesda, MD 20892
(800) 575-9355
(301) 592-8573
E-mail: nhlbiinfo@nhlbi.nih.gov
www.nhlbi.nih.gov/index.htm

Helping Others

United Way of America
701 N. Fairfax St.
Alexandria, VA 22314-2045
(703) 836-7100
www.unitedway.org

Hospice

The National Hospice and Palliative Care Organization
1700 Diagonal Rd., Suite 625
Alexandria, VA 22314
(703) 837-1500
(800) 646-6460
E-mail: info@nhpco.org
www.nhpco.org

Immunization

National Immunization Program
Centers for Disease Control
Mail Stop E-05
1600 Clifton Rd., N.E.
Atlanta, GA 30333
(404) 639-3311
(800) 232-2522
www.cdc.gov/nip/diseases/adult-vpd.htm

Immunization Action Coalition
(information for children, adolescents, and adults)
1573 Selby Ave., Suite 234
St. Paul, MN 55104
(651) 647-9009
Fax: (651) 647-9131
E-mail: admin@immunize.org
www.immunize.org

Infant Care

La Leche League International
(provides information and support to women interested in breast-feeding)
1400 N. Meacham Rd.
Schaumburg, IL 60168-4079
(800) LA-LECHE (525-3243)
(847) 519-7730
www.lalecheleague.org

Infectious Diseases

Centers for Disease Control and Prevention
1600 Clifton Rd., N.E.
Atlanta, GA 30333
(800) 311-3435
(404) 639-3534
E-mail: cdcinfo@cdc.gov
www.cdc.gov

Infertility

Resolve: The National Infertility Association
(offers counseling, information, and support to people with problems of infertility)
8405 Greensboro Dr., Suite 800
McLean, VA 22102
(703) 556-7172
E-mail: info@resolve.org
www.resolve.org

Kidney Disease

American Kidney Fund (AKF)
(provides information on financial aid to patients, organ transplants, and kidney-related diseases)
110 Executive Blvd., Suite 1010
Rockville, MD 20852
(866) 300-2900
(301) 881-3052
E-mail: Helpline@kidneyfund.org
www.akfinc.org

American Association of Kidney Patients (AAKP)
3505 E. Frontage Rd., Suite 315
Tampa, FL 33607
(800) 749-2257

Fax: (813) 636-8122
E-mail: info@aakp.org
www.aakp.org

National Kidney Foundation (NKF)
30 East 33rd St., Suite 1100
New York, NY 10016
(800) 622-9010
(212) 889-2210
Fax: (212) 689-9261
www.kidney.org

Liver Disease

American Liver Foundation (ALF)
75 Maiden, Suite 603
New York, NY 10038
(800) 465-4837
(212) 668-1000
E-mail: info@liverfoundation.org
www.liverfoundation.org

Lung Disease

American Lung Association
61 Broadway, 6th Floor
New York, NY 10006
(800) LUNG-USA
(800) 548-8252
(212) 315-8700
www.lungusa.org

**National Heart, Lung,
and Blood Institute**
(provides information on cardiovascular
risk factors and disease)
Bldg. 31, Room 5A52
31 Center Dr., MSC 2486
Bethesda, MD 20892
(800) 575-9355
E-mail: nhlbiinfo@nhlbi.nih.gov
www.nhlbi.nih.gov/index.htm

Lupus Erythematosus

Lupus Foundation of America (LPA)
2000 L Street, N.W., Suite 710
Washington, DC 20036
(202) 349-1155
(800) 558-0121
Fax: (202) 349-1156
E-mail: info@lupus.org
www.lupus.org

Marriage and Family

**Women Work! The National Network
for Women's Employment**
(national advocacy group for women over
35 who have lost their primary means
of support through death, divorce, or
disabling of spouse)
1625 K St. N.W., Suite 300

Washington, DC 20006
(202) 467-6346
E-mail: Info@womenwork.org
www.womenwork.org

Alliance for Children & Families
11700 West Lake Park Dr.
Milwaukee, WI 53224-3099
(414) 359-1040
Fax: (414) 359-1074
E-mail: info@alliance1.org
www.alliance1.org

Stepfamily Association of America
(provides information and publishes
quarterly newsletter)
650 J St., Suite 205
Lincoln, NE 68508
(800) 735-0329
(402) 477-7837
Fax: (402) 477-8317
E-mail: stepfamfs@aol.com
www.saafamilies.org

Medications

(Prescriptions and Over-the-Counter)

Food and Drug Administration (FDA)
Office of Consumer Affairs Public
Inquiries
5600 Fishers Lane (HFE-88)
Rockville, MD 20857-0001
(888) 463-6332 (INFO-FDA)
www.fda.gov

Mental Health

American Psychiatric Association
1000 Wilson Blvd., Suite 125
Arlington, VA 22209
(888) 357-7924
(703) 907-7300
E-mail: apa@psych.org
www.psych.org

American Psychological Association
750 First St., N.E.
Washington, DC 20002-4242
(800) 374-2721
(202) 336-5510
TDD/TTY: (202) 336-6123
http://www.apa.org

American Psychoanalytic Foundation
309 East 49th Street
New York, NY 10017
(212) 752-0450
E-mail: APF@cyberpsych.org
www.cyberpsych.org/apf

**National Alliance for the
Mentally Ill (NAMI)**
(self-help advocacy organization for
persons with schizophrenia and depressive
disorders and their families)
Colonial Place Three
2107 Wilson Blvd., Suite 300
Arlington, VA 22201
(703) 524-7600
HelpLine: (800) 950-NAMI (950-6264)
www.nami.org

National Institute of Mental Health
Information Resources and Inquiries
Branch
6001 Executive Blvd., Room 8184
MSC 9663
Bethesda, MD 20892-9663
(301) 443-4513 (local)
866) 615-6464
Fax: (301) 443-4279
TTY: (301) 443-8431
(866) 415-8051 (TTY toll-free)
E-mail: nimhinfo@nih.gov
www.nimh.nih.gov

**National Mental Health Association
(NMHA)**
2000 N. Beauregard St., 6th Floor
Alexandria, VA 22311
(800) 969-NMHA (969-6642)
(703) 684-7722
Fax: (703) 684-5968
www.nmha.org

Mental Retardation

The ARC
1010 Wayne Ave., Suite 650
Silver Spring, MD 20910
(301) 565-3842
E-mail: info@thearc.org
www.thearc.org

Missing and Runaway Children

Child Find of America
(800) I-AM-LOST (426-5678)
Runaway Hotline
(800) 621-4000
www.childfindofamerica.org

**National Center for Missing and
Exploited Children (NCMEC)**
699 Prince St., Suite 550
Alexandria, VA 22314
(703) 274-3900
Fax: (703) 274-2200
4-hour Hotline:
(800) THE-LOST (843-5678)
www.missingkids.org

Neurological Disorders

National Institute of Neurological Disorders and Stroke
P.O. Box 5801
Bethesda, MD 20892
(800) 352-9424
(301) 496-5751
Fax: (301) 402-2186
E-mail: braininfo@ninds.nih.gov
www.ninds.nih.gov

Nutrition

American Dietetic Association
120 South Riverside Plaza, Suite 2000
Chicago, IL 60606-6995
(800) 877-1600
www.eatright.org

American Society for Nutritional Sciences
9650 Rockville Pike, Suite 4500
Bethesda, MD 20814-3990
(301) 530-7050
Fax: (301) 634-7892
E-mail: sec@nutrition.org
www.asnutrition.org

Food and Drug Administration (FDA)
Office of Consumer Affairs
Public Inquiries
5600 Fishers Lane (HFE-88)
Rockville, MD 20857
(888) 463-6332 (INFO-FDA)
www.fda.gov

Food and Nutrition Information Center
U.S. Dept. of Agriculture
National Agricultural Library
10301 Baltimore Ave.
Beltsville, MD 20705-2351
(301) 504-5719
Fax: (301) 504-6409
TTY: (301) 504-6856
E-mail: fnic@nal.usda.gov
www.nal.usda.gov/fnic

Center for Nutrition in Sport and Human Performance
206A Chenoweth Lab
University of Massachusetts
Amherst, MA 01002
413) 545-1076
Fax: (413) 545-1074
E-mail: volpe@nutrition.umass.edu
www.umass.edu/cnshp/

National Dairy Council
10255 W. Higgins Rd., Suite 900
Rosemont, IL 60018-5616
(800) 426-8271
E-mail: ndc@dairyinformation.com
www.nationaldairycouncil.org

Occupational Safety and Health

Occupational Safety and Health Administration (OSHA)
U.S. Dept. of Labor
Office of Public Affairs, Room N3647
200 Constitution Ave.
Washington, DC 20210
(202) 693-1999
(800) 321-OSHA (6742)
TTY: (877) 889-5627
www.osha.gov

Organ Donations

The Living Bank (TLB)
(provides information and acts as registry and referral service for people wanting to donate organs for research or transplantation)
P.O. Box 6725
Houston, TX 77265
(800) 528-2971
E-mail: info@livingbank.org
www.livingbank.org

Osteopathic Medicine

American Osteopathic Association (AOA)
142 East Ontario St.
Chicago, IL 60611
(800) 621-1773
312) 202-8000
Fax: (312) 202-8200
E-mail: info@osteotech.org
www.osteopathic.org

Parent Support Groups

National Organization of Mothers of Twins Clubs (NOMOTC)
P.O. Box 700860
Plymouth, MI 48170-0955
(877) 540-2200
248) 231-4480
E-mail: Info@NOMOTC.ORG
www.nomotc.org

Parents Anonymous
(self-help group for abusive parents)
675 W. Foothill Blvd., Suite 220
Claremont, CA 91711-3475

(909) 621-6184
Fax: (909) 625-6304
E-mail: parentsanonymous@parentsanonymous.org
www.parentsanonymous.org

Parents Without Partners, Inc.
1650 South Dixie Highway, Suite 510
Boca Raton, FL 33432
(561) 391-8833
Fax: (561) 395-8557
E-mail: pwp@jti.net
www.parentswithoutpartners.org

Parenting

National Parent Information Network
ERIC Clearinghouse on Elementary and Early Childhood Education
University of Illinois at Urbana-Champaign
Children's Research Center
51 Gerty Dr.
Champaign, IL 61820-7469
(800) 583-4135
(217) 333-1386
Fax: (217) 333-3767
www.npin.org

Phobias

Anxiety Disorders Association of America (ADAA)
(provides information about phobias and referrals to therapists and support groups)
8730 Georgia Ave., Suite 600
Silver Spring, MD 20910
(240) 485-1001
Fax: (240) 485-1035
www.adaa.org

TERRAP Programs
(headquarters for national network of treatment clinics for agoraphobia)
932 Evelyn St.
Menlo Park, CA 94025
(415) 327-1312
(800) 2-PHOBIA (274-6242)
www.terrap.com

Physical Fitness

See local yellow and white pages of telephone directory for listing of local health clubs and YMCAs, YWCAs, and Jewish Community Centers

Cooper Institutes for Aerobics Research
12330 Preston Rd.
Dallas, TX 75230
(972) 341-3200

Fax: (972) 341-3227
E-mail: courses@cooperinst.org
www.cooperinst.org

President's Council on Physical Fitness and Sports
Dept. W 200 Independence Ave., S.W.
Room 738 H
Washington, DC 20201
(202) 690-9000
Fax: (202) 690-5211
www.fitness.gov

American College of Sports Medicine
ACSM National Center
P.O. Box 1440
Indianapolis, IN 46206-1440
(317) 637-9200
www.acsm.org

Center for Nutrition in Sport and Human Performance
206A Chenoweth Lab
University of Massachusetts
Amherst, MA 01002
(413) 545-1076
Fax: (413) 545-1074
E-mail: volpe@nutrition.umass.edu
www.umass.edu/cnshp/

Poisoning

See emergency numbers listed in the front of your local phone directory

National Poison Hotline
(800) 222-1222

Pregnancy

National Institute of Child Health & Human Development
Bldg. 31, Room 2A32, MSC 2425
31 Center Dr.
Bethesda, MD 20892-2425
(800) 370-2943
E-mail: NICHDInformationResource
Center@mail.nih.gov
www.nichd.nih.gov

Product Safety

U.S. Consumer Product Safety Commission
4330 East West Hwy.
Bethesda, MD 20814
(800) 638-CPSC (638-2772)
(301) 504-7923
www.cpsc.gov

Radiation Control and Safety

Center for Devices and Radiological Health
U.S. Food and Drug Administration
Office of Consumer Affairs
1350 Piccard Drive, HFZ-210
Rockville, MD 20850
(800) 638-2041
(301) 827-3990
www.fda.gov/cdrh/

National Institute of Environmental Health Sciences

National Institutes of Health
P.O. Box 12233
Research Triangle Park, NC 27709
(919) 541-3345
www.niehs.nih.gov

Rape, Victimization

See white pages of telephone directory for listing of local rape crisis and counseling centers

National Center for Victims of Crime
2000 M St., N.W., Suite 480
Washington, DC 20010
(202) 467-8700
Fax: (202) 467-8701
www.ncvc.org

National Organization for Victim Assistance (NOVA)
NOVA
510 King Street, Suite 424
Alexandria, VA 22314
(800) TRY-NOVA (879-6682)
(703) 535-NOVA
Fax: (703) 535-5500
www.trynova.org

National Sexual Violence Resource Center
123 North Enola Dr.
Enola, PA 17025
(877) 739-3895
(717) 909-0710
Fax: (717) 909-0714
TTY: (717) 909-0715
E-mail: resources@nsvrc.org
www.nsvrc.org

Reye's Syndrome

National Reye's Syndrome Foundation
P.O. Box 829
Bryan, OH 43506-0829

(800) 233-7393 (U.S. only)
(419) 636-2679
Fax: (419) 636-9897
E-mail: nrsf@reyessyndrome.org
www.reyessyndrome.org

Self-Care/Self-Help

National Self-Help Clearinghouse (NSHC)
(provides information about self-help groups)
365 5th Ave., Suite 3300
New York, NY 10016
(212) 817-1822
http://selfhelpweb.org

Sex Education

American Association of Sex Educators, Counselors and Therapists (AASECT)
P.O. Box 1960
Ashland, VA 23005-1960
(804) 752-0026
Fax: (804) 752-0056
E-mail: aasect@aasect.org
www.aasect.org

Advocates for Youth
(develops programs and material to educate youth on sex and sexual responsibility)
2000 M Street N.W., Suite 750
Washington, DC 20005
(202) 419-3420
Fax: (202) 419-1448
E-mail: information@advocatesfor
youth.org
www.advocatesforyouth.org

Planned Parenthood Federation of America (PPFA)
434 West 33rd St.
New York, NY 10001
(212) 541-7800
www.plannedparenthood.org

Sexuality Information and Education Council of the U.S. (SIECUS)
(maintains an information clearinghouse on all aspects of human sexuality)
130 West 42nd St., Suite 350
New York, NY 10036-7802
(212) 819-9770
Fax: (212) 819-9776
E-mail: siecus@siecus.org
www.siecus.org

Sexual Abuse and Assault

National Center for Assault Prevention
(provides services to children, adolescents, mentally retarded adults, and elderly)
606 Delsea Dr.
Sewell, NJ 08080
(800) 258-3189
(908) 369-8972
www.ncap.org

Prevent Child Abuse America
500 N. Michigan Ave., Suite 200
Chicago, IL 60611
(312) 663-3520
Fax: (312) 939-8962
E-mail: mailbox@preventchildabuse.org
www.preventchildabuse.org

Sexually Transmitted Diseases

Centers for Disease Control and Prevention
1600 Clifton Rd. N.E.
Atlanta, GA 30333
(800) CDC-INFO
(404) 639-3534
(800) 311-3435
E-mail: cdcinfo@cdc.gov
www.cdc.gov

American Social Health Association
P.O. Box 13827
Research Triangle Park, NC 27709
(919) 361-8400
Fax: (919) 361-8425
E-mail: info@ashastd.org
www.ashastd.org

National Herpes Resource Center
American Social Health Association
P.O. Box 13827
Research Triangle Park, NC 27709-3827
(919) 361-8488
E-mail: hsvnet@ashastd.org
www.ashastd.org/hrc/index.html

National STD Hotline
(800) 227-8922

Sexuality Information and Education Council of the U.S. (SIECUS)
(maintains an information clearinghouse on all aspects of human sexuality)
130 West 42nd St., Suite 350
New York, NY 10036-7802
(212) 819-9770
Fax: (212) 819-9776
E-mail: siecus@siecus.org
www.siecus.org

Sickle-Cell Disease

Sickle Cell Disease Association of America
231 East Baltimore St., Ste 800
Baltimore, MD 21202
(800) 421-8453
410) 528-1555
E-mail: scdaa@sicklecelldisease.org
www.sicklecelldisease.org

The Sickle Cell Information Center
The Georgia Comprehensive Sickle Cell Center at Grady Health System
P.O. Box 109, Grady Memorial Hospital, 80 Jesse Hill Jr. Dr.
Atlanta, GA 30303
(404) 616-3572
Fax: (404) 616-5998
E-mail: aplatt@emory.edu
www.scinfo.org

Skin Diseases

American Academy of Dermatology
P.O. Box 4014
Schaumburg, IL 60168-4014
(888) 503-SKIN (7546)
(847) 330-0230
Fax: (847) 330-0050
www.aad.org

University of Iowa Hospitals and Clinics Department of Dermatology
200 Hawkins Drive BT 2045-1
Iowa City, IA 52242-1090
(319) 356-SKIN (7546)
(319) 384-6012
Fax: (319) 356-8317
www.tray.dermatology.uiowa.edu

National Psoriasis Foundation
6600 SW 92nd Ave., Suite 300
Portland, OR 97223-7195
(800) 723-9166
(503) 244-7404
Fax: (503) 245-0626
E-mail: getinfo@psoriasis.org
www.psoriasis.org

Sleep and Sleep Disorders

American Sleep Apnea Association
1424 K St., N.W., Suite 302
Washington, DC 20005
(202) 293-3650
Fax: (202) 293-3656
E-mail: asaa@sleepapnea.org
www.sleepapnea.org

American Academy of Sleep Medicine
One Westbrook Corporate Center, Suite 920
West Chester, IL 60154
(708) 492-0930
Fax: (708) 492-0943
www.aasmnet.org

Better Sleep Council
501 Wythe St.
Alexandria, VA 22314
(703) 683-8371
E-mail: spali@sleepproducts.org
www.bettersleep.org

National Sleep Foundation
1522 K St., N.W., Suite 500
Washington, DC 20005
(202) 347-3471
Fax: (202) 347-3472
E-mail: nsf@sleepfoundation.org
www.sleepfoundation.org

Smoking and Tobacco

Action on Smoking and Health (ASH)
(provides information on nonsmokers' rights and related subjects)
2013 H St., N.W.
Washington, DC 20006
(202) 659-4310
http://ash.org

American Cancer Society
(provides information about quitting smoking and smoking cessation programs)
2200 Lake Blvd.
Atlanta, GA 30319
(800) 227-2345
(404) 816-7800
www.cancer.org

American Heart Association
(provides information about quitting smoking and smoking cessation programs)
7272 Greenville Ave.
Dallas, TX 75231
(800) 242-8721
(214) 373-6300
www.americanheart.org

American Lung Association
(provides information about quitting smoking and smoking cessation programs)
61 Broadway, 6th Floor
New York, NY 10006

(212) 315-8700

To reach your local American Lung Association: (800) LUNG-USA (586-4872)

www.lungusa.org

Americans for Nonsmokers' Rights

2530 San Pablo Ave., Suite J

Berkeley, CA 94702

(510) 841-3032

Fax: (510) 841-3071

E-mail: anr@no-smoke.org

www.no-smoke.org

Stress Reduction

American Institute of Stress

124 Park Ave.

Yonkers, NY 10703

(914) 963-1200

Fax: (914) 965-6267

E-mail: stress125@optonline.net

www.stress.org

American Psychological Association

750 First St., N.E.

Washington, DC 20002-4242

(800) 374-2721

(202) 336-5500

TDD/TTY: 202-336-6123

www.apa.org

**Association for Applied
Psychophysiology and Biofeedback**

10200 W. 44th Ave., Suite 304

Wheat Ridge, CO 80033

(800) 477-8892

(303) 422-8436

E-mail: aapb@resourcenter.com

www.aapb.org

Stroke

Council on Stroke

American Stroke Association

National Center

7272 Greenville Ave.

Dallas, TX 75231

AHA: (800) AHA-USA-1 (800-242-8721)

ASA: (888) 4-STROKE (888-478-7653)

www.strokeassociation.org

**National Institute of Neurological
Disorders and Stroke**

National Institutes of Health

P.O. Box 5801

Bethesda, MD 20824

(800) 352-9424

(301) 496-5751

www.ninds.nih.gov

Stuttering

National Center for Stuttering

200 East 33rd St.

New York, NY 10016

Hotline: (800) 221-2483

(212) 532-1460

www.stuttering.com

Sudden Infant Death Syndrome (SIDS)

First Candle/SIDS Alliance

(provides information and referrals to
families who have lost an infant because
of SIDS)

1314 Bedford Ave., Suite 210

Baltimore, MD 21208

(800) 221-7437

410) 653-8226

Fax: (410) 653-8709

E-mail: info@firstcandle.org

www.sidsalliance.org

Suicide Prevention

**American Association
of Suicidology (AAS)**

5221 Wisconsin Avenue, NW

Washington, DC 20015

(202) 237-2280; hotline

(800) 273-TALK (8255)

Fax: (202) 237-2282

E-mail: info@suicidology.org

www.suicidology.org

American Psychoanalytic Foundation

309 East 49th Street

New York, NY 10017

(212) 752-0450

www.cyberpsych.org/apf

Terminal Illness

**Make-A-Wish Foundation
of America (MAWFA)**

(dedicated to granting the special wishes
of terminally ill children)

3550 North Central Ave., Suite 300

Phoenix, AZ 85012-2127

(800) 722-WISH (722-9474)

(602) 279-WISH (279-9474)

Fax: (602) 279-0855

E-mail: mawfa@wish.org

www.wish.org

Make Today Count (MTC)

(self-help group for persons with terminal
illness)

St. Johns Hospital

1235 E. Cherokee St.

Springfield, MO 65804

(800) 909-8326

(417) 885-3324

Fax: (417) 820-2587

E-mail: Info@stjohns.com

www.stjohns.com

Victimization

National Center for Victims of Crime

2000 M St., N.W., Suite 480

Washington, DC 20036

(202) 467-8700

Fax: (202) 467-8701

www.ncvc.org

**National Coalition Against
Domestic Violence**

1120 Lincoln Street, Suite 1603

Denver, CO 80203

(303) 839-1852

Fax: (303) 831-9251

E-mail: mainoffice@ncadv.org

www.ncadv.org

**National Coalition
Against Sexual Assault**

125 N. Enola Dr.

Enola, PA 17025

(717) 728-9764

Fax: (717) 728-9781

http://dreamingdesigns.com/other/
indexncasa.html

**National Organization for Victim
Assistance (NOVA)**

NOVA

510 King Street, Suite 424

Alexandria, VA 22314

(800) Try-NOVA (879-6682)

(703) 535-NOVA

Fax: (703) 535-5500

www.trynova.org

Weight Control

Overeaters Anonymous (OA)

P.O. Box 44020

Rio Rancho, NM 87174-4020

(505) 891-2664

Fax: (505) 891-4320

E-mail: info@overeatersanonymous.org

www.oa.org

Weight-Control Information Network (WIN)
National Institute of Diabetes and Digestive and Kidney Diseases
1 WIN Way
Bethesda, MD 20892-3665
(877) 946-4627
(202) 828-1025
Fax: (202) 828-1028
E-mail: win@info.niddk.nih.gov
www.win.niddk.nih.gov

Take Off Pounds Sensibly (TOPS)
P.O. Box 07360
4575 S. Fifth St.
Milwaukee, WI 53207-0360
(800) 932-8677
(414) 482-4620
www.tops.org

Weight Watchers International
175 Crossways Park West
Woodbury, NY 11797
(516) 390-1657
www.weight-watchers.com

Wellness

National Wellness Institute, Inc.
1300 College Court
P.O. Box 827

Stevens Point, WI 54481-0827
(800) 243-8694
(715) 342-2969
Fax: (715) 342-2979
E-mail: nwi@nationalwellness.org
www.nationalwellness.org

Wellness Associates of Chicago
(publishes *The Wellness Inventory*)
4250 Marine Dr., Suite 200
Chicago, IL 60613
(773) 935-6377
Fax: (773) 929-4446
E-mail: wellness-info@wellnessof
chicago.com
www.wellness-associates.com

Women's Health

National Women's Health Network (NWHN)
514 10th St., N.W., Suite 400
Washington, DC 20004
(202) 347-1140
Health Info: (202) 628-7814
Fax: (202) 347-1168
E-mail: nwhn@nwhn.org
www.womenshealthnetwork.org

National Women's Health Information Center

U.S. Public Health Service on Women's Health
8270 Willow Oaks Corporate Drive
Fairfax, VA 22031
(800) 994-WOMAN (994-9662)
www.4women.gov

GenneX Healthcare Technologies, Inc.

Estronaut: A Forum for Women's Health
GenneX Healthcare Technologies, Inc.
207 E. Ohio, 186
Chicago, IL 60611
(312) 335-0095
E-mail: ask@gennexhealth.com
www.estronaut.com

Planned Parenthood
434 West 33rd St.
New York, NY 10001
(212) 541-7800
Fax: (212) 245-1845
www.plannedparenthood.org
See also white or yellow pages of telephone directory for listing of local chapter

By definition, an emergency is a situation in which you have to think and act fast. Start by assessing the circumstances. Shout for help if you're in a public place. Look for any possible dangers to you or the victim, such as a live electrical wire or a fire. Seek medical assistance as quickly as possible. Dial 911 or a local emergency phone number. Don't attempt rescue techniques, such as cardiopulmonary resuscitation (CPR), unless you are trained. If you have a car, be sure you know the shortest route from your home to the nearest 24-hour hospital emergency department.

Supplies

Every home should have a kit of basic first aid supplies kept in a convenient location out of the reach of children. Stock it with the following:

- Bandages and sterile gauze pads
- Adhesive tape
- Scissors
- Cotton balls or absorbent cotton
- Cotton swabs
- Thermometer
- Antibiotic ointment
- Sharp needle
- Safety pins
- Calamine lotion

Keep a similar kit in your car or boat. You might want to add some extra items from your home, such as a flashlight, soap, blanket, paper cups, and any special equipment that a family member with a chronic illness may need.

Bleeding

Blood loss is frightening and dangerous. Direct pressure stops external bleeding. Since internal bleeding can also be life-threatening, you must be aware of the warning signs.

For an Open Wound

1. Apply direct pressure over the site of the wound. Cover the entire wound.
2. Use sterile gauze, a sanitary napkin, a clean towel, sheet, or handkerchief or, if necessary, your washed bare hand. Ice or cold water in a pad will help stop bleeding and decrease swelling.
3. Apply firm, steady pressure for five to fifteen minutes. Most wounds stop bleeding within a few minutes.
4. If the wound is on a foot, hand, leg, or arm, use gravity to help slow the flow of blood. Elevate the limb so that it is higher than the victim's heart.
5. If the bleeding doesn't stop, press harder.
6. Seek medical attention if the bleeding was caused by a serious injury, if stitches will be needed to keep the wound closed, or if the victim has not had a tetanus booster within the last ten years.

For Internal Bleeding

1. Suspect internal bleeding if a person coughs up blood, vomits red or brown material that looks like coffee grounds, passes blood in urine or stool, or has black, tarlike bowel movements.
2. Do not let the victim take any medication or fluids by mouth until seen by a doctor, because surgery may be necessary.
3. Have the victim lie flat. Cover him or her lightly.
4. Seek immediate medical attention.

For a Bloody Nose

1. Have the victim sit down, leaning slightly forward so the blood does not run down his or her throat. The person should spit out any blood in his or her mouth.
2. Use the thumb and forefingers to pinch the nose. If the victim can do the pinching, apply a cold compress to the nose and surrounding area.
3. Apply pressure for ten minutes without interruption.
4. If pinching does not work, gently pack the nostril with gauze or a clean strip of cloth. Do not use absorbent cotton, which will stick. Let the ends hang out so you can remove the packing easily later. Pinch the nose, with the packing in place, for five minutes.
5. If a foreign object is in the nose, do not attempt to remove it. Ask the person to blow gently. If that does not work, seek medical attention.
6. The nose should not be blown or irritated for several hours after a nosebleed stops.

Breathing Problems

If a person appears to be unconscious, approach carefully. The victim may be in contact with electrical current. If so, make sure the electricity is shut off before touching the victim. The first function you should check is respiration. Tap or shake the victim's shoulder gently, shouting, "Are you all right?" Look for any signs of breathing: Can you hear breath sounds? Can you feel breath on your cheek? If the person is breathing, do not perform mouth-to-mouth resuscitation.

If you aren't certain if the victim is breathing, or if there are no signs of breath, follow these steps:

1. Lay the person on his or her back on the floor or ground. Roll the victim over if necessary, being careful to turn the head with the remainder of the body as a unit to avoid possible neck injury. Loosen any tight clothing around the neck or chest.
2. Check for any foreign material in the mouth or throat and remove it quickly.
3. Open the airway by tilting the head back and lifting the chin up.
4. Pinch the nostrils shut with your thumb and index finger.
5. Take a deep breath, open your mouth wide and place it securely over the victim's, and give two slow breaths, each lasting 1 to 10 seconds. Remove your mouth, turn your head, and check to see if the victim's chest rises and falls. If you hear air escaping from the victim's mouth and see the chest fall, you know that you are getting air into the lungs.

6. Repeat once every five seconds (twelve breaths per minute) until professional help takes over, or the victim begins breathing on his or her own. It may take several hours to revive someone. If you stop, the victim may not be able to breathe on his or her own. Once the person does begin to breathe independently, always get professional help.

7. If air doesn't seem to be entering the chest, or the chest doesn't fall between breaths, tilt the head further back. If that doesn't work, follow the directions for choking emergencies later in this section.

8. If the victim is a child, do not pinch the nose shut. Cover both the mouth and nose with your mouth, and place your free hand very lightly on the child's chest. Use small puffs of air rather than big breaths. Feel the chest inflate as you blow, and listen for exhaled air. Repeat once every three seconds (twenty breaths per minute).

Broken Bones

If you suspect that a person has broken a leg, do not move him or her unless there is immediate danger.

1. Check for signs of breathing. If there is none or breathing is very weak, administer mouth-to-mouth resuscitation.

2. If the person is bleeding, apply direct pressure on the site of the wound.

3. Try to keep the victim warm and calm.

4. Do not try to push a broken bone back into place if it is sticking out of the skin. You can apply a moist dressing to prevent it from drying out.

5. Do not try to straighten out a fracture.

6. Do not allow the victim to walk.

7. Splint unstable fractures to prevent painful motion.

Burns

1. If fire caused the burn, cool the affected area with water to stop the burning process.

2. Remove the victim's garments and jewelry and cover him or her with clean sheets or towels.

3. Call for help immediately.

4. If chemicals caused the burn, wash the affected area with cool water for at least 20 minutes. Chemical burns of the eye require immediate medical attention after flushing with water for 20 minutes.

Choking

A person with anything stuck in the throat and blocking the airway can stop breathing, lose consciousness, and die within four to six minutes. A universal signal of distress because of choking is clasping the throat with one or both hands. Other signs are an inability to talk and noisy, difficult breathing. You need to take immediate action, but NEVER slap the victim's back. This could make the obstruction worse.

If the victim can speak, cough, or breathe, do not interfere. Coughing alone may dislodge the foreign object. If the choking continues without lessening, call for medical help.

If the victim cannot speak, cough, or breathe but is conscious, use the Heimlich maneuver, as follows

1. Stand behind the victim (who may be seated or standing) and wrap your arms around his or her waist.

2. Make a fist with one hand and place the thumb side of your fist against the victim's abdomen, just above the navel. Grasp your fist with your other hand and press into his or her abdomen with a quick, upward thrust. Do not exert any pressure against the rib cage with your forearms.

3. Repeat this procedure until the victim is no longer choking or loses consciousness.

4. If the person is lying face down, roll the victim over. Facing the person, kneel with your legs astride his or her hips. Put the heel of one hand below the rib cage and place your other hand on top. Press into the abdomen with a quick, upward thrust. Repeat thrusts as needed.

5. If you start choking when you're by yourself, place your fist below your rib cage and above your navel. Grasp this fist with your other hand and press into your abdomen with a quick, upward thrust. You also can lean over a fixed, horizontal object, such as a table edge or chair back, and press your upper abdomen against it with a quick, upward thrust. Repeat as needed until you dislodge the object.

If the Victim Is Unconscious

1. Place him or her on the ground and give mouth-to-mouth resuscitation as described earlier.

2. If the victim does not start breathing and air does not seem to be going into his or her lungs, roll the victim onto his or her back and give one or more manual thrusts: Place one of your hands on top of the other with the heel of the bottom hand in the middle of the abdomen, slightly above the navel and below the rib cage. Press into the abdomen with a quick, upward thrust. Do not push to either side. Repeat six to ten times as needed.

3. Clear the airway. Hold the victim's mouth open with one hand and use your thumb to depress the tongue. Make a hook with the index finger of your other hand and, using a gentle, sweeping motion, reach into the victim's throat and feel for a swallowed foreign object in the airway.

4. Repeat the following steps in this sequence:

   - Six to ten abdominal thrusts
   - Probe in mouth
   - Try to inflate lungs
   - Repeat

5. If the victim suddenly seems okay, but no foreign material has been removed, take him or her directly to the hospital. A foreign object, such as a fish or chicken bone or other jagged object, could do internal damage as it passes through the victim's system.

If the Victim Is a Child

1. If the child is coughing, do nothing. The coughing alone may dislodge the object.

2. If the airway is blocked and the child is panicky and fighting for breath, do *NOT* probe the airway with your fingers to clear an unseen foreign object. You might push the material

back into the airway, worsening the obstruction.

3. For an infant younger than a year, hang the child over your arm so that the head is lower than the trunk. Using the heel of your hand, administer four firm blows high on the back between the shoulder blades. For a bigger child, follow the same procedure, but invert the child over your knee rather than your arm.

4. After four back blows, perform four chest thrusts (the Heimlich maneuver as described above).

Drowning

A person can die of drowning four to six minutes after breathing stops. Although prevention is the wisest course, follow these steps in case of a drowning emergency:

1. Get the victim out of the water fast. Be extremely cautious, because a drowning person may panic and grasp at a rescuer, endangering that individual as well. If possible, push a branch or pole within the victim's reach.

2. If the victim is unconscious, use a flotation device if at all possible. Carefully place the person on the device. Once out of the water, place the victim on his or her back.

3. If the victim is not breathing, start mouth-to-mouth resuscitation. Continue until the person can breathe unassisted or help arrives. (Note that it may take an hour or two for a drowning victim to resume independent breathing.) Do not leave the victim alone for any reason.

4. Once the person is breathing without assistance, even if he or she is still coughing, you need only stay nearby until professional help arrives.

Electrical Shock

1. If you suspect that an electrical shock has knocked a person unconscious, approach very carefully. Do not touch the victim unless the electricity has been turned off.

2. Shut off the power at the plug, circuit breaker, or fuse box. Simply shutting off an appliance does not remove the shock hazard. Use a dry stick to move

a wire or downed power line from the victim. Keep in mind that you also are in danger until the power is off.

3. If the person's breathing is weak or has stopped, follow the steps for mouth-to-mouth resuscitation.

4. Even if the victim returns to consciousness, call for medical help. While waiting, cover the victim with a blanket or coat to keep him or her warm. Place a blanket underneath the body if the surface is cold. Be sure the person lies flat if conscious, with legs raised. If the victim is unconscious, place him or her on one side, with a pillow supporting the head. Do not give the victim anything to eat or drink.

5. Electrical burns can extend deep into the tissue, even when they appear minor. Do not put butter, household remedies, or sprays on burns without a doctor's instruction. Do not use ice or cold water on an electrical burn that is more than 2 inches across.

Heart Attack

Chest pain can be caused by indigestion, strained muscles, or lung infections. The warning signs of a heart attack are:

- Intense pain that lasts for more than two minutes, produces a tight or crushing feeling, is centered in the chest, or spreads to the neck, jaw, shoulder, or arm
- Shortness of breath that is worse when the person lies flat and improves when the person sits
- Heavy sweating
- Nausea or vomiting
- Irregular pulse
- Pale or bluish skin or lips
- Weakness
- Severe anxiety, feeling of doom

If an individual develops these symptoms:

1. Call for emergency medical help immediately.

2. Have the person sit up or lie in a semi-reclining position. Loosen tight clothing. Keep him or her comfortably warm.

3. If the person loses consciousness, turn on his or her back and check for breathing and pulse. If vomiting

occurs, turn the victim's head to one side and clean the mouth.

4. If the person has medicine for angina pectoris (chest pain) and is conscious, help him or her take it.

5. If the person is unconscious, and you are trained to perform cardiopulmonary resuscitation (CPR), check for a pulse at the wrist or neck. If there is none, begin CPR in conjunction with mouth-to-mouth resuscitation. Do not attempt CPR unless you are trained. It is not a technique you can learn from a book.

Poisoning

Many common household substances, including glue, aspirin, bleaches, and paint, can be poisonous. If you think someone has been poisoned, call the National Poison Control Center: (800) 222-1222. Be prepared to provide the following information:

- The kind of substance swallowed and how much was swallowed
- If a child or adult swallowed the substance
- Symptoms
- Whether or not vomiting has occurred
- Whether you gave the person anything to drink
- How much time it will take to get to an emergency room

The Poison Control Center will tell you whether or not to induce vomiting or neutralize a swallowed poison. Here are some additional guidelines:

1. Always assume the worst if a small child has swallowed or might have swallowed something poisonous. Keep the suspected item or container with you to answer questions.

2. Do not give any medications unless a physician or the Poison Control Center instructs you to do so.

3. Do not follow the directions for neutralizing poisons on the container unless a doctor or the Poison Control Center confirms that they are appropriate measures to take.

4. If the child is conscious, give moderate doses of water to dilute the poison.

5. If a poisoning victim is unconscious, make sure he or she is breathing. If

not, give mouth-to-mouth resuscitation. Do not give anything by mouth or attempt to stimulate the person. Call for emergency help immediately.

6. If the person is vomiting, make sure he or she is in a position in which he or she cannot choke on what is brought up.

7. While vomiting is the fastest way to expel swallowed poisons from the body, never try to induce vomiting if the person has swallowed any acid or alkaline substance, which can cause burns of the face, mouth, and throat (examples include ammonia, bleach, dishwasher detergent, drain and toilet cleaners, lye, oven cleaners, or rust removers), or petroleum-like products, which produce dangerous fumes that can be inhaled during vomiting (examples include floor polish, furniture wax, gasoline, kerosene, lighter fluid, turpentine, and paint thinner)

A CONSUMER'S GUIDE TO MEDICAL TESTS

✓ **What They Tell the Doctor**
✓ **How Often You Need Them**
✓ **What to Do About Abnormal Results**

Do you wonder what the doctor sees when he looks into your eyes with that little light or what it means when your blood or urine test is normal? In this section we cover some of the most common tests your doctor does, what they tell, and how often they should be done.

General Information

- Always ask your doctor what tests are being done, why they are being ordered, what they involve, and what the results mean.
- No test is foolproof. If a result is unexpected, whether normal or abnormal, your doctor should repeat the test before making any decisions.
- Modern X-ray machines expose you to a minuscule amount of radiation. Nevertheless, be sure to tell the physician or X-ray technician if there is even a chance you may be pregnant.
- Often a doctor orders a test because that is the only way to prove you do not have a disease.

Allergy Skin Testing

- Skin testing is still the most reliable method.
- The physician either pricks your skin 20 to 40 or more times to introduce a tiny bit of potentially allergic material or injects a small amount.
- Children who are frightened by multiple needle sticks and are unlikely to sit still for as long as necessary may have blood (RAST) tests instead.

What the results mean. If you develop redness or a hivelike bump around an area, you are probably allergic to the injected substance. Sometimes you can avoid the offending material, but things like pollen and dust are everywhere. Your allergist may recommend desensitizing shots to reduce your reaction. The results of skin tests won't be reliable if you take antihistamines within 48 hours of the test.

How often to be tested. Skin tests are necessary only if you cannot get allergy relief from other measures such as over-the-counter medications, reducing mold and dust in the house, and staying away from animals.

Blood Pressure Reading

- High blood pressure, a major cause of stroke and heart attacks, usually causes no symptoms.
- The upper number in a reading—the systolic—refers to peak amount of pressure generated when your heart pumps blood, the lower number—the diastolic—measures the least amount of pressure.

What the results mean. Most doctors today think the lower the pressure the better, which means a reading of 120/80 or less. Because the mere anxiety of having your blood pressure taken can cause a mild elevation, your doctor will want to repeat an abnormal test, ideally on a different day, before diagnosing high blood pressure.

How often to be tested. Everyone—no matter how healthy—should have a blood-pressure reading taken at least once a year, more often if you have high blood pressure.

Blood Tests

- Blood may be taken from either a finger prick or, more commonly, a vein in your arm.
- See below for information on cholesterol testing, which is also done from a blood sample.

Complete Blood Count (CBC)

This is the most commonly performed of all blood tests.

What the results mean. A low red-cell count, called anemia, can be caused by something as simple as too little iron in your diet, as complex as an abnormality in your digestion, or as serious as a bone marrow problem or silent bleeding. Iron deficiency is the most frequent cause, with women who menstruate and limit their intake of red meat at the greatest risk. If your doctor diagnoses this problem, ask about making dietary changes as well as taking iron supplements.

A high white-cell count, a measure of the body's defenses against infection, usually indicates some kind of infection. Depending on the type of cell that predominates, your doctor may be able to identify whether you have a bacterial or viral infection.

Platelets, the first participants in blood clotting, may be decreased because of a viral infection, abnormal bleeding, or for no identifiable reason.

Chemistry Panels (Chem 12 or 18, SMA 12 or 24)

Kidney, bone, liver, pancreas, prostate, and some glandular functions are screened by these tests.

What the results mean. An abnormality may signal a problem that needs treatment. Because accuracy decreases when many tests are run together, any specific abnormal test should be repeated, especially if unexpected.

CAT (Computerized Axial Tomography) Scan

- A CAT scan is 100 times more sensitive than an X ray.
- You lie as motionless as possible in a large tube while an X-ray beam travels 360 degrees around you. The test takes about an hour.

What the results mean. The test can help diagnose such conditions as tumors, blood clots, cysts, and bleeding in the brain as well as in various other organs.

Cholesterol Test/ Lipoprotein Profile

- Anyone can have a high cholesterol level, but you are more apt to be at risk if there is a family history of early heart attacks, strokes, or high blood cholesterol.

- Your doctor will look at total blood cholesterol, high-density lipoprotein (HDL, the "good" cholesterol that prevents cholesterol from sticking to your blood vessels), low-density lipoprotein (LDL, the "bad" cholesterol that does the reverse), and triglycerides.

What the results mean. Experts today think optimum total cholesterol levels are below 200 mg/dL of blood. Persistently high cholesterol values will prompt your doctor to advise dietary and lifestyle changes—less fat intake, more exercise—and perhaps medication. Optimal LDL levels depend on your risk factors for heart disease, and optimal HDL levels are 60 mg/dL or higher.

How often to be tested. If your cholesterol level is under 200 and your LDL level is under 130, repeat the test every five years. If your test is borderline, repeat it annually. (Note that the test should be taken when you have not eaten for at least twelve hours.)

   If you have a family history of cholesterol problems, have your children tested annually from age 2; if you don't, have them tested around age 10 and every few years thereafter. Children under 2 should not be given a low-cholesterol diet; they need extra fat to make brain tissue and hormones for growth.

Fundoscopy

The doctor looks into your eye with a little light.

What the results mean. The beginnings of cataracts may be visible, as well as irregularities in the blood vessels that indicate damage from high cholesterol (fatty deposits in the blood vessels), high blood pressure (narrowing and notching), diabetes, or other diseases. If the optic nerve is swollen, there may be excess pressure inside your skull.

   What your doctor *cannot* see are the early signs of glaucoma, which can lead to blindness if not treated. Over age 20, have a pressure check for glaucoma from an ophthalmologist or optometrist every three years—or every year if you have a family history of glaucoma.

Heart Tests

- The following tests are listed from the simplest through the most complicated.
- Also see listings for blood pressure readings, cholesterol tests, and pulse.

Electrocardiogram (ECG, EKG)

A machine amplifies the electrical signals from your heart and records them on paper.

What the results mean. An EKG can detect such things as an enlarged heart, abnormal levels of potassium or calcium, disease of the small vessels of the heart, or the source of an abnormal heart rhythm. It is a nonspecific test, however, and more advanced studies should be done if serious disease is suspected.

Echocardiogram

In this painless test sound waves are used to produce a picture of the heart in action on a TV-type screen.

What the results mean. The test investigates the size of the heart chambers, the thickness of the walls, how the four heart valves are working, and the condition of the membrane surrounding the heart. Mitral valve prolapse, a common minor abnormality, often shows up on this test, as well as more serious problems.

Stress Test

Your heart rate, blood pressure, and EKG are constantly monitored as you exercise on a treadmill that goes faster and faster with a steeper and steeper incline. This test—also called an exercise tolerance test or treadmill test—should be performed in the presence of a cardiologist and in or near a hospital in case the strain causes heart problems that need emergency treatment. The test should be stopped immediately if you experience any light-headedness, chest pain, nausea, or palpitations.

What the results mean. The increasing strain on the heart causes changes that can tell your doctor if you are at risk of a heart attack. This is because a blockage in the coronary arteries—the blood vessels that feed your heart muscle—may show up only during exercise.

Angiography

A dye is injected into various arteries, and X rays are taken.

What the results mean. The doctor can detect blockages in the blood vessels that can lead to heart attack or stroke, as well as aneurysms (weakened spots in the blood-vessel walls). The test carries some risk of causing stroke.

Kidney Tests

The two tests listed here involve taking X rays. Ultrasound (similar to an echocardiogram) can also be used to outline the kidneys.

Intravenous Pyelogram (IVP)

After an iodine-containing substance is injected into a vein, X rays are taken at five-minute intervals to show the outlines of the kidney, ureter, and bladder.

What the results mean. Tumors, kidney stones, and swelling of the kidney tissue can be seen, as well as blockage to urine flow or a mass that may be pressing on the kidney. A kidney that is not functioning will not appear on the X ray, and one in an abnormal position can be found.

Voiding Cystourethrogram (VCUG)

A technician will fill your bladder with a dye injected through a catheter and take X rays while you urinate.

What the results mean. If you have recurrent urinary-tract infections, the test will show if there is a significant backup of urine from the bladder into the ureter, in which case daily antibiotics may be needed to prevent infection. Investigating recurrent urinary tract infections is particularly important for children.

Magnetic Resonance Imaging (MRI)

MRI uses no radiation but produces pictures of the brain that are much more detailed than those of a CAT scan.

What the results mean. In addition to locating bleeding or tumors, as a CAT scan does, the test picks up subtle signs such as those of Parkinson's disease and multiple sclerosis in the brain or a herniated disc in the spinal column.

Mammography

- Only a small amount of radiation is used to take the mammogram. You usually stand up and put your breast on a photographic plate where it is compressed with a plastic shield or balloon-like device. It shouldn't hurt. If your breasts are tender at certain times in your menstrual cycle, schedule your mammogram when they are least sensitive.
- Mammograms can detect breast abnormalities at easily treated stages before you can feel them, but they are not foolproof. Examine your breasts monthly.

What the results mean. Mammograms can detect cysts, abscesses, and tumors. Whether a mass is benign or malignant is hard to tell in the early stages, so abnormalities usually need to be biopsied or removed totally to determine treatment.

How often to be tested. Although there is controversy over the benefits of mammography for women under 50, many experts still recommend having a first mammogram between ages 35 and 40, followed by one every two years between 40 and 50, and yearly thereafter. If your mother or sister has had breast cancer, consult your doctor for an appropriate schedule. And if you have a lump, pain, or nipple discharge, have a mammogram right away, no matter what your age.

You also should have a breast examination by a doctor at least every three years between ages 20 and 40, and every year after 40.

Pap Smear

- A routine part of every gynecological examination.
- Your doctor takes a painless swab from the cervix and vaginal walls and sends it to a lab for analysis.

What the results mean. Pap smears can detect not only cervical cancer but also inflammation and many infections, minor and more serious; they also provide important information about the state of your female hormones. A normal test is termed class I, and abnormal results are graded by degree into four classifications, with only the most severe—a class V test—signifying outright cancer. Treatment depends on the diagnosis and may range from doing nothing for a minor inflammation to, in rare cases, a hysterectomy for cancer. Because the error rate of Pap smears is high, the doctor should always repeat an abnormal test.

How often to be tested. Women who are on birth control pills and are sexually active should have a Pap smear every six months; other women should be checked every year.

Physical Examination

The routine physical exam generally includes a pulse and blood-pressure reading, measure of height and weight, blood tests (including a lipoprotein profile), fundoscopy, and sometimes other tests as well, such as a fecal occult blood test.

What the results mean. A physical exam serves as a general measure of health and sometimes picks up early signs of disease.

How often to have a physical exam. Most doctors no longer recommend yearly physicals for everybody. A good schedule to follow instead is to have a complete checkup every four or five years under age 40, every three years between 40 and 50, every two years between 50 and 60, and every year after that. At any age, you should have more frequent examinations if you have chronic medical problems such as diabetes or high blood pressure, are obese, or smoke cigarettes.

Pulse

To take your own pulse, press two fingertips over the artery in your wrist, just below the base of the thumb. Count the beats in 20 seconds, then multiply by 3.

What the results mean. The normal pulse rate—the speed at which your heart pumps blood—is 60–80 beats a minute; it should be regular, without skipped or extra beats. Abnormal rates can be due to thyroid problems (too high causes a fast rate, too low a slow one), heart problems, anxiety (even the stress of a physical exam), or weakness from an illness such as the flu or other problems.

The character of your pulse is also important. A discrepancy between the strength of the pulse on one side of the neck and the other may mean you are in danger of a stroke. A pulse that is abnormally strong and bounding can signal a problem with a heart valve. If the pulse is weak, you may have blockages in your blood vessels from diabetes, atherosclerosis (hardening of the arteries), or a variety of other disorders.

Stomach and Intestinal Tests

Though most of these tests are uncomfortable, they generally are not painful.

Barium Enema

Barium, a radioactive material, is instilled in your large intestine through a tube inserted into your anus. Because barium is constipating, drink fluids afterward. Don't be alarmed if you have white stools for a day or two.

What the results mean. The doctor will be able to see tumors or polyps, any obstructions, and other abnormalities.

Colonoscopy and Sigmoidoscopy

In colonoscopy, for which you will be sedated, the doctor looks into the colon with a flexible tube inserted into your anus. The procedure is essentially the same for sigmoidoscopy, except that the doctor looks only into the lower third of the intestine.

What the results mean. Your doctor can see where bleeding comes from, remove a polyp, or biopsy a mass.

Upper GI Series

You will be asked to down a drink of barium so that X rays can be taken of the esophagus, stomach, duodenum, and sometimes the small intestine.

What the results mean. Your doctor can diagnose swallowing disorders, hiatus hernias, ulcers, tumors, and some inflammations of the stomach and small bowel.

Fecal Occult Blood Test (FOBT)

A small sample of stool that remains on the doctor's glove after a rectal exam or that is collected by you at home is tested for blood that is invisible to the eye.

What the results mean. This test is done routinely as part of a regular checkup to detect the earliest sign of cancer of the colon. It is also part of an investigation of anemia or abdominal pain. If your test is positive, tell your doctor if you recently ate radishes, turnips, or red meat, took large doses of vitamin C or iron pills, or had a nosebleed. All of these things can produce misleading results.

Urinalysis

Urine can tell about the health not only of the kidneys but also of other organ systems.

What the results mean. Specific gravity is the degree to which your urine is concentrated or diluted. If it is persistently too dilute, your doctor may ask for a first morning sample to see how well your kidneys concentrate your urine overnight. Urine that is too concentrated may indicate poor fluid intake, decreased kidney function, or dehydration from vomiting and diarrhea.

Acidity or alkalinity (pH) is useful information when there is a history or possibility of kidney stones, urinary tract infection, or kidney disease.

Glucose or sugar in the urine may mean you have diabetes. You will need a blood test to confirm the diagnosis, as some families filter sugar easily through their kidneys but do not have any disease. Inflammation of the pancreas and thyroid problems also may cause sugar in the urine.

Blood in the urine may mean infection, a stone, or an inflammation of the kidney. Excessive exertion such as running sometimes causes some blood to leak into the urine; this usually disappears after resting.

Protein molecules are large and under normal conditions should not filter into the urine. However, they may appear in small amounts in the urine after strenuous exercise or an illness, especially one with a fever. In large amounts, protein in the urine warrants a search for an underlying kidney problem.

Nitrites, substances produced when bacteria multiply, may be the earliest or only sign of an infection.

White blood cells may be present because of a urinary tract or vaginal infection.

X Ray

The simple X ray is a nonspecific test that is being replaced more and more by CAT scans, magnetic resonance imaging, and other tests.

What the results mean. An X ray can detect such things as an enlarged heart, a broken bone, a sinus infection, or pneumonia.

Glossary

A

abscess A localized accumulation of pus and disintegrating tissue.

absorption The passage of substances into or across membranes or tissues.

abstinence Voluntary refrainment from sexual intercourse.

acquired immune deficiency syndrome (AIDS) The final stages of HIV infection, characterized by a variety of severe illnesses and decreased levels of certain immune cells.

active stretching A technique that involves stretching a muscle by contracting the opposing muscle.

acupuncture A Chinese medical practice of puncturing the body with needles inserted at specific points to relieve pain or cure disease.

acute injuries Physical injuries, such as sprains, bruises, and pulled muscles, which result from sudden traumas, such as falls or collisions.

adaptive response The body's attempt to reestablish homeostasis or stability.

addiction A behavioral pattern characterized by compulsion, loss of control, and continued repetition of a behavior or activity in spite of adverse consequences.

additive Characterized by a combined effect that is equal to the sum of the individual effects.

adoption The legal process for becoming the parent to a child of other biological parents.

advance directives Documents that specify individual's preferences regarding treatment in a medical crisis.

aerobic exercise Physical activity in which sufficient or excess oxygen is continually supplied to the body.

affirmation A single positive sentence used as a tool for behavior change.

aging The characteristic pattern of normal life changes that occur as humans grow older.

alcohol abuse Continued use of alcohol despite awareness of social, occupational, psychological, or physical problems related to its use, or use of alcohol in dangerous ways or situations, such as before driving.

alcohol dependence Development of a strong craving for alcohol due to the pleasurable feelings or relief of stress or anxiety produced by drinking.

alcoholism A chronic, progressive, potentially fatal disease characterized by impaired control of drinking, a preoccupation with alcohol, continued use of alcohol despite adverse consequences, and distorted thinking, most notably denial.

allergy A hypersensitivity to a particular substance in one's environment or diet.

altruism Acts of helping or giving to others without thought of self-benefit.

Alzheimer's disease A progressive deterioration of intellectual powers due to physiological changes within the brain; symptoms include diminishing ability to concentrate and reason, disorientation, depression, apathy, and paranoia.

amenorrhea The absence or suppression of menstruation.

amino acids Organic compounds containing nitrogen, carbon, hydrogen, and oxygen; the essential building blocks of proteins.

amnion The innermost membrane of the sac enclosing the embryo or fetus.

amphetamine Any of a class of stimulants that trigger the release of epinephrine, which stimulates the central nervous system; users experience a state of hyper-alertness and energy, followed by a crash as the drug wears off.

anabolic steroids Drugs derived from testosterone and approved for medical use, but often used by athletes to increase their musculature and weight.

anaerobic exercise Physical activity in which the body develops an oxygen deficit.

androgyny The expression of both masculine and feminine traits.

angina pectoris A severe, suffocating chest pain caused by a brief lack of oxygen to the heart.

angioplasty Surgical repair of an obstructed artery by passing a balloon catheter through the blood vessel to the area of disease and then inflating the catheter to compress the plaque against the vessel wall.

anorexia nervosa A psychological disorder in which refusal to eat and/or an extreme loss of appetite leads to malnutrition, severe weight loss, and possibly death.

antagonistic Opposing or counteracting.

antibiotics Substances produced by micro-organisms, or synthetic agents, that are toxic to other types of micro-organisms; in dilute solutions, used to treat infectious diseases.

antidepressant A drug used primarily to treat symptoms of depression.

antioxidants Substances that prevent the damaging effects of oxidation in cells.

antiviral drug A substance that decreases the severity and duration of a viral infection if taken prior to or soon after onset of the infection.

anxiety A feeling of apprehension and dread, with or without a known cause; may range from mild to severe and may be accompanied by physical symptoms.

anxiety disorders A group of psychological disorders involving episodes of apprehension, tension, or uneasiness, stemming from the anticipation of danger and sometimes accompanied by physical symptoms, which cause significant distress and impairment to an individual.

aorta The main artery of the body, arising from the left ventricle of the heart.

appetite A desire for food, stimulated by anticipated hunger, physiological changes within the brain and body, the availability of food, and other environmental and psychological factors.

arteriosclerosis Any of a number of chronic diseases characterized by degeneration of the arteries and hardening and thickening of arterial walls.

artificial insemination The introduction of viable sperm into the vagina by artificial means for the purpose of inducing conception.

assertive Behaving in a confident manner to make your needs and desires clear to others in a nonhostile way.

asthma A disease or allergic response characterized by bronchial spasms and difficult breathing.

atherosclerosis A form of arteriosclerosis in which fatty substances (plaque) are deposited on the inner walls of arteries.

atrium) (plural **atria**) Either of the two upper chambers of the heart, which receive blood from the veins.

attention deficit/hyperactivity disorder (ADHD) A spectrum of difficulties in controlling motion and sustaining attention, including hyperactivity, impulsivity, and distractibility.

autoimmune disorder Resulting from the attack on body tissue by an immune system that fails to recognize the tissue as self.

autonomy The ability to draw on internal resources; independence from familial and societal influences.

autoscopy The sensation of one's self being outside its body, often experienced by individuals in near-death medical crises.

aversion therapy A treatment that attempts to help a person overcome a dependence or bad habit by making the person feel disgusted or repulsed by that habit.

axon The long fiber that conducts impulses from the neuron's nucleus to its dendrites.

axon terminal The ending of an axon, from which impulses are transmitted to a dendrite of another neuron.

ayurveda A traditional Indian medical treatment involving meditation, exercise, herbal medications, and nutrition.

B

bacteria (singular, **bacterium**) One-celled microscopic organisms; the most plentiful pathogens.

bacterial vaginosis A vaginal infection caused by overgrowth and depletion of various microorganisms living in the vagina, resulting in a malodorous white or gray vaginal discharge.

ballistic stretching Rapid bouncing movements.

barbiturates Antianxiety drugs that depress the central nervous system, reduce activity and induce relaxation, drowsiness, or sleep; often prescribed to relieve tension and treat epileptic seizures or as a general anesthetic.

barrier contraceptives Birth-control devices that block the meeting of egg and sperm, either by physical barriers, such as condoms, diaphragms, or cervical caps, or by chemical barriers, such as spermicide, or both.

basal metabolic rate (BMR) The number of calories required to sustain the body at rest.

behavioral activation A technique in which depressed people discover and do the things that give them a sense of accomplishment.

behavioral therapy Psychotherapy that emphasizes application of the principles of learning to substitute desirable responses and behavior patterns for undesirable ones.

benzodiazepines Antianxiety drugs that depress the central nervous system, reduce activity and induce relaxation, drowsiness, or sleep; often prescribed to relieve tension, muscular strain, sleep problems, anxiety, and panic attacks; also used as an anesthetic and in the treatment of alcohol withdrawal.

bidis Skinny, sweet-flavored cigarettes.

binge drinking For a man, having five or more alcoholic drinks at a single sitting; for a woman, having four drinks or more at a single sitting.

binge eating The rapid consumption of an abnormally large amount of food in a relatively short time.

biofeedback A technique of becoming aware, with the aid of external monitoring devices, of internal physiological activities in order to develop the capability of altering them.

bipolar disorder Severe depression alternating with periods of manic activity and elation.

bisexual Sexually oriented toward both sexes.

blended family A family formed when one or both of the partners bring children from a previous union to the new marriage.

blood-alcohol concentration (BAC) The amount of alcohol in the blood, expressed as a percentage.

body composition The relative amounts of fat and lean tissue (bone, muscle, organs, water) in the body.

body mass index (BMI) A mathematical formula that correlates with body fat; the ratio of weight to height squared.

botulism Possibly fatal food poisoning, caused by a type of bacterium that grows and produces its toxin in the absence of air and is found in improperly canned food.

bulimia nervosa Episodic binge eating, often followed by forced vomiting or laxative abuse, and accompanied by a persistent preoccupation with body shape and weight.

burnout A state of physical, emotional, and mental exhaustion resulting from constant or repeated emotional pressure.

C

caesarean delivery The surgical procedure in which an infant is delivered through an incision made in the abdominal wall and uterus.

calorie The amount of energy required to raise the temperature of 1 gram of water by 1 degree Celsius. In everyday usage related to the energy content of foods and the energy expended in activities, a calorie is actually the equivalent of a thousand such calories, or a kilocalorie.

candidiasis An infection of the yeast *Candida albicans,* commonly occurring in the vagina, vulva, penis, and mouth and causing burning, itching, and a whitish discharge.

capillary A minute blood vessel that connects an artery to a vein.

carbohydrates Organic compounds, such as starches, sugars, and glycogen, that are composed of carbon, hydrogen, and oxygen, and are sources of bodily energy.

carbon monoxide A colorless, odorless gas produced by the burning of gasoline or tobacco; displaces oxygen in the hemoglobin molecules of red blood cells.

carcinogen A substance or agent that produces cancerous cells or enhances their development and growth.

cardiac muscle Heart muscle.

cardiometabolic Referring to the heart and to the biochemical processes involved in the body's functioning.

cardiopulmonary resuscitation (CPR) A method of artificial stimulation of the heart and lungs; a combination of mouth-to-mouth breathing and chest compression.

cardiorespiratory fitness The ability of the heart and blood vessels to circulate blood through the body efficiently.

celibacy Abstention from sexual activity; can be partial or complete, permanent or temporary.

certified social worker A person who has completed a two-year graduate program in counseling people with mental problems.

cervical cap A thimble-sized rubber or plastic cap that is inserted into the vagina to fit over the cervix and prevent the passage of sperm into the uterus during sexual intercourse; used with a spermicidal foam or jelly, it serves as both a chemical and a physical barrier to sperm.

cervix The narrow, lower end of the uterus that opens into the vagina.

chanchroid A soft, painful sore or localized infection usually acquired through sexual contact.

chiropractic A method of treating disease, primarily through manipulating the bones and joints to restore normal nerve function.

chlamydia A sexually transmitted infection caused by the bacterium *Chlamydia trachomatis,* often asymptomatic in women, but sometimes characterized by urinary pain; if undetected and untreated, may result in pelvic inflammatory disease (PID).

chlorinated hydrocarbons Highly toxic pesticides, such as DDT and chlordane, that are extremely resistant to breakdown; may cause cancer, birth defects, neurological disorders, and damage to wildlife and the environment.

cholesterol An organic substance found in animal fats; linked to cardiovascular disease, particularly atherosclerosis.

chronic fatigue syndrome (CFS) A cluster of symptoms whose cause is not yet known; a primary symptom is debilitating fatigue.

circumcision The surgical removal of the foreskin of the penis.

clitoris A small erectile structure on the female, corresponding to the penis on the male.

club drugs Illegally manufactured psychoactive drugs that have dangerous physical and psychological effects.

cocaine A white crystalline powder extracted from the leaves of the coca plant which stimulates the central nervous system and produces a brief period of euphoria followed by a depression.

codependency An emotional and psychological behavioral pattern in which the spouses, partners, parents, children, and friends of individuals with addictive behaviors allow or enable their loved ones to continue their self-destructive habits.

cognitive therapy A technique used to identify an individual's beliefs and attitudes, recognize negative thought patterns, and educate in alternative ways of thinking.

cohabitation Two people living together as a couple, without official ties such as marriage.

coitus interruptus The removal of the penis from the vagina before ejaculation.

coma A state of total unconsciousness.

companion-oriented marriage A marital relationship in which the partners share interests, activities, and domestic responsibilities.

complementary and alternative medicine (CAM) A term used to apply to all health-care approaches, practices, and treatments not widely taught in medical schools, not generally used in hospitals, and not usually reimbursed by medical insurance companies.

complementary proteins Incomplete proteins that, when combined, provide all the amino acids essential for protein synthesis.

complete proteins Proteins that contain all the amino acids needed by the body for growth and maintenance.

complex carbohydrates Starches, including cereals, fruits, and vegetables.

computer vision syndrome A condition caused by computer use marked by tired and sore eyes, blurred vision, headaches, and neck, shoulder, and back pain.

conception The merging of a sperm and an ovum.

condom A latex sheath worn over the penis during sexual acts to prevent conception and/or the transmission of disease; the female condom lines the walls of the vagina.

contraception The prevention of conception; birth control.

corpus luteum A yellowish mass of tissue that is formed, immediately after ovulation, from the remaining cells of the follicle; it secretes estrogen and progesterone for the remainder of the menstrual cycle.

Cowper's glands Two small glands that discharge into the male urethra; also called bulbourethral glands.

culture The set of shared attitudes, values, goals, and practices of a group that are internalized by an individual within the group.

cunnilingus Sexual stimulation of a woman's genitals by means of oral manipulation.

cystitis Inflammation of the urinary bladder.

D

daily values (DV) Reference values developed by the FDA specifically for use on food labels.

decibel (dB) A unit for measuring the intensity of sounds.

decisional balance Weighting the positive and the negative consequences of change to yourself and to others.

defense mechanism A psychological process that alleviates anxiety and eliminates mental conflict; includes denial, displacement, projection, rationalization, reaction formation, and repression.

delirium tremens (DTs) The delusions, hallucinations, and agitated behavior following withdrawal from long-term chronic alcohol abuse.

dementia Deterioration of mental capability.

dendrites Branching fibers of a neuron that receive impulses from axon terminals of other neurons and conduct these impulses toward the nucleus.

depression In general, feelings of unhappiness and despair; as a mental illness, also characterized by an inability to function normally.

dermatitis Any inflammation of the skin.

detoxification The supervised removal of a poisonous or harmful substance (such as a drug) from the body; a therapy for alcoholics in which they are denied alcohol in a controlled environment.

diabetes mellitus A disease in which the inadequate production of insulin leads to failure of the body tissues to break down carbohydrates at a normal rate.

diagnostic-related group (DRG) A category of conditions requiring hospitalization for which the cost of care has been determined prior to a client's hospitalization.

diaphragm A bowl-like rubber cup with a flexible rim that is inserted into the vagina to cover the cervix and prevent the passage of sperm into the uterus during sexual intercourse; used with a spermicidal foam or jelly, it serves as both a chemical and a physical barrier to sperm.

diastole The period between contractions in the cardiac cycle, during which the heart relaxes and dilates as it fills with blood.

diastolic blood pressure Lowest blood pressure between contractions of the heart.

dietary fiber The nondigestible form of carbohydrates found in plant foods, such as leaves, stems, skins, seeds, and hulls.

dilation and evacuation (D and E) A medical procedure in which the contents of the uterus are removed through the use of instruments.

distress A negative stress that may result in illness.

do-not-resuscitate (DNR) An advance directive expressing an individual's preference that resuscitation efforts not be made during a medical crisis.

drug Any substance, other than food, that affects bodily functions and structures when taken into the body.

drug abuse The excessive use of a drug in a manner inconsistent with accepted medical practice.

drug misuse The use of a drug for a purpose (or person) other than that for which it was medically intended.

dynamic flexibility The ability to move a joint quickly and fluidly through its entire range of motion with little resistance.

dysfunctional Characterized by negative and destructive patterns of behavior between partners or between parents and children.

dysmenorrhea Painful menstruation.

dyspareunia A sexual difficulty in which a woman experiences pain during sexual intercourse.

dysthymia Frequent, prolonged mild depression.

E

eating disorders Bizarre, often dangerous patterns of food consumption, including anorexia nervosa and bulimia nervosa.

ecosystem A community of organisms sharing a physical and chemical environment and interacting with each other.

ecstasy (MDMA) A synthetic compound, also known as methylenedioxymethamphetamine, that is similar in structure to methamphetamine and has both stimulant and hallucinogenic effects.

ectopic pregnancy A pregnancy in which the fertilized egg has implanted itself outside the uterine cavity, usually in the fallopian tube.

ejaculation The expulsion of semen from the penis.

ejaculatory duct The canal connecting the seminal vesicles and vas deferens.

electromagnetic fields (EMFs) The invisible electric and magnetic fields generated by an electrically charged conductor.

embryo An organism in its early stage of development; in humans, the embryonic period lasts from the second to the eighth week of pregnancy.

emergency contraception Types of oral contraceptive pills usually taken within 72 hours after intercourse that can prevent pregnancy.

emotional health The ability to express and acknowledge one's feelings and moods.

emotional intelligence A term used by some psychologists to evaluate the capacity of people to understand themselves and relate well with others.

enabling To unwittingly contribute to a person's addictive or abusive behavior. Components of enabling include shielding or covering up for an abuser/addict; controlling them; taking over responsibilities; rationalizing addictive behavior; or cooperating with them.

enabling factors The skills, resources, physical and mental capabilities that shape our behavior.

endocrine disruptors Synthetic chemicals that interfere with the ways that hormones work in humans and wildlife.

endocrine system The group of ductless glands that produce hormones and secrete them directly into the blood for transport to target organs.

endometrium The mucous membrane lining the uterus.

endorphins Mood-elevating, pain-killing chemicals produced by the brain.

environmental tobacco smoke Secondhand cigarette smoke; the third leading preventable cause of death.

epididymis That portion of the male duct system in which sperm mature.

epilepsy A variety of neurological disorders characterized by sudden attacks (seizures) of violent muscle contractions and unconsciousness.

erectile dysfunction (ED) The consistent inability to maintain a penile erection sufficient for adequate sexual relations.

erogenous   Sexually sensitive.

essential nutrients   Nutrients that the body cannot manufacture for itself and must obtain from food.

estrogen   The female sex hormone that stimulates female secondary sex characteristics.

ethyl alcohol   The intoxicating agent in alcoholic beverages; also called ethanol.

eustress   Positive stress, which stimulates a person to function properly.

F

failure rate   The number of pregnancies that occur per year for every 100 women using a particular method of birth control.

fallopian tubes   The pair of channels that transport ova from the ovaries to the uterus; the usual site of fertilization.

family   A group of people united by marriage, blood, or adoption, residing in the same household, maintaining a common culture, and interacting with one another on the basis of their roles within the group.

fellatio   Sexual stimulation of a man's genitals by means of oral manipulation.

fertilization   The fusion of the sperm and egg nuclei.

fetal alcohol effects (FAE)   Milder forms of FAS, including low birthweight, irritability as newborns, and permanent mental impairment as a result of the mother's alcohol consumption during pregnancy.

fetal alcohol syndrome (FAS)   A cluster of physical and mental defects in the newborn, including low birthweight, smaller-than-normal head circumference, intrauterine growth retardation, and permanent mental impairment caused by the mother's alcohol consumption during pregnancy.

fetus   The human organism developing in the uterus from the ninth week until birth.

fiber   Indigestible materials in food that lower blood cholesterol or facilitate digestion and elimination.

FITT   A formula that describes the frequency, intensity, type, and length of time for physical activity.

flexibility   The range of motion allowed by one's joints; determined by the length of muscles, tendons, and ligaments attached to the joints.

folate   Various chemical forms of a water-soluble B vitamin that can be obtained from a diet high in vegetables and citrus fruit.

folic acid   A form of folate used in vitamin supplements and fortified foods.

functional fiber   Isolated, nondigestible carbohydrates with beneficial effects in humans.

functional fitness   The ability to perform real-life activities, such as lifting a heavy suitcase.

fungi (singular, **fungus**)   Organisms that reproduce by means of spores.

G

gamma globulin   The antibody-containing portion of the blood fluid (plasma).

GBL gamma butyrolactone   The main ingredient in gamma hydroxybutyrate (GHB), also known as the "date rape drug"; once ingested, GBL converts to GHB and can cause the ingestor to lose consciousness.

gender   Maleness or femaleness, as determined by a combination of anatomical and physiological factors, psychological factors, and learned behaviors.

general adaptation syndrome (GAS)   The sequenced physiological response to a stressful situation; consists of three stages: alarm, resistance, and exhaustion.

generalized anxiety disorder (GAD)   An anxiety disorder characterized as chronic distress.

generic   Refers to products without trade names that are equivalent to other products protected by trademark registration.

GHB gamma hydroxybutyrate   A brain messenger chemical that stimulates the release of human growth hormone; commonly abused for its high and its alleged ability to trim fat and build muscles. Also known as "blue nitro" or the "date rape drug."

gingivitis   Inflammation of the gums.

glia   Support cells for neurons in the brain and spinal cord that separate the brain from the bloodstream, assist in the growth of neurons, speed transmission of nerve impulses, and eliminate damaged neurons.

global warming   Increase in Earth's surface and atmospheric temperature due to increased levels of greenhouse gases (carbon dioxide, methane, and nitrous oxide) that trap heat in the atmosphere.

gonadotropins   Gonad-stimulating hormones produced by the pituitary gland.

gonorrhea   A sexually transmitted infection caused by the bacterium *Neisseria gonorrhoeae;* symptoms include discharge from the penis; women are generally asymptomatic.

guided imagery An approach to stress control, self-healing, or motivating life changes by means of visualizing oneself in the state of calmness, wellness, or change.

gum disease Inflammation of the gum and bones that hold teeth in place.

H

hallucinogen A drug that causes hallucinations.

hashish A concentrated form of a drug, derived from the cannabis plant, containing the psychoactive ingredient TCH, which causes a sense of euphoria when inhaled or eaten.

health A state of complete well-being, including physical, psychological, spiritual, social, intellectual, and environmental components.

health belief model (HBM) A model of behavioral change that focuses on the individual's attitudes and beliefs.

health maintenance organization (HMO) An organization that provides health services on a fixed-contract basis.

health promotion An educational and informational process in which people are helped to change attitudes and behaviors in an effort to improve their health.

heart rate The number of heartbeats per minute.

helminth A parasitic roundworm or flatworm.

hepatitis An inflammation and/or infection of the liver caused by a virus, often accompanied by jaundice.

herbal medicine An ancient form of medical treatment using substances derived from trees, flowers, ferns, seaweeds, and lichens to treat disease.

herpes simplex A condition caused by one of the herpes viruses and characterized by lesions of the skin or mucous membranes; herpes virus type 2 is sexually transmitted and causes genital blisters or sores.

heterosexual Primary sexual orientation toward members of the other sex.

holistic An approach to medicine that takes into account body, mind, emotions, and spirit.

holographic will A will wholly in the handwriting of its author.

home health care Provision of medical services and equipment to patients in the home to restore or maintain comfort, function, and health.

homeopathy A system of medical practice that treats a disease by administering dosages of substances that would in healthy persons produce symptoms similar to those of the disease.

homeostasis The body's natural state of balance or stability.

homosexual Primary sexual orientation toward members of the same sex.

hormone Substance released in the blood that regulates specific bodily functions.

hormone therapy (HT) The use of supplemental hormones during and after menopause.

hospice A homelike health-care facility or program committed to supportive care for terminally ill people.

host A person or population that contracts one or more pathogenic agents in an environment.

human immunodeficiency virus (HIV) A type of virus that causes a spectrum of health problems, ranging from a symptomless infection to changes in the immune system, to the development of life-threatening diseases because of impaired immunity.

human papilloma virus (HPV) A pathogen that causes genital warts and increases the risk of cervical cancer.

hunger The physiological drive to consume food.

hypertension High blood pressure occurring when the blood exerts excessive pressure against the arterial walls.

hypothermia An abnormally low body temperature; if not treated appropriately, coma or death could result.

I

immune deficiency Partial or complete inability of the immune system to respond to pathogens.

immunity Protection from infectious diseases.

immunotherapy A series of injections of small but increasing doses of an allergen, used to treating allergies.

implantation The embedding of the fertilized ovum in the uterine lining.

incomplete proteins Proteins that lack one or more of the amino acids essential for protein synthesis.

incubation period The time between a pathogen's entrance into the body and the first symptom.

indemnity insurance A form of insurance that pays a major portion of medical expenses after a deductible amount is paid by the insured person.

infertility The inability to conceive a child.

infiltration A gradual penetration or invasion.

inflammation A localized response by the body to tissue injury, characterized by swelling and the dilation of the blood vessels.

influenza Any of a type of fairly common, highly contagious viral diseases.

informed consent Permission (to undergo or receive a medical procedure or treatment) given voluntarily, with full knowledge and understanding of the procedure or treatment and its possible consequences.

inhalants Substances that produce vapors having psychoactive effects when sniffed.

integrative medicine An approach that combines traditional medicine with alternative/complementary therapies.

intercourse Sexual stimulation by means of entry of the penis into the vagina; coitus.

interpersonal therapy (IPT) A technique used to develop communication skills and relationships.

intimacy A state of closeness between two people, characterized by the desire and ability to share one's innermost thoughts and feelings with each other either verbally or nonverbally.

intoxication Maladaptive behavioral, psychological, and physiologic changes that occur as a result of substance abuse.

intramuscular Into or within a muscle.

intrauterine device (IUD) A device inserted into the uterus through the cervix to prevent pregnancy by interfering with implantation.

intravenous Into a vein.

ionizing radiation A form of energy emitted from atoms as they undergo internal change.

irradiation Exposure to or treatment by some form of radiation.

isokinetic Having the same force; exercise with specialized equipment that provides resistance equal to the force applied by the user throughout the entire range of motion.

isometric Of the same length; exercise in which muscles increase their tension without shortening in length, such as when pushing an immovable object.

isotonic Having the same tension or tone; exercise requiring the repetition of an action that creates tension, such as weight lifting or calisthenics.

L

labia majora The fleshy outer folds that border the female genital area.

labia minora The fleshy inner folds that border the female genital area.

labor The process leading up to birth: effacement and dilation of the cervix; the movement of the baby into and through the birth canal, accompanied by strong contractions; and contraction of the uterus and expulsion of the placenta after the birth.

lacto-vegetarians People who eat dairy products as well as fruits and vegetables (but not meat, poultry, or fish).

Lamaze method A method of childbirth preparation taught to expectant parents to help the woman cope with the discomfort of labor; combines breathing and psychological techniques.

laparoscopy A surgical sterilization procedure in which the fallopian tubes are observed with a laparoscope inserted through a small incision, and then cut or blocked.

licensed clinical social worker (LCSW) *See* certified social worker.

lipoprotein A compound in blood that is made up of proteins and fat; a high-density lipoprotein (HDL) picks up excess cholesterol in the blood; a low-density lipoprotein (LDL) carries more cholesterol and deposits it on the walls of arteries.

listeria A bacterium commonly found in deli meats, hot dogs, and soft cheeses that can cause an infection called listeriosis.

living will A written statement providing instructions for the use of life-sustaining procedures in the event of terminal illness or injury.

locus of control An individual's belief about the source of power and influence over his or her life.

lumpectomy The surgical removal of a breast tumor and its surrounding tissue.

Lyme disease A disease caused by a bacterium carried by a tick; it may cause heart arrhythmias, neurological problems, and arthritis symptoms.

lymph nodes Small tissue masses in which some immune cells are stored.

M

macronutrients Nutrients required by the human body in the greatest amounts, including water, carbohydrates, proteins, and fats.

mainstream smoke The smoke inhaled directly by smoking a cigarette.

major depression Sadness that does not end.

mammography A diagnostic X-ray exam used to detect breast cancer.

managed care Health-care services and reimbursement predetermined by third-party insurers.

marijuana The drug derived from the cannabis plant, containing the psychoactive ingredient THC, which causes a mild sense of euphoria when inhaled or eaten.

marriage and family therapist A psychiatrist, psychologist, or social worker who specializes in marriage and family counseling.

mastectomy The surgical removal of an entire breast.

masturbation Manual (or nonmanual) self-stimulation of the genitals, often resulting in orgasm.

medical abortion Method of ending a pregnancy within 9 weeks of conception using hormonal medications that cause expulsion of the fertilized egg.

medical history The health-related information collected during the interview of a client by a health-care professional.

meditation A group of approaches that use quiet sitting, breathing techniques, and/or chanting to relax, improve concentration, and become attuned to one's inner self.

menarche The onset of menstruation at puberty.

meningitis An extremely serious, potentially fatal illness that attacks the membranes around the brain and spinal cord; caused by the bacterium *Neisseria meningitis.*

menopause The complete cessation of ovulation and menstruation for twelve consecutive months.

menstruation Discharge of blood from the vagina as a result of the shedding of the uterine lining at the end of the menstrual cycle.

mental disorder Behavioral or psychological syndrome associated with distress or disability or with a significantly increased risk of suffering death, pain, disability, or loss of freedom.

mental health The ability to perceive reality as it is, to respond to its challenges, and to develop rational strategies for living.

meta-analysis Summarization and review of research in a particular area to evaluate the results of several large clinical trials in a uniform manner.

metabolic syndrome A cluster of disorders of the body's metabolism that make diabetes, heart disease, or stroke more likely.

metastasize To spread to other parts of the body via the bloodstream or lymphatic system.

micronutrients Vitamins and minerals needed by the body in very small amounts.

microwaves Extremely high frequency electromagnetic waves that increase the rate at which molecules vibrate, thereby generating heat.

mindfulness A method of stress reduction that involves experiencing the physical and mental sensations of the present moment.

minerals Naturally occurring inorganic substances, small amounts of some being essential in metabolism and nutrition.

minipill An oral contraceptive containing a small amount of progestin and no estrogen, which prevents contraception by making the mucus in the cervix so thick that sperm cannot enter the uterus.

miscarriage A pregnancy that terminates before the twentieth week of gestation; also called spontaneous abortion.

mononucleosis An infectious viral disease characterized by an excess of white blood cells in the blood, fever, bodily discomfort, a sore throat, and kidney and liver complications.

monophasic pill *See* constant-dose combination pill.

mons pubis The rounded, fleshy area over the junction of the female pubic bones.

mood A sustained emotional state that colors one's view of the world for hours or days.

motivational interviewing A nonjudgmental but directive method for supporting motivation to change.

multiphasic pill An oral contraceptive that releases different levels of estrogen and progestin to mimic the hormonal fluctuations of the natural menstrual cycle.

multiple chemical sensitivity (MCS) A sensitivity to low-level chemical exposures from ordinary substances, such as perfumes and tobacco smoke, that results in physiological responses such as chest pain, depression, dizziness, fatigue, and nausea. Also known as environmentally triggered illness.

muscular endurance The ability to withstand the stress of continued physical exertion.

muscular strength Physical power; the maximum weight one can lift, push, or press in one effort.

mutagen An agent that causes alterations in the genetic material of living cells.

myocardial infarction (MI) A condition characterized by the dying of tissue areas in the myocardium, caused by interruption of the blood supply to those areas; the medical name for a heart attack.

N

naturopathy An alternative system of treatment of disease that emphasizes the use of natural remedies such as sun, water, heat, and air. Therapies may include dietary changes, steam baths, and exercise.

neuron A nerve cell—the basic working unit of the brain, which transmits information from the senses to the brain and from the brain to specific body parts; each neuron consists of a cell body, an axon terminal, and dendrites.

neuropsychiatry The study of the brain and mind.

neurotransmitters Chemicals released by neurons that stimulate or inhibit the action of other neurons.

nicotine The addictive substance in tobacco; one of the most toxic of all poisons.

nocturnal emissions Ejaculations while dreaming; wet dreams.

nonexercise activity thermogenesis (NEAT) Nonvolitional movement that can be an effective way of burning calories.

nongonococcal urethritis (NGU) Inflammation of the urethra caused by organisms other than the *Gonococcus* bacterium.

nonopioids Chemically synthesized drugs that have sleep-inducing and pain-relieving properties similar to those of opium and its derivatives.

nonvolitional sex Sexual behavior that violates a person's right to choose when and with whom to have sex and what sexual behaviors to engage in.

nucleus The central part of a cell, contained in the cell body of a neuron.

nutrition The science devoted to the study of dietary needs for food and the effects of food on organisms.

O

obesity The excessive accumulation of fat in the body; class 1 obesity is defined by a BMI between 30.0 and 34.9; class 2 obesity by a BMI between 35.0 and 39.9; class 3 or severe obesity by a BMI of 40 or higher.

obsessive-compulsive disorder (OCD) An anxiety disorder characterized by obsessions and/or compulsions that impair one's ability to function and form relationships.

opioids Drugs that have sleep-inducing and pain-relieving properties, including opium and its derivatives and nonopioid, synthetic drugs.

optimism The tendency to seek out, remember, and expect pleasurable experiences.

oral contraceptives Preparations of synthetic hormones that inhibit ovulation; also referred to as birth control pills or simply the pill.

organic Term designating food produced with, or production based on the use of, fertilizer originating from plants or animals, without the use of pesticides or chemically formulated fertilizers.

organic phosphates Toxic pesticides that may cause cancer, birth defects, neurological disorders, and damage to wildlife and the environment.

orgasm A series of contractions of the pelvic muscles occurring at the peak of sexual arousal.

osteoporosis A condition common in older people in which the bones become increasingly soft and porous, making them susceptible to injury.

outcomes The ultimate impacts of particular treatments or absence of treatment.

ovary The female sex organ that produces egg cells, estrogen, and progesterone.

overload principle Providing a greater stress or demand on the body than it is normally accustomed to handling.

overloading Method of physical training involving increasing the number of repetitions or the amount of resistance gradually to work the muscle to temporary fatigue.

over-the-counter (OTC) drugs Medications that can be obtained legally without a prescription from a medical professional.

overtrain Working muscles too intensely or too frequently, resulting in persistent muscle soreness, injuries, unintended weight loss, nervousness, and an inability to relax.

overuse injuries Physical injuries to joints or muscles, such as strains, fractures, and tendinitis, which result from overdoing a repetitive activity.

overweight A condition of having a BMI between 25.0 and 29.9.

ovo-lacto-vegetarians People who eat eggs, dairy products, and fruits and vegetables (but not meat, poultry, or fish).

ovulation The release of a mature ovum from an ovary approximately 14 days prior to the onset of menstruation.

ovum (plural, **ova**) The female gamete (egg cell).

ozone A form of oxygen that is a harmful component of air pollution.

P

panic attack A short episode characterized by physical sensations of light-headedness, dizziness, hyperventilation, and numbness of extremities, accompanied by an inexplicable terror, usually of a physical disaster such as death.

panic disorder An anxiety disorder in which the apprehension or experience of recurring panic attacks is so intense that normal functioning is impaired.

Pap smear A test in which cells removed from the cervix are examined under a microscope for signs of cancer; also called a Pap test.

passive stretching A stretching technique in which an external force or resistance (your body, a partner, gravity, or a weight) helps the joints move through their range of motion.

pathogen A microorganism that produces disease.

PCP (phencyclidine) A synthetic psychoactive substance that produces effects similar to other psychoactive drugs when swallowed, smoked, sniffed, or injected, but may also trigger unpredictable behavioral changes.

pelvic inflammatory disease (PID) An inflammation of the internal female genital tract, characterized by abdominal pain, fever, and tenderness of the cervix.

penis The male organ of sex and urination.

perimenopause The period from a woman's first irregular cycles to her last menstruation.

perineum The area between the anus and vagina in the female and between the anus and scrotum in the male.

periodontitis Severe gum disease in which the tooth root becomes infected.

persistent vegetative state A state of being awake and capable of reacting to physical stimuli, such as light, while being unaware of pain or other environmental stimuli.

phobia An anxiety disorder marked by an inordinate fear of an object, a class of objects, or a situation, resulting in extreme avoidance behaviors.

physical dependence The physiological attachment to, and need for, a drug.

physical fitness The ability to respond to routine physical demands, with enough reserve energy to cope with a sudden challenge.

phytochemicals Chemicals such as indoles, coumarins, and capsaicin, which exist naturally in plants and have disease-fighting properties.

placenta An organ that develops after implantation and to which the embryo attaches, via the umbilical cord, for nourishment and waste removal.

plaque The sludgelike substance that builds up on the inner walls of arteries; the sticky film of bacteria that forms on teeth.

pollutant A substance or agent in the environment, usually the by-product of human industry or activity, that is injurious to human, animal, or plant life.

polyabuse The misuse or abuse of more than one drug.

posttraumatic stress disorder (PTSD) The repeated reliving of a trauma through nightmares or recollection.

potentiating Making more effective or powerful.

preconception care Health care to prepare for pregnancy.

precycling The use of products that are packaged in recycled or recyclable material.

predisposing factors The beliefs, values, attitudes, knowledge, and perceptions that influence our behavior.

preferred provider organization (PPO) A group of physicians contracted to provide health care to members at a discounted price.

prehypertension A condition of slightly elevated blood pressure, which is likely to worsen in time.

premature ejaculation A sexual difficulty in which a man ejaculates so rapidly that his partner's satisfaction is impaired.

premature labor Labor that occurs after the twentieth week but before the thirty-seventh week of pregnancy.

premenstrual dysphoric disorder (PMDD) A disorder that causes symptoms of psychological depression during the last week of the menstrual cycle.

premenstrual syndrome (PMS) A disorder that causes physical discomfort and psychological distress prior to a woman's menstrual period.

prevention Information and support offered to help healthy people identify their health risks, reduce stressors, prevent potential medical problems, and enhance their well-being.

primary care Ambulatory or outpatient care provided by a physician in an office, emergency room, or clinic.

progesterone The female sex hormone that stimulates the uterus, preparing it for the arrival of a fertilized egg.

progestin-only pill See minipill.

progressive overloading Gradually increasing physical challenges once the body adapts to the stress placed upon it to produce maximum benefits.

progressive relaxation A method of reducing muscle tension by contracting, then relaxing certain areas of the body.

proof The alcoholic strength of a distilled spirit, expressed as twice the percentage of alcohol present.

prostate gland A structure surrounding the male urethra that produces a secretion that helps liquefy the semen from the testes.

protection Measures that an individual can take when participating in risky behavior to prevent injury or unwanted risks.

protein A substance that is basically a compound of amino acids; one of the essential nutrients.

protozoa Microscopic animals made up of one cell or a group of similar cells.

psychiatric drugs Medications that regulate a person's mental, emotional, and physical functions to facilitate normal functioning.

psychiatric nurse A nurse with special training and experience in mental health care.

psychiatrist Licensed medical doctor with additional training in psychotherapy, psychopharmacology, and treatment of mental disorders.

psychoactive Mood-altering.

psychodynamic Interpreting behaviors in terms of early experiences and unconscious influences.

psychological dependence The emotional or mental attachment to the use of a drug.

psychologist Mental health-care professional who has completed doctoral or graduate programs in psychology and is trained in a variety of psychotherapeutic techniques, but who is not medically trained and does not prescribe medications.

psychoprophylaxis *See* Lamaze method.

psychotherapy Treatment designed to produce a response by psychological rather than physical means, such as suggestion, persuasion, reassurance, and support.

Q

quackery Medical fakery; unproven practices claiming to cure diseases or solve health problems.

R

range of motion The fullest extent of possible movement in a particular joint.

rape Sexual penetration of a female or a male by means of intimidation, force, or fraud.

rapid-eye-movement (REM) sleep Regularly occurring periods of sleep during which the most active dreaming takes place.

Rating of Perceived Exertion (RPE) A self-assessment scale that rates symptoms of breathlessness and fatigue.

receptors Molecules on the surface of neurons on which neurotransmitters bind after their release from other neurons.

recycling The processing or reuse of manufactured materials to reduce consumption of raw materials.

refractory period The period of time following orgasm during which the male cannot experience another orgasm.

reinforcing factors Rewards, encouragement, and recognition that influence our behavior in the short run.

relapse prevention An alcohol recovery treatment method that focuses on social skills training to develop ways of preventing or minimizing a relapse.

relative risk The risk of developing cancer in persons with a certain exposure or trait compared to the risk in persons who do not have the same exposure or trait.

rep (or repetition) In weight training, a single performance of a movement or exercise.

repetitive motion injury (RMI) Inflammation of or damage to a part of the body due to repetition of the same movements.

rescue marriage A marital relationship in which one partner has had a traumatic childhood and views marriage as a way of healing the past.

resting heart rate The number of heartbeats per minute during inactivity.

reuptake Reabsorption by the originating cell of neurotransmitters that have not connected with receptors and have been left in synapses.

reversibility principle The physical benefits of exercise are lost through disuse or inactivity.

rhythm method A birth-control method in which sexual intercourse is avoided during those days of the menstrual cycle in which fertilization is most likely to occur.

romantic marriage A marital relationship in which sexual passion never fades.

rubella An infectious disease that may cause birth defects if contracted by a pregnant woman; also called German measles.

S

same-sex marriage Governmentally, socially, or religiously recognized marriage in which two people of the same sex live together as a family.

satiety A feeling of fullness after eating.

saturated fat A chemical term indicating that a fat molecule contains as many hydrogen atoms as its carbon skeleton can hold. These fats are normally solid at room temperature.

schizophrenia A general term for a group of mental disorders with characteristic psychotic symptoms, such as delusions, hallucinations, and disordered thought patterns during the active phase of the illness, and a duration of at least six months.

scrotum The external sac or pouch that holds the testes.

secondary sex characteristics Physical changes associated with maleness or femaleness, induced by the sex hormones.

self-actualization A state of wellness and fulfillment that can be achieved once certain human needs are satisfied; living to one's full potential.

self-disclosure Sharing personal information and experiences with another that he or she would not otherwise discover; self-disclosure involves risk and vulnerability.

self-efficacy Belief in one's ability to accomplish a goal or change a behavior.

self-esteem Confidence and satisfaction in oneself.

semen The viscous whitish fluid that is the complete male ejaculate; a combination of sperm and secretions from the prostate gland, seminal vesicles, and other glands.

seminal vesicles Glands in the male reproductive system that produce the major portion of the fluid of semen.

sets In weight training, the number of repetitions of the same movement or exercise.

sex Maleness or femaleness, resulting from genetic, structural, and functional factors.

sexual coercion Sexual activity forced upon a person by the exertion of psychological pressure by another person.

sexual dysfunction The inability to react emotionally and/or physically to sexual stimulation in a way expected of the average healthy person or according to one's own standards.

sexual harassment Uninvited and unwanted sexual attention, either verbal or physical.

sexual health The integration of the physical, emotional, intellectual, social, and spiritual aspects of sexual being in ways that are positively enriching and that enhance personality, communication, and love.

sexual orientation The direction of an individual's sexual interest, either to members of the opposite sex or to members of the same sex.

sexuality The behaviors, instincts, and attitudes associated with being sexual.

sexually transmitted disease (STD) A disease that is caused by a sexually transmitted infection that produces symptoms.

sexually transmitted infection (STI) The presence in the human body of an infectious agent that can be passed from one sexual partner to another.

sidestream smoke The smoke emitted by a burning cigarette and breathed by everyone in a closed room, including the smoker; contains more tar and nicotine than mainstream smoke.

simple carbohydrates Sugars; like all carbohydrates, they provide the body with glucose.

social isolation A feeling of unconnectedness with others caused by and reinforced by infrequency of social contacts.

social norms The unwritten rules regarding behavior and conduct expected or accepted by a group.

social phobia A severe form of social anxiety marked by extreme fears and avoidance of social situations.

solution-focused therapy A technique that accentuates the positive and focuses on goals and implementation of alternatives.

specificity principle Each part of the body adapts to a particular type and amount of stress placed upon it.

sperm The male gamete produced by the testes and transported outside the body through ejaculation.

spermatogenesis The process by which sperm cells are produced.

spiritual health The ability to identify one's basic purpose in life and to achieve one's full potential.

spiritual intelligence The capacity to sense, understand, and tap into ourselves, others, and the world around us.

spirituality A belief in someone or something that transcends the boundaries of self.

static flexibility The ability to assume and maintain an extended position at one end point in a joint's range of motion.

static stretching A gradual stretch held for a short time of 10 to 30 seconds.

sterilization A surgical procedure to end a person's reproductive capability.

stress The nonspecific response of the body to any demands made upon it; may be characterized by muscle tension and acute anxiety, or may be a positive force for action.

stressor Specific or nonspecific agents or situations that cause the stress response in a body.

stroke A cerebrovascular event in which the blood supply to a portion of the brain is blocked.

subcutaneous Under the skin.

suction curettage A procedure in which the contents of the uterus are removed by means of suction and scraping.

sustainability A method of using a resource so that the resource is not depleted or permanently damaged.

synapse A specialized site at which electrical impulses are transmitted from the axon terminal of one neuron to a dendrite of another.

synergistic Characterized by a combined effect that is greater than the sum of the individual effects.

syphilis A sexually transmitted infection caused by the bacterium *Treponema pallidum,* and characterized by early sores, a latent period, and a final period of life-threatening symptoms including brain damage and heart failure.

systemic disease A pathologic condition that spreads throughout the body.

systole The contraction phase of the cardiac cycle.

systolic blood pressure Highest blood pressure when the heart contracts.

T

tar A thick, sticky dark fluid produced by the burning of tobacco, made up of several hundred different chemicals, many of them poisonous, some of them carcinogenic.

target heart rate Sixty to eighty-five percent of the maximum heart rate; the heart rate at which one derives maximum cardiovascular benefit from aerobic exercise.

terminal illness An illness in which death is inevitable.

testes (singular, **testis**) The male sex organs that produce sperm and testosterone.

testosterone The male sex hormone that stimulates male secondary sex characteristics.

toxic shock syndrome (TSS) A disease characterized by fever, vomiting, diarrhea, and often shock, caused by a bacterium that releases toxic waste products into the bloodstream.

toxicity Poisonousness; the dosage level at which a drug becomes poisonous to the body, causing either temporary or permanent damage.

traditional marriage A marital relationship in which the roles of the partners are distinct; defined by gender-based cultural norms and expectations.

transcendence The sense of passing into a foreign region or dimension, often experienced by a person near death.

trans-fat Fat formed when liquid vegetable oils are processed to make table spreads or cooking fats, and also found in dairy and beef products; considered to be especially dangerous dietary fats.

transgender Having a gender identity opposite one's biological sex; transsexual.

transient ischemic attack (TIA) A cerebrovascular event in which the blood supply to a portion of the brain is blocked temporarily; repeated attacks are predictors of more severe strokes.

transtheoretical model of change A model of behavioral change that focuses on the individual's decision making; it states that an individual progresses through a sequence of six stages as he or she makes a change in behavior.

trichomoniasis An infection of the protozoan *Trichomonas vaginalis;* females experience vaginal burning, itching, and discharge, but male carriers may be asymptomatic.

triglyceride A blood fat that flows through the blood after meals and is linked to increased risk of coronary artery disease.

tubal ligation The suturing or tying shut of the fallopian tubes to prevent pregnancy.

tubal occlusion The blocking of the fallopian tubes to prevent pregnancy.

tuberculosis A highly infectious bacterial disease that primarily affects the lungs and is often fatal.

twelve-step programs Self-help group programs based on the principles of Alcoholics Anonymous.

U

ulcer A lesion in, or an erosion of, the mucous membrane of an organ.

unsaturated fat A chemical term indicating that a fat molecule contains fewer hydrogen atoms than its carbon skeleton can hold. These fats are normally liquid at room temperature.

urethra The canal through which urine from the bladder leaves the body; in the male, also serves as the channel for seminal fluid.

urethral opening The outer opening of the thin tube that carries urine from the bladder.

urethritis Infection of the urethra.

uterus The female organ that houses the developing fetus until birth.

V

vagina The canal leading from the exterior opening in the female genital area to the uterus.

vaginal contraceptive film (VCF) A small dissolvable sheet saturated with spermicide that can be inserted into the vagina and placed over the cervix.

vaginal spermicide A substance that kills or neutralizes sperm, inserted into the vagina in the form of a foam, cream, jelly, suppository, or film.

vaginismus A sexual difficulty in which a woman experiences painful spasms of the vagina during sexual intercourse.

values The criteria by which one makes choices about one's thoughts and actions and goals and ideals.

vas deferens Two tubes that carry sperm from the epididymis into the urethra.

vasectomy A surgical sterilization procedure in which each vas deferens is cut and tied shut to stop the passage of sperm to the urethra for ejaculation.

vector A biological or physical vehicle that carries the agent of infection to the host.

vegans People who eat only plant foods.

ventricle Either of the two lower chambers of the heart, which pump blood out of the heart and into the arteries.

virus A submicroscopic infectious agent; the most primitive form of life.

visualization An approach to stress control, self-healing, or motivating life changes by means of guided, or directed, imagery.

vital signs Measurements of physiological functioning; specifically, temperature, blood pressure, pulse rate, and respiration rate.

vitamins Organic substances that are needed in very small amounts by the body and carry out a variety of functions in metabolism and nutrition.

W

waist-to-hip ratio The proportion of one's waist circumference to one's hip circumference.

wellness A state of optimal health.

withdrawal Development of symptoms that cause significant psychological and physical distress when an individual reduces or stops drug use.

Z

zygote A fertilized egg.

References

Chapter 1

1. "Constitution of the World Health Organization." *Chronicle of the World Health Organization,* Geneva, Switzerland: WHO, 1947.
2. Travis, John, and Regina Sara Ryan. *The Wellness Workbook* 3rd ed. Berkeley, CA: Celestial Arts, 2004.
3. Travis, John. Personal interview.
4. Travis and Ryan, *The Wellness Workbook.*
5. Benson, Herbert, et al. "Study of the Therapeutic Effects of Intercessory Prayer (STEP) in Cardiac Bypass Patients: A Multicenter Randomized Trial of Uncertainty and Certainty of Receiving Intercessory Prayer." *American Heart Journal* Vol. 151, No. 4, April 2006, pp. 934–942.
6. Krucoff, Mitchell, et al. "From Efficacy to Safety Concerns: A STEP Forward or a Step Back for Clinical Research and Intercessory Prayer? The Study of Therapeutic Effects of Intercessory Prayer (STEP)." *American Heart Journal,* Vol. 151, No. 4, April 2006, p. 762.
7. Goleman, Daniel. Personal interview.
8. Kashdan, Todd. Personal interview.
9. American College Health Association. "American College Health Association National College Health Assessment Spring 2006 Reference Group Data Report (Abridged)." *Journal of American College Health,* Vol. 55, No. 4, January–February 2007, pp. 195–206.
10. Harris, Kathleen Mullan, et al. "Longitudinal Trends in Race/Ethnic Disparities in Leading Health Indicators from Adolescence to Young Adulthood." *Archives of Pediatric and Adolescent Medicine,* Vol. 160, No. 1, January 2006, p. 74.
11. Donaldson, Joe, and Barbara Townsend. "Higher Education Journal's Discourse about Adult Undergraduate Students," *Journal of Higher Education,* 2007, Vol. 78, No. 1, January–February p. 27(24).
12. U.S. Department of Education, Higher Education Center, www.higheredcenter.org/socialnorms.
13. American College Health Association. *American College Health Association National College Health Assessment: Reference Group Data Report Spring 2006.* Baltimore: American College Health Association, 2006.
14. Lewis, Melissa, and Clayton Neighbors. "Optimizing Personalized Normative Feedback: The Use of Gender-Specific Referents." *Journal of Studies on Alcohol and Drugs,* Vol. 68, 2007, pp. 228–237.
15. American College Health Association. *American College Health Association National College Health Assessment: Reference Group Data Report Spring 2006.* Baltimore: American College Health Association, 2006.
16. Reyna, Valerie F. & Farley, Frank. "Risk and Rationality in Adolescent Decision Making: Implication for Theory, Practice, and Public Policy." *Psychological Science in the Public Interest* Vol. 7, No. 1, pp. 1–44.
17. Adams, P. F., et al. "Summary health statistics for the U.S. population: National Health Interview Survey, 2005." *Vital and Health Statistics.* Ser. 10, No. 233. Hyattsville, MD: U.S. Department of Health and Human Services, 2007.
18. Ibid.
19. *HP 2010 Midcourse Review,* http://www.healthypeople.gov/data/midcourse/default.htm#pubs.
20. Adams, et al.
21. "Eliminating Racial & Ethnic Health Disparities," http://www.cdc.gov/omh/AboutUs/disparities.htm.
22. Blackstock, A. William, et al. "Similar Outcomes Between African American and Non-African American Patients with Extensive-Stage Small-Cell Lung Carcinoma: Report from the Cancer and Leukemia Group B." *Journal of Clinical Oncology,* Vol. 24, No. 3, January 2006, p. 407.
23. Rust, George and Lisa Cooper. "How Can Practice-based Research Contribute to the Elimination of Health Disparities?" *The Journal of the American Board of Family Medicine* Vol. 20, No. 2, 2007, pp. 105–114.
24. Hales, Dianne and Kenneth W. Christian. *An Invitation to Personal Change.* Belmont: Thomson Publishing, 2009.
25. Prochaska, James, et al. *Changing for Good.* New York: Quill, 1994.
26. Christian, Kenneth W. Personal interview.

Chapter 2

1. Seligman, Martin. *Authentic Happiness.* New York: Free Press, 2002.
2. Seligman, Martin. Personal interview.
3. Goodstein, Charles. Personal interview.
4. Lyubomirsky, Sonja. *The How of Happiness: A Scientific Approach to Getting the Life You Want.* In press.
5. Lyubomirsky, Sonja. Personal interview.
6. Seligman, *Authentic Happiness.*
7. Larsen, Randy. Personal interview.
8. Hale, Cara, et al. "Social Support and Physical Health: The Importance of Belonging." *Journal of American College Health,* Vol. 53, No. 6, May–June 2005, p. 276.
9. Hermann, Karen, and Nancy Betz. "Path Models of the Relationships of Instrumentality and Expressiveness to Social Self-Efficacy, Shyness, and Depressive Symptoms." *Sex Roles: A Journal of Research,* Vol. 51, No. 1–2, July 2004, p. 55(12).
10. Wilson, K. A. et al. "The Developmental Psychopathology of Social Anxiety in Adolescents," *Depression and Anxiety,* 2007, pp. 1–7.
11. Ornish, Dean. *Love & Survival: The Scientific Basis for the Healing Power of Intimacy.* New York: HarperCollins, 1999.
12. Robinson, E. A. et al. "Six-Month Changes in Spirituality, Religiousness, and Heavy Drinking in a Treatment-Seeking Sample." *Journal of Studies on Alcohol and Drugs.* Vol. 68, No. 2, March 2007, pp. 282–290.
13. Curlin, F. A. et al. "Physicians' Observations and Interpretations of the Influence of Religion and Spirituality on Health." *Archives of Internal Medicine,* Vol. 167, No. 7, April 2007, pp. 649–654.
14. Storch, Eric, et al. "Religiosity and Depression in Intercollegiate Athletes." *College Student Journal,* Vol. 36, No. 4, December 2002, p. 526.
15. Edwards, Paul. Personal interview.
16. Pryor, John, et al. *The American Freshman: National Norms for Fall 2005.* Los Angeles: Higher Education Research Institute, UCLA, December 2005.
17. Koenig, Harold. Personal interview.
18. McCaffrey A. M., et al. "Prayer for Health Concerns: Results of a National Survey on Prevalence and Patterns of Use." *Archives of Internal Medicine,* Vol. 164, No. 8, April 26, 2004, pp. 858–862.
19. Krucoff, Mitchell, et al. "Music, Imagery, Touch, and Prayer as Adjuncts to Interventional Cardiac Care: The Monitoring and Actualisation of Noetic Trainings (MANTRA) II Randomised Study." *Lancet,* Vol. 366, July 15, 2005, pp. 211–217.
20. Aaronson, Lauren. "Make a Gratitude Adjustment: Feeling Thankful Is One Key to Happiness." *Psychology Today,* March–April 2006, Vol. 39, No. 2, p. 60(2).
21. McCullough, Michael. Personal interview.
22. Colten, Harvey, and Altevogt, Bruce (eds.), Committee on Sleep Medicine and Research of the Institute of Medicine. *Sleep Disorders and Sleep Deprivation: An Unmet Public Health Problem.* Washington, DC: National Academies Press, 2006.
23. National Sleep Foundation. *2006 Sleep In America Poll,* www.sleepfoundation.org.
24. "Sleep: Snooze or Lose," University of Michigan Health Service, www.uhs.umich.edu/wellness/other/sleep.html.
25. Law, Daniel. "Exhaustion in University Students and the Effect of Coursework Involvement," *Journal of American College Health,* Vol. 55, No. 4, January–February 2007, p. 239(7).
26. Rolston, Emily, et al. "Power Napping: Effects on Cognitive Ability and Stress Levels Among College Students," *Research Quarterly for Exercise and Sport,* Vol. 78, No. 1, February 2007, p. A-36(1).
27. Gau, S. S., et al. "Association Between Sleep Problems and Symptoms of Attention-Deficit/Hyperactivity Disorder in Young Adults," *Sleep,* Vol. 30, February 2007, Vol. 30, No. 2, pp. 195–201.

28. Brown, Franklin, et al. "Development and Evaluation of the Sleep Treatment and Education Program for Students (STEPS)." *Journal of American College Health,* Vol. 54, No. 4, January–February 2006, p. 201.

29. Ellenbogen, J. M., et al. "Human Relational Memory Requires Time and Sleep," *Proceedings of the National Academy of Science USA,* April 20, 2007.

30. Buysse, Daniel, et al. "Sleep Disorders." *Textbook of Clinical Psychiatry,* Washington, D.C.: American Psychiatric Press, 2008.

31. "The Importance of Sleep and Health: Six Reasons Not to Scrimp on Sleep," Harvard Health Publications, http://www.health.harvard.edu.

32. Millman, Richard. "Excessive Sleepiness in Adolescents and Young Adults: Causes, Consequences, and Treatment Strategies." *Pediatrics,* Vol. 115, No. 6, June 2005, p. 774.

Chapter 3

1. American College Health Association. "American College Health Association National College Health Assessment Spring 2006 Reference Group Data Report (Abridged)." *Journal of American College Health,* Vol. 55, No. 4, January–February 2007, pp. 195–206.

2. Lazarus, R., and R. Launier. "Stress-Related Transactions Between Person and Environment." *Perspectives in Interactional Psychology.* New York: Plenum, 1978.

3. Schmeelk-Cone, K. H., et al. "The Buffering Effects of Active Coping on the Relationship Between SES and Cortisol Among African American Young Adults." *Behavioral Medicine,* Vol. 29, No. 2, Summer 2003, p. 85.

4. Sastry, K. S., et al. "Epinephrine Protects Cancer Cells from Apoptosis via Activation of PKA and BAD Phosphorylation." *Journal of Biological Chemistry,* March 2007.

5. Jones, M. P. "The Role of Psychosocial Factors in Peptic Ulcer Disease: Beyond *Helicobacter pylori* and NSAIDs." *Journal of Psychosomatic Research,* Vol. 60, No. 4, April 2006, pp. 407–412.

6. Freeman, L. M., and K. M. Gil. "Daily Stress, Coping, and Dietary Restraint in Binge Eating." *International Journal of Eating Disorders,* Vol. 36, No. 2, September 2004, p. 204.

7. Yosipovitch, G., et al. "Study of Psychological Stress, Sebum Production and Acne Vulgaris in Adolescents." *Acta dermato-venereologica,* Vol. 87, No. 2, 2007, 135–139.

8. "Stressed Out: A New Study Explains Why Female Professors Have Added Stress." *University Business,* Vol. 8, No. 4, April 2005, p. 26.

9. Uhart, M., et al. "Hormonal Responses to Psychological Stress and Family History of Alcoholism." *Neuropsychopharmacology.* March 22, 2006.

10. "In Case You Haven't Heard. . . ." *Mental Health Weekly,* Vol. 15, No. 3, January 17, 2004, p. 8.

11. Pryor, John, et al. *The American Freshman: National Norms for Fall 2006.* Los Angeles: Higher Education Research Institute, 2006.

12. Reed, Verona, et al. "Gender Differences in Emotional and Overt/Covert Aggressive Responses to Stress." *Aggressive Behavior,* Vol. 33, No. 3, April 2007, pp. 261–271.

13. Evans, Sybil. Personal interview.

14. Bushman, Brad. Personal interview.

15. Moons, W. G., and D. M. Mackie, "Thinking Straight While Seeing Red: The Influence of Anger on Information Processing." *Personality and Social Psychology,* April 17, 2007.

16. Clays, E., et al. "High Job Strain and Ambulatory Blood Pressure in Middle-Aged Men and Women from the Belgian Job Stress Study." *Journal of Occupational and Environmental Medicine,* Vol. 49, No. 4, April 2007, pp. 360–367.

17. Maslach, Christina. Personal interview.

18. Goleman, Daniel. Personal interview.

19. Utay, Joe, and Megan Miller. "Guided Imagery as an Effective Therapeutic Technique: A Brief Review of Its History and Efficacy Research." *Journal of Instructional Psychology,* Vol. 33, No. 1, March 2006, p. 40.

20. Archer, Shirley. "Tangible Proof of Brain Changes Associated with Meditation." *IDEA Fitness Journal,* Vol. 3, No. 3, March 2006, p. 88(1).

21. Jayadevappa, R., et al. "Effectiveness of Transcendental Meditation on Functional Capacity and Quality of Life of African Americans with Congestive Heart Failure: A Randomized Control Study." *Ethnicity and Disease,* Vol. 17, No. 1, Winter 2007, pp. 72–77.

22. "The Risk for PTSD: New Findings." *Harvard Mental Health Letter,* Vol. 23, No. 8, February 2007, p. 4.

23. Schnurr, Paula, et al. "Cognitive Behavioral Therapy for Posttraumatic Stress Disorder in Women." *Journal of the American Medical Association,* Vol. 297, No. 8, February 28, 2007, pp. 820–830.

24. Seal, K. H., et al. "Bringing the War Back Home: Mental Health Disorders Among 103,788 U.S. Veterans Returning from Iraq and Afghanistan Seen at Department of Veterans Affairs Facilities." *Archives of Internal Medicine,* Vol. 167, No. 5, March 2007, pp. 476–482.

25. Kubzansky, L. D., et al. "Prospective Study of Posttraumatic Stress Disorder Symptoms and Coronary Heart Disease in the Normative Aging Study." *Archives of General Psychiatry,* Vol. 64, January 2007, pp. 109–116.

26. Finn, Robert. "Undergrads' Words After Trauma Can Predict PTSD." *Clinical Psychiatry News,* Vol. 35, No. 2, February 2007, p. 16(1).

Chapter 4

1. Messias, Erick, et al. "Psychiatrists' Ascertained Treatment Needs for Mental Disorders in a Population-Based Sample." *Psychiatric Services,* Vol. 58, March 2007, pp. 373–377.

2. Kobau, R., et al. "Sad, Blue, or Depressed Days, Health Behaviors and Health-Related Quality of Life, Behavioral Risk Factor Surveillance System, 1995–2000." *Health Quality of Life Outcomes,* Vol. 2, No. 1, July 30, 2004, p. 40.

3. Hales, Robert E. et al (editors). *Textbook of Clinical Psychiatry.* Washington, D.C.: American Psychiatric Press, 2008.

4. Messias, et al. "Psychiatrists' Ascertained Treatment Needs for Mental Disorders in a Population-Based Sample."

5. Ibid.

6. Mojtabai, Raibin. "Americans' Attitudes Toward Mental Health Treatment Seeking: 1990–2003." Psychiatric Services, Vol. 58, 2007 , pp. 642–651.

7. Brea, L. et al. "Comparison of Public Attributions, Attitudes, and Stigma in Regard to Depression Among Children and Adults." *Psychiatric Services,* Vol. 58, 2007, pp. 632–635.

8. Schilling, E. A., et al. "Adverse Childhood Experiences and Mental Health in Young Adults: A Longitudinal Survey." *BMC Public Health,* Vol. 7, No. 1, March 2007, p. 30.

9. Insel, Thomas, and Wayne S. Fenton. "Psychiatric Epidemiology: It's Not Just About Counting Anymore." *Archives of General Psychiatry,* Vol. 62, No. 6, June 2005, p. 590.

10. Schwartz, Allan. "Are College Students More Disturbed Today? Stability in the Acuity and Qualitative Character of Psychopathology of College Counseling Center Clients: 1992–1993 through 2001–2002." *American Journal of College Health,* Vol. 54, No. 6, May–June 2006, pp. 327–337.

11. American College Health Association. "American College Health Association National College Health Assessment Spring 2006 Reference Group Data Report (Abridged)." *Journal of American College Health,* Vol. 55, No. 4, January–February 2007, pp. 195–206.

12. Wart, Paula. "Why Be Happy?" *Health Plus,* Vanderbilt University, January 3, 2005.

13. Miller, Michael Craig. "Is Exercise a Good Treatment for Depression?" *HEALTHBeat,* July 6, 2005, www.health.harvard.edu/mental.

14. Joska, John et al. "Mood Disorders." **Textbook of Clinical Psychiatry.** Washington, D.C.: American Psychiatry Press, 2008.

15. Williams, D. R., et al. "Prevalence and Distribution of Major Depressive Disorder in African Americans, Caribbean Blacks, and Non-Hispanic Whites: Results from the National Survey of American Life." *Archives of General Psychiatry,* Vol. 64, No. 3, March 2007, pp. 305–315.

16. Turner, R. J., and D. A. Lloyd. "Stress Burden and the Lifetime Incidence of Psychiatric Disorder in Young Adults: Racial and Ethnic Contrasts." *Archives of General Psychiatry,* Vol. 61, No. 5, May 2004, p. 481.

17. Franko, Debra, et al. "Self-Reported Symptoms of Depression in Late Adolescence to Early Adulthood: A Comparison of African-American and Caucasian Females." *Journal of Adolescent Health,* Vol. 37, No. 6, December 2005, pp. 526–529.

18. Jensen, Peter. Personal interview.

19. Kuehn, Bridget. "Link Between Smoking and Mental Illness May Lead to Treatments." *The Journal of the American Medical Association,* Vol. 295, No. 5, February 1, 2006, p. 483.

20. Soares, Claudio. "Antidepressants During Pregnancy: Treating the Condition While Acknowledging the Risks." *Journal Watch Women's Health,* April 26, 2007.

21. Kendler, Kenneth, et al. "Sex Differences in the Relationship between Social Support and Risk for Major Depression: A Longitudinal Study of Opposite-Sex Twin Pairs." *American Journal of Psychiatry,* Vol. 162, No. 2, February 2005, p. 250.

22. Dubovsky, Steven. "Do Antidepressants Make Patients Suicidal?" *Journal Watch Psychiatry,* January 29, 2007.

23. Bridge, J. A., et al. "Clinical Response and Risk for Reported Suicidal Ideation and Suicide Attempts in Pediatric Antidepressant Treatment: A Meta-Analysis of Randomized Controlled Trials." *Journal of the American Medical Association,* Vol. 297, No. 8, April 2007, pp. 1683–1696.

24. Gibbons, R. D., et al. "Relationship between antidepressants and suicide attempts: an analysis of the veterans health administration data sets." *American Journal of Psychiatry,* Vol. 164, No. 7, July 2007, pp. 1044–1049; Simon G. E., Savarino J. "Suicide attempts among patients starting depression treatment with medications or psychotherapy." *American Journal of Psychiatry,* Vol. 164, No. 7, July 2007, pp. 1029–1034.

25. Shern, David. "Antidepressants and the Risk of Suicide: Additional Warning Labels Create Treatment Barriers." *Psychiatry 2007,* Vol. 4, No. 2, February 2007, p. 15.

26. Trivedi, M. H., et al. "Medication Augmentation After the Failure of SSRIs for Depression." *New England Journal of Medicine,* Vol. 354, No. 12, March 23, 2006, pp. 1243–1252.

27. "Electroconvulsive Therapy," *Harvard Mental Health Letter,* Vol. 23, No. 8, February 2007, pp. 1–4.

28. Greden, John. Personal interview.

29. Swann, Alan. "What Is Bipolar Disorder?" *American Journal of Psychiatry,* Vol. 163, No. 1, February 2006, p. 177.

30. Kroenhke, Kurt, et al. "Anxiety Disorders in Primary Care: Prevalence, Impairment, Comorbidity, and Detection." *Annals of Internal Medicine,* Vol. 146, No. 5, March 2007, pp. 317–325.

31. Katon, Wayne, and Peter Roy-Byrne. "Anxiety Disorders: Efficient Screening Is the First Step in Improving Outcomes." *Annals of Internal Medicine,* Vol. 146, March 2007, pp. 390–392.

32. Milrod, B., et al. "A Randomized Controlled Clinical Trial of Psychoanalytic Psychotherapy for Panic Disorder." *American Journal of Psychiatry,* Vol. 164, February 2007, pp. 265–272.

33. Dusseldorp, E., et al. "Which Panic Disorder Patients Benefit from Which Treatment: Cognitive Therapy or Antidepressants?" *Psychotherapy and Psychosomatics,* Vol. 76, No. 3, 2007, pp. 154–161.

34. Frazier, Thomas, et al. "ADHD and Achievement: Meta-Analysis of the Child, Adolescent, and Adult Literatures and a Concomitant Study with College Students." *Journal of Learning Disabilities,* Vol. 40, No. 1, January–February 2007, p. 49(17).

35. "Ritalin Abuse Poses Risk during College Exam Week," University of Florida Health Sciences Center news release, May 10, 2007.

36. Kollins, S. H., "Abuse Liability of Medications Used to Treat Attention-Deficit/Hyperactivity Disorder." *American Journal of Addictions,* Vol. 16, 2007, pp. 35–44.

37. Stroup, T. Scott, et al. "Effectiveness of Olanzapine, Quetiapine, and Risperidone in Patients with Chronic Schizophrenia After Discontinuing Perphenazine: A CATIE Study." *American Journal of Psychiatry,* Vol. 164, March 2007, pp. 415–427.

38. Gold, Lisa. "Suicide and Gender." *Textbook of Suicide Assessment and Management,* Simon, Robert and Robert Hales, (eds.). Washington, DC: American Psychiatric Publishing, 2006, p. 77.

39. Ash, Peter. "Children and Adolescents." *Textbook of Suicide Assessment and Management,* Simon, Robert and Robert Hales, (eds.). Washington, DC: American Psychiatric Publishing, 2006, p. 35.

40. Schwartz, Allan. "College Student Suicide in the United States: 1990–1991 through 2003–2004." *American Journal of College Health,* Vol. 54, No. 6, May–June 2006, pp. 341–352.

41. Schwartz, Allan. "Four Eras of Study of College Student Suicide in the United States: 1920–2004." *American Journal of College Health,* Vol. 54, No. 6, May–June 2006, pp. 353–366.

42. Gould, Madelyn. Personal interview.

43. Horton, Leslie. "Social, Cultural, and Demographic Factors in Suicide." *Textbook of Suicide Assessment and Management,* Simon, Robert and Robert Hales, (eds.). Washington, DC: American Psychiatric Publishing, 2006, p. 107.

44. Ash, "Children and Adolescents."

45. Hammad, T. A., et al. "Suicidality in Pediatric Patients Treated with Antidepressant Drugs." *Archives of General Psychiatry,* Vol. 63, No. 3, March 2006, pp. 332–339.

46. Hirsch J. K., et al. "Optimism and Suicide Ideation Among Young Adult College Students," *Archives of Suicide Research,* Vol. 11, No. 2, 2007, pp. 177–185.

47. Miller, Matthew, et al. "Household Firearm Ownership and Rates of Suicide Across the 50 United States." *Journal of Trauma-Injury Infection & Critical Care,* Vol. 62, No. 4, April 2007, pp. 1029–1035.

48. Pompili, M., et al. "Body Uneasiness and Suicide Risk in a Non-Clinical Sample of University Students," *Archives of Suicide Research,* Vol. 11, No. 2, 2007, pp. 193–202.

49. American College Health Association, "American College Health Association National College Health Assessment Spring 2006 Reference Group Data Report (Abridged)."

50. Frankenberger, Kristi, et al. "Effects of Information on College Students' Perceptions of Antidepressant Medication." *Journal of American College Health,* Vol. 53, No. 1, July–August 2004, p. 35.

51. Wu, Ping, et al. "Use of Complementary and Alternative Medicine among Women with Depression: Results of a National Survey." *Psychiatric Services,* Vol. 58, March 2007, pp. 349–356.

Chapter 5

1. American College Health Association. "American College Health Association National College Health Assessment Spring 2006 Reference Group Data Report (Abridged.)" *Journal of American College Health,* Vol. 55, No. 4, January-February 2007, pp. 195–206.

2. "Top Trends Predicted in an American College of Sports Medicine Survey —Health and Fitness Solutions Sought for Young and Old." *Journal of Musculoskeletal Medicine,* Vol. 24, No. 1, January 1, 2007, p. 8.

3. Wall, Sarah, et al. "Gender Differences in Cortical Response to Physical Activity: Comparing Young Children with Adults." *Research Quarterly for Exercise and Sport,* Vol. 78, No. 1, February 2007, p. A-22(2).

4. Keller, Joy. "U.S. to Introduce New Physical Activity Guidelines: IDEA Members Share Their Visions for What the Recommendations Should Include." *IDEA Fitness Journal,* Vol. 4, No. 1, January 2007, p. 16(1).

5. Carnation, M. R., et al. "Prevalence and Cardiovascular Disease Correlates of Low Cardiorespiratory Fitness in Adolescents and Adults." *Journal of the American Medical Association,* Vol. 294, No. 23, December 21, 2005, pp. 2981–2988.

6. Keller, Joy. "U.S. to Introduce New Physical Activity Guidelines."

7. Behrens, Timothy, et al. "Vigorous Physical Activity Among College Students: Findings from the 2005 Utah Higher Education Health Behavior Survey." *Research Quarterly for Exercise and Sport,* Vol. 78, No. 1, February 2007, p. A-89(1).

8. Alman, Robert E., et al. "Impact of the First Semester College Experience on Cardiovascular Risk Factor Development." *Research Quarterly for Exercise and Sport,* Vol. 78, No. 1, February 2007, p. A-23(1).

9. Zhang, Tao, et al. "Examining Environmental Influences on College Students' Participation in Physical Activity." *Research Quarterly for Exercise and Sport,* Vol. 78, No. 1, February 2007, p. A-38(1).

10. Reed, Julian. "Perceptions of the Availability of Recreational Physical Activity Facilities on a University Campus." *Journal of American College Health,* Vol. 55, No. 4, January–February 2007, pp. 189–194.

11. "Physical Activity May Help Protect Aging Eyes." *Tufts University Health & Nutrition Letter,* Vol. 24, No. 9, January 2007, p. 8(1).

12. Wright, Hillary. "Getting Physically Active May Increase Your Chances of Surviving Cancer." *Environmental Nutrition,* Vol. 30, No. 3, March 2007, p. 1.

13. Ibid.

14. Leung, Raymond, et al. "Preventing and Treating Type 2 Diabetes Through a Physically Active Lifestyle," *JOPERD—The Journal*

of *Physical Education, Recreation & Dance,* Vol. 78, No. 4, April 2007, p. 38(5).

15. Bauer, Jeff. "Regular Exercise May Help Ward Off Dementia." *RN,* Vol. 69, No. 3, March 2006, p. 20.

16. "Fitness and Cognitive Ability in Elderly." *The Futurist,* Vol. 41, No. 1, January–February 2007, p. 2(1).

17. "Step Up to Denser Bones." *Science News,* Vol. 167, No. 17, April 23, 2005, p. 270.

18. "Physical Activity for Lifelong Bone Health: The American College of Sports Medicine Promotes Osteoporosis Prevention." *Journal of Musculoskeletal Medicine,* Vol. 22, No. 1, January 2005, p. 6.

19. Penhollow, Tina, and Michael Young. "Sexual Desirability and Sexual Performance: Does Exercise and Fitness Really Matter?" *Electronic Journal of Human Sexuality,* Vol. 7, October 5, 2004, www.ejhs.org.

20. Penhollow, Tina, et al. "Impact of Physical Fitness on Older Adult Sexual Desirability and Sexual Performance." *Research Quarterly for Exercise and Sport,* Vol. 78, No. 1, February 2007, p. A-35(1).

21. Keller, Joy. "U.S. to Introduce New Physical Activity Guidelines."

22. Mitchell, Murray, et al. "Living the Physically Active Lifestyle: A Profile of College Students Enrolled in Elective Physical Activity Courses." *Research Quarterly for Exercise and Sport,* Vol. 78, No. 1, February 2007, p. A-68(1).

23. Screws, Doris, et al. "Exploring Perceptual Gender Differences Toward Lifetime Fitness and Wellness Classes Among College Students." *Research Quarterly for Exercise and Sport,* Vol. 78, No. 1, February 2007, p. A-21(2).

24. Liu, Xinian, et al. "Value-Based Motivation for Physical Activity and Physical Education: A Case of College Students in China." *Research Quarterly for Exercise and Sport,* Vol. 78, No. 1, February 2007, p. A-66(1).

25. Huang, Ming-Xue, et al. "College Female Students' Fitness Levels, Learning Motivation, and Attitudes in a Physical Education Setting." *Research Quarterly for Exercise and Sport,* Vol. 78, No. 1, February 2007, p. A-18(2).

26. Beauchamp, Mark, et al. "Older Adults' Preferences for Exercising Alone Versus in Groups: Considering Contextual Congruence." *Annals of Behavioral Medicine,* Vol. 33, No. 2, April 2007.

27. Haskell, William, et al. "Physical Activity and Public Health: Updated Recommendations for Adults from the American College of Sports Medicine and the American Heart Association." *Medicine and Science in Sports and Exercise,* August 2007, www.acsm-msse.org.

28. www.acsm.org.

29. "Moderate Exercise: No Pain, Big Gains." *Harvard Men's Health Watch,* May 2007, p. NA.

30. Church, Timothy, et al. "Effects of Different Doses of Physical Activity on Cardiorespiratory Fitness Among Sedentary, Overweight or Obese Postmenopausal Women with Elevated Blood Pressure: A Randomized Controlled Trial." *Journal of the American Medical Association,* Vol. 297, No. 19, May 16, 2007, pp. 2053–2158.

31. "Women with Pedometers Step Up Exercise Levels." American College of Sports Medicine, News Release, April 5, 2005.

32. Keller, Joy. "Does Stretching Improve Performance?" *IDEA Fitness Journal,* Vol. 2, No. 1, January 2005, p. 16.

33. Mosca, Lorie, et al. "Waist Circumference Predicts Cardiometabolic and Global Framingham Risk among Women Screened during National Women's Heart Day." *Journal of Women's Health,* Vol. 15, No. 1, January 2006, pp. 24–34.

34. Serpico, Robert, et al. "Vigorous Physical Activity and Fruit and Vegetable Consumption in a Large Cohort of College Students." *Research Quarterly for Exercise and Sport,* Vol. 78, No. 1, February 2007, p. A-36(2).

35. "Hydration Tips for Runners: American College of Sports Medicine Clarifies Balancing of Fluid Loss/Intake." Journal of Musculoskeletal Medicine, Vol. 22, No. 6, June 2005, p. 320.

36. Hartman, Joseph, et al. "Consumption of fat-free fluid milk after resistance exercise promotes greater lean mass accretion than does consumption of soy or carbohydrate in young, novice, male weightlifters." *American Journal of Clinical Nutrition,* Vol. 86, August 2007, pp. 373–81.

37. Garman, F., et al. "Occurrence of Exercise Dependence in a College-Aged Population." *Journal of American College Health,* Vol. 52, No. 5, March–April 2004, p. 221.

Chapter 6

1. Pierce, John, et al. "Influence of a Diet Very High in Vegetables, Fruit, and Fiber and Low in Fat on Prognosis Following Treatment for Breast Cancer." *Journal of the American Medical Association,* Vol. 298, No. 3, July 18, 2007, pp. 289–298.

2. Schulze, M.B., et al. "Fiber and Magnesium Intake and Incidence of Type 2 Diabetes: A Prospective Study and Meta-analysis." *Archives of Internal Medicine,* Vol. 167, No. 9, May 14, 2007, pp. 956–965.

3. Mellen, P. B., et al. "Whole Grain Intake and Cardiovascular Disease: A Meta-analysis." *Nutrition, Metabolism and Cardiovascular Disease,* April 19, 2007, [Epub ahead of print].

4. University of Sydney, Australia, Glycemic Index Testing Service, Human Nutrition Unit, www.glycemicindex.com.

5. Hooper, Lee, et al. "Risks and Benefits of Omega 3 Fats for Mortality, Cardiovascular Disease, and Cancer: Systematic Review." *British Medical Journal,* Vol. 332, No. 7544, April 1, 2006, pp. 752–760.

6. Brunner, Eric. "Oily Fish and Omega 3 Fat Supplements." *British Medical Journal,* Vol. 332, No. 7544, April 1, 2006, pp. 739–740.

7. *Dietary Guidelines for Americans 2005,* USD-HHS, USDA.

8. Jackson, R. D., et al. "Calcium Plus Vitamin D Supplementation and the Risk of Fractures." *New England Journal of Medicine,* Vol. 354, February 16, 2006, pp. 669–683.

9. Bjelakovic, Goran, et al. "Mortality in Randomized Trials of Antioxidant Supplements for Primary and Secondary Prevention." *Journal of the American Medical Association,* Vol. 297, No. 8, February 28, 2007, pp. 842–855.

10. Lester, Greg. "No Magic Tomato? Study Breaks Link between Lycopene and Prostate Cancer Prevention." American Association for Cancer Resarch, news release, May 16, 2007.

11. "Vitamin E Gets an F." *Harvard Health Letter,* June 2005.

12. "The Riddle of MyPyramid." *Harvard Heart Letter,* April 2006.

13. "One Year Later: Lessons from New Guidelines and Pyramid." *Tufts University Health & Nutrition Letter,* Vol. 23, No. 12, February 2006, p. 4(2).

14. "Prevalence of Fruit and Vegetable Consumption and Physical Activity by Race/Ethnicity—United States, 2005." *MMWR Weekly,* Vol. 56, No. 13, April 6, 2007, pp. 301–304.

15. "Rebuilding the Pyramid: The Government's New Food Pyramid Replaces 'One Size Fits All' with a Customizable Eating and Exercise Plan." *Tufts University Health & Nutrition Letter,* Vol. 23, No. 4, June 2005, p. 1.

16. Vartanian, Lenny, et al. "Consumption StereotypeWhat You Eat." *Appetite,* Vol. 48, 2007, pp. 265–277.

17. Gray, L. E., et al. "Assessment of Dietary Fiber Intake Among University Students." *Journal of the American Dietetic Association,* Vol. 104, No. 8, August 2004, p. A26.

18. Vartanian, L.R., et al. "Effects of Soft Drink Consumption on Nutrition and Health: A Systematic Review and Meta-analysis." *American Journal of Public Health.* Vol. 97, No. 4, April 2007, pp. 667–675.

19. Brody, Jane. "You Are Also What You Drink." *New York Times,* March 27, 2007.

20. Vartanian, et al., "Effects of Soft Drink Consumption on Nutrition and Health."

21. Dhingra, Ravi, et al. "Soft Drink Consumption and Risk of Developing Cardiometabolic Risk Factors and the Metabolic Syndrome in Middle-Aged Adults in the Community." *Circulation,* 2007, [Epub ahead of print July 23, 2007].

22. Worcester, Sharon. "Sales of Energy Drinks Top $3 Billion—But at What Cost?" *Clinical Psychiatry News,* Vol. 35, No. 3, March 2007, p. 42(1).

23. "The Problem with Energy Drinks." *MMR,* Vol. 24, No. 1, January 8, 2007, p. 73.

24. Worcester, Sharon. "Sales of Energy Drinks Top $3 Billion—But at What Cost?"

25. Ibid.

26. "Mediterranean Diet Protects Against Asthma." *GP,* April 20, 2007, p. 18. Elec. Coll.: A162286922.

27. Varraso, Raphaelle, et al. "Prospective Study of Dietary Patterns and Chronic Obstructive Pulmonary Disease among U.S. Men." *Thorax,* www.tiraxjnl.com, May 2007.

28. Conklin, Martha, et al. "Nutrition Information at Point of Selection Could Benefit College Students." *Topics in Clinical Nutrition*, Vol. 20, No. 2, April–June 2005, p. 90(7).
29. Chapman, Jean, et al. "Food Allergy: A Practice Parameter." *Annals of Allergy, Asthma and Immunology*, Vol. 96, No. 3, Supp. 2, March 2006, pp. 1–68.

Chapter 7

1. "Global Strategy on Diet, Physical Activity and Health." World Health Organization, www.who.int/dietphysicalactivity/publications/facts/obesity/en/.
2. Ogden, Cynthia, et al. "Prevalence of Overweight and Obesity in the United States, 1999–2004." *Journal of the American Medical Association*, Vol. 295, No. 13, April 5, 2006, pp. 1549.
3. "Weigh Less, Live Longer." *Harvard Health Letter*, January 3, 2007. Online.
4. Vartanian L.R., et al. "Effects of Soft Drink Consumption on Nutrition and Health: A Systematic Review and Meta-analysis." *American Journal of Public Health*, Vol. 97, No. 4, April 2007, pp. 667–675.
5. Pereira, M. A., et al. "Fast-food Habits, Weight Gain, and Insulin Resistance (The CARDIA Study): 15-year Prospective Analysis." *Lancet*, Vol. 365, No. 9453, January 1, 2005, pp. 36–42.
6. Frayling, T. M., Timpson, N. J. Weedon, M. N., et al. "A Common Variant in the FTO Gene Is Associated with Body Mass Index and Predisposes to Childhood and Adult Obesity." *Science*, Vol. 316, 2007, pp. 889–894.
7. Christakis, N. A., and J. H. Fowler. "The Spread of Obesity in a Large Social Network over 32 Years." *New England Journal of Medicine*, Vol. 357, No. 4, July 26, 2007, pp. 370–379.
8. Barabási, Albert-László. "Network Medicine—From Obesity to the Diseasome." *New England Journal of Medicine*, Vol. 357, No. 4, July 26, 2007, pp. 404–407.
9. Davison, Tany, and Marita McCabe. "Relationships Between Men's and Women's Body Image and Their Psychological, Social, and Sexual Functioning." *Sex Roles: A Journal of Research*, Vol. 52, No. 7–8, April 2005, p. 463.
10. Roy, Jane, et al. "Percent Body Fat Is Related to Body Shape Perception and Dissatisfaction." *Research Quarterly for Exercise and Sport*, Vol. 78, No. 1, February 2007, p. A-84.
11. Wing, Rena. Presentation, Obesity Society, Boston, October 2006.
12. Houston, Denise, et al. "The Association Between Weight History and Physical Performance in the Health, Aging and Body Composition Study." *International Journal of Obesity*, May 22, 2007 [Epub ahead of print].
13. "Trimmer Waistline May Mean a Sharper Mind." *Tufts University Health & Nutrition Letter*, Vol. 24, No. 12, February 2007, p. 8(1).
14. Simons-Morton, Denise, et al. "Obesity Research—Limitations of Methods, Measurements, and Medications." *Journal of the American Medical Association*, Vol. 295, No. 7, February 15, 2006, p. 826.

15. Yan, Lijing, et al. "Excessive Adiposity, Calorie Restriction, and Aging." *Journal of the American Medical Association*, Vol. 295, No. 13, April 5, 2006, p. 1577.
16. Eisenberg, Marla, et al. "Weight-Related Issues and High-Risk Sexual Behaviors among College Students." *Journal of American College Health*, Vol. 54, No. 2, September–October 2005, p. 95.
17. American College Health Association. "American College Health Association National College Health Assessment Spring 2006 Reference Group Data Report (Abridged)." *Journal of American College Health*, Vol. 55, No. 4, January–February 2007, pp. 195–206.
18. Redman, Leeanne, et al. "Effect of Calorie Restriction with or without Exercise on Body Composition and Fat Distribution." *Journal of Clinical Endocrinology & Metabolism*, Vol. 92, No. 3, March 2007, pp. 867–872.
19. Dansinger, Michael, et al. "Meta-analysis: The Effect of Dietary Counseling for Weight Loss," *Annals of Internal Medicine*, Vol. 147, No. 1, July 3, 2007, pp. 41–50.
20. Gardner, Christophere, et al. "Comparison of the Atkins, Zone, Ornish, and LEARN Diets for Change in Weight and Related Risk Factors among Overweight Premenopausal Women." *Journal of the American Medical Association*, Vol. 297, No. 9, March 7, 2007, pp. 969–977.
21. "Low-Carbohydrate Diets: A Place in Health Promotion?" *Family Practice News*, Vol. 37, No. 10, p. 30(1).
22. "What the Latest Diet Trial Really Means: Any Diet That Helps You Take in Fewer Calories Will Help You Shed Pounds." *Harvard Heart Letter*, Vol. 17, No. 9, p. 5.
23. Ebbeling, Cara, et al. "Effects of a Low-Glycemic Load vs. Low-Fat Diet in Obese Young Adults." *Journal of the American Medical Association*, Vol. 297, No. 19, May 16, 2007, pp. 2092–2102.
24. Thomas, D. E., E. J. Elliott, and L. Baur. "Low Glycaemic Index or Low Glycaemic Load Diets for Overweight and Obesity," *Cochrane Database of Systematic Reviews*, Issue 3, 2007.
25. Blanck, H. M., et al. "Use of Nonprescription Dietary Supplements for Weight Loss Is Common among Americans." *Journal of the American Dietetic Association*, Vol. 107, No. 3, March 2007, pp. 441–447.
26. Levine, James, et al. "Interindividual Variation in Posture Allocation: Possible Role in Human Obesity." *Science*, Vol. 307, No. 5709, January 28, 2005, p. 584.
27. Voelker, Rebecca. "Losers Can Win at Weight Maintenance." *Journal of the American Medical Association*, Vol. 298, No. 3, pp. 272–273.
28. Simons-Morton, Denise, et al. "Obesity Research—Limitations of Methods, Measurements, and Medications."
29. Tsai, Wilson, et al. "Bariatric Surgery in Adolescents: Recent National Trends in Use and In-Hospital Outcome," *Archives of Pediatrics & Adolescent Medicine*, Vol. 161, No. 3, March 2007, pp. 217–221.

30. Singh, Sonal, et al. "Wernicke Encephalopathy after Obesity Surgery: A Systematic Review." *Neurology*, Vol. 68, March 2007, pp. 807–811.
31. Hunt, J. S. and A. J. Rothman, "College Students' Mental Models for Recognizing Anorexia and Bulimia Nervosa." *Appetite*, Vol. 48, No. 3, May 2007, pp. 289–300.
32. Frank, Guido, et al. "Increased Dopamine D2/D3 Receptor Binding After Recovery from Anorexia Nervosa Measured by Positron Emission Tomography and [(11)C] Raclopride." *Biological Psychiatry*, June 28, 2005.
33. Dominguez, J., et al. "Treatment of Anorexia Nervosa Is Associated with Increases in Bone Mineral Density, and Recovery Is a Biphasic Process Involving Both Nutrition and Return of Menses." *Journal of Clinical Nutrition*, Vol. 86, No. 1, July 2007, pp. 92–99.
34. Levine, D., et al. "A Self Psychological and Relational Approach to Group Therapy for University Students with Bulimia." *International Journal of Group Psychotherapy*, Vol. 57, No. 2, April 2007, pp. 167–185.

Chapter 8

1. Hale, Cara. "Social Support and Physical Health: The Importance of Belonging." *Journal of American College Health*, Vol. 53, No. 6, May–June 2005, p. 276.
2. Maple, Marilyn. Personal interview.
3. Goulston, Mark. Personal Interview.
4. Hall, Judith. Personal interview.
5. Stepp, Laura Sessions. *Unhooked*. New York: Riverhead, 2007.
6. Carroll, Janell. *Sexuality Now*, 2nd edition. Belmont: Thomson-Wadsworth, 2007.
7. Lito, Mie. "Self-Disclosure in Romantic Relationships and Friendships Among American and Japanese College Students." *The Journal of Social Psychology*, Vol. 145, No. 2, April 2005, p. 127.
8. Billingham, Robert. Personal interview.
9. Yager, Jan. Personal interview.
10. Miller, Laura. "Physical Abuse in College Dating Relationships." *Research Quarterly for Exercise and Sport*, Vol. 78, No. 1, February 2007, p. A-33.
11. Laumann, Edward. Personal interview.
12. Luo, Shanhong, and Eva Klohnen. "Assortative Mating and Marital Quality in Newlyweds: A Couple-Centered Approach." *Journal of Personality and Social Psychology*, Vol. 88, No. 2, February 2005.
13. Buss, David. *The Evolution of Desire*. New York: Basic Books, 1994.
14. Fisher, Helen. Personal interview.
15. U.S. Census Bureau, Washington, DC, www.census.gov.
16. U.S. Census Bureau.
17. Dnes, Antony. "Marriage, Cohabitation, and Same-Sex Marriage." *Independent Review*, Vol. 12, No. 1, Summer 2007, p. 85(15).
18. Ibid.
19. Crooks, Robert, and Karla Baur. *Our Sexuality*, 8th ed. Pacific Grove, CA: Wadsworth, 2002.
20. Sternberg, Robert. Personal interview.
21. National Center for Health Statistics, Washington, DC, www.cdc.gov/nchs.

22. Davidson, Jon. "Fundamental Rights for All." *National Law Journal,* June 11, 2007.
23. Crooks and Baur. *Our Sexuality.*
24. The Gottman Institute, Seattle, WA, www.gottman.com.
25. Neff, L. A., and B. R. Karney. "Gender Differences in Social Support: A Question of Skill or Responsiveness?" *Journal of Personality and Social Psychology,* Vol. 88, 2005, p. 79.
26. U.S. Census Bureau.
27. Dnes, "Marriage, Cohabitation, and Same-Sex Marriage."

Chapter 9

1. Herman-Giddens, Marcia. Personal interview.
2. Bertone-Johnson, Elizabeth, et al. "Calcium and Vitamin D Intake and Risk of Incident Premenstrual Syndrome." *Archives of Internal Medicine,* Vol. 165, June 2005, p. 1246.
3. "Adult Male Circumcision Significantly Reduces Risk of Acquiring HIV." *NIH News,* December 13, 2006.
4. Crooks, Robert, and Karla Baur. *Our Sexuality,* 8th ed. Pacific Grove, CA: Wadsworth, 2002.
5. Centers for Disease Control and Prevention, Washington, DC, www.cdc.gov.
6. "National Survey of Adolescents and Young Adults: Sexual Health Knowledge, Attitudes, and Experiences." Menlo Park, CA: Kaiser Family Foundation, 2003.
7. Ibid.
8. Carroll, Janell L. *Sexuality Now: Embracing Diversity,* 2nd ed. Belmont, CA: Thomson-Wadsworth, 2007.
9. Martens, Matthew, et al. "Differences Between Actual and Perceived Student Norms: An Examination of Alcohol Use, Drug Use, and Sexual Behavior." *Journal of American College Health,* Vol. 54, No. 5, March–April 2006, p. 295.
10. Raffaelli, Marccela, et al. "Acculturation Status and Sexuality among Female Cuban American College Students." *Journal of American College Health,* Vol. 54, No. 1, July–August 2005, p. 7
11. Ibid.
12. Meston, Cindy, and David Buss. "Why Humans Have Sex." *Archives of Sexual Behavior,* August 2007, Vol. 36; pp. 477-507.
13. Ford, C. L., et al. "Black Sexuality, Social Construction, and Research Targeting 'The Down Low.'" *Annals of Epidemiology,* Vol. 17, No. 3, March 2007, pp. 209-216.
14. Caroll, *Sexuality Now.*
15. Kenagy, Gretchen. "Transgender Health: Findings from Two Needs Assessment Studies in Philadelphia." *Health and Social Work,* Vol. 30, No. 1, February 2005, p. 19.
16. Trenholm, Christopher, et al. "Impacts of Four Title V Section 520 Abstinence Education Programs: Final Report." Princeton: Mathematica Policy Research, 2007.
17. Selvin, E., et al. "Prevalence and Risk Factors for Erectile Dysfunction in the U.S." *American Journal of Medicine,* Vol. 120, No. 2, February 2007, pp. 151-157.
18. O'Leary, Michael Philip. *What to Do about Erectile Dysfunction.* Boston: Harvard Health Publications, 2007.

Chapter 10

1. Guttmacher Institute, www.guttmacher.org.
2. American College Health Association. "American College Health Association National College Health Assessment Spring 2006 Reference Group Data Report (Abridged)." *Journal of American College Health,* Vol. 55, No. 4, January–February 2007, pp. 195–206.
3. American College Health Association. American College Health Association-National College Health Assessment (ACHA-NCHA) Web Summary, www.acha.org/projects_programs/ncha_sampledata.cfm.
4. Crosby, Richard, et al. "Condom Discomfort and Associated Problems with Their Use among University Students." *Journal of American College Health,* Vol. 54, No. 3, November–December 2005, p. 143.
5. James, Chris. "Prevalence of Erectile Dysfunction and Use of ED Medications Among Teens, Young Men." News Release, Children's Memorial Hospital and Northwestern University, April 24, 2006.
6. Macaluso, M., et al. "Efficacy of the Male Latex Condom and of the Female Polyurethane Condom as Barriers to Semen during Intercourse: A Randomized Clinical Trial." *American Journal of Epidemiology.* Vol. 166, No. 1, July 2007, pp. 88–96.
7. Roberts, J. N., et al. "Genital Transmission of HPV in a Mouse Model is Potentiated by Nonoxynol-9 and Inhibited by Carrageenan." *Nature Medicine,* Vol. 13, No. 7, July 2007 pp. 857–861.
8. U.S. Food and Drug Administration, www.fda.gov.
9. "FDA Approves Contraceptive for Continuous Use." *FDA News,* May 22, 2007.
10. "Birth Control Patch-Wearers at Higher Risk of Blood Clots." *Contemporary OB/GYN,* Vol. 5, No. 1, January 2006, p. 17.
11. Ibid.
12. "Birth Control and Weight Gain." *Family Practice News,* Vol. 36, No. 5, March 1, 2006, p. 21(1).
13. Fennell, Reginald. "The Emperor Has No Clothes": Emergency Contraception Should Be Available Over-the-Counter." *Journal of American College Health,* Vol. 54, No. 5, March–April 2006, p. 257(3).
14. "Plan B for Consumers," www.gotoplanb.com.
15. Foster, D.G., et al. "Trends in Knowledge of Emergency Contraception among Women in California, 1998–2004." *Women's Health Issues,* Vol 17, No. 1, January–February 2007, pp. 22–28.
16. American College Health Association. "ACHA-NCHA Spring 2004 Reference Group Data Report."
17. Miller, Laura McKeller, and Robin Sawyer. "Emergency Contraceptive Pills: A 10-Year Follow-Up Survey of Use and Experiences at College Health Centers in the Mid-Atlantic United States." *Journal of American College Health,* Vol. 54, No. 5, March–April 2006, p. 257(3).
18. Michels, Karin, et al. "Induced and Spontaneous Abortion and Incidence of Breast Cancer Among Young Women: A Prospective Cohort Study." *Archives of Internal Medicine,* Vol. 167, 2007, pp. 814–820.
19. "A Question of Life and Death," *The Economist* (US), Vol. 383, No. 8529, May 19, 2007 p. 66.
20. ACOG Committee on Practice Bulletins. "Screening for Fetal Chromosomal Abnormalities." *Obstetrics & Gynecology,* Vol. 109, January 2007, pp. 217–228.
21. Wright V. C., et al. "Assisted Reproductive Technology Surveillance—United States, 2004." *MMWR Surveillance Summary,* Vol. 56, No. 6, June 8 2007, pp. 1–22.
22. Ibid.

Chapter 11

1. *2007 World Drug Report.* New York: United Nations Office on Drugs and Crime, 2007.
2. "Prescription Drugs: Abuse and Addiction," National Institute on Drug Abuses (NIDA), www.nida.gov.
3. Kuehn, Bridget. "Prescription Drug Abuse Rises Globally," *Journal of the American Medical Association,* Vol. 297, No. 12, March 28, 2007, p. 1306.
4. *Wasting the Best and the Brightest: Substance Abuse at America's Colleges and Universities.* New York: National Center on Addiction and Substance Abuse at Columbia University, March 2007.
5. Ibid.
6. Platz, Laurie, et al. "Gambling by Underage College Students: Preferences and Pathology." *College Student Journal,* Vol. 39, No. 1, March 2005, p. 3.
7. Califano, Joseph. "Wasting the Best and the Brightest: Alcohol and Drug Abuse on College Campuses." *America,* Vol. 196, No. 19, May 28, 2007, p. 16(3).
8. *Wasting the Best and Brightest: Substance Abuse at America's Colleges and Universities.*
9. Ibid.
10. Ibid.
11. Ibid.
12. Ibid.
13. Ibid.
14. Institute for Safe Medication Practices, www.ismp.org.
15. "Expert Warns of Overdose of Over-the-Counter Pain Medication." News release, University of Michigan Health System, March 6, 2006.
16. "National Institutes of Health State-of-the-Science Conference Statement: Manifestations and Management of Chronic Insomnia in Adults." Bethesda, MD: National Institutes of Health, 2005.
17. McCabe, Sean, et al. "Medical Use, Illicit Use, and Diversion of Abusable Prescription Drugs." *Journal of American College Health,* Vol. 54, No. 5, March–April 2006, p. 269.
18. Labig, Chalmer, et al. *Journal of American College Health,* Vol. 54, No. 3, November–December 2005, p. 177.
19. Kuehn, "Prescription Drug Abuse Rises Globally."
20. National Institute on Drug Abuse, www.nida.gov.

21. "Prescription Drug Abuse Still Rising, Illicit Drug Abuse Still Falling.(Monitoring the Future survey)," *Alcoholism & Drug Abuse Weekly,* Vol. 19, No. 1, January 2007, p. p4(2).

22. Moon, Mary Ann. "Tenfold increase seen in abuse of OTC Cold Drug." *Clinical Psychiatry News,* Vol. 35, No. 1, January 2007, p. 31(1).

23. Kuehn, "Prescription Drug Abuse Rises Globally."

24. Schneider, Mary Ellen. "Motivations of Opioid and Stimulant Abusers Differ." *Clinical Psychiatry News,* Vol. 35, No. 2, February 2007, p. 36(1).

25. White, Barbara, et al. "Stimulant Medication Use, Misuse, and Abuse in an Undergraduate and Graduate Student Sample." *Journal of American College Health,* Vol. 54, No. 5, March–April 2006, p. 261.

26. McCabe, S. E., et al. "Nonmedical Use of Prescription Opioids Among U.S. College Students: Prevalence and Correlates from a National Survey." *Addiction Behavior,* May 2005, Vol. 30, No. 4, pp. 789–805.

27. Leamon, Martin, et al. "Substance-Related Disorders," *Textbook of Clinical Psychiatry.* Washington, DC: American Psychiatric Press, 2008.

28. Duncan, Greg, et al. "Peer Effects in Drug Use and Sex Among College Students." *Journal of Abnormal College Psychology,* Vol. 33, No. 3, June 2005, p. 375.

29. "A Third of 21–25-Year-Old Drivers Drank or Used Drugs in First Year." *Alcoholism & Drug Abuse Weekly,* Vol. 17, No. 26, July 11, 2005, p. 7(1).

30. "Marijuana and Mental Health Problems." *Drug Detection Report,* Vol. 15, No. 13, June 30, 2005, p. 104.

31. Hayatbakhsh, Mohammad, et al. "Cannabis and Anxiety and Depression in Young Adults: A Large Prospective Study." *Journal of the American Academy of Child and Adolescent Psychiatry,* Vol. 46, No. 3, March 2007, p. 408(10).

32. Moore, Theresa, et al. "Cannabis Use and Risk of Psychotic or Affective Mental Health Outcomes: A Systematic Review." *The Lancet,* Vol. 370, 2007, pp. 319–328.

33. Messinis, L., et al. "Neuropsychological Deficits in Long-Term Frequent Cannabis Users." *Neurology,* Vol. 66, No. 5, March 14, 2006, pp. 737–739.

34. Colyar, Margaret, and Tracy Call-Schmidt. "Methamphetamine Abuse in the Primary Care Patient." *Clinician Reviews,* Vol. 16, No. 3, March 2006, p. 55.

35. Curtis, E. K. "Meth Mouth: A Review of Methamphetamine Abuse and Its Oral Manifestations." *General Dentistry,* Vol. 54, No. 2, March–April, 2006, pp. 125–129.

36. Williams, Janet, and Michael Storck. "Inhalant Abuse." *Pediatrics,* Vol. 119, No. 5, May 2007, p. 1009(9).

37. National Institute on Drug Abuse, www.nida.nih.gov.

38. White, Helene, et al. "Evaluating Two Brief Substance-Use Interventions for Mandated College Students." *Journal of Studies on Alcohol,* Vol. 67, No. 2, March 2006, p. 309(9).

39. MacNeil, Jane. "Medications for Addictions Are Safer and More Effective." *Family Practice News.* April 1, 2007.

Chapter 12

1. National Institute on Alcohol Abuse and Alcoholism, www.niaaa.nih.gov.

2. Ibid.

3. American College Health Association. "American College Health Association National College Health Assessment Spring 2006 Reference Group Data Report (Abridged)." *Journal of American College Health,* Vol. 55, No. 4, January–February 2007, pp. 195–206.

4. Timberlake, D. S., et al. "College Attendance and Its Effect on Drinking Behaviors in a Longitudinal Study of Adolescents." *Alcoholism: Clinical and Experimental Research,* Vol. 31, No. 6, June 2007.

5. LaBrie, Joseph, et al. "Classifying Risky-Drinking College Students: Another Look at the Two-Week Drinker-Type Categorization," *Journal of Studies on Alcohol,* Vol. 68, No. 1, January 2007, p. 86(5).

6. *Wasting the Best and the Brightest: Substance Abuse at America's Colleges and Universities.* New York: National Center on Addiction and Substance Abuse at Columbia University, March 2007.

7. American College Health Association. "American College Health Association National College Health Assessment Spring 2006 Reference Group Data Report."

8. *Wasting the Best and the Brightest.*

9. Westmaas, Johann, et al. "Validation of a Measure of College Students' Intoxicated Behaviors: Associations with Alcohol Outcome Expectancies, Drinking Motives, and Personality." *Journal of American College Health,* Vol. 55, No. 4, January–February 2007, p. 227(11).

10. Eisenbarth, Chris. "Psychological Distress, Coping Deficits, and the Tendency to Drink Alcohol to Cope in a College Population." *Research Quarterly for Exercise and Sport,* Vol. 78, No. 1, February 2007, p. A-26(1).

11. Neighbors, Clayton, et al. "Are Social Norms the Best Predictor of Outcomes Among Heavy-Drinking College Students?" *Journal of Studies on Alcohol and Drugs,* Vol. 68, No. 4, July 2007, p. 556(10).

12. Sessa, Frances. "Peer Crowds in a Commuter College Sample: The Relation Between Self-Reported Alcohol Use and Perceived Peer Crowd Norms." *Journal of Psychology,* Vol. 141, No. 3, May 2007, p. 293(13).

13. Neighbors, Clayton, et al. "Social Anxiety as a Moderator of the Relationship Between Perceived Norms and Drinking." *Journal of Studies on Alcohol and Drugs,* Vol. 68, 2007, pp. 91–96.

14. College Drinking Prevention, www.collegedrinkingprevention.gov.

15. *Wasting the Best and the Brightest.*

16. Ibid.

17. Ford, Jason. "Substance Use Among College Athletes: A Comparison Based on Sport/Team Affiliation." *Journal of American College Health,* Vol. 55, No. 6, May–June 2007, p. 367(7).

18. Ransdell, Lynda, et al. "Higher, Faster, Stronger, Drunker? The Need for Effective Strategies to Prevent Alcohol Abuse Among Female Athletes." *JOPERD—The Journal of Physical Education, Recreation & Dance,* Vol. 78, No. 3, March 2007, p. 5(4).

19. Grossbard, Joel, et al. "Are Drinking Games Sports? College Athlete Participation in Drinking Games and Alcohol-Related Problems." *Journal of Studies on Alcohol,* Vol. 68, No. 1, January 2007, p. 97(9).

20. Wallenstein, Gene, et al. "Results of National Alcohol Screening Day: College Demographics, Clinical Characteristics, and Comparison with Online Screening." *Journal of American College Health,* Vol. 55, No. 6, May–June 2007, p. 341(9).

21. Misch, Donald. "'Natural Recovery' from Alcohol Abuse Among College Students." *Journal of American College* Health, Vol. 55, No. 4, January–February 2007, p. 215(4).

22. Williams, Ronald, and Donald Belcher. " Alcohol-Related Social and Personal Problems of Undergraduate College Students," *Research Quarterly for Exercise and Sport,* Vol. 78, No. 1, February 2007, p. A-37(1).

23. American College Health Association. "American College Health Association National College Health Assessment Spring 2006 Reference Group Data Report."

24. McCabe, Sean, et al. "Alcohol-Use Disorders and Nonmedical Use of Prescription Drugs Among U.S. College Students." *Journal of Studies on Alcohol and Drugs,* Vol. 68, No. 1, July 2007, p. 543(5).

25. Westmaas, et al., "Validation of a Measure of College Students' Intoxicated Behaviors."

26. Singleton, Royce. "Collegiate Alcohol Consumption and Academic Performance," *Journal of Studies on Alcohol and Drugs,* Vol. 68, No. 4, July 2007, p. 548(8).

27. *Wasting the Best and the Brightest.*

28. Ibid.

29. Ibid.

30. Ibid.

31. Ibid.

32. NIAAA, College Drinking Prevention, www.collegedrinkingprevention.gov/NIAAACollegeMaterials/TaskForce/CallToAction_02.aspx#CallToAction_02_a.

33. Bersamin, Melina, et al. "Effectiveness of a Web-Based Alcohol-Misuse and Harm-Prevention Course Among High- and Low-Risk Students," *Journal of American College Health,* Vol. 55, No. 4, January–February 2007, p. 247(8).

34. Marlatt, G. Alan, and Neharika Chawla. "Meditation and Alcohol Use." *Southern Medical Journal,* Vol. 100, No. 4, April 2007, p. 451(3).

35. Martens, Matthew, et al. "Do Protective Behavioral Strategies Mediate the Relationship Between Drinking Motives and Alcohol Use in College Students?" *Journal of Studies on Alcohol and Drugs,* Vol. 68, No. 4, July 2007, pp. 106–114.

36. Weitzel, Jessica, et al. "Using Wireless Hand-held Computers and Tailored Text Messaging to Reduce Negative Consequences of Drinking Alcohol," *Journal of Studies on Alcohol and Drugs*, Vol. 68, No. 4, July 2007, p. 534(4).

37. Thombs, Dennis, et al. "Outcomes of a Technology-Based Social Norms Intervention to Deter Alcohol Use in Freshman Residence Halls." *Journal of American College Health*, Vol. 55, No. 6, May–June 2007, p. 325(8).

38. Bass, Martha, and Rosanne Keathley. "Effectiveness of Social Marketing Poster Campaigns on a University Campus." *Research Quarterly for Exercise and Sport*, Vol. 78, No. 1, February 2007, p. A-23(2).

39. White, A. M., et al. "College Students Lack Knowledge of Standard Drink Volumes: Implications for Definitions of Risky Drinking Based on Survey Data." *Alcoholism, Clinical and Experimental Research*, Vol. 29, No. 4, April 2005, pp. 631–663.

40. Nelson, T. F., et al. "'Binge' Drinking and Blood Alcohol Concentration." *Journal of Studies on Alcohol*, Vol. 66, No. 3, May 2005, pp. 438–439.

41. American Heart Association, www.americanheart.org.

42. Nichol, P. E., R. F. Krueger, and W. G. Iacono "Investigating Gender Differences in Alcohol Problems: A Latent Trait Modeling Approach." *Alcoholism: Clinical and Experimental Research*, Vol. 31, No. 5, 2007.

43. "Some Minorities Less Likely to Seek Alcohol Treatment." *Alcoholism & Drug Abuse Weekly*, Vol. 19, No. 3, January 15, 2007, p. 8(1).

44. Krantzler, Henry. "Evidence-Based Treatments for Alcohol Dependence." *Journal of the American Medical Association*, Vol. 295, No. 17, May 3, 2006, p. 2075.

45. Tonigan, J. Scott. "Spirituality and Alcoholics Anonymous." *Southern Medical Journal*, Vol. 100, No. 4, April 2007, p. 437(4).

46. Kirkpatrick, Jean. Personal interview.

47. Helping Others Stay Sober Leads to Positive Outcomes for Recovering Alcoholics." *The Brown University Digest of Addiction Theory and Application*, Vol. 24, No. 6, June 2005, p. 2(2).

48. Marlatt and Chawla, "Meditation and Alcohol Use."

Chapter 13

1. National Health Interview Survey 2007, www.cdc.gov/nchs/nhis.htm.

2. Ibid.

3. Monitoring the Future Study (Institute for Social Research, University of Michigan, www.monitoringthefuture.org.

4. American College Health Association, College Health Association National College Health Assessment (ACHA–NCHA) Web Summary, Fall 2006, www.acha-ncha.org/data_highlights.html.

5. *Wasting the Best and the Brightest: Substance Abuse at America's Colleges and Universities.*

New York: National Center on Addiction and Substance Abuse at Columbia University, March 2007.

6. Ibid.

7. Ibid.

8. Ibid.

9. Ibid.

10. "Economic Facts about U.S. Tobacco Use and Tobacco Production," Smoking & Tobacco Use Fact Sheet, www.cdc.gov.

11. *Wasting the Best and the Brightest.*

12. Connolly, Gregory, et al. *Trends in Smoke, Nicotine Yield, and Relationship to Design Characteristics among Popular U.S. Cigarette Brands.* Boston: Tobacco Research Program, Harvard School of Public Health, January 2007.

13. *Wasting the Best and the Brightest.*

14. National Health Interview Survey, 2007.

15. *Wasting the Best and the Brightest.*

16. Gullu, Hakan, et al. "Light Cigarette Smoking Impairs Coronary Microvascular Functions as Severely as Smoking Regular Cigarettes," *Heart*, Vol. 0, May 2007, pp. 1–4, www.heartjnl.com.

17. "Smokeless Tobacco," Smoking & Tobacco Use Fact Sheet, CDC, www.cdc.gov.

18. *Wasting the Best and the Brightest.*

19. Mitchell, Amy, and Thomas Parish. "Using Combination Therapy for Smoking Cessation." *Clinician Reviews*, Vol. 15, No. 5, May 2005, p. 39(8).

20. "Study Finds Online Smoking Cessation Treatments Fall Short." *The Brown University Digest of Addiction Theory and Application*, Vol. 24, No. 5, May 2005, p. 5(1).

21. Aveyard, Paul. "Managing Smoking Cessation," *BMJ*, Vol. 335, No. 7609, July 2007, pp. 37–41.

22. "Nicotine Replacement Use on the Rise." *Alcoholism & Drug Abuse Weekly*, Vol. 17, No. 31, August 15, 2005, p. 7(1).

23. Nicotrol, www.nicotrol.com.

24. "Cigarettes: The Lung Cancer Risk Lingers." *Harvard Health Letter*, July 2005.

25. "Secondhand Smoke," Smoking & Tobacco Use, CDC, www.cdc.gov.

26. Wilson, Stephen, et al. "The Role of Air Nicotine in Explaining Racial Differences in Cotinine among Tobacco-Exposed Children." *Chest*, Vol. 131, March 2007, pp. 856–862.

27. Oh, Sang Woo, et al. "Association Between Cigarette Smoking and Metabolic Syndrome." *Diabetes Care*, Vol. 28, No. 8, August 2005, p. 2064(3).

28. O'Hegarty, Michelle, et al. "Young Adults' Perceptions of Cigarette Warning Labels in the United States and Canada." *Preventing Chronic Disease*, Vol. 4, No. 2, April 2007, p. A27.

29. "Decline in Smoking Prevalence—New York City, 2002–2006," *Morbidity and Mortality Weekly Reports (MMWRs)*, Vol. 56, No. 24, June 22, 2007.

30. "Reduced Secondhand Smoke Exposure After Implementation of a Comprehensive State-wide Smoking Ban—New York." *Morbidity and Mortality Weekly Reports (MMWRs)* Vol. 56, No. 28, July 20, 2007.

Chapter 14

1. Ford, Earl, et al. "Explaining the Decrease in U.S. Deaths from Coronary Disease, 1980–2000," *New England Journal of Medicine*, Vol. 356, June 7, 2007, pp. 2388–2398.

2. Hu, Frank. "Obesity and Mortality: Watch Your Waist, Not Just Your Weight." *Archives of Internal Medicine*, Vol. 167, May 14, 2007, pp. 875–876.

3. See, Raphael, et al. "The Association of Differing Measures of Overweight and Obesity with Prevalent Atherosclerosis." *Journal of the American College of Cardiology*, Vol. 50, August 2007, p. 33-3.

4. Ardern, C. I., and I. Janssen, "Metabolic Syndrome and Its Association with Morbidity and Mortality." *Applied Physiology, Nutrition and Metabolism*, Vol. 32, No. 1, February 2007, pp. 33–45.

5. Vartanian, L.R., et al. "Effects of Soft Drink Consumption on Nutrition and Health: A Systematic Review and Meta-analysis." *American Journal of Public Health*, Vol. 97, No. 4, April 2007, pp. 667–675.

6. Torpy, Janet. "The Metabolic Syndrome." *Journal of the American Medical Association*, Vol. 295, No. 7, February 15, 2006, p. 850.

7. Fernandez, M. I., "The Metabolic Syndrome." *Nutrition Reviews*, Vol. 65, No. 6, Pt. 2, June 2007, pp. 530–534.

8. Franco, Oscar, et al. "Associations of Diabetes Mellitus with Total Life Expectancy and Life Expectancy with and without Cardiovascular Disease." *Archives of Internal Medicine*, Vol. 167, June 11, 2007, p. 1111.

9. "U.S. Predicts Diabetes Epidemic to Go on Unchecked." *HealthDay*, June 24, 2007, www.nim.nih.gov/medlineplus/news.

10. Mitka, Mike. "Report Quantifies Diabetes Complications." *Journal of the American Medical Association*, Vol. 297, No. 21, June 6, 2007, p. 2337–2338.

11. Schulze, Matthias, et al. "Fiber and Magnesium Intake and Incidence of Type 2 Diabetes: A Prospective Study and Meta-analysis." *Archives of Internal Medicine*, Vol. 167, May 14, 2007, pp. 956–965.

12. Hampton, Tracy. "Studies Probe Value of Lifestyle Changes for Preventing Type 2 Diabetes." *Journal of the American Medical Association*, Vol. 298, No. 6, August 8, 2007, p. 617.

13. Keymeulen, B., et al. "Insulin Needs After CD3-Antibody Therapy in New-Onset Type 1 Diabetes." *New England Journal of Medicine*, Vol. 352, No. 25, June 23, 2005, pp. 2642–2644.

14. Robertson, Rose Marie. Personal interview.

15. Thom, T., N. Haas, and R. Wayne. "Heart Disease and Stroke Statistics—2006 Update: A Report from the American Heart Association Statistics Committee and Stroke Statistics

Subcommittee." *Circulation,* Vol. 113, No. 6, Feb 14, 2006, pp. 85–151.

16. "Prevalence of Heart Disease, 2005." *Journal of the American Medical Association,* Vol. 297, No. 12, August 8, 2007, p. 1308.

17. Alman, Robert, et al. "Impact of the First Semester College Experience on Cardiovascular Risk Factor Development." *Research Quarterly for Exercise and Sport,* Vol. 78, No. 1, February 2007, p. A-23.

18. "High Job Strain Linked to Increased Blood Pressure." American College of Occupational and Environmental Medicine News Release, April 10, 2007.

19. De Vogli, Roberto, et al. "Unfairness and Health: Evidence from the Whitehall II Study." *Journal of Epidemiology and Community Health,* Vol. 61, May 2007, pp. 513–518.

20. Smith, Timothy, et al. "Hostile Personality Traits and Coronary Artery Calcification in Middle-Aged and Older Married Couples: Different Effects for Self-Reports Versus Spouse Ratings." *Psychosomatic Medicine,* Vol. 69, August 2007, pp. 441–448.

21. "Anger: Heartbreaking at any age." *Harvard Mens Health Watch,* Sept 2006.

22. Mosca, Lori, et al. "Evidence-Based Guidelines for Cardiovascular Disease Prevention in Women: 2007 Update." *Circulation,* 2007. www.circulationaha.org.

23. Ibid.

24. Opotowsky, A.R., et al. "Gender Differences in Aspirin Use Among Adults with Coronary Heart Disease in the United States." *General Internal Medicine,* Vol. 22, No. 1, January 2007, pp. 55–61.

25. Manson, JoAnn, et al. "Estrogen Therapy and Coronary-Artery Calcification." *New England Journal of Medicine,* Vol. 356, No. 25, June 21, 2007, pp. 2591–2602.

26. Cook, Nancy, et al. "A Randomized Factorial Trial of Vitamins C and E and Beta Carotene in the Secondary Prevention of Cardiovascular Events in Women." *Archives of Internal Medicine,* Vol. 167, No. 15, August 13–27, 2007, pp. 1610–1618.

27. Baron, John. "Can Aspirin Keep Mortality at Bay?" *Archives of Internal Medicine* Vol. 167, No. 6, March 16, 2007, pp. 535–536.

28. Mitka, Mike. "Studies Explore Stroke's Gender Gap." *Journal of the American Medical Association,* Vol. 295, No. 15, April 19, 2006, p. 1755.

29. Deng, Y. Z., et al. "IV Tissue Plasminogen Activator Use in Acute Stroke: Experience from a Statewide Registry." *Neurology,* Vol. 63, No. 3, February 14, 2006, pp. 66(3): 306–312.

30. Elkind, M. S., et al. "Sex as a Predictor of Outcomes in Patients Treated with Thrombolysis for Acute Stroke," *Neurology,* Vol. 68, March 13, 2007, pp. 842–848.

31. American Cancer Society. *Cancer Facts & Figures 2007.* Atlanta: American Cancer Society, 2007.

32. Ibid.

33. McCracken, Melissa, et al. "Cancer Incidence, Mortality, and Associated Risk Factors Among Asian Americans of Chinese, Filipino, Vietnamese, Korean, and Japanese Ethnicities." *CA: Cancer Journal for Clinicians,* Vol. 57, July 2007, pp. 190–205.

34. Hornung, Robin, et al. "UV Light Abuse and High-Risk Tanning Behavior among Undergraduate College Students." *Journal of the American Academy of Dermatology,* March 2007.

35. "Indoor Tanning Contributes to Increased Incidence of Skin Cancer." News Release, American Academy of Dermatology, January 12, 2006.

36. Warthan, M. M., et al. "UV Light Tanning as a Type of Substance-Related Disorder." *Archives of Dermatology,* Vol. 141, No. 8, August 2005, pp. 963–966.

37. Michels, Karin, et al. "Induced and Spontaneous Abortion and Incidence of Breast Cancer among Young Women." *Archives of Internal Medicine,* Vol. 167, 2007, pp. 814–820.

38. Hampton, Tracy. "Research Findings Point to Advances in Breast Cancer Screening and Treatment." *Journal of the American Medical Association,* Vol. 98, No. 4, July 25, 2007, pp. 389–390.

39. Saslow, Debbi. "American Cancer Society Guidelines for Breast Screening with MRI as an Adjunct to Mammography." *CA: A Cancer Journal for Clinicians,* Vol. 57, 2007, pp. 75–89.

40. Lehman, Constance, et al. "MRI Evaluation of the Contralateral Breast in Women with Recently Diagnosed Breast Cancer." *New England Journal of Medicine,* Vol. 337, No. 13, March 29, 2007, p. 1295.

41. Saules, Karen, et al. "Actual Versus Perceived Risk of Cervical Cancer Among College Women Smokers." *Journal of American College Health,* Vol. 55, No. 4, January–February 2007, p. 207(7).

42. Markowitz, Lauri, et al. "Quadrivalent Human Papillomavirus Vaccine Recommendations of the Advisory Committee on Immunization Practices (ACIP)." *MMWR,* Vol. 56, March 12, 2007, pp. 1–24.

43. Saslow, Debbie, et al. "American Cancer Society Guidelines for the Early Detection of Cervical Neoplasia and Cancer," *CA: A Cancer Journal for Clinicians,* Vol. 52, January 22, 2007, pp. 342–362.

44. U.S. Preventive Services Task Force. "Routine Aspirin or Nonsteroidal Anti-inflammatory Drugs for the Primary Prevention of Colorectal Cancer." *Archives of Internal Medicine.*

45. "Statin Drugs and the Risk of Advanced Prostate Cancer." *UroToday,* March 22, 2007.

Chapter 15

1. American College Health Association. "American College Health Association National College Health Assessment Spring 2006 Reference Group Data Report (Abridged)." *Journal of American College Health,* Vol. 55, No. 4, January–February 2007, pp. 195–206.

2. Ibid.

3. National Institute of Allergy and Infectious Diseases, www.niaid.nih.gov.

4. Mitka, Mike. "Age Range Widens for Pertussis Vaccine." *Journal of the American Medical Association,* Vol. 295, No. 8, February 22, 2006, p. 871.

5. Chaves, Sandra, et al. "Loss of Vaccine-Induced Immunity to Varicella over Time." Vol. 356, No. 11, March 15, 2007, pp. 1121–1129.

6. Douglas R. M., et al. "Vitamin C for Preventing and Treating the Common Cold," *Cochrane Report,* July 2007.

7. Shah, Sachin, et al. "Evaluation of Echinacea for the Prevention and Treatment of the Common Cold: A Meta-analysis." *The Lancet Infectious Diseases,* Vol. 7, No. 7, July 2007, pp. 473–480.

9. "Meningococcal Vaccines: What You Need to Know," www.cdc.gov.

10. "STOP Meningitis," National Foundation for Infectious Diseases, http://66.11.193.178.

11. "Meningococcal Vaccines: What You Need to Know."

12. "FDA Clears Rapid Test for Meningitis," March 16, 2007, www.fda.gov/bbs/topics/NEWS/2007/NEW01588.htm.

13. "Meningococcal Vaccines: What You Need to Know."

14. Sullivan, Michele. "Hepatitis A and B Incidence Hits All-Time Low." *Pediatric News,* Vol. 41, No. 5, May 2007, p. 10(2).

15. Chang, T. T., et al. "A Comparison of Entecavir and Lamivudine for HBeAg-Positive Chronic Hepatitis B." *New England Journal of Medicine,* Vol. 354, No. 10, March 9, 2006, pp. 1001–1010.

16. Bereket-Yucel, S. "Risk of Hepatitis B Infections in Olympic Wrestling," *British Journal of Sports Medicine,* 2007, 0: 1–4, www.bjsportmed.com.

17. "Hep C Ups Cancer Risk." *GP,* May 11, 2007, p. 02.

18. Boreham, Helen. " MRSA: Four Letters, Big Problem." *Chemist & Druggist,* April 21, 2007, p. S20.

19. Klevens, R. M., et al. "Invasive Methicillin-Resistant Staphylococcus aureus Infections in the United States." *Journal of the American Medical Association,* Vol. 298, No. 15, October 17, 2007, pp. 1763–1771.

20. "1.2 Million U.S. Patients Get Resistant Staph Each Year." *NIH Healthday,* June 26, 2007.

21 Consumers Union, www.stophospital infections.org.

22. "CA-MRSA Skin Infections: Coming to a Patient Near You." *JAAPA-Journal of the American Academy of Physicians Assistants,* Vol. 20, No. 1, January 2007, p. 14(2).

23. Zeller, John. "MRSA Infections." *Journal of the American Medical Association,* Vol. 298, No. 15, October 17, 2007, p. 1826.

24. Zeller, John, et al. "Lyme Disease." *Journal of the American Medical Association,* Vol. 297, No. 23, June 20, 2007, p. 2664.

25. Mechcatie, Elizabeth. "First Avian Flu Vaccine Approved for U.S. Stockpile." *Pediatric News,* Vol. 41, No. 5, May 2007, p. 8(1).

26. Richardson, Zachary. "FDA's New Preparedness Plan Outlines Efforts to Fight Avian Flu." *Food Chemical News,* Vol. 49, No. 6, March 26, 2007, p. 15(3).

27. U.S. Department of Health and Human Services, Washington, DC, www.pandemicflu.gov.

28. Taubenberger, J. K., et al. "The Next Influenza Pandemic: Can It Be Predicted?" *Journal of the American Medical Association,* Vol. 297, No. 18, May 9, 2007, pp. 2025–2027.

29. Schwebke, Jane and Renee Desmond. "A Randomized Trial of Metronidazole in Asymptomatic Bacterial Vaginosis to Prevent the Acquisition of Sexually Transmitted Diseases." American Journal of Obstetrics and Gynecology, Vol. 196, No. 6, June 2007, pp. 517.e1–517.e6.

Chapter 16

1. American College Health Association. *American College Health Association National College Health Assessment Reference Group Executive Summary Fall 2006.* Baltimore: American College Health Association, 2007.

2. Robinson, June. "Anatomical and Hormonal Influences on Women's Dermatologic Health." *Journal of the American Medical Association,* Vol. 295, No. 12, March 22/29, 2006, p. 1443.

3. Markowitz, Lauri, et al. "Quadrivalent Human Papillomavirus Vaccine Recommendations of the Advisory Committee on Immunization Practices (ACIP)." *MMWR,* Vol. 56, March 12, 2007, pp. 1–24.

4. D'Souza, Gypsyamber, et al. "Case–Control Study of Human Papillomavirus and Oropharyngeal Cancer." *New England Journal of Medicine,* Vol. 356; No. 19, May 2007, pp. 1944–1956.

5. Weller, Susan, and Lawrence Stanberry. "Estimating the Population Prevalence of HPV." *Journal of the American Medical Association,* Vol. 297, No. 8, February 2007, pp. 876–878,

6. Dunne, Eileen, et al. "Prevalence of HPV Infection Among Females in the United States." *Journal of the American Medical Association,* Vol. 297, February 2007, pp. 813–819.

7. LeMar, Catherine, and Larry Olsen. "Knowledge and Attitudes of Selected College Students About HPV and Cervical Cancer," *Research Quarterly for Exercise and Sport,* Vol. 78, No. 1, February 2007, p. A-31(1).

8. Wagner, Donald, et al. "College Women's Sexual Knowledge, Beliefs and Behaviors Related to the Prevention of Human Papilloma Virus." *Research Quarterly for Exercise and Sport,* Vol. 78, No. 1, February 2007, p. A-37(1).

9. "Human Papillomavirus (HPV) Vaccine," CDC, www.cdc.gov/std/hpv.

10. FUTURE II Study Group. "Quadrivalent Vaccine Against Human Papillomavirus to Prevent High-Grade Cervical Lesions. *New England Journal of Medicine,* Vol. 356, May 2007, pp. 1915–1927.

11. Garland, S. M., et al. "Quadrivalent Vaccine Against Human Papillomavirus to Prevent Anogenital Diseases. *New England Journal of Medicine,* Vol. 356, May 2007, pp. 1928–1943.

12. Sawaya, G. F., and K. Smith-McCune, "HPV Vaccination—More Answers, More Questions." *New England Journal of Medicine,* May 2007, Vol. 356, pp. 1991–1993.

13. Charo, R. A., "Politics, Parents, and Prophylaxis—Mandating HPV Vaccination in the United States." *New England Journal of Medicine,* Vol. 356, May 2007, pp. 1905–1908.

14. McPartland, Tara, et al. "Men's Perceptions and Knowledge of Human Papillomavirus (HPV) Infection and Cervical Cancer." *Journal of American College Health,* Vol. 53, No. 5, March–April 2005, p. 225.

15. Tavé van Zyl, Eric Wooltorton, and Noni MacDonald, "Public Health Fact Sheet: Patient Information about HPV and the HPV Vaccine." *Canadian Medical Association Journal.* Vol. 177, No. 5, August 2007, p. 462.

16. "Human Papillomavirus (HPV) Vaccine."

17. "Human Papillomavirus (HPV) Vaccine."

18. "African Americans and HIV/AIDS." *Kaiser Family Foundation HIV/AIDS Fact Sheet,* February 2006, www.kff.org.

19. "Women and HIV/AIDS in the United States." *Kaiser Family Foundation HIV/AIDS Fact Sheet,* February 2006, www.kff.org.

20. "Adult Male Circumcision Significantly Reduces Risk of Acquiring HIV." *NIH News,* December 13, 2006.

21. Centers for Disease Control and Prevention, www.cdc.gov.

Chapter 17

1. Rothstein, William, and Sushama Rajapaksa. "Health Beliefs of College Students Born in the United States, China, and India." *Journal of American College Health,* Vol. 51, No. 5, March 2003, p. 189.

2. Bard, Mark. Personal interview.

3. Michaud, Dominique, et al. "A Prospective Study of Periodontal Disease and Pancreatic Cancer in U.S. Male Health Professionals." *Journal of the National Cancer Institute,* Vol. 99, January 2007, pp. 171–175.

4. Prochazka, Allan, et al. "Support of Evidence-Based Guidelines for the Annual Physical Examination: A Survey of Primary Care Providers." *Archives of Internal Medicine,* Vol. 165, No. 12, June 27, 2005, pp. 1347–1352.

5. "20 Tips to Help Prevent Medical Errors," Agency for Healthcare Research and Quality, www.ahrq.gov.

6. Questions Are the Answer," Agency for Healthcare Research and Quality, http://www.ahrq.gov/questionsaretheanswer/.

7. American Society of Plastic Surgeons, www.plasticsurgery.org.

8. National Center for Complementary and Alternative Medicine, http://nccam.nih.gov/health/backgrounds/mindbody.htm

9. Grzywacz, J.G., et al. "Age, Ethnicity, and Use of Complementary and Alternative Medicine in Health Self-Management." *Journal of Health and Social Behavior,* Vol. 48, No. 1, 2007.

10. Hsieh, Lisa Li-Chen, et al. "Treatment of Low Back Pain by Acupressure and Physical Therapy: Randomized Controlled Trial," *British Medical Journal,* Vol. 332, No. 7543, March 25, 2006, pp. 696–700.

11. Bardia, Aditya, et al. "Use of Herbs Among Adults Based on Evidence-Based Indications: Findings from the National Health Interview Survey." *Mayo Clinic Proceedings,* Vol. 82, No. 5, May 2007, pp. 561–566.

12. Shah, Sachin, et al. "Evaluation of Echinacea for the Prevention and Treatment of the Common Cold: A Meta-Analysis." *The Lancet Infectious Diseases,* Vol. 7, No. 7, July 2007, pp. 473–480.

13. Gardner, Christopher, et al. "Effect of Raw Garlic vs Commercial Garlic Supplements on Plasma Lipid Concentrations in Adults with Moderate Hypercholesteriemia." *Archives of Internal Medicine,* Vol. 167, No. 4, February 2007, pp. 346–353.

14. Torpy, Janet. "Health Care Insurance: The Basics." *Journal of the American Medical Association,* Vol. 297, No. 10, March 2007, pp. 1031.

15. Hadley, Jack. "Insurance Coverage, Medical Care Use, and Short-Term Health Changes Following an Unintentional Injury or the Onset of a Chronic Condition," *Journal of the American Medical Association,* Vol. 297, No. 10, March 2007, pp. 1073–1084.

Chapter 18

1. National Center for Health Statistics, http://www.cdc.gov/nchs.

2. National Highway Traffic Safety Administration, www.nhtsa.dot.gov.

3. Allen, Shane, et al. "A Comprehensive Statewide Analysis of Seatbelt Non-use with Injury and Hospital Admissions: New Data, Old Problem." *Academic Emergency Medicine,* Vol. 13, 2006, pp. 427–434.

4. Nerenberg, Arnold. Personal interview.

5. "Cell Phones and Driving," Insurance Information Institute, February 2007, www.iii.org/media/hottopics/cellphones.

6. Ibid.

7. Prothrow-Stith, Deborah. "Keynote Address: Making Campuses Safer Communities for Students." *Journal of American College Health,* Vol. 55, No. 5, March/April 2007, pp. 261–266.

8. Carr, Joetta, et al. "Campus Violence White Paper." *Journal of American College Health,* Vol. 55, No. 5, March/April 2007, pp. 304–319.

9. Ibid.

10. Ibid.

11. Thompson, Marie, et al. "Reasons for Not Reporting Victimizations to the Police: Do They Vary for Physical and Sexual Incidents?"

Journal of American College Health, Vol. 55, No. 5, March/April 2007, pp. 277–282.

12. Carr, et al. "Campus Violence White Paper."

13. Ibid.

14. Ibid.

15. *Drawing the Line: Sexual Harassment on Campus.* Washington, DC: American Association of University Women, January 2006.

16. Ibid.

17. Oswald, Debra, and Brenda Russell. "Perceptions of Sexual Coercion in Heterosexual Dating Relationships: The Role of Aggressor Gender and Tactics." *The Journal of Sex Research,* Vol. 43, No. 1, February 2006, p. 87(9).

18. Loiselle, Marci, and Wayner Fuqua. "Alcohol's Effects on Women's Risk Detection in a Date-Rape Vignette." *Journal of American College Health,* Vol. 55, No. 5, March/April 2007, pp. 261–266.

19. Gips, Michael. "Campus Rape Still Not Well Reported." *Security Management,* Vol. 50, No. 3, March 2006, p. 22(1).

20. Rothman, Emily, and Jay Silverman. "The Effect of a College Sexual Assault Prevention Program on First-year Students' Victimization Rates." *Journal of American College Health,* Vol. 55, No. 5, March/April 2007, pp. 283–290.

Chapter 19

1. "Climate Change 2007," Intergovernmental Panel on Climate Change, www.ipcc.ch/.

2. Ibid.

3. American Association for the Advancement of Science, www.aaas.org/climate.

4. Wilson, Jennifer. "Facing an Uncertain Climate." *Annals of Internal Medicine,* Vol. 146, No. 2, January 16, 2007, pp. 153–156.

5. Watston, R. Climate Change Is Likely to Affect the Health of Millions, Report Warns." *British Medical Journal,* Vol. 334, No. 7597, April 14, 2007, p. 768.

6. Chuang, K. J., et al. "Urban Air Pollution on Inflammation, Oxidative Stress, Coagulation and Autonomic Dysfunction." *American Journal of Respiratory and Critical Care Medicine,* April 26, 2007.

7. *American Lung Association State of the Air: 2007,* http://lungaction.org/reports/stateoftheair2007.html.

8. Gauderman, W. J., et al. "Effect of Exposure to Traffic on Lung Development from 10 to 18 Years of Age: A Cohort Study." *Lancet,* Vol. 369, No. 9561, February 2007, pp. 571–577.

9. Egan, Timothy. "The Greening of America's Campuses." *New York Times,* January 8, 2006.

10. U.S. Office of Health and Human Services. *The Health Consequences of Involuntary Exposure to Tobacco Smoke.* Washington, DC: Office of the Surgeon General, 2006.

11. Becklake, M. R., et al. "Asbestos-Related Diseases of the Lungs and Pleura: Uses, Trends and Management over the Last Century." *International Journal of Tuberculosis and Lung Disease,* Vol. 11, No. 4, April 2007, pp. 356–369.

12. Johansson, C., et al. "Neurobehavioural and Molecular Changes Induced by Methylmercury Exposure During Development." *Neurotoxicology Research,* Vol. 11, No. 3–4, April 2007, pp. 241–260.

13. Portnoy, Jay, et al. "Health Effects of Indoor Fungi." *Annals of Allergy, Asthma & Immunology,* Vol. 94, No. 3, March 2005, p. 313.

14. Hales, Dianne. "New Help for Hearing Loss." *Parade,* May 14, 2006, p. 16.

15. "Cranked Up Music on Headphones Can Lead to Hearing Loss." University of Michigan Health System, January 3, 2006.

16. "Environmental Cancer Risks." *Cancer Facts & Figures 2006,* American Cancer Society, 2006.

17. Cooper, C. "Multiple Chemical Sensitivity in the Clinical Setting." *American Journal of Nursing,* Vol. 107, No. 3, March 2007, pp. 40–47.

18. Tahvanainen, K., et al. "Effects of Cellular Phone Use on Ear Canal Temperature Measured by NTC Thermistors." *Clinical Physiology and Functional Imaging,* Vol. 27, No. 3, May 2007, pp. 162–172.

Chapter 20

1. *A Profile of Older Americans: 2006.* Washington, DC: Administration on Aging, 2007. www.aoa.gov/prof/Statistics/statistics.asp.

2. Ibid.

3. Ibid.

4. Knox, David, et al. "College Student Views of the Elderly: Some Gender Differences." *College Student Journal,* Vol. 39, No. 1, March 2005, p. 14(3).

5. Roizen, Michael. Personal interview.

6. Schonfeld, Amy. "More Data Show Positive Effects of Aspirin on Brain Matter." *Clinical Psychiatry News,* Vol. 35, No. 3, March 2007, p. 21(1).

7. Kang, Jae Hee, et al. "Low Dose Aspirin and Cognitive Function in the Women's Health Study Cognitive Cohort," *British Medical Journal,* April 27, 2007, ONLINE First, dol: 10.1136/bmj.39166.597836.BE.

8. ADAPT Research Group. "Naproxen and Celebcoxib Do Not Prevent AD in Early Results from a Randomized Controlled Trial." *Neurology,* April 2007 (epub prior to publication).

9. Sherman, Sherry. Personal interview.

10. Speller, Marsha. Personal interview.

11. "Depression at Menopause," *Harvard Mental Health Letter,* April 2007 p. NA.

12. Pinkerton, JoAnn. Personal interview.

13. Elavsky, S. and McAuley, E. "Physical Activity and Mental Health Outcomes During Menopause: A Randomized Controlled Trial." *Annals of Behavioral Medicine,* Vol. 33, No. 2, April 2007, pp. 132–142.

14. Chen, W. Y., et al. "Unopposed Estrogen Therapy and the Risk of Invasive Breast Cancer." *Archives of Internal Medicine,* Vol. 166, No. 9, May 8, 2006, pp. 1027–1032.

15. "Estrogen and Progestogen Use in Peri- and Postmenopausal Women: March 2007 Position Statement of the North American Menopause Society." *Menopause,* Vol. 14, No. 2, 2007, 168–182.

16. "Black Cohosh Fails to Relieve Menopause Symptoms." *Tufts University Health & Nutrition Letter,* Vol. 25, No. 1, March 2007, p. 6(1).

17. *Alzheimer's Disease Facts and Figures 2007.* Washington, DC: Alzheimer's Association, 2007.

18. Prentice, Ross, et al. "Low-Fat Dietary Pattern and Risk of Invasive Breast Cancer." *Journal of the American Medical Association,* Vol. 295, No. 6, February 8, 2006, p. 629.

19. Duffy, S. A., et al. "Racial/Ethnic Preferences, Sex Preferences, and Perceived Discrimination Related to End-of-Life Care." *Journal of the American Geriatrics Society,* Vol. 54, No. 1, January 2006, pp. 150–157.

20. Cuende, N., et al. "Effect of Population Aging on the International Organ Donation Rates and the Effectiveness of the Donation Process." *American Journal of Transplantation,* April 8, 2007 (epub).

21. Siminoff, L., et al. "The Reasons Families Donate Organs for Transplantation: Implications for Policy and Practice." *Journal of Trauma,* Vol. 62, No. 4, April 2007, pp. 969–978.

22. *World Health Statistics 2007.* Geneva: World Health Organization, 2007.

23. Kübler-Ross, Elisabeth. *Death: The Final Stage of Growth.* Englewood Cliffs, NJ: Prentice-Hall, 1975.

24. Marcoux, I., et al. "Withdrawing an Explicit Request for Euthanasia or Physician-Assisted Suicide: A Retrospective Study on the Influence of Mental Health Status and Other Patient Characteristics." *Psychological Medicine,* Vol. 35, No. 9, September 2005, p. 1265.

25. Maciejewski, Paul, et al. "An Empirical Examination of the Stage Theory of Grief." *Journal of the American Medical Association,* Vol. 297, No. 7, February 21, 2007, pp. 716–723.

26. Ringold, Sarah. "Grief." *Journal of the American Medical Association,* Vol. 293, No. 21, June 1, 2005, p. 2686.

Index